Volume One

Mouth Rehabilitation

Volume one

Mouth Rehabilitation

CLINICAL AND LABORATORY PROCEDURES

Max Kornfeld, D.D.S, F.A.C.D., F.I.C.D.

Former Professor and Director of the Department of Crown and Bridge Prosthodontics, St. Louis University School of Dentistry, St. Louis, Mo.
Former Lecturer and Instructor in Dental Materials and Comparative Dental Anatomy, Washington University School of Dental Medicine, St. Louis, Mo.
Professor of Advanced Restorative Dentistry, Washington University School of Dental Medicine, St. Louis, Mo.
Clinical Professor of Orthodontics, Department of Occlusion, Graduate School of Orthodontics, St. Louis University Medical Center, St. Louis, Mo.
American Academy of Crown and Bridge Prosthodontics
American Academy of Restorative Dentistry
International Academy of Gnathology

SECOND EDITION

with 3,866 illustrations, including 9 in color and two full-color plates

The C. V. Mosby Company

ST. LOUIS 1974

Second edition

Printed in the United States of America

Distributed in Great Britain by Henry Kimpton, London

Library of Congress Cataloging in Publication Data

Kornfeld, Max.
Mouth rehabilitation.
Includes bibliographies.
1. Dentistry. I. Title. [DNLM: 1. Mouth rehabilitation. 2. Prosthodontics. WU500 K84m]
RK51.K62 617.6 74-10681
ISBN 0-8016-2726-5

TS/VH/B 9 8 7 6 5 4 3 2 1

Dedicated to my beloved wife

RUTH

for her ever-present help, devotion, and encouragement

PREFACE to second edition

This book endeavors to provide a good foundation in the concept of jaw function and in the practical techniques of reproducing it. But, as in all scientific advancement, the coming of the new techniques has brought its own responsibility, for it embodies powers for destruction equal to its powers of construction. We must exercise greater vision and vigilance.

Coordination of all phases of dentistry for the maintenance of proper function and good periodontal health is our objective. The mouth is a functioning organ that is subject to the same physiologic laws that govern other parts of the body.

I have made an extreme effort to organize the material in these volumes so as to give the subject a unified approach—its rationale of therapy and its methodology. Also, whenever possible, illustrations have been added to augment or emphasize various points in procedures and to effect a process more or less of visual instruction. Important new facts and concepts that have emerged since the publication of the first edition have been incorporated, and inevitable errors of the first edition have been sought out and corrected. Simplification is always the desire of an author, but what may appear complicated or complex to some cannot always be rectified in a simple manner. Some of the content is a reorganization of existing knowledge and, in a few instances, a shift of emphasis.

Dentistry is rapidly changing from a profession of techniques alone to one requiring application of techniques based on an understanding of complexities of the basic sciences and superimposed on a philosophical backdrop. An effort has been made in this book to avoid untested maxims and to accept good, sound research findings as truths. Research, well conceived and executed, can measure the validity of concepts. The procedures offered in these volumes are not necessarily theoretical—they have been proved clinically, and they are practical and routinely reproducible.

In other words, with the addition of four new chapters (Chapters 2, 7, 15, 16) and some important considerations of adult orthodontics, the second edition follows the outline of the first edition, with an enhancement and expansion of its original thought, including all necessary revisions and additions to bring subject matter up to date. Many new drawings and photographs have been added, and some have been improved for easier comprehension. A number of new and interesting case histories have been added, and all the latest clinical and related research findings have been incorporated.

Chapter 3, Diagnosis and Treatment Planning, has been almost completely rewritten. Chapter 6, Prosthetic-Periodontal Interrelationships, has been updated, and vividly shows that if proper form and function are not attained for restorations and splintage and other restorative measures are not implemented, when indicated, such procedures as removal of diseased gingival tissues and changing of architectural form of the involved osseous structures would come to naught.

Chapter 2, Principles, Objectives, and Terminology, was added because it is desirable to understand at the outset that within the strictly disciplined contexts of the sciences exact or almost exact agreements about terminology can be established. I am not presuming that any reader of these volumes does not have enough of a common background of controlled experience in the field of dentistry to have real difficulties about understanding the terms used, but I am desirous of conveying that they mean the same thing to both of us. I have endeavored to use terms in such a way and with sufficient illustrative examples so that their specific meaning will emerge from their context.

Chapter 7, Essential and Fundamental Factors Involved in Crown and Bridge Prosthodontics, is of great importance. Mechanical and engineering principles have been properly related to our daily tasks in the practice of dentistry, and emphasis on these mechanical and engineering aspects has been balanced by and correlated with the biologic requirements. Materials, concepts, and techniques presented have been carefully evaluated in the light of tried and proven fundamental principles, past and present clinical experiences (over a long number of years), and objective appraisals. In other words, only fundamental principles and methods that have been proved sound, both biologically and mechanically, have been presented. An occasional return to fundamentals is a good habit for all of us to cultivate. We must master the elementary principles of biologics, mechanics, and engineering to become good and reputable practitioners of dentistry. It is advisable to learn fundamental principles so as to be able to introduce change, especially when function dictates deviation; by so doing it will be possible to attain successful results in the more complex problems of mouth rehabilitation.

The subject of porcelain fused to metal has received extensive treatment—by the profuse use of illustrations and by detailed description. Oral-systemic relationships have been considered, especially in the treatment of older patients, because tissue changes are brought about by hormone changes incident to aging and reduced saliva flow. The adaptive capacity of the individual patient for resistance and repair must be taken into consideration.

Chapter 15, dealing with temporomandibular joint dysfunction, was written by Dr. John Vincelli. He has a new and fresh approach to this most aggravating problem, and his treatise deserves serious consideration. I have a great regard for Vincelli's work but am still of the opinion that the psychologic component that triggers the muscle spasm is what, in most instances, "sets off" the syndrome. However, the type of appliance Dr. Vincelli has designed for the alleviation of the severe pain in these cases is excellent.

Chapter 16, Precision Removable Partial Dentures, was written because I was asked by many colleagues to include a more detailed discussion of these very valuable adjuncts to treatment. Precision attachments must not be used indiscriminately, but only where specifically indicated after a thorough study of the case at hand. Keep in mind that the type of attachment must be chosen effectively, and limiting oneself to one type of attachment for all cases is wrong. Various types of precision attachments are discussed and profusely illustrated in this chapter—the internal precision attachment, the removable telescopic external attachment with an axial-rotational joint, the C & L spring attachment, the Thompson dowel (an intracoronal semiprecision retainer), and the resilient hinge-action stressbreaker. Another important feature is the E.M. Attachment Selector, which is a compendium of the attachments and connecting units available throughout the world.

Chapter 19, Emotional Aspects of Extended Restorative Procedures, assumes more importance because the increased tempo of living may be expected to increase the number of "stress patients" in our practice.

Emphasis has been placed on the need of a thorough knowledge of the physiology of occlusion as an important basis for the diagnosis and treatment of dysfunctional disturbances of the masticatory system.

The relationship between occlusal anatomy and mandibular movements has been emphasized from several viewpoints. New and fresh concepts of instrumentation have been shown graphically for the reader's serious consideration.

The field of oral implantology has been touched upon. Great strides have been made in this area, but more scientific research must be done and different materials must be tried. If this is done the profession will accept it with less skepticism, and it will take its place as an important adjunct in mouth rehabilitation procedures.

Some important phrases have been repeated on several occasions in these volumes, and this approach may be criticized as redundant but, after many years of teaching and lecturing, I feel that repetition, properly used and applied, can be a very valuable teaching aid.

I most fervently hope that the end result of this endeavor will be an edition of organized and applicable knowledge of the subject matter discussed in these volumes. In ending this preface the verse written by L. M. Alcott seems apropos: "Far away there in the sunshine are my highest aspirations; I may not reach them, but I can look up and see their beauty, believe in them, and try to follow where they lead."

Max Kornfeld

PREFACE to first edition

To write a book on clinical and laboratory procedures in mouth rehabilitation calls for at least a clinical familiarity with most established concepts in this particular field. Experience with only one concept is not enough to evaluate properly the good or bad of the other concepts of mouth rehabilitation. I have been most fortunate to have had the opportunity to be exposed to these various philosophies long enough and to have treated and completed a sufficient number of cases in each of these disciplines so that results could be evaluated properly; that is, how did restorations function, how were they accepted by the oral tissues, what was their longevity, and so forth. It is true that clinical evaluation, which can be nothing more than opinion, can have no justification for support without controls and therefore is not scientific. However, I have been able to apply the knowledge accumulated over the years, and there is no substitute for experience and mature clinical judgment.

Although some areas of the book will deal with certain specific techniques and materials used in restoring teeth with cast restorations, a primary objective in this book is to emphasize fundamental principles that are the basis for the application of any technique or material. Since it is not feasible to assume that all readers are familiar with the techniques, in a way one should be in performing this type of work with so-called routine crown and bridge prosthodontics, details of these procedures have been included. It is advisable to learn the fundamental principles that enable us to introduce change, especially when function dictates deviation. A knowledge of anatomy, physiology, periodontics, orthodontics, and endodontics is essential to a full understanding of the problems of full-mouth treatment. Laboratory procedures must be understood (by having done them) to control the laboratory situation. Control does not mean only the date of delivery of the restoration but also the knowledge to recognize whether all steps have been executed correctly and, if not so executed, to be able to detect the flaws and suggest or make necessary corrections.

Too much energy and effort are extravagantly wasted in futile attempts to seek an easier, quicker solution to a problem. Such an easy, single solution to a full-mouth rehabilitation is not always available, but there must be a logical, sound, clinically proved (at least) method with sequential procedures to allow for an end result commensurate with our present knowledge of the basic sciences and advanced dental technology.

There is nothing easy about restoring the oral mechanism to proper form and function. Procedural methods and instruments that appear at first to be difficult to understand and apply are not difficult if one is willing to give thought, effort, and time to their use. Shouldn't this really be part of a professional man's obligation to himself and his patients?

To rehabilitate the mouth to proper function and effectiveness it is believed that the principles of gnathology are sound for clinical purposes, even if not completely proved scientifically. The function of the temporomandibular joint, a major and unalterable factor in diagnosis, treatment planning, and therapy, gives us the information as to condylar guidance. It is necessary to comprehend the fixed biologic factors, as well as those subject to change by the dentist, that are involved in the occlusion of the teeth. The cusps, ridges, grooves, and fossae of the teeth that will function properly in any given mouth are the result of these fixed and variable factors. It is our job and responsibility to record them and to make restorations accordingly, if the restorations are to be successful.

I believe that one should be at the same time a believer and a skeptic and always keep in mind that, as scientific and technologic advances are made, resistance to change cannot be tolerated. Greatly increased research in the basic sciences and in clinical practice is providing the dentist with new approaches to old problems in diagnosis, treatment planning, and therapy. The practitioner should preserve the best of the old, but should try new ideas and apply current research to the treatment of the patient.

A word should be said about the format of the book. Its main purpose is to convey to the reader the chair and laboratory procedures encountered in this type of work. This is done not only by the narrative method but also by liberal use of illustrations. In some instances they are presented in detailed step-by-step sequences designed to illustrate a particular procedure. Photographs and roentgenograms of case histories are submitted as clinical evidence of the feasibility and applicability of the selected technique with which it is possible to achieve consistent, positive results that are long lasting and beneficial to the patient. The scope and needs of general clinical dental practice have been seriously considered.

Chapter 19 on emotional aspects of extended restorative procedures is very important in full-mouth treatment. Without a good working knowledge and understanding of this subject life can become miserable for both the patient and the dentist, and the end result of treatment, however well executed, will come to naught. A few case histories are included in this chapter.

Human life has only such ends as we set up for it, individually and collectively, and these are dependent on good health, on joy in our work, and on an intelligent appreciation of the durable values of life.

Max Kornfeld

ACKNOWLEDGEMENTS

I wish to express my thanks and appreciation to those individuals from whom I have obtained bits of information from lectures, by word of mouth, and from articles that are incorporated in this book, but whose names and exact source of reference I cannot remember so that proper credit could be given.

"No one has of himself become what he is; everyone stands on the shoulders of his predecessors."

I also wish to express my great indebtedness and appreciation to my friends and colleagues who contributed chapters or sections of a chapter, or imparted important information, in specific areas in which they are experts: *Victor O. Lucia, Harold R. Schreiber, James W. Bynum, Anthony J. DePietro, Earl E. Shepard, John Vincelli, Morton Amsterdam, Peter K. Thomas, Charles J. Welter, William R. Dykins, Alex Koper, William R. Scott, Merrill C. Mensor, Jr., Leonard Abrams, Richard W. Huffman, John W. Regenos, Edwin S. Smyd, Martin Henry Berman, Gerard L. Courtade, Ralph A. Youdelis, Harold F. Eissmann, Peter Dawson, Herbert T. Shillingburg, Jr., Clifford Sturdevant,* and *George E. Myers.*

Also, my sincere thanks go to those friends and colleagues from whose excellent articles I have gathered some important information or adapted illustrations with their permission, graciously given, and to whom due credit is noted in these volumes.

My thanks and grateful appreciation to the allied dental companies—*The J. M. Ney Co., J. F. Jelenko & Co., Inc., Kerr Dental Mfg. Co., Whaledent, Inc., American Thermocraft Corp., Ceramco, Inc., Star Dental Mfg. Co., Stern Dental Co., Inc., S. S. White Co., The Denar Corp., TMJ Instrument Co., Inc., American Precision Metals,* and *J. Aderer, Inc.*—for supplying important data unselfishly which was most helpful in making this book more complete and practical.

I also wish to express my deep appreciation to *my children, Frances, Rosalind, Stuart,* and *Bernard,* who offered constructive criticism and encouragement; to *Elsie Riddles,* for the many services rendered to me during the writing of this manuscript; to the individuals who participated in the development and quality of the art and photographic illustrative material, *Bill Briggs, Annette Porter,* and *Dennis Kreps;* to *Harriet Stuernagel,* librarian at Washington University School of Dental Medicine, who was always willing to assist me in obtaining references; to *the fine typists at Superior Office Service, Inc.,* for their excellent efforts in typing the manuscript; and to *John Johannessen,* my dental technologist of many years, a man who works with his hands, his head, and his heart—an artist.

And my warmest thanks and appreciation to *my wife, Ruth,* whose understanding of the many problems involved in this undertaking not only helped me in writing, proofreading, and art and photographic work, to which she contributed many new fine photographs for the second edition of these volumes, but, above all, whose counsel, encouragement, devotion, and steadfastness made the completion of this task possible.

In closing this section I feel compelled to quote from Winston Churchill, because that is exactly what I experienced: "Writing a book is an adventure. To begin with it is a joy, an amusement. Then it becomes a mistress. And then, it becomes a master. Then, it becomes a tyrant. And in the last phase, when you are reconciled to your servitude you kill the monster."

Max Kornfeld

CONTENTS

Volume One

Volume Two

Color plates

Volume One

Mouth Rehabilitation

CHAPTER 1

MY PHILOSOPHY OF PRACTICE

As I seriously considered the subject of mouth rehabilitation I vividly recalled the many conversations that I had with my father during my early youth and adolescence which have helped me so much in the development of my philosophy of practice.

He stressed the importance of humility—the ability to really feel and to practice it. He taught me to assume responsibilities without complaint, to be patient, conscientious, understanding, and sincere, and to never compromise for second best if one's capabilities and knowledge point toward the best. He felt that to realize independence one must be a creative man. One must be stimulated to independent learning, to be a continuous student, and to work hard to keep out in front, accomplishing this without harm to, or disrespect for, your fellow man.

In other words, what he truly wanted me to know is that through study, reflection, and the development of interests in the arts, sciences, and humanities, I would develop into a good citizen, would be self-sufficient and feel worthy, and thereby would do a good job at anything that I undertook. He urged the widest development possible and, above all, the broadening of my intellectual horizons. He always stressed the fact that success was not always measured in material worth, but rather in self-expression and personal excellence.

This was a lot of philosophizing, and I have sincerely tried to follow his advice. Being somewhat self-effacing, I leave how successful I have been for others to judge. But wholeheartedly I can advise my friends and colleagues to do their best to measure up to these human factors.

Percy Phillips has aptly said: "To fulfill its responsibilities to society and to survive as a profession, dentistry must call on all its priceless ingredients—honesty, integrity, professional independence, maintenance of the high quality of dental service, continuing study, expansion of dental research, the clinical application of the findings of research, and observance of our code of ethics."*

It does not take very much imagination to know that these basic ingredients are the heart and soul of the practice of dentistry and must be taken seriously. In fact, we must live and practice by them.

Today's changing socioeconomic conditions present many perplexing problems and, with them, responsibilities. In dentistry we must assume these responsibilities in relationship to ourselves, to our colleagues, and to our public.

Our patients are only interested in a longer and healthier life. For our profession to exist as a private enterprise we must have moral and professional responsibility. We must start to think positively and to do something about solving these socioeconomic problems that face us today. Otherwise, instead of our own efforts and initiative, some governmental agency will solve these problems for us.

In my travels around the country attending

*From Phillips, Percy T.: The priceless ingredients of our profession, J.A.D.A. **60:**282-284, 1960.

meetings and conferences, giving lectures and clinics, and studying with individuals and groups, I am appalled at the apathy and ignorance of many men in our profession, especially as to the scientific and technical advances in dentistry. I am really concerned because ours is a most noble and honorable profession rendering a service of great physiologic and psychologic value.

My creed always has been to be a perpetual student, to perfect myself in the latest proved techniques, and to conduct, study, and apply basic and clinical research in my practice. I have never been interested in any narrow individual aggrandizement or the development or pushing of one's own narrow ideas. Also I have felt the necessity to know myself, my inner drives, motivations, etc. so that I could have the ability to understand the peculiarities of people whom I am called upon to serve, turning their oddities into an asset of goodwill. Since it is always necessary to deal with the human equation, an intimate knowledge of the varying temperaments of people is very important for application in practice. By developing myself to the best of my abilities along cultural and professional lines, and by being able to have more rapport with patients, I am able to fulfill the aforementioned basic ingredients of our profession and also to help my patients to a longer and healthier life. One must be a teacher and a friend as well as a good technician.

Another cardinal factor in conducting a dental practice is that of the most scrupulous and constant cleanliness.

I am known as a perfectionist, but by knowing myself, my drives and motivations, I can afford to be a perfectionist without injury to my soma or psyche and thereby be of help to my patients.

It is argued that more and more dental services for more people are needed and that there should be more personnel and better trained personnel who are legally able to render services to the patient. It is true that more dental services for more people are needed, but only well-trained dentists should do any operative or restorative work for the patient regardless of the nature of the operation. The inherent dangers of the legalizing of auxiliary help are great. Following the specific duties that are indicated by the nature of her training, the dental hygienist is the only exception to this rule. Delegation of authority to legalized auxiliary help, even types of procedures considered somewhat simple, can get out of hand, and many operations that are not in their realm of authority will be performed with or without the consent of the dentist.

Auxiliary personnel are of the utmost importance in a busy dental practice, but their functions must not include any operative procedures in the mouth.

The dentist must be knowledgable, and he must learn to be efficient and skillful. By so doing he will become more productive. A profitable dental practice cannot be conducted without making the minutes count, and truthfully there is altogether too much waste motion in the average practice. The basis of time conservation is efficiency and precision of technique and also the training and experience to know precisely what to do and the most expeditious manner of doing it. We must follow the old adage: "Plan your work, and then work your plan." And, above all, we always must remember that patients must be taught a greater respect for the value of dental services, and they will never be taught this until dentists assume a greater respect for their own service. We must always keep in mind the quality, not the quantity of our services.

Although the business side of dentistry is very important, professional competence must come first. The selling of dental services in the same manner that is used in Madison Avenue advertising cannot be condoned—it is deplorable. The new fad of "time and motion" has a lot of merit, provided this form of automation is not carried to the extreme that the dentist and his staff become some kind of a machine or automaton. We must not sacrifice any of the fine details of operative procedures and even of remakes when indicated because of the factor of time. It is not necessary to constantly want to make our gross income larger and larger since the net return because of the higher percentage of overhead costs does not warrant an ulcer, a coronary, or an anxiety neurosis.

Before any professional man can exact a just fee for his services, he must first have the conviction in his own mind that his training warrants this fee.

A certain amount of confidence is necessary, but overconfidence is fatal. One must have humility—must be able to say "I don't know," when necessary, or "I would like for you to consult with Dr. X who has had more training or experience in this or that type of work." The greatest majority of dentists seem to be reluctant to admit these facts, but until this is done we will not reach the true status of professional men.

We must not have narrowness of vision and always must be willing to experiment with new ideas and new equipment. A willingness to listen and to have an open mind and a keen appreciation of the other fellow's ideas and beliefs is also worthy of consideration.

We must attend dental meetings regularly. We must take graduate and postgraduate courses and read the dental literature—and, in fact, be an avid reader and a continuous student. We must serve organized dentistry in whatever capacity we can. Service and consideration of the patient must be a guiding principle. We must fight legislation that endangers the health of the public.

All of us—practitioners and dental educators—must make a determined effort to attract many more of the dedicated type of student who is being lost to the engineering profession, to research, and to public service. We have been accused of attracting more of the business type of person.

To be successful professional men in the true sense, we must make at least a limited study of affairs outside our profession and be able to discuss intelligently some of the important issues of national and international policies. We must participate in community affairs and have an interest in the arts.

We must surely take cognizance of the need of accumulating material worth, but this, in itself, does not necessarily mean success or happiness. We must involve ourselves in a type of development that will give us a breadth of vision and in the culture, ethics, and morals that will not overlook the finer aspirations of life. A successful dentist must be more than a fine operator.

CHAPTER 2

PRINCIPLES, OBJECTIVES, AND TERMINOLOGY

"For whenever man makes a great, new forward step in learning, his duties and responsibilities increase by that much. But men are loath to take up an increment of duty or responsibility. They prefer to exploit new learning, and only for such increment as it may furnish in comfort, luxury, a higher living standard. But they know deep within themselves that their exploitation is irresponsible. So they grow guilty, and guilt is a constant eroding river of anxiety. Anxious, they take the last wrong step. To quench their worry they turn back to the 'old faiths' that soothed them before the new learning brought their gains, the responsibilities they evaded—and the guilt for that. They pretend that the new learning offers only physical benefits for them, and does not demand the new duty, the new responsibility of rethinking everything; of changing themselves. The prior faiths are always there: obsolete, now, but ready to shore up nervousness for all who will blind themselves. And that is easy: one becomes blind by ceasing to look ahead honestly. Then one sees only that which lies behind—and is no longer the whole truth."

PHILIP WYLIE

Every effort has been expended in these volumes not to rally around the use of a specific articulator or analog or even to belong to any specific cult, because, in spite of the fact that my philosophy and methodology, properly conceived and executed, have proved themselves in clinical cases over a period of years, I am cognizant of a wide and complex variation of known and unknown factors, which possibly accounts for the honest differences of opinion and lack of agreement as to what is the best treatment or procedure for any given patient. The objective is to stress the need of a familiarity with the biomechanical aspects of the teeth and their supporting structures and to present procedures that fulfill what practice consists of and theory comprises.

The facts and findings, gathered from study, investigation, research, and experimentation (clinical and laboratory), have been classified and correlated. By analyzing the theoretical aspects and applying them in a practical manner, by making clinical observations, by applying the laws and principles of engineering as they pertain to restorative dentistry, by perfecting technical procedures, and by keeping an "open mind" to other viewpoints, I have endeavored to present a sound application of proven principles. How a mouth should be rehabilitated depends on training, skills, experience, knowledge, and attitude. It is directly proportional to the individual's understanding and appreciation of oral physiology and his conception of what constitutes a normal function of the jaws and their component parts.

It also means that one must have, to be more specific, a thorough knowledge of anatomy, histology, and physiology of the jaws and associated structures and must understand the function of the temporomandibular joint and that of the muscles responsible for its motivation. An understanding of the harmony that should exist between cuspal interdigitation and mandibular centricity and the ability to recognize this lack of harmony and predict its possible effect on the temporomandibular joints, the teeth, and the associated structures are most important.

A number of years ago, the members of the Gnathological Society of California gave to the dental profession proof of the existence of the transverse axis, along with an accurate device for locating it. They demonstrated the difference between mandibular centric and so-called "acquired centric," proved the importance of the Bennett movement, and devised a way to construct anatomic occlusal surfaces that would be harmonious with its influence.[1] A recording apparatus (pantograph) and an articulator (analog) were developed whereby a dentist could not only accurately determine the functional movement of the jaw but could diagnose the various abnormalities of mandibular function or occlusal disharmony and subsequently restore it to its best physiologic function. Application of these principles will show that teeth in malfunction do not "wear in" but "wear out" of occlusion. Flat teeth exert increased stress on the periodontium, as well as on the temporomandibular structures.

We swallow many, many times every 24 hours. When we swallow, the teeth are brought together with force. This points up the fact that chewing and swallowing forces must be equally and properly distributed for maximum longevity of the teeth and their supporting structures.

A knowledge of all systemic and psychologic factors that influence the health of the oral cavity is also of the utmost importance. The mouth is a functioning organ subject to the same physiologic laws that govern other parts of the body.

To reach a stage of development that would be very helpful in our professional endeavors, it might be wise to pause and reflect on some thoughts that a philosopher[2] conveyed to me some time ago. Movement creates change, and change necessitates the adjustments that can result in suffering. The inescapable pain of adaptation to new conditions is intrinsic to the personality. It is questionable whether even the concept of complete achievement is tenable—the perfect state must present a condition where change would be unwelcome indeed. There would be no more to accomplish, and none willing to accept any deviations. And yet without change, life itself must disappear. Absorption in the process of creation and self-enlightenment may help to develop within you the condition you sought.

A mental attitude can reduce pain; it cannot eliminate it. Elimination has been confused with reduction. In the field of mouth rehabilitation I have followed a number of paths that I thought would lead to salvation and have in my disillusionment with some of these paths failed to appreciate the reductions that I gained. The better parts of various concepts have been welded together to attain the best possible results with our present knowledge of the subject.

The clinical phase has been correlated with the basic sciences. The dentist must utilize the available basic science knowledge but must not allow himself to be hoodwinked into underestimating the importance of technical skills and adequate clinical training—he must become biomechanically oriented.

In other words, the purpose of a book of this nature is to impart to the student of mouth rehabilitation an analysis of phases of theory and research and its practical applications that will bring to the fore the "why" and the "how" of the science and art of rehabilitative procedures, whose important objective is the restoration and maintenance of the function of the dental mechanism. Our purpose is to restore the vital function and characteristic beauty of the masticatory apparatus by an intelligent application of the basic requirements such as the anatomic, physiologic, mechanical, hygienic, and esthetic which show that no superstructure can be more enduring than its foundation. Occlusal stress and foundation resistance are reciprocal forces, and these forces must be properly balanced to obtain efficiency in occlusal performance and durability. Tissue response and tolerance varies from one individual to another.

Therefore, we must make keen clinical observations, perfect our techniques, and apply engineering principles that would pertain to restorative dentistry, the development of art and workmanship, a knowledge of dental materials, etc. This will allow us to (1) maintain the health of the supporting tooth or teeth and the investing and environmental tissues that will help in the resistance of the forces developed by the oral mechanism; (2) restore proper anatomic form including coronal form, cusps, ridges, grooves, fossae, interproximal embrasures (keeping in mind the normal deflection in the gingival half of the proximal surface to avoid periodontal complications), approximal contact areas, etc.; (3) meet all the requirements of articulation and occlusion and thereby good function (the stresses will be properly distributed); (4) obtain a peripheral continuity between the retainer and supporting tooth, and also adaptation of pontic to tissue, with a degree of accuracy that will offer no mechanical irritation to the investing and surrounding tissues and will ensure protection from subsequent caries; and (5) maintain vitality of abutment teeth.

A degree of inherent strength adequate to the requirements of stress must be obtained.[3] It is necessary to understand and apply engineering principles to avoid failures in our splints, fixed and removable partial dentures, etc.—lack of sufficient rigidity in these types of appliances is a frequent cause of failure. Abutment parallelism, removal of adequate tooth structure, and the use of the proper materials arranged in the correct shape, form and thickness in regard to the forces acting upon them will obtain this rigidity and thereby adequate retention of the retainers, which will prevent dislodgment of the finished restorations. Flexure can cause damage to the abutments and may result in the eventual loosening of the retainers and fatigue of the metal. The pontic must be properly designed and must be of adequate strength to provide stability to the fixed partial denture. The connector also requires sufficient strength to prevent breakage of the joint between the retainer and its suspended member, the pontic.

The finished restoration must be correctly finished and polished, thereby keeping the adherence of food particles to a minimum. The abutment teeth must be properly positioned, free of pathosis, and with sufficient supporting structures to hold the fixed partial denture or splint. Teeth tilted beyond 25 degrees can only be used as abutments if orthodontic intervention can return them to a more favorable position, otherwise they must be ruled out.

Retainers and pontics must preserve the symmetrical alignment of the adjacent teeth and, if within the range of vision, must match them closely in size, type, and color. All unnecessary display of gold should be avoided. However, if an appliance of proper strength cannot be made because of esthetic considerations, esthetics must take second place. A combination of the fixed and removable partial dentures must be used in many cases to preserve the integrity of the dental arch and to restore its proper function.

The question of art in dentistry must not be overlooked. It is an oft-repeated saying that "the highest form of art is to conceal art." Art is a talent that may be acquired by training and application, but as an inherent quality it is a gift from heaven. The expression of art in dentistry is the expression of the dentist or technician: "Fortunate is he who is so endowed, for within his hands, mind, and eyes repose untold powers to restore the beauty, character, and harmony of human form." The importance of good workmanship or skilled craftsmanship plays a major role in restorative dentistry. It brings to fruition all the efforts concentrated toward an efficient piece of work.[4]

The student or practitioner must place himself in the proper frame of mind to receive the various viewpoints with respect to his professional responsibilities. He must continue to read, study, and make accurate clinical and laboratory observations. In other words, he must be a continuous student.

TERMINOLOGY*

A *fixed partial denture* is attached to the abutment teeth by means of retainers and replaces the missing teeth by means of pontics, thereby establishing good function, comfort, esthetics, and health to the supporting structures (Fig. 2-1).

Component parts of a fixed partial denture:

The components of a fixed partial denture are (1) abutment, (2) retainer, (3) pontic, and (4) connector (Fig. 2-2).

1. An *abutment* is a tooth or root that furnishes the support for the bridge. It is a tooth to which the fixed prosthesis is attached by means of a retainer (Fig. 2-3).

2. A *retainer* is that part of the fixed prosthesis that is attached to the abutment tooth and to the pontic or suspended portion of the bridge (Fig. 2-4). *There are several types of retainers—intracoronal and extracoronal.*

   a. A *full veneer crown* is a restoration that restores all surfaces of the coronal portion of the tooth (Fig. 2-5).
   b. A *partial veneer crown* is a restoration that restores all surfaces of the coronal portion of a tooth except its facial surface (Fig. 2-6).
   c. A *dowel crown* is a restoration that restores all or a large portion of the coronal part of an endodontically treated tooth by adding a post or dowel for retention (Fig. 2-7). A *pinledge or dowel pin crown* (partial veneer) is a restoration that restores from one to three surfaces of the coronal portion of a tooth and is retained by means of dowel pins or lock grooves and dowel pins (Fig. 2-8).
   d. An *inlay or onlay* is a restoration that is usually modified in one form or another for added retention and resistance to displacement (Figs. 2-9 and 2-10).

---

*The terminology generally used in these volumes is the same as the accepted terms in Boucher, Carl O., editor: Current clinical dental terminology, St. Louis, 1974, The C. V. Mosby Co.

A

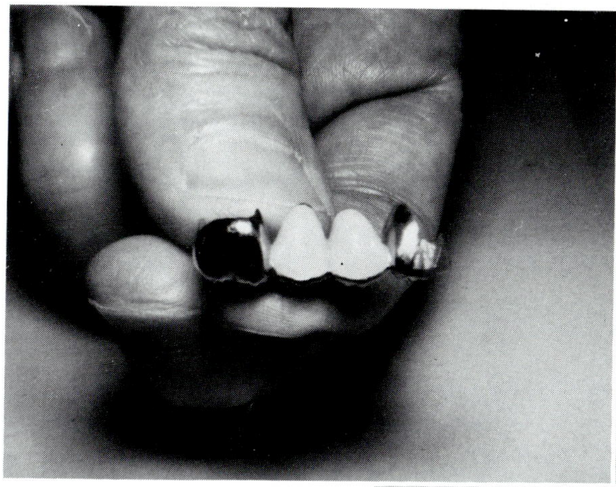

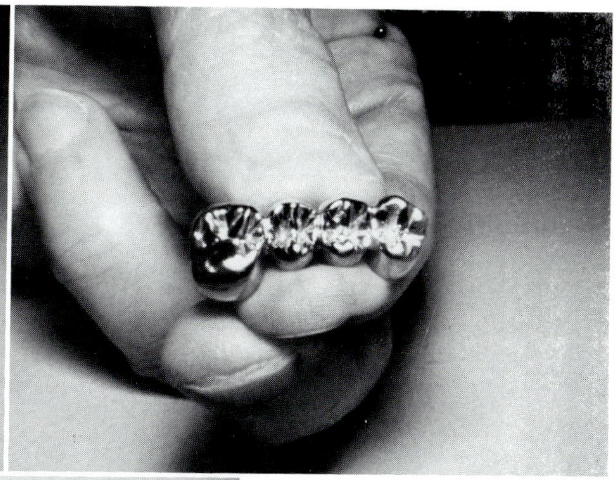

B

C

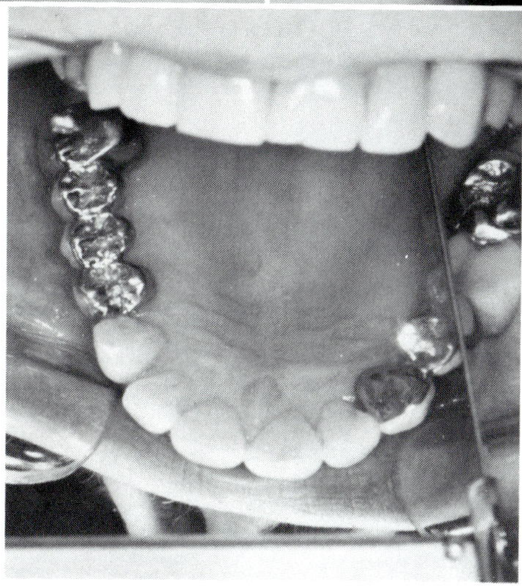

Fig. 2-1. A, A fixed partial denture. **B,** Occlusal view. **C,** As it appears in the mouth.

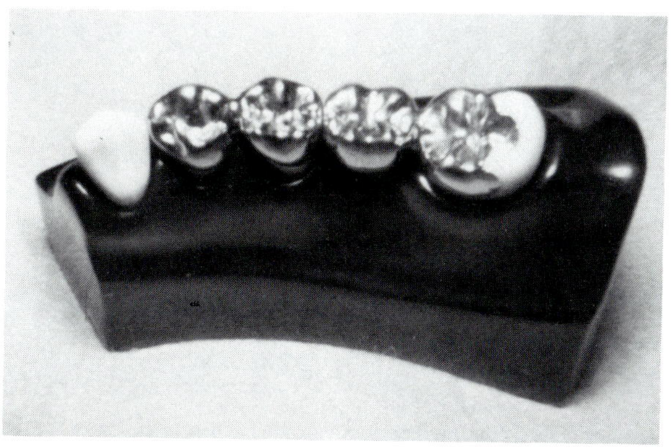

Fig. 2-2. Components of a fixed partial denture: three-quarter crown (bicuspid) and half-crown (molar) abutment preparations, partial veneer crown and half-crown retainers, veneered pontics, and rigid connectors.

A

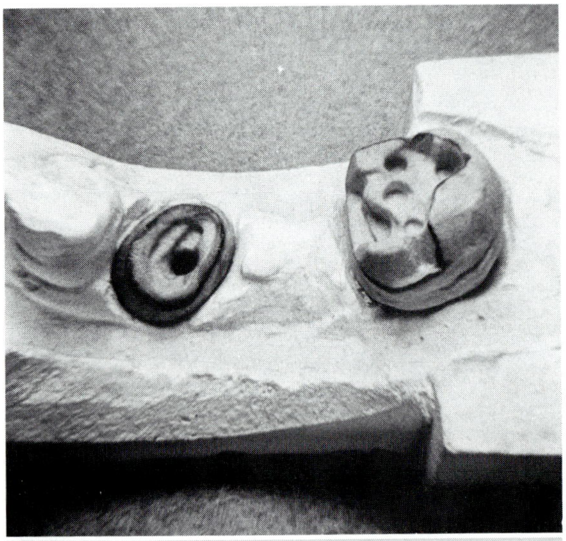

B

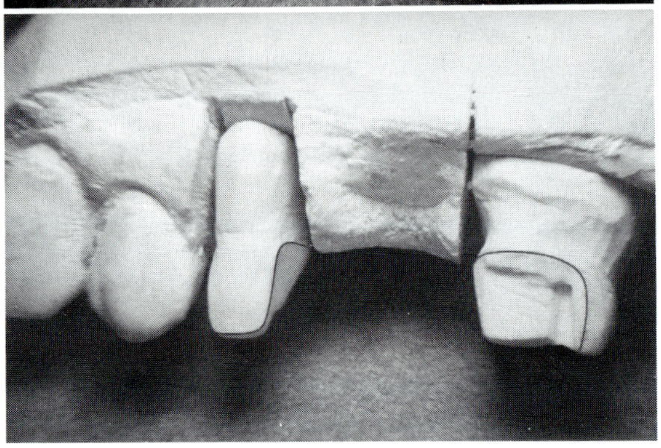

Fig. 2-3. Various types of abutments. **A,** Root support by means of post anchorage support and modified half-crown; **B,** half-crown and three-quarter crown.

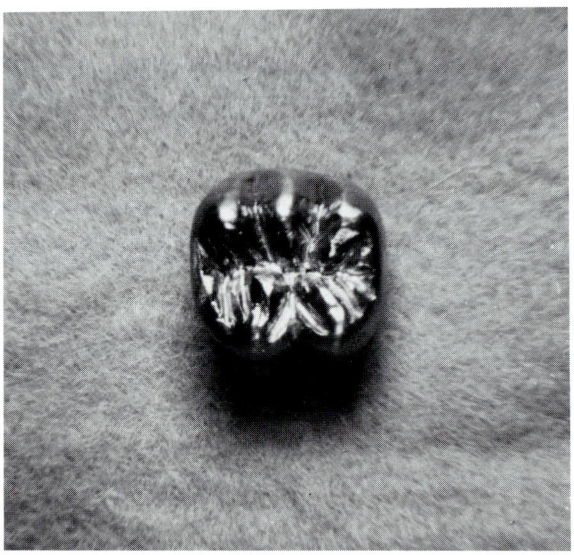

Fig. 2-4. A full crown retainer.

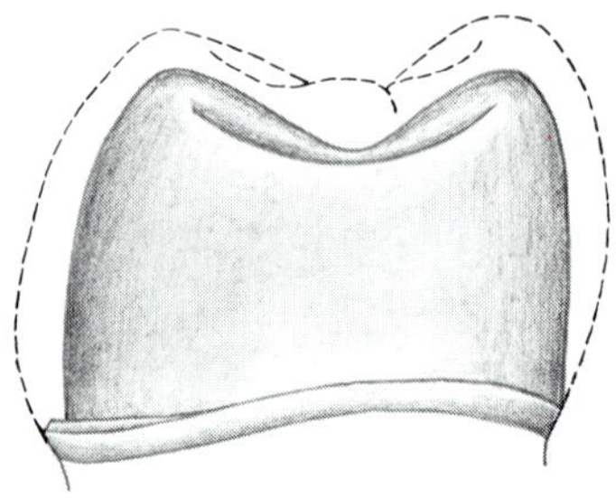

A

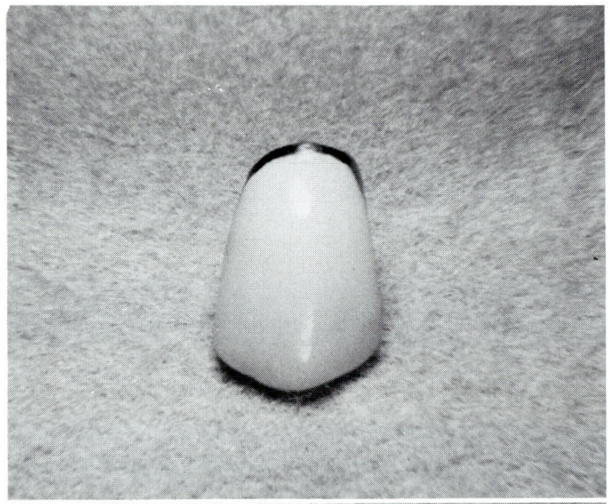

B

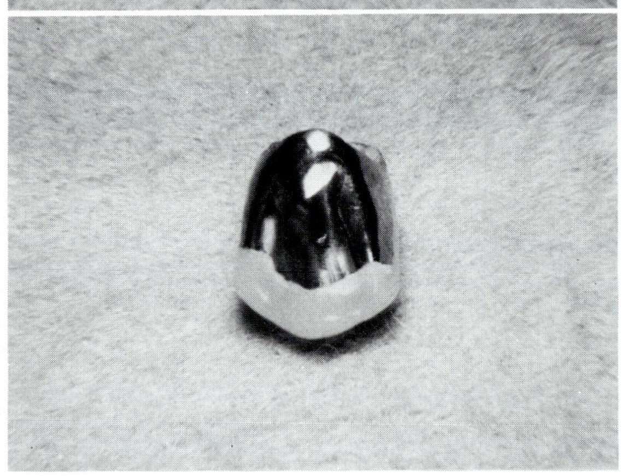

C

Fig. 2-5. **A,** Type of preparation for a posterior full veneer crown to be used as a retainer. **B,** Labial view of a porcelain veneer retainer. **C,** Lingual view of same retainer.

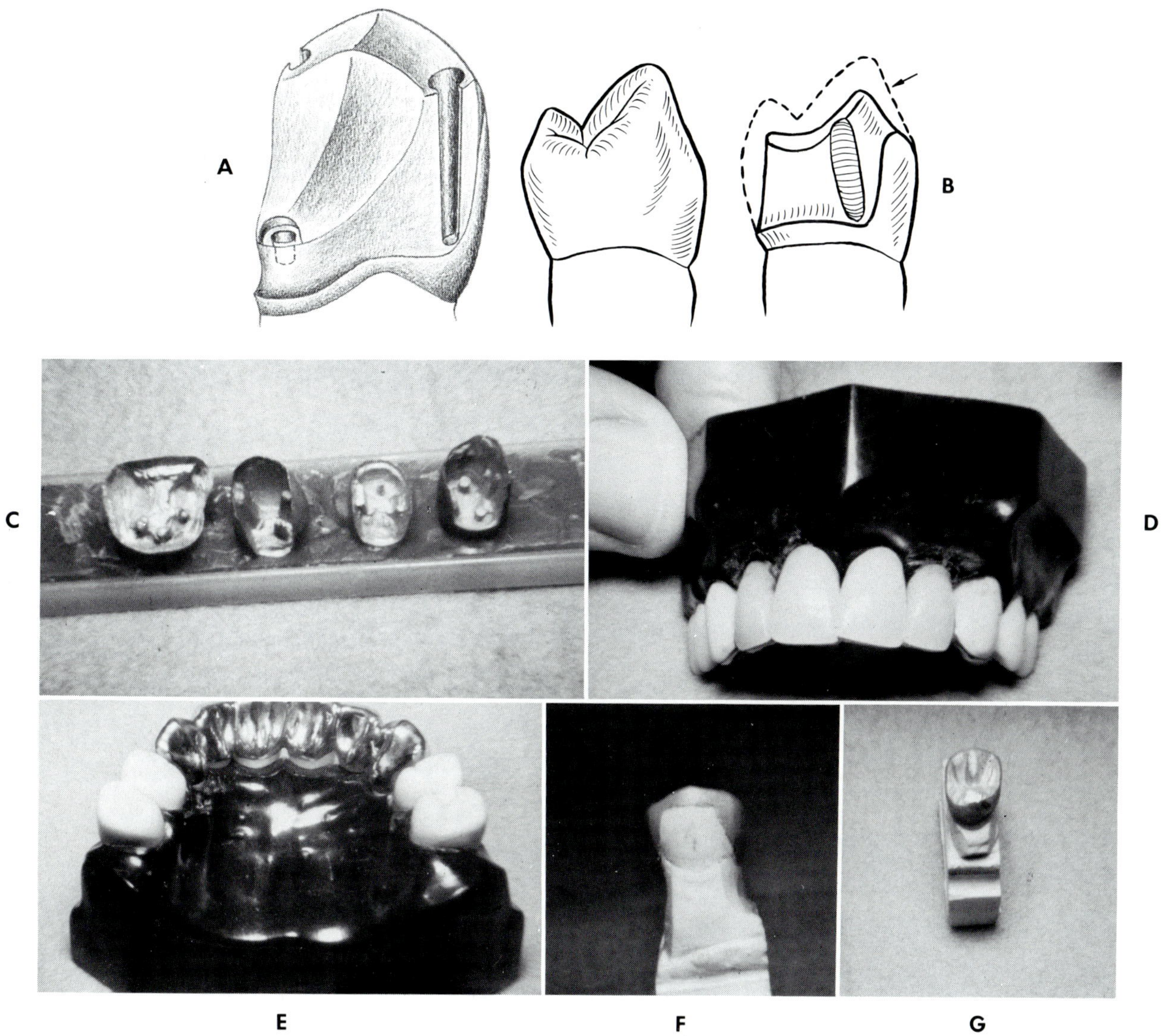

Fig. 2-6. Various views of the partial veneer crown from preparation to completion.

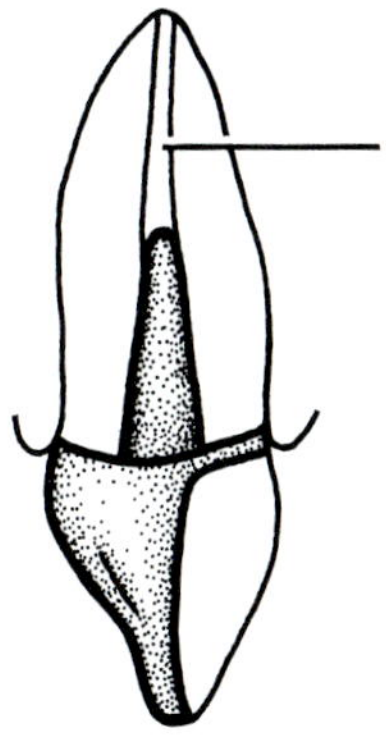

Fig. 2-7. A dowel crown.

A

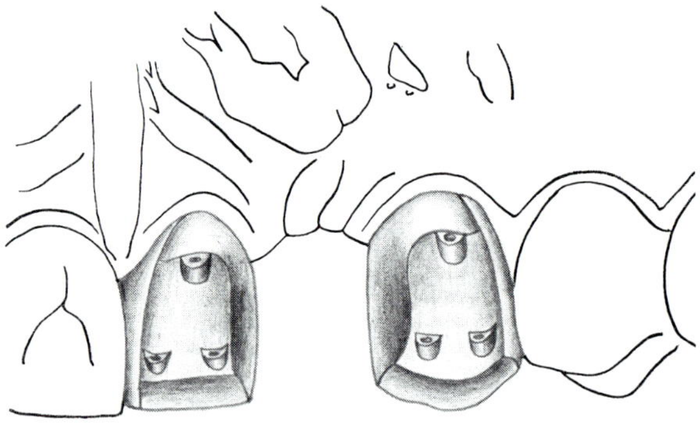

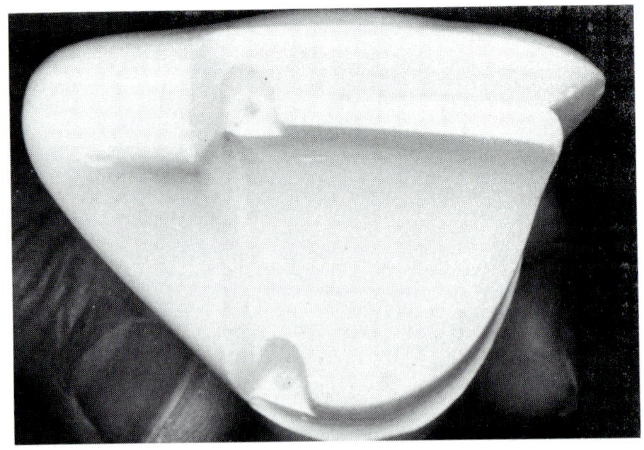

B

Fig. 2-8. Pinledge or dowel pin crown (partial veneer).

A

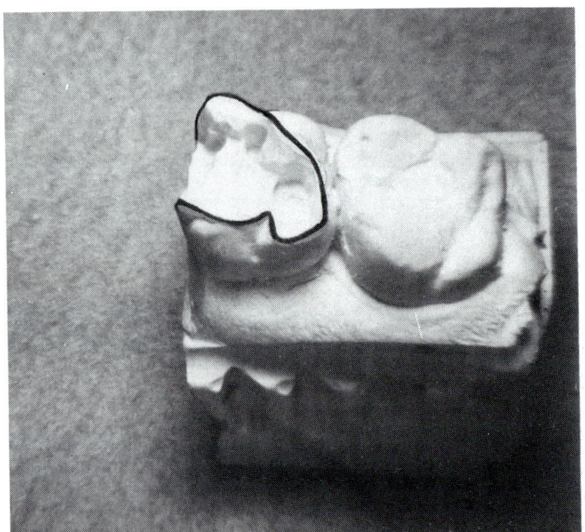

B

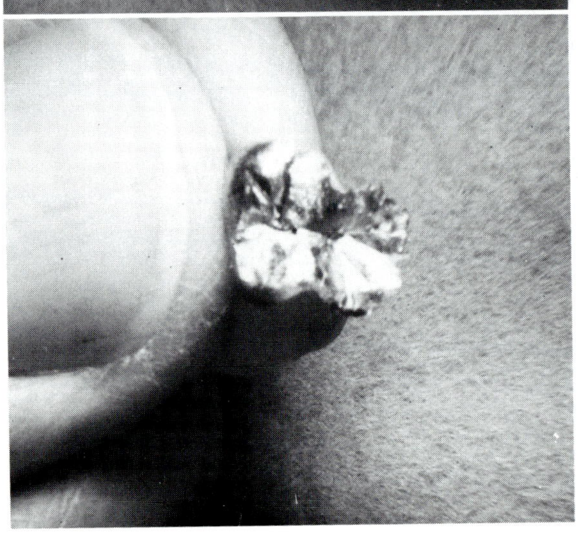

Fig. 2-9. A, Inlay preparation; **B,** the casting.

3. A *pontic* is the suspended member of a fixed prosthesis; it replaces the lost natural tooth and restores both its function and its esthetics (Fig. 2-11).

4. A *connector* is that part of the fixed prosthesis that joins the pontic, or suspended member, to the retainer. It is of two types: (1) rigid (soldered joint) or (2) nonrigid (tapered key and keyway or subocclusal connector) (Figs. 2-12 to 2-14).

A *removable partial denture* replaces one or more teeth and depends primarily upon the mucosa underlying its base(s) for its major support, and for its secondary support and retention it relies on clasps and rests or one of several types of precision attachments (Figs. 2-15 and 2-16).

In *a cantilever fixed partial denture* a missing tooth is suspended from a single or multiple abutment teeth (Figs. 2-17 to 2-19).

A *fixed splint* (unilateral and bilateral) joins two or more teeth by means of crowns for stabilization and reorientation of forces and stresses (Figs. 2-20 to 2-23).

Physiologic occlusion is an occlusion that operates in harmony and presents no pathologic manifestation in the supporting structures of the teeth. The stresses placed on the teeth are dissipated normally, with a balance existing between the stresses and the adaptive capacity of the supporting tissues—in other words, an occlusion in harmony with functions of the masticatory system. It implies a balance between occlusal stress and tissue resistance.

Pathogenic occlusion is an occlusal relationship capable of producing pathologic changes in the supporting tissues.

Balanced occlusion is the simultaneous contacting of the upper and lower teeth on the right and left sides

Text continued on p. 16.

A

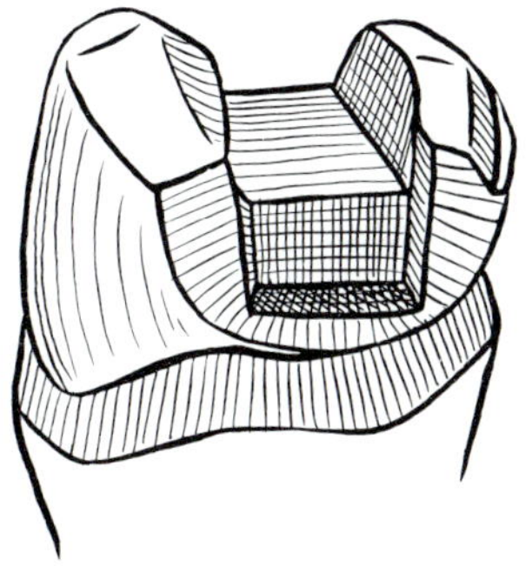

B

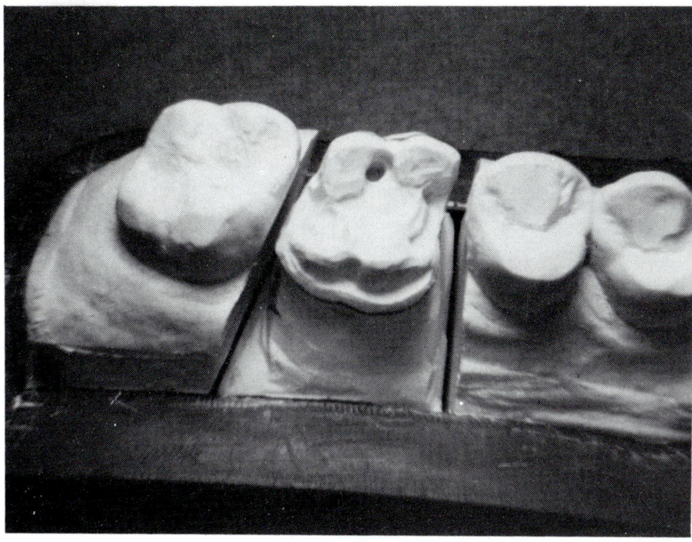

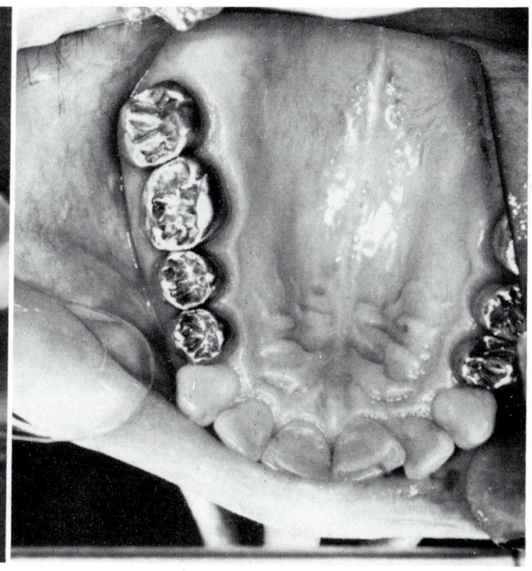

C

Fig. 2-10. A and **B,** The onlay preparation; **C,** as it appears in the mouth.

A

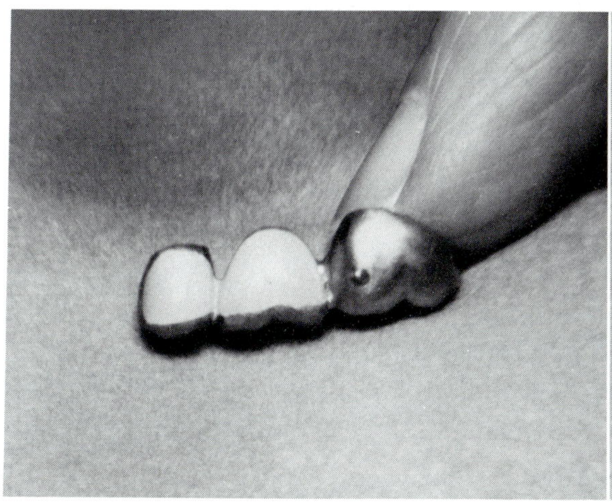

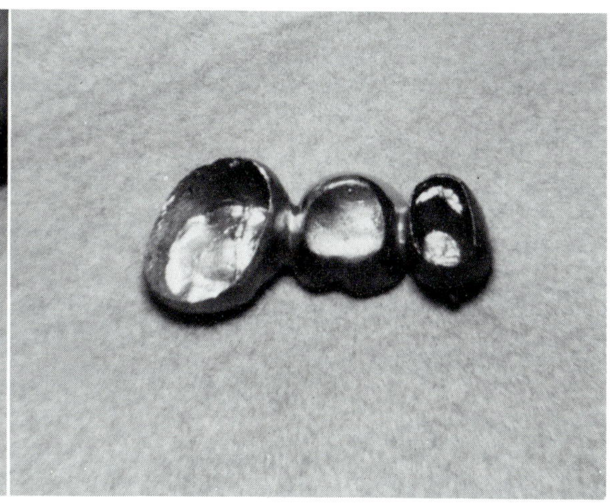

B

Fig. 2-11. The pontic.

A

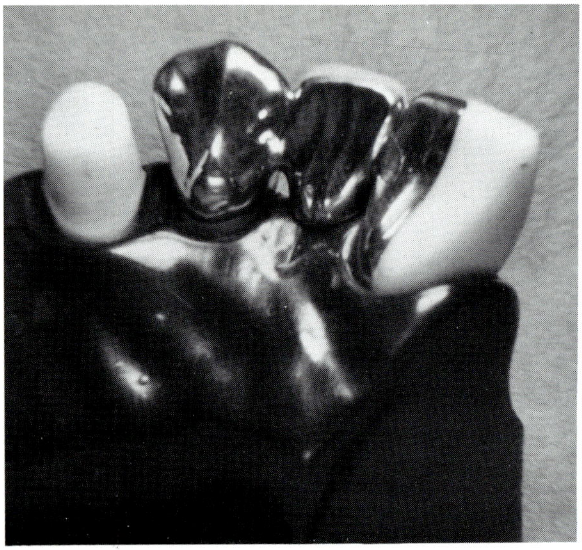

B

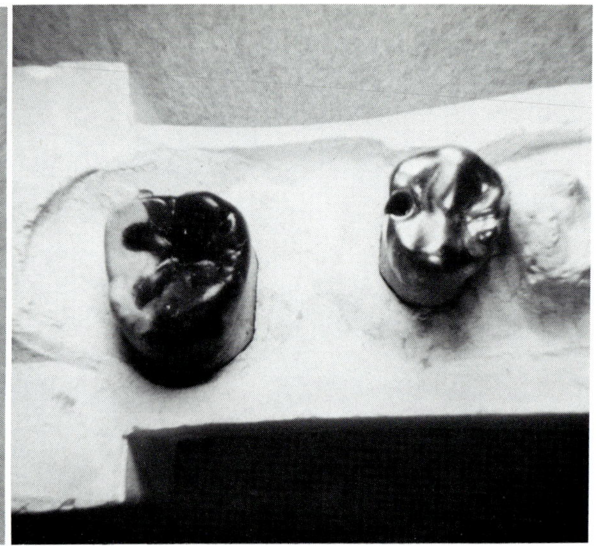

Fig. 2-12

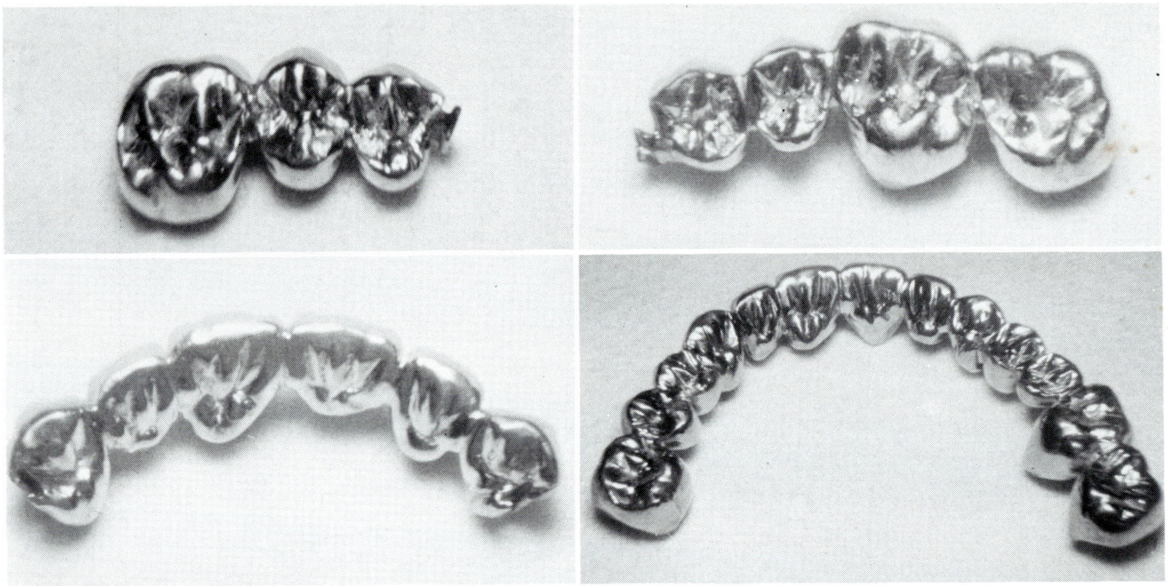

Fig. 2-13

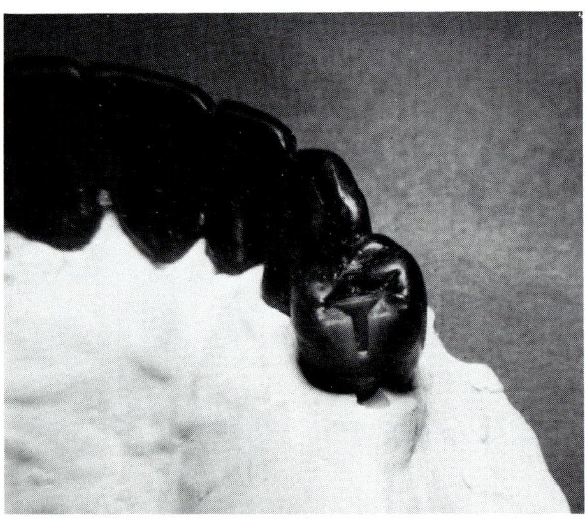

Fig. 2-14

Figs. 2-12 to 2-14. The rigid and nonrigid connector.

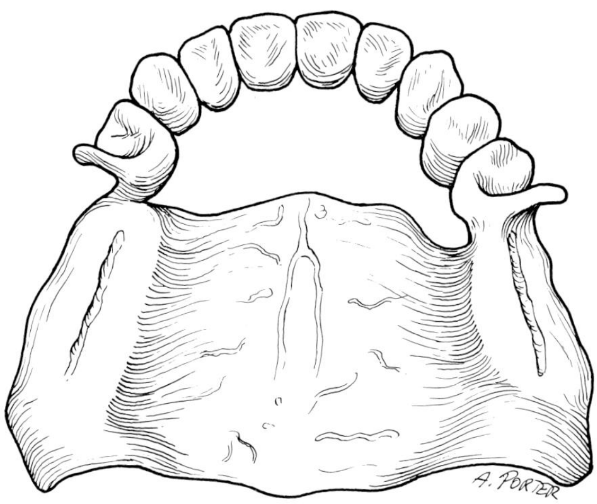

Fig. 2-15

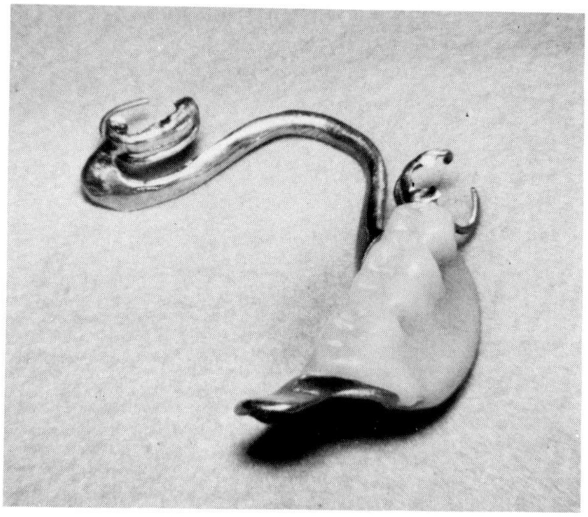

Fig. 2-16

Figs. 2-15 and 2-16. The precision attachment removable partial denture and the modified clasp removable partial denture. (Note the use of the wire clasp below cast clasp section on lower left molar.)

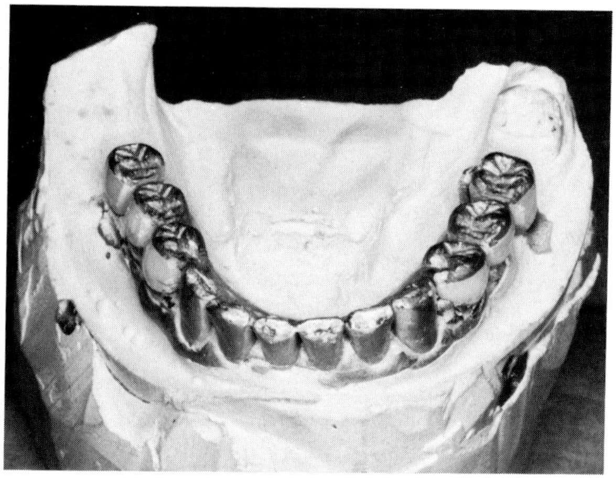

Fig. 2-17

Figs. 2-17 to 2-19. The cantilevered fixed partial denture or splint.

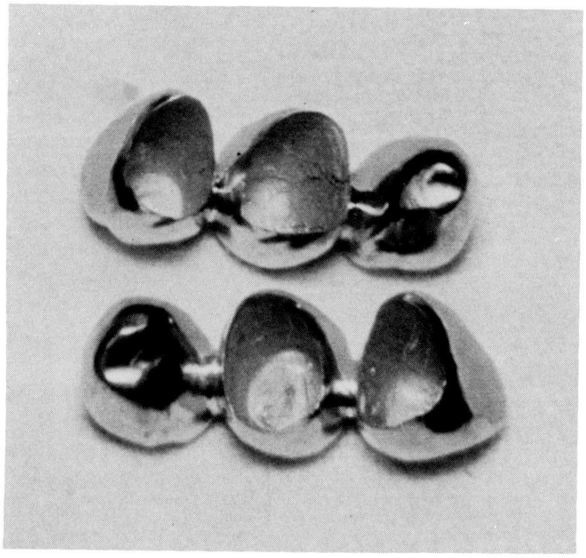

Fig. 2-18

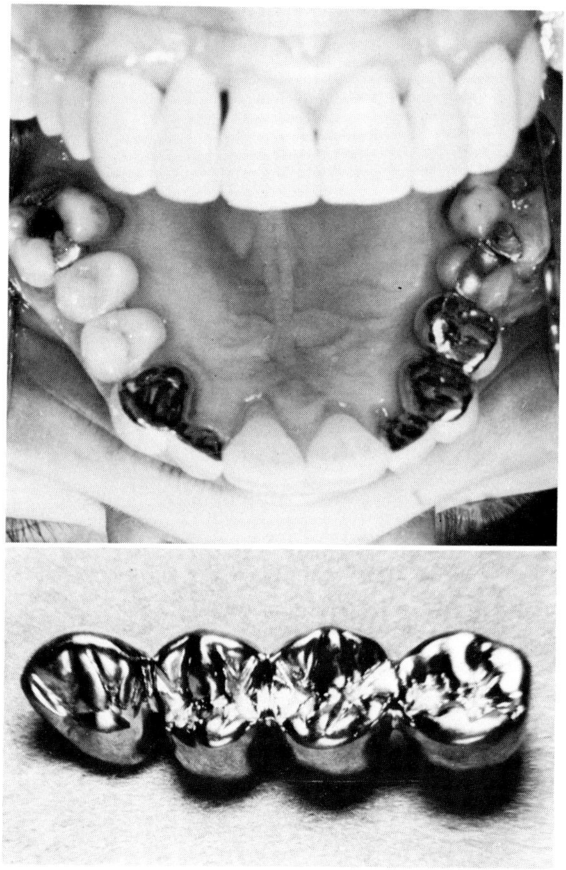

A

B

Fig. 2-19

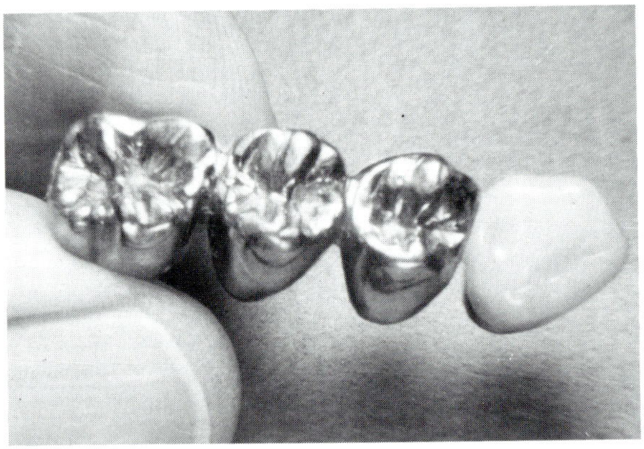

Fig. 2-20

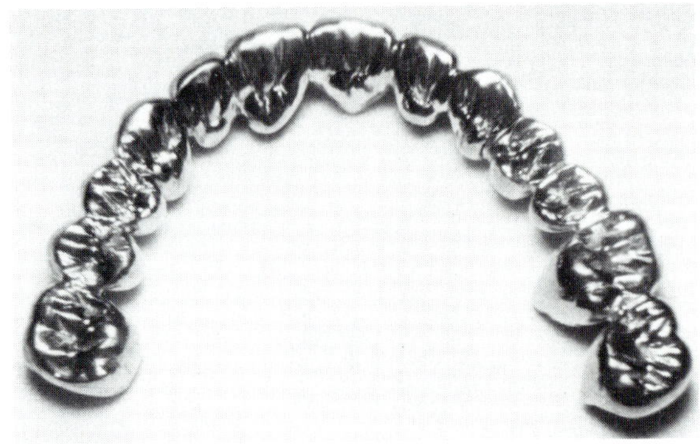

Fig. 2-21

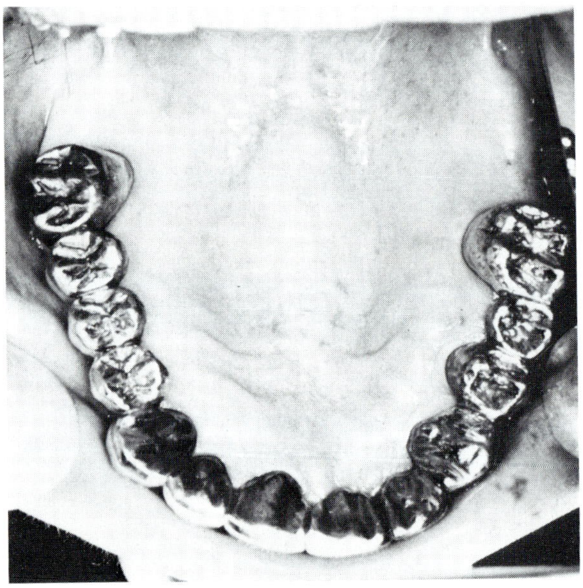

Fig. 2-22

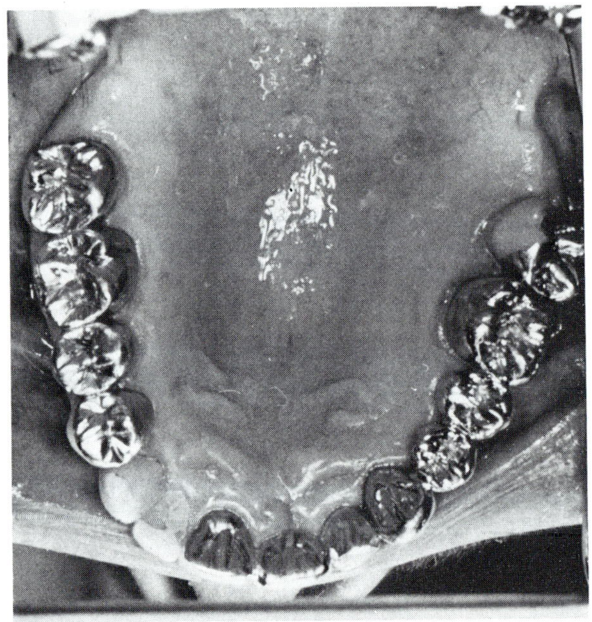

Fig. 2-23

Figs. 2-20 to 2-23. Types of unilateral and bilateral fixed splints.

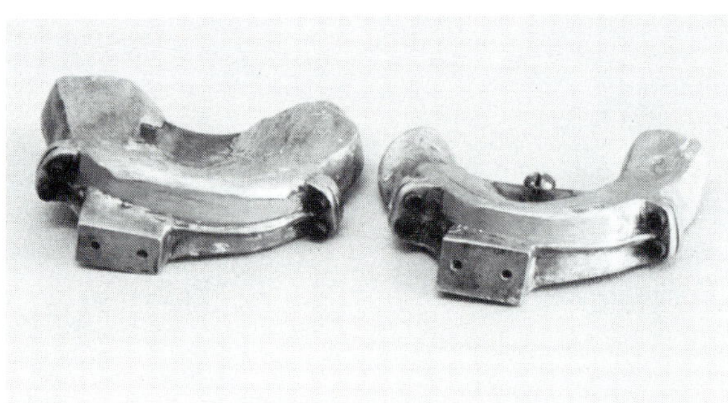

Fig. 2-24. Clutches.

A

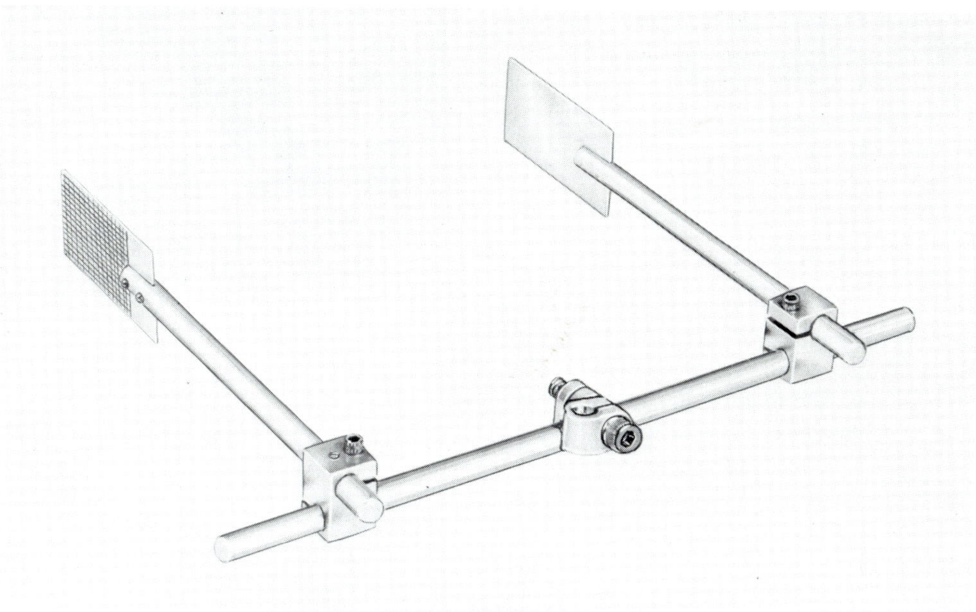

B

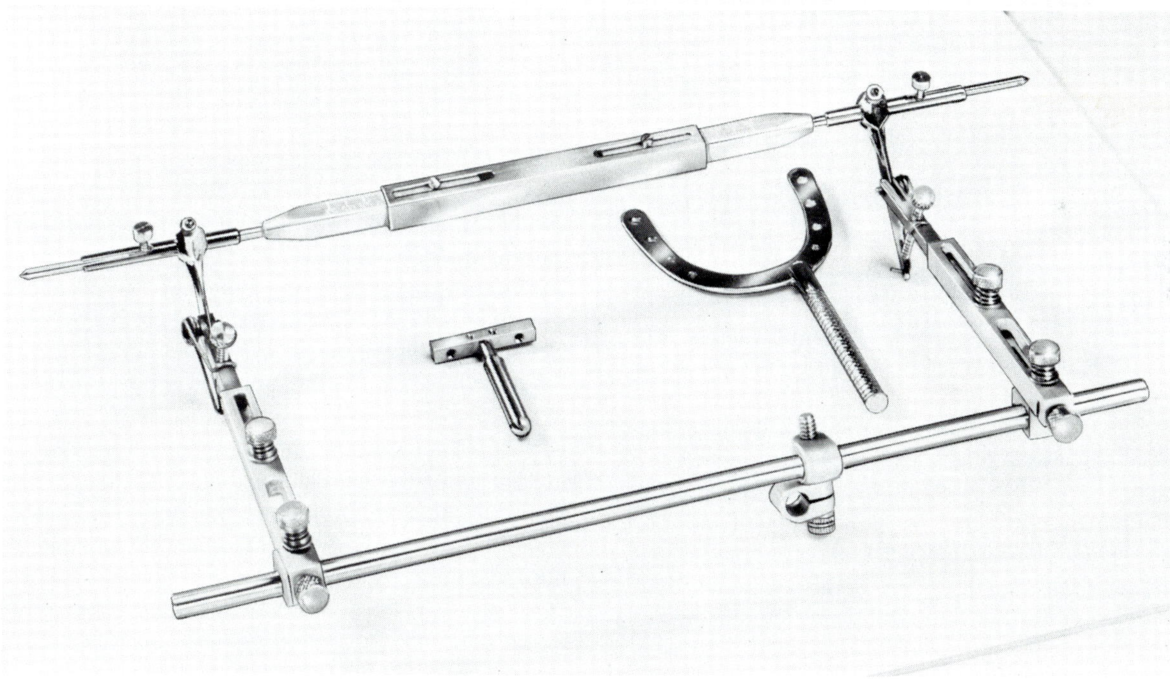

Fig. 2-25. The kinematic face-bow. **A,** Thin aluminum plates attached to the side arms, covered with a ruled surface; **B,** the hinge-bow also showing the hinge-bow holder, the bite fork, and the intercondylar gauge. (Courtesy J. Aderer, Inc., New York, N.Y.)

(during excursive movements) and in the anterior and posterior occlusal areas of the jaws.

The *working side* is the lateral segment of a dentition toward which the mandible is moved.

The *balancing side* is the side opposite the working side of the dentition; it is usually the side toward which the mandible is moved.

Clutches (or trays attached to the teeth with temporary cement) are necessary appendages for holding the devices used in recording jaw relations (Fig. 2-24).

Centric relation "of the mandible is its rearmost, midmost, untranslated hinged position. It is a strained relation as are all border relations. It is the only maxillo-mandibular relation that can be statically repeated."* It is the terminal posterior, superior position of the mandibular condyles in their fossae.

Centric occlusion is the occlusion of the teeth that is the result of mandibular closure, the condyles remaining in their terminal hinge position.

Gnathology "is the sum total knowledge required to successfully treat the complex organ of chewing and includes all the ramifications of dentistry."†

A *face-bow* is a caliper-like device that is used to record the relationship of the jaws to the temporomandibular joints (or opening axis of the jaws) and to orient the casts in this same relationship to the opening axis of the articulator.

A *kinematic face-bow* (hinge-bow) is a face-bow whose caliper ends (condyle rods) can be adjusted to permit the accurate location of the axis of rotation of the mandible by observation of the movement of the condyle rods while the mandible is moved up and down in its most posterior, superior position (Fig. 2-25).

Hinge axis (transverse axis) is an imaginary line between the mandibular condyles around which the mandible can rotate without translatory movement. The kinematic face-bow is the instrument used to locate the hinge axis (transverse axis).

Bennett movement is the bodily lateral movement or lateral shift of the mandible resulting from the movements of the condyles along the lateral inclines of the mandibular fossae during lateral jaw movement. Bennett movement, or lateral motion of the head of the condyle, is very powerful. It is a lateral bodily shift of the mandible. Articulators that do not have a vertical axis on which the Bennett movement can be registered are considered to be inaccurate. In taking a Gothic arch tracing, the repeated appearance of a blunted apex is not due to faulty technique but is an expression of the Bennett movement. The lines should therefore not be arbitrarily extended to arrive at a "true" centric position (Fig. 2-26).

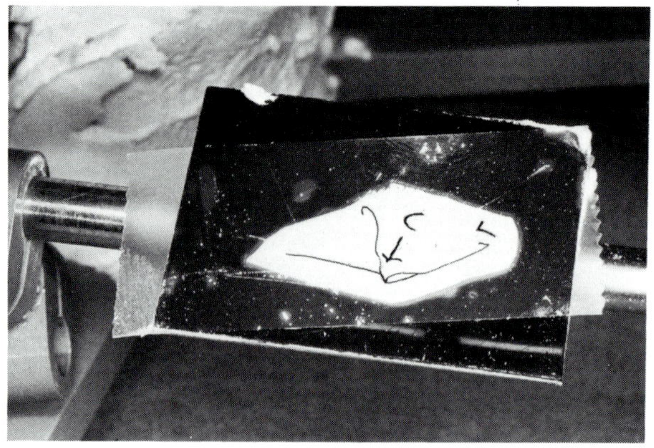

Fig. 2-26. Repeated appearance of a blunted or peculiar apex is sometimes not due to faulty technique but is an expression of the Bennett movement.

Condylar guidance is the mechanical device on an articulator. It is intended to produce similar guidance in articulator movement as is produced by the paths of the condyles in the temporomandibular joints. The *condyle path* is the path traveled by the mandibular condyle in the temporomandibular joint during the various mandibular movements.

Incisal guidance is the influence on mandibular movements by the contacting surfaces of the mandibular and maxillary anterior teeth.

Rest position is the position of the mandible when the jaws are in rest relation. It is a postural position of the mandible under the influence of the resting length of the muscles that elevate or depress the mandible or, we may say, the position that the mandible passively assumes when the mandibular musculature is relaxed.

A *pantograph* is an extraoral tracing device that traces the paths of motion of the transverse axis. It consists of a maxillary and mandibular face-bow to carry recording plates and writing styli (Fig. 2-27). With the pantograph it is possible to determine on the patient the full characters of the condyle paths, their inclinations and shape, the amount of Bennett movement, the centric position of the mandible, the transverse axis and the maxillomandibular dimensions, and the plane of the dimensional reference, the axis-orbital plane. It definitely shows what the mandible actually

*From Stuart, Charles E.: Personal communication.

†From Stallard, Harvey: Personal communication.

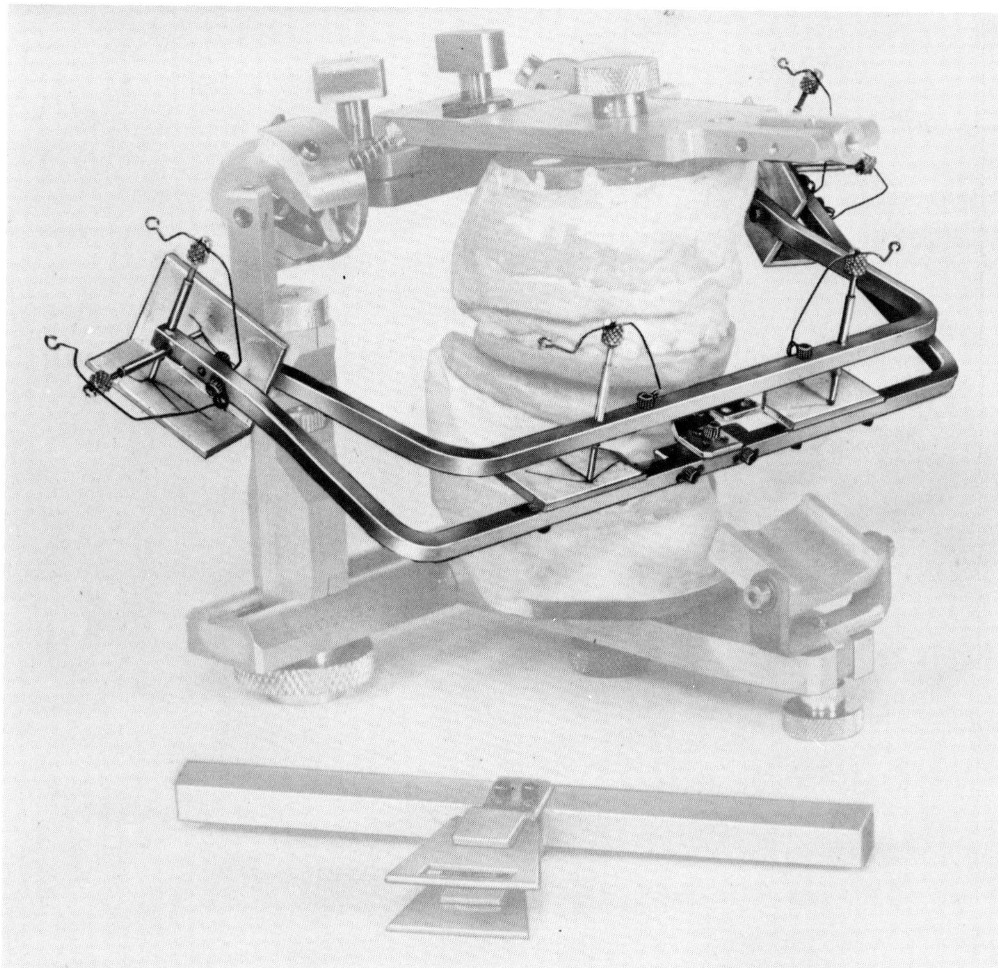

Fig. 2-27. The Simulator pantograph. (Courtesy J. Aderer, Inc., New York, N.Y.)

does. The fixed biologic factors of articulation are determined. Movements of the mandible that bring about the ever-changing relation of tooth contacts result from paths of motion of the transverse axis. These functional relations can be recorded and reproduced by means of a suitable pantograph or writing apparatus.

An *adjustable articulator* is an articulator that may be adjusted to permit movement of the casts into recorded eccentric relationships. This articulator is capable of adjustment to more than one eccentric position (Fig. 2-28). It orients the casts as to their relations to the face, and it discloses the fixed elements of articulation; it admits of a positive diagnosis of the conditions presented by the patient in regard to his articulation in the minutest detail.

The articulator settings must be oriented to the plane of reference by means of an orbital rest on the upper bow. Herein lies the need for an articulator in which the condyle path and the Bennett movement are a part of the upper bow, just as in the skull, and the axis in the lower bow, just as in the mandible. Otherwise the settings cannot be oriented to the plane of reference (Fig. 2-29).

In other words, by means of the hinge-bow and the pantograph one is able to record accurately the opening and closing axis and the protrusive, the lateral protrusive, and the basic lateral positions, with or without the Bennett movement, as the joints dictate.[8]

In the analog we have an instrument that can reproduce not only the relative positions of the mandible to the maxillae but all paths of motion to a definite and precise degree. Also, because of the accuracy of the method of transfer, it is possible to make diagnostic casts, working casts, and remount casts of the restorations and examine the occlusion on

A

B

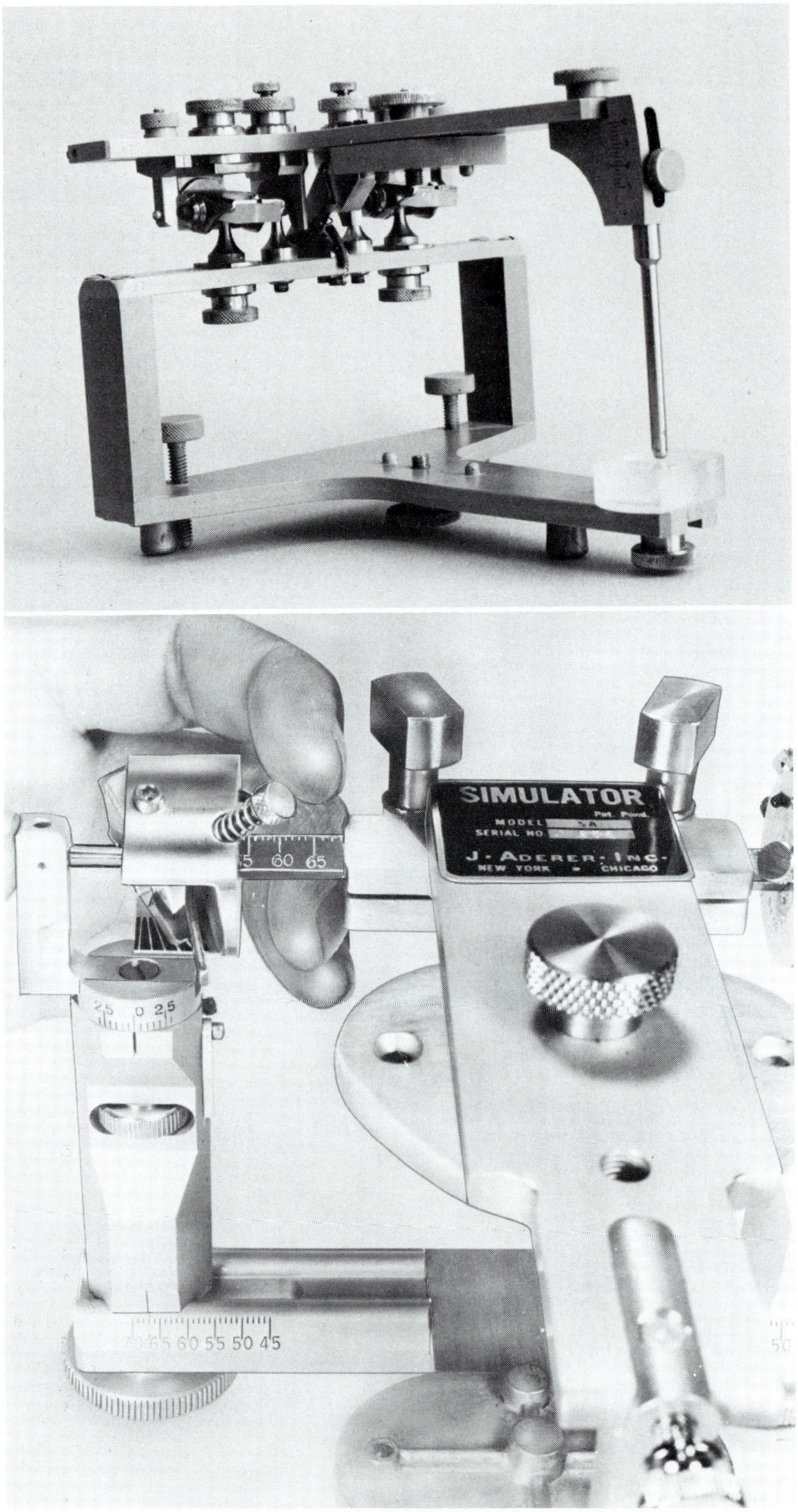

Fig. 2-28. A, The Stuart Computer; **B,** making the intercondylar adjustment on the Simulator articulator.

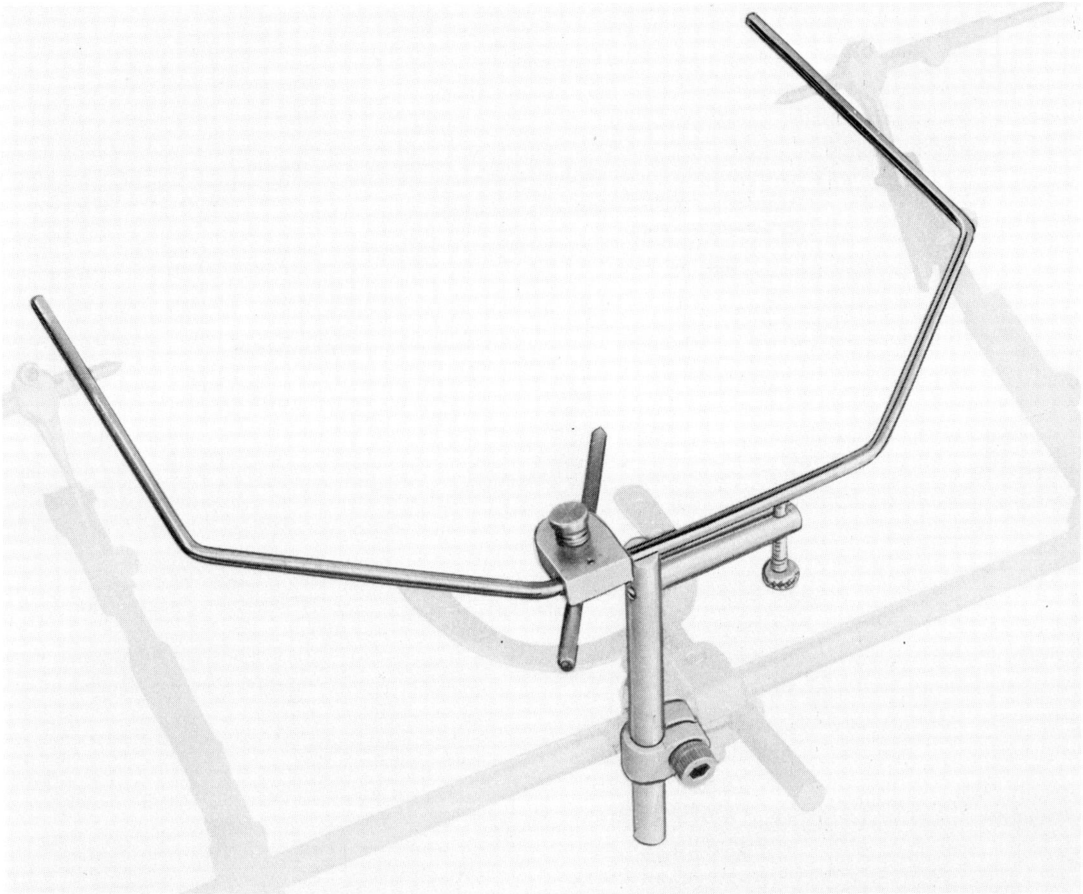

Fig. 2-29. Articulator settings must be oriented to the plane of reference by means of an orbital rest on the upper bow. (Courtesy J. Aderer, Inc., New York, N.Y.)

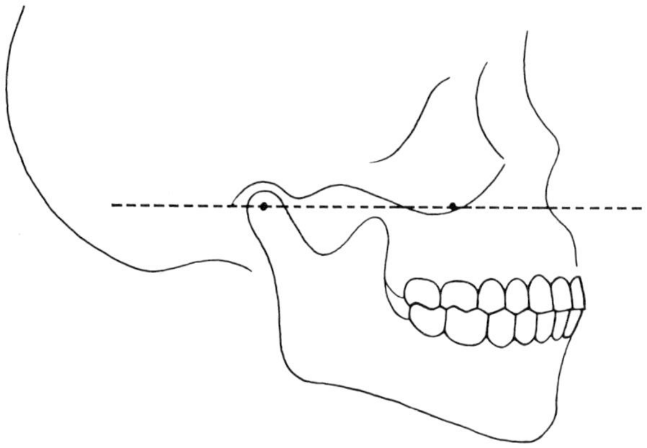

Fig. 2-30. Plane of reference (axis-orbital plane).

the analog. A thorough knowledge of the way the mouth functions is necessary.

The problem seems to resolve itself into a very important fact, which is that it is necessary to comprehend the "fixed biologic factors," and also those subject to change by the dentist (plane of occlusion, curve of Spee, curve of Wilson, anterior guidance, cusp height, compensating occlusal curve), that are involved in the occlusion of the teeth.

Fixed and variable factors of occlusion must be determined accurately in order to create and maintain a physiologic occlusion because, under any given fixed set of these factors, there is only one set of cusps that can function in harmony with jaw movement.

In the *plane of reference* (axis-orbital plane) the transverse axis is constant to the mandible. The terminal hinge position, which is actually centric relation, is constant to both mandible and maxillae. All our mountings are made in this relation. Therefore, the only practical way to maintain constant relationships throughout treatment is to use the axis points and a fixed third point at the base of the right orbit (or on the nose) as the plane of reference (Fig. 2-30).

Thus the axis-orbital plane will give a constant position for the upper jaw, and a correct interocclusal record will establish the position of the lower jaw to the constant upper jaw. In this way repeated mountings will have a constant relation to the records and to the patient's centers of rotation.

The axis-orbital plane is used to maintain approximate relationship of occlusal plane to condylar angulation in mounting casts on the articulator.

Convenience occlusion (acquired, habitual) is the assumed position of maximum intercuspation when there is occlusal interference in the centric path of closure. The convenience occlusion may be anterior, lateral, anterolateral, etc. to the true centric occlusion.

Bruxism is a clenching of the teeth associated with forceful lateral or protrusive jaw movements that results in rubbing, gritting, or grinding together of the teeth, usually during sleep. It is a pathologic condition.

To attain a working knowledge of all that has been presented in this chapter, to correct a mouth in dysfunction to normal function with a high degree of harmony existing between the form and function of the parts, is a lofty ideal. It implies not only a knowledge of scientific facts and technical procedures but hard work, unusual effort, and an understanding that disappointments, difficulties, and obstacles are to be encountered and surmounted. The profession of dentistry has developed a philosophy that transcends the mere filling of holes and spaces—the dentist is a physician to the mouth. However, the dentist must keep in mind at all times that attaining mouth health is one thing, but maintaining it is another thing. Why? It is because all our treatments and procedures are affected and influenced by many known and unknown systemic factors—heredity, diet, metabolism, glandular function, psychologic factors, parafunctions, etc. And let us not overlook iatrogenic factors and patient home care. It is necessary to analyze and learn from our failures as well as our successes.

REFERENCES

1. Coomer, O. B.: Attaining and maintaining mouth health, J. Prosthet. Dent. **3**:500-505, 1953.
2. Rosenkranz, Samuel: Personal communication.
3. Reynolds, J. Marvin: Abutment selection for fixed prosthodontics, J. Prosthet. Dent. **19**:483-488, 1968.
4. Schwartz, Jacob R.: Modern methods of tooth replacement, Brooklyn, N. Y., 1948, Dental Items of Interest Publishing Co., Inc.
5. Boucher, Carl O.: Current clinical dental terminology, St. Louis, 1974, The C. V. Mosby Co.
6. Stallard, Harvey: Personal communication.
7. Stuart, Charles E.: Personal communication.
8. Kornfeld, Max: The problem of function in restorative dentistry, J. Prosthet. Dent. **5**:670-676, 1955.

CHAPTER 3

DIAGNOSIS AND TREATMENT PLANNING

DIAGNOSIS

General considerations

A thorough oral diagnosis is the first order of business if one is to treat the dental patient completely. Diagnosis precedes and dictates the plan of treatment. Examination of the dental patient must be an orderly, detailed, and comprehensive evaluation of the patient's oral, dental, and orofacial structures. It forms the basis on which an accurate diagnosis and logical treatment plan can be formulated. In other words, a thorough examination of the patient and an evaluation of all available data are the essential elements necessary for comprehensive diagnosis and treatment planning, and they determine the success or failure of restorative procedures. The most meticulous techniques may fail if the case is not correctly diagnosed and properly planned.

It is necessary to make a detailed study of the physiologic and pathologic conditions of the masticatory mechanism to determine how, if necessary, to intercept any pathologic processes or to eliminate conditions conducive to disease or injury. The oral cavity often reveals a systemic condition before the patient is aware of one; therefore, recognition of not only dental and oral diseases but any indication of a change from normal in the systemic status of the patient is of the utmost importance.

Diagnostic data are obtained by (1) visual and digital examination of the oral cavity and associated structures, which must be performed in an organized and logical manner, (2) medical and dental histories, (3) clinical and laboratory diagnostic aids, (4) a complete series of roentgenograms, and (5) properly oriented casts on an adjustable articulator.

The data obtained by these means must be all-inclusive and detailed both in observation and recording, because with this information the dentist may proceed to definitive treatment planning and therapy. No dental service can be of value unless the entire mouth is studied and treated as an integral unit.

Consideration of the total personality makeup of the patient is also essential, especially if extensive restorative procedures are being considered, because of the possibility of psychotherapeutic component, the importance of which must never be overlooked.

The dentist must apply his biomechanical and psychologic training to the fullest extent, always keeping in mind the whole person. Never hesitate to ask for a consultation with specialists in the fields of dentistry and medicine.

Diagnostic procedures

MEDICAL AND DENTAL HISTORY

The first appointment with a new patient should consist of what may be designated as the interview and preliminary examination. The chief complaint, if any, is ascertained, and the asking of questions pertaining to the medical and dental histories bring to the fore, among other things, the mood, manner, and anxiety of the patient. Close observation of the patient at this time points up the chances of rapport between the involved individuals and also any semblance of the presence of psychogenic factors. The dentist can get an impression of the psychologic makeup of the patient—his fears, anxieties, and thoughts about his oral and bodily ailments. During the interview it is usually possible to determine whether the patient's teeth are really important to him, whether he is willing to undergo the necessary therapeutic treatment, whether he desires to devote sufficient time in home care, and whether he is willing and able to spend the time and money for the proper type of treatment. Insight is also gathered into the reasons for the patient's lack of attention to his mouth or his compulsive attention to his teeth, his attitude toward dentists and dentistry, and whether it is possible to fulfill the needs of this particular patient. A history of any unusual reactions to local anesthetics or medicaments of any kind should be obtained at this time.

If a complete medical history is available, many unfortunate situations can be prevented. Prior serious systemic diseases may dictate certain modifications of any contemplated oral or dental treatment. Patients with cardiovascular disease may be on a regimen of anticoagulant therapy, which requires precautionary measures. Oral manifestations of systemic diseases—allergies, metabolic disturbances, nutritional disturbances, blood dyscrasias, and many others—may be insidious factors often overlooked as the reason for prosthodontic failures. The oral cavity is an accurate mirror of systemic health or disease. Do not overlook the fact that many a beautiful and well-executed biomechanical dental result has not maintained itself because of the failure to obtain a good medical history. Such history should include the patient's age, occupation, drug intake, information concerning cardiovascular diseases, blood dyscrasias, bleeding time, nutritional or metabolic disturbances, endocrine dysfunction, pain in or around the face, head, and neck, if any, history of a neurosis or psychosis, and other pertinent information. The patient should be questioned concerning systemic conditions that might affect the mouth or his ability to respond well to dental procedures. To avoid reactions, special precautions must be taken by the dentist when he is treating a patient who is taking diuretics and antihypertensive drugs, nitroglycerin, or ganglionic blocking agents. The type of diet is and always will be of such importance that it cannot be overlooked. This detailed general health history allows one to ascertain possible correlations that may exist between oral symptoms and a medical problem. Consultation with the patient's physician is the best source of desired information.

Several well-worded questions will bring out (1) possible reasons for excessive attrition of the teeth, if present, or parafunctions such as bruxism, clenching, picking on teeth, tongue, lip, or cheek biting, and chewing on foreign objects, (2) success or failure of past dental restorations, (3) feelings about former dentists, (4) acute or chronic infections about the mouth, and (5) professional and home care oral hygiene procedures. A detailed history of the patient's dental and periodontal complaints is recorded.

ORAL EXAMINATION

If the patient is desirable from the therapist's viewpoint or amenable to treatment, the oral examination is now undertaken. To make this thorough study, the dentist must employ every available diagnostic measure to the finest detail of each and every tooth and its supporting and surrounding tissues. All the tissues in the oral cavity should be carefully looked at and examined.

The dental and oral tissues are examined visually and digitally. A meticulous scrutiny of the oral tissues by inspection and palpation is very important. It provides the opportunity for studying the tissue conditions of the entire oral mucosa, which includes the soft tissues immediately adjacent to the teeth and the tissues remote from the teeth. The external and internal aspects of the lips, the tongue (its dorsum, lateral borders, and underside), the frenulum and sublingual gland area, the hard and soft palates, the floor of the mouth, the buccal mucosa, and the throat and tonsillar region should be examined by inspection and palpation. Any changes in color, topographic consistency, surface characteristics, etc. should be noted. This part of the examination can also detect oral manifestations of systemic disease (Fig. 3-1).

Unusually large freni and tori are recorded since they can influence appliance design. Aberrant manifestations such as deviations from normal gingival form, color, and pocket depth and fistulas or neoplasms are important findings. A dentist must be stimulated, by making use of diagnostic instrumentation combined with his visual and tactile faculties, to observe oral lesions so that a greater number of patients with early symptoms of oral cancer will be guided toward accurate pathologic diagnosis and specific early treatment. Every effort should be made to detect oral neoplasms long before subjective symptoms appear. Any departures from normal in this area should be referred to the physician for definitive diagnosis.

Examination of the gingival tissues requires detailed inspection and probing to determine its health status. The dentist must be alert to changes in gingival color, texture, and form. If the gingivae are not anatomically normal with proper surface characteristics, this is indicative of pathologic changes. Local and systemic influences upon the gingival tissues, and also gingival changes from the effects of calcareous deposits and plaque, drugs, pregnancy, puberty, menopause, and systemic diseases with gingival manifestations, should be kept in mind. The calibrated periodontal probe for measurement of pocket depth is an important tool in our armamentarium (Fig. 3-2). The depths of all periodontal pockets are measured with this millimeter probe and are recorded as to depth and character of the periodontal pocket, degree of

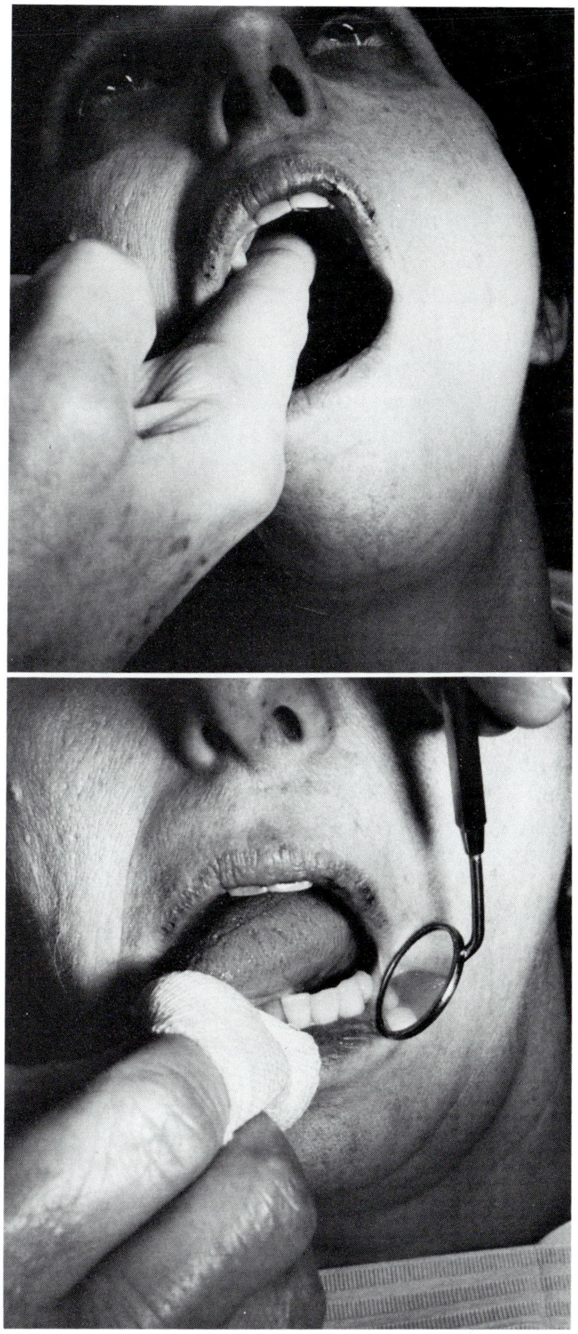

Fig. 3-1. Oral tissues being examined by palpation and inspection.

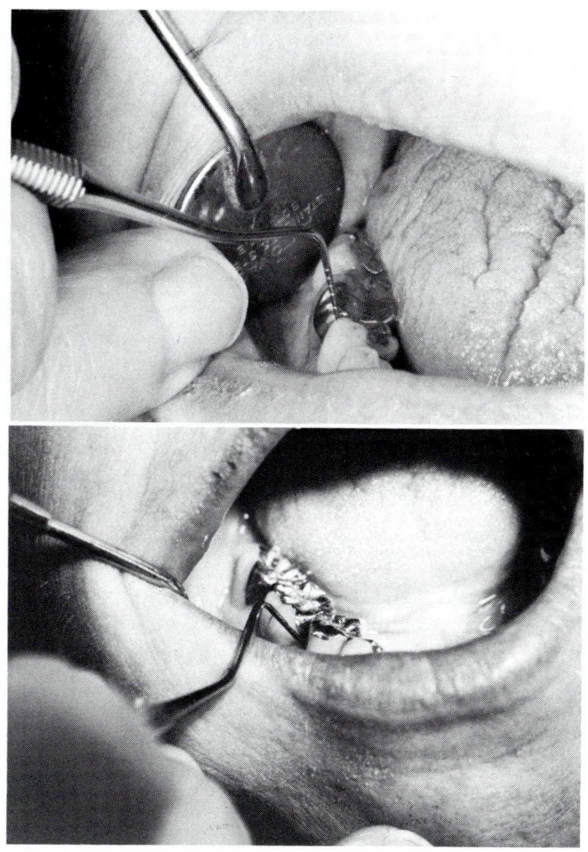

Fig. 3-2. Calibrated periodontal probe for measurement of pocket depth.

gingival detachment, and presence and extent of subgingival deposits. Detection of bifurcation and trifurcation involvements are also noted. Before making use of a tooth with a furcation involvement as an abutment tooth, we should apply Ante's law in estimating the remaining support of the tooth. Ante's law states: "In fixed bridgework the combined pericemental area of the abutment teeth should be equal to or greater in pericemental area than the tooth or teeth to be replaced."[1] The periodontal condition also must be studied in relation to the function of the mouth.

We must observe and evaluate the following:

1. Swallowing pattern—whether it is a closed or an open one. Swallowing ideally occurs with even distribution of pressure and maximum interdigitation of cusps with the condyles in their terminal hinge position. If this pattern does not occur, perverted movements are precipitated. Also, deviations in swallowing patterns, especially thrusting of tongue during deglutition should be noted.
2. Chewing habits—whether unilateral or bilateral
3. Diastemas and migrations
4. Physiologic rest position
5. Free-way space (distance between occlusal and rest vertical dimension)

Valuable diagnostic information can be obtained by means of transillumination, percussion, pulpal vitality tests, laboratory tests, and examination of the temporomandibular joints.

TRANSILLUMINATION

Transillumination is a fine adjunct in the oral examination (Fig. 3-3). It consists of the passage of light through tissues by interposing the object to be examined between the light source and the examiner. The area thus examined appears variably opaque to the transmission of light. The extent of subgingival calcareous deposits, interproximal caries, the presence of opaque foreign objects embedded in soft tissues, etc. can often be evaluated with transillumination.

PERCUSSION

Percussion is the tapping of teeth for indication of pulpal and periapical inflammation. This is accomplished with the handle end of the mouth mirror; a healthy tooth responds with a bell-like sound, while one contained within inflamed tissues sounds dull. A positive reaction to percussion confirms, as a rule, pulpal degeneration.

PULPAL VITALITY TESTS

Thermal and electrical tests should be utilized to obtain more detailed information relative to the integrity of the pulp and tissues surrounding the apices of the teeth.

All teeth in the suspected area are tested initially by percussion, and then vitality tests are run with an electric vitalometer* (Fig. 3-4), ice, and heat.

Ice is the most useful single aid that is available to locate the offending tooth in early acute pulpitis. A small piece of ice is held with a cotton pliers and tapered to a point against the hot shield of a bunsen burner (Fig. 3-5, *A*). The teeth are tested by placing the point of the ice against the labial or buccal surface of the teeth near the cervical region (Fig. 3-5, *B*), and

*Burton Medi-Quip Co., Van Nuys, Calif.

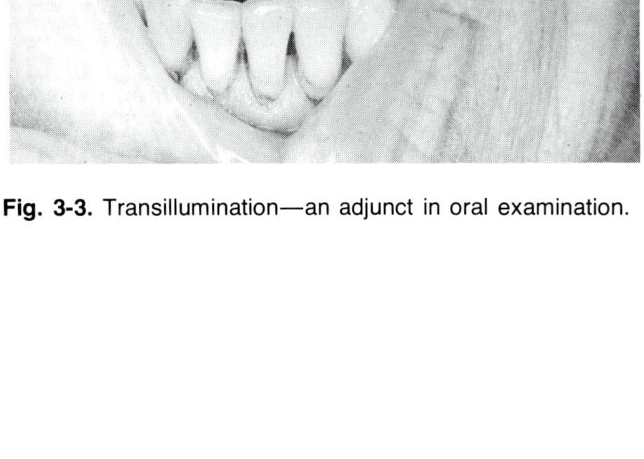

Fig. 3-3. Transillumination—an adjunct in oral examination.

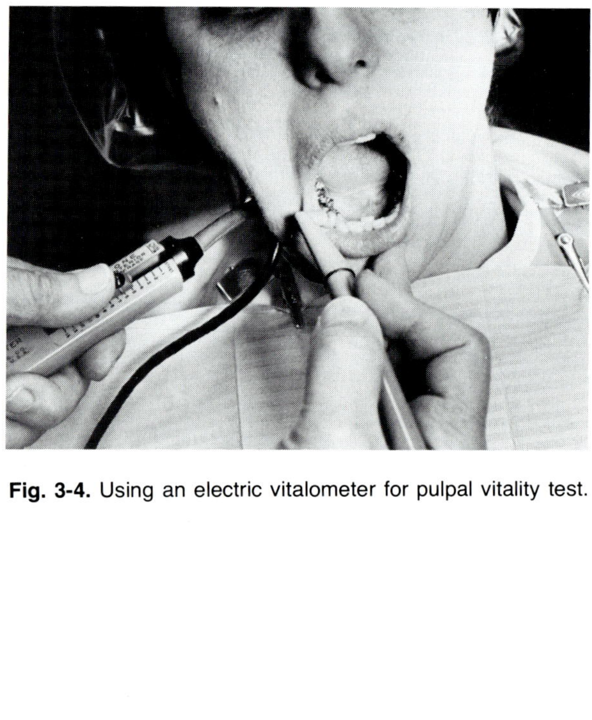

Fig. 3-4. Using an electric vitalometer for pulpal vitality test.

the patient is asked to signal as soon as he feels a definite sensation in the tooth. (The patient must understand the difference in a normal and abnormal response to the test. It is wise to spend a little time explaining the tests to the patient and to test two or three teeth in an uninvolved quadrant before going to the region in doubt so as to help the patient give an accurate response.) When the patient signals, the ice is removed immediately. The recovery period is the time required for the tooth to be relieved of all abnormal sensation after the ice has been removed from the tooth. A normal recovery period will range from 1 to 10 seconds. In early pulp hyperemia the recovery period will be from 10 to 25 seconds, while in acute pulpitis the recovery period may vary from 25 seconds to several minutes. Those teeth that fall within the range of hyperemia must be classified and treated as having irreversible pulpitis if there is a history of spontaneous pain or carious exposure. Others may be tested 48 to 72 hours later and the response compared. Sometimes it is necessary to isolate one tooth at a time with a rubber dam for the series of tests.

The electric vitalometer is of little value in determining the tooth with an early or serous acute pulpitis, but a slow or negative response often will help to isolate the tooth in later stages where considerable pulp tissue is necrotic.

Ice is necessary to determine the involved tooth in early acute pulpitis, since the tooth with respond quickly and the elicited pain will last much longer than it does in the adjacent normal teeth.

Heat (a heated ball burnisher or hot gutta-percha) will elicit pain in later stages of acute pulpitis, and in many instances it will confirm the diagnosis that was suspected from the poor or negative response elicited from the electric vitalometer. When the pulpitis reaches this stage, suppuration is present, and the pain often is spontaneous, penetrating, and severe.

Vitality of abutment teeth should always be checked. Those with a history of a pulpal problem must be resolved before the fixed partial denture is constructed, because pulpitis and periapical infection are more difficult to treat when the fixed partial denture has been cemented into place.

In many instances it is necessary to make a differential diagnosis between causes originating in the pulp and those emanating from severe inflammatory periodontal lesions.

Roentgenographic examination often reveals areas of periapical radiolucencies around apices of asymptomatic teeth, indicating the possibility of pulpal disease.

Any evidence of fistulas, sinus tracts, and swellings should also be noted during the examination.

LABORATORY TESTS

At times the clinical symptoms presented by the patient make it necessary to perform tests that are usu-

A

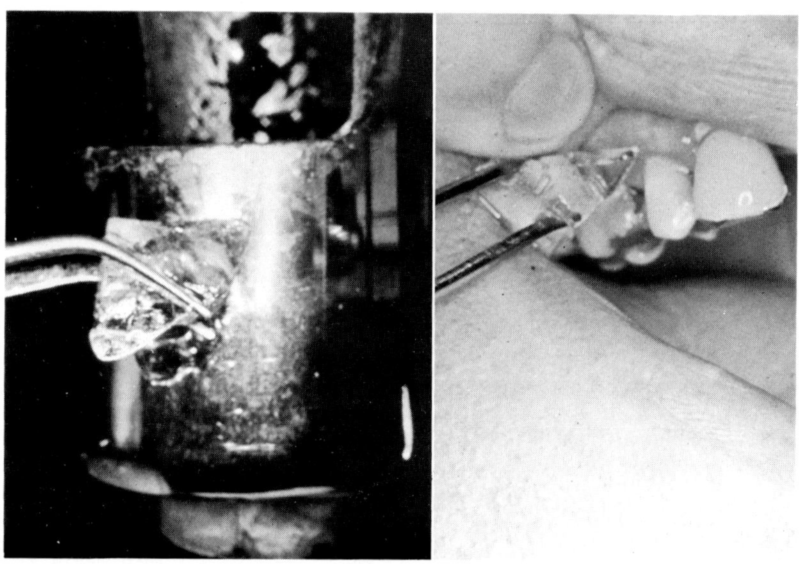

B

Fig. 3-5. A, Ice is held with forceps and tapered to a point by rotating it against the shield of a lighted bunsen burner. **B,** In testing vitality of teeth with this pointed ice it is most effective to apply it to buccal or labial surfaces of teeth near cervical line.

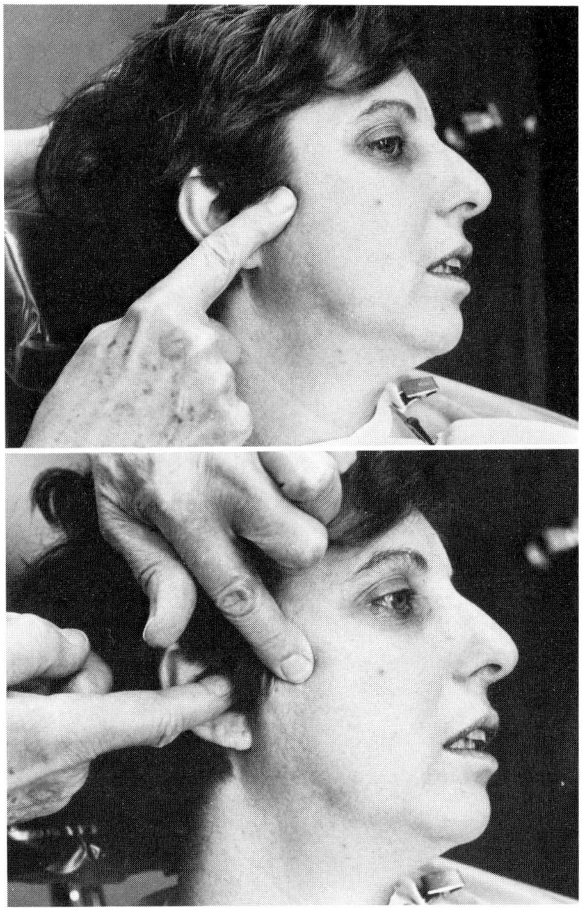

Fig. 3-6. Area of the temporomandibular joint being palpated during the opening and closing phases.

ally not in the domain of the dental office. Therefore, specific additional clinical or laboratory procedures should be performed, when indicated. These may include biopsy, urinalysis, blood chemistry, and bacteriologic and pathologic examinations. At times it has been advisable in advanced periodontal disease to secure complete blood count, blood calcium, blood phosphorus, alkaline phosphatase, sugar tolerance test, and urinalysis.

EXAMINATION OF TEMPOROMANDIBULAR JOINT

The area of the temporomandibular joints should be observed visually and should be palpated during the opening and closing phases. Evidences of subluxation, clicking, and deviations from the midline opening can be assessed (Fig. 3-6).

If the patient complains of pain or discomfort in this area, palpation of the musculature may elicit muscle spasm and tenderness. A stethoscope placed over

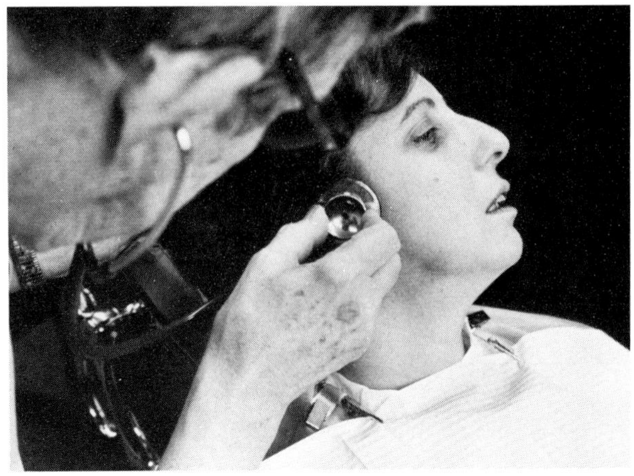

Fig. 3-7. Using the stethoscope in the temporomandibular joint examination.

the temporomandibular articulature, on opening and closing, will amplify the sounds produced by the movement of the condyle within the fossa of the temporal bone. The sounds heard by this means can be helpful in the determination of the extent of the dysfunction (Fig. 3-7).

If it is believed that the problem is one other than functional, radiography of the joint is indicated. By this means such possibilities as osteoarthritic changes in the joint, condylar fractures, organic disease of the disk, etc. can be ascertained or ruled out.

Presence or absence of inhibited mandibular movements that may be caused by degenerative or inflammatory changes in the temporomandibular joints should be noted.

EXAMINATION OF HARD TISSUES

Next comes the examination and recording of the condition of the hard tissues. The skillful use of the mirror and explorer point, coupled with good illumination and a dry field, should not be overlooked in the examination for caries. All observations should be correlated with adequate roentgenograms. The examination starts at the most posterior tooth in the maxillary right quadrant and proceeds to the maxillary anterior teeth and left quadrant, and then this procedure is repeated in the mandibular arch. Each tooth should be observed on all surfaces for evidence of caries, chalky white areas without cavitation (does this represent decalcified or deficiently calcified areas?), areas of abrasion and erosion (is it caused by improper toothbrushing, salivary composition, acid juices, occlusal factors?), and character of dental work in the mouth, carefully observing marginal fit, contact

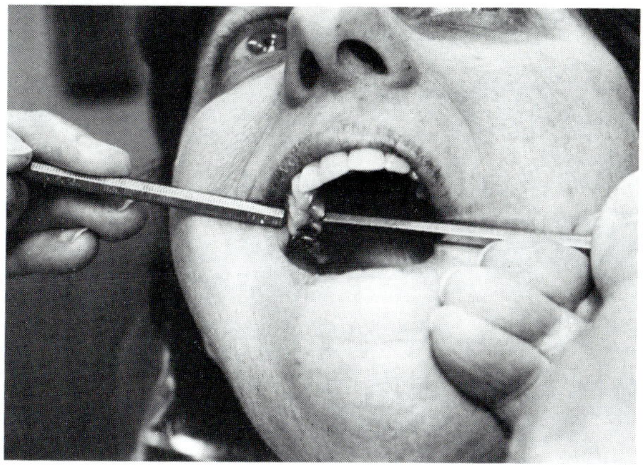

Fig. 3-8. Utilizing handles of two instruments to assess extent of tooth mobility.

areas or loss of proximal tooth contacts, form, and function. Also any malformations of the teeth, missing teeth, migration of teeth, tooth fractures, edentulous areas, occlusal interferences, tooth and arch alignment, exposed root surfaces, and esthetics should be noted.

During this definitive examination the dentist should observe whether there is any unusual amount of sensitivity to hot or cold, the degree and location of both hard and soft accretions on the tooth surfaces, as well as plaque and stains (which can be an important etiologic factor in caries and periodontal disease), presence of furcations (will a tooth so affected be able to be used as an abutment tooth?), pocket depth and gingival inflammation, spontaneous or persistent bleeding or suppuration, facial neuralgias, foci of infection (pulpal, periodontal, oral, or paraoral site), the quality of the surface tooth structure, and tolerance of mouth tissues to restorations.

A dietary survey may be essential in patients who have extensive caries; the results will determine the need for dietary correction.

A record of tooth mobility is of great importance in diagnosis as well as in observation of the progress of treatment. The mobility pattern of teeth should be carefully tested in all directions and degrees of mobility recorded, such as 1, 2, or 3 degrees (some skilled clinicians use half degrees for a more accurate evaluation of mobility). The operator should do it instrumentally rather than with his fingers. Handles of two instruments should be utilized to assess extent of tooth mobility (Fig. 3-8).

A mobility of 1 degree means that the tooth is just barely movable. Its most facial position is about 1 mm. from its most lingual position when it is rocked from the labial or buccal side to the lingual side with the instruments. Two degrees means that the tooth has a 2 mm. range of movement and that it must be considered a problem tooth. Three degrees means that the tooth has a 3 mm. range of movement and carries with it the connotation that the tooth is very loose.

Even though some dentists are of the opinion that such judgments are subjective, all agree that they are of value for assessing changes in mobility patterns before and following therapy and that the extent of tooth mobility is a critical factor in evaluating the degree of periodontal destruction and subsequently its prognosis.

INTRAORAL OCCLUSAL EXAMINATION

In making an intraoral occlusal examination, the dentist must keep in mind that more accurate information can be obtained by a study of occlusal relationships under dynamic conditions rather than static ones.

The operator should inquire of the patient whether he is conscious of his teeth; does he grind, clench, or clamp his teeth (day or night or both), or does he have a "negative occlusal perception"?

The patient should open and close his mouth and any presence of clicking or "popping" or subluxation in the region of the temporomandibular joints, presence or absence of inhibited mandibular movements (may be caused by degenerative or inflammatory changes in the temporomandibular joints), presence of trismus, tongue thrust during deglutition, and presence or absence of simultaneous even contact of the teeth in terminal hinge closure should be observed. The dentist should look for premature contacts when guiding the patient into terminal hinge closure.

The following should be noted:

1. The manner in which the mandibular teeth interdigitate with the maxillary teeth (by applying slight retrusive pressure on the mandible and "jiggling" the jaw); is there a correct cusp-fossa relationship and are the excursive movements (diagnostic slides) within the range of "norm" (Fig. 3-9)?
2. Presence or absence of mobility or fremitus during occlusal contacts
3. Symmetry or asymmetry of jaw relationships
4. Presence or absence of cross-bite relationships
5. Position of teeth on basal bone
6. Relationship of midlines during closure to complete occlusal contact
7. Marginal ridge relationships

A

B

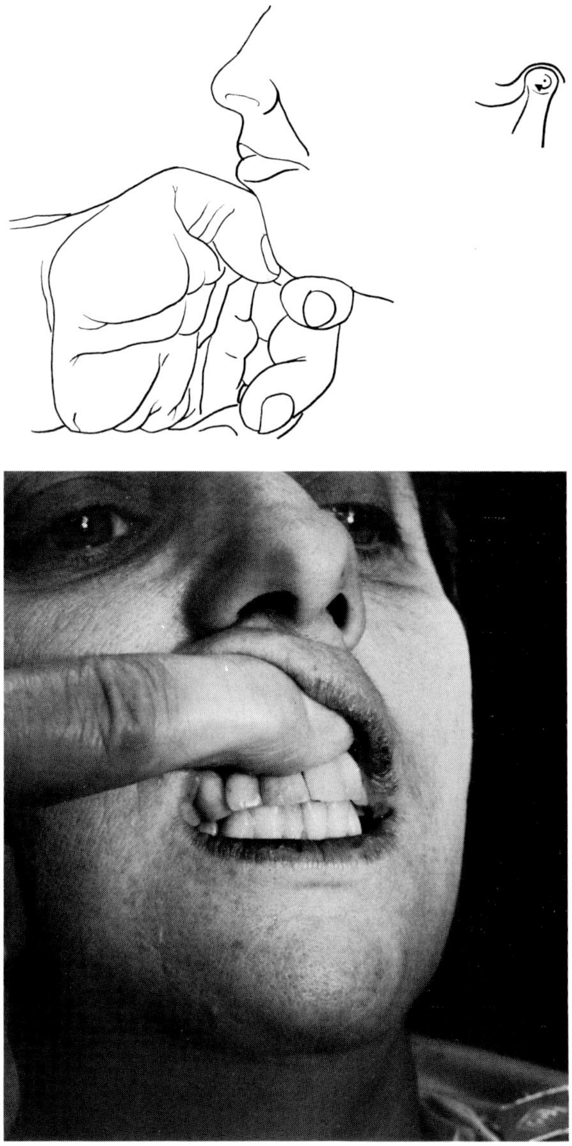

Fig. 3-9. A, Guiding the patient into terminal hinge closure. **B,** Examining for presence or absence of fremitus during occlusal closure.

8. Presence or absence of wear facets (occlusal and proximal surfaces)
9. Overbite, overjet, incisal guidance, and freeway space evaluations
10. The lip line and the "smile" line
11. Shade of teeth (determined by use of a suitable shade guide) and any special characteristics of the teeth
12. A solid, clear sound on closure of mandibular teeth against maxillary teeth (gives us some idea of coincidence of centric relation and centric occlusion). A dull sound usually indicates premature occlusal contact.

In some instances, exploration of the carious or extensively restored tooth or teeth to be used as an abutment or abutments is a "must," because of the possibility of pulpal involvement and the need to know the proportion of remaining tooth substance.

Consideration should also be given, in some cases, to the feasibility of orthodontic repositioning of abutment or opposing teeth (see Chapter 6).

EVALUATION OF NONFUNCTIONAL MOVEMENTS

Observation and evaluation of tensional or pernicious habits, if present, are of the utmost importance in making a diagnosis and in evaluating the treatment plan. Patients under emotional stress clench and grind their teeth for hours at night, and some even carry out this damaging habit during the day. When it is practiced during their sleeping hours, they awaken in the morning with soreness of the teeth and masticatory muscles.

Besides the patient exhibiting these grinding and gnashing habits, there is the patient who develops biting habits. Tongue, lip, and cheek biting, biting on fingernails, and biting on foreign objects such as bobby pins, toothpicks, and pipes are common to this type of patient.

Such habits (nonfunctional movements) as just mentioned may transmit light or heavy pressures, depending on the hardness or softness of the intermediate object, but the constant application of these forces can and does cause migration of the teeth, temporomandibular joint difficulties, and periodontal destruction. Other habits such as mouth breathing and tongue thrust warrant close observation.[2]

Mouth breathing may be caused by inadequate nasal passageways, which need the attention of the E.N.T. (ear, nose, and throat) physician, or it may be a result of habit, which may have a psychologic component.

Tongue thrusting is the child's way of using the tongue as a nipple and of sucking on the tongue. This leads to abnormal swallowing habits. In normal swallowing the teeth are brought together in centric relation, and the tongue is pressed against the palate in the area of the anterior palatine papilla. In abnormal swallowing the tongue places heavy pressure on the anterior teeth or may even be forced between them, causing an open-bite condition in this area. Myofunctional therapy methods may be used to treat these patients, but this type of condition has a bad prognosis.

Fig. 3-11

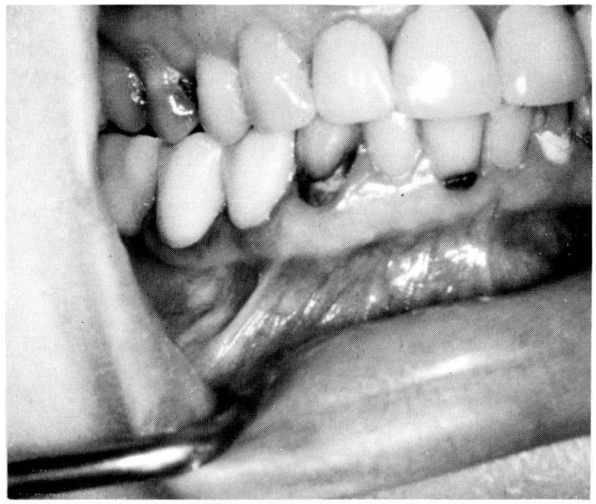

Fig. 3-10

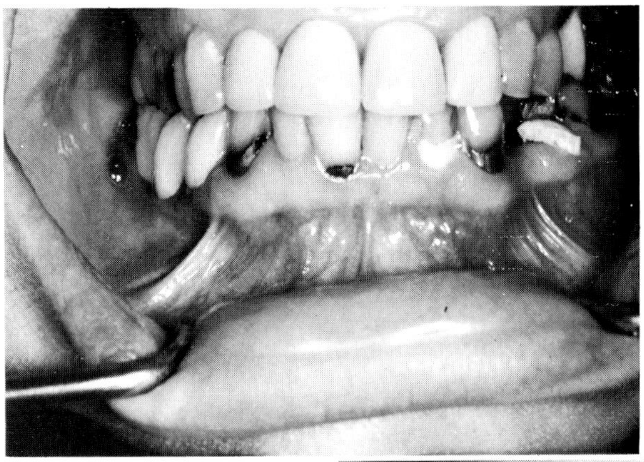

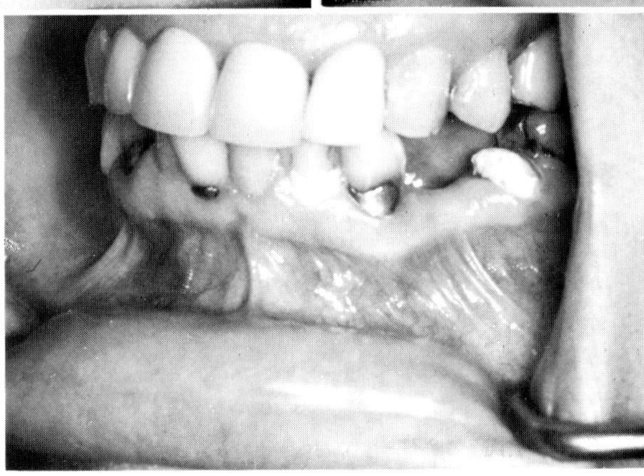

Fig. 3-12

Figs. 3-10 to 3-12. Preoperative centric relation views.

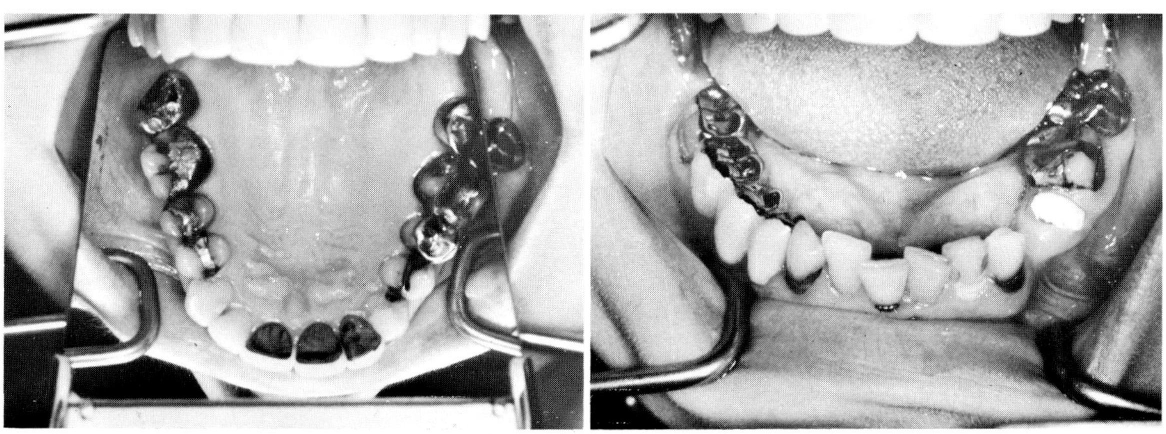

Fig. 3-13. Preoperative occlusal views of upper and lower teeth.

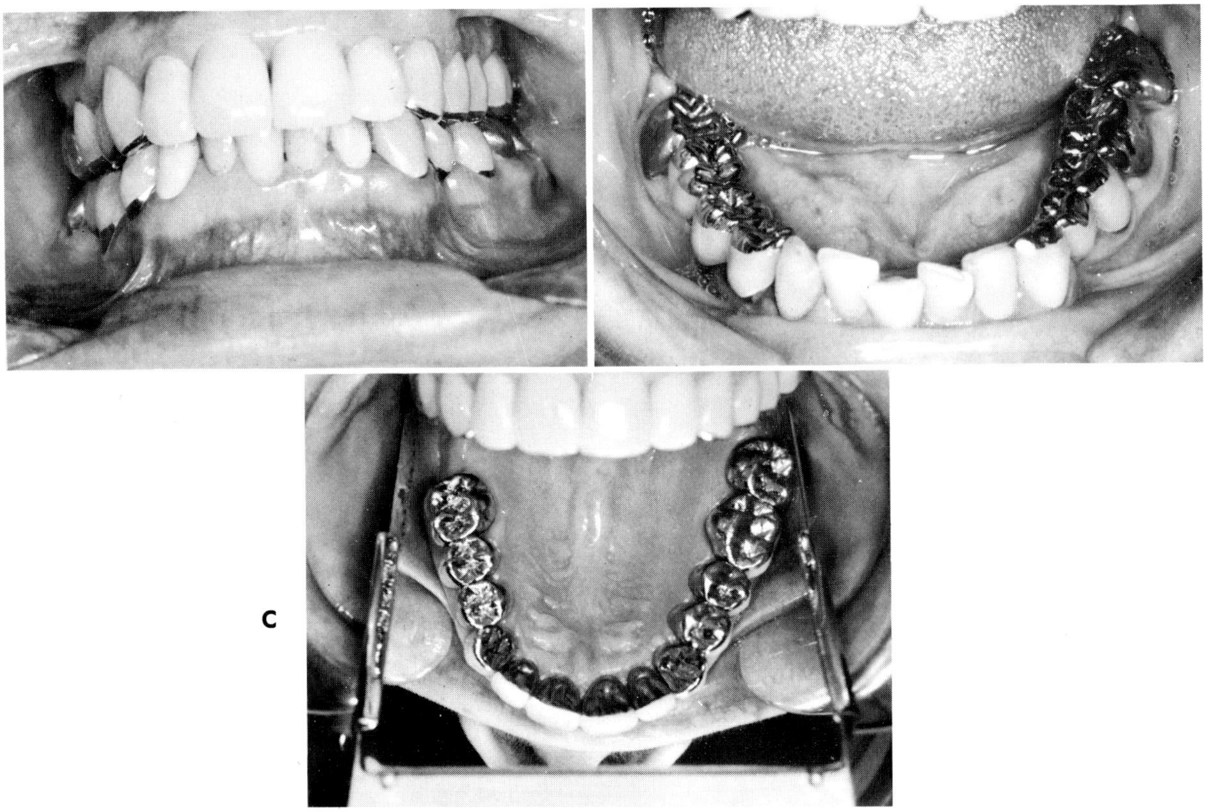

A B C

Fig. 3-14. A, Postoperative centric relation view. **B** and **C,** Postoperative occlusal views of lower **(B)** and upper **(C)** teeth.

PHOTOGRAPHS

Intraoral photography (black and white or color photographs) should be routinely taken in all dental offices. Photographs should be taken to document the preoperative and intermediate treatment phases and postoperative conditions (Figs. 3-10 to 3-14). They supplement the study casts and other records. They will provide a lasting record of the patient's teeth, soft tissues, and other oral structures from which comparisons can be made from time to time. Projection of such photographs often reveals subtle changes not readily apparent during the visual examination.

Intraoral photography is a very valuable adjunct in the presentation of future cases of a somewhat similar nature. It also carries with it a great psychologic impact as regards the esthetic and functional improvements that can easily be seen by the patient.

ROENTGENOGRAPHIC EXAMINATION

Since the basis for therapy is a comprehensive diagnosis established on the accumulation and the evaluation of all pertinent information, complete roentgenographic documentation is an essential part of this information.

This documentation is important preoperatively and postoperatively (every year or two) for evaluation of whether our diagnostic, treatment planning, and therapeutic techniques are adequate to restore functional requirements within the metabolic activity of the bone for the patient. Will his stomatognathic system be relatively immune to disease, or will there be a return of pathology?

The objective of an intraoral examination, as aptly pointed out by Simpson,[3] is disclosing for diagnostic purposes the following structures:

1. "An extensive periapical area to observe histologic changes, and reveal foreign or anomalous bodies;
2. "The roots of the teeth with approximate accuracy, to determine the number, size, form, and location;
3. "The lamina dura entirely around the profile of

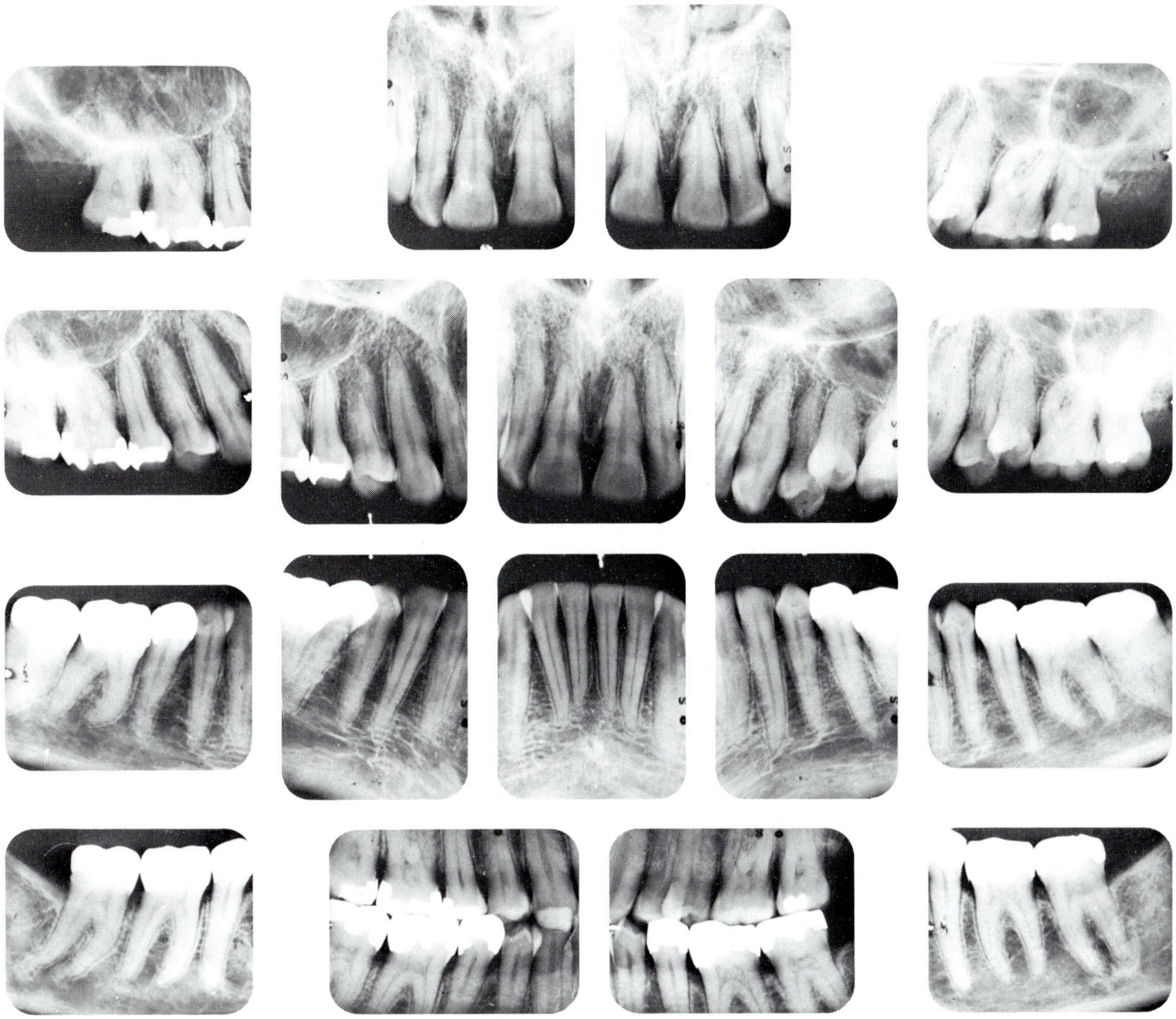

A_1

Continued.

Fig. 3-15. A, Good roentgenograms from a diagnostic and photographic viewpoint. **B,** Long cone and panoramic roentgenograms.

the roots, which is a significant diagnostic index often indistinguishable because of technical deficiencies;

4. "The crest of the alveolar process to reveal marginal destruction earlier and more accurately than by clinical inspection;
5. "The pulp chambers and canals to determine the relation of the pulp to cavities and restorations, the access and course of canals for operations, and the relative efficiency of canal operations; and
6. "The proximal surfaces of the teeth to detect caries and deposits, and to observe the relative contact of the teeth and the contour of restorations."*

To obtain this objective and verify the evidence requires, in some instances, two or more views of a region.

A complete set of roentgenograms, including bite-wing and panoramic films, is usually taken at the first appointment, and although this procedure is an adjunct to diagnosis, it must not supplant it. Roent-

*From Simpson, Clarence O.: Technic of oral radiography, ed. 2, St. Louis, 1928, The C. V. Mosby Co.

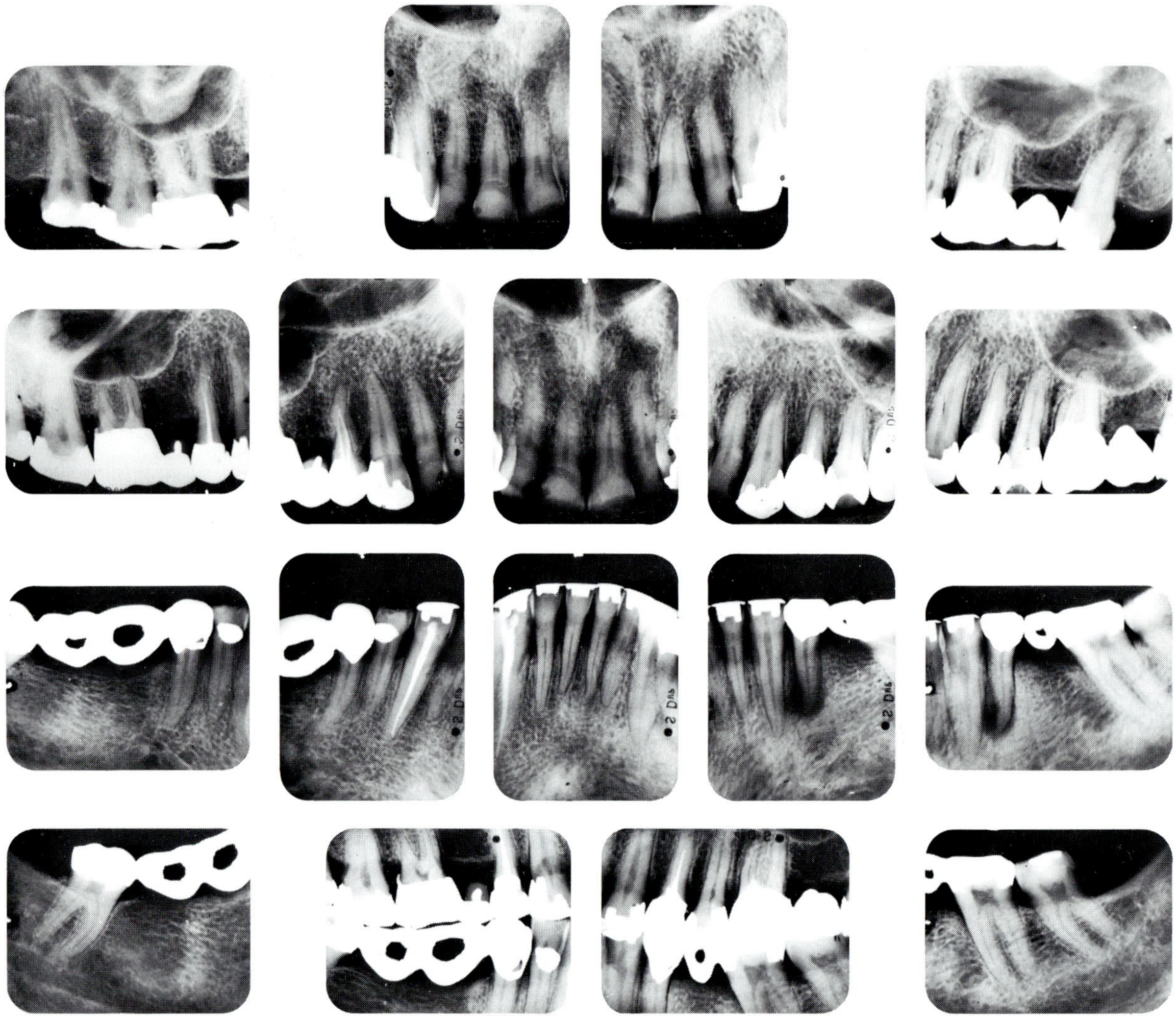

A_2

Fig. 3-15, cont'd. For legend see p. 31.

genograms help in recognizing pathologic conditions, which must be either removed or restored to a state of health capable of supporting normal function.

The roentgenograms must be good from a diagnostic as well as a photographic standpoint (Fig. 3-15). In the roentgenograms the teeth should never be elongated or foreshortened, and they should be clear, well angulated, and properly processed. Technical skill and diagnostic acuity are of the utmost importance.

Roentgenograms must be studied and related to the patient being examined, which includes visual and tactile procedures, because they are meaningless unless correlated to the clinical findings in the oral cavity. One should observe carefully whether any destruction has accrued in the area that receives the force in the form of a rebound from prematurities that prevent the occurrence of a normal path of closure of the mandible.

The roentgenograms, which should be accurate reproducible images, will reveal the following information:

1. Extent of carious lesions.
2. Type, amount, and distribution of alveolar bone. It should be noted whether the alveolar process in the edentulous area is well filled.
3. Presence or absence of apical infection.
4. Furcation involvements. In many instances teeth with furcation involvement can be successfully treated by periodontal techniques which include, when indicated, hemisection. They can also be used as abutment teeth. Oral hygiene habits must be carried out

B

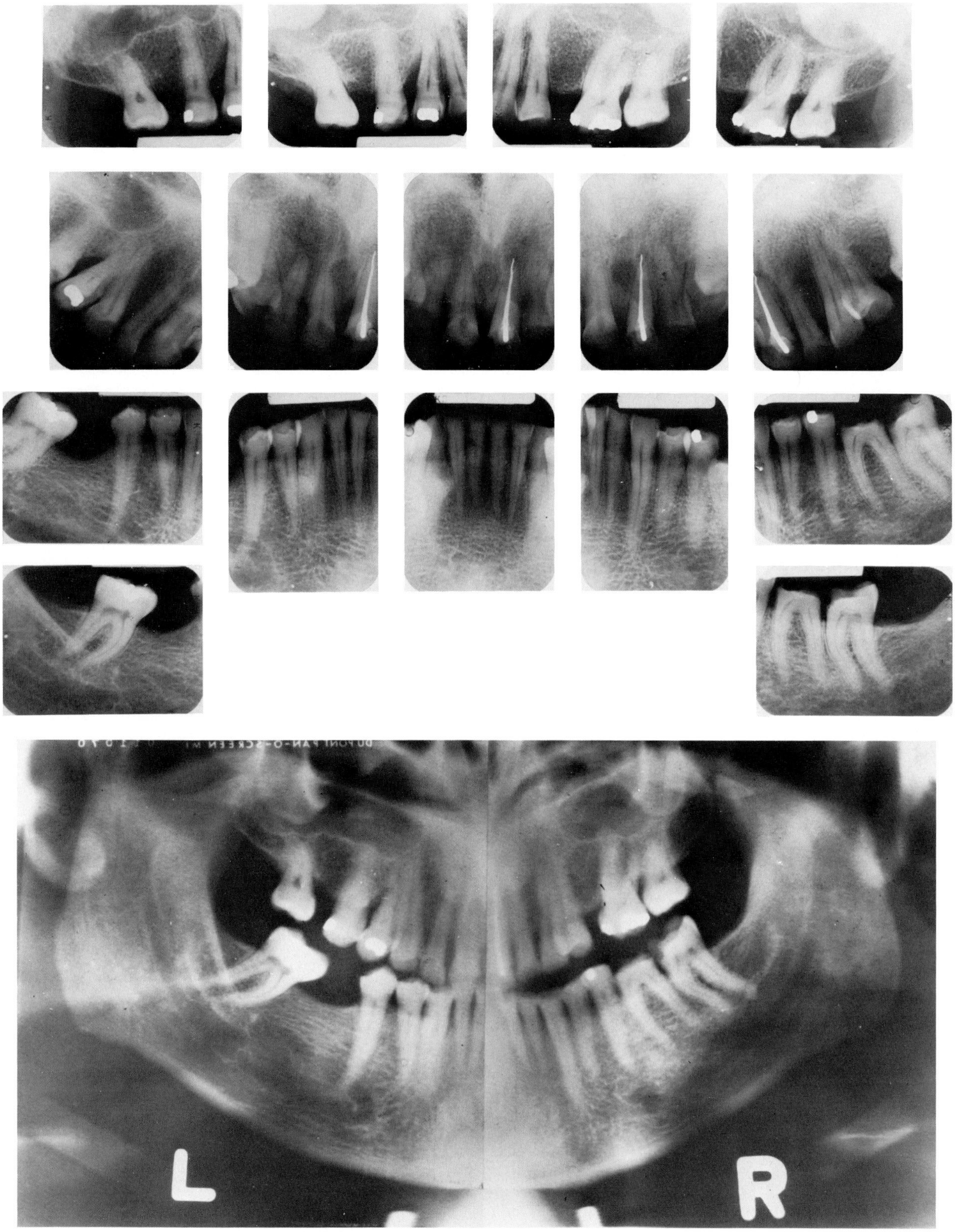

Fig. 3-15, cont'd. For legend see p. 31.

properly and with great care. However, maxillary molar furcations call for a guarded prognosis.

5. Root resorption or apposition. The proximity or relationship of the root of one tooth with the other should be determined.

6. Size, shape, number, inclination, and position of the roots. Conically shaped roots and fused roots do not offer the resistance to forces that may dislodge them as do widely divergent bifurcated and trifurcated roots.

Root length within the alveolus should be equal to or greater than combined lengths of coronal and root portion outside it. If it is not, the principle of splintage should be used.

Long roots that are well supported by bone make the most ideal abutment. One must use his clinical judgment whether to use a tooth with short roots that is well supported by bone as an abutment singly or as part of a double abutment. A lot depends on the ratio of remaining alveolar bone to the length and width of the roots and the stress-bearing ability of the periodontium.

7. Condition of the supporting structures of the teeth. The presence or absence of abnormal pocket depth and, if the abutment tooth is periodontally involved, whether it can be treated successfully are questions that have to be resolved.

8. Impactions and retained roots.

9. Cysts and granulomas.

10. Status of endodontically treated teeth.

11. Crown-to-root ratio. An accurately projected roentgenogram is important for this determination. The extent of the effective periodontal support must be determined, especially if there is a mobility pattern. A root covered its full length with dense alveolar bone is ideal for abutment purposes, but a bone loss of one half or more of the length of the root may contraindicate its use as an abutment unless adjacent teeth with adequate periodontal support can be used according to the principle of splintage. In many instances, root-end resection will adversely alter the crown-to-root ratio.

12. Conditions of the coronal portion of the tooth.

13. Pulps of the teeth. Any evidence of pulp stones should be noted. Position and size of the pulp horns help in our determination of whether to use an intra- or extracoronal retainer with or without pin retention.

14. Periodontal ligament space. Is the periodontal ligament space normal or thickened? Changes in its width may reflect problems related to excessive trauma.

Another problem to be considered is whether there are any changes in the lamina dura. The lamina dura is the most important feature in the diagnosis of periapical disease. The first evidence of periapical infection is the distension of the lamina dura by a thickening of the periodontal ligament. The next stage is a break in some part of the lamina dura, which occurs before there is destruction of the surrounding bone. Its loss or lack of continuity may be a significant clue to the presence of excessive occlusal forces.

15. Long-axis relationship of abutment teeth. Are they within the acceptable 25 to 30 degree relationship of parallelism?

16. Horizontal and vertical bone loss. Patterns of horizontal and vertical osseous resorption are easily visible (Figs. 3-16 to 3-19).

The bite-wing roentgenograms provide much-needed information relative to carious lesions and the proximity of these lesions and of old restorations to the pulp, deficiencies in contact areas (open contacts lead to food impaction, and difficulty in removal of debris may cause subsequent periodontal breakdown), shape of restorations interproximally, the gingival marginal fit of restorations, and often the crestal bone involvement (apparent levels of crestal alveolar bone interproximally) attending periodontal inflammation.

Simpson[3] has said that a good, readable dental roentgenogram should (1) cover the field of examination to the best advantage, (2) show no evidence of mobility during exposure, (3) show a diagnostic view of the region with a minimum distortion of the image, (4) show maximum definition and contrast consistent with penetration of the structure, (5) be free from stains and abrasions, and (6) present a symmetrical projection of the image on the film.

TYPES OF DENTAL ROENTGENOGRAPHIC SURVEY

Intraoral periapical series. This series consists of sixteen or more exposures including bite-wing roentgenograms, using either the bisecting-angle technique or the long cone paralleling technique.

Panoramic roentgenographic surveys (Fig. 3-15, *B*). I am of the opinion that a competent diagnostician can obtain the same amount of information from a film taken of an identical area using either the bisecting-angle or long cone paralleling technique. In some instances both techniques have been used during a roentgenographic examination of a patient to get the best results (Fig. 3-20). However, Wuehrmann[4] and other competent radiologists are of the opinion that it is more difficult to extract all important information from films taken by the bisecting-angle technique

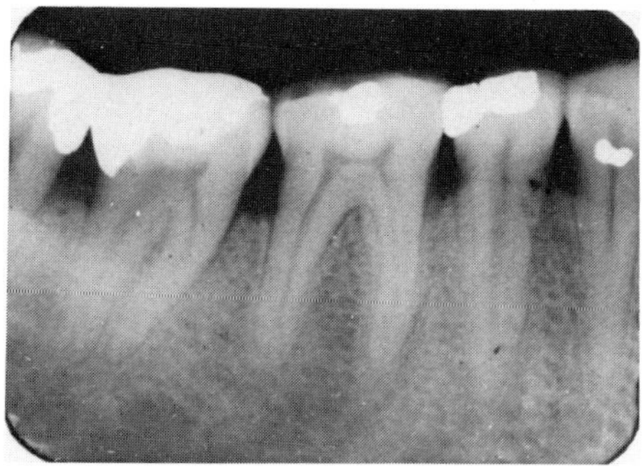

Fig. 3-16

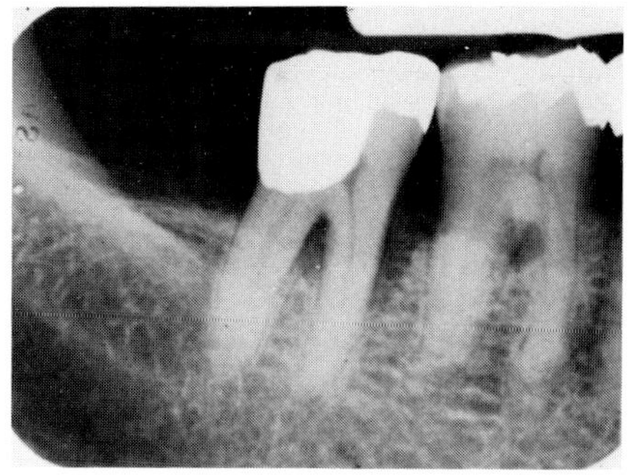

Fig. 3-18

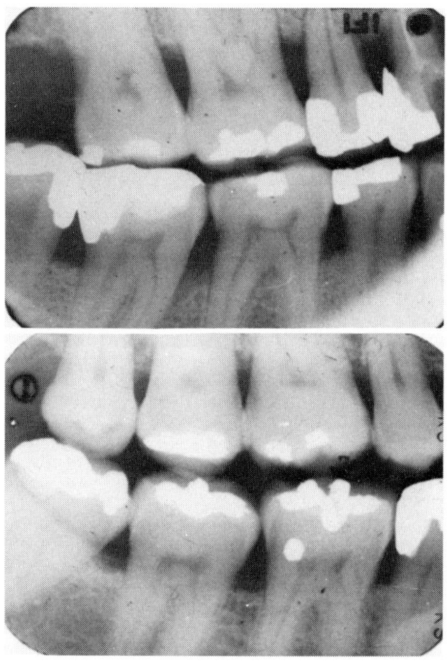

Fig. 3-17

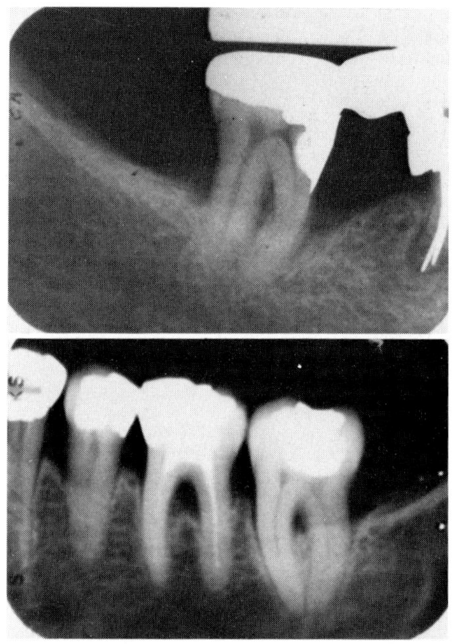

Fig. 3-19

Figs. 3-16 to 3-19. Patterns of horizontal and vertical osseous resorption.

because of technical factors that cause distortion and poor definition. The long cone paralleling technique has gained the ascendency.

By utilizing a long cone paralleling technique (16 to 20 inch focal film distance), a minimal amount of structural distortion is induced. A film positioner, such as XCP,* used with this technique is an excellent device designed to align the film packet correctly and to minimize the amount of error associated with a method that uses the patient's finger to hold the film (Fig. 3-21).

The long cone paralleling technique necessitates an increased focal spot–film distance so that the paths of the x-rays are practically parallel. This increased distance is used so that the dental films can be placed parallel with the long axes of the teeth. The central beam of radiation is thereby directed at a right angle to the teeth and to the film, which results in images of the teeth that approach anatomical accuracy and have fine sharpness of detail of tooth and bone (Figs. 3-22 to 3-24).

We must keep in mind that 16 inches is double the normal anode-film distance as used in the bisecting-angle technique. This means that the exposure time

---

*Rinn Corp., Elgin, Ill.

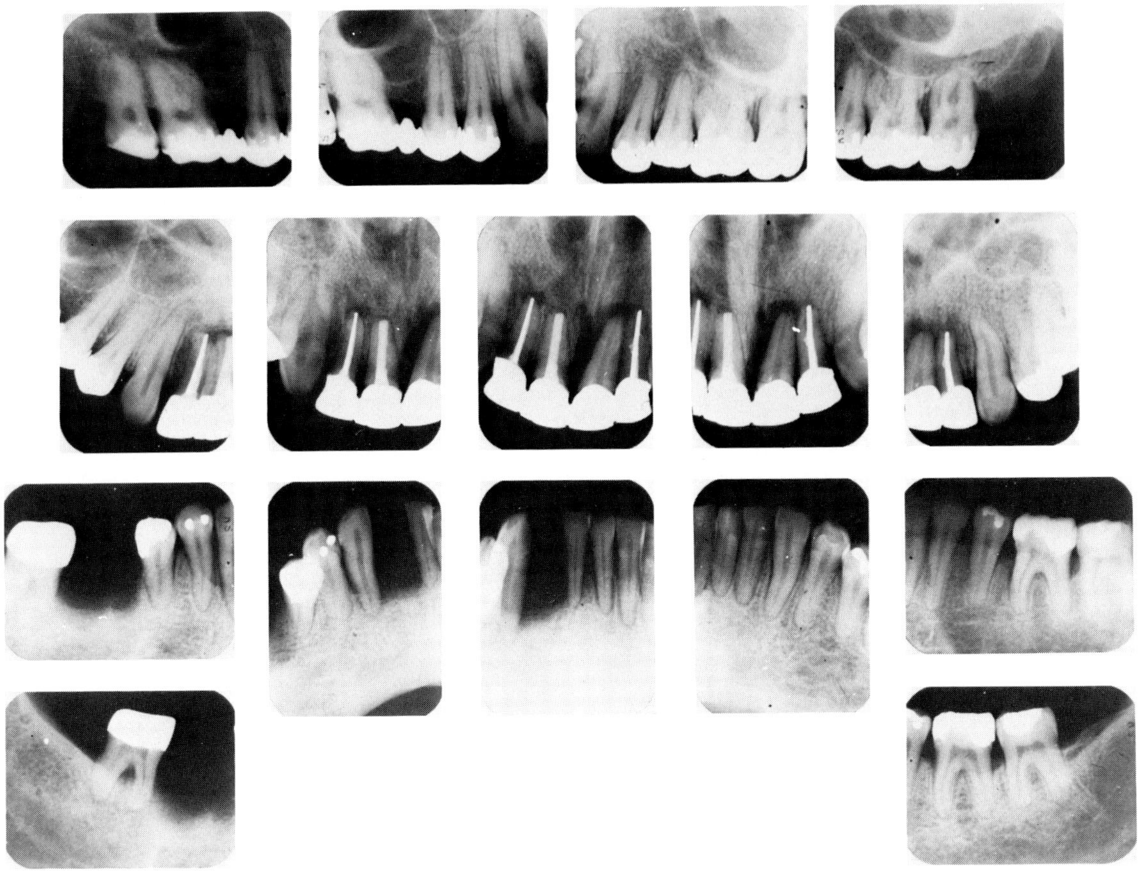

Fig. 3-20. The long cone technique and bisecting-angle technique (used on upper teeth because of shallow vault) was utilized in the roentgenographic examination of the patient.

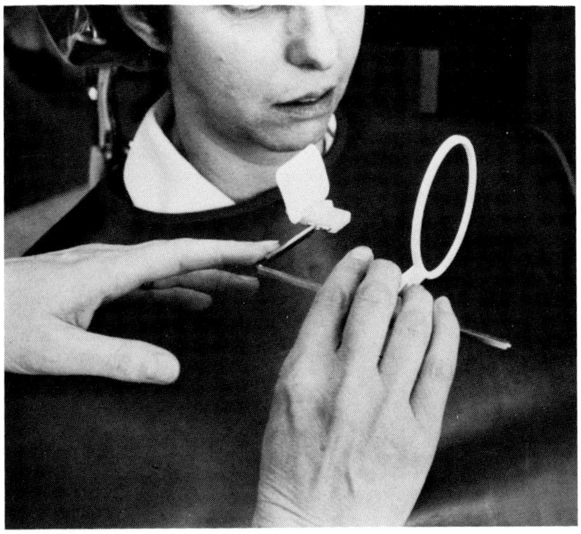

Fig. 3-21. The XCP film positioner, an excellent device designed to align the film packet correctly.

must be increased, but any danger from excess radiation can be overcome by using a faster emulsion film and modifying the kilovoltage and milliamperage to suite the technique.

Close examination of properly exposed (long cone paralleling technique) and processed dental films will show[5]:

1. Greater anatomic accuracy—truer shape and size of the dental structures
2. Sharpness of details
3. Better alignment of the teeth and more definitively detailed roentgenograms for diagnostic purposes
4. Minimal enlargement and control of shadow of malar bone
5. No elongation or foreshortening. This is especially important in regard to upper molar roots.
6. Much less chance of overlapping teeth. Interdental spaces are opened up.

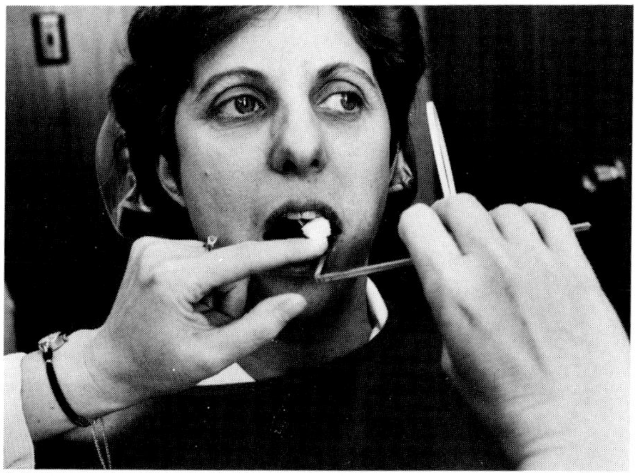

Fig. 3-22

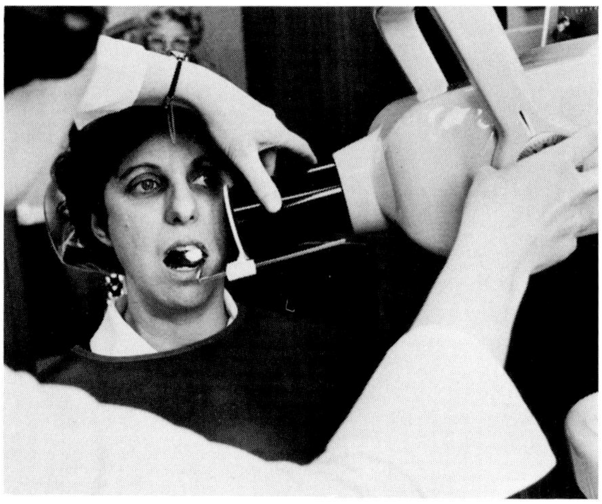

Fig. 3-23

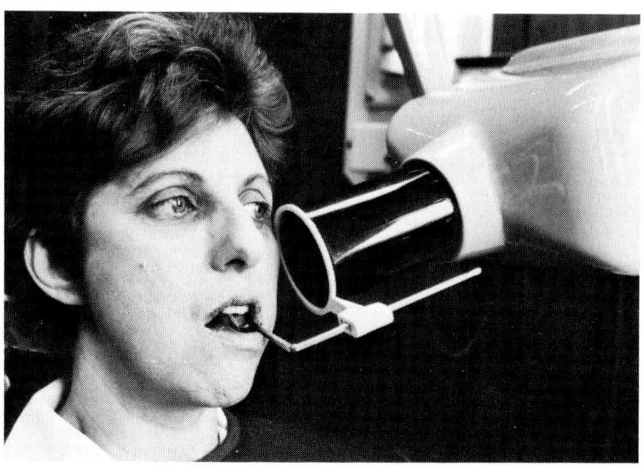

Fig. 3-24

Figs. 3-22 to 3-24. The correct positioning of the film and film positioner and the long cone tube for obtaining a roentgenogram by the long cone technique.

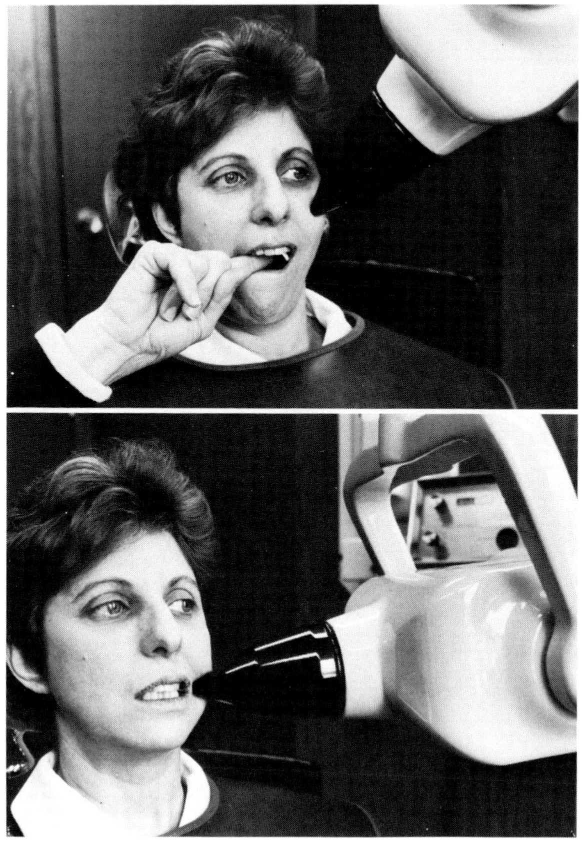

Fig. 3-25. Positioning the pointed or short cone for obtaining a roentgenogram by the bisecting-angle technique.

7. True relationship of crest of alveolar bone to the teeth. The extent of alveolar atrophy can be readily seen.
8. Clarity and increased definition and contrast

The bisecting-angle technique projects the central beam of radiation perpendicular to the bisecting angle formed by the long axis of the tooth and the plane of the film.[6] Variations in tooth alignment require good technical skill and judgment in establishing proper angulations to be used, so as not to make this fine method a hit-or-miss operation (Fig. 3-25).

When using the bisecting-angle technique, many capable dentists believe that it is advantageous to place the film as close as possible to the object to avoid distortion. With this technique linear or longitudinal distortion (the projection of an image that is either larger or smaller than the object) will in all probability be eliminated, but it will also produce a dimensional distortion (the distortion caused by projecting three-dimensional objects on two-dimensional surfaces), which may not always be recognized. This dimen-

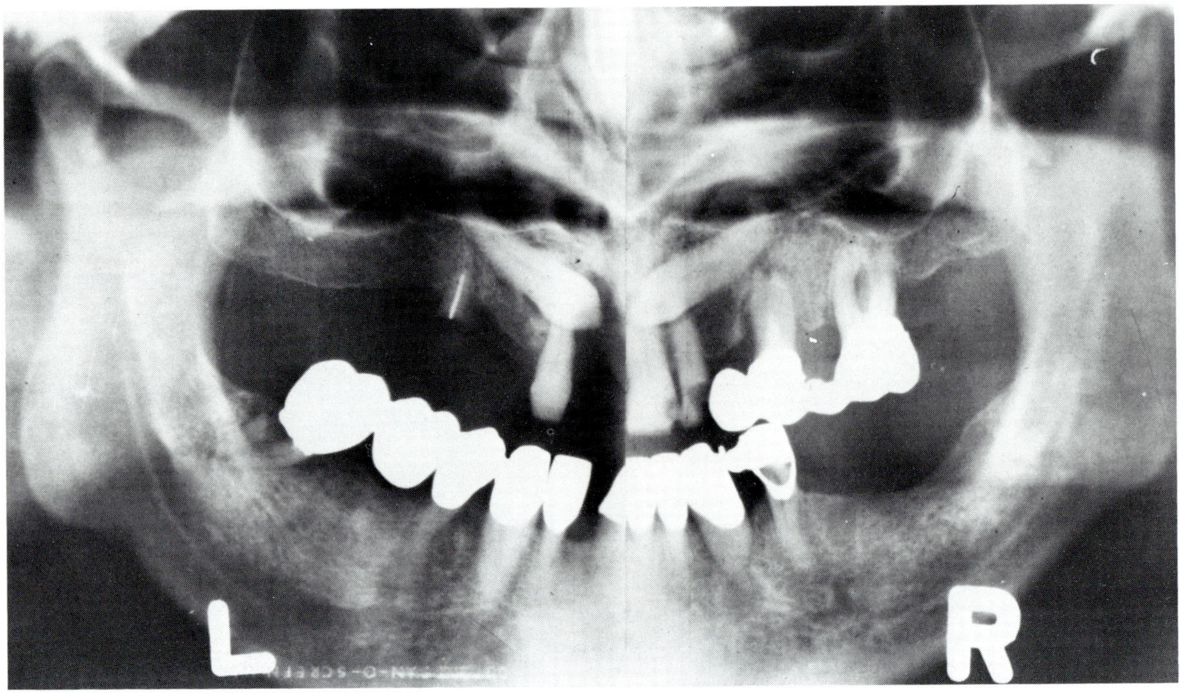

Fig. 3-26. A panoramic roentgenogram.

sional distortion becomes accentuated as the angulation is increased; roentgenograms of the maxillary molars will, in some instances, show buccal roots foreshortened.

ROENTGENOGRAPHIC MODIFICATION IN CASES OF PERIODONTAL DISEASE

Hutchinson[7] has called attention to periodontists' need for roentgenograms that can be technically described as "thin."

"The periodontist considers, in many instances, roentgenograms of normal contrast do not give a true picture of the condition of the interdental spines and tables or, in some instances, even of the bone between the roots of multirooted teeth, as there is a tendency to show a greater destruction of the bone than is actually the case.

"The answer to this problem of producing 'thin' roentgenograms is to cut down on the exposure time and, where practicable, to reduce the kilovoltage to a minimum."*

PANORAMIC ROENTGENOGRAMS

Panoramic roentgenograms should not supplant, but be adjunctive to, the periapical and bite-wing series of roentgenograms. They have certain advanges in that they are easier on the patient because the film is placed outside the mouth, the amount of total radiation received by the patient is reduced, and the procedure is fast (Fig. 3-26).

In summation of this phase of the subject, it can be said that a complete understanding of the technique of film exposure, which includes placement of the film, angulation of the roentgen rays, time of exposure, understanding of the difference in effect of changes in milliamperage and voltage, and the varying results to be obtained by the quality and type of film used, is essential. If films are properly placed and exposed, the early destruction of the investing tissue can be detected, as can the breakdown of the cortical plate in the interdental spaces.

RADIATION HAZARDS

It is of the utmost importance to protect the patient, office personnel, and the dentist from all unnecessary radiation. The x-ray machine must meet the recommendations for filtration and collimation so as to reduce radiation exposure.

There are two chief hazards of radiation—the somatic and the genetic. It is the opinion of some authorities in dental roentgenography that there is no known somatic hazard, if necessary precautions are taken, but that a measurable amount of radiation does

*From Hutchinson, A. C. W.: Dental radiology, Dent. Progr. **3:**19-27, 1962.

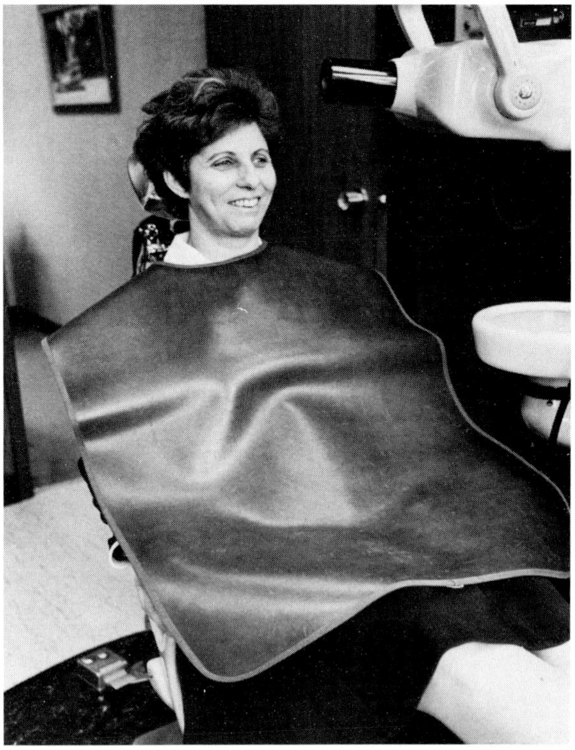

Fig. 3-27. A leaded apron should be used as a shield to reduce irradiation.

reach the gonadal region. Richards[8] has said that there is no radiation scatter to the gonads through the torso of the patient. Gonadal exposure is largely due to scatter of secondary radiation through air from the mandible and skull of the patient.

The following protective measures should be taken:

1. Use a shield (a leaded apron) to reduce somatic and gonadal irradiation (Fig. 3-27). This is also psychologically reassuring to the patient.
2. With patients in the first 3 months of pregnancy, the shield offers a means of minimizing irradiation of the fetus. In this period only take roentgenograms that are absolutely necessary.
3. Use only that amount of radiation that is necessary.
4. Never hold the film in the patient's mouth.
5. Never stand unprotected in the path of the useful x-ray beam that passes through the cone of the x-ray machine. X-rays scatter in all directions from the patient's face while x-ray machine is in operation.
6. Never hold the pointer cone during exposures.
7. During each exposure stand at least 6 feet or

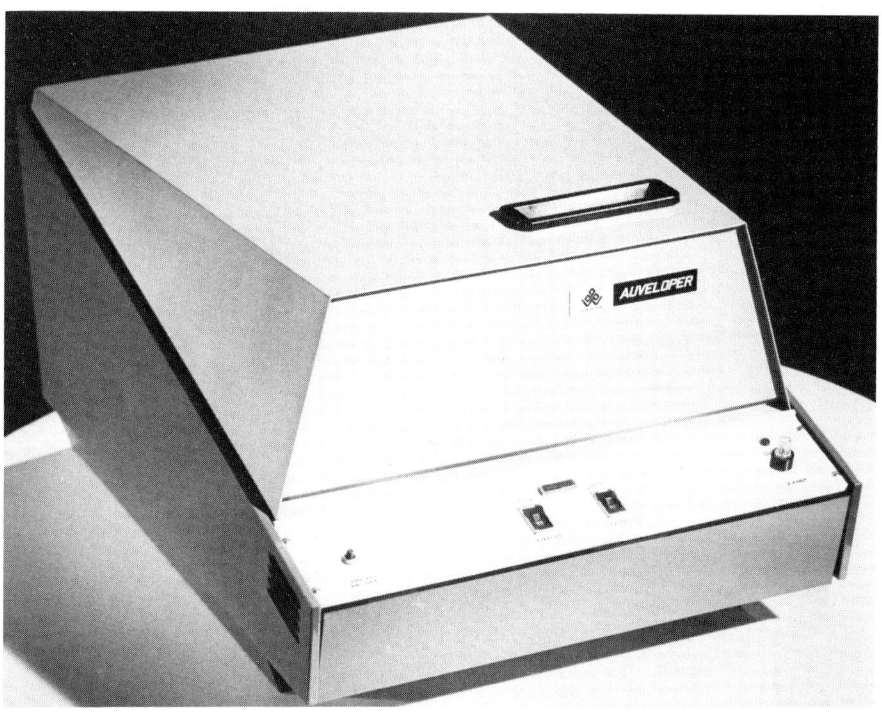

Fig. 3-28. The S. S. White Auveloper is a device that automatically processes roentgenograms.

more from the patient or behind a protective barrier.

8. Reduce the amount of primary radiation by using a restricting diaphragm at the outlet of the tube head, bearing in mind that the smaller the field, the less is the volume dose received by the patient from primary and secondary rays.
9. Use an added filter of aluminum at least 1 mm. thick for intraoral films and a slightly thicker filter for extraoral films.
10. Use as high a kilovoltage as possible, being sure it is compatible with adequate contrast. Also use the fastest films compatible with adequate detail.

There are definitive rules for exposure times and developing procedures that come with most packets of films. If these instructions are followed the examination can be made with very small amounts of radiation, and the resultant roentgenograms will provide the information needed for a roentgenographic diagnosis.

DARKROOM TECHNIQUE

In order to provide roentgenograms with optimal diagnostic and lasting value, proper laboratory processing is absolutely essential or, in other words, darkroom technique is of prime importance in film development.

Improperly developed films are the basis of many errors of interpretation. This accentuates the need of proper developing, fixing, and washing of films. Fresh solutions, proper processing times, correct temperatures, and proper handling of the films should be used to produce films of high quality. The fast films are most susceptible to darkroom deficiencies. Such critical points as (1) a light-tight darkroom, (2) position of the safelights, (3) bulb size in the safelights, and (4) recommended safelight filters should be checked.

Devices that automatically process roentgenograms are now available (Fig. 3-28).

ROENTGENOGRAPHIC PITFALLS*

1. *Exposure pitfalls*
   a. Thin image
   b. Dense image
   c. Blurred image
   d. Partial image
2. *Processing pitfalls*
   a. Thin image
   b. Dense image
   c. Partial image
3. *Fog*
   a. Age fog
   b. Storage
   c. White-light fog
   d. Safelight fog
   e. Chemical fog
4. *Handling pitfalls*
   a. Black lines
   b. Static
   c. Glass chips in the cone
   d. Air bubbles
   e. Fixer splashes
   f. Rough handling
   g. Packet-tube side
   h. Clip lines
   i. High temperature
   j. Packet placement
   k. Double exposure
   l. Fog

BITE-WING ROENTGENOGRAMS

Bite-wing roentgenograms are particularly valuable for the determination of the presence of proximal carious lesions. This type of roentgenogram made with the short cone technique is as good as one made

*I recommend that "Radiodontic Pitfalls" by A. Porter S. Sweet and published by the Eastman Kodak Co., X-ray Division, Rochester, N. Y., be read with great care for definitive elaboration of the topics being mentioned.

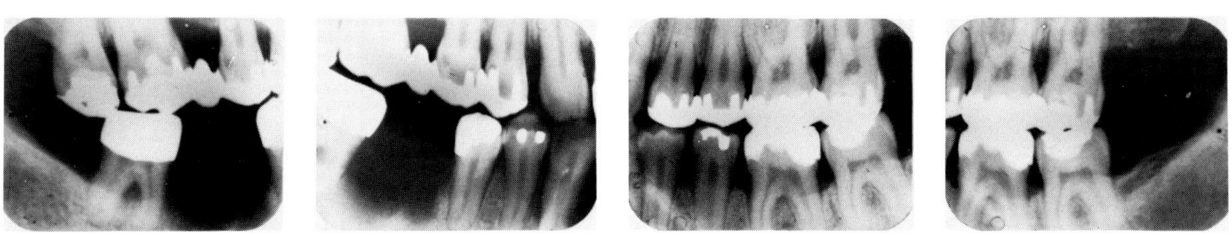

Fig. 3-29. An acceptable bite-wing roentgenogram.

with the long cone technique. I use the short cone technique for bite-wing roentgenograms using 65 kvp instead of 90 kvp because it seems to have "greater visual differences between the blacks and whites with fewer shades of gray"[9] (Fig. 3-29).

It is now known that the sum of primary and secondary radiation is almost identical for exposures made at both high and low kilovoltage.[10]

It is necessary to familiarize oneself with the various appearances that these proximal carious lesions may assume. Images that appear on the roentgenograms are the result of the action of caries demineralization and cavitation and assume several forms.

Buchholz[9] classifies these forms as follows:

"One form is the classic triangular shape, the base of the triangle being the original contour of the surface of the tooth with the apex pointing toward the dentino-enamel junction.

"If further penetration into the dentin has taken place, another form is seen, i.e., another triangle is formed with the base on the dentino-enamel junction, and the apex pointing toward the pulp following the path of the dentinal tubules."*

The carious lesion is more radiolucent than the adjoining tissue. Experience shows that the actual lesion is further advanced than the radiograph indicates. Wuehrmann[11] says this is due to an increase in the ratio of the enamel thickness to caries volume through which the x-rays must pass as the carious lesion approaches the dentino-enamel junction. The amount of destroyed tooth structure is minimized and never exaggerated in a radiograph. The small V-shaped area of decalcification that reaches the dentinoenamel junction should be filled, but if decalcification has only partially penetrated the thickness of enamel, the patient should be kept under periodic roentgenographic observation.

*From Buchholz, Robert E.: Radiographic interpretation of proximal carious lesions, Dent. Radiogr. Photogr. **38**:9-12, 1965.

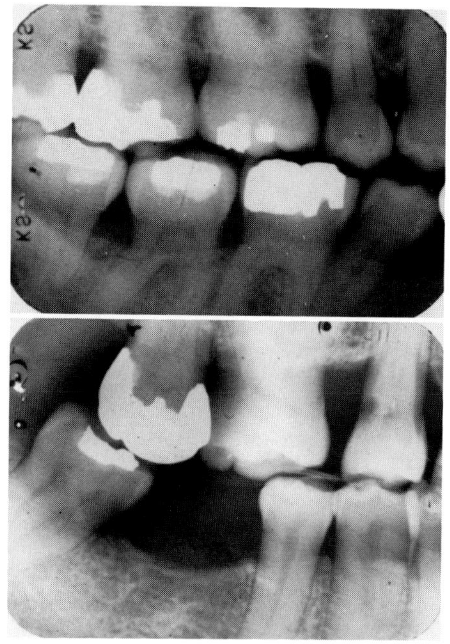

Fig. 3-30. A root concavity mesially or distally at the cervical line usually creates a radiolucency that can be interpreted as a carious lesion.

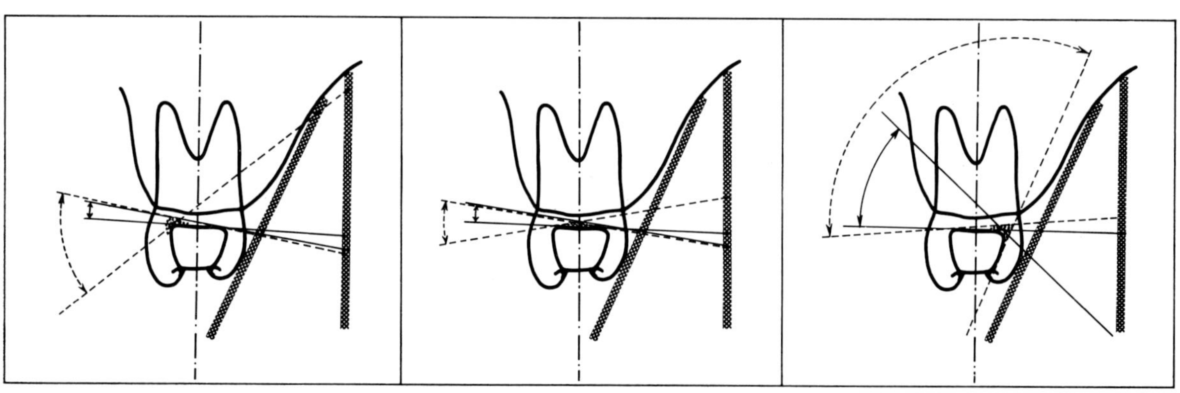

Fig. 3-31. Diagrammatic views of changes in vertical angulation when carious lesions are located at the buccogingival midway and linguogingival areas on the gingival seat of a proximal restoration. Films are positioned for the bisecting angle and paralleling techniques. The practical arc is indicated by solid black lines; the theoretical arc, by broken black lines. (From Buchholz, Robert E.: Radiographic interpretation of proximal carious lesions, Dent. Radiogr. Photogr. **38**[1]: 9-12, 1965.)

Cemental caries appear cup shaped. A root concavity mesially or distally at the cervical line usually creates a radiolucency and, in some instances, a wrong interpretation is made indicating this condition as caries (Fig. 3-30).

In making a bite-wing x-ray the operator must change the angulation of the x-ray beam on the second exposure, because a restoration may obliterate a carious lesion located midway between the buccogingival and linguogingival line angles (Fig. 3-31). A good image is absolutely necessary for correct interpretation. The anatomy of the particular area, the size of the lesion, and the roentgenographic technique will determine whether the lesion can be seen on the roentgenogram.

VIEWING

The roentgenograms should be properly mounted to facilitate examination under the most ideal conditions.

One must not be careless in the manner of viewing the roentgenograms. If the roentgenograms are held up to the window, shadows made by any object in the line of vision cause confusion in interpretation. A further handicap to accurate interpretation is the variation in the light intensity affected by the time of day and weather conditions.[9]

Use should be made of an x-ray illuminator and magnifier (Fig. 3-32). The value of the illuminator is amplified when the room is darkened so that the only light is that passing through the roentgenogram. The

A

B

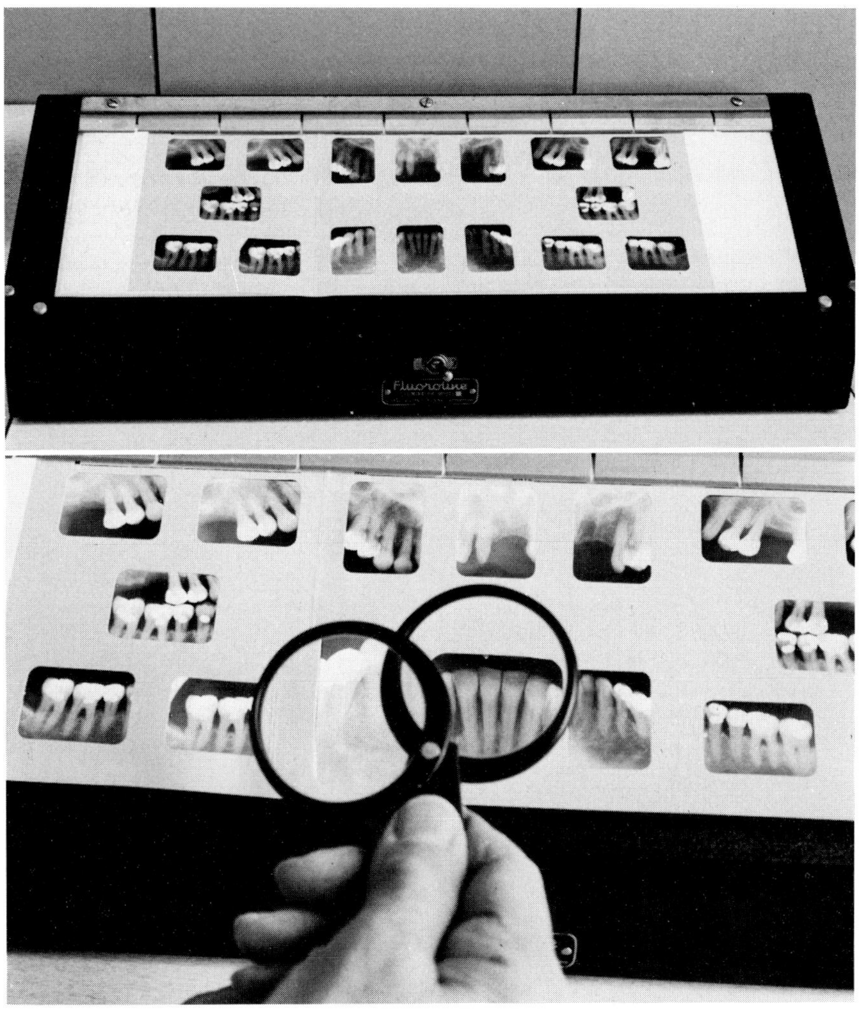

Fig. 3-32. Use should be made of **A,** an x-ray illuminator and **B,** a magnifier.

actual study of the dental roentgenograms is best accomplished by first viewing the entire roentgenogram before focusing on finer details.

INTERPRETATION

Roentgenographic interpretation is made difficult by the variations of normal anatomy, the abnormal nonpathologic conditions, and the changes caused by pathologic processes of local or systemic origin. Changes in the periodontal ligament, lamina dura, and alveolar bone may occur as a result of both local and systemic factors. One must be thoroughly familiar with the appearance of the normal as well as the abnormal.

In dental roentgenography we are dealing with the interpretation of variations in calcified hard structures and with images that are the result of various densities. Keep in mind that the images produced are two-dimensional projections of three-dimensional structures.

Refined roentgenography projects accurate images, minimizes superimposition, registers sharp definitions, and records a maximum range of shade gradation. It identifies the anatomic landmarks, observes the structural detail, compares the variations in radiability, and makes logical deductions.

By combining refined roentgenography and refined interpretation, the wonderful possibilities are utilized in the correct diagnosis of disorders and in preventive service.

The information obtainable from a roentgenogram is in proportion to the visibility of the images, which is increased many fold by enlargement or magnification. Magnification is imperative for refined interpretation, because the unaided vision cannot discern all the evidence in roentgenograms. The structures upon which the interpretation is based are, in many instances, too fine and too closely associated for abnormalities to be distinguished without enlargement.[12]

The popular conception that dark areas in roentgenograms always indicate the presence of infection is responsible for many mistakes. Circumscribed dark areas in roentgenograms are produced not only by destruction of bone but also by variations in density and form. Be careful not to mistake anatomic radiolucencies for the evidence of disease.

The first consideration in viewing a roentgenogram should be to identify the anatomic landmarks. This can be done by knowing the landmarks of each region and being familiar with the variations in the roentgenographic images of them. The interpretation should begin in the part of the roentgenogram farthest from the teeth, so that conclusions will not be influenced by dental repairs. After locating the landmarks, the dentist should proceed in order to the periapical bone, the roots, the crest of the alveolar process, and the crowns of the teeth. Never interpret by a hasty glance at a wet film.

LAMINA DURA AND PERIODONTAL LIGAMENT

The lamina dura is the most important feature in the diagnosis of periapical disease. The first evidence of periapical infection is the distension of the lamina dura by a thickening of the periodontal ligament. The next stage is a break in some part of the lamina dura, which occurs before there is destruction of the surrounding bone. The thickening of the periodontal ligament and breaks in the lamina dura are often invisible without magnification. The thickness of the normal periodontal ligament is approximately 0.2 mm., and only a trace of the lamina dura is registered in some aspects.[13] Therefore, considerable enlargement, by magnification, is necessary to detect pathologic changes in these structures.

PULPLESS TEETH

The only preoperative means of determining whether or not a pulpless tooth is disease producing is roentgenographic evidence. When the lamina dura is unbroken, it can be assumed that the tooth is not a source of infection. Sharp roentgenograms, different views, and magnification are necessary to trace the lamina dura around teeth.

In summation, it can be said that in many instances a general roentgenographic examination exposes some unsuspected abnormality or pathologic alteration and leads to the correction of these conditions. The discovery of obscure caries or incipient marginal destruction before irreparable damage has occurred is of the greatest service to a patient.[3] Also, when disturbances arise, roentgenographic records of a patient over a period of time are most helpful in distinguishing histologic changes, in deciding upon the treatment to apply, and in judging the prognosis. The dentist must realize, however, the limitations of roentgenograms and be able to properly use all the diagnostic aids (verbal, ocular, instrumental, roentgenographic, etc.) in order to reach the decision that is best for the patient (Figs. 3-33 to 3-38).

CAST ORIENTATION

The proper use of study casts in diagnosis and treatment planning is of the utmost importance in the evaluation of the patient's occlusion and also in the determination of necessary occlusal changes, if any.

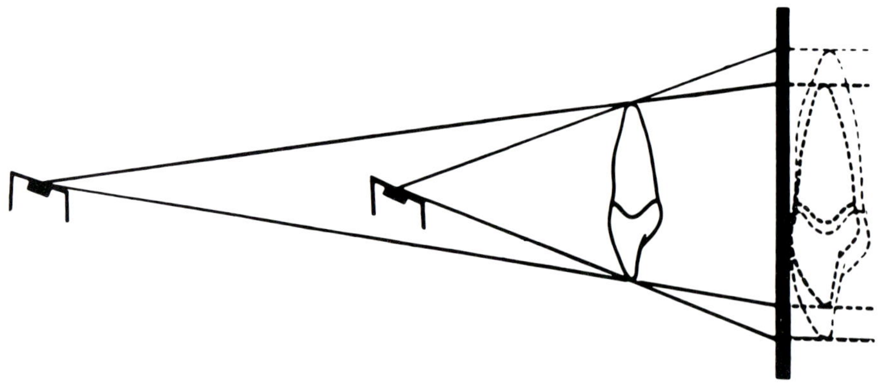

Fig. 3-33. Comparison of 8 inch and 16 inch focal film distances, with demonstration of divergent rays and effect on image. (From Grieder, Arthur, and Cinotti, William R.: Periodontal prosthesis, vol. 1, St. Louis, 1968, The C. V. Mosby Co.; courtesy Rinn Corp., Elgin, Ill.)

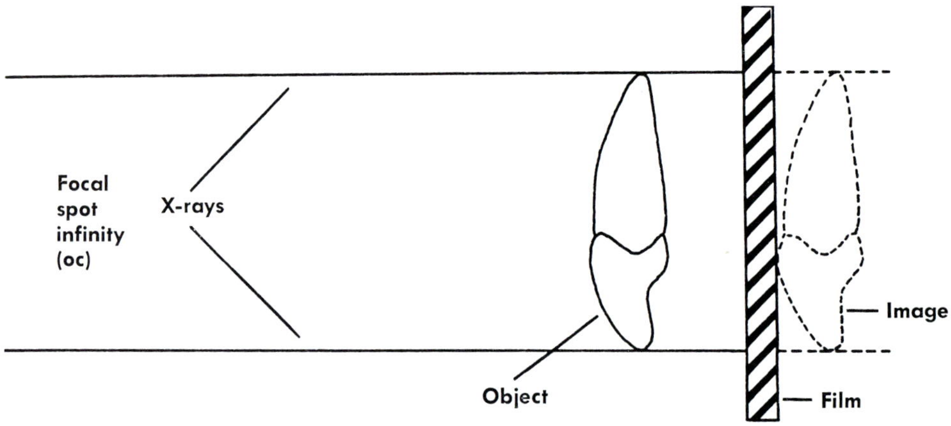

Fig. 3-34. All rays from focal spot parallel at infinity. (From Grieder, Arthur, and Cinotti, William R.: Periodontal prosthesis, vol. 1, St. Louis, 1968, The C. V. Mosby Co.; courtesy Rinn Corp., Elgin, Ill.)

A

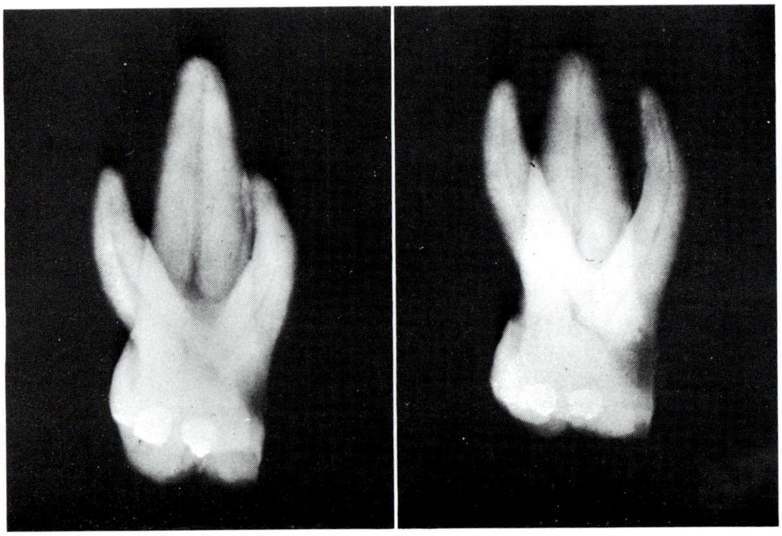

B

Fig. 3-35. A, Distorted relationship of molar roots. **B,** Normal relationship of molar roots. (From Grieder, Arthur, and Cinotti, William R.: Periodontal prosthesis, vol. 1, St. Louis, 1968, The C. V. Mosby Co.; courtesy Rinn Corp., Elgin, Ill.)

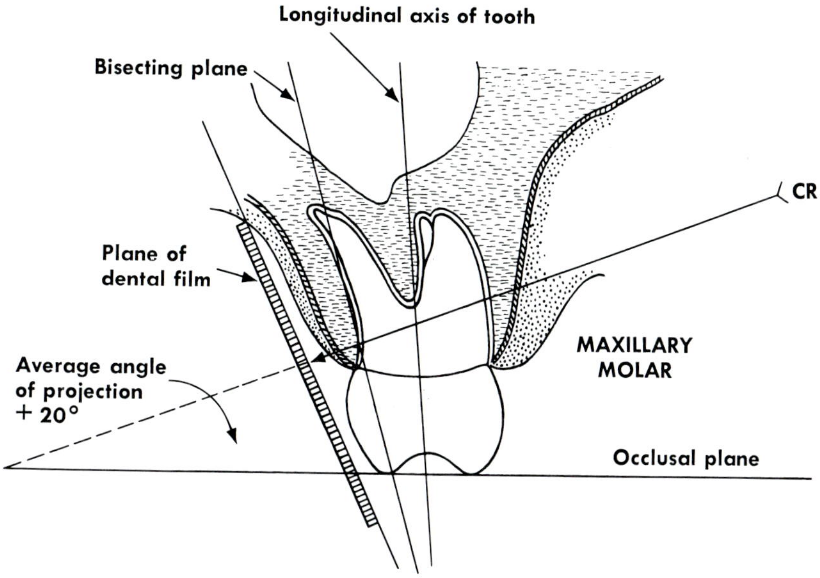

Fig. 3-36. Diagram illustrating proper bisecting technique for x-ray film of maxillary molar. (From Grieder, Arthur, and Cinotti, William R.: Periodontal prosthesis, vol. 1, St. Louis, 1968, The C. V. Mosby Co.; courtesy Eastman Kodak Co., Rochester, N.Y.)

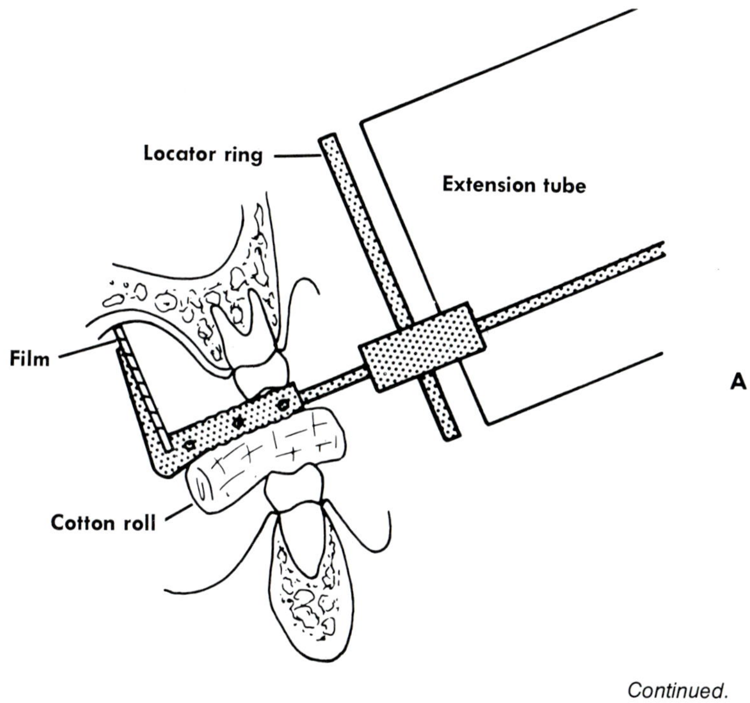

Continued.

Fig. 3-37. Diagram illustrating proper paralleling technique for maxillary molar. **A,** Faciolingual view; **B,** anteroposterior view. (From Grieder, Arthur, and Cinotti, William R.: Periodontal prosthesis, vol. 1, St. Louis, 1968, The C. V. Mosby Co.; courtesy Rinn Corp., Elgin, Ill.)

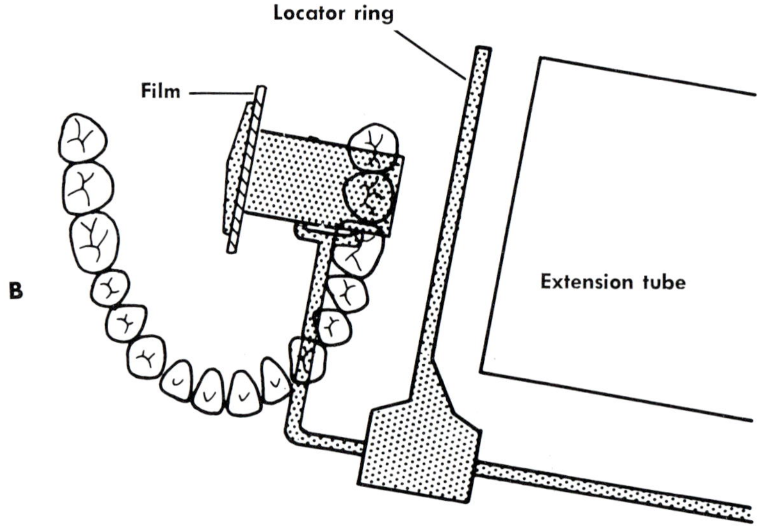

Fig. 3-37, cont'd. For legend see p. 45.

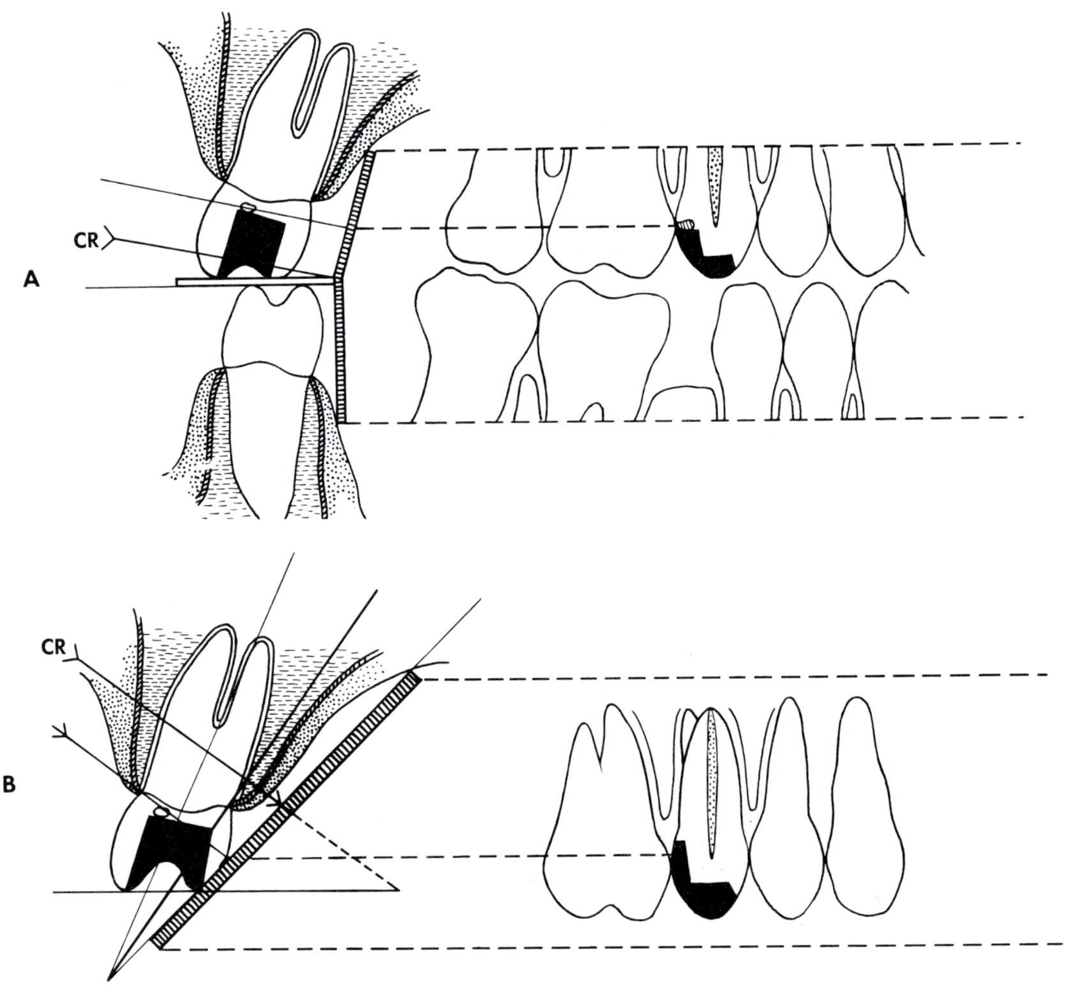

Fig. 3-38. A, Bite-wing projection demonstrates defective restoration. **B,** Periapical projection does not demonstrate defective restoration. (From Grieder, Arthur, and Cinotti, William R.: Periodontal prosthesis, vol. 1, St. Louis, 1968, The C. V. Mosby Co.; courtesy Eastman Kodak Co., Rochester, N. Y.)

It not only permits evaluation of the coronal portion (form, contour, alignment, contacts) of the individual teeth but also of the arch form, arch relationship, and functional movements.

For a functional diagnosis, casts must be mounted on an adjustable articulator with some semblance of order. Unmounted casts are of limited value because they may reveal centric occlusion but not centric relation and because tooth contacts in working and balancing positions cannot be determined. This points up the importance of a careful mounting of the patient's dental casts on an instrument that copies his mandibular movements, so that a diagnosis of the functional relations may be made by studying them in connection with clinical and roentgenographic findings.

Mounted casts on an articulator must reproduce proper mouth relations to reproduce the correct movements of the mandible. Stallard aptly said: "What should be expected of an articulator is the individual expression of the condylar movements of a patient, something that may differ from all other patients."* In other words, we must refer to the controlling mandibular axes, and only by so doing can diagnostic casts be of any value in arriving at a diagnosis and correct plan of treatment. With correctly articulator-oriented casts, disharmonies or interferences can be readily recognized. By modifying the occlusal surfaces of the casts, the dentist can make a better judgment as to whether restorations with reshaped occlusal surfaces or orthodontic repositioning of teeth or selective grinding or a combination of all of these is indicated for the production of more favorable forces. This in turn will help decrease the trigger areas of bruxism and functional disturbances of the temporomandibular joints, which Ramfjord[14] says are located in the range of mandibular movements between centric relation and centric occlusion. Steep inclines that deflect terminal hinge closure and interfere with gliding movements can also be studied and corrected.

A consideration of these facts makes it obvious that the location of occlusal interferences by direct observation has many limitations. Conditioned-reflex avoidance patterns allow patients to bypass occlusal interferences. An understanding of the proprioceptive feedback phenomenon is essential.[15]

A thorough knowledge of occlusion, which is the common denominator of all dental practice, is of the utmost importance in diagnosis and treatment planning. It guides us in understanding the "why" and "how" of the fabrication of our restorations, which not only involves mechanics but also a knowledge of neuromuscular physiology.

*From Contino, R. M., and Stallard, Harvey: Instruments essential for obtaining data needed in making a functional diagnosis of the human mouth, J. Prosthet. Dent. **7**:66-77, 1957.

IMPRESSIONS AND CASTS

In cast orientation accurate study casts of the patient's mouth should be made from well-taken impressions making use of an elastic impression material such as alginate, hydrocolloid, silicone, or rubber base (see Chapter 9). This type of impression should be poured immediately for accuracy, using a hard artificial stone (Fig. 3-39).

If possible, two sets of impressions are taken to provide the following:

1. A set of preoperative casts for the study of occlusal relations for diagnosis, treatment planning, and method of therapy. This set should be preserved as a permanent preoperative record for future documentation.

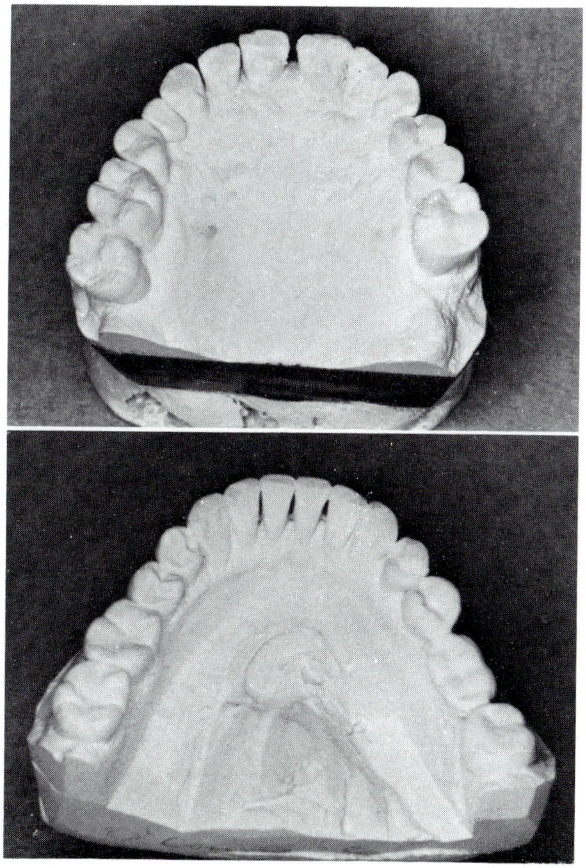

Fig. 3-39. Preoperative study casts made from alginate impressions.

2. A set for the construction of clutches. These are necessary in the location of the hinge axis and in the recording of a three-dimensional pantographic tracing of the controlling mandibular axes.
3. A set for preoperative study. This is used for the determination of types of tooth preparations, for location and amount of tooth structure to remove, and for the development of the articulation in wax, which is required to properly restore the patient's mouth to good function.

However, with great care, a second and third set of casts can be poured from the original impression when alginate material has been used. Be very careful in the removal of the first or second set of casts so that tears and distortion are avoided.

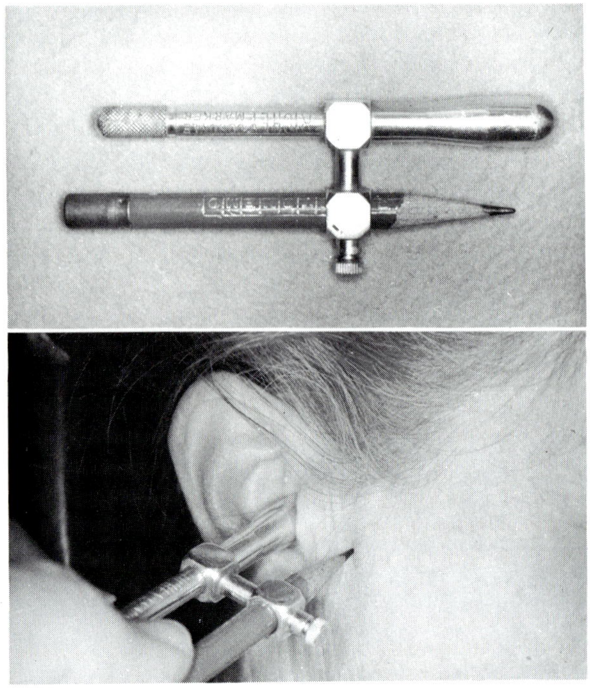

Fig. 3-40. Location of arbitrary axis points, making use of Ritchey pencil.

FACE-BOW TRANSFER

In addition, a conventional face-bow mounting and a centric relation record for mounting the study casts in a fairly accurate relationship to each other must be taken. The face-bow transfer is taken so that the upper cast on the adjustable articulator can be oriented to the same plane of occlusion as is found in the patient's mouth.

The transverse axis is generally accepted as the most stable reproducible point from which maxillary casts can be mounted. However, the arbitrary location for preliminary diagnostic and treatment planning studies, construction of clutches, etc. is the most common method of determining the axis.

A simple method for locating the arbitrary axis points is to locate the ala-tragus line or a line from the tragus to the outer canthus of the eye on both sides of the face and, making use of a Ritchey pencil or flexible millimeter rule, to mark a point approximately 13 mm. anterior to the tragus of the ear (Figs. 3-40 to 3-42). To use the face-bow transfer properly we must have a third reference point to establish a plane of reference, the axis-orbital plane. This third point is marked on the right side of the nose 2⅛ inches from the incisal edge of a central incisor tooth, or it is determined by locating the inferior border of the orbit on the right side and, for convenience, recording a mark on the same plane on the side of the nose (Fig. 3-43).

An ear type face-bow for mounting the maxillary cast has proved simple to use (Whip-Mix "Quick Mount" Face Bow).* It is designed as a self-centering

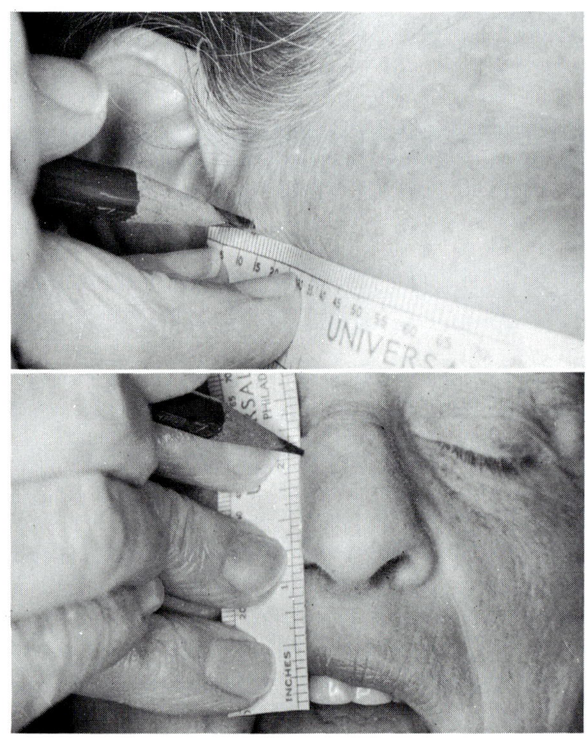

Fig. 3-41. Location of arbitrary axis points and of third reference point on nose by means of millimeter rule.

*Whip-Mix Corp., Louisville, Ky.

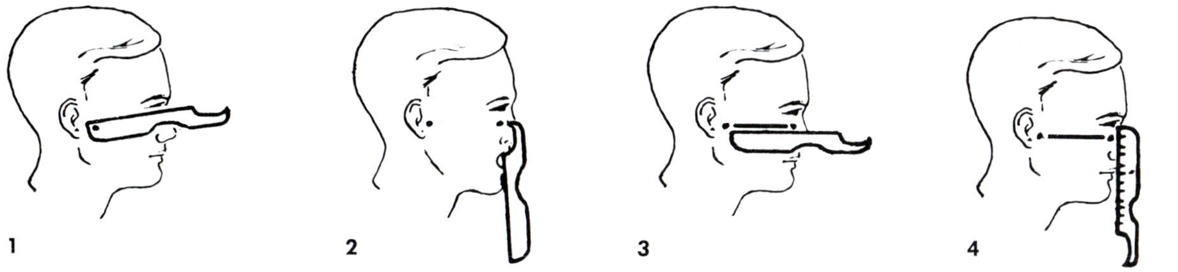

Fig. 3-42. Location and marking of anterior and posterior reference points. Reference plane is also marked.

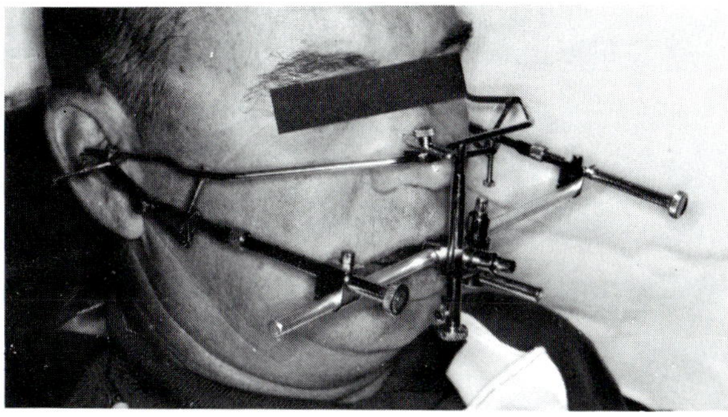

Fig. 3-43. Face-bow transfer for orientation of upper cast on articulator to same plane of occlusion as found in mouth.

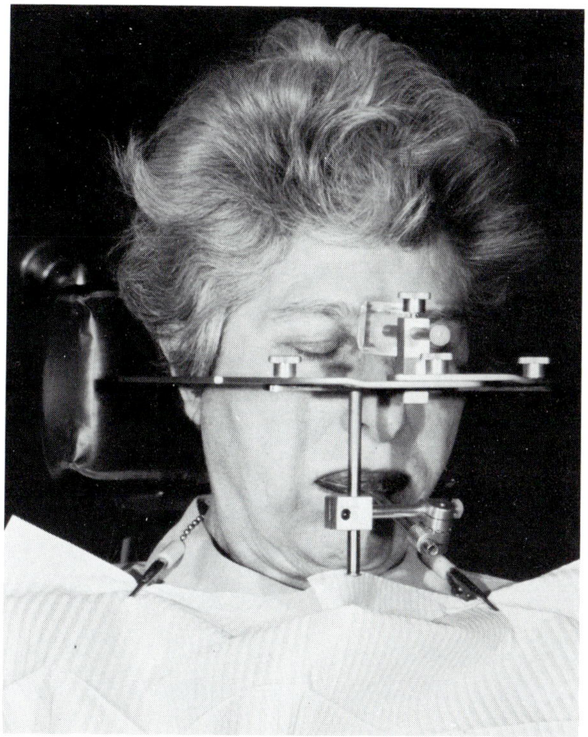

Fig. 3-44. The use of an ear type face-bow for mounting the maxillary cast has proved simple to use. The external auditory meati are used for the posterior reference points, and the nasion is used as the anterior reference point.

caliper, thereby eliminating extra time required to center and align the articulator to conventional type face-bows. It does not require measuring and marking of reference points on the skin. The external auditory meati are used for the posterior reference points as a means of relating the maxillary cast to an arbitrary hinge axis location. The nasion is used as the anterior reference point (Fig. 3-44).

The orientation of the face-bow to the articulator is managed quickly by the holes in the plastic ear posts of the face-bow over the lateral pins on the condylar guidance housings of the Whip-Mix articulator* (Figs. 3-45 and 3-46). Next the lower cast is mounted with centric relation record and the articulator ''set'' with positional wax records.

This particular method allows us to mount casts with an accuracy acceptable for a preliminary diagnostic and treatment planning study and also can be used for routine restorative procedures with better end results. Teteruck and Lundeen[16] have concluded after exhaustive studies that 56.4% of the arbitrary points achieved by the ear face-bow fell within a 6 mm. radius of the true hinge axis, whereas 33% of conventional axis locations were within 6 mm. of the true axis. They also concluded that with a simple modifi-

*Whip-Mix Corp., Louisville, Ky.

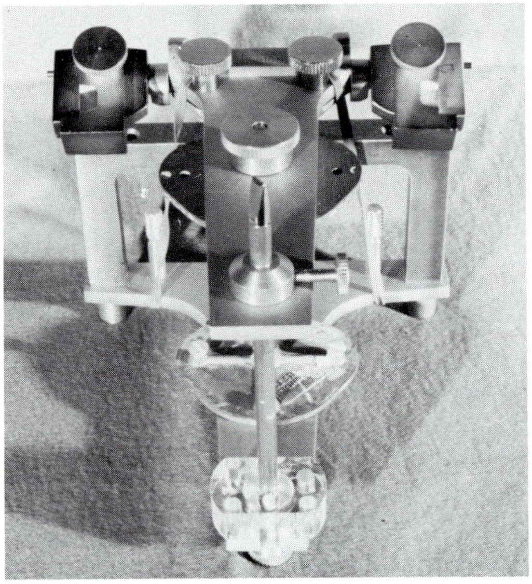

Fig. 3-45

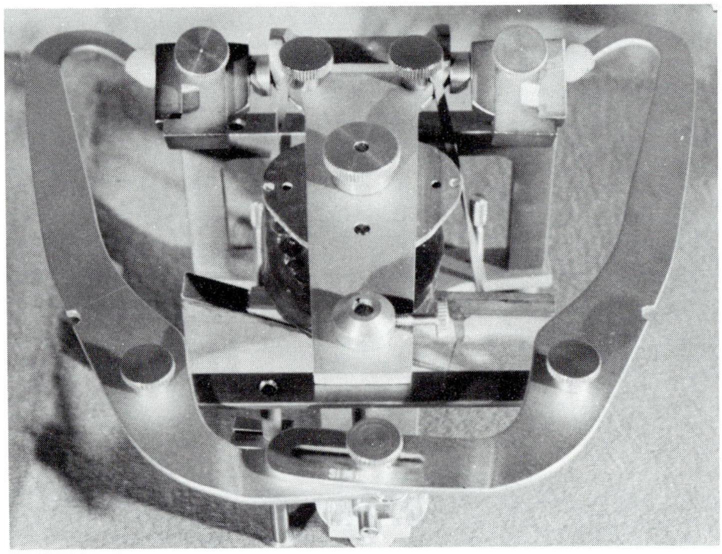

Fig. 3-46

Figs. 3-45 and 3-46. The orientation of the face-bow to the Whip-Mix Articulator is managed quickly by the holes in the plastic ear posts of the face-bow over the lateral pins on the condylar guidance housings of the articulator.

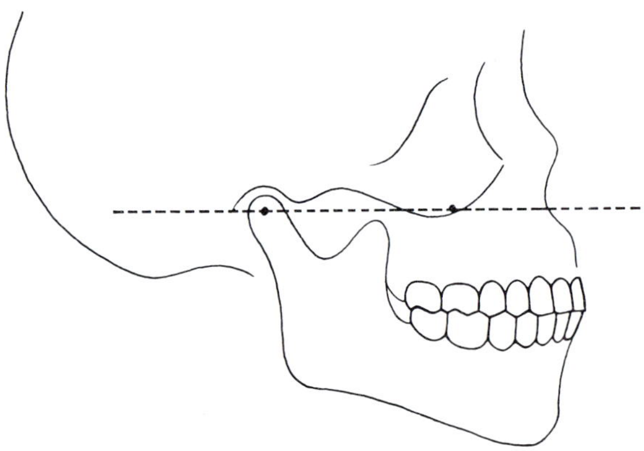

Fig. 3-47. Plane of reference (axis-orbital plane).

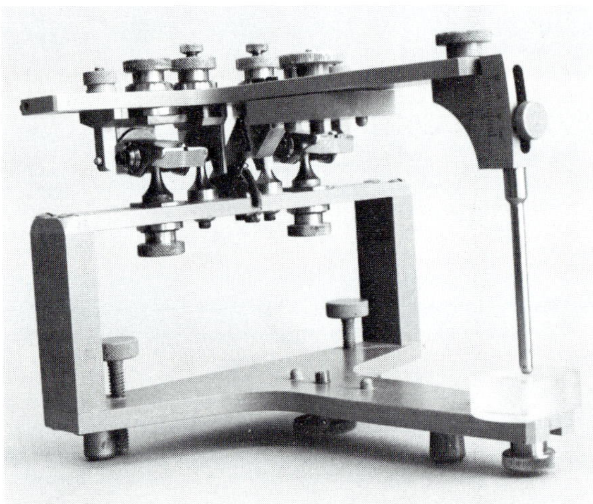

Fig. 3-48. A fully adjustable articulator.

cation of the ear face-bow the figure of 56.4% could be increased to 75.5%.

For more definitive diagnostic and treatment planning studies the axis-orbital line must be used for the mounting of the upper cast. This plane is virtually the same as the Frankfort plane used by anthropologists. It was first used by Simon, an orthodontist, to establish the positions of the teeth in the facial plane. This is the same reason it is used in gnathology in preference to the ala-tragus line or a line from the tragus of the ear to the outer canthus of the eye (Fig. 3-47).

Definitive accuracy in reproducing mandibular movements can only be done on a fully adjustable articulator (Figs. 3-48 and 3-49). What we observe in making the occlusal analysis on correctly oriented casts (among many things) are interferences between centric relation and centric occlusion position, as well as those located on the nonworking side. Not only can

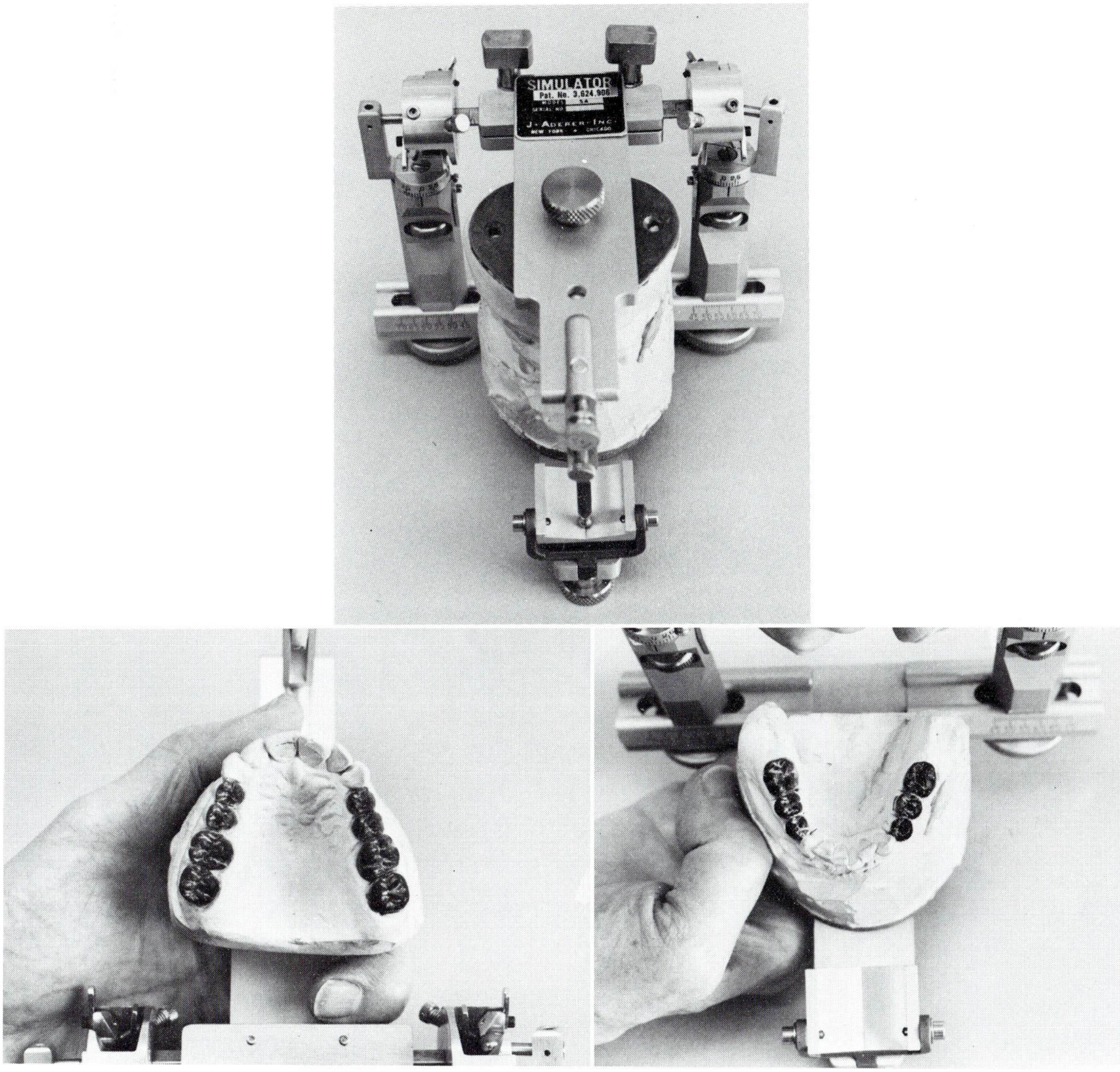

Fig. 3-49. Definitive accuracy in reproducing mandibular movements and, thereby, accurate practical or clinical results can only be done on a fully adjustable analog.

these interferences be revealed and identified, but cusp pathways during eccentric mandibular movements can probably interpret the "why" of wear facets, etc., and corrective measures can also be formulated. All this is a help in the planning of the restorations.

A knowledge of the initial side shifting of the mandible and its influence on occlusal anatomy is of the utmost importance, because with this knowledge one is cognizant of the fact that this particular motion must be accurately recorded and reproduced in proper laboratory equipment upon which the restorations are to be constructed and, by so doing, overcome the necessity of extensive occlusal corrections in the mouth in order to avoid possible resultant disease.

The pantograph and the adjustable articulator are important tools in this determination. The pantograph graphically reflects anatomic characteristics of the temporomandibular articulations that influence mandibular paths of motion, and the articulator should be capable of adjusting for those essential elements of the determinants of mandibular movement which are of clinical importance (Fig. 3-50).

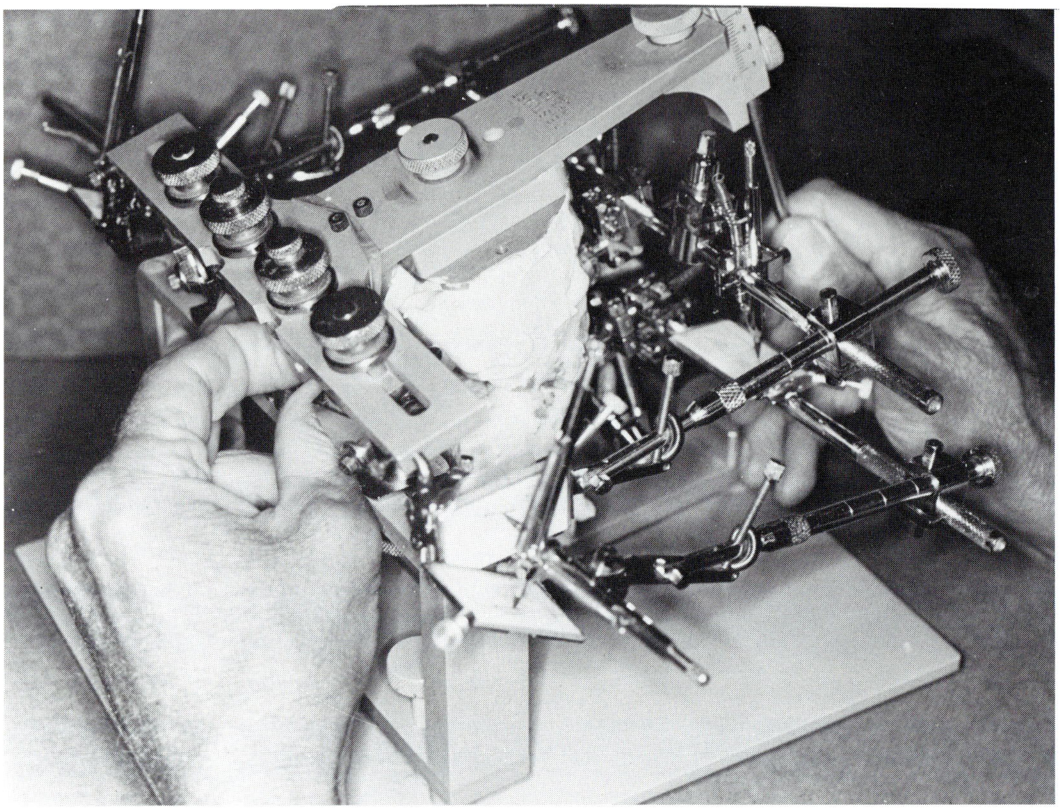

Fig. 3-50. Using the pantograph and the analog properly.

Fig. 3-5l. A, Cohen trainer. **B,** Cohen trainer left on patient for 5 to 10 minutes to prevent protruding of jaw.

A

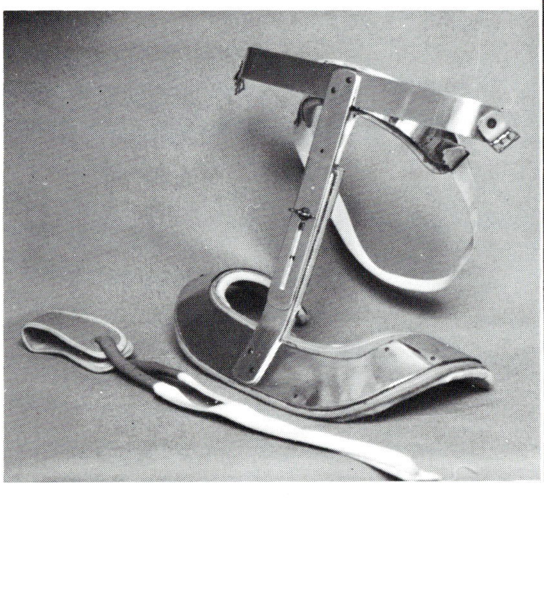

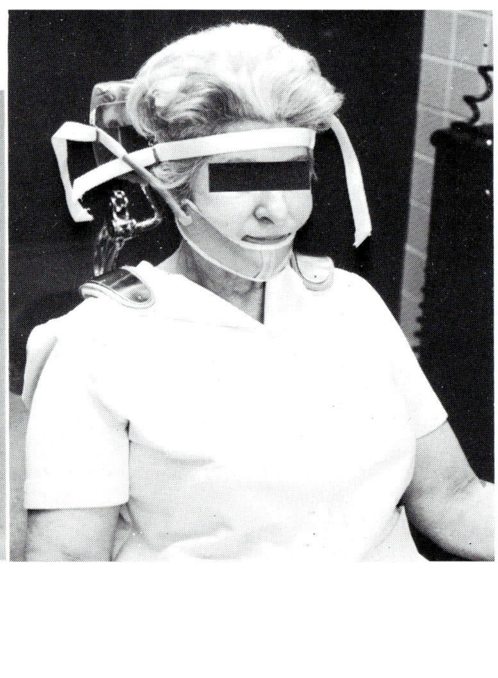

B

CENTRIC RELATION RECORD

The next order of business in this preliminary diagnostic procedure in cast orientation is the conditioning of the patient for a centric relation record. This conditioning can be done by means of a trainer (Cohen or Hickok type) or the use of some form of anterior resistance, which tends to overcome the translating contractions of the external pterygoid muscle (Fig. 3-51).

The centric relation record must be registered at an increased vertical dimension (within the limits of pure rotation of the condyles) so that the guidance provided by the teeth is removed. Some form of anterior resistance must be provided. This resistance tends to act as a fulcrum, which aids in obtaining a registration of the condyles in the posterior and superior positions—rearmost, uppermost, and midmost.

In all preliminary diagnostic procedures a wax form (made with "Sure-Set Wax"*) is accurately adapted to the occlusal and incisal surfaces of the upper cast (which has been lubricated) and down the facial and lingual surfaces to the height of contour of the teeth. This makes a wax form that can be seated firmly and definitely on the upper teeth (Fig. 3-52). Use is then made of a piece of "air chamber metal."† It provides the anterior resistance and acts as a fulcrum, thereby preventing penetration of the wax by the teeth and interference from habit patterns and also allowing for enough clearance in the posterior region for the recording material. Breaking the reflex pattern of closure will permit a normal closure. Only a few lower anterior teeth contact this piece of "air chamber metal" (Fig. 3-53).

During the exact positioning and adjustment of the metal form to the wax form for proper contact with a few lower teeth and posterior clearance for the recording material, the patient is not allowed to bring his teeth together in order to keep blocking out the proprioceptive reflex. A saliva ejector is inserted into the mouth every time the wax form is removed for adjustment of the metal form.

Use is made of a soft wax, Aluwax,‡ for the recording of shallow occlusal indentations. The well-adapted wax form with the softened Aluwax on the underside is seated on the upper teeth and is held in place with the operator's left thumb and forefinger. With the right thumb on the patient's chin, the opera-

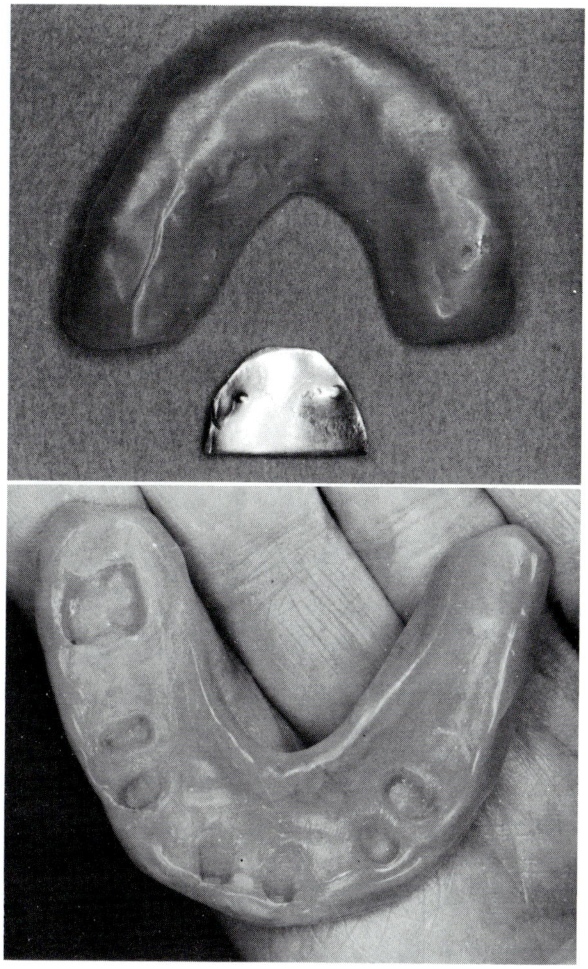

Fig. 3-52. Prepared wax form and "air chamber metal" form. This form can be definitely seated on upper teeth, and with provision made for anterior resistance to act as a fulcrum, it serves well as a preliminary interocclusal record.

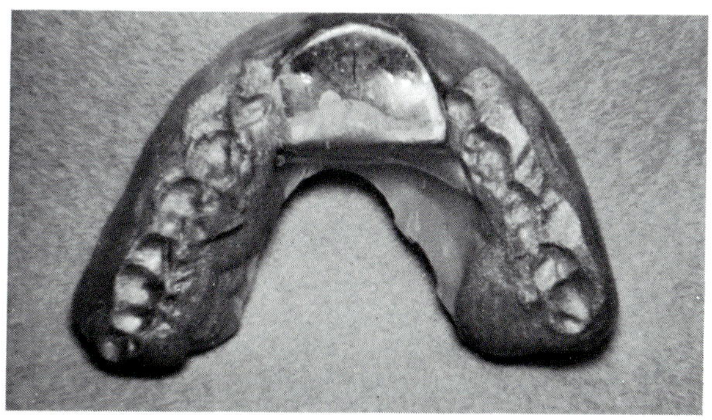

Fig. 3-53. Completed preliminary centric relation record.

*Kerr Mfg. Co., Detroit, Mich.

†Dixon Mfg. Co., Newark, N. J.

‡Hickok Specialties Co., Grand Rapids, Mich.

tor guides the patient into the terminal hinge closure. The mandible is guided, not pushed or forced, into repeated closures. The wax record is removed and placed in cool water. The excess wax is removed with a Bard-Parker* knife, leaving only the cusp tip indentations so that the cast may be accurately seated when the mounting is made. This wax record is again seated on the upper teeth, and the patient closes his mouth once again. The operator guides the mandible to position to eliminate any warpage that may have resulted from the chilling in cool water or from the trimming of the excess wax. If no distortion can be detected on closure, the record is accepted. Two other centric relation records are taken to check the accuracy of the records by checking one record against the other, making use of the Lauritzen split-cast method (for detailed accounts of technique see Chapters 4 and 17).

Dawson[17] has described a method of manipulation for centric relation that has been enthusiastically accepted by me.

The following procedures are used:

1. Lay the patient back flat, chin pointed up.
2. While working from a seated position behind the patient, firmly stabilize his head between your forearm and rib cage.
3. Place the last three fingers of each hand on the lower border of the mandible. This is for exerting pressure *up* on the condyles. *Keep the pressure on bone.* Do not let the fingers push into the soft tissue of the neck.
4. Grasp the symphysis with thumb and forefinger of each hand. *Thumbs should touch each other.*
5. Thumbs and index fingers should form a small diamond. Grasp should be on bone. If thumbs get separated too far, too much pressure is exerted on soft tissue.
6. Now, with a gentle touch, manipulate the open jaw *lightly* into terminal hinge position and then apply pressure *back* with the thumbs and forefingers and *up* with the other three fingers. This produces a kind of up-back torque to the whole mandible, which allows a free axis rotation of the condyle without letting it off the terminal axis.
7. The assistant holds the wax form (or ribbon, etc.) while the dentist does step 6 (Fig. 3-54).

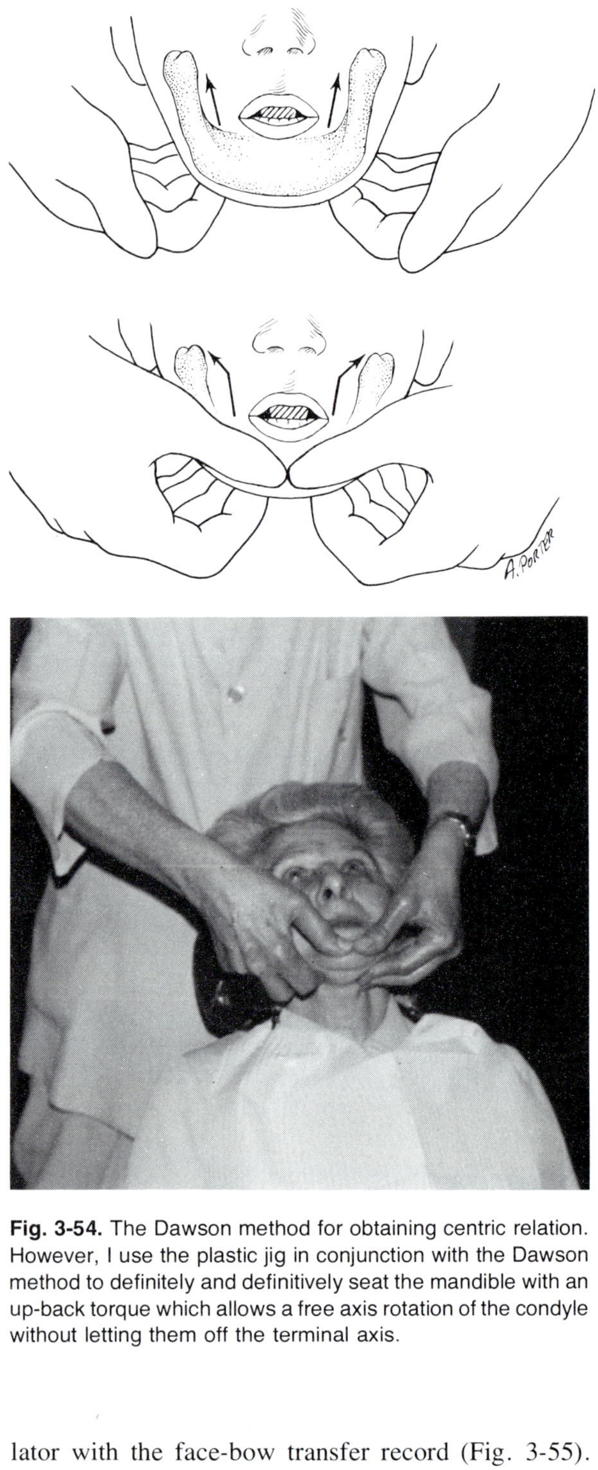

Fig. 3-54. The Dawson method for obtaining centric relation. However, I use the plastic jig in conjunction with the Dawson method to definitely and definitively seat the mandible with an up-back torque which allows a free axis rotation of the condyle without letting them off the terminal axis.

MOUNTING THE CASTS IN ARTICULATOR

The upper cast, which has been prepared for the split-cast method, is mounted on an adjustable articulator with the face-bow transfer record (Fig. 3-55). After this step has been completed, the articulator is inverted and the centric relation record is placed on the occlusal surface of the upper cast. Then the lower cast is placed on the centric relation record, held firmly in this record and against the upper cast, and attached by means of a stone with a low setting expan-

*Bard-Parker Co., Danbury, Conn.

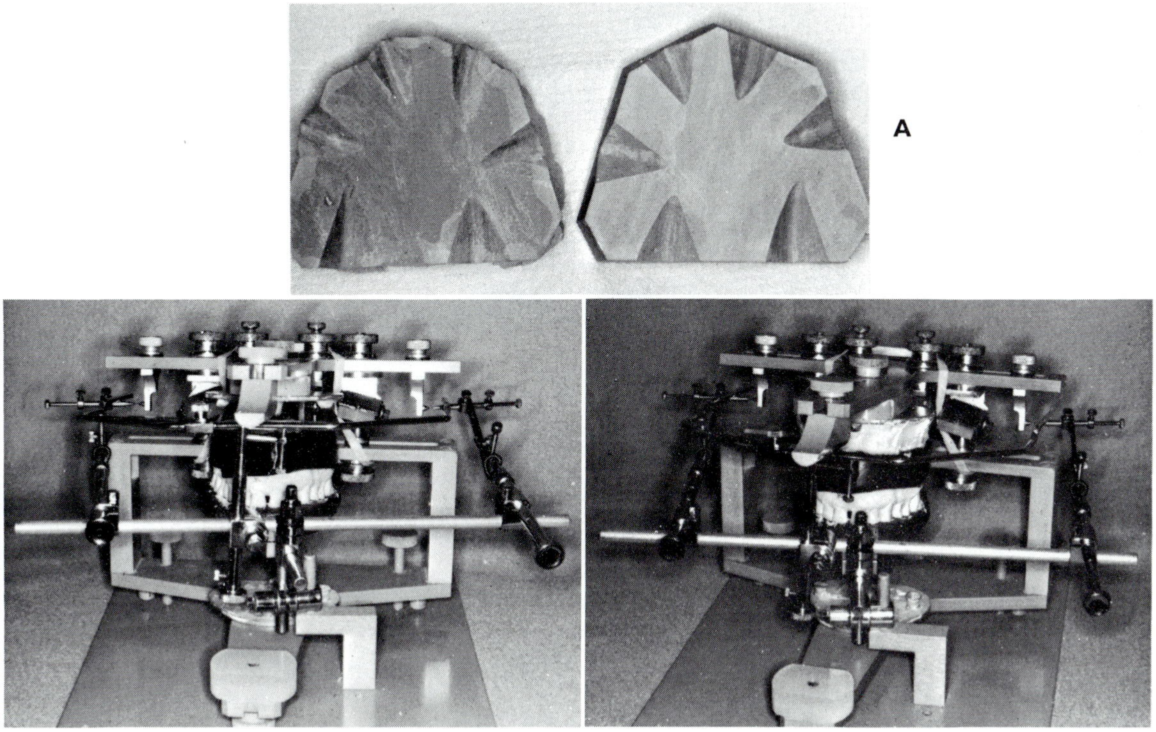

A

B

C

Fig. 3-55. A, Upper cast prepared for split-cast method. B, Upper cast being readied for mounting to upper frame of articulator. C, Upper cast mounted to upper bow of articulator.

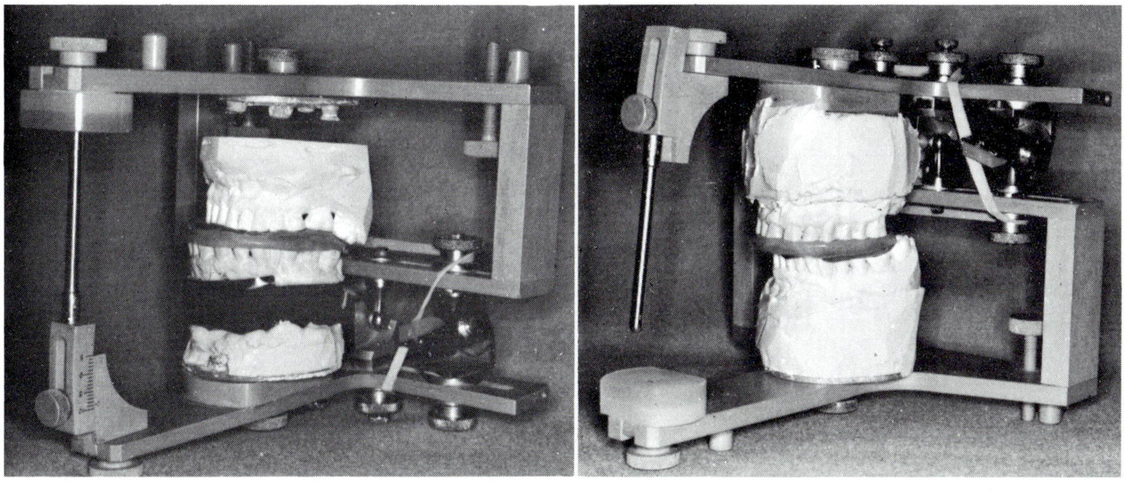

Fig. 3-56. Articulator inverted, centric relation record positioned, and lower cast then attached to lower bow of articulator.

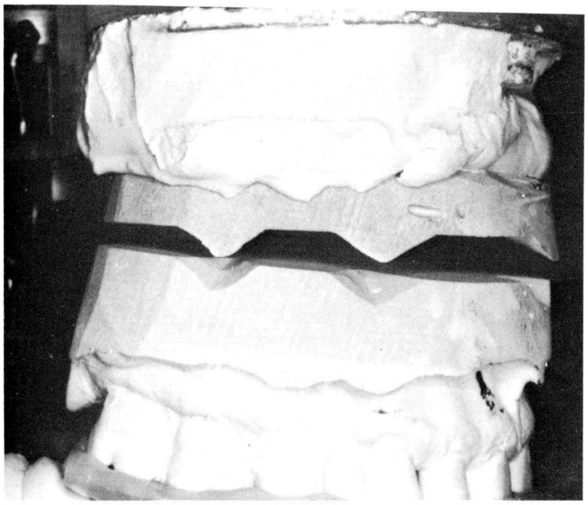

Fig. 3-57. Verification of centric relation records: separation of grooved upper primary base cast from secondary base cast, which is attached to upper bow of articulator.

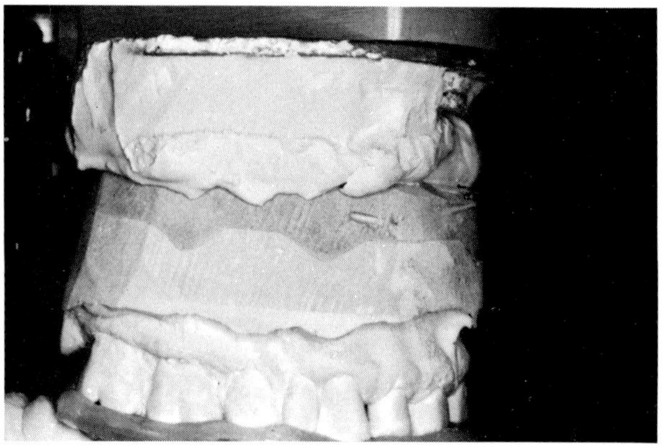

Fig. 3-58. Verification of centric relation records completed: secondary base fits accurately into primary base; no discrepancies are visible.

sion to the lower bow of the articulator. The upper and lower members of the articulator must be in centric relation (Figs. 3-56 and 3-57).

The second and third centric relation records are verified by separating the grooved upper primary base cast from the secondary base cast (which is attached to the upper member of the articulator), placing the primary base cast into the second or third record (which is carefully held in position), and closing the secondary base cast against and into the primary base cast. If the secondary base cast fits accurately into the primary base cast and no discrepancies are visible, the centric relation records have been proved to be correct and the casts are correctly mounted in terminal hinge relation (Figs. 3-58 and 3-59).

In this type of cast orientation, where an arbitrary axis has been located for preliminary study of occlusal relations and the construction of clutches, if necessary, for the recording and the transferring of mandibular relations, some discrepancies will result. However, the discipline required in making a hinge-bow transfer, centric relation records, and mounting procedures by the split-cast method will be very helpful in the steps that are to follow (see Figs. 3-60 to 3-66).

RECORDING AND TRANSFERRING OF MANDIBULAR RELATIONS

Importance of mandibular relation. Function is the prime object of restorative dentistry. The proper care and treatment of the oral organ should be the concern of all practitioners of dentistry, and of necessity this requires a knowledge of the form and function of this organ—its parts, how it can be, at least figuratively, taken apart and put back together, how it is made, and how it works in health and disease. In other words, a complete knowledge and understanding of the anatomy and physiology of this most important organ is a "must."

The accurate recording and transferring of mandibular relations is possible now, provided certain principles are understood and executed carefully.

The ability to treat and save mouths is directly related to the ability to capture and transfer jaw function to the restoration.

Although I am thoroughly in accord with the modern concept of periodontics, I also firmly believe that complete pocket elimination, as important as it is, comes to naught if stability in function is not attained.

We must concern ourselves with a *center* that can be easily located and useful for our procedures—a *center* that will enable us to reproduce the patient's movements on a suitable articulator.

The dentist must be able to recognize and distinguish between normal and abnormal occlusion and joint function. It is therefore necessary (1) to have a knowledge of mandibular function, since the temporomandibular joint bears an almost unbelievably precise relation to the teeth, and (2) to keep in mind that there must be a harmony between centric occlusion and centric relation, which can only occur if the occlusal surfaces of the teeth can be

A

B

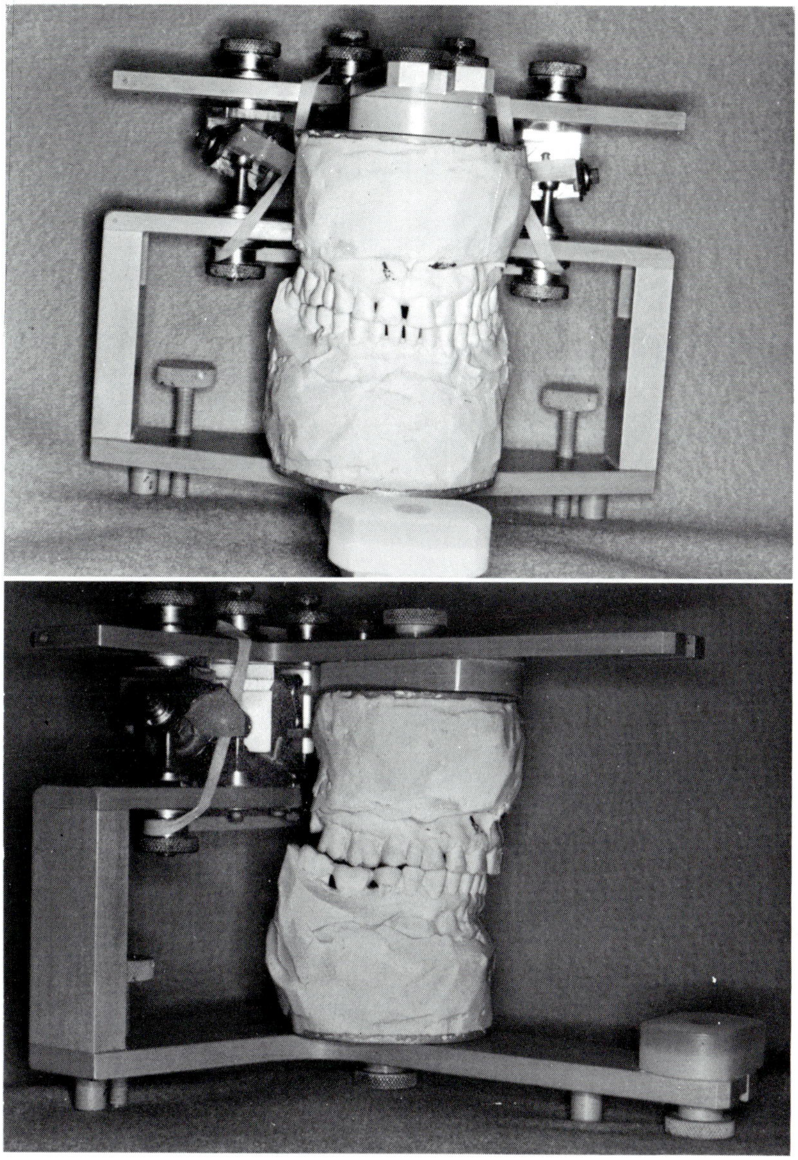

Fig. 3-59. A, Mounted casts in centric relation, anterior view. **B,** Mounted casts in centric relation, right posterior view.

brought into maximum contact without cuspal interference as the mandible assumes its terminal hinge position.

Existing conditions must be analyzed by means of a functional method. The mere relation of teeth to each other is not enough. Unless the relationship satisfies the functional requirements of the whole mouth, it becomes a destructive function, creating a metabolic demand in excess of the normal requirements of the mouth. Functional relations that will make it possible for the natural metabolic processes of the body to come to our aid must be created.

We now have the instruments and knowledge to make good functional examinations and diagnoses leading to proper treatment planning, prognosis, and therapy.

We must be able to duplicate the variety of patterns of mandibular motion, realizing that the musculature motivates the movement of the man-

Fig. 3-60

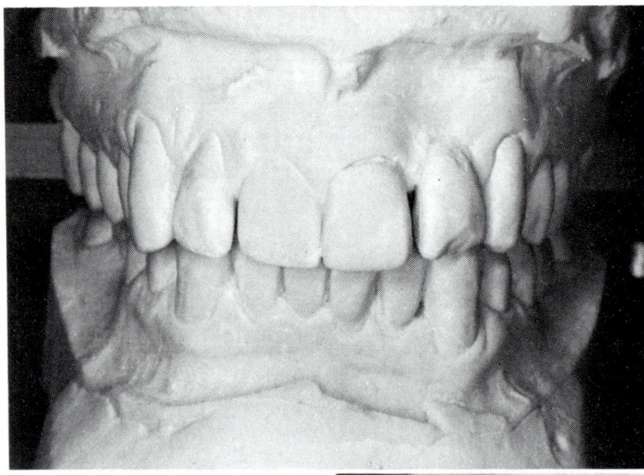

Fig. 3-61

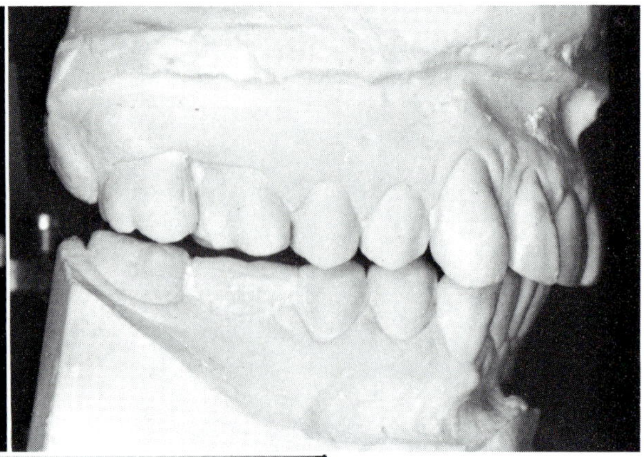

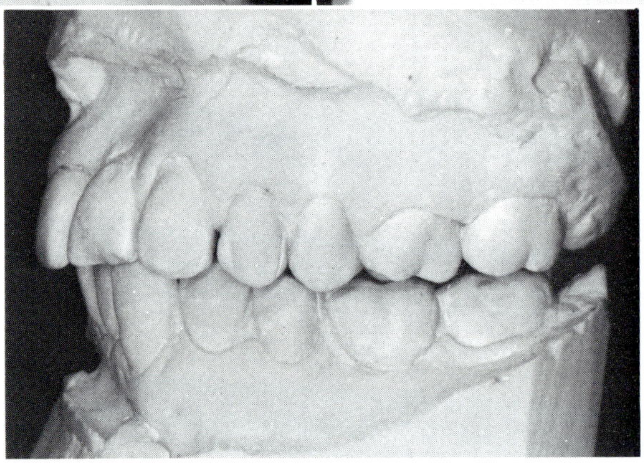

Fig. 3-62

Figs. 3-60 to 3-62. Cast orientation on arbitrary axis for preliminary study of occlusal relations, construction of clutches, and preoperative wax up.

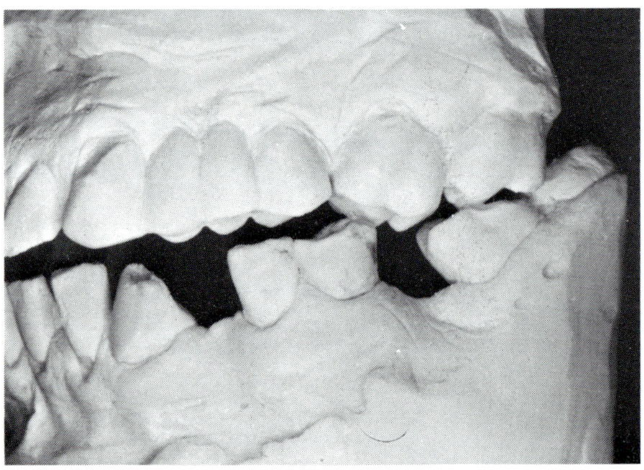

Fig. 3-63. Diagnostic casts correctly oriented on adjustable articulator revealing initial occlusal contacts.

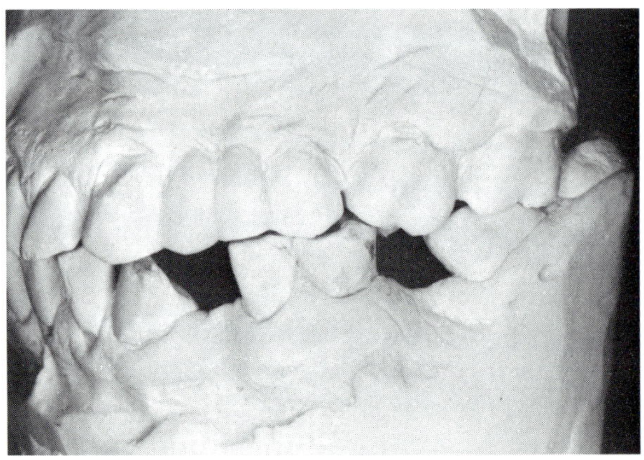

Fig. 3-64. Diagnostic casts forced into maximum occlusal contact (acquired centric occlusion) by displacement of condyle forward (see Figs. 3-65 and 3-66).

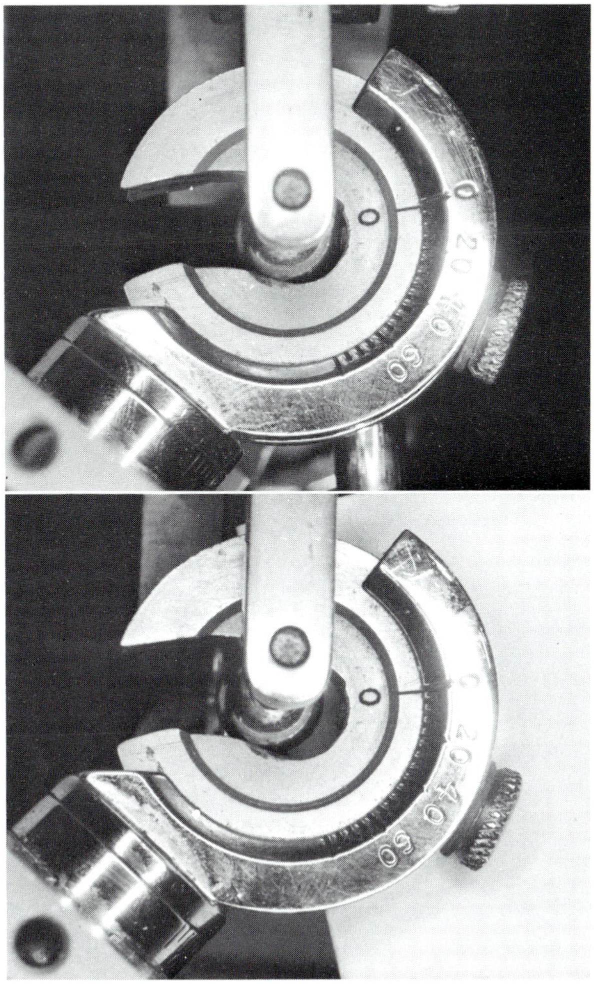

Fig. 3-65

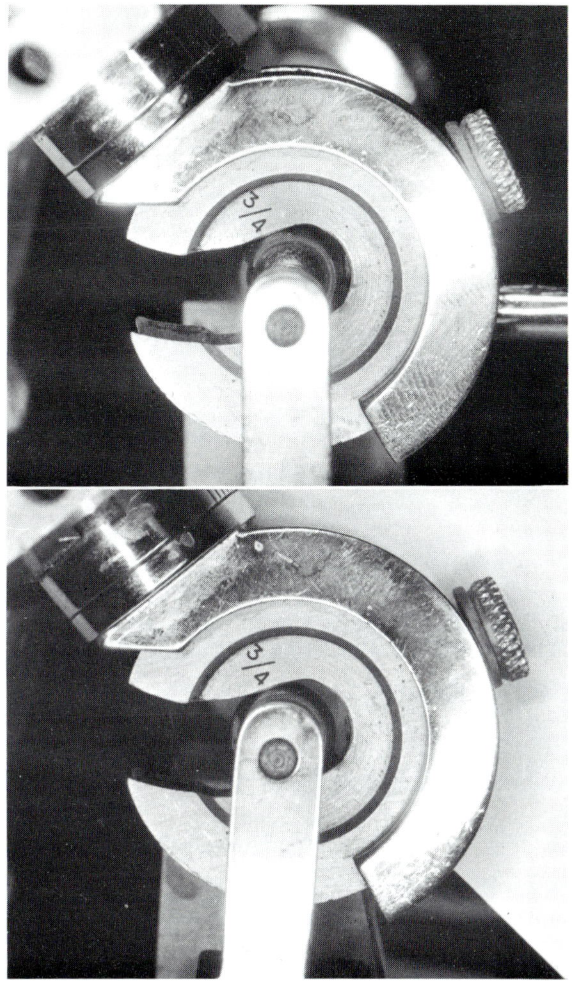

Fig. 3-66

Figs. 3-65 and 3-66. A, The condyle (ball) when teeth are occluded in centric occlusion. **B,** The condyle (ball) pulled forward to allow meshing of occlusal surfaces out of centric relation.

dible and the temporomandibular joint determines the nature of the movements. To generate a proper occlusal form it is necessary to know how and why the mandible moves. Casts must be oriented properly upon an adjustable articulator so that occlusal relationships will be reproduced correctly. The determinants of mandibular movements that dictate the occlusal morphology must be possible of attainment. But how can all this be accomplished?

To begin with, a set of clutches must be made using the casts of the preliminary mounting. With these clutches, a hinge-bow, and a pantograph the hinge axis can be located, registrations or "jaw writings" taken, the articulator adjusted to these registrations, and the study casts remounted to the correct axis.

The first step is the accurate location of the hinge axis of the mandibular articulation. Many investigators have shown that a hinge axis does exist and can be precisely located in its terminal position with the use of mechanical aids. A fixed point of rotation can be obtained clinically and utilized in restorative procedures.

In vivo the only axial centers that can function independently in mandibular motion are the horizontal axial centers of rotation. In a limited degree of mandibular opening (about 12 degrees) the condylar element, because of the limiting effect of the superior and anterior slopes of the glenoid fossa and the temporomandibular ligament, can brace itself superiorly, medially, and at its posterior limit. Thereby the condylar element can enable the horizontal centers of rotation to be located. An imaginary line connecting both horizontal axial centers of rotation is termed the *horizontal axis*. This may be referred to as the hinge axis, or the transverse axis (Chapter 14).

Tooth relations on the articulator will not be the same as in the mouth unless the opening-closing hinge and centric relations are the same on the articulator as in the patient's mouth. We must reproduce on the articulator the same relation of the casts to the axis of the instrument that the teeth have to the axis of the mandible. Unless casts can be occluded by closing them on the same arc of closure as that exhibited by the patient, erroneous conclusions may be drawn concerning existing occlusal patterns and the need for restorative procedures for the patient.

The rotational centers of the condyles can be determined and transposed to the rotational centers of an adjustable articulator. Therefore, we must locate the hinge axis and record and transfer the three basic paths that it follows. These paths can be recombined to create every possible movement of the teeth and mandible, that is, we must reproduce on the instrument the paths of motion of the axis.

Granger[18] so aptly pointed out that "we cannot deal with one compartment of the temporomandibular joint by a simple hinge-axis mounting or a centric relation record and ignore the paths of motion of the axis, because this is something the patient cannot do. The patient is compelled to use both compartments of the temporomandibular joint every time he moves the jaw. Therefore, we cannot ignore the precise location and paths of motion of the center of rotation."*

Why use the hinge axis?† Use of the hinge axis permits us to accomplish the following:

1. It provides a definite point of reference (a constant) for all procedures necessary in reconstruction. This permits a similar relation of the parts as they are constructed and corrected.

2. By recording the various relations of the axis and by transferring these to an adjustable articulator, we are able to reproduce the patient's mandibular movements with *fidelity*. If we wish to work on a laboratory instrument that is a mechanical and relational likeness of the mouth, we must have it open and close on the same axis as the mouth.

3. It permits us to accurately *record* and *check* the centric relation of each patient.

   a. We can then arrange the cusps of the teeth so that the closure can be made in centric relation without striking opponents on the way.
   b. We can then register our centric relation with enough opening between the teeth to avoid any deflective malocclusion that might be present in the dentition, and we can diagnose it.

4. It affords us the privilege of being able to alter the vertical dimension on an articulator with the certainty that any such alterations will be identical to such changes in the patient's mouth.

5. Adjustments (remounts) that may be necessary in the completed work can be accomplished on the articulator. This permits the completion of an extensive restorative procedure on an articulator without the need for very much adjustment in the mouth.

6. The hinge axis is a component of every masticatory movement of the mandible and therefore cannot be disregarded. The hinge axis of the articulating instrument must be a duplicate of the hinge axis of the jaw, or there can be no mechanical reproduction of jaw motions.

7. The hinge axis permits duplication of all the arcs of closure of the mandible on an instrument, and thus the cusps can be tailored to harmonize with these arcs.

8. If we do not locate an axis, we ignore the laws of geometry, physics, and mechanics.

9. a. If we could transfer the centric relation to articulated mounted casts and could finish our work without changing the opening component, then we would not need an axis.
   b. If we have no cusps on teeth around and over which closures are made, we would need no axis determination unless we want to diagnose the ills of the occlusion.

Because of the previously mentioned reasons, the location on a patient and the transference to an articulator of the hinge axis are well worth the effort involved.

We feel the hinge axis is imperative—yes, mandatory.

Mandibular movements are three dimensional in character, and a competent articulator is a three-dimensional pantograph. Therefore, a primary law of mechanics must be satisfied—to pantograph in three dimensions one axis must be duplicated, in this case, the hinge axis. In mandibular movements there is a fourth dimension of time sequence; that is the amount and character of movement in one plane in relation to the other two planes.

Instantaneous axes. When rotation and translation

---

*From Granger, E. R.: Functional relations of the stomatognathic system, J.A.D.A. **48:**638-647, 1954.

†With the assistance of Charles E. Stuart and Harvey Stallard.

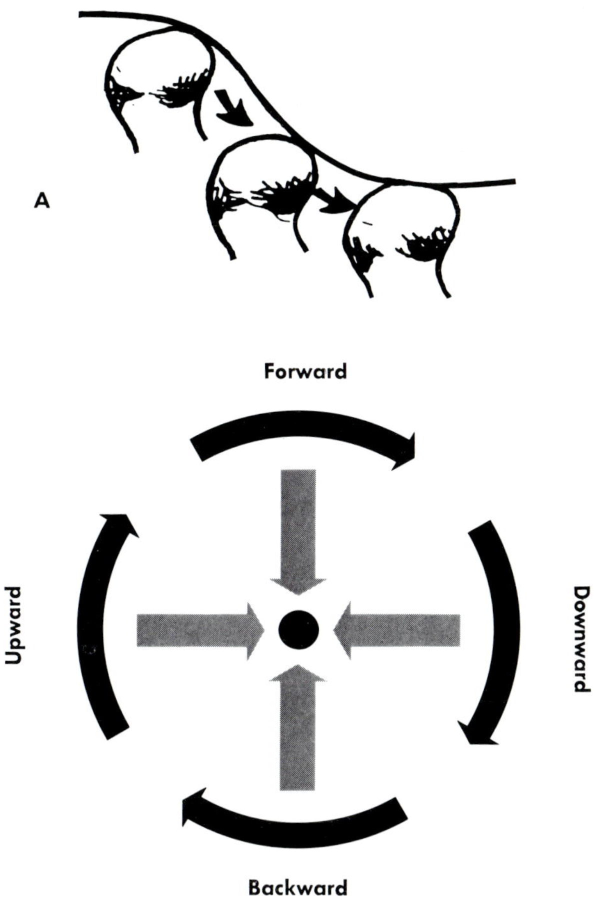

Fig. 3-67. A, Instantaneous axis of rotation. **B,** The bold dot in the center of this illustration represents the location of the terminal hinge axis. The outer black arrows illustrate the direction of migration of a stylus. The lighter inner arrows indicate the direction in which the stylus would have to be readjusted in order to locate the terminal hinge position of the horizontal axis. (Courtesy Niles F. Guichet.)

are combined, there is no constant axes of control. Picture a body rotating about an axis and then translating. As soon as translation takes place the axis changes; then when rotation begins again, a new axis is in control, and this goes on and on. *The axis that changes is called the instantaneous axis of rotation* (Fig. 3-67, *A*). It is only in control for an instant and it can be located only when motion is stopped, and then only mathematically. In the physiologic function of the mandible this is precisely what is happening. Because we cannot locate the instantaneous centers, we have no way of plotting the functional envelope of motion. Therefore, we are forced to use the border paths of the complete envelope. Much of the confusion of the profession centers about this area. When we masticate, we do not do so with the hinge axis in control; instead it is the instantaneous axis or more properly axes. Also when we close from physiologic rest to centric relation, again it is the instantaneous axis in control. This is why we must avoid *rest* in taking our records and also why we do not need it. The hinge axis then has control only along the border paths.

What I am trying to emphasize is that many axes having to do with mandibular motion can be plotted. However, most of them cannot be used, and so we must utilize only those with which we can work. Because of some inaccuracies in our technical procedures, we must use an axis more than once. Therefore, we must choose one that is constant. We use the axis that is in control in the terminal position. Because this is also centric relation, the hinge axis is not only convenient but mandatory.[19]

Unless the opening-closing hinge and centric relation are the same on the articulator as in the patient, tooth relations on the articulator will not be the same in the mouth.

The mandible should be allowed to reach all its border limits freely without any restrictions by cusp interference.

Locating the hinge axis. The hinge axis can be located accurately by trial and error with a hinge-bow, which is rigidly attached to the lower teeth by an aluminum clutch or clamped to the edentulous ridge. The side arms of the bow are adjustable, horizontally and vertically, and carry pointed styluses, which are directed at the positions of the condyles. The patient is coached to open and close the mouth with a pure hinge movement, using the thumb and index finger to guide this movement and avoiding translation of the mandible. Attention is directed to the action of the *tip of the stylus* as the patient executes the hingelike movement. The tip of the stylus will arc in a definite direction, depending upon its relation to the actual centers of rotation. By close observation of the arc scribed by the stylus, an adjustment is made to approach the center of rotation. The nature of the adjustment is determined by the direction and the size of the arc. Use is made of the geometric principle that if a secant intersects an arc of a circle, its perpendicular bisector will coincide with the radius of the circle. In other words, when the tip of the stylus describes an arc, the axis will always be toward its radius.

1. If the stylus moves backward with the opening, it means that it is below the axis.
2. If the stylus moves forward with the opening, it is above the axis.

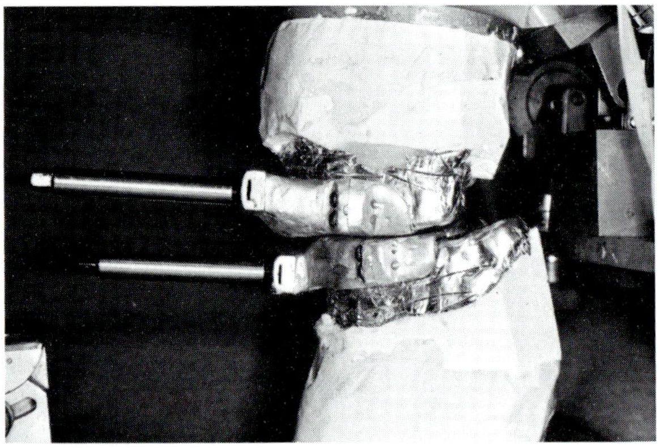

Fig. 3-68. Clutches on casts on articulator and center bearing screw adjusted so that no contact exists in centric, protrusive, and lateral positions except on screw.

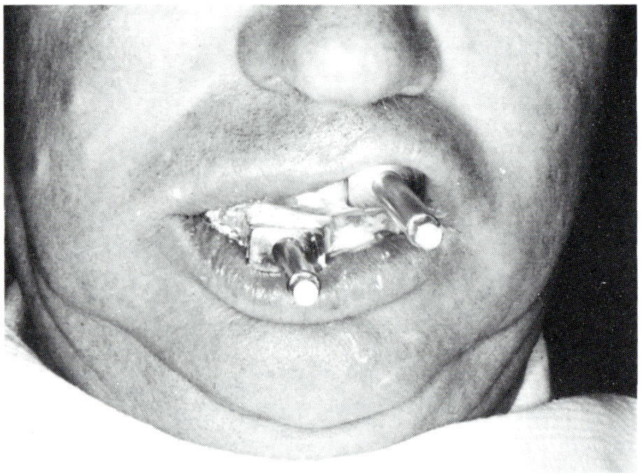

Fig. 3-70

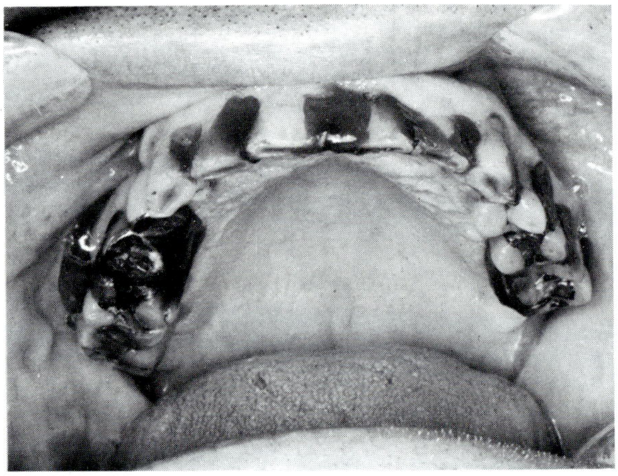

Fig. 3-69. Interproximal spaces and undercut areas around restorations and under pontics are blocked out with a soft wax before cementation of clutches for ease of removal. Be careful to have enough relief around teeth showing a high degree of mobility.

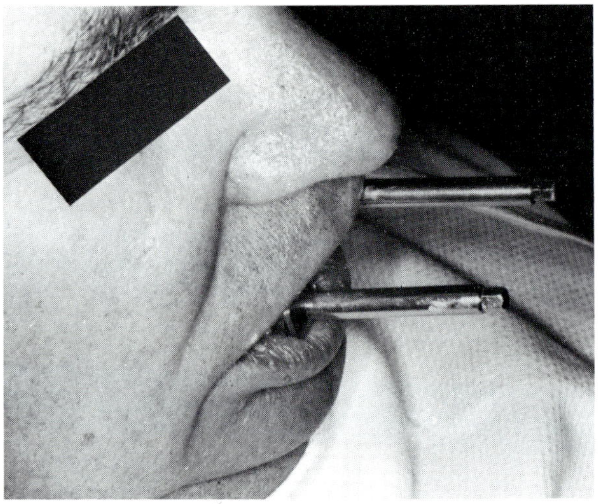

Fig. 3-71

Figs. 3-70 and 3-71. Clutches cemented. Observe alignment of separable studs from both front and side views to "eye" the studs properly for parallelism to each other during cementation of the clutches.

3. If the stylus moves downward with the opening, it is in front of axis.
4. If the stylus moves upward with the opening, it is behind the axis (Fig. 3-67, *B*).

By trial and error and repeated adjustments it is possible to arrive quite readily at the exact center of rotation (as the patient executes the pure vertical rotational motion of the condyle on the meniscus), which is indicated *when the tip of the stylus will no longer arc; it will merely rotate*. A magnifying glass is now used to help see that the stylus tip is definitely rotating.

This procedure is carried out on both sides simultaneously, and the points so located are transferred to the skin. The dental practitioner must remember to move the patient's head out of the headrest, which will eliminate any possible skin displacement that would occur from pressure against the headrest. The stylus tip is rubbed with an indelible pencil and gently pushed against the face to transfer the point to the skin, after which the hinge-bow and clutches are removed. (See Figs. 3-68 to 3-77.)

By locating the center of rotation for each condyle and joining these with an imaginary line, we locate the hinge axis.

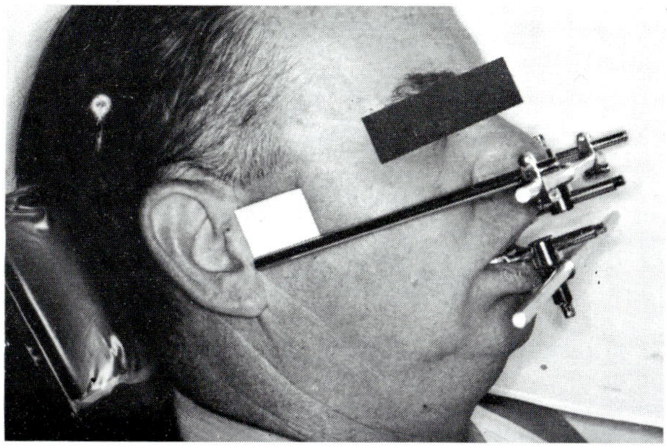

Fig. 3-72. Front bars and side arm with graph paper on flag positioned to provide a stationary background against which axis can be located.

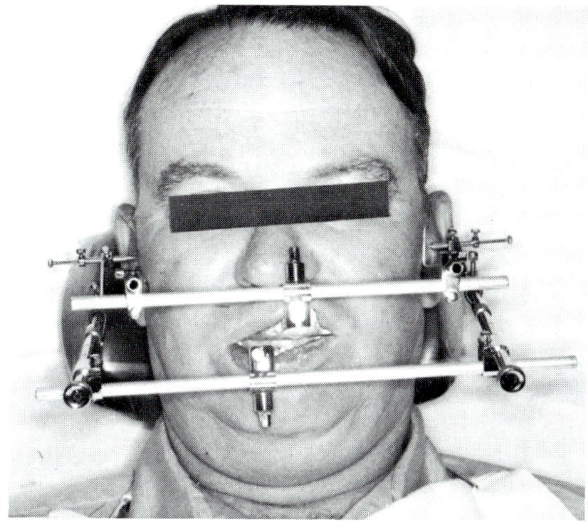

Fig. 3-73

We must also keep in mind the following:

1. The Cohen or Hickok trainer should be used for 5 to 10 minutes before positioning the hinge-bow for location of the axis.
2. The hinge action actually is being located in the facial plane (on the side of the face).
3. This is not the true center of vertical motion for that is located in the condyle.
4. A point on a line that has been extended from the centers of vertical motion is being located.
5. Centers of hinge action can be located only when the condyle is in a position where it can repeatedly scribe these arcs—when it is in the most retruded position in the glenoid fossa.[20]

The axis points are now related to a third point on the side of the nose. This point is usually placed on the right side of the nose 2⅛ inches from the incisal edge of a central incisor tooth, or it is determined by locating the inferior border of the orbit on the right side and, for convenience, recording with a mark on the same plane on the side of the nose. These three points are on the axis-orbital plane, which is a plane of reference. They are used to make a conventional face-bow transfer so that the casts will be oriented on the articulator in the same relation to its axis as the jaws are to the hinge axis.

This axis-orbital plane will give a constant position for the upper jaw, and a correct interocclusal record will establish the position of the lower jaw to the constant upper jaw. In this way repeated mountings will have a constant relation to the records and the patient's centers of rotation.

The three points (marks) are made permanent by

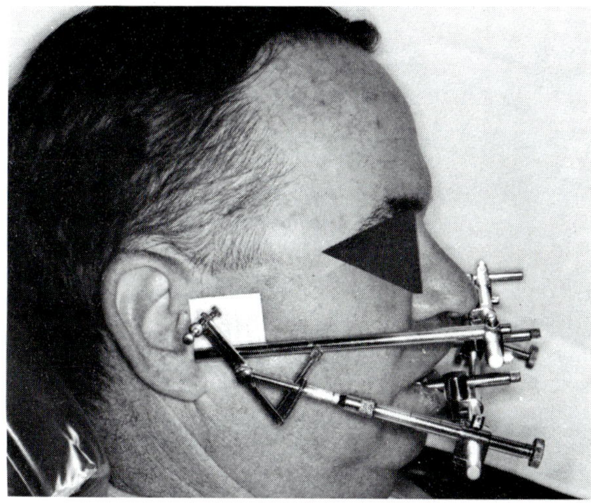

Fig. 3-74

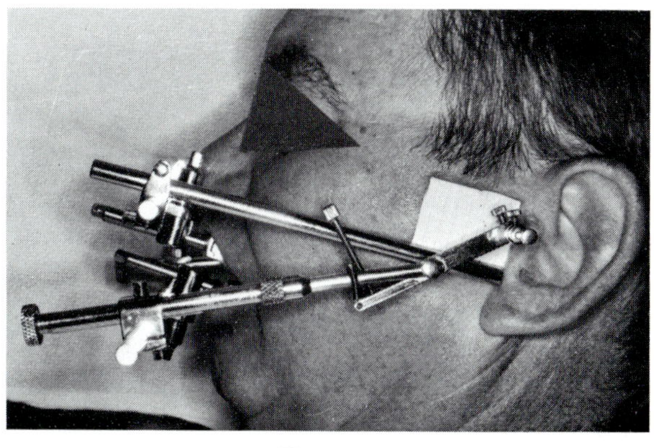

Fig. 3-75

Figs. 3-73 to 3-75. Stylus arms (adjustable horizontally and vertically) placed on lower front bar with stylus in vicinity of condyle.

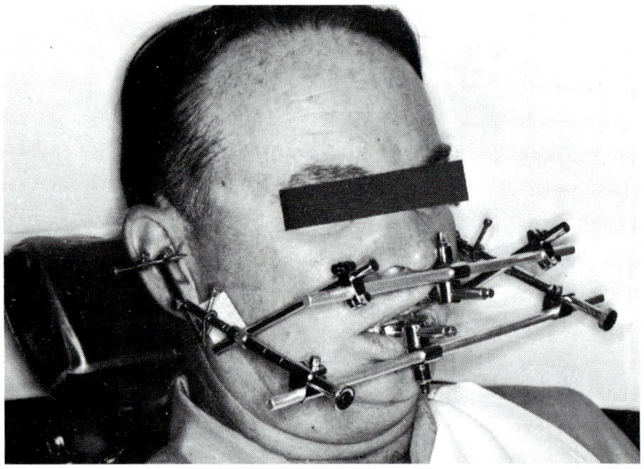

Fig. 3-76. After tip of stylus will no longer arc but merely rotate (carried out on both sides simultaneously) upper arm is dropped and points so located are transferred to skin.

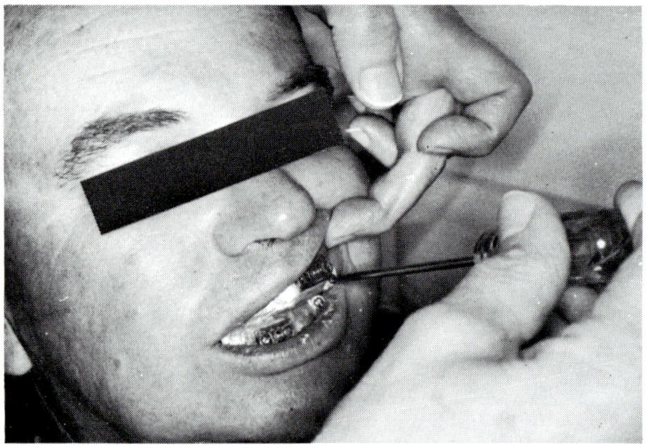

Fig. 3-77. Removal of clutches. Removal of screws holding two parts of clutch together and positioning screwdriver in "pry slot" for easy displacement of anterior section.

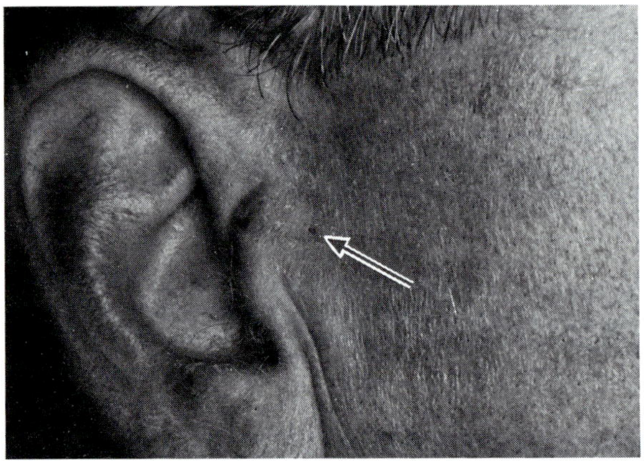

Fig. 3-78. Axis point on right side made permanent by using a special tattoo ink.

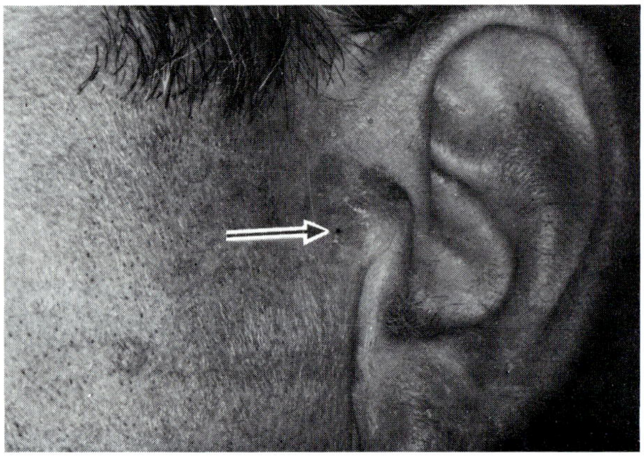

Fig. 3-79. Axis point on left side made permanent by using a special tattoo ink.

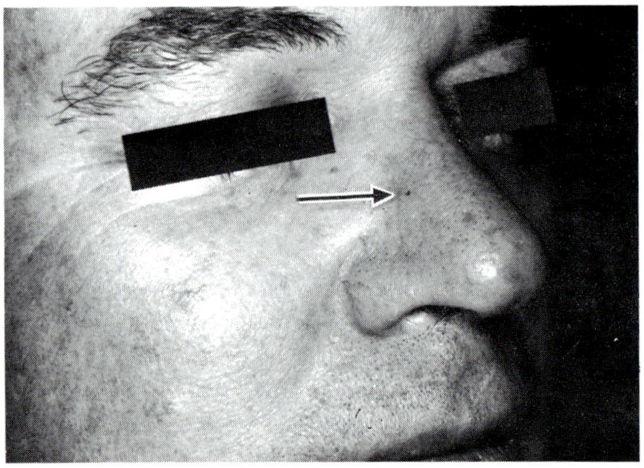

Fig. 3-80. Nose reference point made permanent by using tattoo ink.

using a special tattoo needle and a little pink marking dye (sulfide of mercury) (Figs. 3-78 to 3-80). India ink, which is used in conjunction with a disposable hypodermic needle, is also used very successfully. Tattoo marks should be examined at intervals, and re-inked if any of them start to fade out.

The axis is constant to the mandible, and it determines the arc of closure upon which the cusps of the teeth meet in any contacting position. For convenience, the hinge axis is located and reproduced in centric relation. It can be said, therefore, that the hinge-axis position is a physiologically acceptable maxillomandibular relationship.

Use of pantograph in recording of jaw movements. The procedure so far permits the correct apposition of the casts on an instrument in the opening and closing component, but only in the terminal hinge position. It is necessary to transfer the centers of lateral motion to an articulator if the other movements of the mandible are to be faithfully reproduced. This is accomplished by the use of twin Gothic arch (needle point) tracings. On a suitable articulator that can be adjusted for intercondylar width, the centers of lateral movement are located from the twin Gothic arches (Fig. 3-81). All that remains now is to duplicate the paths of these centers, and all possible jaw relationships will have been duplicated. It can be used as a means of creating occlusal forms that will be in harmony with the joint and also the supporting structures of the teeth.

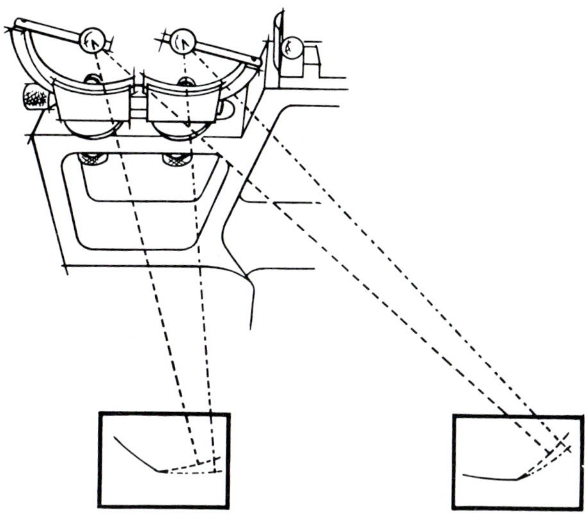

Fig. 3-8l. Diagrams showing how the wings of the Gothic arches determine the correct centers of rotation for each patient. (Courtesy Victor O. Lucia.)

The most accurate practical method of recording jaw movements is the use of an extraoral tracing device. Actually this is a pantograph, which consists of two face-bows with six recording slides and six styli (Fig. 3-82), that scribes the paths of the centers of rotation of the mandible. The tracings are made in three dimensions simultaneously.

Pantograph registrations should be used for the following reasons:

1. They permit us to accurately record the border movements of our patients and to duplicate these movements on an articulator. This makes it possible to conveniently design and construct the occlusal surfaces of the restorations so that they will be in harmony with the patient's jaw movements.

2. Copying mandibular movements on an articulator is necessary if we are going to produce an organic occlusion that fits the masticatory organ.

3. The direction, shape, and depth of the occlusal grooves can be carved accurately so that the cusps that travel in these grooves can arrive at their destinations (fossae) without trauma. They can be on the right "track," or let us put it this way:

A

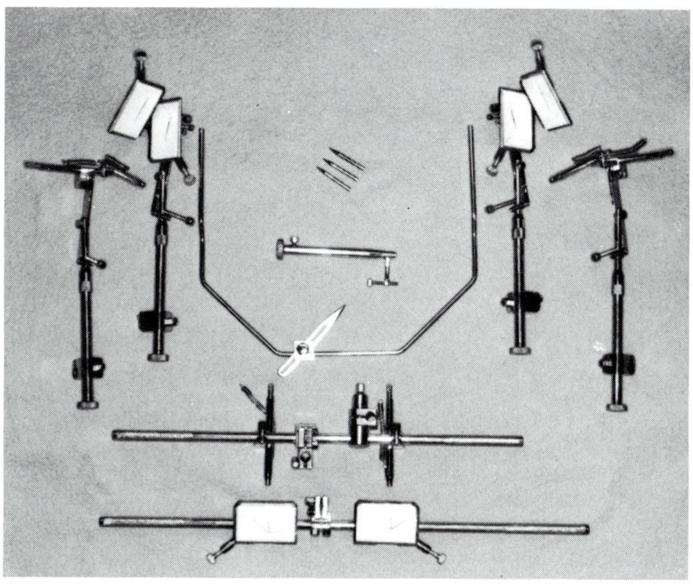

Continued.

Fig. 3-82. A, Various parts of a pantograph. It consists of two face-bows with six recording slides and six styli. **B,** The Denar pantograph. **C,** The Simulator pantograph.

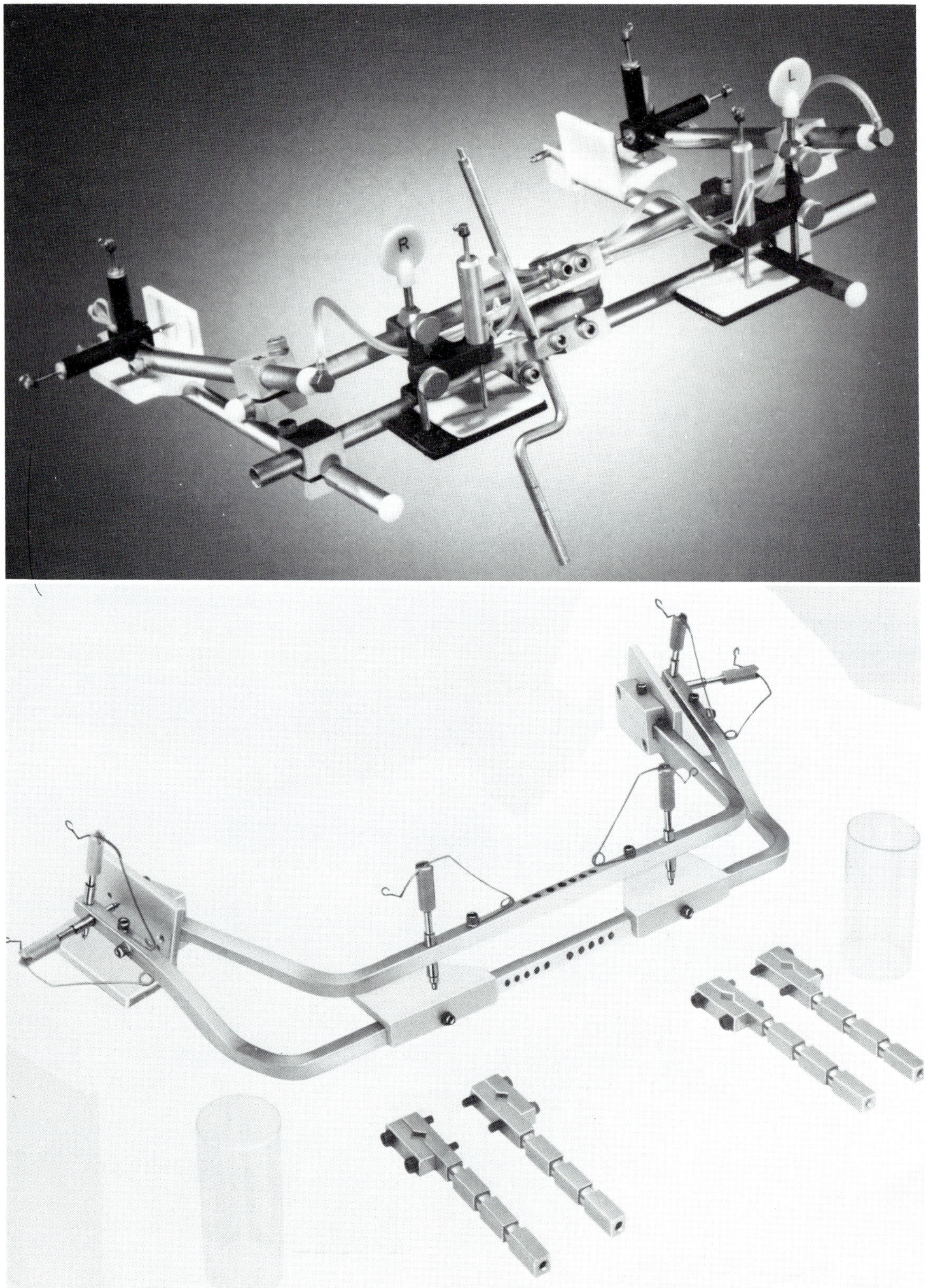

B

C

Fig. 3-82, cont'd. For legend see p. 65.

a. The ridge and groove directions are determined as a result of the movement of the condyles.
b. In the main, the cusp height and fossa depth are determined as a result of mandibular movements.
c. The proper concavity of the lingual surface of the upper anterior teeth is determined by the movements of the condyles.

(These determinants can be applied in the fabrication of the occlusion of the teeth if we will record the mandibular movements of the patient and then cause the articulator to reproduce the same border and intermediate movements.)

4. Cuspal elements (cusps, marginal ridges, triangular ridges, developmental grooves, supplemental grooves, fossae) are necessary to maintain the vertical stability of the teeth by distributing the forces of occlusion in the long axis of the teeth.

(Pantograph registrations permit us to accurately determine the height, position, and relation of the cuspal elements so that they will efficiently perform their functions without creating lateral stresses on the supporting structures.)

5. The centric relation intercusping is built by first consulting the eccentric paths of mandibular travel. If we do not consult the eccentric travel, the cusps will not be free to travel in and out of centric relation closure without conflict. The result will be trauma, wear, and loss of the centric relation contacts.

6. *So, by logic we believe the only way we can work accurately and measure our work is to use a faithful substitute for the jaws, an articulator in which all the occlusal determinants and the opening and closing axis relations are precisely incorporated.*

This method of employing the pantograph graphically records the various positions and movements of the mandible. These graphs are then utilized to adjust the articulator to reproduce the same relations and the actual path of the movements found in the patient.

In making these records the clutches have to be separated vertically so that there will be no tooth guidance during the registrations, and the minimum amount of separation that will ensure this is desired.

When an accurate and complete record of the jaw movements has been registered and the orbital guide set (if this step is forgotten, the registrations will be useless), the upper and lower arms of the pantograph are firmly locked together with a fast-setting stone making use of four vise grips. (See Figs. 3-83 to 3-95.)

Transference to an adjustable articulator. The entire assembly is removed intact from the patient (not including the clutches, which are subsequently removed) and is transferred to the mounting frame. The mounting frame is a jig that conveniently holds a face-bow in proper relation to an articulator. It permits accurate relationship of the clutch or cast to the articulator while the attaching stone sets.

The leveling device is in position on the front of the upper bow and rests on the axis-orbital plane. This arrangement automatically makes the upper bow parallel to the axis-orbital plane. (See Fig. 3-96.) The lower clutch is attached to the lower bow, the vise grips are removed, the articulator is adjusted or set, and the adjustments are recorded on a suitable card (Figs. 3-97 to 3-108).

By means of a face-bow transfer and a correct centric interocclusal record, study casts, working casts, and remount casts can be mounted on this set

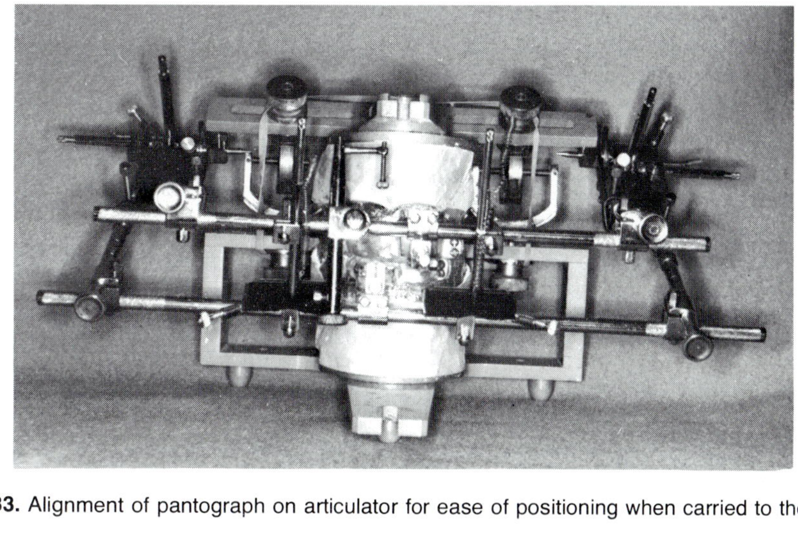

Fig. 3-83. Alignment of pantograph on articulator for ease of positioning when carried to the patient.

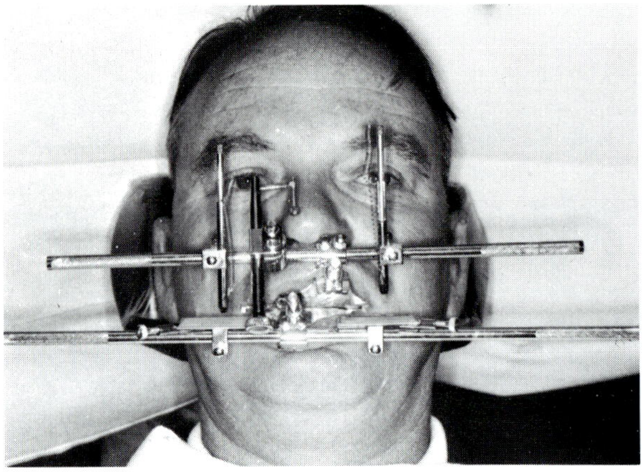

Fig. 3-84. Upper and lower crossbars of pantograph positioned.

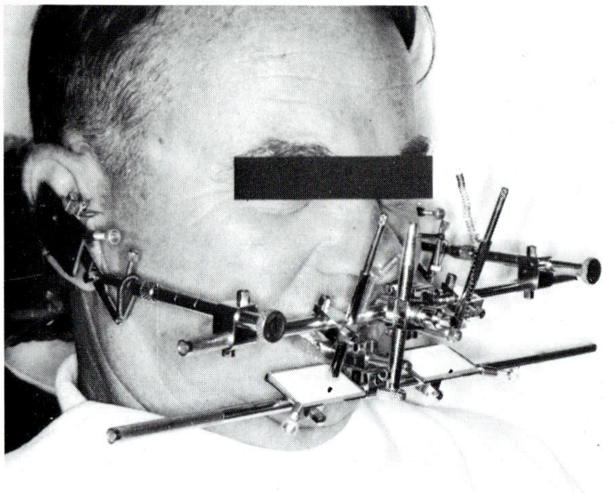

Fig. 3-85. Side arms with slide holders placed on each end of upper crossbar. Position axis stylus pins on axis tattoo marks, barely touching skin.

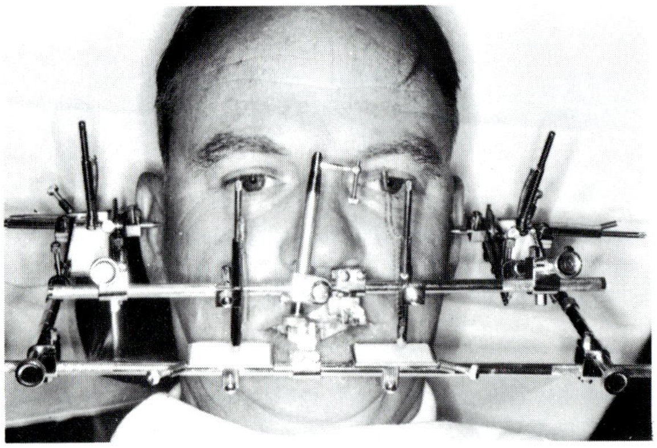

Fig. 3-86. Lower lateral arms placed on lower front crossbar. Adjust them so as to put horizontal styli on hinge with patient in centric relation.

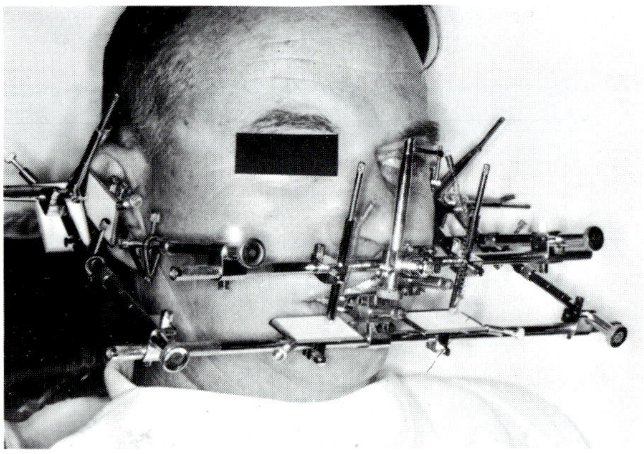

Fig. 3-87. Vertical styli placed about ¼ inch inside horizontal recording plate.

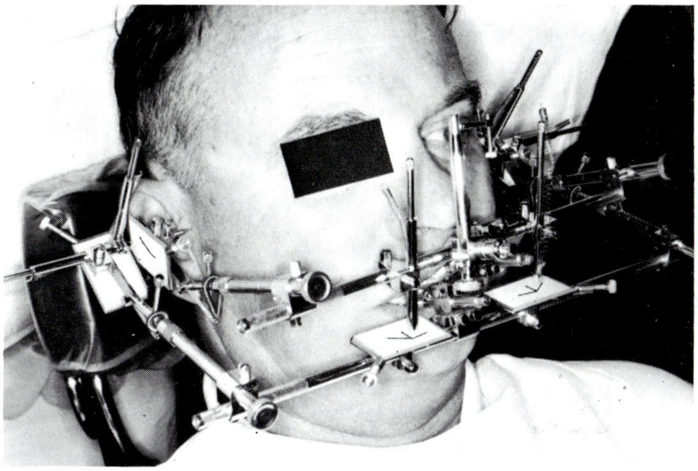

Fig. 3-88

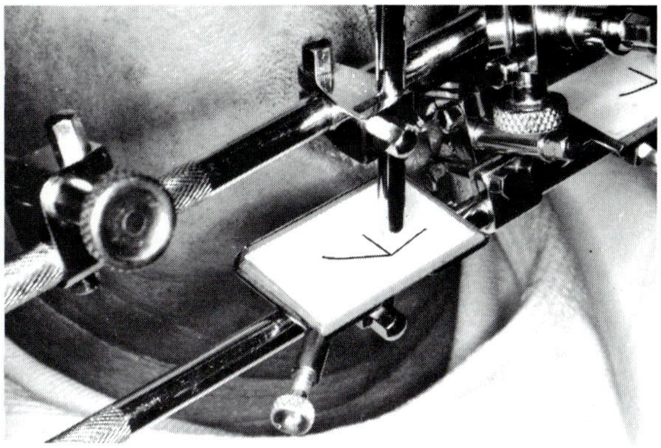

Fig. 3-89

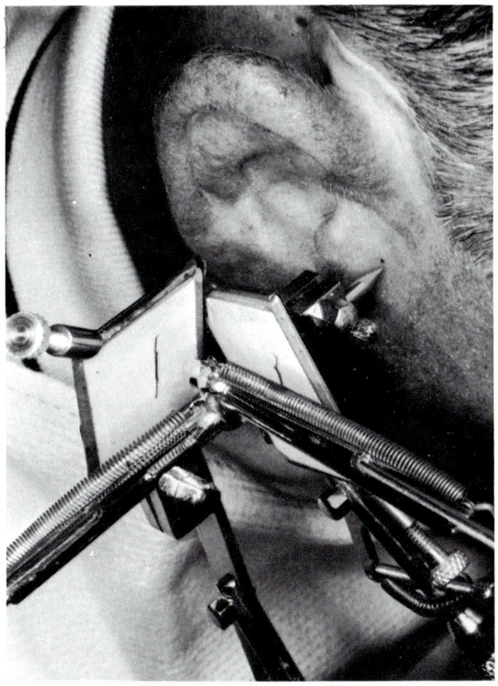

Fig. 3-90

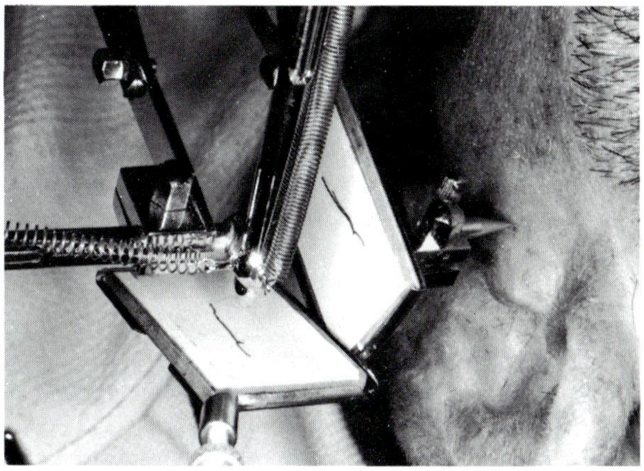

Fig. 3-91

Figs. 3-88 to 3-91. A series of completed tracings—centric, protrusive, and lateral.

adjustable articulator, which is capable of duplicating the patient's jaw movements (Figs. 3-109 to 3-117).

FIXED AND VARIABLE FACTORS OF OCCLUSION

The factors utilized in properly orienting the casts were all *fixed factors of occlusion,* which were accurately recorded and reproduced and which cannot be changed or altered. These factors are Bennett movement, lateral angulation and curvature, protrusive angulation and curvature, intercondylar distance, and horizontal axis. They exert the greatest amount of control in the posterior region, and the effect of the fixed factors diminishes gradually toward the anterior portion of the arch.

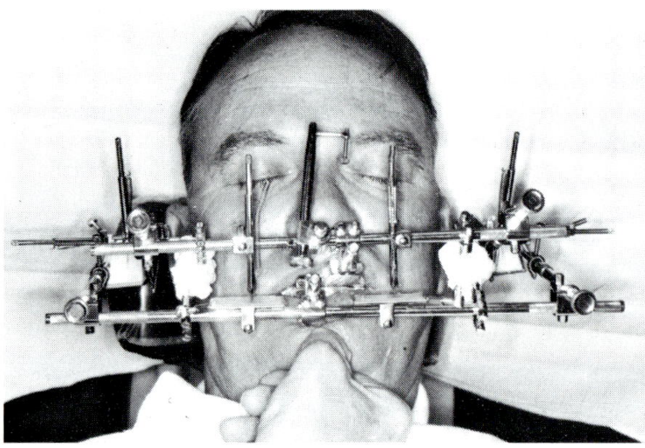

Fig. 3-92. Fast-setting stone applied around crossed studs of vise grips. Patient held in centric position until stone sets.

There are other factors, not anatomically fixed, that can be altered to restore the mouth to normal function. These are known as the *variable factors of occlusion* and are anterior guidance, plane of occlusion, curve of Spee, cusp height, etc. This effect manifests itself primarily in the anterior region, and there is a gradual diminution of this control toward the posterior region. They can be altered, provided one knows how they are related to the fixed factors of occlusion, giving us the possibility of a physiologic articulation. Under any given fixed set of factors of occlusion only one set of cusps can function in harmony with jaw movement.[21]

The fixed and variable factors of occlusion functioning simultaneously form the complete spaciotemporal continuum in all excursions that directly influence the morphology of the occlusal forms to be constructed (Chapter 14).

CENTRIC RELATION

Dykins has said that the most important task in dentistry is to get the two jaws to come together correctly.

Granger has said that regardless of our beliefs with respect to cusps, articulators, materials, or methods, there is no single factor in all dentistry equal in importance to centric relation.

Therefore, a thorough understanding of centric relation is essential to the proper practice of dentistry.

Centric relation defined. Despite the fact that some authorities contend that there is not such a thing as "centric relation" and that maybe, from a purely sci-

Text continued on p. 78.

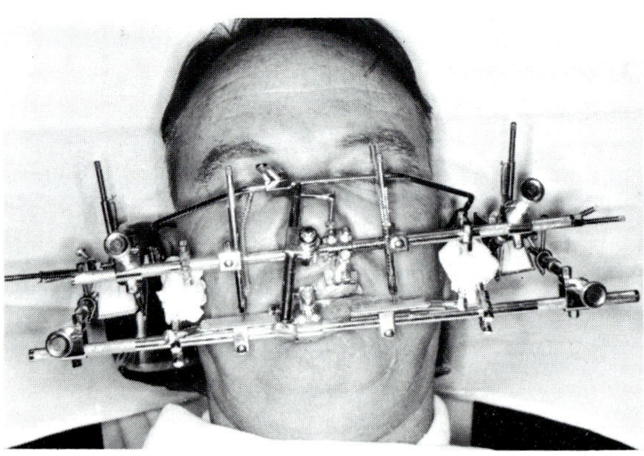

Fig. 3-93

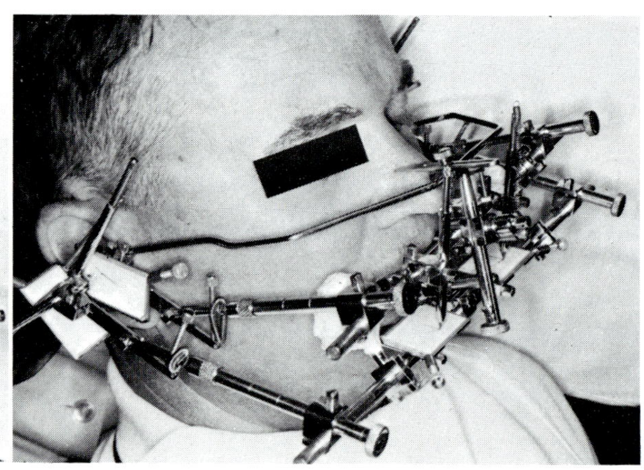

Fig. 3-94

Figs. 3-93 and 3-94. Axis-orbital indicator bow placed on support. Lays across axis indicator pins posteriorly and indicator point on bow is on nose tattoo mark. Don't forget this step!

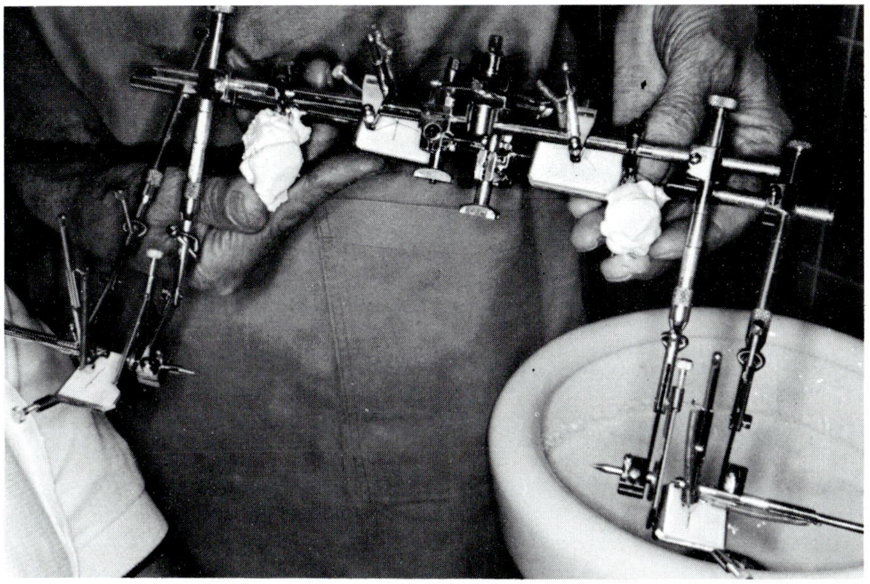

Fig. 3-95. Pantograph removed intact from patient and ready for mounting on articulator.

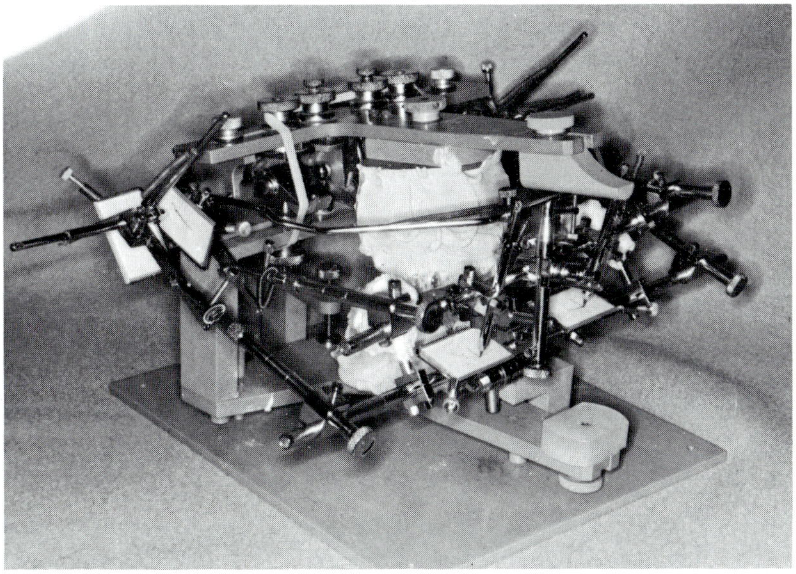

Fig. 3-96. Pantograph mounted on articulator. Leveling device in position on front of upper bow, resting on axis-orbital plane (making upper bow parallel to axis-orbital plane).

Fig. 3-97

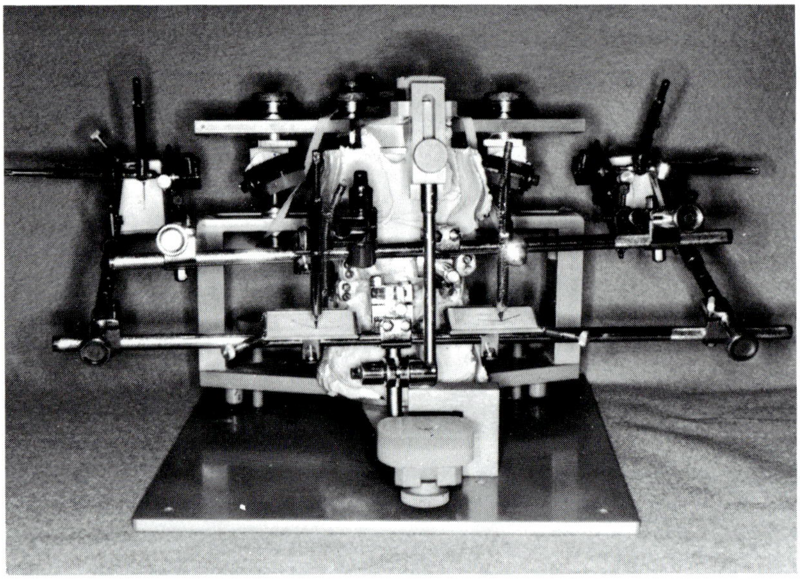

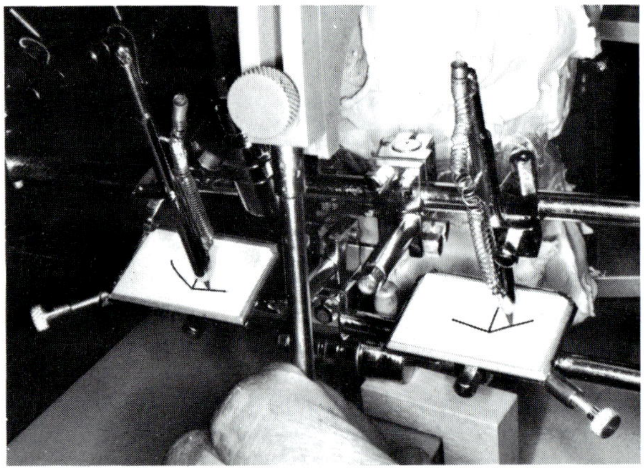

Fig. 3-98

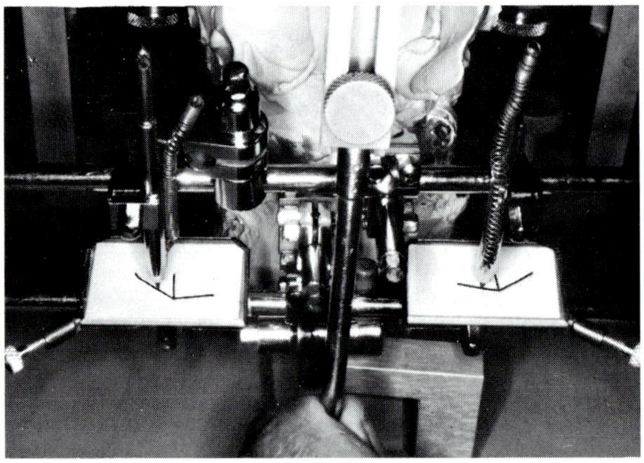

Fig. 3-99

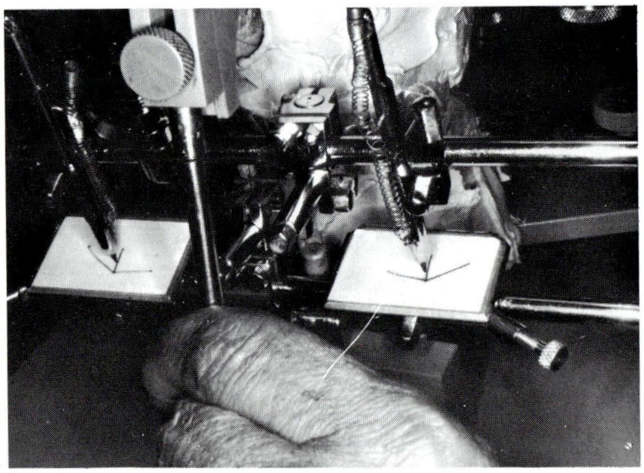

Fig. 3-100

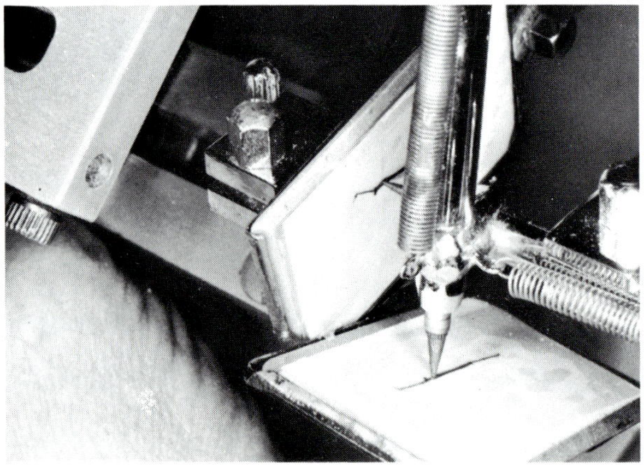

Fig. 3-101

Figs. 3-97 to 3-105. Vise grips removed and articulator set to recorded registrations. Styli following tracings in all mandibular excursions.

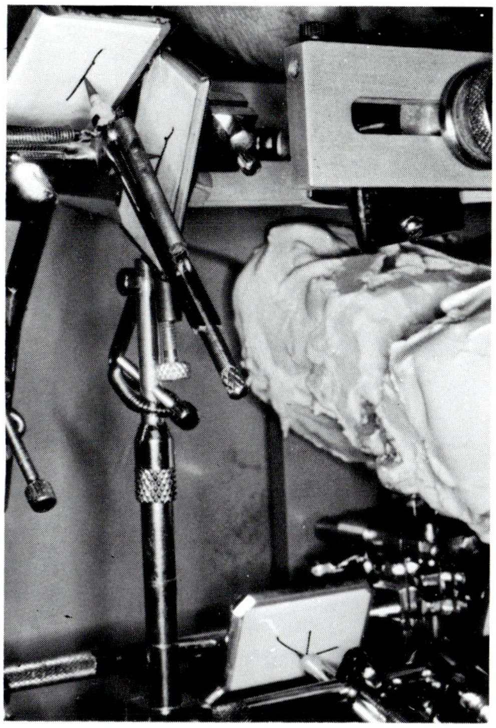

Fig. 3-102

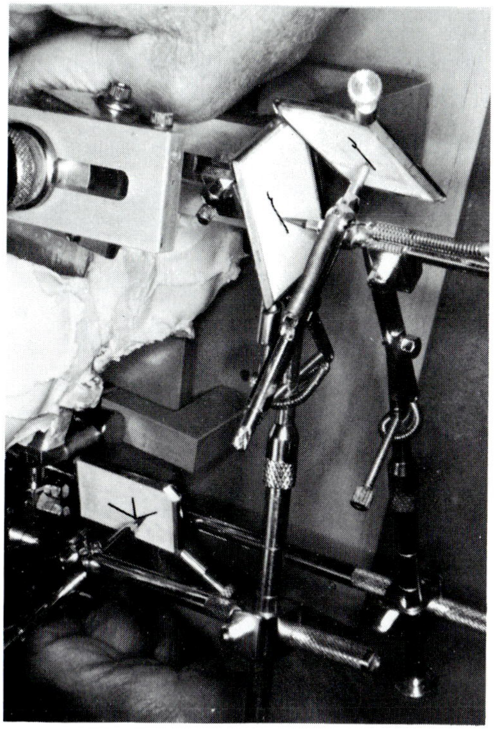

Fig. 3-103

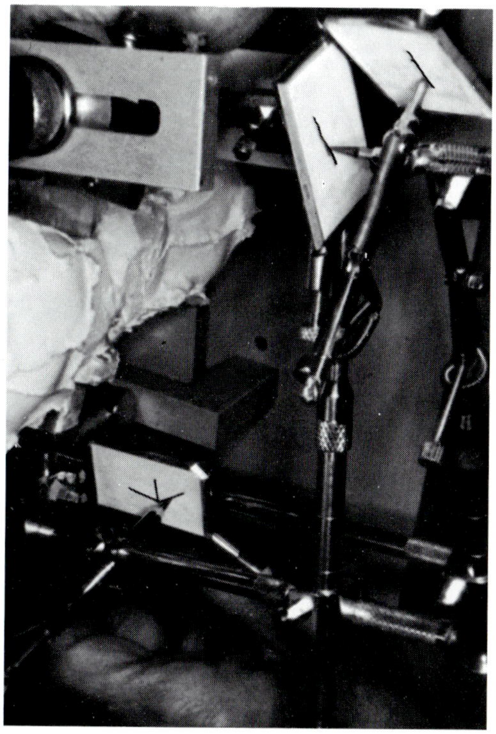

Fig. 3-104

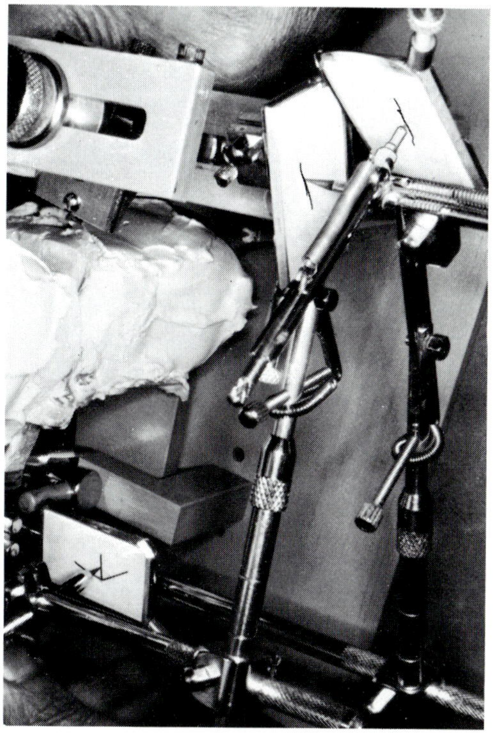

Fig. 3-105

Figs. 3-102 to 3-105. For legend see opposite page.

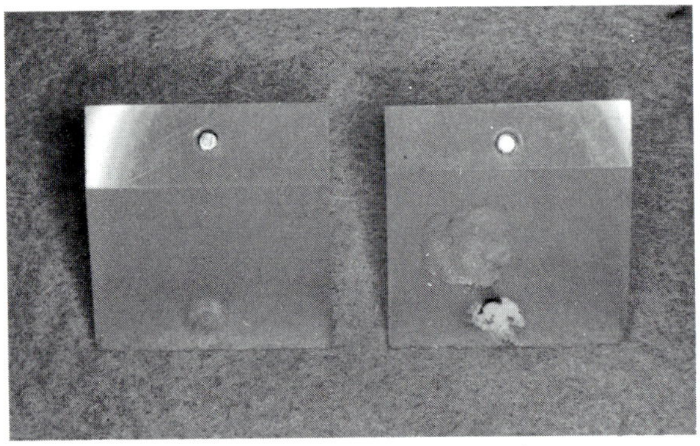

Fig. 3-106. Ground eminentiae.

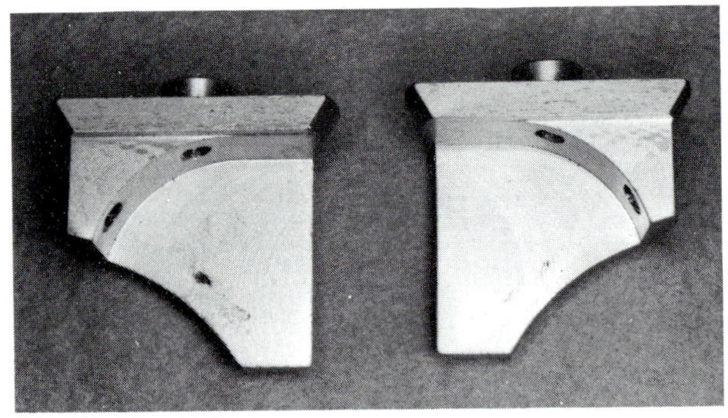

Fig. 3-107. Side shifts (in this case, straight or unground).

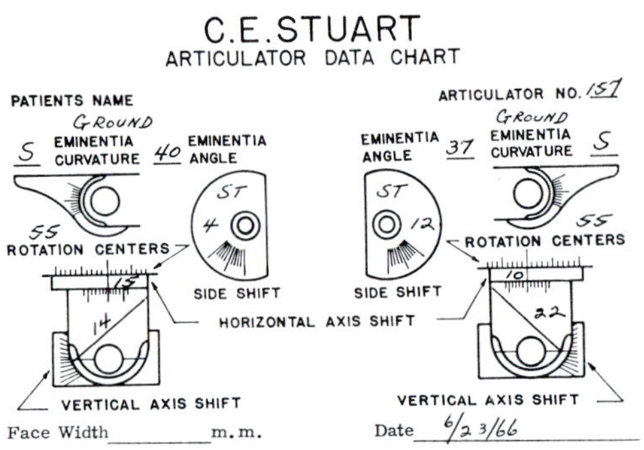

Fig. 3-108. Adjustments recorded on a suitable card.

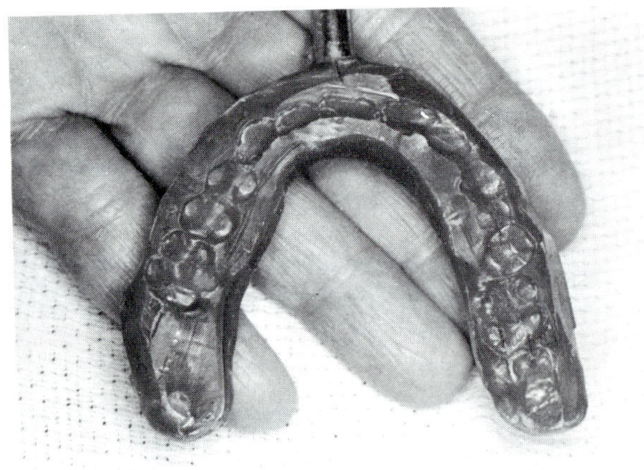

Fig. 3-109. Face-bow fork showing tips of cusp indentation of maxillary teeth.

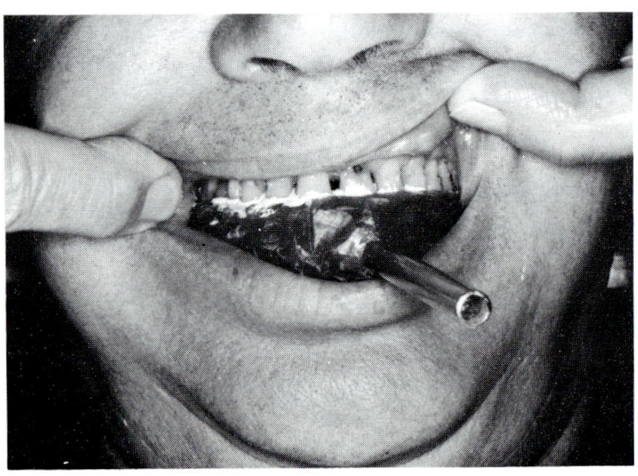

Fig. 3-110

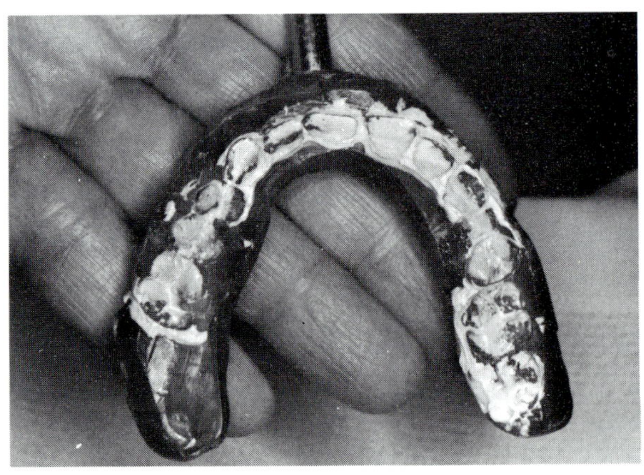

Fig. 3-111

Figs. 3-110 and 3-111. Bite fork cusp tip indentations rebased with Temp-Bond (zinc oxide–eugenol paste) for greater accuracy in cast positioning and avoidance of rocking of cast.

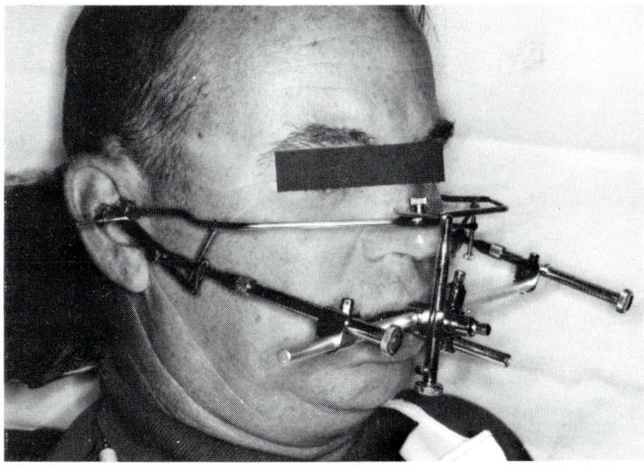

Fig. 3-112. Hinge-bow transfer for mounting casts to correct axis.

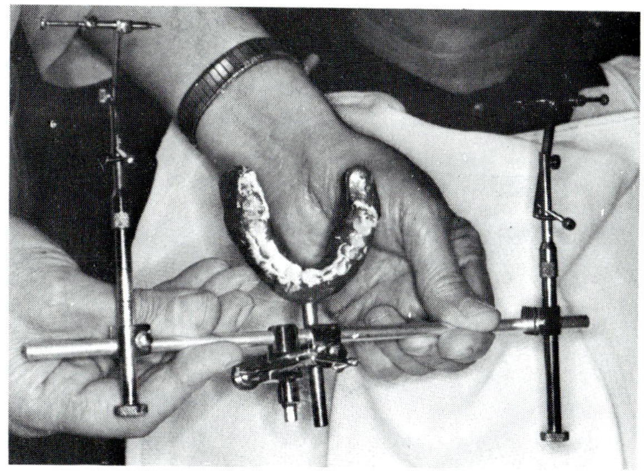

Fig. 3-113. Hinge-bow and bite fork removed.

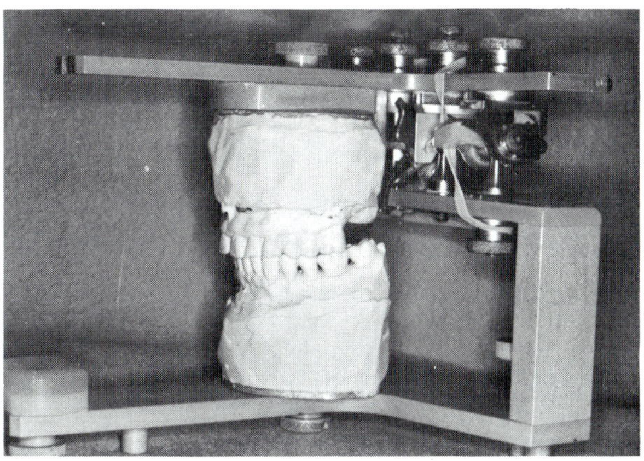

Fig. 3-114

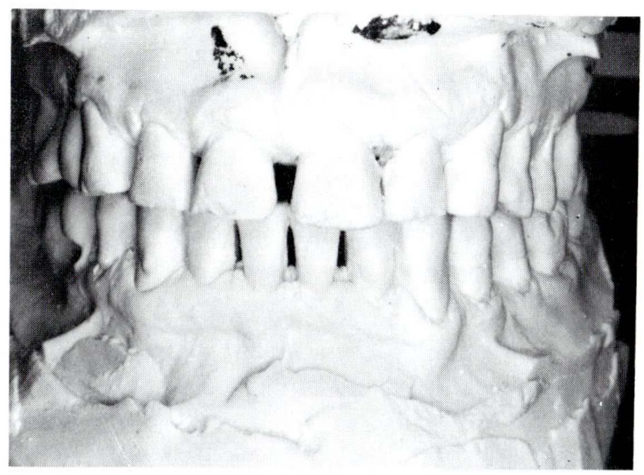

Fig. 3-115

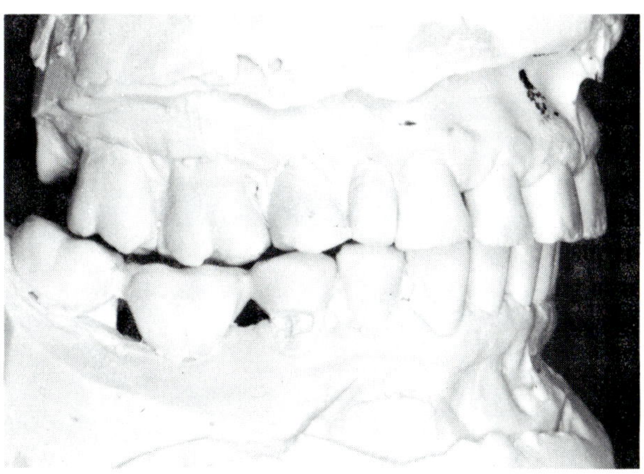

Fig. 3-116

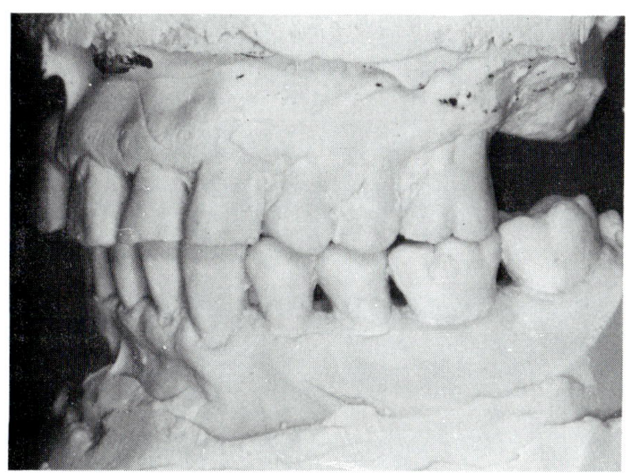

Fig. 3-117

Figs. 3-114 to 3-117. Study casts mounted to correct axis, anterior and right and left posterior views.

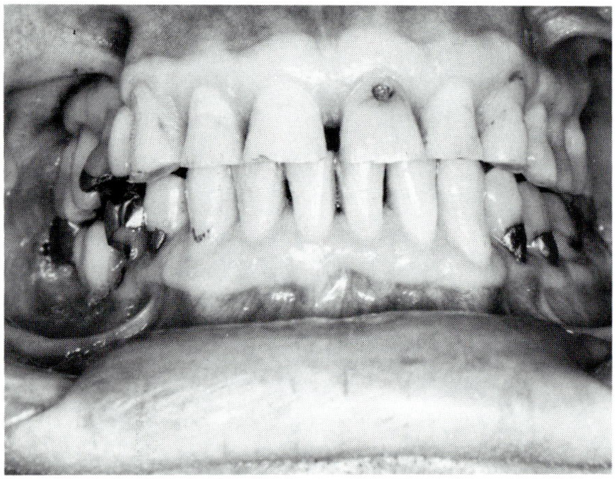

Fig. 3-118. Anterior view in centric position.

Figs. 3-118 to 3-126. Preoperative and postoperative views of case under consideration.

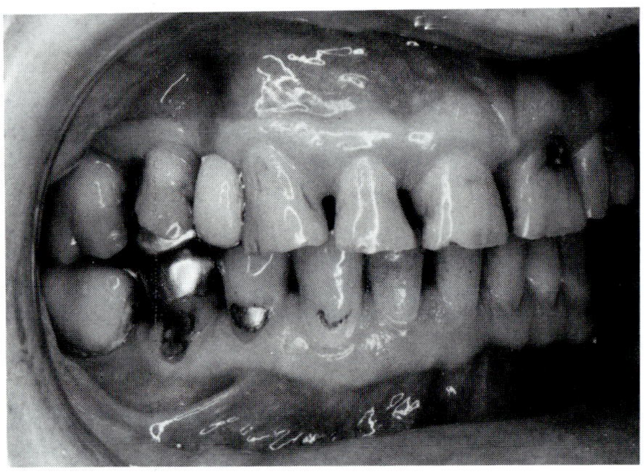

Fig. 3-119. Right side view in centric position.

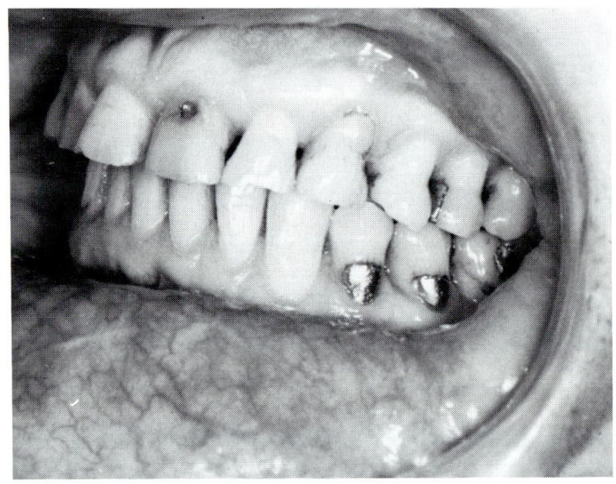

Fig. 3-120. Left side view in centric position.

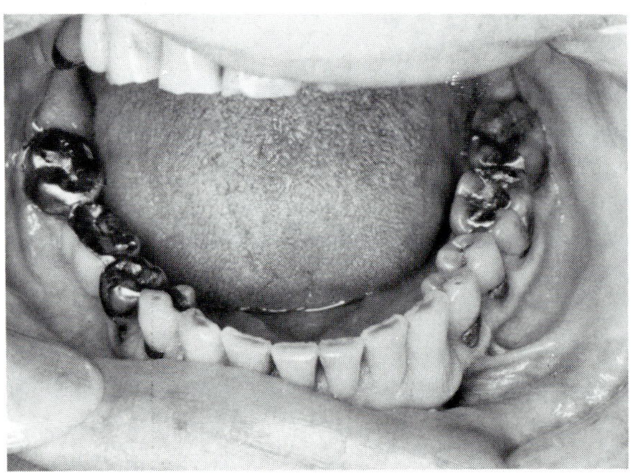

Fig. 3-121. View of lower occlusal surfaces.

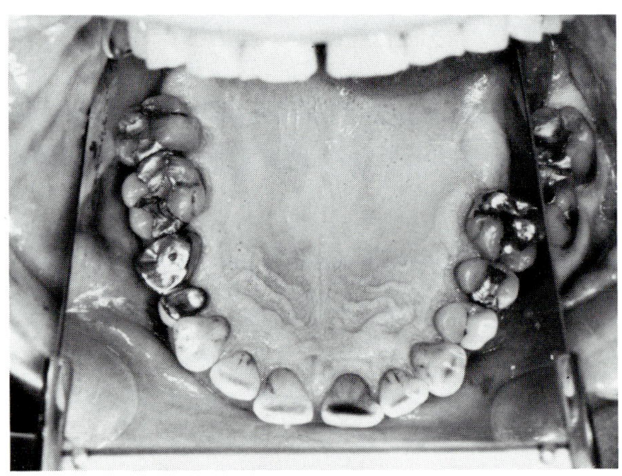

Fig. 3-122. View of upper occlusal surfaces.

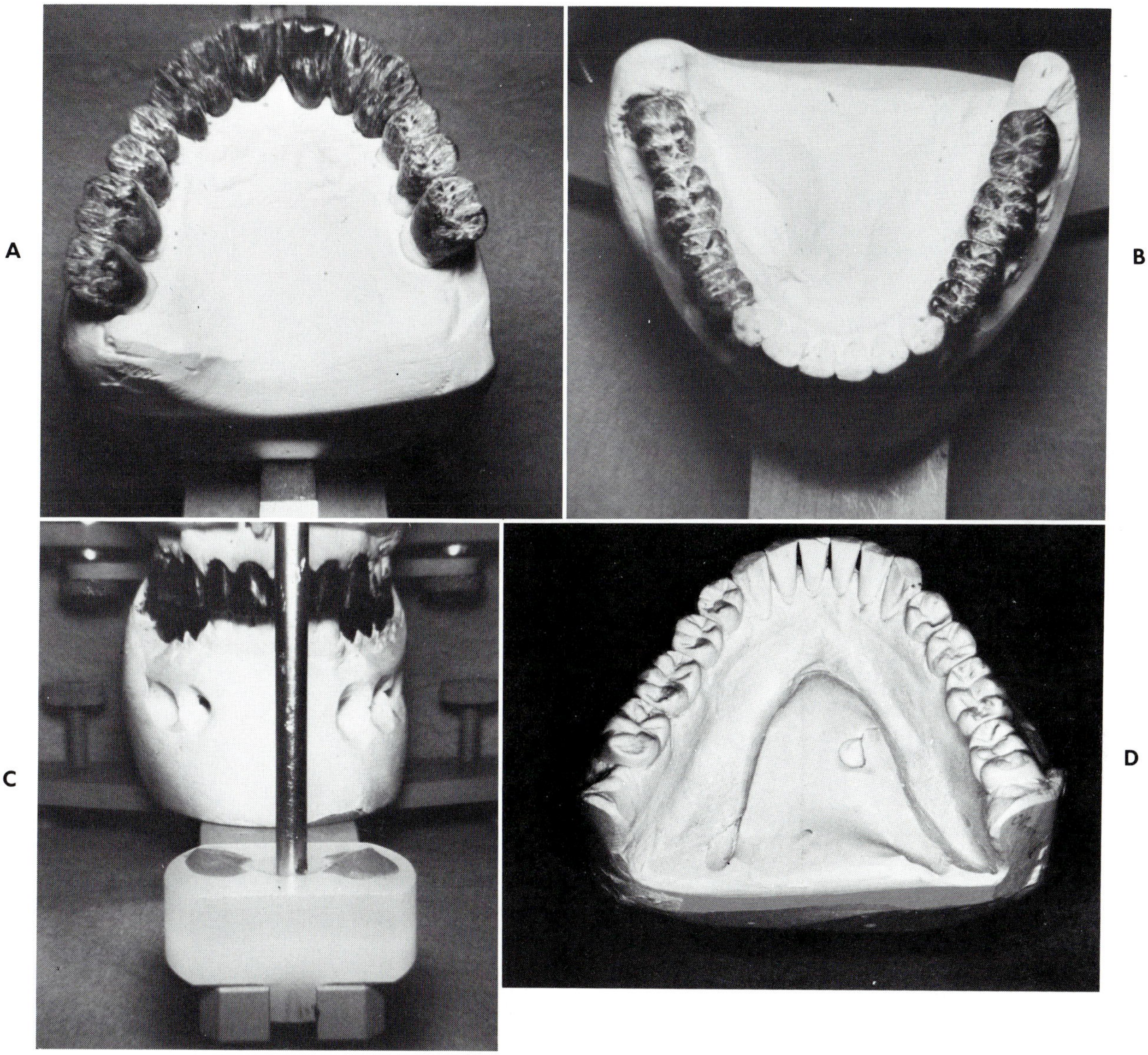

Fig. 3-123. A, Wax up of the upper arch; **B,** wax up of the lower arch; **C,** personalized incisal table; **D,** postoperative cast of lower arch.

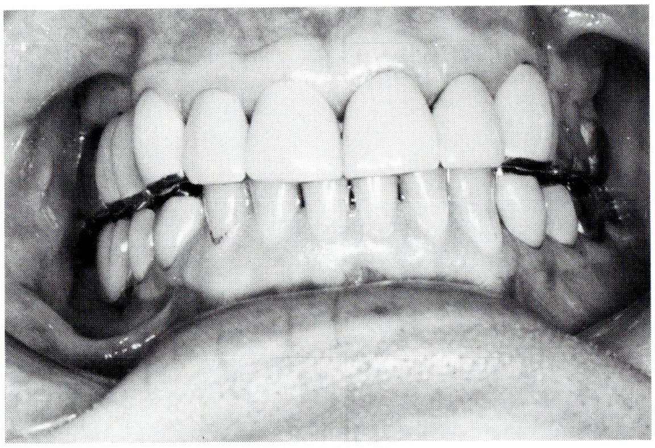

Fig. 3-124. Postoperative anterior view.

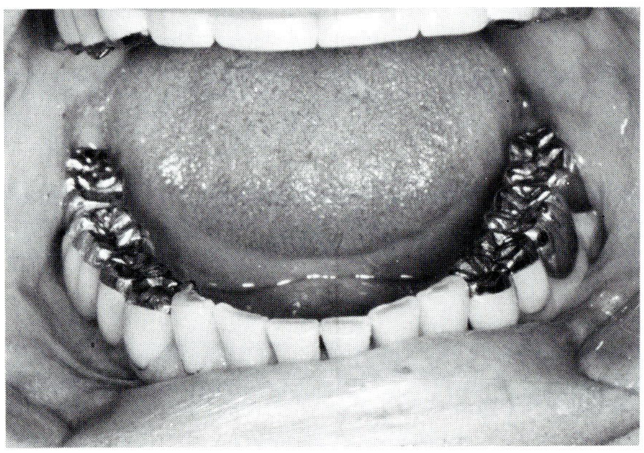

Fig. 3-125. Postoperative occlusal view of lower teeth.

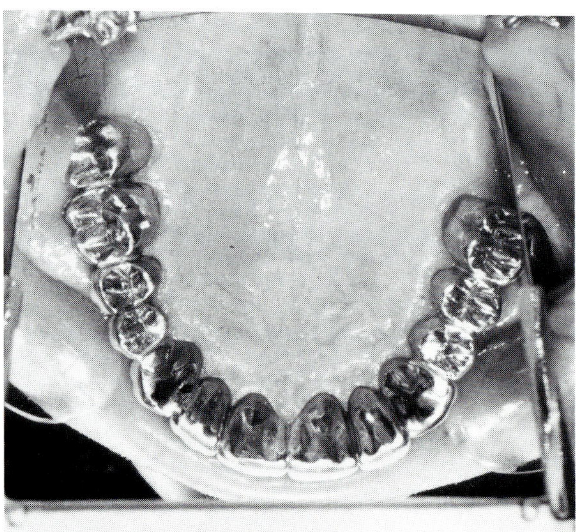

Fig. 3-126. Postoperative occlusal view of upper teeth.

entific standpoint, they are right, dentists doing clinical procedures must have it defined and must have a method of correctly registering jaw relations. This condition must exist until such time that a truly scientific approach is given to the profession.

"Centric relation of the mandible is its rearmost, midmost, untranslated hinged position. It is a strained relation as are all border relations. It is the only maxillo-mandibular relation that can be statically repeated."*

"We may define temporomandibular centricity as that terminal hinge fossae relationship necessary for the establishment of a fulcral seat toward which the condyles rotate and translate in the dynamics of function. Or it may be expressed by saying the opposing occlusal surfaces of the teeth bear a reciprocal dependence to the temporomandibular joint. Centric relation denotes both condyles in their firmest bracing contact and the only motion possible in this relationship is vertical rotation."†

Actually, establishing centric relation is the orienting of horizontal centers of motion, which are identical with the vertical centers of rotation to the maxilla. When the exact centers of lateral rotation have been located and this has been done in conjunction with the location of the centers of vertical rotation (hinge action), then we have truly found centric relation.

The following must be done: (1) location of the hinge axis, (2) location of the centers of lateral rotation, and (3) transference of the casts to the axis, which entails face-bow transfer of the upper cast to the axis and relation of the lower cast to the upper cast by a correct centric relation record. *The lower cast must be oriented to these centers.*[22]

In other words, *geometrically,* the problem of centric relation is one of relating the position of the hinge axis and rotational centers to the maxilla.

Anatomically, the problem of centric relation becomes one of employing ways and means whereby the physiology of the involved anatomic parts is utilized to establish a correct joint-fossae relationship.[23]

It can be said that the criterion of centric relation acceptability is its capability of reproduction.

Reproduction of centric relation using the Lucia method. Fundamentally, the problem of joint-fossae relationship involves directed joint positioning, application of patient bilateral muscular effort, and means of joint stabilization.

---

*From Stuart, Charles E.: Personal communication.

†From Dykins, William R.: Personal communication.

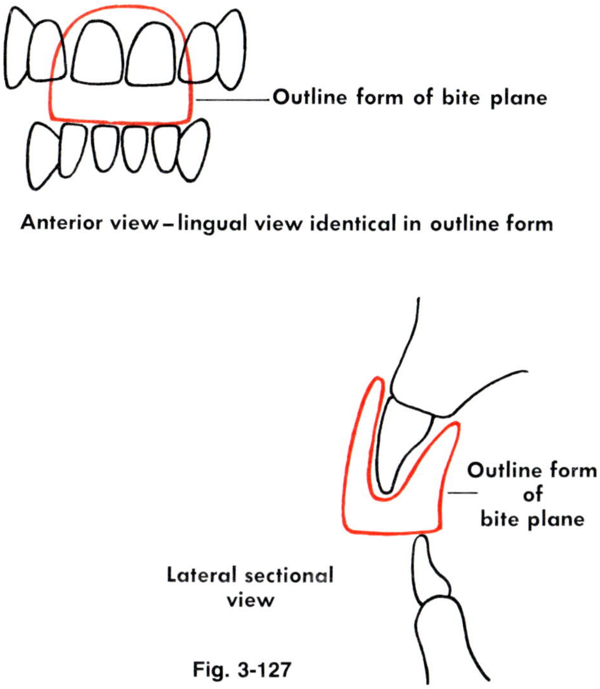

Fig. 3-127

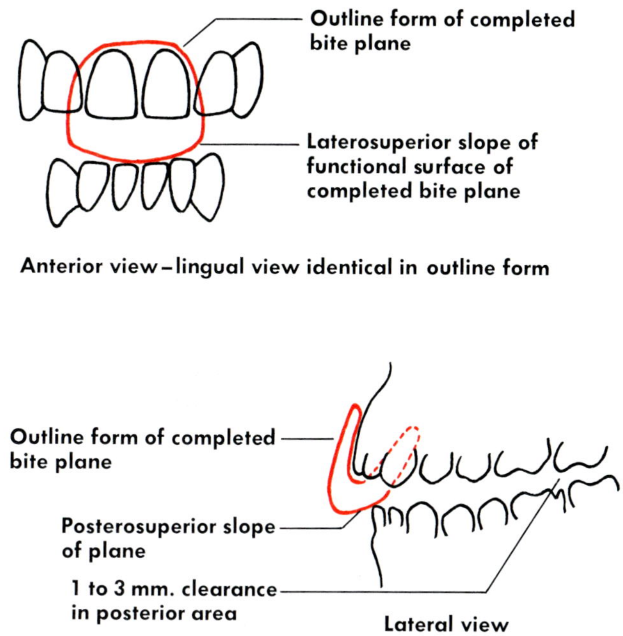

Fig. 3-128

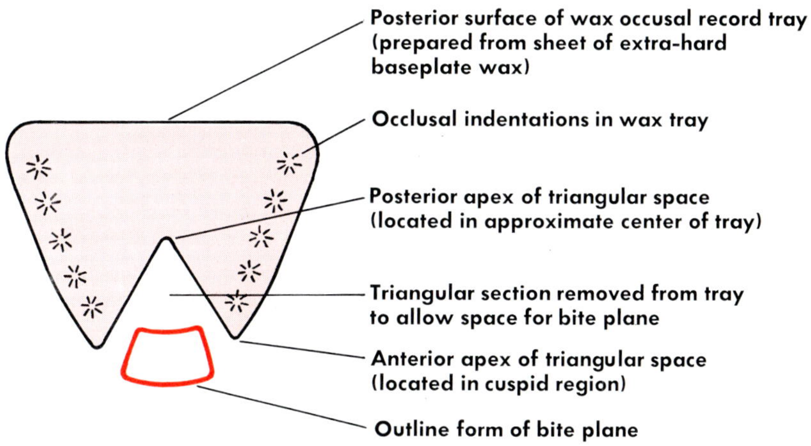

Fig. 3-129

Figs. 3-127 to 3-129. Graphic representations of principles of Lucia's method of registering centric relation record.

Operator guidance serves as the means of orienting the posterior relation of the condyles to the fossae, while the musculature is interpreted as the factor in placing the condyles in their correct superior relationship. To utilize bilateral muscular balance an anterior stop, as suggested by Victor O. Lucia of New York, must be provided as close to the desired vertical dimension as possible. An absolute requirement of the stop is that it must not be capable of any movement for constancy in its relation to the supporting teeth; neither should it be designed so that the backward and upward movement of the condyles is influenced. For convenience and form it is fabricated from quick-setting acrylic on models mounted on an articulator by means of a preliminary centric bite.

One or more layers of Sure-Set wax is the vehicle that is employed to carry the recording medium, such as Kerr's Temp-Bond,* between the teeth. The wax

*Kerr Dental Mfg. Co., Detroit, Mich.

wafer should not be in contact with the posterior teeth when the jaw is closed against the anterior stop. If it comes in contact, it may invite displacement because of the stretching of the ligaments.

Two or more wafer recordings are necessary. The criterion of acceptance of correct condylar centricity is their capability of reproduction demonstrated by the split-cast idea as presented by Lauritzen. With this technique the objective of recording centric relation at a predetermined, vertical dimension can be fulfilled.[24]

A step-by-step description of *Lucia's method* is in order. A small anterior self-curing acrylic bite plane is first constructed on the maxillary master model of the patient, the design of which can be seen in Fig. 3-127.

The bite plane is then placed in position in the patient's mouth and the teeth closed in centric relation onto the plane. In this position there must be enough lingual extension of the plane to allow firm contact with the lower anterior teeth, and there must be enough height or thickness to the plane to allow a 1 to 3 mm. clearance of the posterior maxillary and mandibular cusps.

After any necessary preliminary corrections are made, the plane is again placed in the patient's mouth. A piece of articulating paper is placed between the plane and the lower incisors, and the patient is guided into protrusive, centric, and lateral movements. The plane is then removed from the mouth, and the resulting Gothic arch tracing is observed. Any interferences on the plane are corrected, and it is shaped in such a manner as to render it ineffective as a lateral or protrusive guide for the mandible upon closure against the plane. In most patients this would necessitate sloping the plane's occlusal surface in a slightly upward direction, both posteriorly and laterally from a central ridge, which would now have but minimum contact with a single lower central incisor or with at most two incisors. This can be better understood by referring to Fig. 3-128.

Next indentations of the patient's maxillary cusps are made in a sheet of extra-hard base-plate wax. This occlusal pattern is then cut from the sheet and trimmed to within 1 or 2 mm. of the outer edge of the occlusal indentations. A V-shaped section is then removed from the anterior part of the wax form in such a manner and of such size that the wax form and the bite-plane can be placed in the mouth at the same time with some space between them (Fig. 3-129).

Also, the corners of the wax tray are turned up in the region of the cuspids. This ensures the reseating of the wax tray in its proper position after the Temp-Bond has been placed on the tray.

Thus a wax impression tray is formed for the centric relation record. The wax tray is then softened in warm water, enough to allow further occlusal indentations and yet not enough to cause the tray to lose its general shape while being handled. In this state the tray is positioned properly in the mouth, and the patient's mandible is guided into a centric closure and then is opened prior to complete penetration of the wax. The wax tray then is removed and chilled and is repositioned in the mouth to check for distortion.

With the wax tray still in position, the bite plane is inserted (some denture powder may have to be used to secure the plane in the mouth), and the patient's mandible is closed in the centric arc onto the bite plane. When in this position, the wax tray should be freely movable between the occlusal surfaces of the maxillary and mandibular teeth. The freedom of movement of the wax tray is most essential in obtaining the centric relation record. If it comes in contact with the posterior teeth when the jaw is closed against the anterior stop, it may invite displacement because of the stretching of the ligaments.

After completion, the wax tray is dried thoroughly. The patient's teeth are lubricated with a petroleum preparation, and a mix of a zinc oxide– eugenol preparation (Temp-Bond) is prepared properly and placed in the maxillary and mandibular occlusal indentations of the tray. With the bite plane securely in position the wax tray is carried to place and the patient's mandible is guided into a centric closure against the bite plane. At this time the tray is released (i.e., no longer held in place by the dentist) and the patient is instructed to exert pressure in the closure against the bite plane and to retain this pressure until instructed otherwise. The operator should hold the patient's mandible in this centric position until the Temp-Bond has completed its set. The method advocated by Dawson[17] and described on p. 54 of this chapter is used at this point. (See Fig. 3-130.)

The wax tray with the occlusal record is then removed, trimmed, and checked in the mouth without the use of the bite plane.

The study casts, working casts, or remount casts now can be checked with this occlusal recording. This, as well as the subsequent articulator mounting, is done without the bite plane.

Repeating the process and using several similarly constructed wax trays with the same bite plane is essential to verify, by the Lauritzen split-cast method, the accuracy of the centric relation record on the articulator.

It has been shown that it is possible to record the

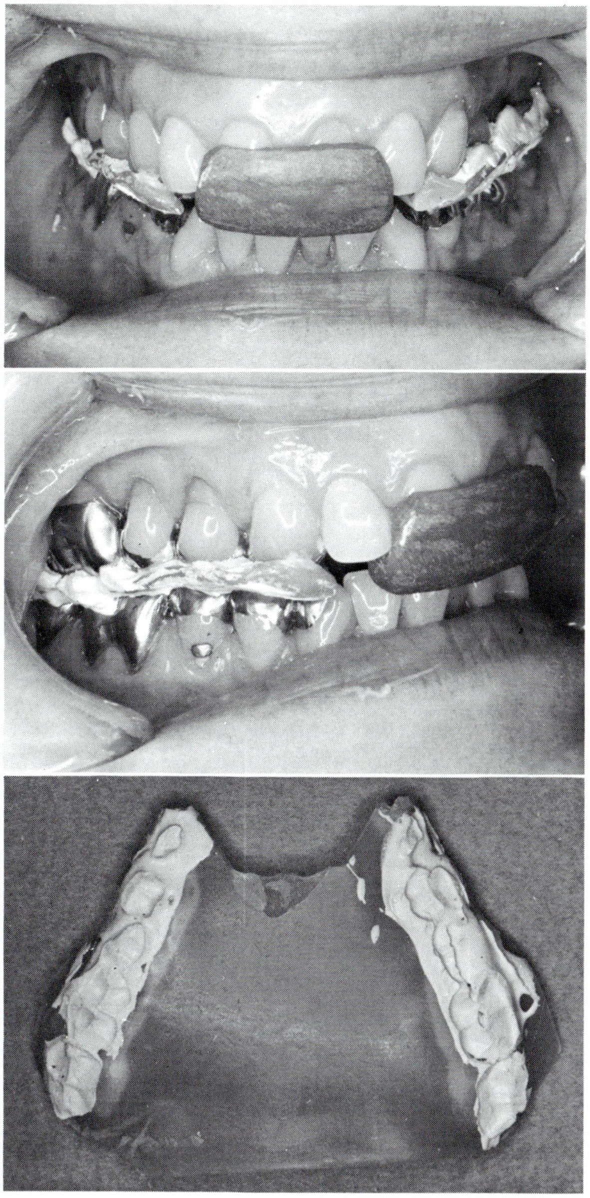

Fig. 3-130. Acrylic resin jig, prepared tray with zinc oxide–eugenol paste (Temp-Bond) carried to place, and patient's mandible guided into centric closure against bite plane.

true, pure, functional movements of a jaw and to transfer those records to an articulator on which they can be duplicated exactly.

The rotational centers control all the movements of the mandible, and they must be located accurately so that centric occlusion can be built at the position of centric relation.

It has been aptly said: "The real problem is recognizing the mouth as a functioning organ, an organ whose condylar function is of such basic importance, that without recognizing it and utilizing its respective quality, restoring a mouth becomes a hit or miss proposition. Taking it into your camp as an ally, dependable and predictable, enhances success. Ignore it and its harmful potential cannot be estimated."*

TREATMENT PLANNING

Objectives

The objective of a treatment plan is to restore the mouth to a healthy, functional condition. Not only must the condition and health of the supporting structures be improved upon, but also the relationship of the teeth. All of this is based on an evaluation of existing conditions and treatment potentials.

The first important consideration in arriving at a plan of treatment is whether there are definite indications for complete mouth rehabilitation and, if so, whether the patient is amenable to this type of treatment—physically, emotionally, and economically. The indications and contraindications of such an important undertaking should be seriously considered.

The second consideration is whether the dentist has not only a good knowledge of mandibular physiology and the basic fundamentals of periodontics, orthodontics, and endodontics (the sequential integration of which is part and parcel of the modus operandi), but also basic and advanced knowledge and the necessary operative skills in the field of crown and bridge prosthodontics.

A coordinated plan of treatment is of the utmost importance. Periodontal, endodontic, surgical, and orthodontic problems should be coordinated with the prosthodontics in treatment planning even though the patient is to be referred to the respective specialists in these fields. The final responsibility of the success or failure of the case in mouth rehabilitation lies with the prosthodontist. This makes it imperative that he know what is being done by the specialist and why and that he be in accord with the procedural objectives.

It is essential to be very well trained not only in the operative phases of prosthodontics but also in all laboratory procedures. This holds true regardless of whether the laboratory work is executed by the dentist or by resident or nonresident technicians.

An evaluation of all assembled data must be undertaken before a treatment plan can be recommended and therapy instituted.

---

*From Sloane, Robert B.: Basic principles in mouth reconstruction, Dent. Items Interest **73:**1-10, 1951.

Clinical, laboratory, microscopic, roentgenographic, and medical and dental history findings must be studied carefully, and any recognizable pathologic conditions must be noted and categorized for treatment by self or by referral to a specialist. The length of time that the etiologic factors have been present and the degree of pathology give us some indication of the rate of breakdown.

A study of the occlusion represents a very important aspect of the examination. In evaluating this occlusion the dentist must use the primary objectives of function, form, esthetics, and phonetics as his criteria. Sufficient study of properly oriented casts saves time and effort and prevents errors in treatment planning and therapy.

The following can be noted from the diagnostic casts:

1. Discrepancies between the habitual closure pattern and the centric relation—location, degree, and influence of occlusal prematurities—can be seen.
2. In conjunction with the roentgenograms one can see if any bone destruction has occurred and if centric occlusion and centric relation are not harmonious.
3. The excursive movements can also be studied, and if worn facets of the occlusal surfaces are evident, it is certain that they are produced by stresses in lateral and protrusive mandibular movements.
4. The "why" of mobility patterns of teeth (correlated with the measurement of degree of mobility), spacing or "fanning" of anterior teeth, battered and fractured cusps, etc. are vividly pointed up for observation and study.
5. Relation in size and position of the opposing arches.
6. Jaw-to-jaw relations.
7. Tooth-to-tooth positions.
8. Overbite and overjet relations.
9. Coronal, proximal contacts, embrasure, and occlusal forms of the teeth.
10. Plunger cusps.
11. Edentulous areas—form and size of space. Evaluation of its use for fixed and removable appliances.
12. Cross-bite relations—unilateral or bilateral.
13. Degree of curve of Spee and curve of Wilson. Its effect on the final restorations can be visualized, and any necessary changes can be considered.
14. Tilted, rotated, and extruded teeth. The degree of tipping, rotation, and extrusion of the teeth can be evaluated.
15. Topography of the marginal ridges of the teeth.
16. Temporomandibular malfunction—if it has to do with malrelation of the teeth.
17. Plane of occlusion. Relation of plane of occlusion to condyle path will be apparent; one can alter the occlusal plane somewhat by planning of tooth preparations.
18. Vertical dimension—should it be increased or decreased?
19. Attrition and erosion patterns.
20. Axial positions of the teeth.
21. Type of bite—deep bite, loss of posterior support, prognathic, occlusal attrition, etc.
22. Fixed and variable factors of occlusion.
23. Buccolingual relationship of the posterior teeth. A study of this relationship will be very helpful in determining the type of restoration to be employed—full or partial coverage.
24. Cuspid relations. The path of travel of the

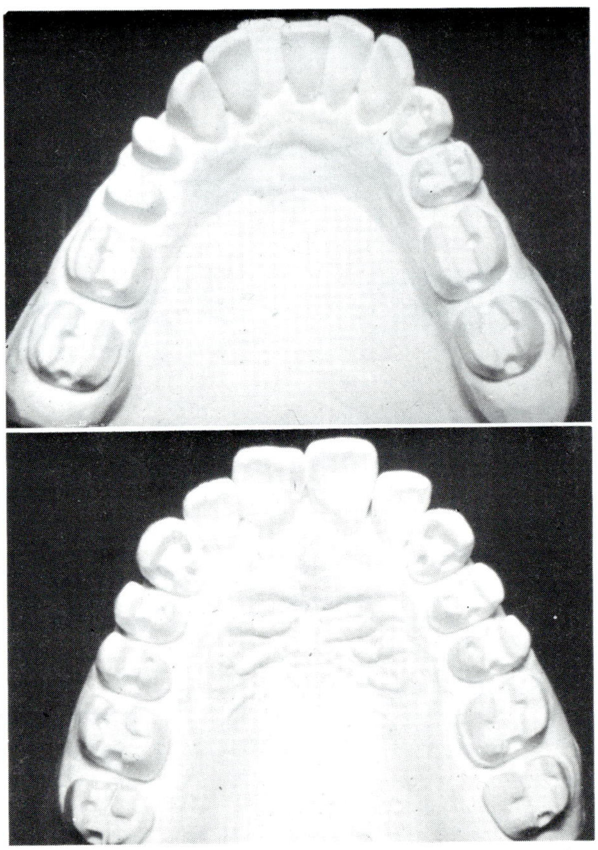

Fig. 3-131. Casts of properly prepared teeth allowing for adequate gold thickness on occlusal surfaces.

lower cuspid is observed, and the complete cuspid relationship is analyzed.

When some question arises as to the successful treatment of the patient or the best method of operative approach to enable recognition of some of the problems that may be encountered, it is exceedingly helpful to make the anticipated preparations in a set of properly oriented study casts. Sufficient tooth structure must be removed to allow for an adequate thickness of gold on the occlusal surfaces in all mandibular excursions (Fig. 3-131).

The next procedure is to work out the coronal and occlusal surfaces in wax. It is possible to study the following determinants of occlusion: (1) the use of cusps and fossae in planning occlusion, (2) ridge and groove direction determinants (axis-orbital horizontal plane), (3) cusp height and fossa depth determinants (sagittal plane), and (4) determinants of the lingual concavity of upper anterior teeth.

Waxing of the case on the preoperative casts (and later on working casts) that were properly oriented on a correctly designed, adjustable articulator allows the cusps (in shapes, placement, and graduated heights) to bear proper relations to the axes of the mandible (Fig. 3-132).

The length or height of the cusps is influenced by the condyle path. The Bennett movement determines the position and form of the cusps. The position and form must be correct to harmonize with the lateral shift; otherwise, the cusps will bump instead of glide around each other as they should.

Where extensive therapy is indicated, the aforementioned procedures create a template of the envisioned completed result, which can also be used as a guide or blueprint during actual treatment.

With all this information available we can also determine whether the teeth in situ can be used as abutments for retainers, appraised on the basis of type

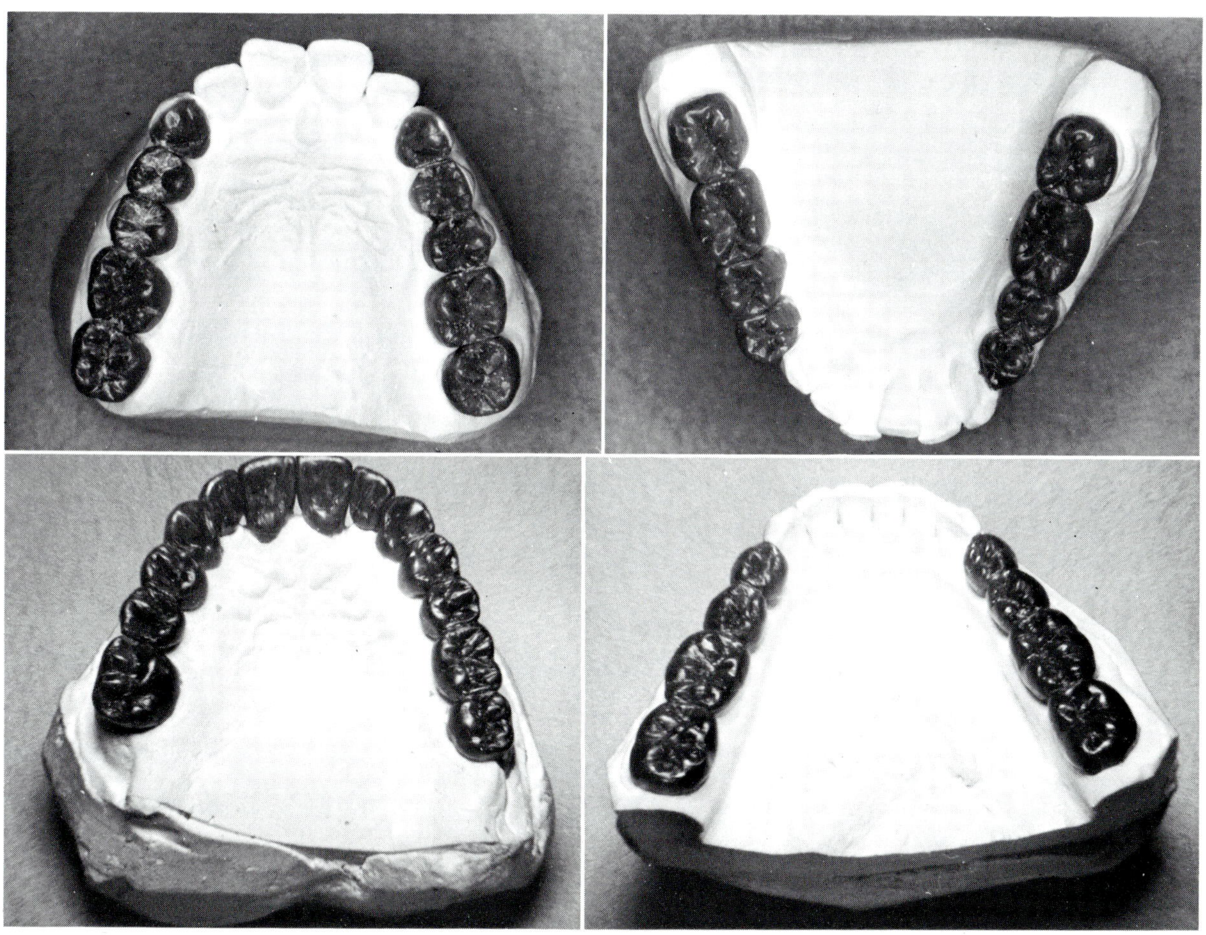

Fig. 3-132. Preoperative wax ups.

of root, coronal form, position of teeth in the arch, amount and quality of supporting bone, and the health status of the periodontium. We can also determine (1) if we should resort to extraction to make the case more ideal, (2) if splinting should be instituted, and (3) if orthodontic treatment, minor or major, can place these teeth in a more favorable position for their use as abutments.

Questionable teeth that are considered clinically expendable should be removed.

Fixed splinting around the arch offsets the potentials of excessive individual tooth leverage. We know that multiple abutments are essential to offset inadequate periodontal support, tooth mobility, or an unfavorable crown-to-root ratio. (See Chapter 6.)

Injudicious use of splinting must be avoided. This type of therapy should never be used as a crutch for proper occlusal forms. Despite the value of fixation, optimum stability depends on the final occlusal and incisal contacts of the teeth.

Malaligned or malposed teeth should be moved orthodontically for better management of abutment teeth or for better relation to the residual ridges. It can often effectively supplement and simplify therapeutic measures. If this is not possible, elective extraction is usually indicated, regardless of the periodontal status.

For minor orthodontic movement some techniques utilized are (1) wire or grassline ligature, (2) rubber dam elastics, (3) removable types such as the Hawley appliance, and (4) various modifications of this type of appliance such as the bite plate. The bite plate can be used as a prerestorative measure. (See Chapter 6.)

If indicated, consideration should be given to the establishment of a closely correct vertical dimension of the dentition to enable a return to a muscularly balanced, maxillomandibular position. The free-way space should not be obliterated.

It seems evident that what is being advocated is a well-executed treatment plan using sound judgment based on scientific fact and clinical experience. All this is formulated from a complete and thorough diagnosis utilizing all necessary aids, which leads to an intelligent and coordinated plan of treatment.

Treatment planning requires the application of all the knowledge one has in attaining and preserving the optimum health of the patient's oral cavity. The dentist must apply his biologic and psychologic training to the fullest extent, always keeping in mind the whole person. He must also remember that the responsibility of the dental profession consists of (1) diagnosis and treatment of all oral lesions which are exclusive to the oral regions and (2) diagnosis of all lesions which, though of systemic origin, present their primary clinical manifestation in the mouth.

It should be kept in mind that in a number of instances a third molar with proper type of roots, bone support, etc. should not be indiscriminately removed because, when necessary, it can be used as an abutment tooth. Also, it is sound practice, in many instances, to use a fixed partial denture or splint as an element of treatment in conjunction with a removable partial denture or a full denture (Fig. 3-133). In some situations it is not necessary or practical to restore the complete dental arch (as to the exact number of restored teeth) in the edentulous areas. The amount of efficiency gained in these situations by using a removable appliance is small compared to the inconvenience or abhorrence of a removable appliance (Figs. 3-134 and 3-135).

Speedy mechanized dentistry is not necessarily of the utmost importance, but, by the same token, one cannot take an unnecessarily prolonged time to get the work done. A "blueprint" (surgical, orthodontic, periodontic, prosthodontic, preventive)—an organization of treatment— should be followed in completing all necessary procedures. The dentist should work with proficiency, keep the office efficiency under strict control, and do the greatest amount of good dentistry per given amount of necessary time for a productive fee that is acceptable and justifiable to both the patient and the dentist.

The business affairs of the dentist are important. If he is not as sound in the business side of his practice as he is in his professional activities, he is headed for failure. Professional competence, however, comes first. The dentist must be proficient in the diagnosis and treatment of disease. If he lacks this kind of ability, all the skills of business administration that he can acquire make him a dim shadow of a professional man. Production line methods are not applicable to the treatment of people and their diseases.[25]

In other words, we should not let the patient assume that a restoration (inlay, crown, fixed partial denture, splint, precision removable appliance, full denture) that has been constructed ends all possibilities of future complications or that a prosthetic appliance keeps adjusting itself to changing conditions or supporting tissues.

Prognosis

Certain patients require some kind of compromise treatment, but it should be an intelligent compromise based on a sound evaluation of all diagnostic findings.

It is impossible to know how certain teeth will

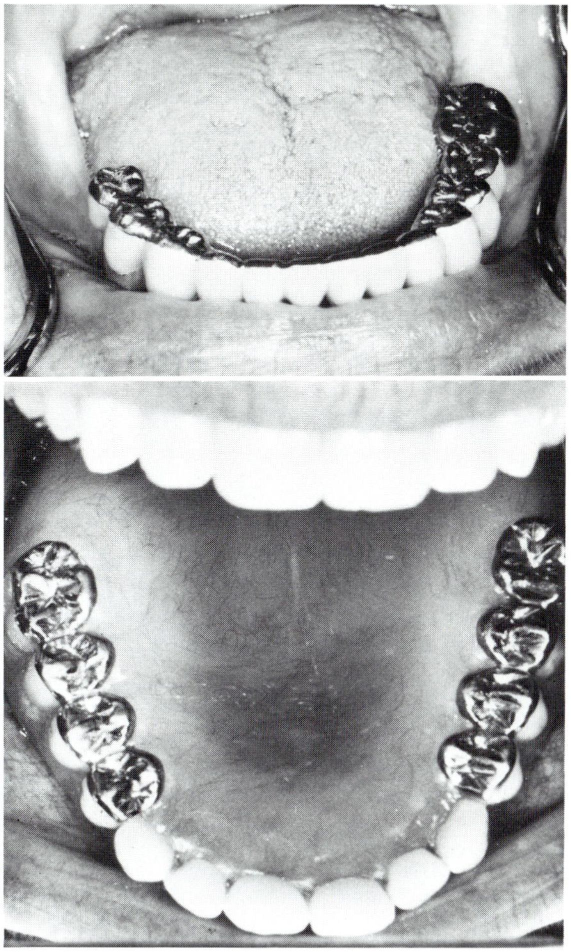

Fig. 3-133. A lower bilateral splint and a full upper denture with posterior gold occlusals.

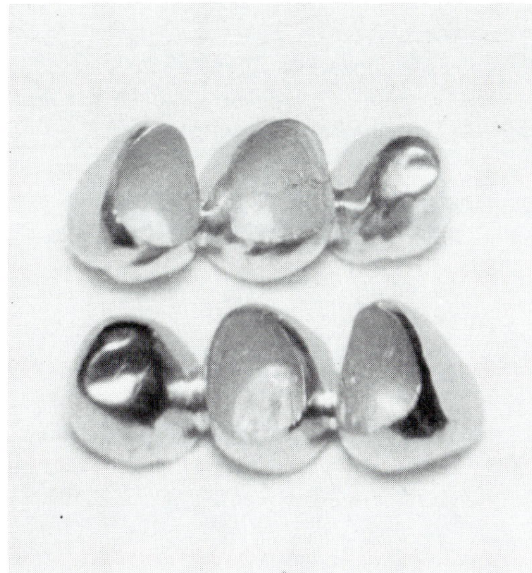

Fig. 3-134

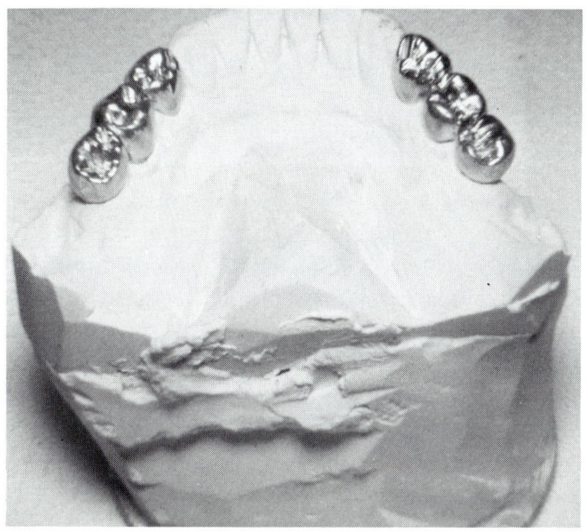

Fig. 3-135

Figs. 3-134 and 3-135. The use of cantilevered splints in the lower arch to avoid the use of a removable appliance.

respond to treatment. Sometimes anticipated failures are resounding successes and vice versa. The patient should be informed of all the inherent advantages, disadvantages, and limitations of this type of work. By all means do not allow your enthusiasm to cause you to overstep the bounds of reason by promising the impossible. One must be on guard especially against the feeling of omnipotence that the excellence of technical skills tends to foster. The operator has to recognize that to the extent he gives the impression of omniscience, to that extent the patient has a right to call on him for omnipotence as well.

Alternative solutions must be in readiness if treatment plans do not work out satisfactorily. The uncontrolled habits of the patient, the possibilities of future periodontal and periapical involvements, and other possible eventualities must always be under constant consideration. Troubleshooting is an important phase in mouth rehabilitation procedures.

Efficient scheduling of appointments for all clinical and laboratory procedures is necessary for the preservation of physical and emotional energies of both patient and dentist and, from an economic standpoint, to make the operation a profitable one. Do not overlook the financial arrangements—inform the patient not only of the cost of the work, but how you expect him to meet his financial obligation. It makes for a more successful relationship.

Prognosis is dependent upon the skills and experience of the dentist in regard to his ability to make a careful and thorough examination and to be able to correctly interpret the findings. Technical ability, laboratory control, and patient dentist rapport (psychologically and economically) are the other necessary ingredients.

The senior citizen

Statistics show that there are more older people living today than at any previous time. Every day in the United States at least 1,000 persons reach their sixty-fifth birthday.[26] Nearly 13 million, or more than 8% of the population, are over the age of 65. Because of these facts, dentists have become very much interested in the problems of aging.

Our elderly patients are most eager to maintain their teeth, oral soft tissues, and jawbones in a state of health. The objective of the dentist caring for the senior citizen is to achieve this goal as effectively for the elderly patient as it can be achieved for the younger patient.

The dentist's attitude toward dental care for the senior citizen is changing. He knows now that advancing age does not necessarily mean the loss of teeth and their replacement with dentures. As a result, he directs his treatment toward the preservation of the teeth and attachment apparatus of the elderly patient. The dentist is attempting to look after the aged with great care, patience, and understanding. Because of the dentist's treatment and attitude, the senior citizen is grateful and appreciative. By enabling him to function adequately and comfortably, the dentist is enabling many older persons to continue their contributions to their associates and their communities.

Ryan[27] has aptly said: "The elderly are not just 'old people'; they are structurally, functionally, and mentally different men and women than they were in the days of their youth and early maturity."*

In treating the aged we must differentiate between senescence, which refers to normal physiologic aging, and senility, which may be defined as pathologic aging. The dentist must approach the problems and the disturbances of the aged with understanding, and he must realize the important role the oral cavity plays in the health of our senior citizens.

*From Ryan, Edward J.: The dental problems of senescence, J. Prosthet. Dent. **1**:64-70, 1951.

Cowdry[28] has this to say: "Some kinds of cells are evidently replaced thousands of times in the human life span, others hundreds of times, and still others not at all. The long-lived cells which are not replaceable accumulate pigments, lipoids and various other relatively inactive materials, which suggest a diminution in physical vigor."*

In the elderly we are confronted with changes in the following:

1. Metabolism. There is a lowering or slowing down of the general metabolism.
2. Vitality of cells. There is retardation of cell division and capacity for cell growth and tissue repair.
3. Glandular balance. There is a decrease in glandular secretions. According to the physiologist, Anton Carlson[29]: "The salivary glands usually show some evidence of atrophy with advancing years; competent investigators have reported definite decrease in salivary volume and in percentage of pytalin with advance in age. To what extent the decrease in saliva or the age changes in the composition of the saliva permit or favor growth of the aciduric flora of the mouth, which in turn may enhance degenerations in teeth and gums, is still an open question."†
4. Speed and strength of neuromuscular reactions. The tonus of the muscles of mastication and deglutition is markedly reduced.
5. Nutritional patterns.

Silverman[30] cautions us not to overlook the biologic aspects of tooth care in relation to the treatment of the periodontium, the bone, and muscle activity of the oral structures. These dental and oral structures depend directly on the systemic effects of the circulation, and the endocrine, neurologic, and metabolic mechanisms of the body.

Another supportive measure for evaluation is the nutritional aspect. Nutrition is the process of providing proper food elements for maintenance of health and growth. A sound nutritional program will do much to maintain the physical vitality and the nervous stability of the older patient. It is also vitally essential to the success of dental restorations.

There is a definite relationship between impaired masticatory function and general nutritive failure. It has been said that there is a definite correlation between what and how a man eats and how long he lives.[26]

*From Cowdry, E. V.: Factors in aging, Sci. Month. **56**:370, 1943.

†From Carlson, Anton: Physiologic changes in normal aging. In Steiglitz, E. J.: Geriatric medicine, ed. 2, Philadelphia, 1949, W. B. Saunders Co.

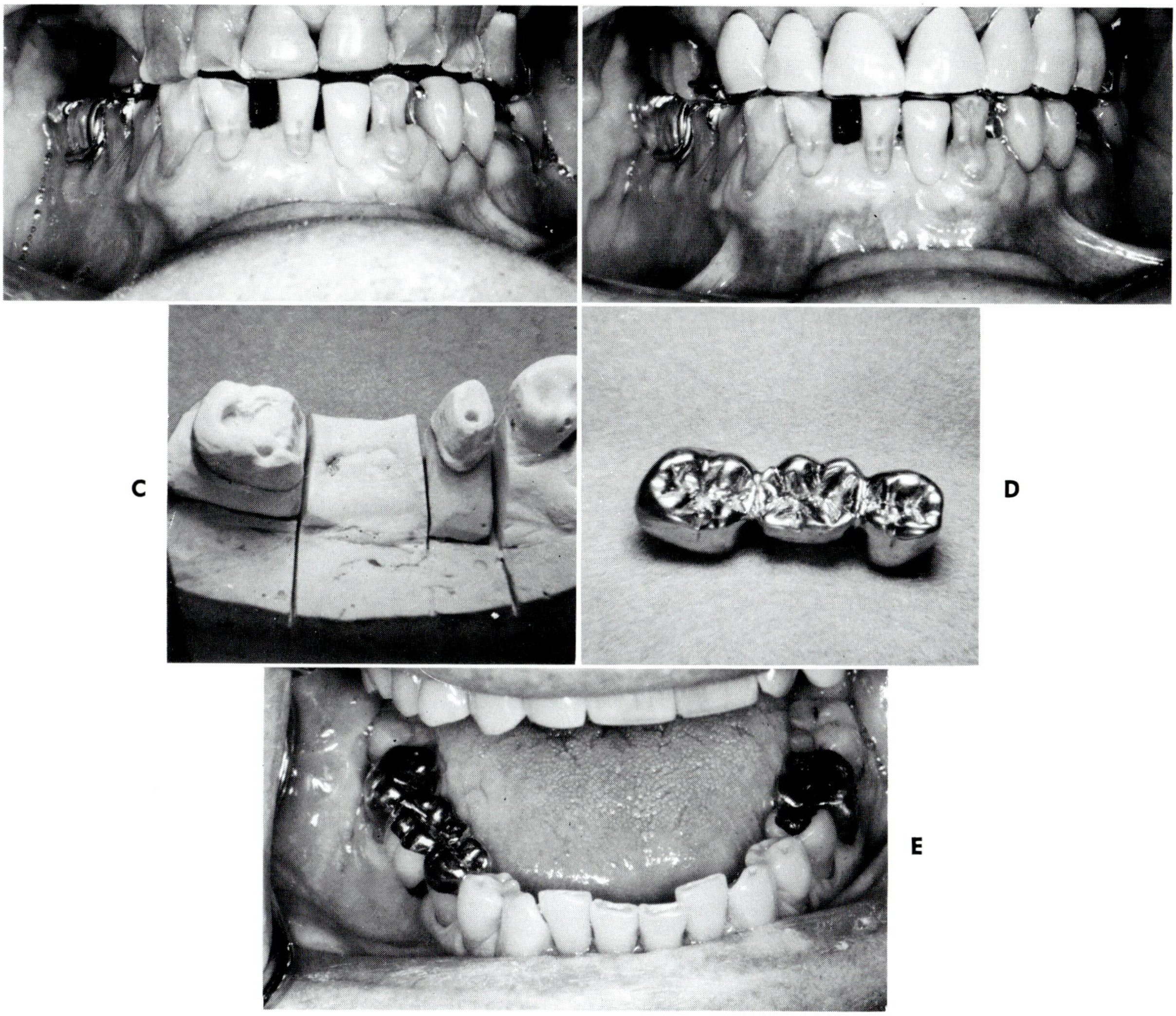

Fig. 3-136. Results of prosthodontic efforts in elderly patients. **A** and **B,** Patient 93 years of age. **C** to **E,** Patient 86 years of age.

According to Stieglitz[31]: "We are what we are today because of our yesterdays."*

Older people require less fat and carbohydrate and more protein. Many diseases and general debilitating states are the result of protein insufficiency. The minerals are also of particular importance to the aged, especially calcium since calcium loss contributes to bone fragility. A negative calcium balance is often found in our senior citizens when rapid ridge resorption is noted.

Stieglitz[31] stated: "Recent studies point out calcium requirements are greatly increased in later years. The older person needs more calcium than the young adult to maintain calcium balance. Calcium loss contributes to bone fragility. The importance of milk (as a source of both protein and calcium) for the elderly is thus once more emphasized. The nutrition of the youth affects his health in maturity, senescence, and old age, but the nutrition of each period of life presents problems peculiar to the period. To age is to change."*

We must not forget that the most nutritious food is of little consequence if the first process of digestion—food preparation in the mouth—is inadequate. Inadequate mechanical preparation of the food results from

*From Stieglitz, Edward J.: Aging as a problem of nutrition, Nutr. News **13:**6, 1949.

*From Stieglitz, Edward J.: Aging as a problem of nutrition, Nutr. News **13:**6, 1949.

A

B

C

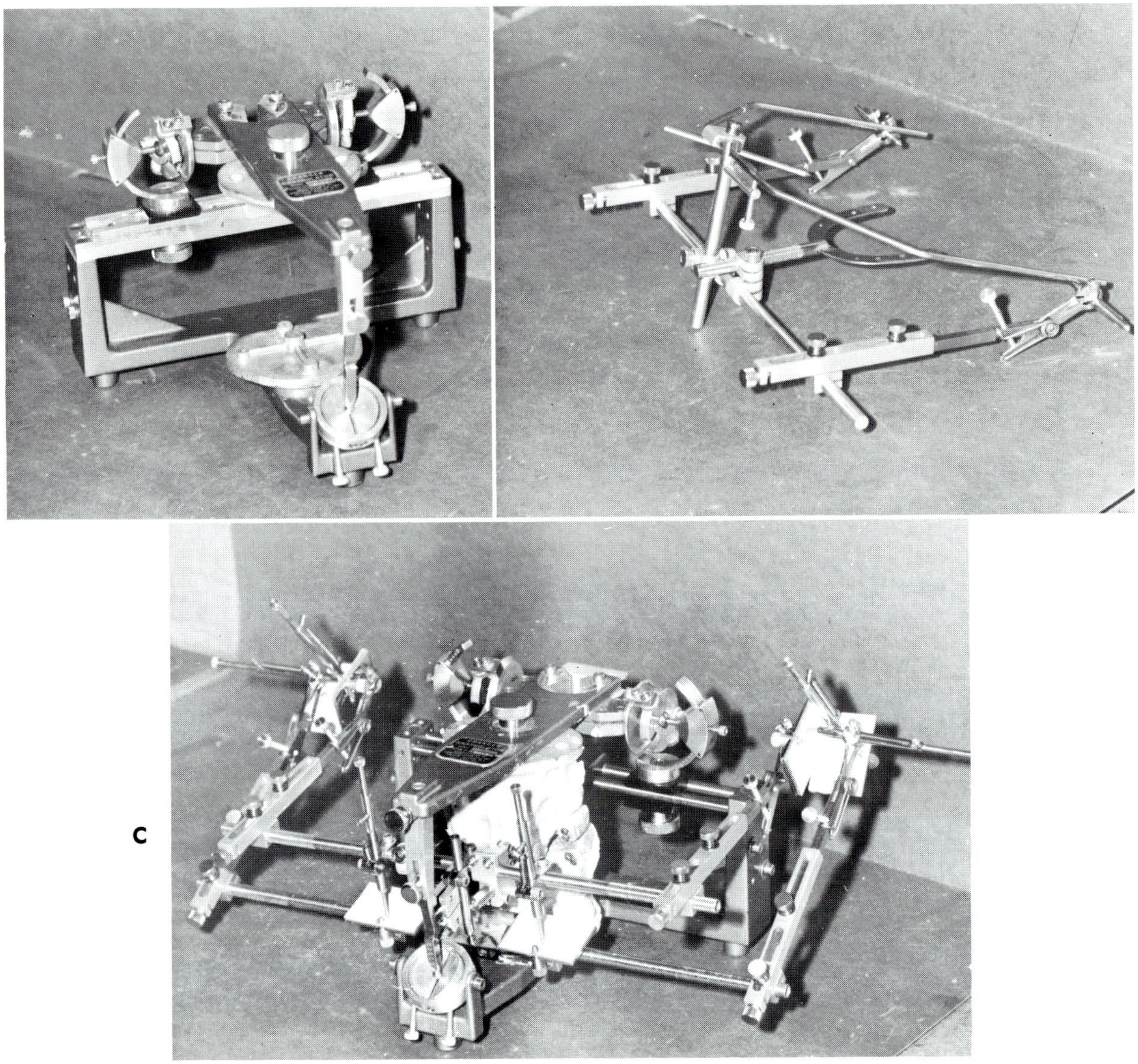

Fig. 3-137. Articulators and face-bows used in mouth rehabilitation procedures. **A,** Granger Gnatholator. **B,** Hinge-bow assembly. **C,** Granger pantograph mounted on Gnatholator.

painful, nonfunctioning, or missing teeth or from faulty dental restorations. Without adequate nutrition the elderly patient cannot do well.

Some investigators recommend multivitamins on a supportive basis, but the possibility of the vitamin therapy masking symptons of chronic, underlying disorders must not be overlooked.

The French have told us that "death enters through the mouth." We might likewise say that so do life, health, and long well-being.[27] We also must not overlook the fact that dental care provides not only nutritional support but also psychologic support for the elderly patient. The desire of older patients to retain and prolong the use of their own teeth is natural and understandable and in many patients must not be discouraged. Advanced age is no deterrent to the construction of limited or extensive crown and bridge prosthodontics provided the patient is in reasonably good health (Fig. 3-136).

Schabel[33] calls attention to the fact that specific oral changes in the geriatric patient are characterized by (1) degenerative mucosa, (2) loss of muscular tone resulting in facial collapse and angular cheilitis, (3) extreme alveolar resorption, (4) decreased vertical

A_1

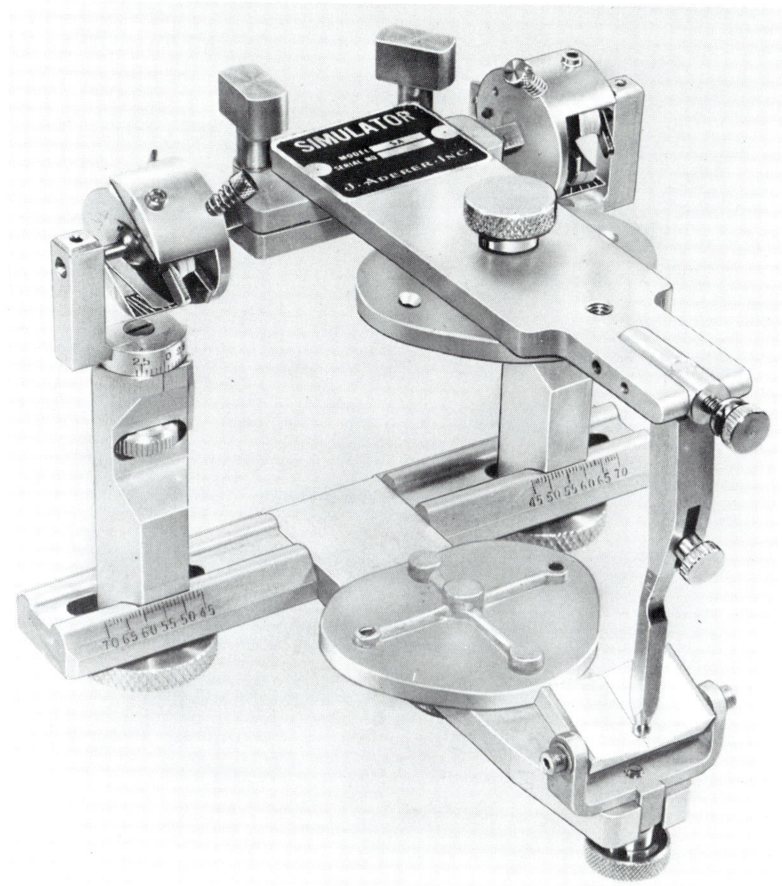

Continued.

Fig. 3-138. A, The Simulator articulator (front $\mathbf{A_1}$, and rear $\mathbf{A_2}$, views); **B,** the Simulator hinge-bow; **C,** the Simulator hinge-bow being used for the precise location of the transverse axis. (Courtesy J. Aderer, Inc., New York, N. Y.)

dimension, (5) enlargement of the tongue, and (6) overall breakdown of the masticatory mechanisms.

The burning tongue syndrome, sore and inflamed mucosa, and mouth dryness are common complaints.

However, the dentist must also be aware of the anxiety, depression, and hostility that many times accompany dental care for the senior citizen. Dental care for these patients should be carefully evaluated as to whether the care should be limited or extensive. By all means do not overtreat or overadjust. Patience and understanding are important to treatment. Establishing rapport with the patient can prevent many problems, but lack of concern and impatience can produce many problems. Even psychiatrists have only limited success unless the patient recognizes his needs and is willing to cooperate.

With advancing age the vitality of the dentin is greatly decreased by sclerosis and obliteration of the tubules and by secondary dentin formation, which cuts off the tubules from the pulp. Old dentin may become entirely insensitive and impermeable. The phenomenon can result in decreased sensitivity during cavity preparation.[32]

However, we also find that many elderly patients lose their teeth from the caries of senescence. Caries in the aged is often rapid and deeply penetrating, with early pulp involvement. This may be caused by the decreased bacteriostatic power of the saliva and the atrophy of the salivary glands. In the aged we are also faced with the degenerations in the dental pulp that may be of blood-borne origin. Emboli and thrombi may affect the blood vessels in the dental pulp in the same manner they affect the vessels of other organs. Pulpitis may also be of hypertensive origin.

As a result of gathering all these findings—that is,

A₂

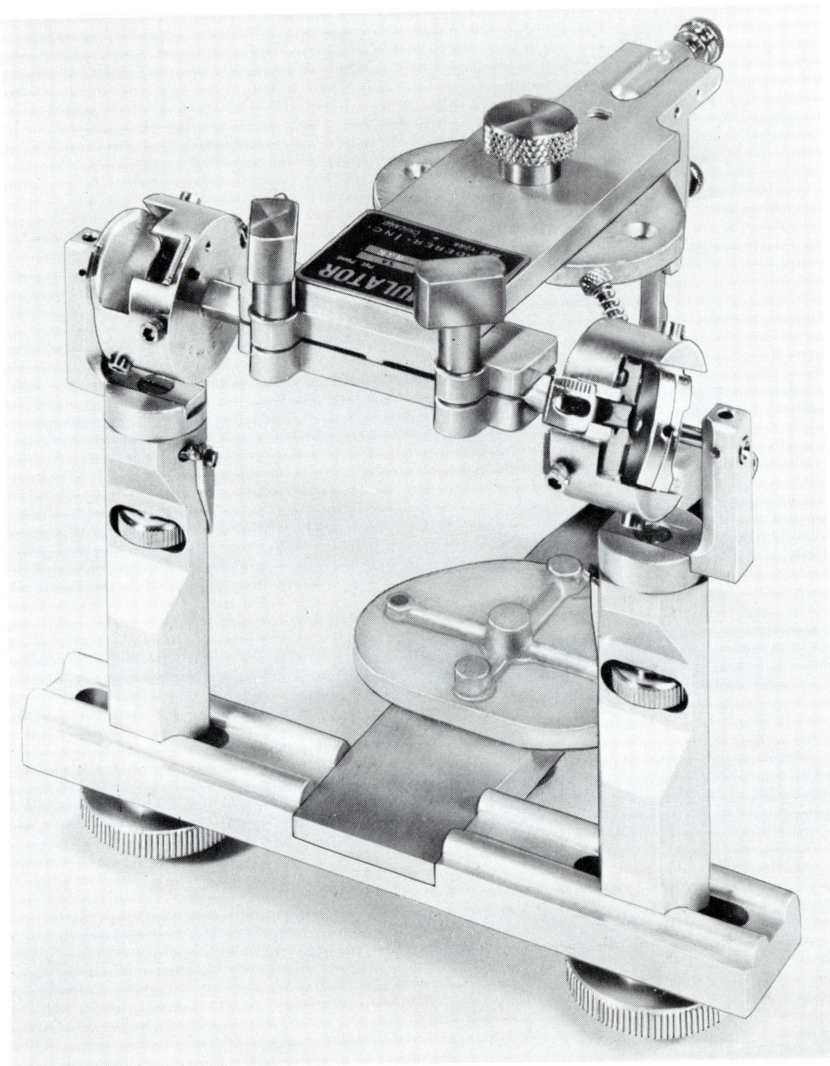

Fig. 3-138, cont'd. For legend see p. 89.

physiologic, nutritional, psychologic, and mechanical —the total problem can be evaluated and the diagnosis and treatment plan made for the senior citizen (Fig. 3-137).

New and fresh designs of desirable instruments for the accurate instrumentation of the recording and transferring of mandibular relations, mounting of study casts, working casts, remount casts, etc. have been developed in the past few years.* A close scrutiny of Figs. 3-138 to 3-150 will show new ideas, improvements, and innovations.

*J. Aderer, Inc., New York, N. Y.; Swanson-Wipf Articulator Co., Inc., Thousand Oaks, Calif.; Denar Corp., Anaheim, Calif.

Text continued on p. 100.

B

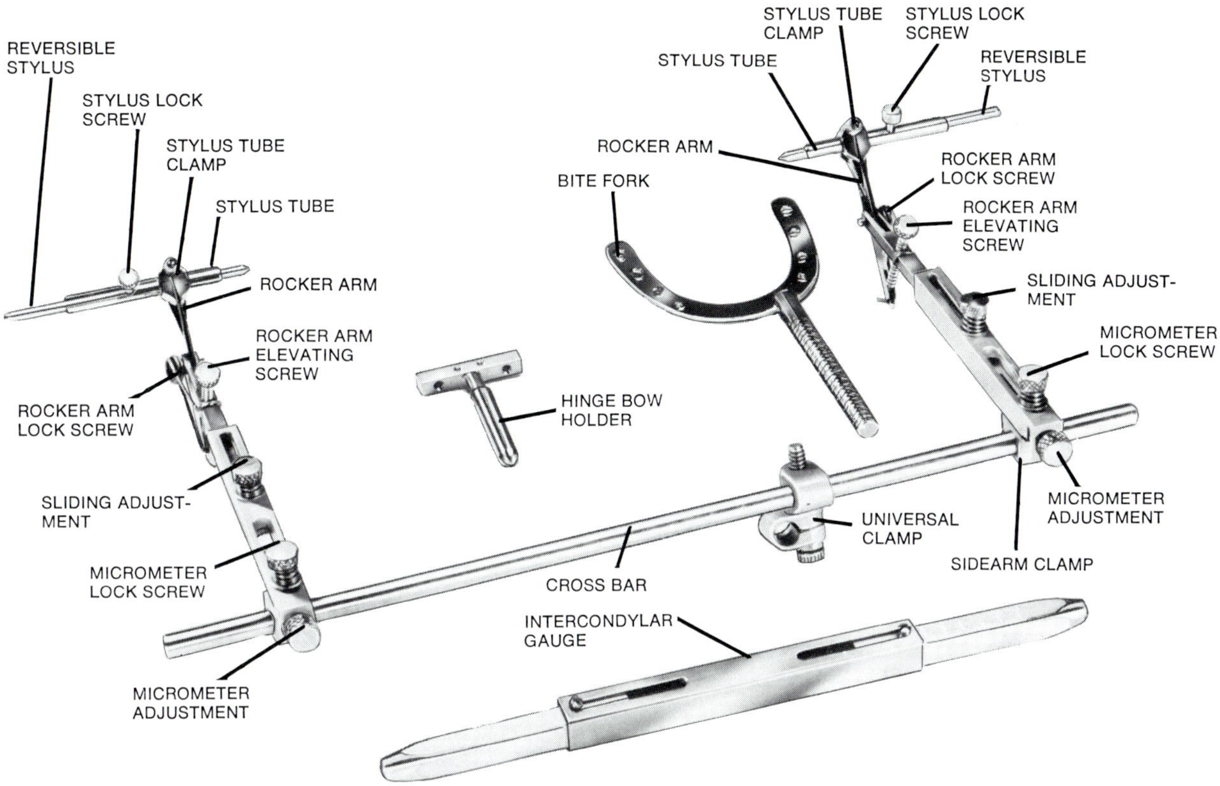

C

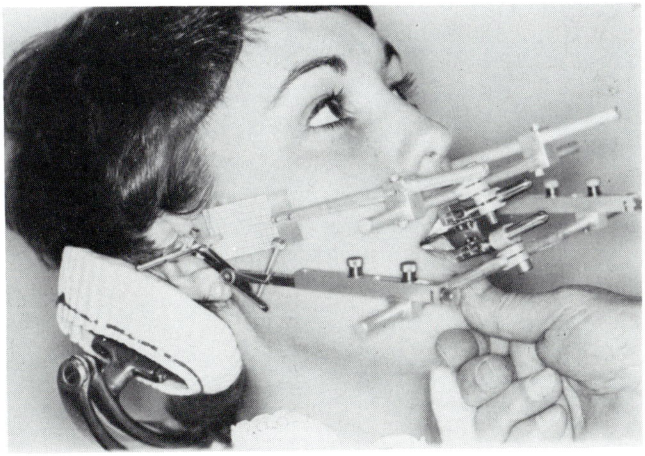

Fig. 3-138, cont'd. For legend see p. 89.

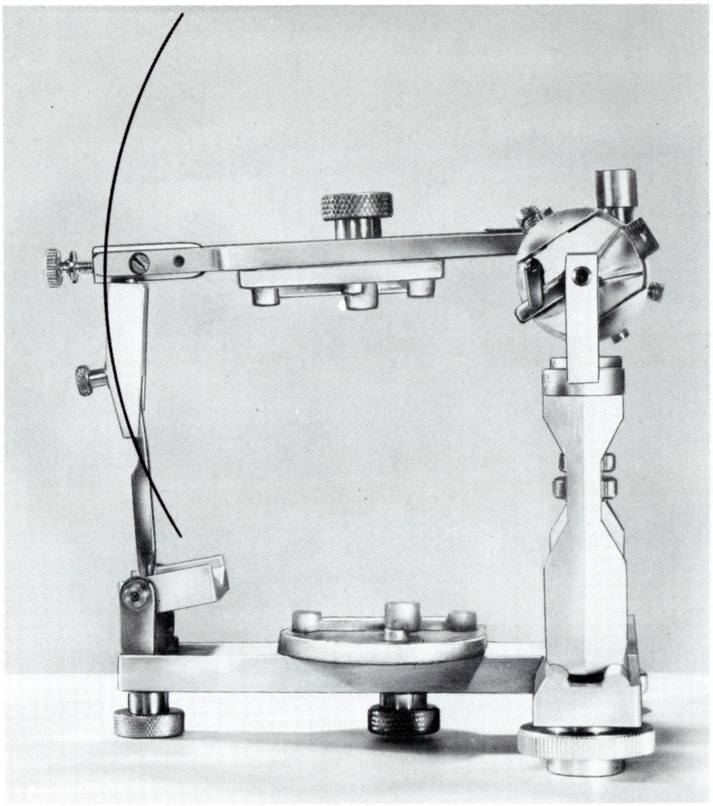

Fig. 3-139. The guide pin holder is machined so that the guide pin moves on a curve as it is raised and lowered. The curve, as illustrated, is made on the radius of the hinge axis. As changes in vertical opening are made, the ball point of the guide pin remains centered on the anterior guide plate. Change in vertical dimension will not alter the anterior guidance. (Courtesy J. Aderer, Inc., New York, N. Y.)

Fig. 3-140

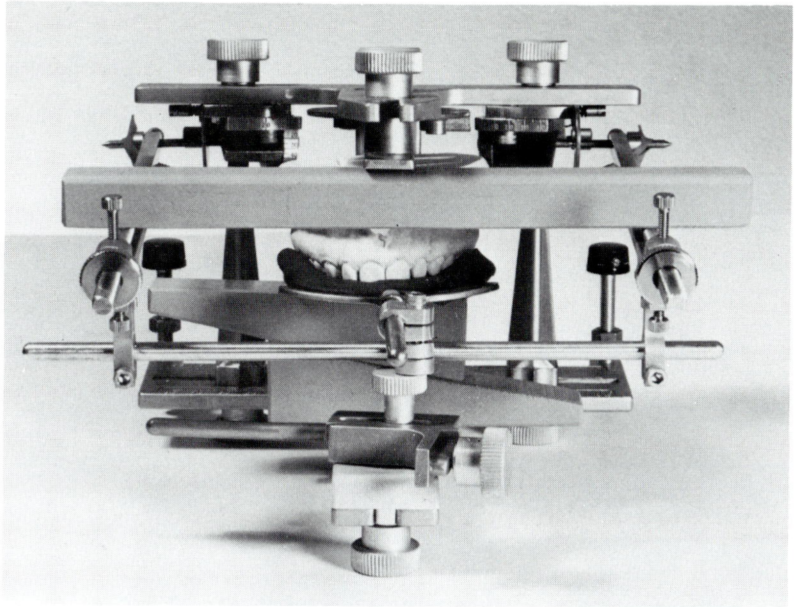

Fig. 3-141

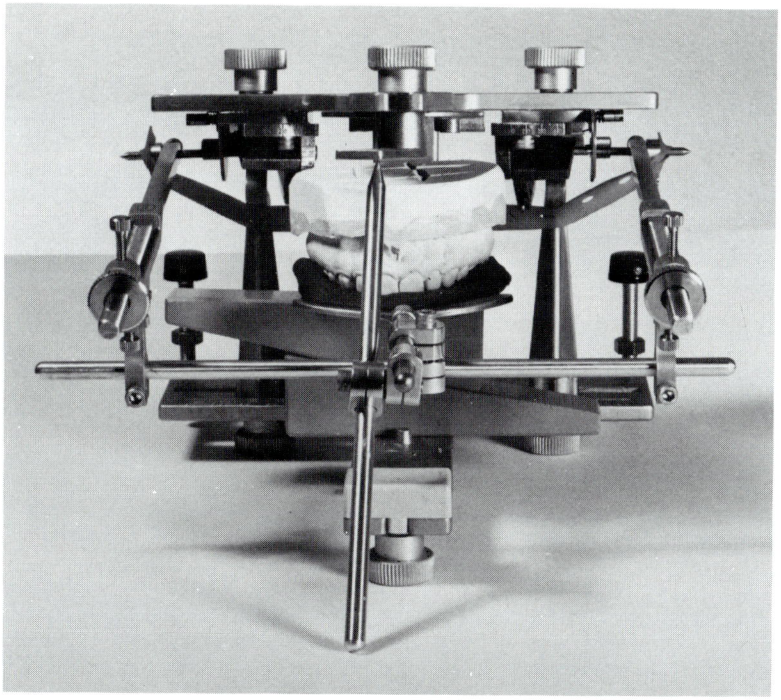

Figs. 3-140 and 3-141. The TMJ kinematic face-bow is utilized with a simple jig to mount the maxillary cast on the TMJ articulator with the mechanical fossa accessory. For a single mount the stick in the TMJ kit is used to relate the cast to the middle of the articulator (Fig. 3-140). If the cast will ever be remounted, it is precisely located on the articulator with the orbital pointer rod (Fig. 3-141). (The illustrations in this series [Figs. 3-140 to 3-148] by courtesy of TMJ Instrument Co., Inc., Thousand Oaks, Calif.)

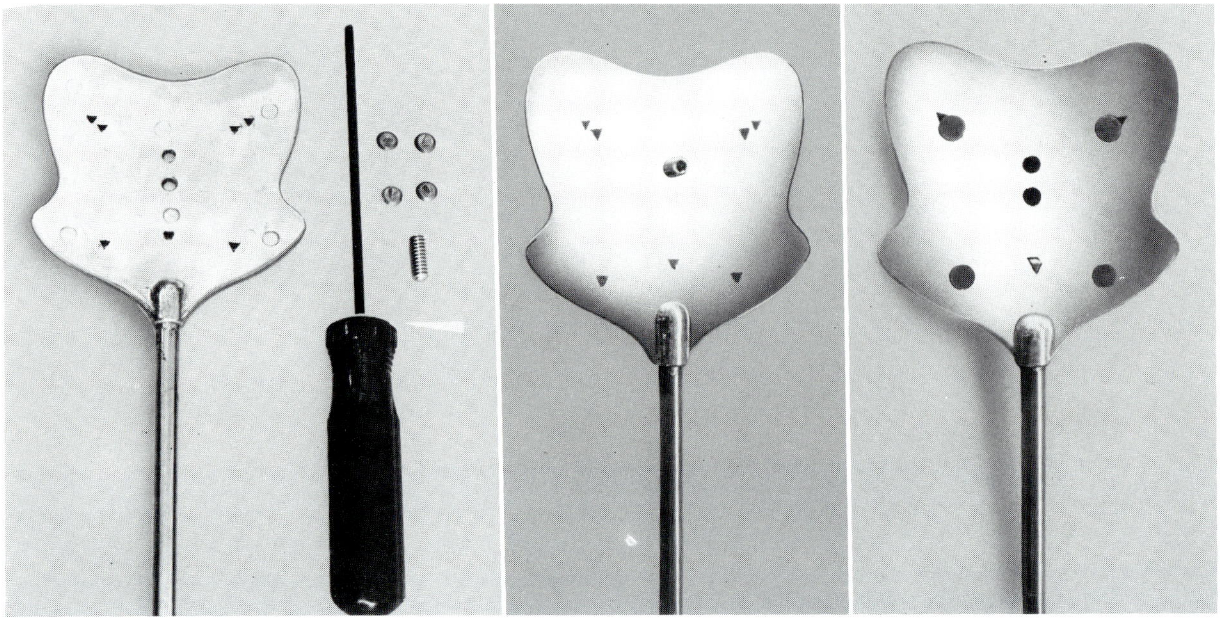

Fig. 3-142. Clutch-forming bite fork. Alternate stud holes are provided for flexibility of positioning. Fill all holes in the clutch-forming bite fork with utility wax, spray with release agent, and seat the studs in the desired hole.

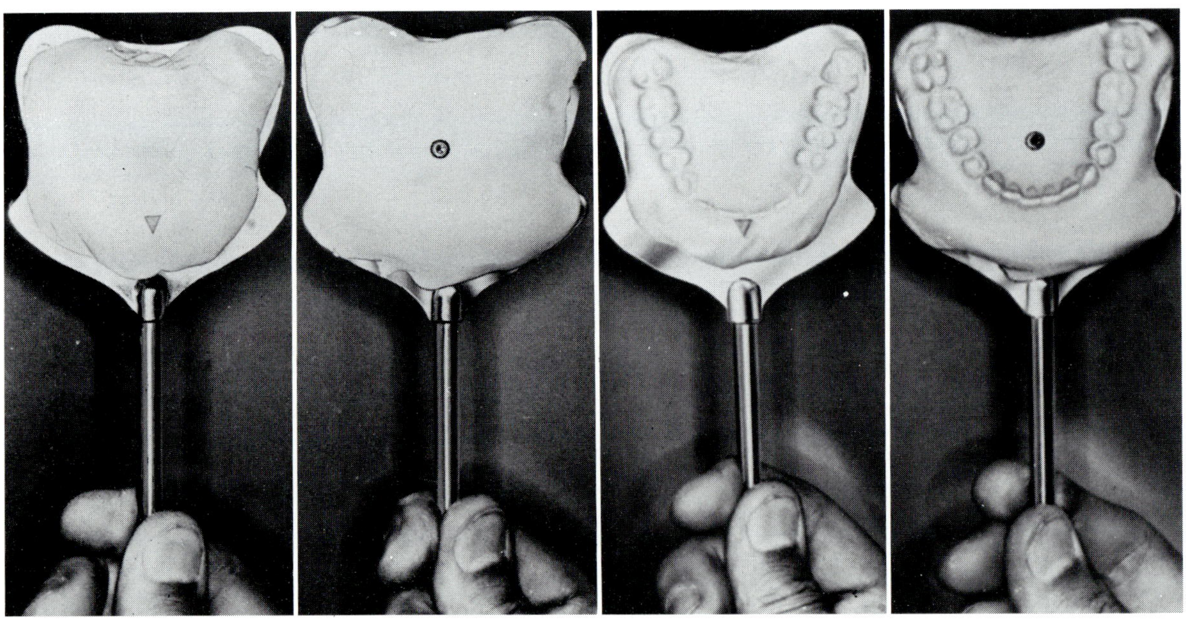

A B

Fig. 3-143. A, Make a double plus mix of TMJ acrylic and place a portion on each side of the clutch former. Be sure to imbed the heads of the studs and the threads of the central bearing screw. **B,** The finished clutches are shown here as the clutch-forming bite fork is removed from the mouth. They should be tested for retention and stability.

A

B

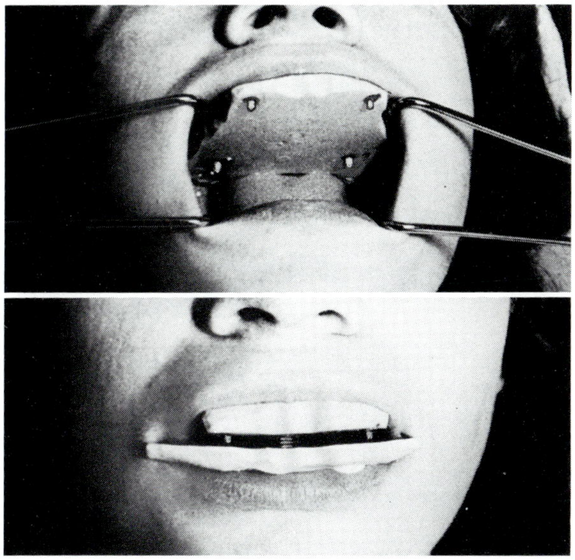

Fig. 3-144. A, The upper clutch positioned on the teeth. **B,** The lower clutch should be tried in the mouth and the clearance of the studs checked in the various jaw movements. There should be about 1 mm. of clearance in any movement at this stage of the operation. Movements should be recorded with the clutches as close together as possible.

A

B

C

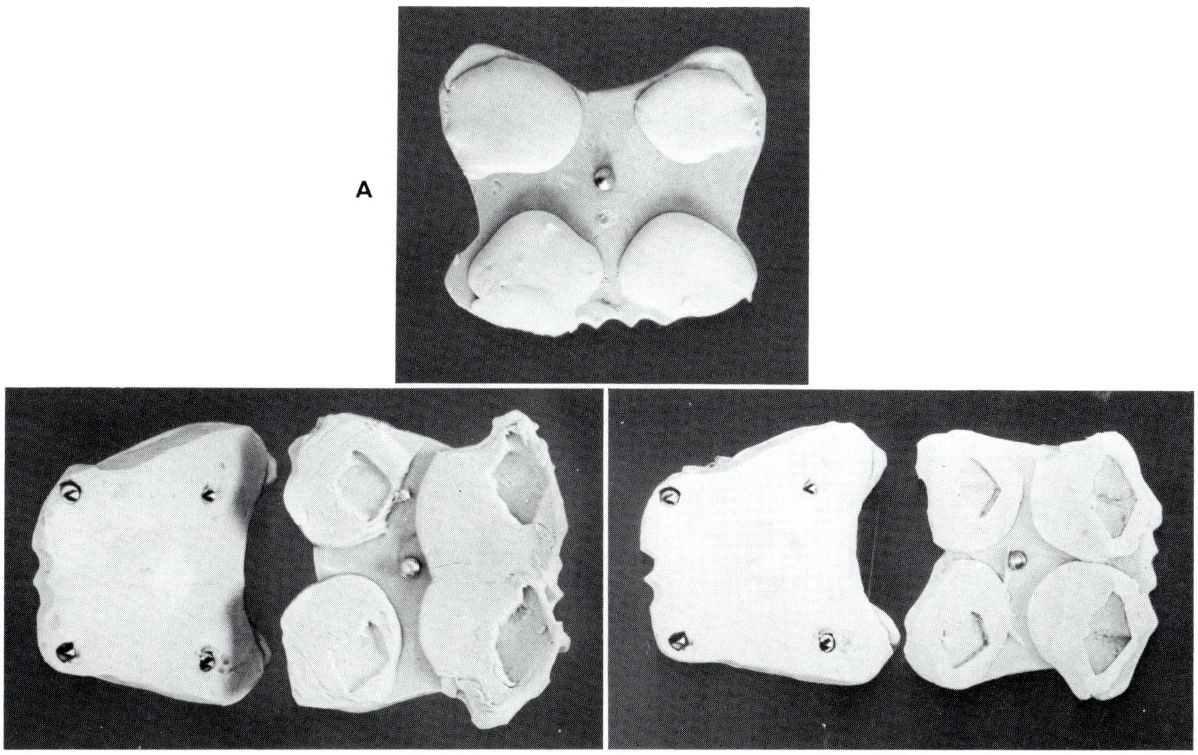

Fig. 3-145. A, Spray the maxillary clutch with silicone release agent or apply petroleum jelly to the convex surface and around the studs. Place the maxillary clutch on the upper teeth. Place a mix of TMJ acrylic on each recording area and wait till it has set to the putty stage. **B,** When the acrylic reaches the putty or dough stage, spray with release agent, place the lower clutch in the mouth, and have patient move into the various mandibular movements. It is essential to record a good protrusive movement and a good right and left lateral border movement including the Bennett shift. **C,** On the lathe wheel, remove all excess material around the recordings of the studs. Taper cuts away from the recorded area. When recording is rechecked in the mouth, nothing must touch but the studs and central bearing screw in any movement. Strive for a smooth free-riding recording.

A B C D E

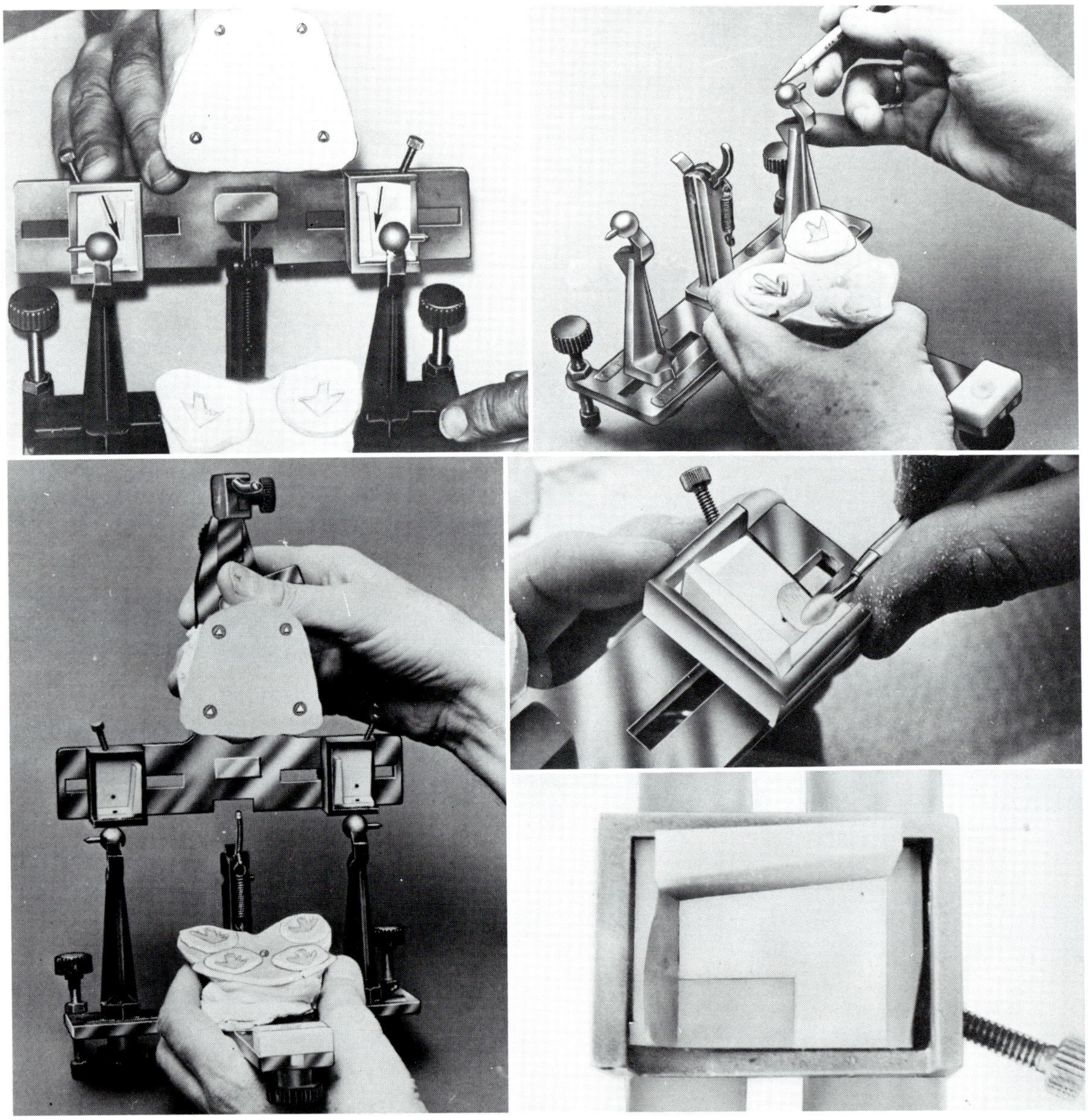

Fig. 3-146. A, When the fossa boxes are positioned at the same millimeter reading as the condyle posts, there is automatically some space allowed for Bennett shift, but check to see if it is sufficient. If not, remove some additional material from the box. **B,** Mark the height of contour of the condyle ball with a soft lead pencil or other coloring agent. **C,** Carefully replace the upper member of the instrument and move it several times in terminal hinge position to mark this position in the fossa box. **D,** Remove a portion of the box laterally from the medial portion of these two marks to allow outward and upward or outward and backward movement of the rotating condyle if it is dictated by the recording. **E,** Newer boxes have been modified so that this cut is already made. It is, however, advisable to check these in the same way.

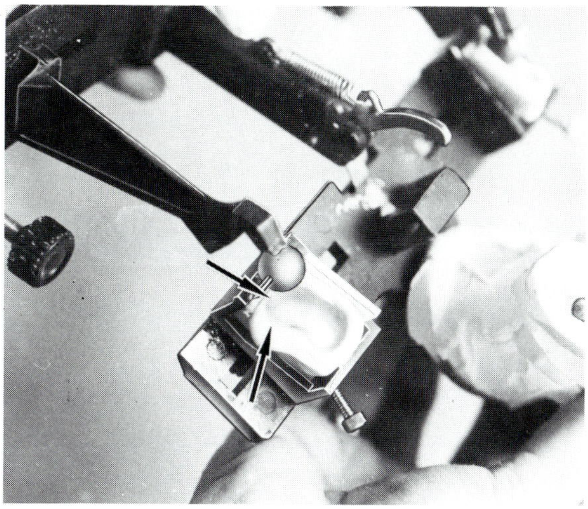

Fig. 3-147. Mix some TMJ acrylic and let it set up until it can be handled in the fingers. Place a small portion in each fossa box (do not use excess), lubricate condyle balls, spray a release agent in the depression, and guide the condyle balls into the filled boxes so that they maintain contact with the posterior interior wall of the fossa box till the hinge position is reached, thus avoiding displacing of anterior material. The studs are drawn over the recordings in protrusive and right and left lateral border movements to form the fossae. The operator may make several passes over the recordings until the acrylic has set. Each time all studs must follow and continually contact their respective paths—this is a "must." Pressure on the forefinger must be directed inward, downward, and forward to assure faithful recording of border movement and working side movement. In lateral movement the thumbs press laterally and downward but not distally. Excess material should be removed from the completed fossa as shown by arrows.

A

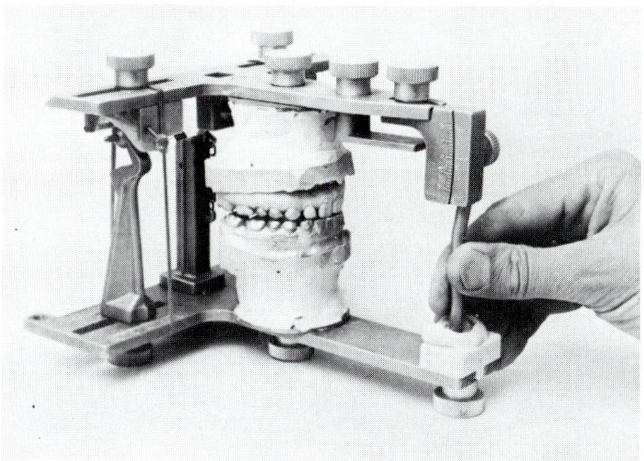

B

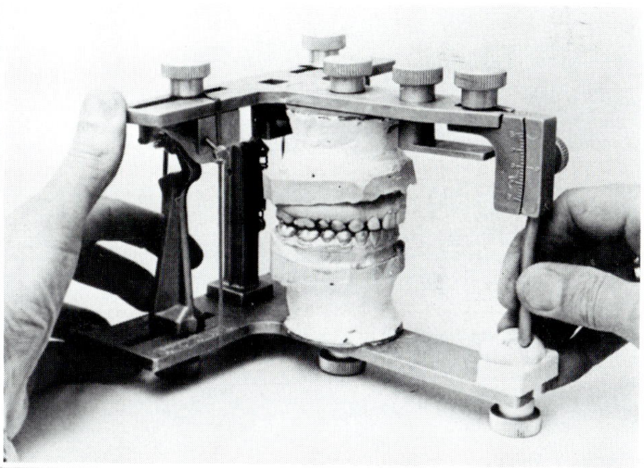

C

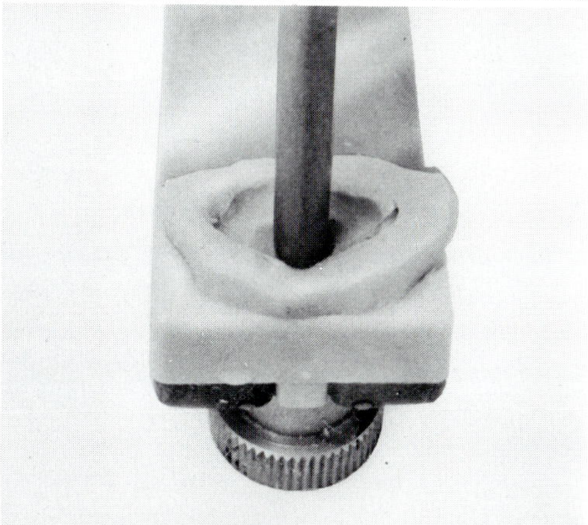

Fig. 3-148. Recording anterior guidance of posterior disclusion. **A,** Protrusive: carefully make the instrument follow the overbite and overjet of the anterior teeth. **B,** Lateral: Follow the cuspid rise on each side, and be certain to incorporate Bennett shift. **C,** Finished incisal table excess can be trimmed away.

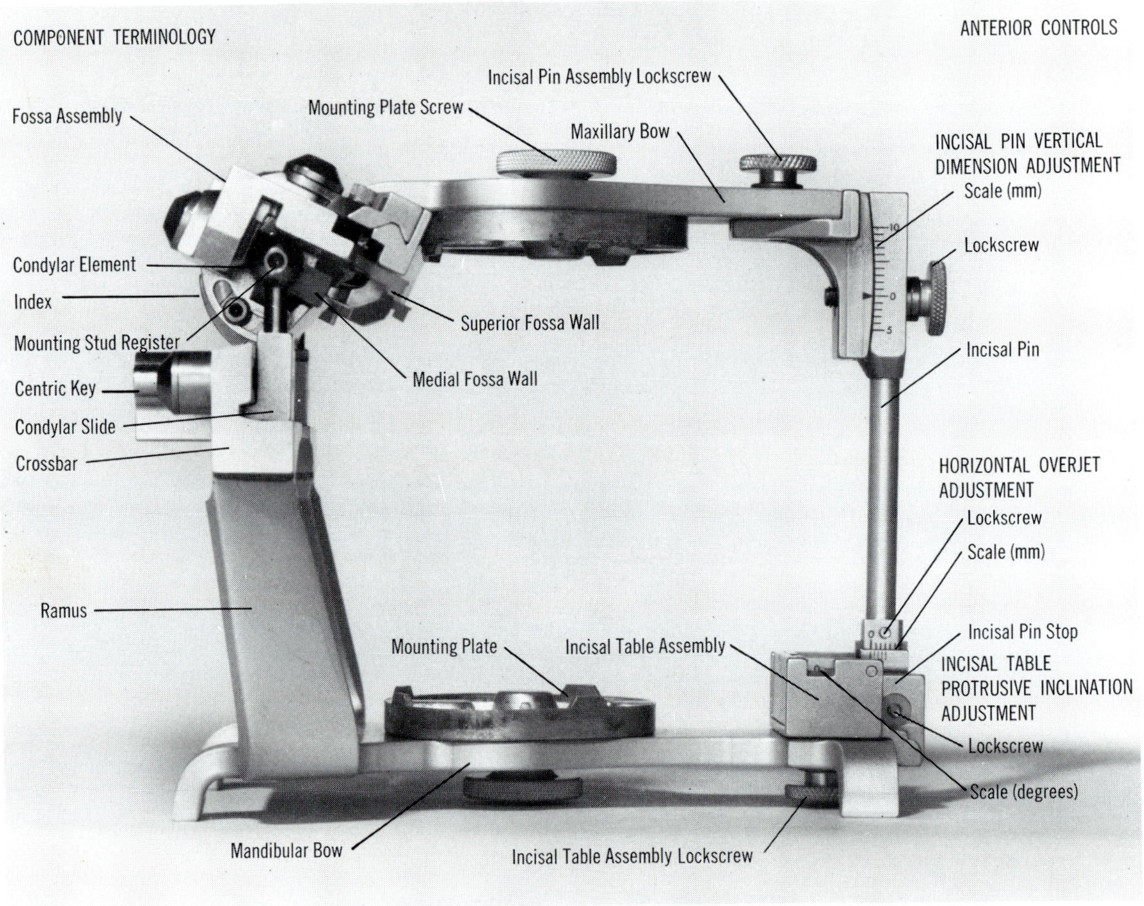

Fig. 3-149. The Denar articulator, a fully adjustable instrument. (Courtesy Denar Corp., Anaheim, Calif.).

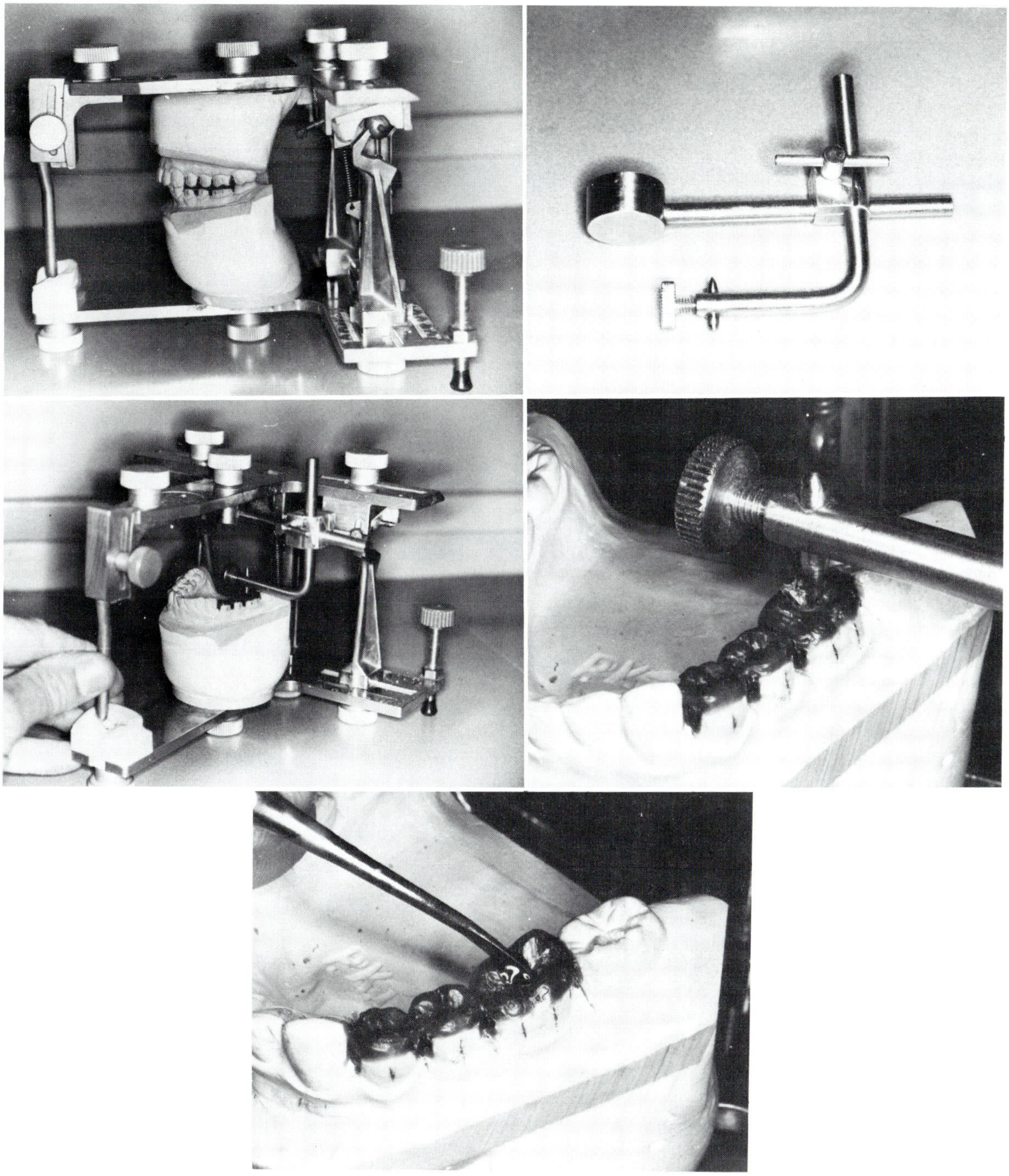

Fig. 3-150. The Automatic Wax Carver. The Automatic Wax Carver gives the dentist or the technician the means for determining cusp height and groove direction in harmony with previously established and clinically acceptable anterior occlusion. The Automatic Wax Carver (available from TMJ Instrument Co., Inc., Thousand Oaks, Calif.) is an instrument which, when secured to the upper member of an articulator, can be adjusted to place a stylus into the center of any selected fossa of a lower wax pattern. When the articulator is then moved through the various excursions as dictated by condylar movement and anterior guidance, the stylus duplicates the path of the upper lingual cusp as it exits from the fossa in the various excursive movements. In order to get the full benefit from this instrument, it is necessary that the articulator be reasonably accurate in duplicating condylar movements and that the anterior teeth present acceptable occlusion. (Courtesy Dr. Alvin J. Fillastre, Lakeland, Fla.)

REFERENCES

1. Ante, I. H.: The fundamental principles of abutments, Mich. State Dent. Soc. Bull. **8:**14, 1926.
2. Goldman, Henry M., and Cohen, D. Walter: Periodontal therapy, ed. 5, St. Louis, 1973, The C. V. Mosby Co., pp. 267-269.
3. Simpson, Clarence O.: Technic of oral radiography, ed. 2, St. Louis, 1928, The C. V. Mosby Co.
4. Wuehrmann, Arthur H.: The long cone technic, Practical Dental Monographs, Chicago, 1957, Year Book Medical Publishers, Inc.
5. Williams, Sam W.: The paralleling technic for intraoral roentgenology, J.A.D.A. **43:**419-434, 1951.
6. Frank, Leonard: A long distance and low penetration technique for dental x-ray units, Dent. Dig. **44:**114, 1938.
7. Hutchinson, A. C. W.: Dental radiology, Dent. Progr. **3:**19-27, 1962.
8. Richards, A. G.: Roentgen ray doses in dental roentgenography, J.A.D.A. **56:**351, 1958.
9. Buchholz, Robert E.: Radiographic interpretation of proximal carious lesions, Dent. Radiogr. Photogr. **38:**9-12, 1965.
10. Wainright, W. W., and Villanyi, A. A.: Film speed—greatest single factor in the reduction of radiation to dentist and patient, J. S. Calif. State Dent. Assoc., **26:**429-430, 1958.
11. Wuehrmann, A. H.: Roentgenographic interpretation of dental caries, Practical Dental Monographs, Chicago, 1959, Year Book Medical Publishers, Inc., pp. 1-46.
12. Simpson, Clarence O.: Personal communication.
13. Simpson, Clarence O.: Notes from seminar lectures delivered in 1951.
14. Ramfjord, S. P., and Ash, Major M., Jr.: Occlusion, ed. 2, Philadelphia, 1971, W. B. Saunders Co.
15. Lucia, Victor O.: Modern gnathological concepts, St. Louis, 1961, The C. V. Mosby Co., pp. 37, 38
16. Teteruck, Walter, R., and Lundeen, Harry C.: The accuracy of an ear face-bow, J. Prosthet. Dent. **16:**1039-1046, 1966.
17. Dawson, Peter E.: Personal communication.
18. Granger, E. R.: Functional relations of the stomatognathic system, J.A.D.A. **48:**638-647, 1954.
19. Celenza, Frank V.: Personal communication.
20. Lucia, Victor O.: Centric relation—theory and practice, J. Prosthet. Dent. **10:**849-856, 1960.
21. Kornfeld, Max: The problem of function in restorative dentistry, J. Prosthet. Dent. **5:**670-676, 1955.
22. Lucia, Victor O.: A technique for recording centric relation, J. Prosthet. Dent. **14:**492-505, 1964.
23. Dykins, William R.: Requirements of partial denture prosthesis, J.A.D.A. **58:**232-236, 1958.
24. Dykins, William R.: Personal communication.
25. Ryan, Edward, J.: Personal communication.
26. Jamieson, Charles H.: Geriatrics and the denture patient, J. Prosthet. Dent. **8:**8-13, 1958.
27. Ryan, Edward J.: The dental problems of senescence, J. Prosthet. Dent. **1:**64-70, 1951.
28. Cowdry, E. V.: Factors in aging, Sci. Mon. **56:**370, 1943.
29. Carlson, Anton: Physiologic changes of normal aging. In Stieglitz, Edward J., editor: Geriatric medicine, ed. 2, Philadelphia, 1949, W. B. Saunders Co., p. 49.
30. Silverman, Sidney: Dental care for the aged; role of the private practitioner, J.A.D.A. **64:**165-172, 1962.
31. Stieglitz, Edward J.: Aging as a problem of nutrition, Nutr. News **13:**6, 1949.
32. Kronfeld, Rudolf: Dental histology and comparative dental anatomy, Philadelphia, 1937, Lea & Febiger.
33. Schabel, Russell: The psychology of aging, J. Prosthet. Dent. **27:**569-573, 1972.

CHAPTER 4

CENTRIC RELATION—THEORY AND PRACTICE*

VICTOR O. LUCIA, D.D.S., F.A.C.D.

DEFINITION

Webster's *Collegiate Dictionary* defines "centric" as follows: "adj. 1. Placed in or at the center or middle: central. 2. Of, pertaining to, or characterized by a center." Is this definition in any way related to what is generally understood by centric in dentistry?

The *Glossary of Prosthodontic Terms*[1] gives this definition of centric relation: "The most retruded relation of the mandible to the maxillae when the condyles are in the most posterior unstrained position in the glenoid fossae from which lateral movement can be made, at any given degree of jaw separation."

The American Dental Association definition of 1955 is not unlike the one in the *Glossary*.

The only inference of a center may be in the phrase, "from which lateral movement can be made," and I doubt whether this was intended. However, I shall endeavor to show that the dictionary definition can very definitely be applied to the centric relation of dentistry.

With which center are we going to be concerned? There are literally millions of centers of mandibular movement. The problem depends on which movements are made and to what they are related. These centers are instantaneous and are changing constantly with each slight movement.

We must concern ourselves with a center that can be located easily, that can be useful for our procedures—a center that will enable us to reproduce the patient's movements on a suitable articulator and to execute our work more intelligently and with greater ease.

The objective of records of centric relation is to relate the mandible to the maxillae (and, in turn, the teeth) so that there can be no fulcrum on the teeth (and periodontal ligaments), but only in the temporomandibular joints. Whether many patients have this condition normally is of no consequence. The important thing is that when the ravages of pathosis are present, the fulcrum must be in the temporomandibular joint if the destruction by the pathosis is to be minimized. This is a mechanical necessity that has

*Modified from Lucia, Victor O.: Centric relation—theory and practice, J. Prosthet. Dent. **10:**849-856, 1960; and Lucia, Victor O.: A technique for recording centric relation, J. Prosthet. Dent. **14:**492-505, 1964.

biologic soundness. Many materials, methods, and devices have been used to fulfill this objective. None of these is universally effective. Yet every sincere dentist doing full mouth rehabilitation has confessed, at one time or another, either publicly or privately, that his lot would be considerably easier if he could be sure of the centric relation record of his patient.

SIGNIFICANCE OF CENTRIC RELATION

Centric relation is a specific relationship of the centers of rotation of the mandible to the maxillae. There is a center of vertical arcing motion in each condyle. These centers of vertical motion are joined by an imaginary line called the hinge axis. In addition, on this hinge axis are two centers of lateral motion—one in each condyle. When the centers of vertical arcing motion and of lateral motion coincide and are in the most posterior terminal position in relation to the maxillae, the mandible and maxillae are in centric relation.

All the movements of the mandible are governed by the centers of rotation. To duplicate these movements on an articulator, the centers of rotation must be located. Moreover, when a patient chews or in any way brings his teeth together, the normal action is to seat the condyles in the rearmost, uppermost position. Unless the condyles are uppermost the restorations made will be in supraocclusion.

All normal swallowing occurs in centric relation. The resultant vector of force of the masticating muscles indicates this relationship. The anatomy dictates this.

Unless centric occlusion occurs when the mandible is in centric relation, there will be a strain on the periodontal tissues of the teeth. Teeth that have lost their supporting structures can least afford to be fulcrums of the masticating mechanism. Lateral forces will be created, and these are destructive.

When pathosis has taken a toll of the supporting structures, it becomes necessary to provide as much "bracing" as possible for the weakened teeth. One means is to set a posterior limit for the movements of the mandible. In this way weakened upper teeth cannot be rocked distally, and weakened lower teeth cannot be rocked mesially. The posterior superior limit of mandibular position, which is maintained by centric relation–holding contacts on the occlusal surfaces, makes possible the stabilization of weakened teeth. When splinting is necessary, additional stability is obtained by the posterior superior position of the mandible.

The upper teeth are like a horseshoe on an anvil. The lower teeth are like the hammer. The anvil and hammer are not damaged in use, but the horseshoe is. The upper teeth can be knocked out of the maxillae by malfunction.

Upper teeth get rocked distally as well as mesially when the mandible is out of centric relation, whereas lower teeth can be rocked only mesially.

Unless the starting point for establishing the anatomy of restorations is correct, the other relationships cannot possibly be right. An improper centric relation record will cause difficulty in the preparation of teeth.

DIFFICULTIES OF RECORDING CENTRIC RELATION

To record the mandible's path of vertical movement in the terminal hinge position the patient must be deceived. The dentist has to block out all the proprioceptive impulses that direct the movements. The proprioceptive impulses are responsible for the awareness of the position of the mandible in space. The impulses guide the mandible in its habitual movements. The reflex actions that take place are reinforced by the proprioceptive stimuli. One of the natural reflex acts of the mandible is to close into a lateral or a lateral protruded position when something is introduced into the mouth (Fig. 4-1). This is what happens when a material such as wax is placed in the mouth and the patient is told to bite. It is necessary to obtain a relationship of the terminal hinge action without any lateral deviation. One practical way of blocking out the proprioception is to prevent the teeth from coming together (Fig. 4-2). The relationship of the mandible to the maxillae in the terminal hinge position without tooth contact must be obtained. Consequently, the patient must be trained and guided to execute the terminal hinge action.

The mechanical procedures necessary to relate the mandible to the maxillae present the problem. Our task would be simple if a magic material that would solidify at a given word could be inserted between the teeth when the lower jaw is executing a perfect terminal hinge closure. Unfortunately, we have no such material! The materials available to us are thermoplastic or chemoset. The thermoplastics have to have some "body" in order to be manipulated. The chemoset materials require some time to undergo their chemical change and thus set. Neither of these qualities or characteristics is at all satisfactory.

One thing should be understood. Any material could be used in some mouths and a satisfactory re-

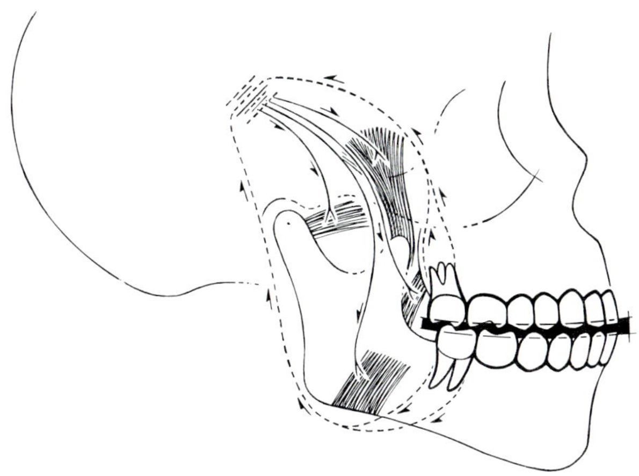

Fig. 4-1. Schematic drawing showing mechanism involved when a proprioceptive stimulus comes into play as second molars penetrate the wax and make a premature contact. This reflex act will preclude possibility of a terminal hinge closure. (From Lucia, Victor O.: J. Prosthet. Dent. **10**:849-856, 1960.)

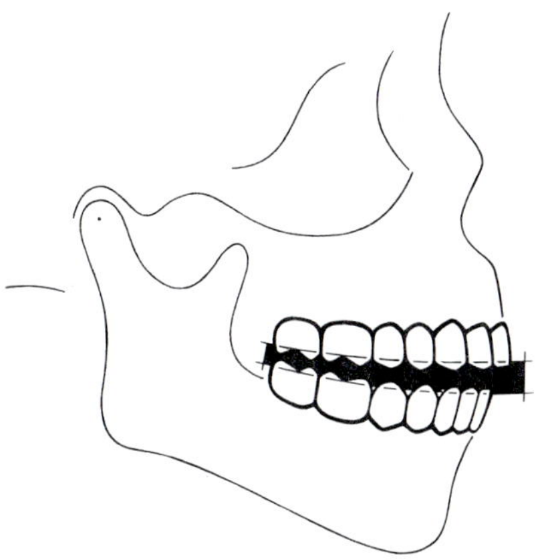

Fig. 4-2. An attempt to block out proprioception is made with a thick wax wafer. Use of such a wafer requires hinge axis—mounted casts. (From Lucia, Victor O.: J. Prosthet. Dent. **10**:849-856, 1960.)

sult could be obtained. However, this cannot be done in many instances in which the patients are more difficult to control.

Most patients have a reflex closure, an engram, determined and guided by the teeth. The proprioceptive mechanism determines the path of mandibular closure. This "meshing" of teeth may or may not take place when the mandible is in centric relation to the maxillae. To determine whether there is coincidence between centric occlusion and centric relation, it is necessary to remove the guidance provided by the teeth. The guidance is eliminated by making the recording at an increased vertical dimension. The proprioceptive reflex must be blocked out to ensure a perfect hinge closure. This is done by the recording medium. Either it is thick enough to "short-circuit" the reflex, or it offers so little resistance (or conduction) that it does not set off the proprioceptive reflex. In either case the recording must be made with the mouth open to the point that the teeth do not touch. This explains the need for a hinge axis location and transfer.

In addition to a peculiar engram, a patient may have what we call a "loose joint," one that, because of improper function, has acquired the habit of "dropping apart" whenever any suggestion of a malrelationship may exist. (This "falling apart" may be experienced when a centric relation record is made.)

Some patients have developed powerful reflexes to avoid injury to their tissues. It requires time and special manipulation to overcome these reflexes and to be able to record the correct relationship.

UNFAVORABLE REFLEX ACTION

A young patient was to be used to demonstrate a new centric relation record method. He had a full complement of teeth and a "good" centric occlusal relationship. The patient was examined by the members of our study group, and all agreed that the relationship of the lower teeth to the upper teeth was excellent.

We proceeded to make a centric relation record. In doing this we had to prepare an anterior "bite block" of cold-curing acrylic resin. It was necessary to adjust the block by having the patient slide his teeth around and bite on the block to mark it with articulating paper. The block was slowly reduced to the desired height in about 20 minutes. Then we made the centric relation records and, by means of a split-cast procedure, checked one record carefully against the other. The two records checked perfectly.

As we admired our results it was suggested that we see how well the teeth occluded on the instrument. What we observed seemed incredible! The cusps of the teeth were almost tip to tip. The contacts were entirely different from the occlusion we had seen in the mouth before we made the recording. We put the patient back in the chair for another examination, and now with very little guidance he closed his teeth together exactly as those on the casts on the articulator.

This same patient with the same guidance now exhibited a horrible centric occlusion! It looked as though we had "fractured the necks" of the condyles. What must have happened was that the strong reflex act of closing eccentrically was broken by our procedure. It fooled four experienced dentists. This experience indicated to us the importance of training a patient before examining him for the location of premature (deflective occlusal) contacts.

LOCATION OF THE CENTERS OF ROTATION

To locate the all-important center of rotation it is necessary to reduce the jaw movements to their simplest form. The jaw can open and close in a hinge movement. This is not a normal movement, but it is one that the patient can be taught for the dentist's convenience. By teaching the patient this hingelike action one can locate the center of this action and make use of it by reproducing the same center on an articulator.

That there is a hinge axis hardly requires any defense. It is now almost universally accepted. We will try to demonstrate its importance. That there is only one axis will have to be accepted for the moment. It has been proved.

LOCATION OF HINGE AXIS

The hinge axis points are located by means of a hinge-bow, which is rigidly attached to the lower teeth. The stylus points in the temporomandibular joint region are adjusted, while the mandible is guided in a terminal hinge closure, until there is no longer any arcing but only pure rotation by the tip of the stylus.

To bring the teeth into contact on the articulator the lower cast must travel toward the upper cast. Thus, unless the closure is made on the same arc as the patient's mandibular closure, the teeth will not contact correctly. The correct mounting of casts on an articulator definitely depends upon the location of the hinge axis of the patient and its transfer to the articulator.

The center of vertical movement of the mandible is found by locating the hinge axis. This enables us to place casts of the mouth on an articulator, which will duplicate the opening and closing component of movement (Figs. 4-3 and 4-4).

The mandible is also capable of lateral movement, and there is a center for this lateral movement. By the use of twin Gothic arch (needle point) tracings in the horizontal plane, which are made outside the patient's mouth on either side of the midline, it is possible to locate the centers of lateral movement. These are located in the condyles and on the hinge axis. These centers can be duplicated on an articulator that has an adjustable intercondylar distance (Figs. 4-5 to 4-7).

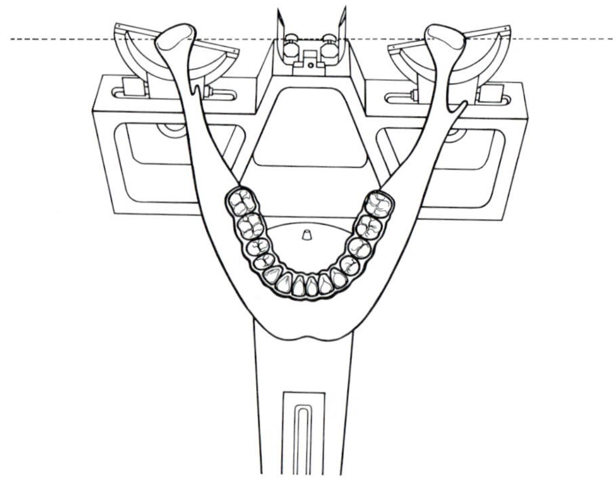

Fig. 4-3. Relation of lower teeth (and mandible) to hinge axis of articulator. (From Lucia, Victor O.: J. Prosthet. Dent. **10:**849-856, 1960.)

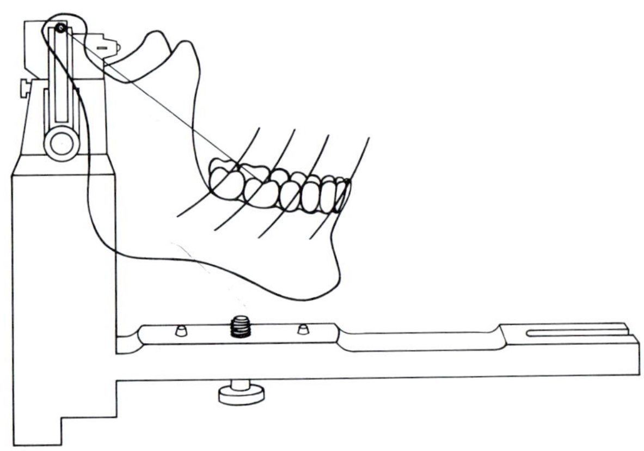

Fig. 4-4. Relation of lower teeth to arc of closure of articulator. Use of hinge axis permits these arcs to be identical with those of patient's mandible. (From Lucia, Victor O.: J. Prosthet. Dent. **10:**849-856, 1960.)

By these two procedures the centers of rotation, both vertical and lateral, have been located and duplicated. When these centers are duplicated on an articulator and the paths of these centers reproduced, all the patient's mandibular movements can be duplicated very easily. All it now requires is a pair of hands to supply the muscular force and a mind to direct those hands.

It becomes necessary to think of the centers of rotation as made of two components, the center of vertical motion and the center of lateral motion. They

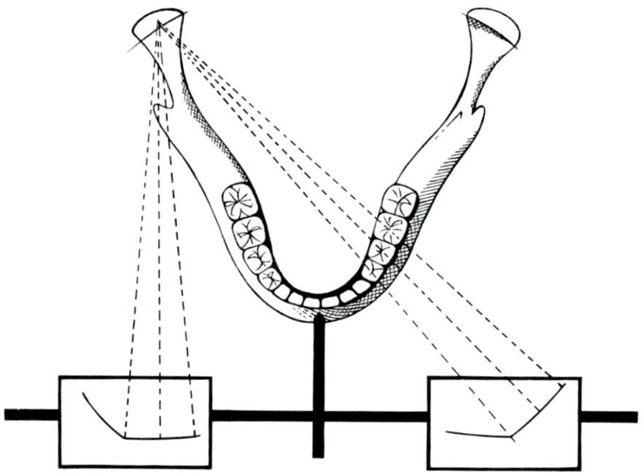

Fig. 4-5. Relation of center of lateral rotation to respective wings of the two tracings. (From Lucia, Victor O.: J. Prosthet. Dent. **10:**849-856, 1960.)

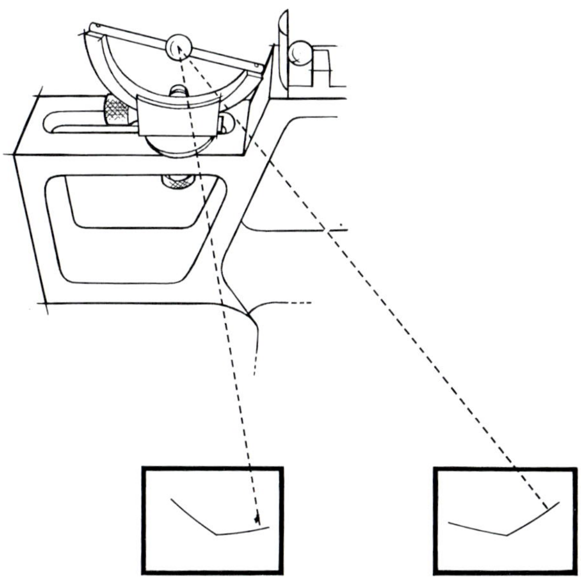

Fig. 4-6. Wings of tracings that were made on a patient are used to locate center of lateral rotation on an articulator. (From Lucia, Victor O.: J. Prosthet. Dent. **10:**849-856, 1960.)

are one and the same center—one in each condyle. These centers determine all the possible movements of the mandible. They are located in the condyles and travel wherever the mandible goes. They are the centers of its every movement. When these centers are in their terminal hinge position, the mandible is in centric relation to the maxillae.

After the centers of lateral motion are recorded

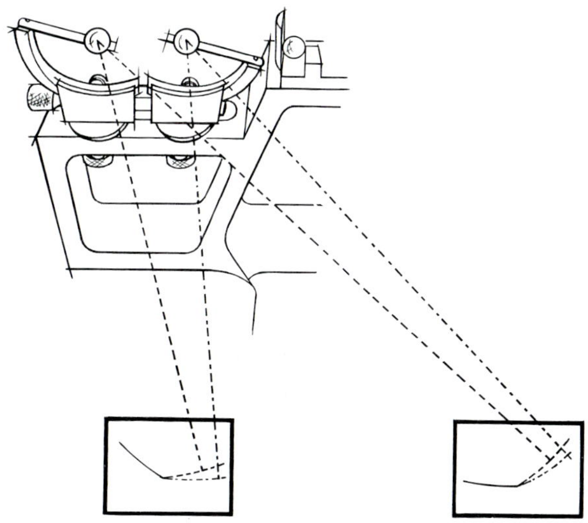

Fig. 4-7. Composite drawing to show different locations of center of lateral rotation as determined by tracings from two different patients. (From Lucia, Victor O.: J. Prosthet. Dent. **10:**849-856, 1960.)

and an articulator adjusted to these centers, the casts of the patient's mouth must be oriented to the articulator. The upper cast is easily related to the upper member of the articulator by means of a transfer bow. Certain precautions are necessary. Care must be taken that the patient is sitting in the same way as when the marks were put on the face and that the imprints of the face-bow fork are accurate for seating the cast.

Now the most difficult part of the procedure has to be undertaken, that is, relating the mandible to the maxillae. Before we discuss the reason why this is so difficult, let us review what has been done.

1. The articulator was set for the centers of lateral rotation by means of the twin Gothic arch (needle point) tracings. (The intercondylar distance has been established.)

2. The hinge axis has been located. If we could "freeze" the *hinge action* used to locate the hinge axis at a convenient vertical relation, the centric relation would have been recorded. The hinge action used to locate the hinge axis had to be in the terminal position; otherwise, the hinge axis could not be located. Thus it would fulfill the requirements of centric relation.

TECHNIQUE FOR SECURING IDENTICAL CENTRIC RELATION RECORDS

The best way to check a centric relation record is to secure two or more identical records. Previously we would insert a second centric relation record between the casts. If the articulator parts were not displaced, we would accept it as a check on the record used to mount the casts. The split-cast technique, which was originated by Needles[2] and used by Lauritzen,[3] is a simple method for comparing interocclusal records. Many *apparently* acceptable records are not correct.

PREPARATION OF UPPER CAST FOR SPLIT-CAST TECHNIQUE

The upper cast is poured very carefully, and the initial set is allowed to occur. The impression is not inverted. The cast is not poured with a very thick base because we must add a smooth base to it. A vacuum mix of stone is made, and a bubble-free base is attached to the cast. The cast is set on a glass slab to form a smooth surface (Fig. 4-8).

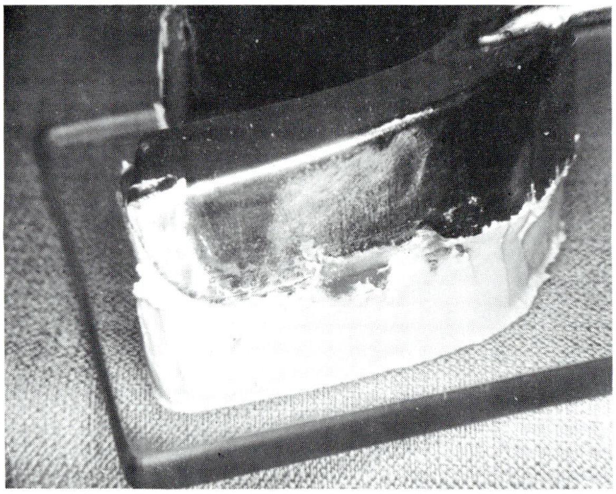

Fig. 4-8. Glass slab produces a smooth surface on base of cast. (From Lucia, Victor O.: J. Prosthet. Dent. **14:**492-505, 1964.)

When the base is set, the cast is separated from the impression and is trimmed in preparation for making the second part of the split cast. Shallow V grooves are cut on the periphery of the base of the cast—about six of them—two on each side and two in back. These grooves must be shallow and cut smoothly so that they will separate freely from the second part of the split cast.

To make the second part of the split cast we wrap some No. 33 Scotch Brand electrical tape around the prepared cast (Fig. 4-9), lubricate the cast with a separating fluid,* and pour into this form a well-spatulated, vacuum-mixed stone. Three knobs of stone are left to serve as a handle for separation after the stone sets. The tape is removed, and the second half is separated from the cast and then put together again. The knobs are ground down to permit clearance with the upper member of the articulator.

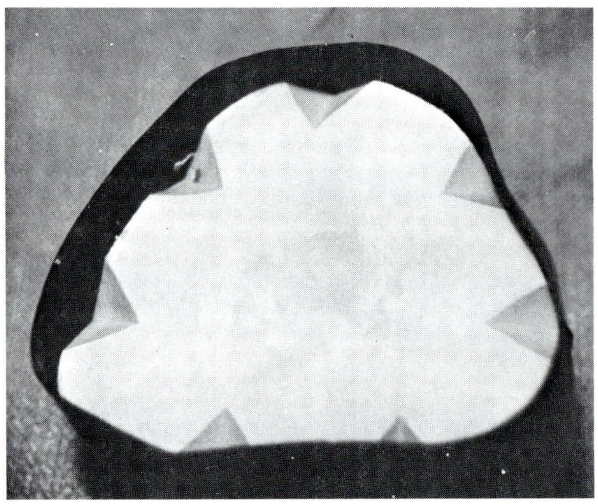

Fig. 4-9. No. 33 Scotch Brand electric tape wrapped around notched upper cast provides a form into which the stone is poured to make split cast. (From Lucia, Victor O.: J. Prosthet. Dent. **14:**492-505, 1964.)

A face-bow transfer is made, and the cast and wafer are related carefully to the centers of rotation of the articulator. The cast and wafer are mounted on the articulator.

Construction and adjustment of the centric relation jig

The centric relation jig is made of DuraLay,† a self-curing plastic. It should be prepared on a set of mounted casts because considerable heat is generated in its construction. If made in the mouth, the oral tissues may be burned.

*Super Sep, Kerr Dental Mfg. Co., Detroit, Mich.

†Reliance Dental Mfg. Co., Chicago, Ill.

Tinfoil is adapted over the upper six anterior teeth and allowed to extend beyond the gingival margin for about a half inch. The incisal pin of the articulator is set so that the bicuspids are about 5 mm. apart.

The DuraLay is mixed in a dappen dish and, when doughy, is placed on the tinfoil covering the upper anterior teeth to cover the labial and lingual surfaces and extend onto the soft tissues (Fig. 4-10).

The DuraLay is molded to form a platform on the lingual surfaces of the upper anterior teeth. While the material is still soft, the articulator is closed so that

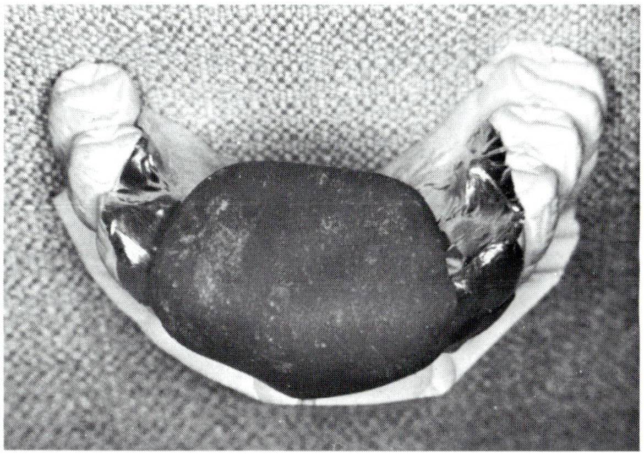

Fig. 4-10. DuraLay in "dough" stage is adapted over tin foil-covered anterior part of upper cast to form an anterior jig. (From Lucia, Victor O.: J. Prosthet. Dent. 14:492-505, 1964.)

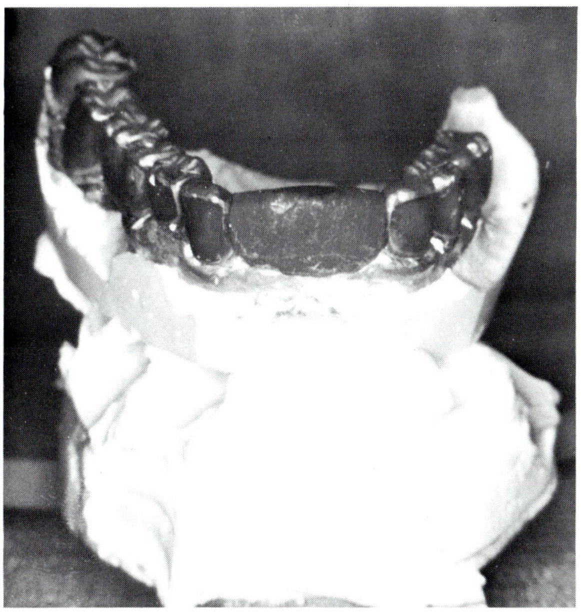

Fig. 4-11. DuraLay "bridge" joins cuspid abutments to replace lower anterior teeth that were missing. (From Lucia, Victor O.: J. Prosthet. Dent. 14:492-505, 1964.)

the lower anterior teeth contact the platform established on the lingual surfaces of the upper anterior teeth. This is done while the DuraLay is still moldable. It can be adjusted approximately to the opening established by the incisal pin. The DuraLay is adapted carefully to the cast to ensure a good fit. Also, periodically, the DuraLay is lifted slightly so that it will not lock into undercuts and break the teeth off the cast. Our object is to have a well-fitting jig that can be removed from the cast.

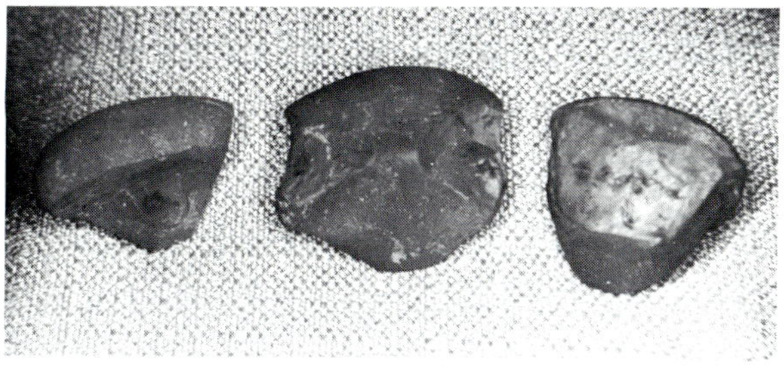

Fig. 4-12. Three variations in shape of jigs for different anterior tooth relation. (From Lucia, Victor O.: J. Prosthet. Dent. 14:492-505, 1964.)

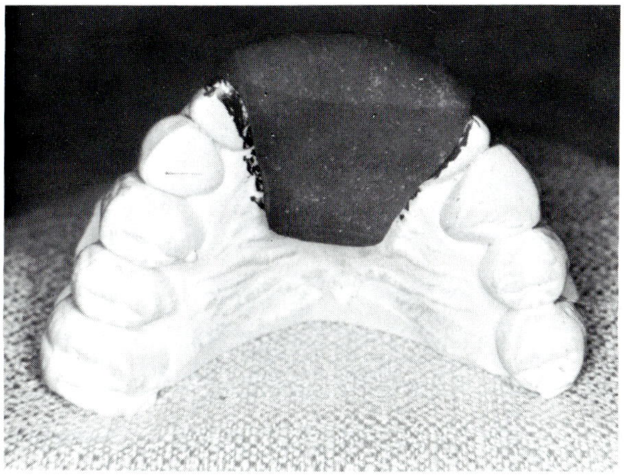

Fig. 4-13. Jig trimmed and ready for use. (From Lucia, Victor O.: J. Prosthet. Dent. 14:492-505, 1964.)

Variations of the jig may be necessary, depending on the number and positions of the anterior teeth as well as the relation of the lower teeth to the upper teeth. In some instances an anterior "bridge" of DuraLay may have to be made (Fig. 4-11). Other situations may call for other modifications (Fig. 4-12).

When the jig is completely "cured," it is trimmed and adjusted. With a straight carborundum disk the jig is cut buccolingually through the incisal surface just lateral to the distal margin of the central incisors (Fig. 4-13). The cut is directed at an angle so that the lingual part of the jig is considerably narrower than the labial part. The labial gingival part is trimmed and contoured until it is narrowed and rounded and does not interfere with the labial frenum. The margin usually extends 1 or 2 mm. beyond the gingival margins of the anterior teeth. This part of the procedure can be done with acrylic trimmers.

The lingual surface of the jig is trimmed to be

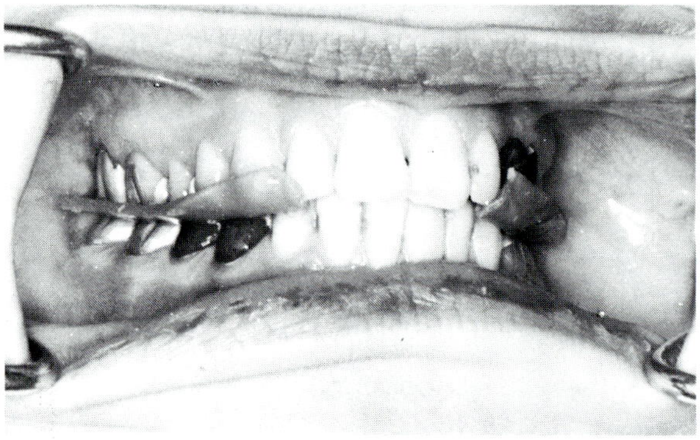

Fig. 4-14. Wax wafer is formed and thinned between teeth so that mandible is approximately in centric relation. (From Lucia, Victor O.: J. Prosthet. Dent. **14:**492-505, 1964.)

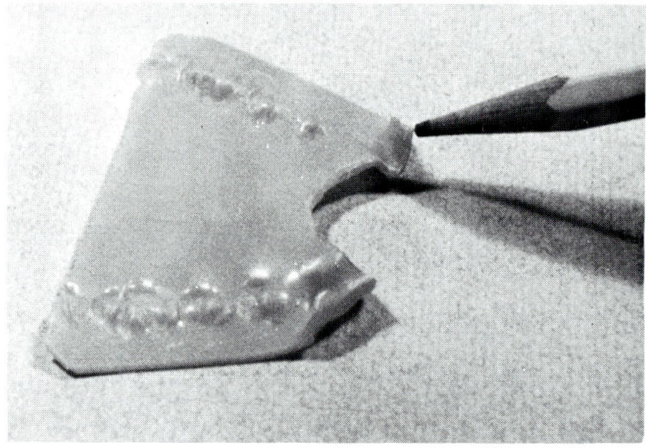

Fig. 4-15. Wax wafer is formed with turned-up corners (ears) to guide its reseating in mouth after Kydac paste has been placed on it. Wax wafer acts as a tray to carry recording medium. (From Lucia, Victor O.: J. Prosthet. Dent. **14:**492-505, 1964.)

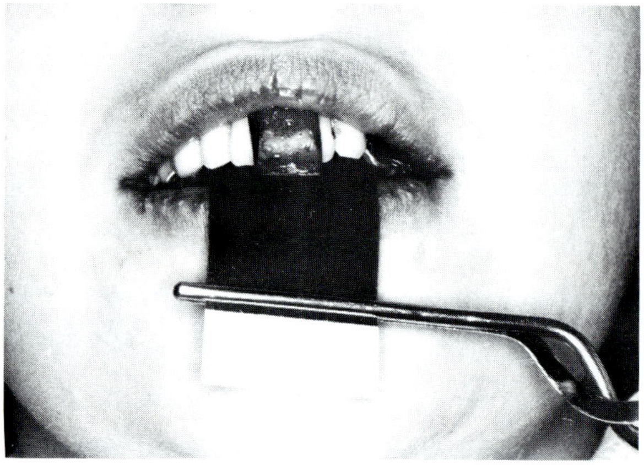

Fig. 4-16. Patient is trained to close in centric relation by sliding the teeth around and marking jig with articulating paper. Height of jig is reduced after marking and sliding motions are repeated to mark jig for further reduction. (From Lucia, Victor O.: J. Prosthet. Dent. **14:**492-505, 1964.)

comfortable to the tongue. It usually extends several millimeters onto the palatal tissues.

A piece of Sure-Set* baseplate wax is held against a maxillary cast to make a wax tray. With a pair of scissors the baseplate wax is trimmed until about ⅜ inch of wax extends beyond the buccal surfaces of the teeth. The wax tray is cut across just anterior to the cuspids, and a U-shaped cut is removed from the anterior part to permit the jig to seat without touching the wax tray when both are in the mouth. Three such trays are prepared by using the first one as a pattern for the others.

The wax is softened in water at 130° F. With the patient's cheeks retracted the wax tray is carefully placed on the upper teeth; one must be sure that the tray is centered as it was cut on the cast. The patient's mandible is guided into a centric closure, and the patient is instructed to hold this position firmly for a second (Fig. 4-14).

During this time the corners of the wax tray are turned up in the cuspid region so that the tray has two little "ears," one in each corner of the mouth (Fig. 4-15). The "ears" will help to reposition the wax tray on the upper teeth in the next step.

The wax tray is removed and chilled. This procedure is repeated with the other two wafers.

Each of the chilled wax trays is placed in position and guided by the "cuspid ears." The patient's mandible is guided into centric relation. This will correct any warpage that may have occurred. The wafers are stored in water.

The jig is placed in position, and its adjustment is started. *This is the most important function of the jig*. The procedures of adjustment seem to break the reflex pattern of closure, thus permitting a normal closure. It is this procedure of adjusting the jig in the mouth that differentiates this application of an anterior stop from previous methods. The adjustment procedure makes this technique work where others have failed in the past. This procedure performs the act of "training" the patient in an easy hinge closure.

By repeated adjustment of the jig the patient will bring the condyles to their uppermost position against the articular eminence and rearmost to the full extension of the temporomandibular ligament. The jig acts to disconnect the reflex circuit, thereby preventing

*Kerr Dental Mfg. Co., Detroit, Mich.

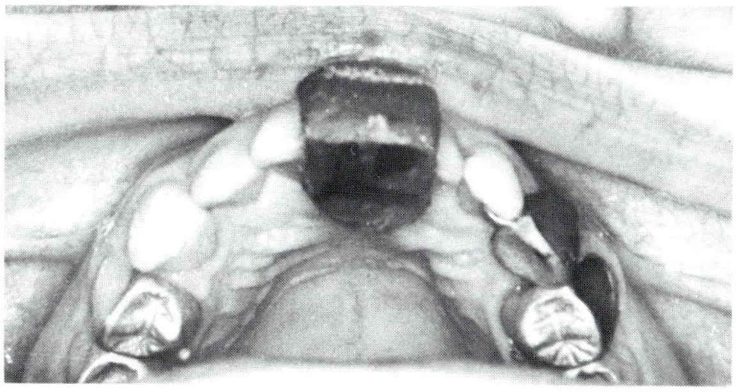

Fig. 4-17. Jig is in place after being adjusted. By the time height of jig is sufficiently reduced, patient is completely trained. (From Lucia, Victor O.: J. Prosthet. Dent. **14:**492-505, 1964.)

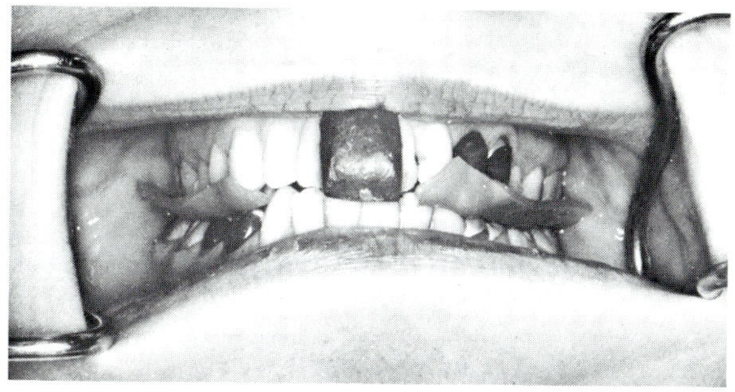

Fig. 4-18. Jig and wafer are in position. Wafer must be free of contact when lower teeth are closed against jig. (From Lucia, Victor O.: J. Prosthet. Dent. **14:**492-505, 1964.)

the patient from making incorrect closures of long-standing habit.

The adjustment is accomplished by marking with carbon paper (Fig. 4-16) and grinding with a rubber abrasive (Cratex*) wheel. The patient is instructed to move the mandible forward and backward and to each side. In so doing he will scribe a Gothic arch (needle point) tracing. (See Fig. 4-17.) With the rubber wheel the "wings" and "tail" of the tracing are carefully removed until only a circle at the apex of the tracing (about 3 mm. in diameter) is left.

The tracing is made by the lower central incisors whenever possible. The object is to have a definite platform on the jig against which a lower anterior tooth will rest without causing any *incorrect guidance* to the mandible. The surface must not incline to the right, or to the left, or forward. We want to establish the third point of the tripod (the two condyles posteriorly and the jig anteriorly). We prefer a *slight* upward and backward slant of the surface to make it easier for the patient to hold this position while the centric relation record is made.

The patient is instructed not to bring his teeth together when the jig is removed for adjustment; otherwise the effect of the training is lost.

Making the centric relation record

A wax wafer is placed in position, and the patient is instructed to close against the jig (Fig. 4-18). *The wax tray must be entirely free of the teeth when the patient is closed in centric relation.* All wax trays are checked for this clearance.

Note: When prepared teeth are involved, as is the case when master casts are to be mounted, it may be necessary to use two or three thicknesses of Sure-Set wax. The reason is that the paste to be used for the next step will not fill too large a space, and, although we desire clearance between the wax tray and the teeth (or restorations), the space must not be too great. We do not want any excessive vertical opening. In other words, there must be a minimum vertical opening, definite clearance, and just enough space between the teeth and the tray.

Once the patient is trained he must not be permitted to bring his teeth together until the procedure is completed. A few closures against his teeth would reestablish his engram.

The occlusal surfaces of the teeth are lubricated with Masque.* The jig is retained in place on the teeth with denture adhesive. There must be no movement of the jig when the patient closes against it.

A small mix of Kerr's Temp-Bond† paste is made. The material is tested to determine how much, if any accelerator is required to allow for ample working time and yet have a short setting time. The Temp-Bond is sparingly applied to the occlusal surfaces of the wax tray. The tray is positioned on the teeth as guided by the "ears." The patient's mandible is guided into centric relation (Fig. 4-19), taking care that he closes *firmly*. The mandible is held firmly in this position until the paste has set.

In removing the centric relation record the dentist must exercise care to avoid distortion. Both of the dentist's thumbs are placed on the patient's chin, and the index fingers are placed on the superior edges of the record. The patient is instructed to separate his

*Cratex Mfg. Co., Inc., Burlingame, Calif.

*Harry J. Bosworth Co., Chicago, Ill.

†Kerr Dental Mfg. Co., Detroit, Mich.

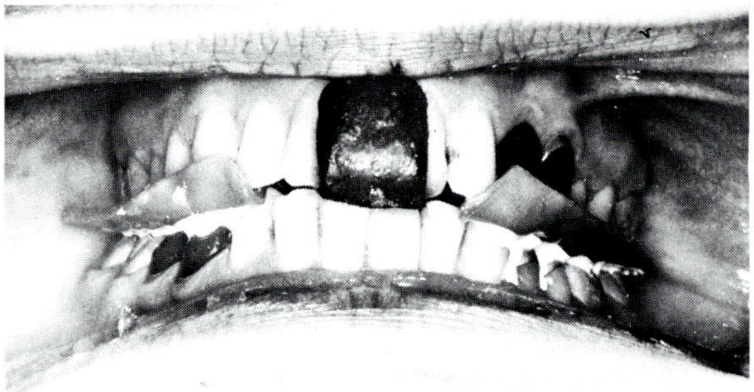

Fig. 4-19. Jig and Kerr's Temp-Bond–surfaced wafer are in position. Kerr's Temp-Bond paste makes contact with teeth to become interocclusal record. (From Lucia, Victor O.: J. Prosthet. Dent. **14:**492-505, 1964.)

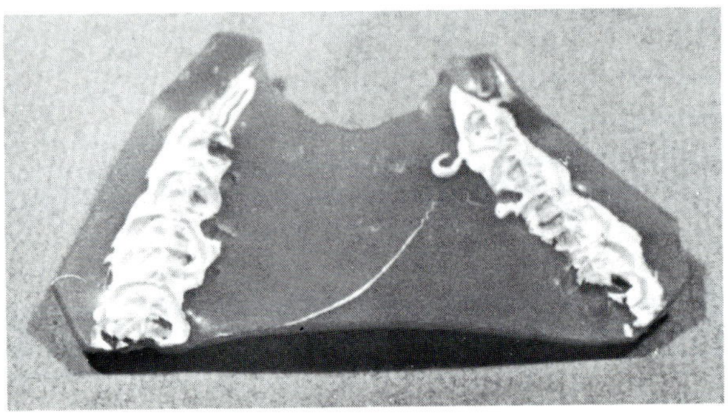

Fig. 4-20. Centric relation record on wax wafer. (From Lucia, Victor O.: J. Prosthet. Dent. **14:**492-505, 1964.)

teeth just slightly. At the same time a slight but firm pressure is exerted with the index fingers to keep the record in position on the lower teeth. This frees the record from the upper teeth. The patient closes again. The thumb and index finger of the left hand are used to hold the record against the upper teeth. The patient's lower jaw is steadied with the right thumb. The patient is instructed to separate his teeth just slightly. This will loosen the record from the lower teeth with a minimum of distortion.

The record is placed in cold water. Then the second and third records are made in a similar manner and placed in cold water.

The first record is trimmed very carefully with a pair of surgical tissue shears. (The one serrated edge helps to trim the Temp-Bond without fracturing it.) All the side extensions that may have been formed by the Temp-Bond are removed. The object of trimming the record at this time is to make it possible to detect any warpage that may have occurred in removal. Trimming is necessary to facilitate the assembly of the casts in mounting, and it also enables one to determine whether or not the casts are completely seated in the record. Only the indentations of the tips of the cusps are required for the accurate seating of the casts in the record (Fig. 4-20).

To test the record the dentist reseats it in the patient's mouth after it is trimmed. With the jig in place the patient is instructed to close the mandible in centric relation. It is important that there are no chips of the Temp-Bond in any of the indentations when the record is reseated. The second and third records are checked in the same manner after trimming. All records are checked again after the jig is removed. Any slight distortion will be corrected if these steps are carefully executed.

Note: By changing the vertical dimension of the DuraLay jig and making additional records at the new vertical relation, the split-cast technique can be used to check the accuracy of the hinge axis location. If the axis has not been located correctly, the centric relation records, which were made at different occlusal vertical dimensions, cannot check out.

Mounting the lower cast

With three centric relation records having been satisfactorily made, the lower cast is mounted in relation to the upper cast, and then the other records are tested to determine whether or not they are duplicates of the first one.

The most accurate way to mount the lower cast on most articulators in proper relation to the upper cast is as follows:

1. The articulator is inverted on a mounting block.
2. The centric relation record is placed on the occlusal surface of the upper cast.
3. The lower cast is placed on the centric relation record.
4. The lower cast is held firmly in the record and against the upper cast (Fig. 4-21).

An assistant mixes the stone and completes the attachment of the lower cast to the lower bow of the articulator. The upper and lower members of the articulator must be in centric relation.

After the attaching stone has set, the inverted articulator is turned over, and the electrical tape that holds together the two parts of the split cast is removed (Fig. 4-22). The upper bow (with the upper half of the split cast) is raised. The upper cast is reseated in the centric relation record (Fig. 4-23). The V grooves of the split cast must go into place accurately (Fig. 4-24). If they do, the mounting was correctly made.

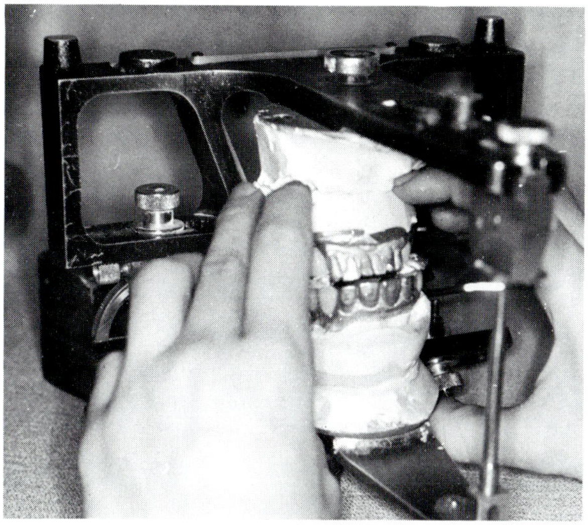

Fig. 4-21. Lower cast is held in position against centric relation record while cast is attached to lower member of articulator. (From Lucia, Victor O.: J. Prosthet. Dent. **14:**492-505, 1964.)

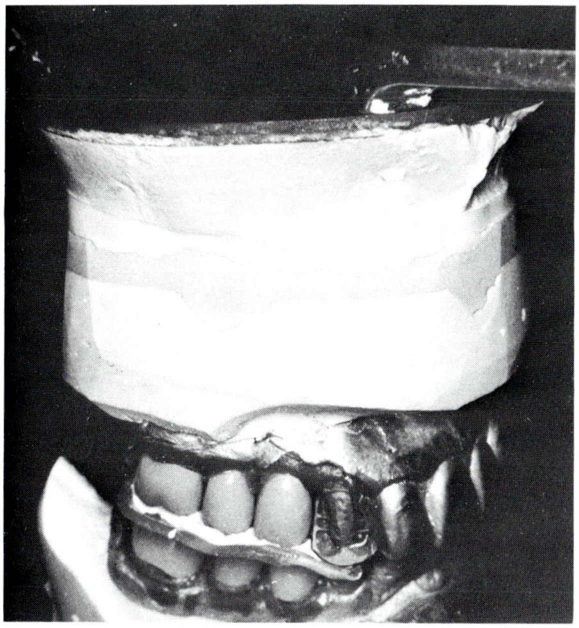

Fig. 4-22. Split cast is in position after articulator is closed in centric relation. Notches of split cast fit accurately. (From Lucia, Victor O.: J. Prosthet. Dent. **14:**492-505, 1964.)

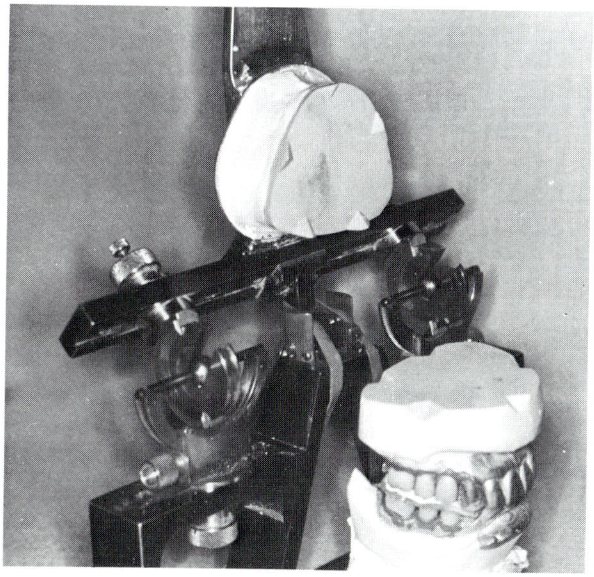

Fig. 4-23. Articulator is opened so that second centric relation record can be used to determine accuracy of records. (From Lucia, Victor O.: J. Prosthet. Dent. **14:**492-505, 1964.)

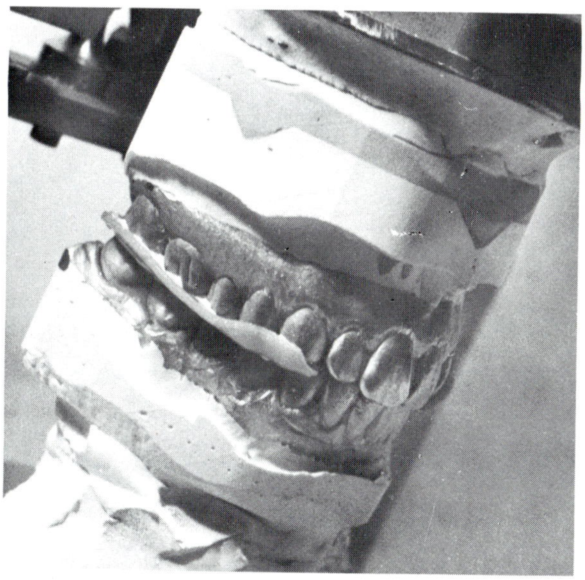

Fig. 4-24. V grooves of split cast fit perfectly together with second record in position. This proves that the two records are identical. (From Lucia, Victor O.: J. Prosthet. Dent. **14:**492-505, 1964.)

Tests to confirm the mounting

The articulator is opened to the first centric relation record, and the upper cast is removed. The second centric relation record is placed in position, and the cast is seated on it. The articulator is closed. If the two parts of the split cast come together perfectly (as they did when the mounting operation was checked), the two records are identical. This procedure is repeated to check the accuracy of the third record. When all three records are identical, the mounting is correct.

This method will produce consistent results when different dentists make the records and tests. To be valuable a procedure must be practical. It must be one that can be performed easily by most dentists. If a technique requires a genius for its execution, then it is not useful in dentistry. By this method it is possible to build and correct restorations on an articulator and to have them check perfectly in the mouth.

SUMMARY AND CONCLUSION

It seems logical, from the anatomy of the temporomandibular joint, that the most stable position of the mandible is that in centric relation. The origin and insertion of the muscles of mastication, the inclination of the glenoid fossae, and the function of the meniscus and synovial membranes—all indicate that any functional movements must seat the condyle in the terminal hinge position. Therefore, centric occlusion should be built to occur at centric relation. Clinical evidence substantiates this belief. The best results are obtained when we succeed in correlating centric occlusion with centric relation.

Regardless of whether we believe that centric occlusion should be slightly anterior to this terminal hinge position, this is the only constant, repeatable position that can be used to check the work as we proceed. It is the only means for accurately relating the casts of the patient so that they can be examined in every detail, with true relationship to each other and without encumbrances of tongue, cheeks, saliva, and the patient's distracting proprioceptive reflexes.

There is nothing new in the principle involved in this technique. Those who are seriously concerned with centric relation have tried, by one means or another, to relate the condyles to the fossae in a specific way. They may not use the same words or terms to describe it, and they may not use the same reasons for their procedures. In the final analysis, however, they want the condyles to be as far up and as far back as *the patient will ever place them when the teeth or restorations are in use;* otherwise there is no justification for being concerned with centric relation.

Many techniques have been developed to accomplish this result. Many techniques resemble the one described here. There is one major difference, however—this procedure enables any dentist to get the same accurate results repeatedly. Having made a great many centric relation records by this procedure, I am convinced that it is the most accurate method in use.

Following are the critical steps in the technique:

1. Locate the centers of rotation, hinge axis, and centers of lateral rotation.
2. Prepare the upper cast for the split-cast technique.
3. Relate the prepared upper cast to the centers of rotation by means of a face-bow transfer.
4. Form the wax wafer tray.
5. Construct and adjust the centric relation jig to interrupt the reflex action of the muscles and to permit a normal closure of the jaws.
6. Check the wafer and jig to make sure there is no tooth impingement against the wax wafer.
7. Make the interocclusal centric relation records.
8. Trim the interocclusal records with a curved tissue shears having serrations on one blade.
9. Replace the records in the mouth to eliminate any possible distortion of them.
10. Relate the lower cast to the upper cast by means of the interocclusal record and attach the cast to the articulator.
11. Check the accuracy of the mounting by using the second and third interocclusal records and observing the fit of the parts of the split cast.

This method has enabled us to consistently and accurately check one centric relation record against another. The important difference between this procedure and others in which anterior stops have been used is that the *adjustment* of the DuraLay jig is responsible for *training the patient* to place his mandible in the centric relation. No special skill is required to carry out the procedure, and it can be accomplished by any dentist.

REFERENCES

1. Academy of Denture Prosthetics: Glossary of prosthodontic terms, J. Prosthet. Dent. **6**(Appendix)**:**11, 1956.
2. Needles, J. W.: Mandibular movements and articulator design, J.A.D.A. **10:**927-935, 1923.
3. Lauritzen, Arne: Postgraduate course, April, 1959, University of Pennsylvania, Philadelphia.

CHAPTER 5

PERIODONTICS

HAROLD R. SCHREIBER, A.B., D.D.S., F.A.C.D.*

ANATOMY AND PHYSIOLOGY OF THE PERIODONTIUM

The practice of modern restorative dentistry depends on a knowledge of the anatomy, physiology, and function of the periodontium. Usually the periodontium is considered to be limited to the gingiva, epithelial attachment, cementum, alveolar bone, and periodontal ligament. The gingiva in turn is bound into a unique, inseparable complex with additional anatomic structures such as the alveolar mucosa, vestibular folds, frena, and muscle attachments. The preservation of the gingivomucosal relationship in periodontal therapy is a prime objective before restorative procedures.

Gross characteristics of gingivomucosal complex

The clinically normal gingiva is light pink or coral in color in Caucasians (Fig. 5-1). In other groups of people gingival color depends on the amount of melanin present and results in varying degrees of brownish pigmentation. The healthy gingiva is firm and resilient.

The gingiva can be divided into the marginal (free, unattached) gingiva, attached gingiva, and interdental gingiva, or papilla. The marginal gingiva surrounds the tooth in a collarlike fashion at the cementoenamel junction, and in health it tapers to a knifelike edge at its crest next to the tooth. The marginal gingiva is demarcated from the adjacent attached gingiva by a depression—the free gingival groove—which is not always visible macroscopically. The width of the marginal gingiva is approximately 1 to 2 mm. and forms the soft tissue wall of the gingival sulcus. The gingival sulcus is the V-shaped depression that is formed by the tooth surface on one side and

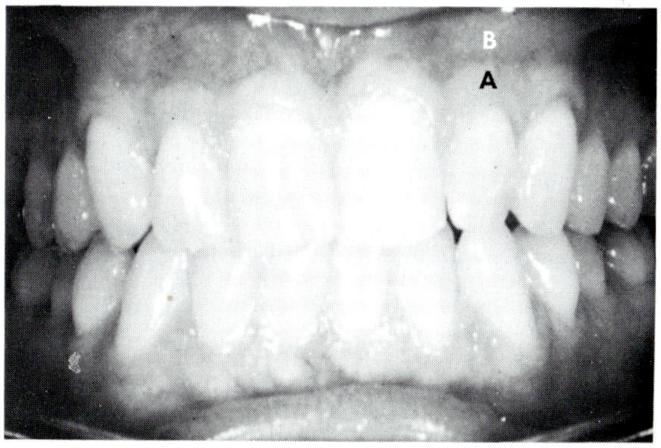

Fig. 5-1. Normal gingiva. *A,* Attached gingiva; *B,* alveolar mucosa.

*Professor and Chairman, Department of Periodontics, Washington University School of Dental Medicine, St. Louis, Mo.

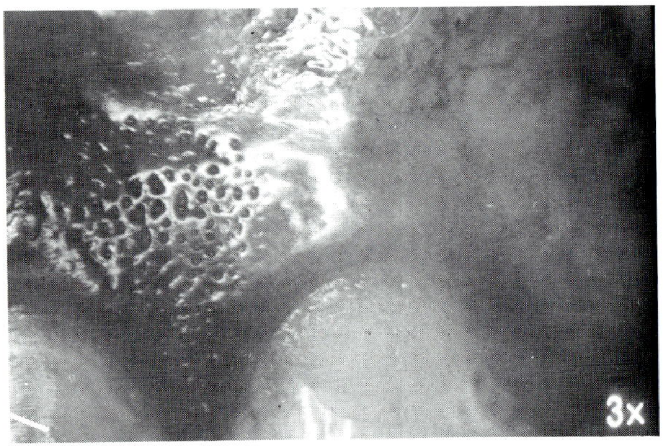

Fig. 5-2. Stippling of gingiva.

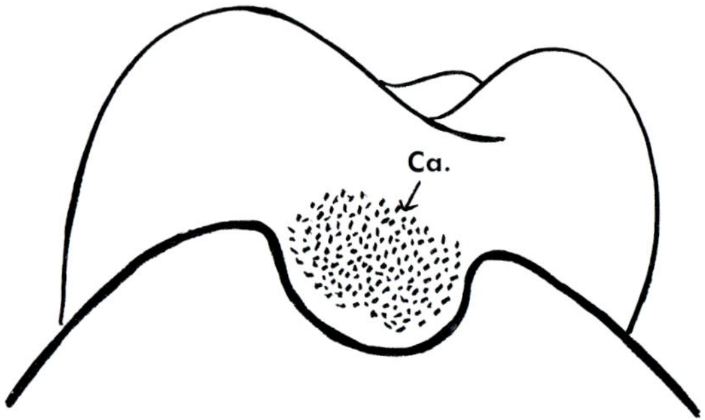

Fig. 5-3. Col. Shape of interdental gingiva between contacting teeth. *Ca.,* Contact area.

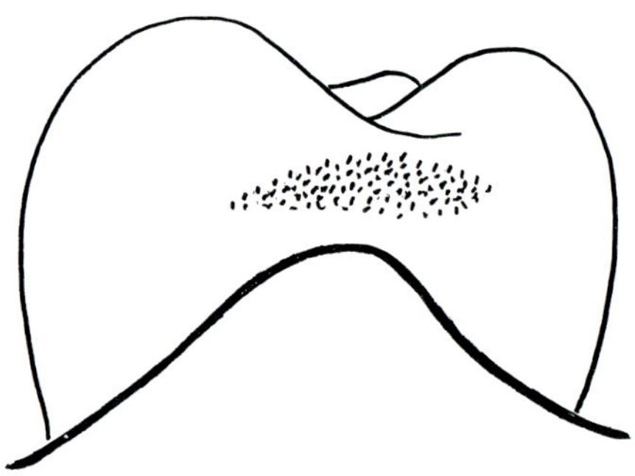

Fig. 5-4. Shape of interdental gingiva where there is space between teeth.

the wall of the marginal gingiva on the other. Its depth in health approximates the width of the marginal gingiva.

The attached gingiva is that portion of the gingiva that is immobile and bound tightly to the underlying cementum and alveolar bone. The width of the attached gingiva on the vestibular aspect is from 1 to 5 mm. The surface of the attached gingiva is characterized by an orange peel–like appearance, or stippling, and may be finely or coarsely grained (Fig. 5-2). The attached gingiva appears slightly depressed between adjacent teeth, corresponding to the depression on the alveolar process between eminences of the sockets.

The interdental gingiva, or interdental papilla, is that part of the gingiva that fills the space between two adjacent teeth up to the contact areas. It lies more coronal to the vestibular and lingual gingivae. It is comprised of marginal gingiva and the adjacent area of attached gingiva. The interdental gingiva is tent shaped and is characterized by a vestibular and lingual peak. The concave depression between these peaks is termed a *col* (Fig. 5-3). The shape of the col is determined by the contact areas of adjoining teeth. In the absence of proximal contacts the col area is replaced by a smooth, rounded surface (Fig. 5-4). The interdental gingiva is of special clinical importance since it is an early and accurate indicator of periodontal pathosis.

The anatomic characteristics of the teeth protect the marginal gingiva. The tooth is formed so that the cervical area is recessed in relation to the greatest contour. The crest of the marginal gingiva lies in contact with the tooth in this recessed area. Food that is forced over the vestibular and lingual contours of the teeth bypass the marginal gingiva. Similarly, the interproximal marginal gingiva is protected by contours in the embrasure areas.

The alveolar mucosa is demarcated from the attached gingiva by a scalloped line, the mucogingival junction. This line of demarcation occurs on the vestibular surfaces of both jaws and on the lingual surface of the mandible. There is no such line on the palate since the gingiva here is continuous with, and similar in structure to, the mucosa of the palate. In contrast to the thick immovable gingiva, the alveolar mucosa is thin, attached loosely to the underlying periosteum of alveolar bone, and movable. The alveolar mucosa is red, smooth, and shiny. It is continuous with the mucosa that lines the vestibular trough or fold, which in turn is reflected as the lining mucosa of the lips and cheeks. On the lingual surface of the mandible the alveolar mucosa is continuous with the mucosa lining the floor of the mouth. In the vestibular fold the thin reddish mucosa is loosely attached to the underlying structures. The position and movements of the alveolar mucosa and vestibular fold mucosa may depend on muscle attachments such as the buccinator, mental, incisive, and nasal. Folds of mucosa in the midline or laterally that connect alveolar mucosa or attached

A

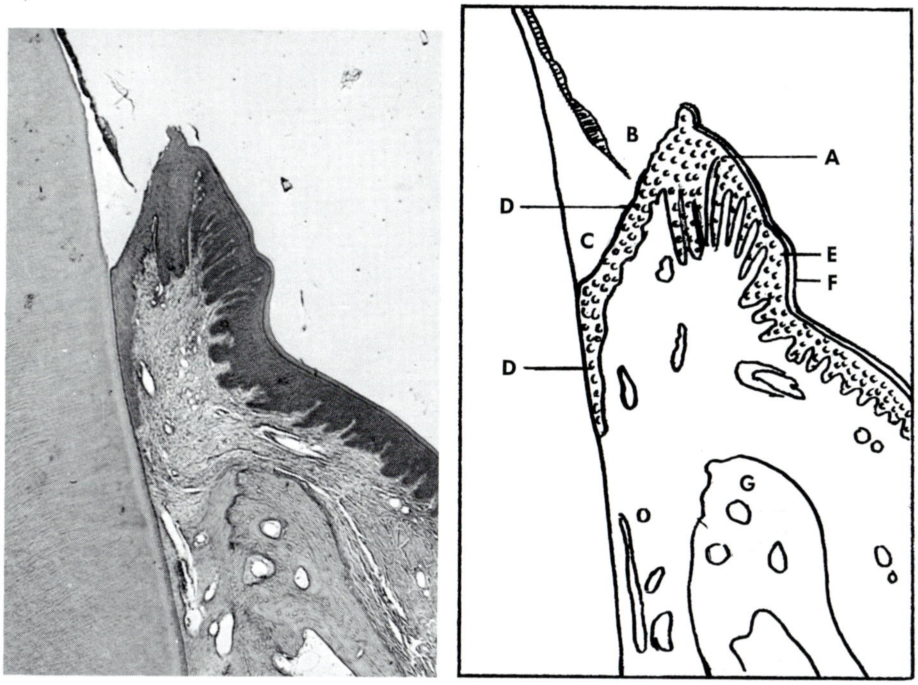

B

Fig. 5-5. A, Histologic section of tooth and gingiva. **B,** Diagram of histologic section. *A,* Marginal gingiva; *B,* gingival sulcus; *C,* enamel space; *D,* epithelial attachment; *E,* attached gingiva; *F,* keratinized layer; *G,* alveolar bone.

gingiva with the mucosa lining the lips or cheeks constitute median vestibular or lateral vestibular frena, respectively. A midline inferior lingual frenum may also be present.

Histologic characteristics of gingivomucosal complex

The outer covering of the gingiva is composed of a stratified, squamous epithelium that usually has a thick keratinized layer. This layer serves as a protection against chemical and bacterial injuries. However, it may be a combination of keratinization or parakeratinization. The epithelium here is characterized by numerous rete pegs. The epithelium on the inner surface of the gingiva is nonkeratinized and lacks rete pegs, and it serves as the lining of the gingival sulcus. From the base of the gingival sulcus the epithelium attaches to the tooth and continues as a collarlike band composed of ten to twenty rows of epithelial cells as the epithelial attachment (Fig. 5-5). The epithelial attachment measures 0.25 to 1.35 mm. in length, with an average length of 1 mm. The function of the epithelial attachment is a biologic one, and it seals off the junction of the gingiva and the tooth.

Supporting the epithelial layer is a dense, inelastic, but resilient connective tissue, the lamina propria. The papillae of the lamina propria are characteristically long and narrow. Into the lamina propria insert strong connective tissue fiber bundles that attach the gingiva to the tooth and the surrounding alveolar bone (Fig. 5-6). These fiber groups are classified as follows:

1. Dentinogingival fibers. These fibers arise from the cementum immediately beneath the epithelial attachment on the vestibular, lingual, and interproximal surfaces. The fibers adjacent to the epithelial attachment project in a fanlike fashion and insert into the lamina propria near the marginal gingiva. The next group of fibers travels directly outward and attaches to the lamina propria of the attached gingiva. Subjacent to the aforementioned group of fibers and seen only on the vestibular and lingual surfaces is a third group of fibers, which passes directly over the alveolar bone and inclines apically between the outer periosteum of the alveolar process and joins with fibers of the outer periosteum and lamina propria of the attached gingiva.

2. Circular fibers. These fibers course through the connective tissue of the gingiva, encircling the tooth and interlacing with other fiber groups.

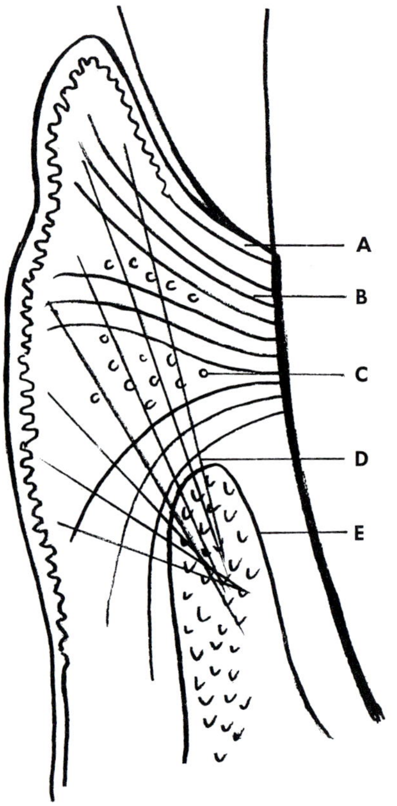

Fig. 5-6. Fiber groups attaching gingiva to tooth and alveolar bone. *A,* Epithelial attachment; *B,* dentinogingival fibers; *C,* circular fibers; *D,* alveogingival fibers; *E,* alveolar bone.

3. Alveogingival fibers. These fibers arise from the alveolar crest and extend to the lamina propria of the gingiva.

4. Transseptal fibers (Fig. 5-7). In the interproximal space and apical to the dentinogingival and circular fibers are prominent connective tissue fibers that arise from the cementum of the tooth, pass directly over the interproximal septum of bone, and attach into the cementum of the adjacent teeth. These fibers form a network to support the interdental gingiva and secure adjacent teeth.

The function of the gingival fibers is to support the gingiva, keeping it closely adapted to the tooth surface and alveolar bone, thus sustaining the gingiva against the forces of mastication. The fibers subjacent to the epithelial attachment prevent apical migration of the epithelial attachment. These fiber groups occupy the area from the apical end of the attached epithelial cuff to the crest of the alveolar bone. This area measures approximately 1 mm. in depth.

At the junction of the gingiva and alveolar mucosa is a change in histologic characteristics (Fig. 5-8). The epithelium of the alveolar mucosa is thinner and nonkeratinized, and the epithelial ridges and connective tissue papilla are insignificant or absent. Since the alveolar mucosa is adapted for mobility, the submucosa is a loosely textured connective tissue containing elastic fibers and glands. The mucosa of

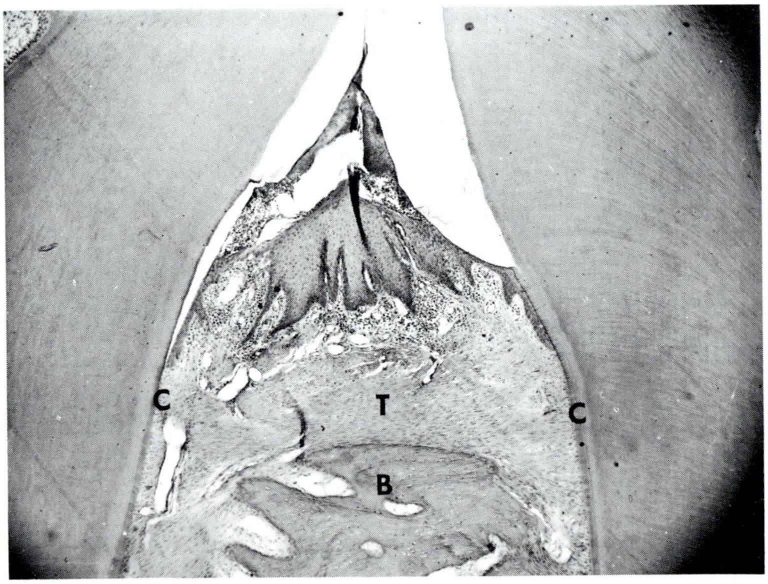

Fig. 5-7. Histologic section of transseptal fibers. *T,* Transseptal fibers; *B,* alveolar bone; *C,* cementum.

A 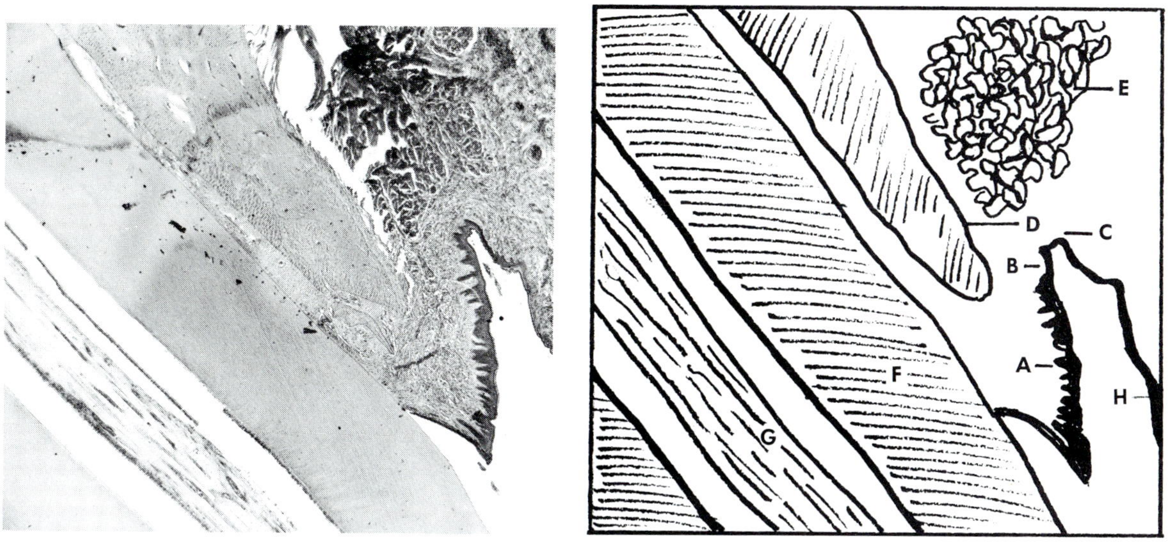 B

Fig. 5-8. A, Histologic section through tooth, gingiva, alveolar mucosa, and vestibular fold. **B,** Diagram of histologic section. *A,* Attached gingiva; *B,* alveolar mucosa; *C,* vestibular fold; *D,* alveolar bone; *E,* muscle; *F,* dentin; *G,* pulp; *H,* buccal mucosa.

the vestibular fold and frena are similar histologically to the alveolar mucosa and are freely movable. Below these submucosal layers will be found striated muscle fibers (buccinator, mental, incisive, nasal) that have attachments to the alveolar bone of maxilla and mandible.

Attachment apparatus

The attachment apparatus consists of the cementum, alveolar bone, and periodontal ligament.

CEMENTUM

Cementum is the hard dental tissue covering the anatomic roots of the teeth. It is light yellow and consists of 45% to 50% of inorganic or calcified substances.

Cementum is deposited in a circumferential pattern about the underlying dentin (Fig. 5-9). Incremental lines separate the layers of cementum and indicate periodontic formation. The surface of cementum is covered by the most recent layer, which is uncalcified cementum or cementoid. The cementoid layer is characterized by a single layer of living cells, cementoblasts, which are responsible for cementoid deposition (Fig. 5-10). Cementum formation is considered to be a continuous process. Under normal conditions resorption of cementum is not significant. Cementum is thinnest at the cementoenamel junction (25 to 50 μ) and thickest at the apex and interradicular areas (150 to 200 μ). Occasionally there is no cementoenamel junction, and a zone of root dentin is devoid of cementum and is exposed.

ALVEOLAR PROCESS

The alveolar process is that part of the maxilla or mandible that forms and supports the sockets of the teeth. The anatomic contour of the alveolar bone generally is dependent on the prominence of the tooth roots (Fig. 5-11). The alveolar bone tapers in thickness as it approaches the cervical area on the vestibular and lingual surfaces. Between the roots the alveolar bone conforms to intervening vertical depressions, which unite from the vestibular and lingual surfaces to form the interdental septum of bone. The crest of the alveolar bone is normally 1 mm. in distance from the apical end of the epithelial attachment or 2 mm. from the cementoenamel junction. The outer wall of the alveolar process is composed of dense cortical plates on the vestibular and lingual surfaces. (See Fig. 5-12.) The inner wall of bone, forming the alveolar socket, is thin and relatively dense. It is termed the *alveolar bone proper,* or *cribriform plate,* since it is perforated by many openings for blood vessels, lymphs, and nerves. Radiographically, the alveolar bone proper appears as a thin, continuous, radiopaque line more commonly known as the *lamina dura* (Fig. 5-13). Between the outer cortical plates and the inner alveolar bone proper are supporting trabeculae of cancellous bone. Alveolar bone is composed of a calcified matrix.

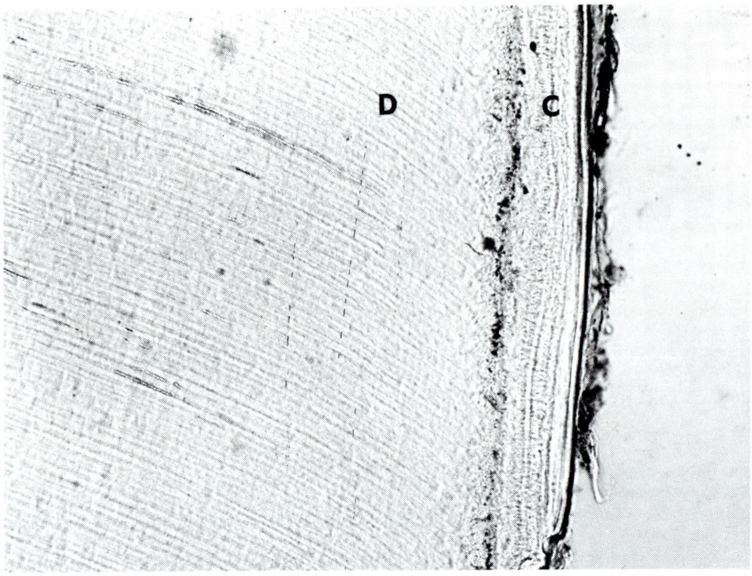

Fig. 5-9. Ground section of tooth. *C,* Cementum; *D,* dentin-incremental pattern of cementum readily visible.

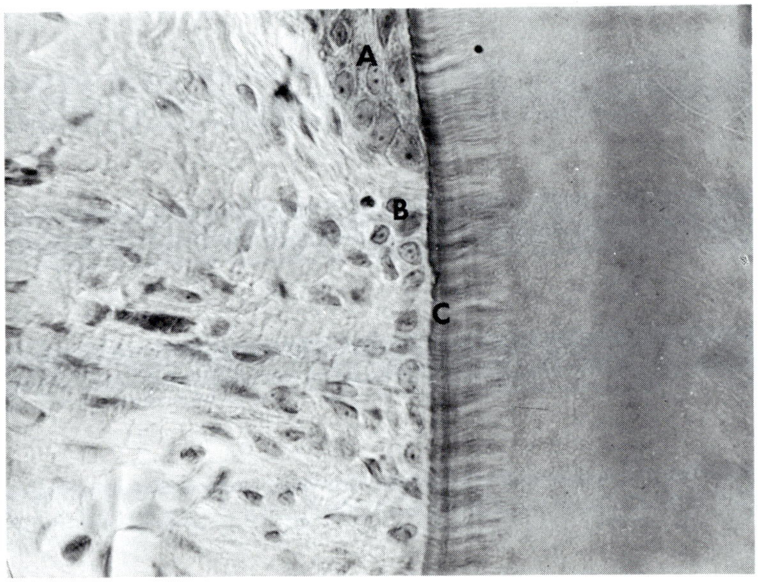

Fig. 5-10. Histologic section. *A,* Apical end epithelial attachment; *B,* cementoblasts; *C,* cementum.

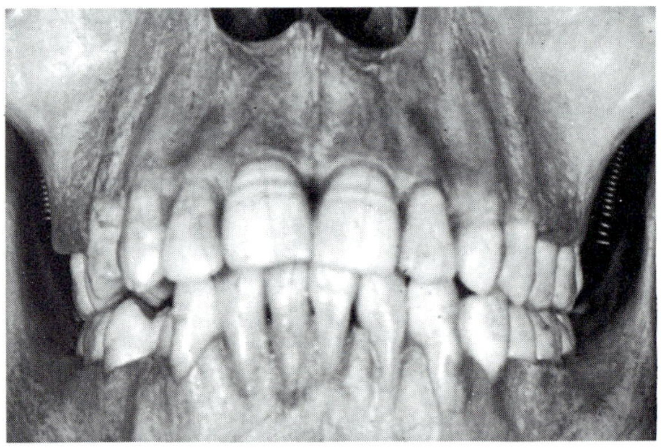

Fig. 5-11. Gross specimen of skull illustrating normal topography of maxillary alveolar bone. (Note alveolar bone resorption in mandibular anterior area.)

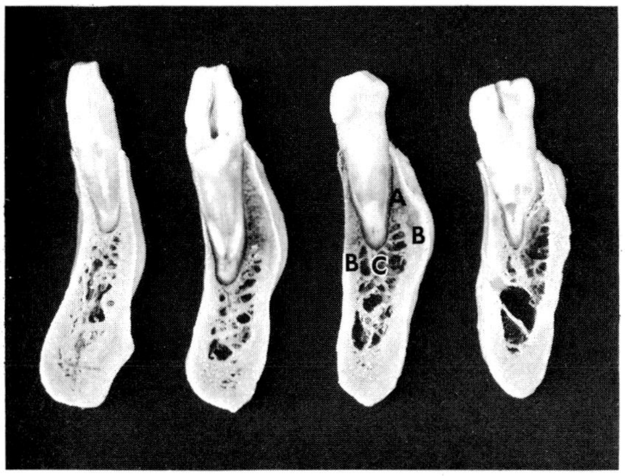

Fig. 5-12. Cross sections through mandible. *A,* Alveolar bone proper; *B,* cortical bone; *C,* cancellous bone.

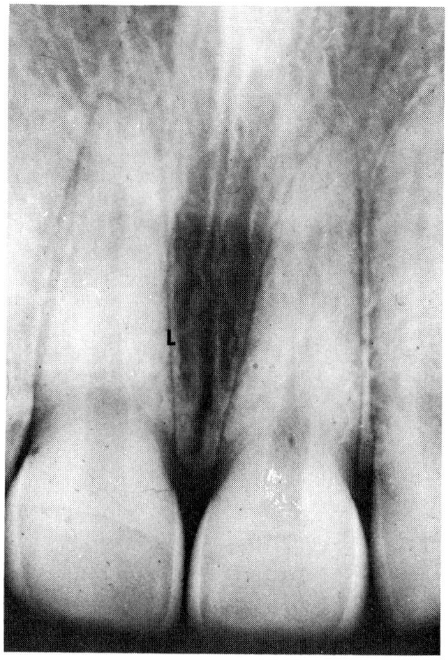

Fig. 5-13. Radiograph of upper central incisor area. *L,* Lamina dura.

Embedded in the matrix are osteocytes lying in lacunae. Extending from each lacuna are minute canals called *canaliculi,* which communicate with canaliculi of adjacent lacunae. The canaliculi form an anastomosing network throughout the intercellular matrix of bone, which brings nutrient material to the osteocyte and removes waste products of metabolism. Since alveolar bone is the least stable component of the attachment apparatus and since it depends upon a functional stimulation for preservation of its structure, it is characterized by areas of

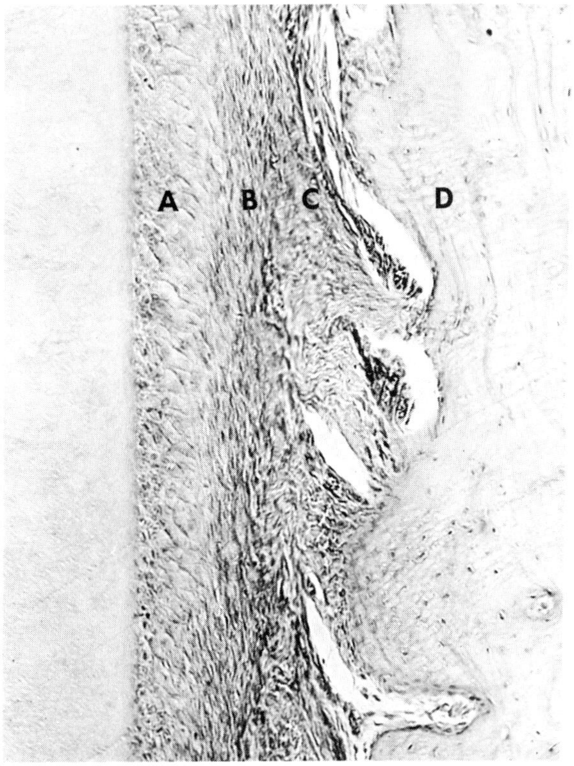

Fig. 5-14. Histologic section through periodontal ligament of rapidly erupting tooth. *A,* Cemental fibers; *B,* intermediate fibers; *C,* alveolar fibers; *D,* alveolar bone.

bone deposition and bone resorption. Whenever bone apposition is occurring, a layer of noncalcified matrix, or osteoid, is present. A lining layer of osteoblasts is responsible for its deposition. Wherever bone is undergoing resorption, large multinucleated cells, osteoclasts, will be seen.

PERIODONTAL LIGAMENT

The periodontal, or alveodental, ligament is the connective tissue that attaches the tooth to the bony alveolus. The principal fibers of the periodontal ligament arise in the cementum as Sharpey's fibers, pass between the layers of cementoblasts as they emerge from the cementum, and continue on to insert into the alveolar bone again as Sharpey's fibers. Near the bone the fibers seem to form larger bundles before their insertion into it. Although the fiber bundles run directly from cementum to bone, single fibers do not span the entire distance. The bundles are spliced or braided together in an intermediate group of fibers midway between the cementum and bone. Eruptive and drifting movements of teeth occur by a rearrangement or resplicing of fibers in the intermediate zone

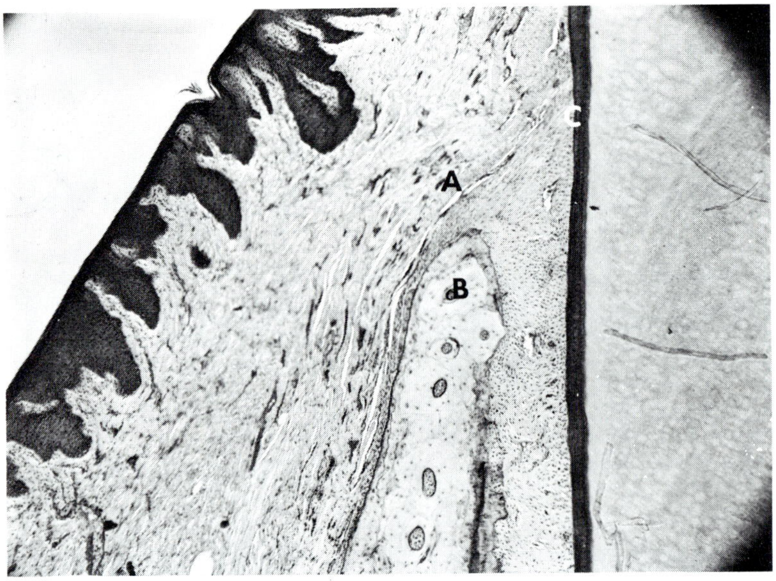

Fig. 5-15. Histologic section through periodontal ligament. *A,* Alveolar crest fibers; *B,* alveolar bone; *C,* cementum.

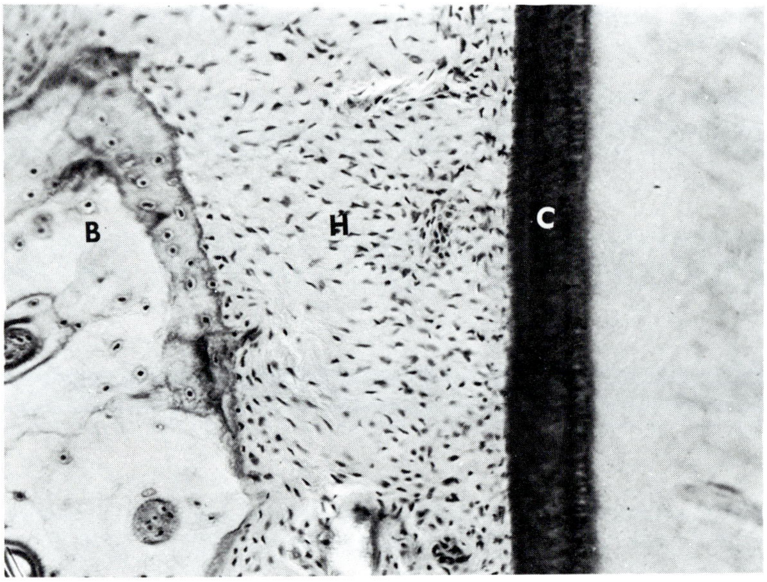

Fig. 5-16. Histologic section through periodontal ligament. *H,* Horizontal fibers; *B,* alveolar bone; *C,* cementum.

(Fig. 5-14). The periodontal ligament consists of the following five groups of fiber bundles, which are functionally arranged.

1. Alveolar crest. These fiber bundles radiate obliquely from the cervical cementum and attach to the crest of the alveolar bone. This is the smallest group of principal fibers. These fibers resist the coronal movements of the teeth, help to retain the tooth within its socket, and resist lateral movements. (See Fig. 5-15.)

2. Horizontal. These bundles originate from the cervical third of the cementum, run at right angles to the long axis of the tooth, and attach to the cervical third of the alveolar bone. This is the next smallest group of fibers. Their function is to resist tooth displacement by lateral pressure. (See Fig. 5-16.)

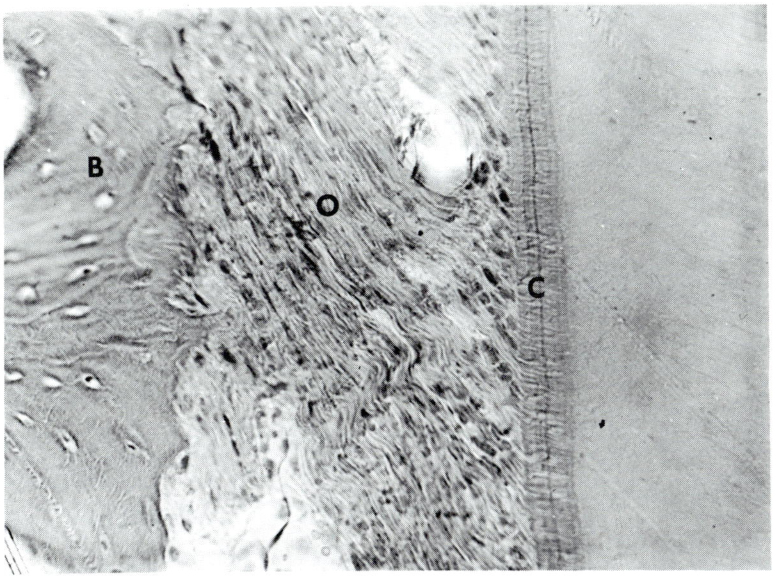

Fig. 5-17. Histologic section through periodontal ligament. *O,* Oblique fibers; *B,* alveolar bone; *C,* cementum.

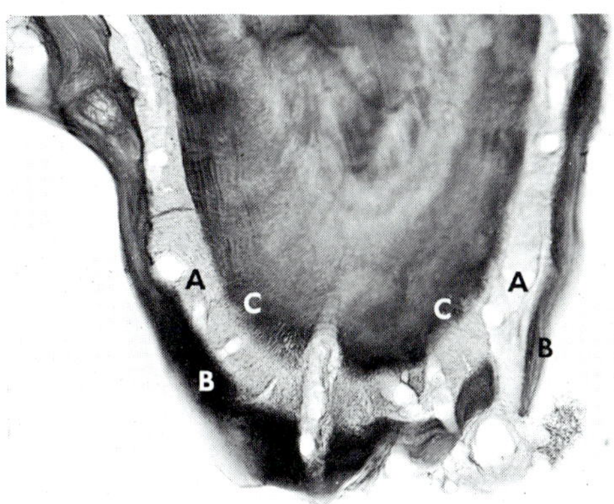

Fig. 5-18. Histologic section through periodontal ligament. *A,* Apical fibers; *B,* alveolar bone; *C,* cementum.

3. Oblique. These fibers arise from the apical two-thirds of the cementum. They radiate coronally and have a broader area of attachment as they insert into the alveolar bone. The oblique fibers are most numerous and constitute the main support of the tooth against masticatory stresses. Their function is to transform vertical pressure exerted on a tooth into tension on the alveolar bone. (See Fig. 5-17.)

4. Apical. These bundles are arranged irregularly and radiate from the apical region of cementum to the apical region of the alveolar socket. They counteract lateral and coronal displacement of the apical portion of the root. (See Fig. 5-18.)

5. Interradicular. From the furcation of multirooted teeth, fiber bundles extend to the bone of the interradicular septum. The most coronal fibers run vertically to the crest of the interradicular bone, whereas the more laterally located fibers radiate obliquely from the cementum to the interradicular septum of bone. These fibers resist tipping and torque in multirooted teeth.

Between the groups of principal fibers is a loose interstitial connective tissue. In this tissue are the blood vessels, lymphatic vessels, and nerves for nutrition and enervation of the tooth, periodontal ligament, and gingiva. Cells found in the interstitial tissue are fibroblasts, histiocytes, undifferentiated mesenchymal reserve cells, and lymphocytes.

The width of the periodontal ligament varies according to the age of the individual and the functional requirements of the tooth. In a tooth in functional occlusion the width varies from 0.25 to 0.2 mm. The width is narrowest below the midroot area, which is the fulcrum of the tooth.

PATHOLOGY OF PERIODONTAL DISEASE
General considerations

In the previous material an attempt has been made to describe the normal gross characteristics of the marginal gingiva, gingival sulcus, attached gingiva, interdental gingiva, alveolar mucosa, and vestibular fornix and their spatial interdependence. The normal histology of these structures as well as that of the

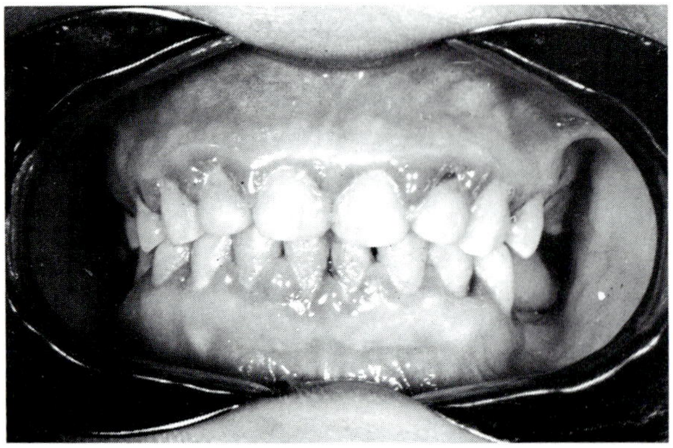

Fig. 5-19. Gingivitis. Changes in surface texture, form, and position of gingiva.

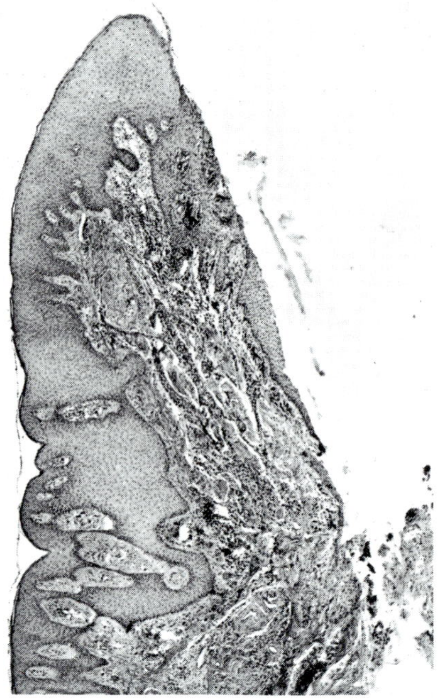

Fig. 5-20. Histologic section of gingiva in gingivitis. Note proliferation of epithelium and accumulation of inflammatory cells.

underlying and interrelated structures such as the epithelial attachment, gingival fibers, cementum, periodontal ligament, and alveolar bone have been presented. Changes in any of the previously mentioned structures or in their relationship to each other may constitute the initiation of periodontal disease.

The tissues are subjected daily to a variety of insults, local and systemic, which may result in either inflammatory or dystrophic conditions or a combination of both. Inflammatory periodontal conditions initially attack the gingiva (i.e., marginal, interdental, or attached gingiva), resulting in some form of gingivitis. Following are clinical manifestations of inflammatory conditions in the gingiva:

1. Change in gingival color. A change from the normal light pink or coral color to varying shades of red to blue occurs.

2. Change in consistency. The normal gingiva is firm and resilient. Inflammation results in a puffiness, softness, and ulceration.

3. Change in surface texture. Normal gingiva is characterized by stippling. Edema and swelling cause a loss of stippling and replacement with a smooth glossy surface.

4. Change in form and position. As a consequence of inflammation the knife-edged and well-contoured appearance of the marginal gingiva may become rounded, enlarged, and irregular (Fig. 5-19). If necrosis should occur, however, portions of the gingiva could be destroyed. The gingiva either can enlarge in height and in bulk and cover a larger portion of the tooth or can recede and denude a portion of the root surface. Gingival enlargements and recession may go on simultaneously.

5. Bleeding. In the normal gingiva the epithelial lining of the gingival sulcus is intact. In inflammatory conditions the epithelium is ulcerated and thinned, allowing for passage of blood from more permeable dilated capillaries through the epithelium into the space betwen the tooth and gingiva.

6. Exudation. Products of necrosis and degeneration in inflammation may form an exudate, which escapes through the ulcerated sulcular epithelium and may be expressed on applying pressure to the gingiva against the tooth. The exudate may be purulent or serous.

7. Increase in depth of gingival sulcus. Increase in bulk of gingival tissue results in an increase in depth of the gingival sulcus and may form a gingival pocket. Increase in sulcular depth because of coronal enlargement of gingival margin may result from edematous accumulation or inflammatory hyperplasia.

8. Pain. Pain may or may not be an accompanying symptom. It is more often present with acute exacerbations of gingival disease.

Histopathology of gingivitis

Inflammatory agents of local etiology or their toxic products invade the nonkeratinized epithelium of the gingival sulcus and penetrate the lamina propria. The initial inflammation is localized in the lamina propria beneath the sulcular epithelium (Fig. 5-20). Here the capillaries will be dilated and en-

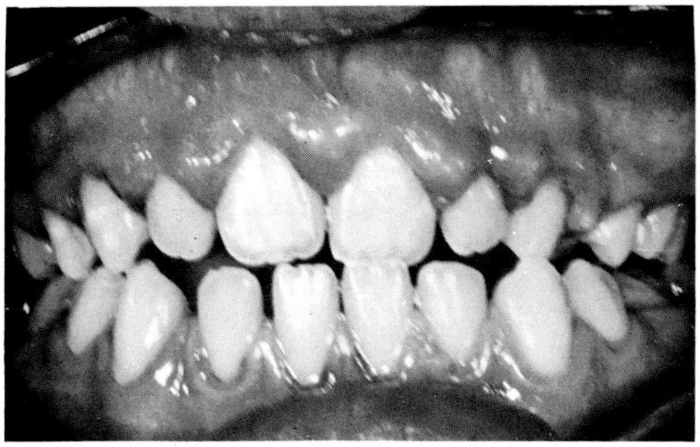

Fig. 5-21. Gingival enlargement caused by inflammation.

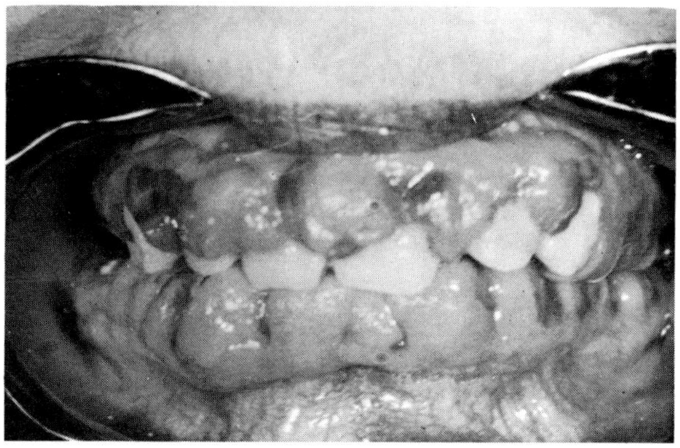

Fig. 5-22. Gingival hyperplasia caused by intake of Dilantin.

gorged. Extravasations of red blood cells into the connective tissue follow. Accumulations of inflammatory cells are present in the lamina propria. The inflammatory cells are mainly plasma cells and lymphocytes. Polymorphonuclear cells may be present, particularly beneath the sulcular epithelium, and macrophages are seen occasionally. The epithelium of the sulcus, the outer gingiva, and the epithelial attachment proliferate into the lamina propria. Concomitant is an influx of inflammatory fluid and cellular exudate in the lamina propria. Degeneration of epithelium and connective tissue occurs, and ulcerations may appear in the epithelium of the sulcus. Polymorphonuclear leukocytes may be seen migrating through these ulcerations. As the inflammatory process progresses, destruction of the connective tissue of the lamina propria and of the dentinogingival fibers takes place. Along with the breakdown, areas of repair may be apparent. Fiber bundles may be replaced by a young proliferating connective tissue, consisting of new capillaries, mesenchymal cells, and inflammatory cells. Because of the increased bulk of the gingiva, the epithelium of the outer gingiva may become thinned. As a result of the inflammatory process and the destruction of gingival fibers, the epithelial attachment may shift apically on the cementum, increasing the depth of the gingival sulcus or pocket. The nature and character of the inflammatory process in the gingiva determines in large measure the extent of the clinical manifestations.

Gingival enlargements

Although enlargements of the gingiva are predominantly of an inflammatory nature, some are true hyperplasias (noninflammatory) of the connective tissue and epithelium (Fig. 5-21). Dilantin hyperplasia illustrates such an enlargement and is of systemic etiology (Fig. 5-22). Other enlargements may be caused by a combination of inflammatory and noninflammatory (hyperplastic) agents, while still other enlargements of the gingiva, such as gingivitis seen in pregnancy, are conditional enlargements; that is, they require local irritating factors to initiate a response under a certain set of systemic conditions.

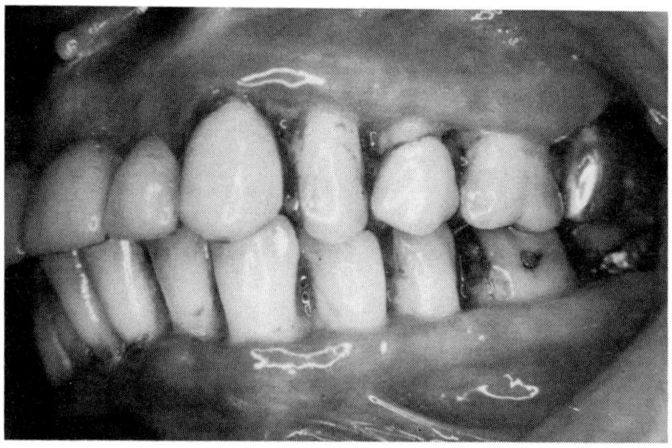

Fig. 5-23. Destruction of interproximal gingiva in necrotizing ulcerative gingivitis.

Gingival atrophy

While inflammatory changes initially exhibit swelling and enlargements, necrosis and degeneration are accompanying features. Recession or atrophy may take place, and a loss of quantity of gingiva may result. Pronounced loss of gingiva is seen in necrotizing ulcerative gingivitis (Vincent's gingivitis) as the interproximal marginal and attached gingivae are destroyed (Fig. 5-23). Interproximal craters may be formed. On the other hand, atrophy may spare the interproximal tissue in patients who use too vigorous toothbrushing techniques, and severe recession

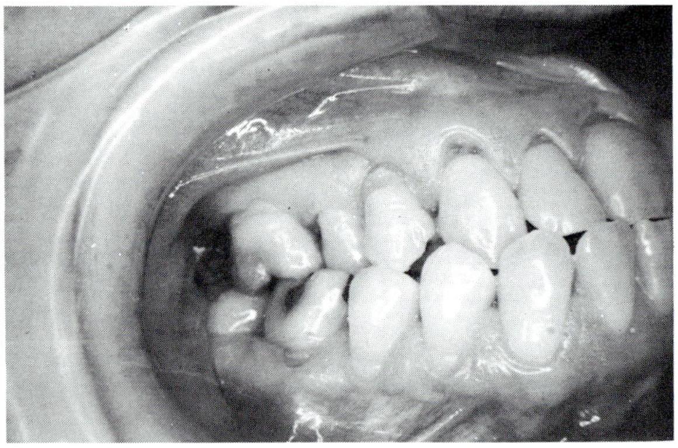

Fig. 5-24. Atrophy of gingiva.

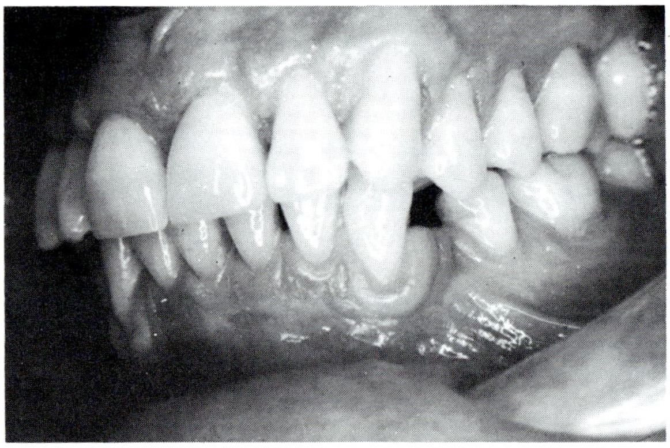

Fig. 5-25. Atrophy of gingiva with rolled margin about lower left cuspid tooth.

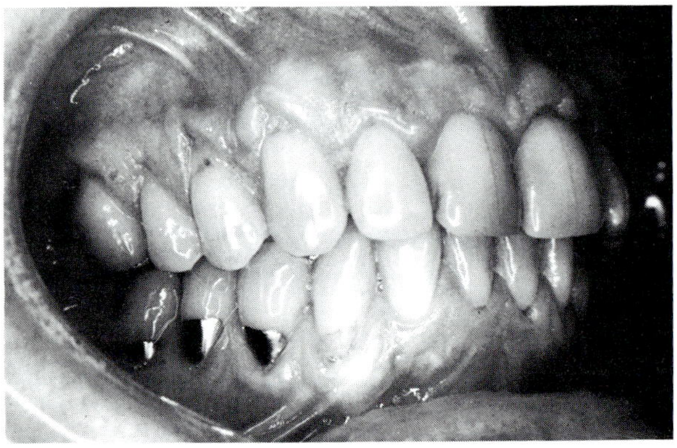

Fig. 5-26. Atrophy of gingiva with cleft formation about upper right cuspid and bicuspid teeth.

may be seen on the vestibular or lingual surfaces with an even destruction of the marginal and portions of the attached gingiva (Fig. 5-24). In this type of recession the gingival sulcus is usually very shallow and without exudate. The remaining gingiva may have a very thin margin or may have a rolled or festooned border (Fig. 5-25). In other instances an uneven atrophy may take place, and formation of clefts may result (Fig. 5-26). In recession the attached epithelial cuff will shift to a more apical position on the cemental surface of the root.

Periodontitis

As the inflammatory process in a gingivitis progresses into the deeper supporting periodontal tissues, a transition from a gingivitis into a periodontitis occurs. The clinical signs and symptoms of a periodontitis are similar to those of gingivitis but with the following variations and additions:

1. Color. Circulatory stagnation will cause a bluish red color of the gingiva to predominate. The color change may extend through the attached gingiva and even into the alveolar mucosa. Occasionally the color will be pink and appear to be clinically normal.

2. Change in consistency and surface texture. The gingiva may present, on pressure, a smooth, shiny surface and pitting (Fig. 5-27). However, a long-standing periodontitis may be undergoing fibrotic changes in the gingival wall and may present a firm, healthy-looking appearance.

3. Change in form and position. As the inflammatory process extends apically, marginal enlargements tend to diminish. The marginal gingiva may present a rolled margin or may revert back to a regular uniform appearance. The interproximal tissue may retain some enlargement and exhibit a convex surface. Separation of the vestibular and oral components of the interproximal papilla may occur. Some marginal recession may take place and cementum may be exposed.

4. Bleeding. Bleeding is usually a constant finding. Again, as fibrosis takes place bleeding may diminish and become less noticeable.

5. Periodontal pocket. Destruction of supporting periodontal tissues transforms a gingival pocket into a periodontal pocket. As more of the dentinogingival fibers are destroyed by progressive inflammation, the epithelial attachment will proliferate apically. As a result, the periodontal probe will enter deeper into the periodontal pocket (Fig. 5-28). The deepest part, or base of the periodontal pocket, will be located at the

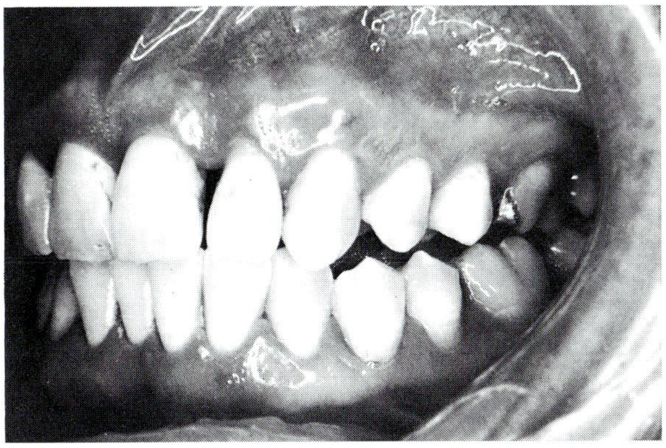

Fig. 5-27. Periodontitis. Gingiva about upper left cuspid and lateral incisor exhibiting smooth, shiny, pitted appearance.

coronal portion of the epithelial attachment. Periodontal pockets may be either suprabony or infrabony. Suprabony pockets comprise the great majority of pockets. The wall of this type of pocket is formed wholly of soft tissue. The soft tissue wall can be gingiva, gingiva and alveolar mucosa, gingiva and palatal mucosa, alveolar mucosa, or palatal mucosa. The wall of the infrabony pocket is composed of the aforementioned soft tissues and a scaffolding of alveolar bone that has survived the resorptive process.

6. Exudation. A purulent exudate is usually a prominent symptom in periodontitis. There is, however, no correlation with the amount of suppuration and the severity of the periodontal condition. (See Fig. 5-29.)

7. Pain. Pain is not a constant finding in periodontal disease, although an awareness of discomfort may be present. Severe pain may be an accompanying symptom in acute conditions such as a periodontal abscess.

8. Bone resorption. The progression of the inflammatory process apically and the destruction of the dentinogingival fibers eventually result in resorption of the alveolar crest of bone (Fig. 5-30). It must be remembered that bone resorption has taken place before it is seen in the radiograph since a sufficient amount of resorption must occur before it can be recorded. Initially, bone resorption would be seen as a cupping out of the interdental septum. Resorption proceeds apically from the alveolar crest and progresses slowly in a horizontal manner along the periosteal aspect of the alveolar bone (Fig. 5-31). Early resorption on vestibular and oral surfaces of alveolar bone will not be seen readily since the tooth overlays these areas in the radiograph. Extension of the inflammatory process along the blood vessels into

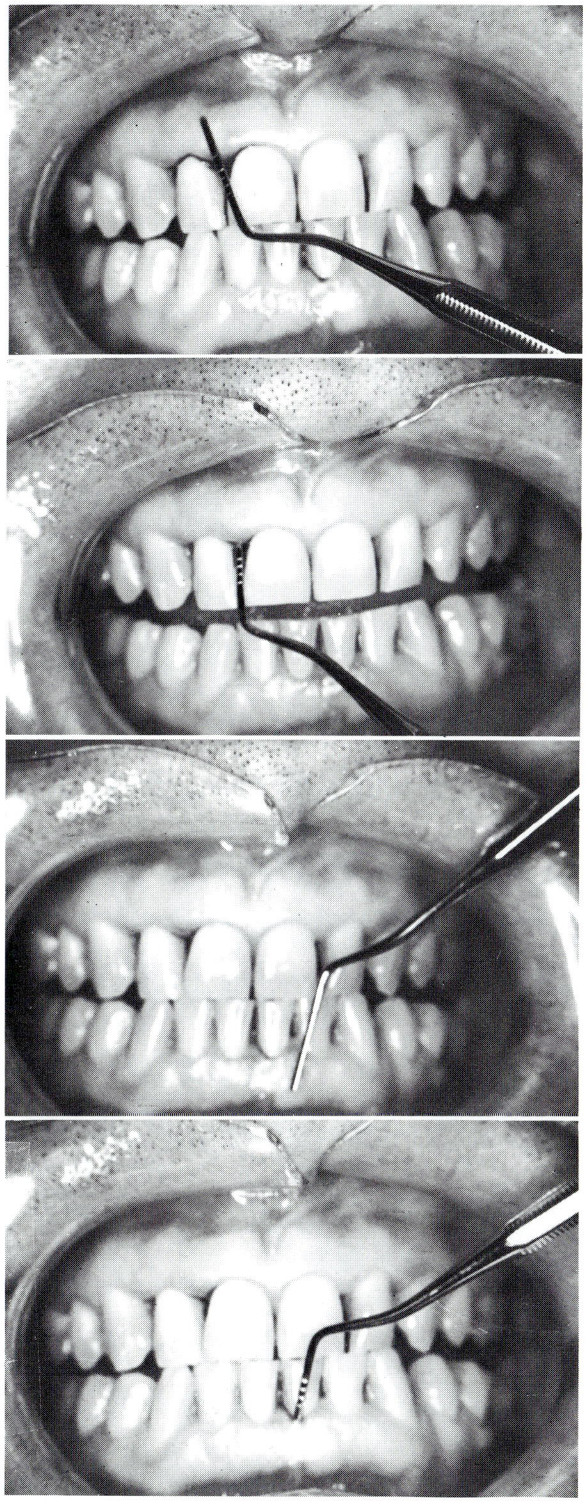

Fig. 5-28. Probe in periodontal pockets of long standing. Periodontitis with gingiva presenting an almost normal appearance in shape and size.

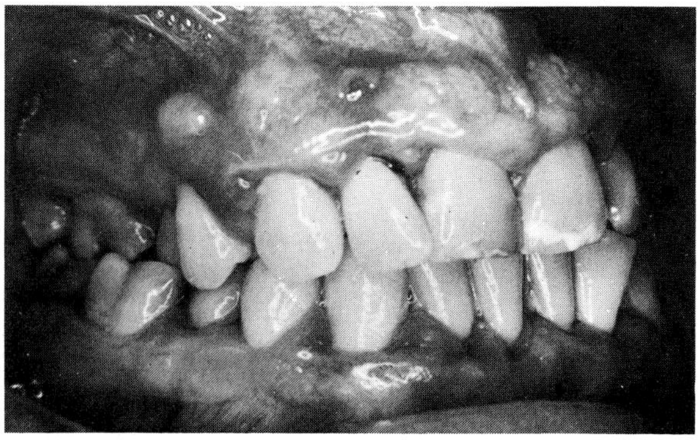

Fig. 5-29. Periodontal abscesses above upper right first biscuspid, cuspid, and lateral incisor teeth in well-advanced periodontitis.

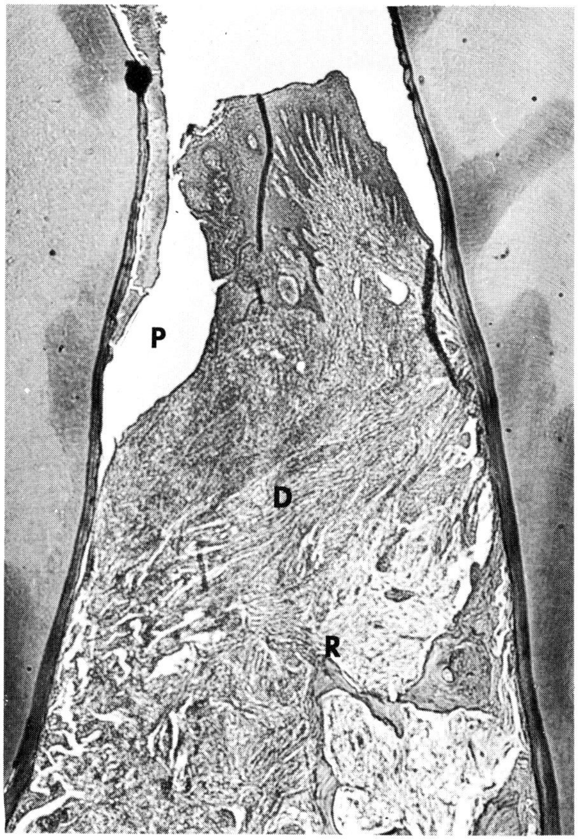

Fig. 5-30. *P,* Histologic section of periodontitis illustrating pocket formation; *D,* destruction of dentinogingival fibers; *R,* resorption of alveolar bone.

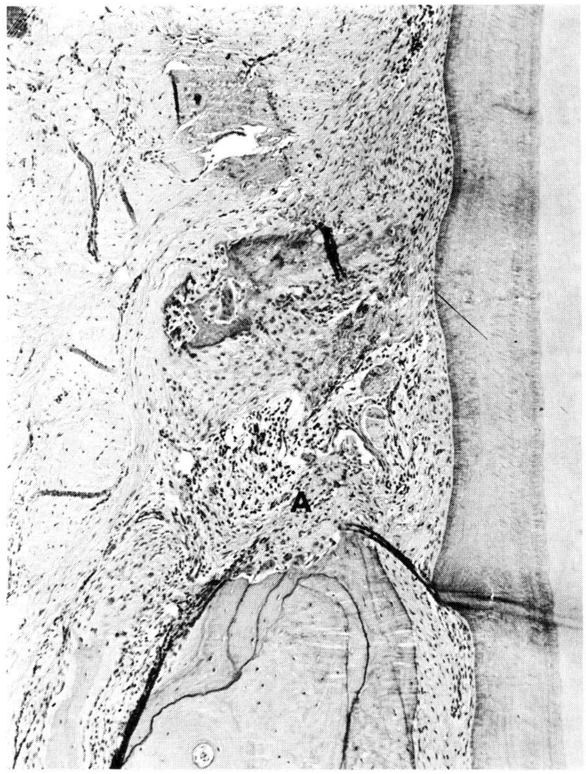

Fig. 5-31. Histologic section showing resorption of bone at alveolar crest, *A.*

the bone marrow spaces will produce further bone resorption and destruction of fibers of the periodontal ligament.

The most common pattern of bone loss that is caused by inflammation is usually a horizontal type of bone resorption (Fig. 5-32). When traumas from occlusion and bruxism or systemic factors are combined with inflammation, a vertical or angular type of bone resorption may take place. Such resorption may result in infrabony defects, craters, ledges, inconsistent margins, hemisepta, or exostoses (Figs. 5-33 to 5-35).

9. Mobility. Resorption of alveolar bone and destruction of fibers of the periodontal ligament eventually will result in varying degrees of looseness of the teeth. On the other hand, teeth subjected to occlusal trauma may exhibit mobility with no apparent loss of supporting structures.

10. Migration. With loss of supporting tissues a tooth may no longer be able to resist normal forces and may elongate, tilt, rotate, or drift into another position (Fig. 5-36). While migration occurs most frequently in the anterior area, posterior teeth may be similarly affected.

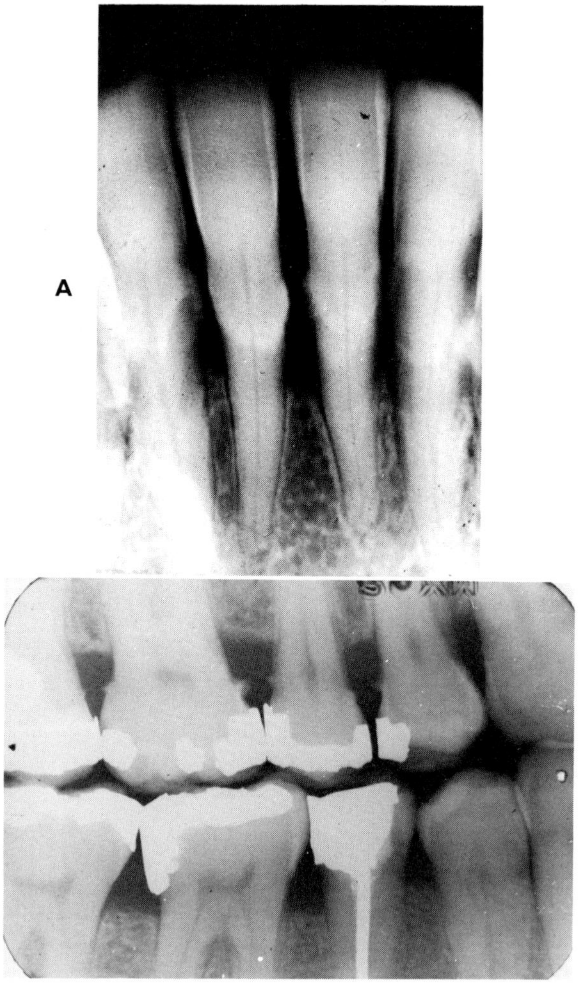

Fig. 5-32. Horizontal bone resorption in periodontitis.

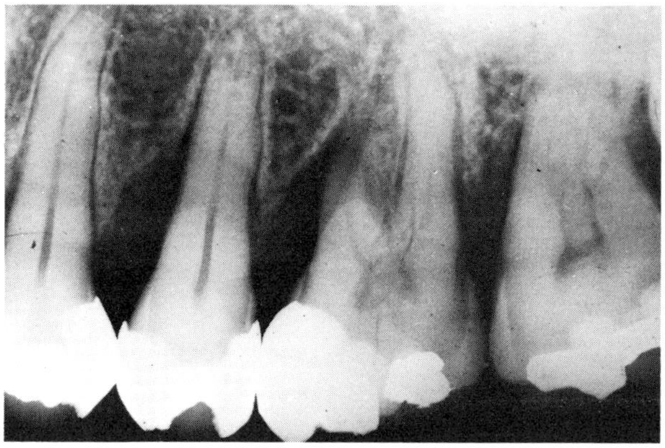

Fig. 5-33. Vertical or angular bone resorption resulting in formation of hemisepta.

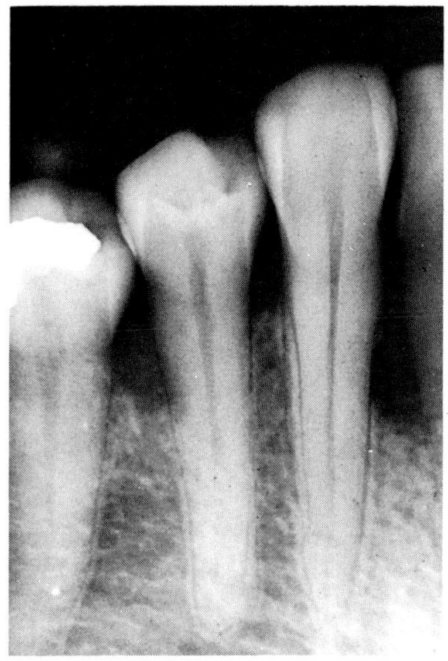

Fig. 5-34. Bone resorption with inconsistent bony margins.

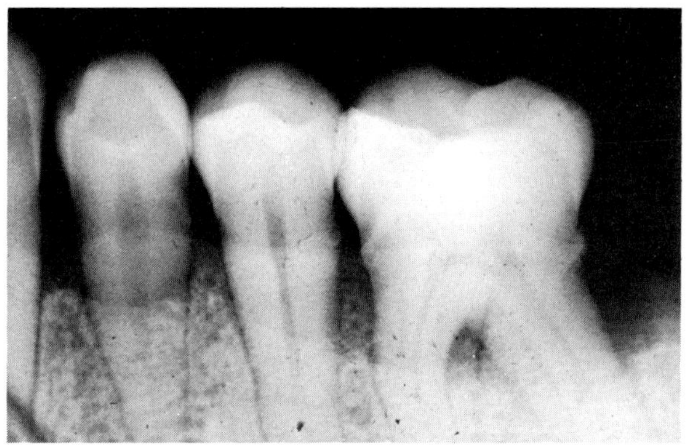

Fig. 5-35. Circular infrabony defect about distal root of lower first molar tooth.

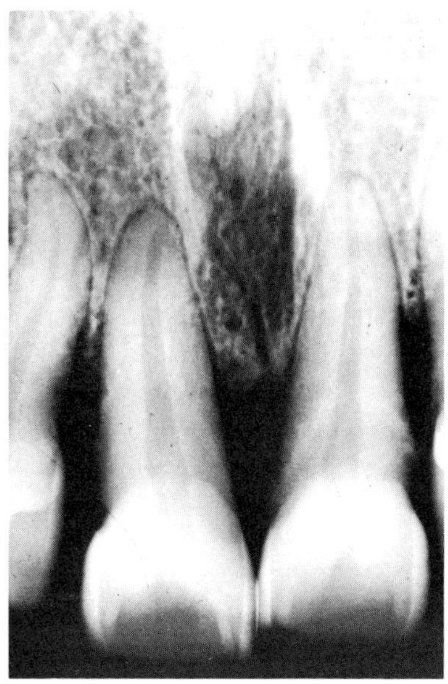

Fig. 5-36. Migration of upper anterior teeth in periodontitis.

A 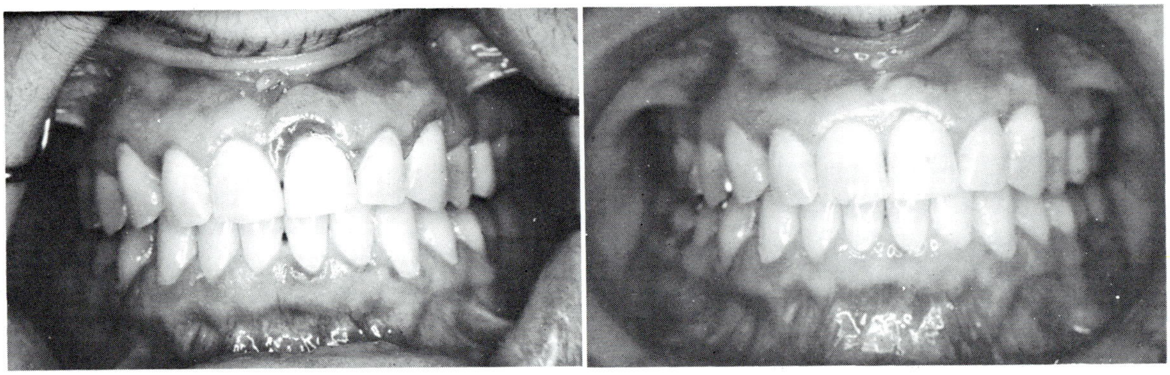 B

Fig. 5-37. **A,** Edematous gingival enlargement of upper left central incisor tooth. **B,** Postoperative view after gingival curettage.

A 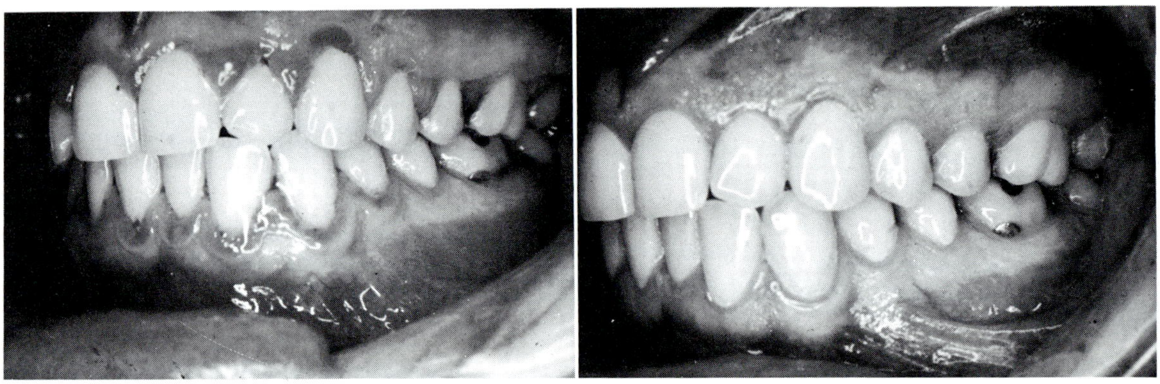 B

Fig. 5-38. **A,** Numerous areas of edematous gingival enlargement. **B,** Postoperative view after gingival curettage.

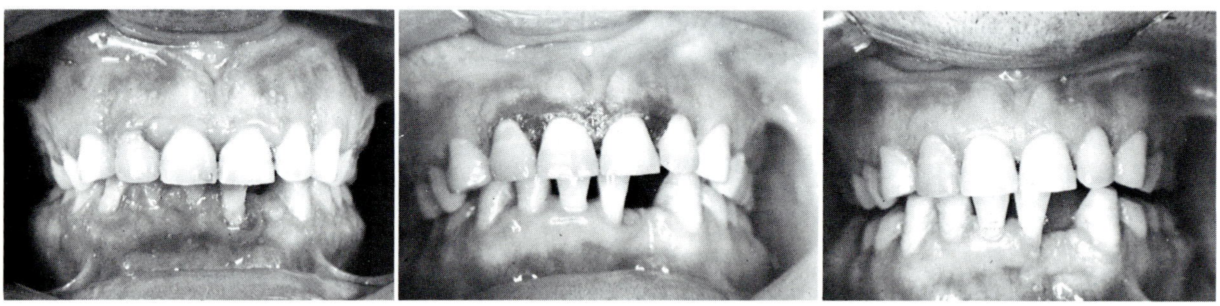

A B C

Fig. 5-39. **A,** Gingival enlargement of upper central incisor teeth. **B,** Gingivoplasty. **C,** Postoperative view after gingivoplasty.

OBJECTIVES OF PERIODONTAL THERAPY

Although it is not within the scope of the chapter to discuss therapy, it is the responsibility of the individual performing advanced restorative procedures not only to recognize periodontal disease in its various forms but also to be well versed in the objectives, attainments, and techniques of periodontal therapy. As in all scientific endeavors these may change as research and newer knowledge make possible a greater insight into the understanding and management of periodontal disease. Before initiating periodontal therapy, a program of plaque control

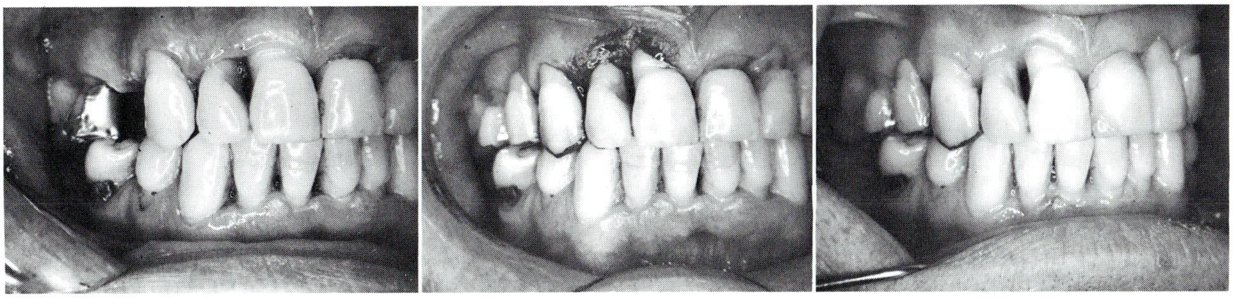

A B C

Fig. 5-40. **A,** Interproximal crater between upper right lateral and central incisor teeth. **B,** Gingivoplasty. **C,** Postoperative view after gingivoplasty.

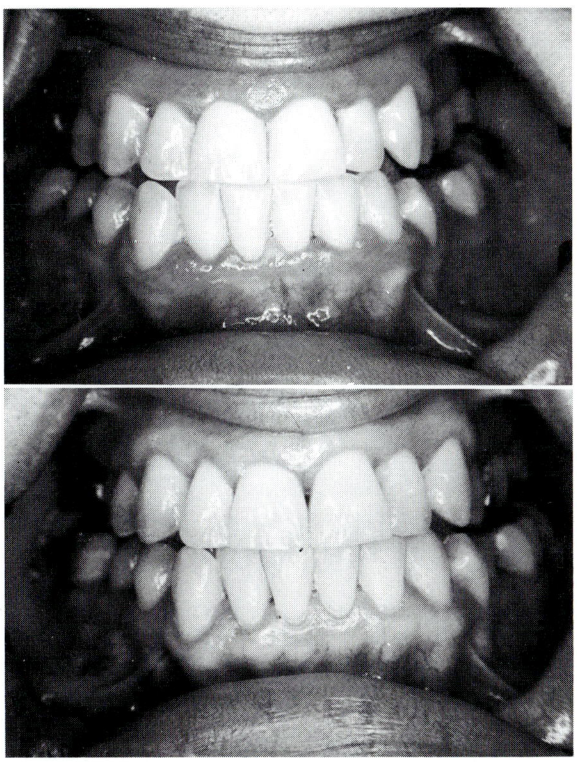

A B

Fig. 5-41. A, Interproximal crater formation in recurrent necrotizing ulcerative gingivitis. **B,** Postoperative view after gingivoplasty.

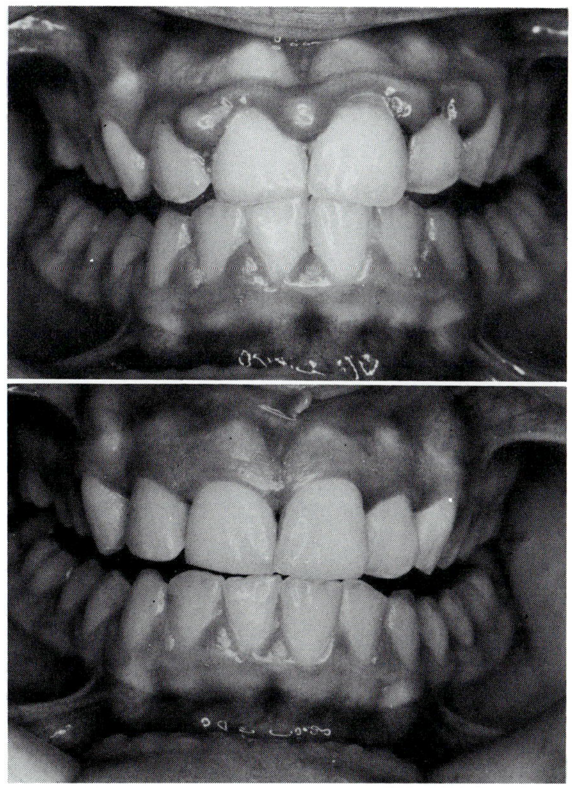

A B

Fig. 5-42. A, Inflammatory hyperplasia of gingiva after orthodontic treatment. **B,** Postoperative view after gingivectomy in upper anterior area.

is mandatory, but it must be tailored to the individual's requirements.

Some of the current-day objectives are as follows:

1. Pink, firm, well-attached gingiva
2. Knife-edged marginal gingiva
3. Minimal depth of gingival sulcus
4. Adequate amount of attached gingiva
5. Elimination of pull of frena and muscle attachments
6. Intact foundation of alveolar bone (elimination of infrabony defects, exostoses)
7. Stability of remaining dentition

The cases that are presented now will attempt to illustrate many of the previously mentioned objectives (Figs. 5-37 to 5-70).

A

B

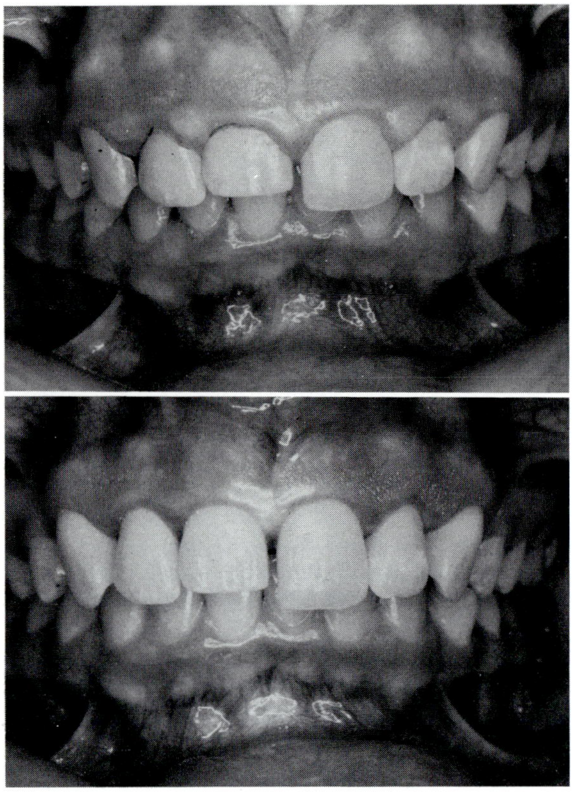

Fig. 5-43. **A,** Gingival enlargement in delayed passive eruption. **B,** Postoperative view after gingivectomy.

A

B

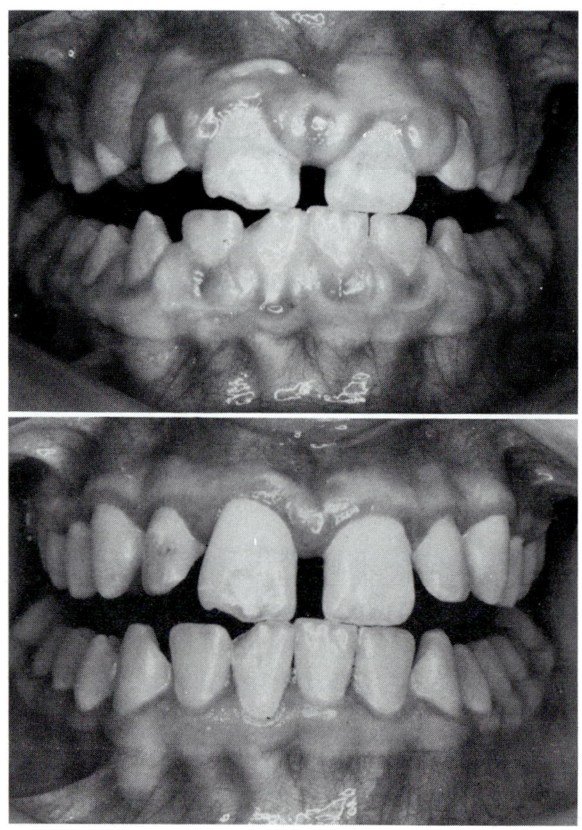

Fig. 5-44. **A,** Hyperplasia of gingiva caused by intake of Dilantin. **B,** Postoperative view after gingivectomy.

A E

B F

C G

D H

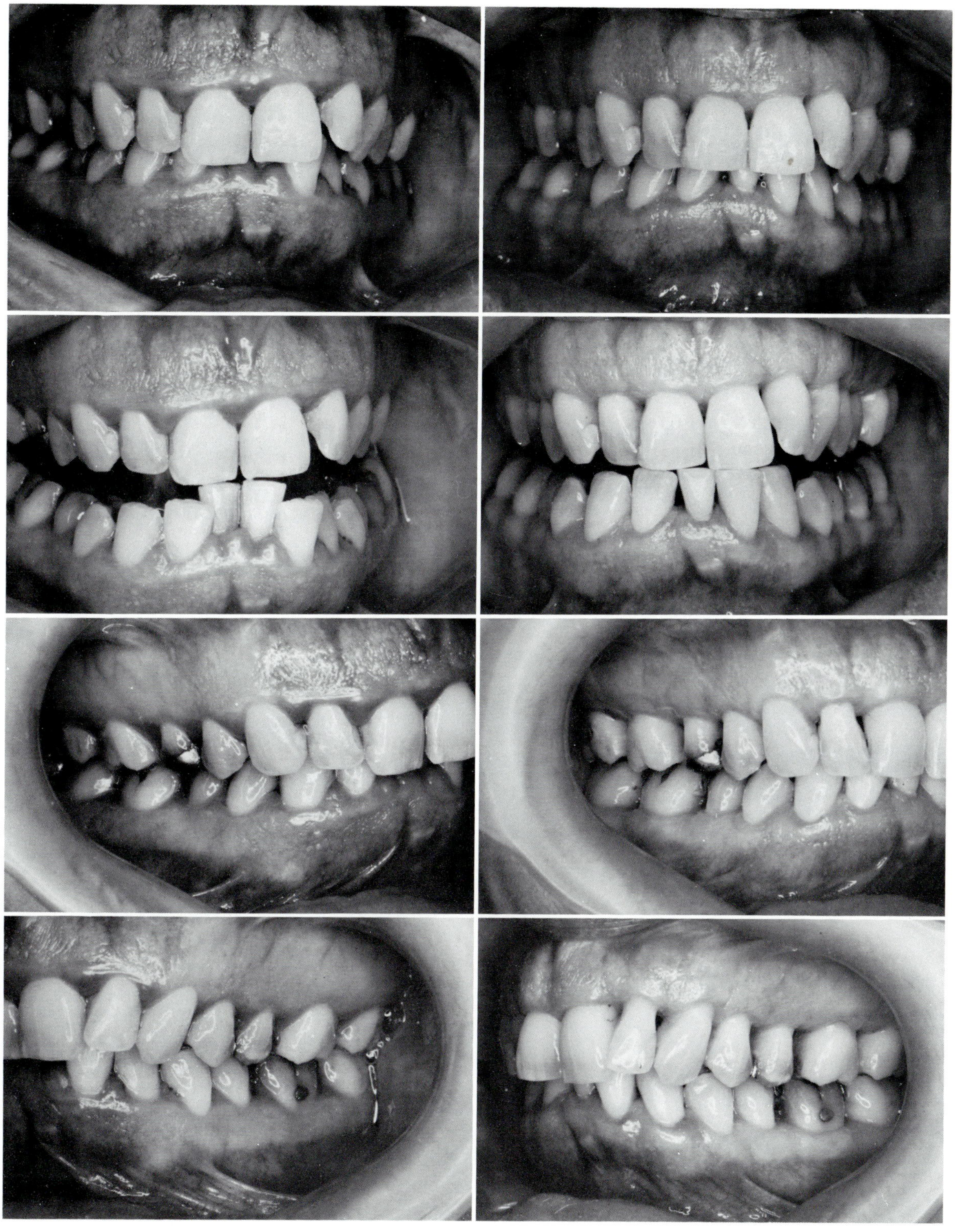

Fig. 5-45. Incipient periodontitis. **A** to **D,** Preoperative views. **E** to **H,** Postoperative views after gingivectomy. Lower right central has been extracted and lower left central has been moved with elastics into proper alignment.

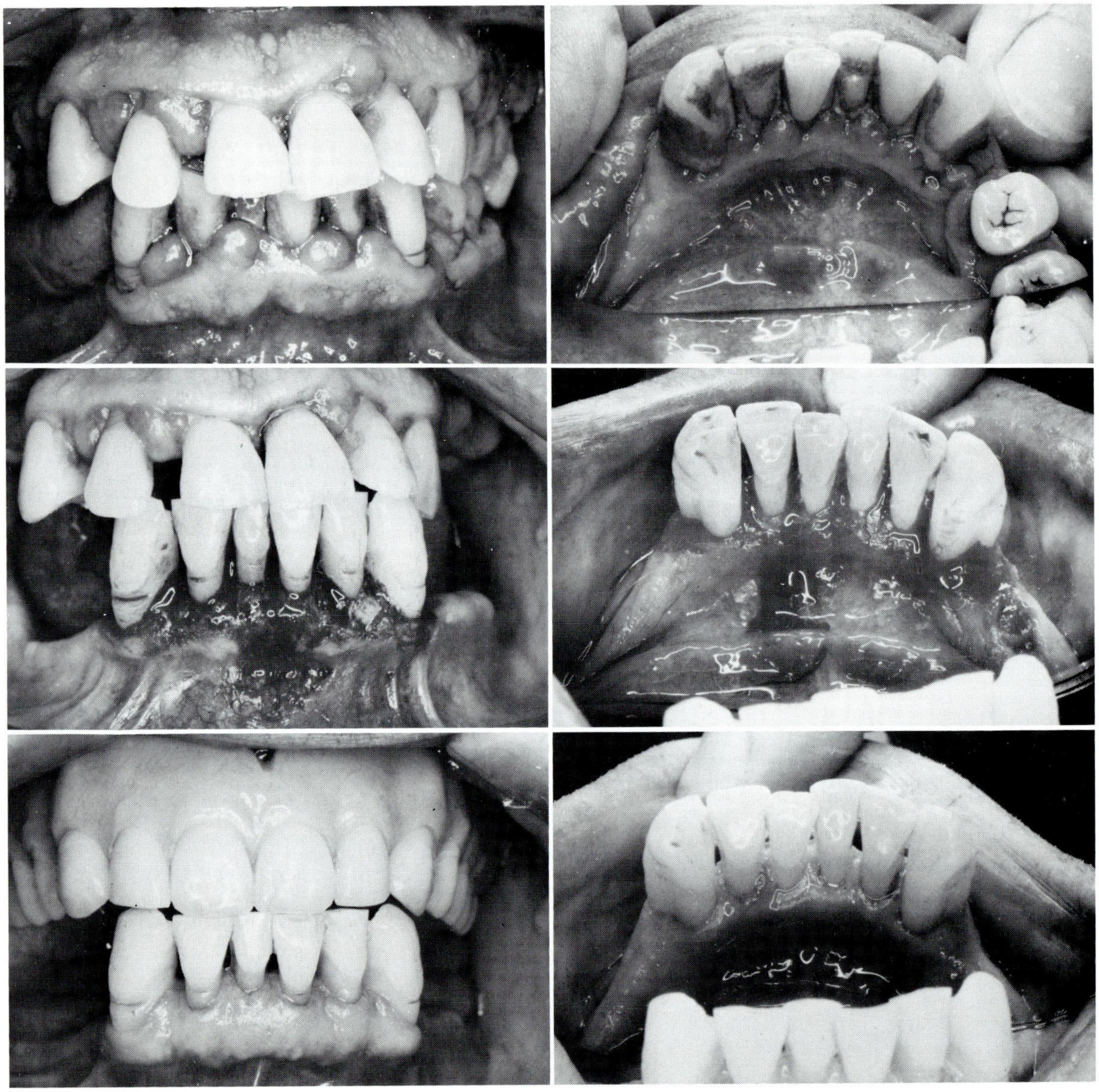

A D

B E

C F

Fig. 5-46. Inflammatory hyperplasia in periodontitis. **A,** Facial view; **D,** Lingual view. **B** and **E,** Gingivectomy. **C** and **F,** Postoperative view after gingivectomy.

A B C D

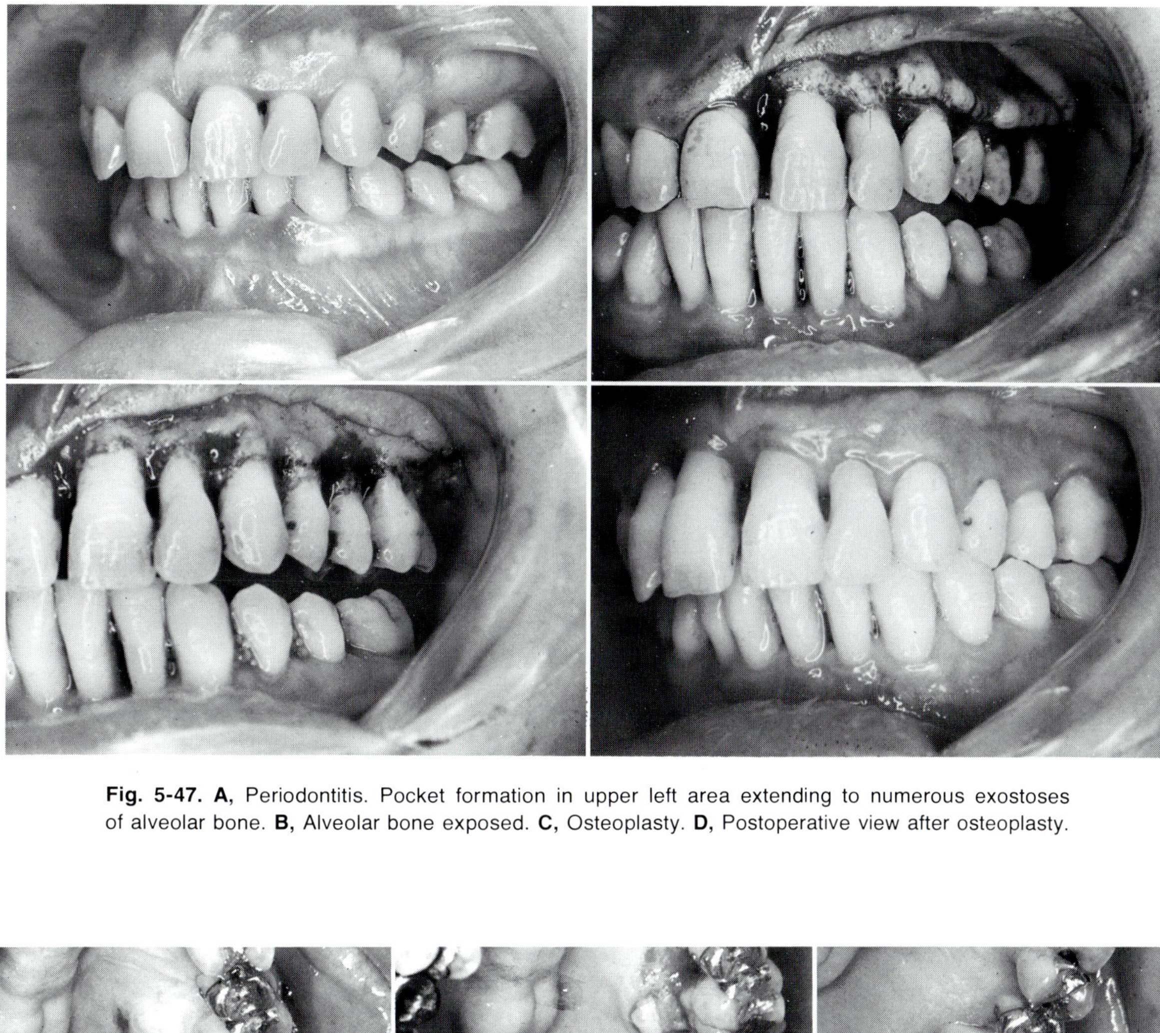

Fig. 5-47. A, Periodontitis. Pocket formation in upper left area extending to numerous exostoses of alveolar bone. **B,** Alveolar bone exposed. **C,** Osteoplasty. **D,** Postoperative view after osteoplasty.

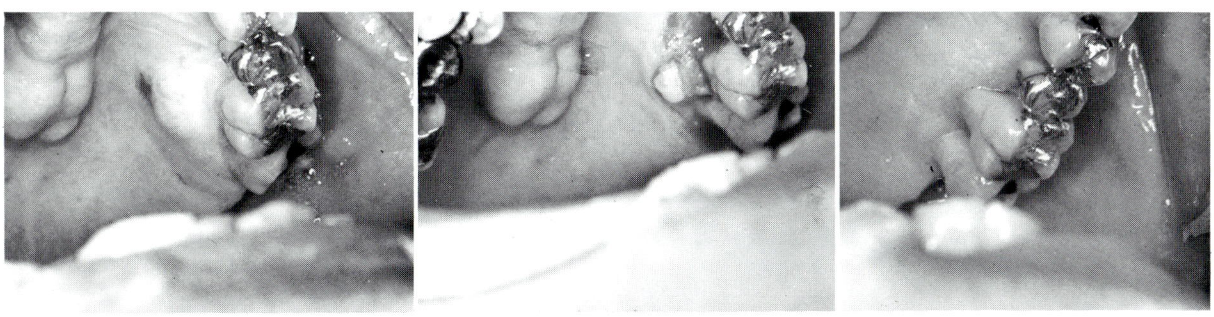

A B C

Fig. 5-48. A, Periodontitis. Pocket formation and large exostosis lingual of upper left first molar tooth. **B,** Exostosis exposed. **C,** Postoperative view after osteoplasty.

A
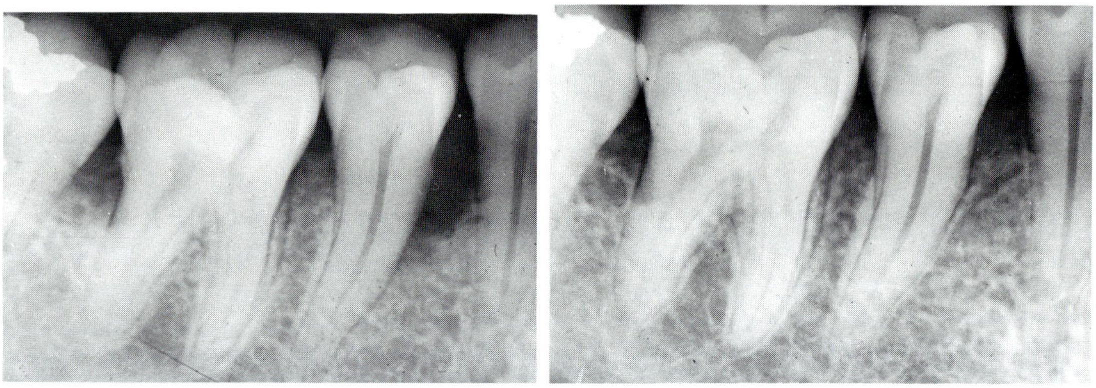
B

Fig. 5-49. A, Intrabony pocket mesial of lower second bicuspid tooth. **B,** Postoperative view after operation for new attachment. (From Schreiber, H. R.: Oral Surg. **17:**161, 1964.)

A
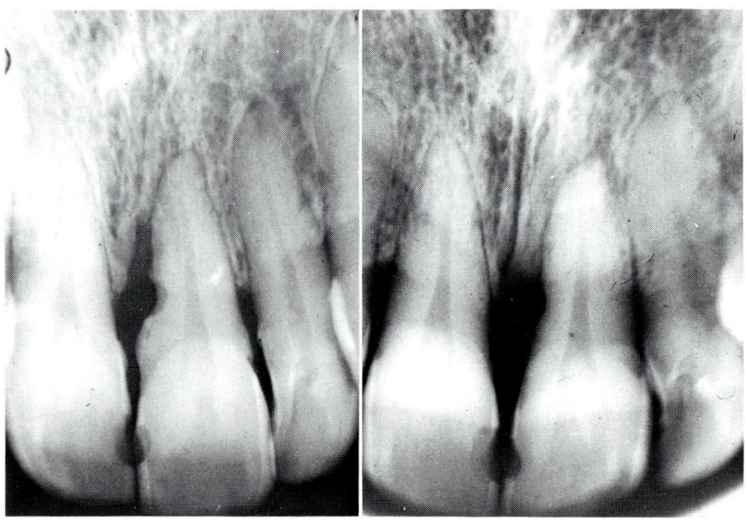
B

Fig. 5-50. A, Intrabony pocket mesial of upper left central incisor tooth. **B,** Postoperative view after operation for new attachment.

A

B

C

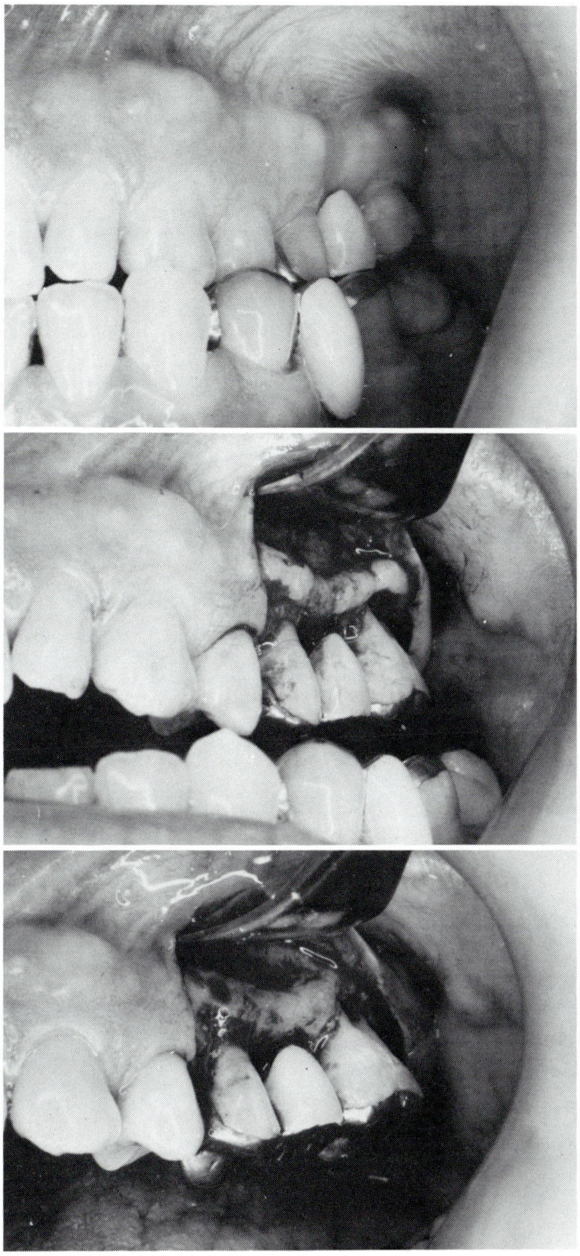

Fig. 5-51. A, Bony enlargements on facial surface. **B,** Infrabony pocket exposed about upper left first molar tooth. **C,** Postoperative view after ostectomy to eliminate infrabony pocket of upper left first molar tooth (osteoplasty performed about bicuspid teeth).

A

B

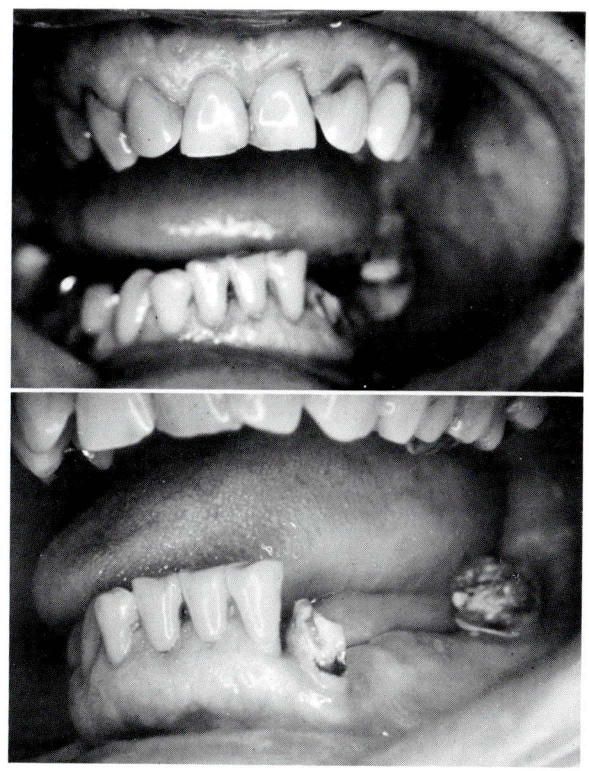

Fig. 5-52. A, Broken-down crowns of lower left first bicuspid and second molar teeth. **B,** Postoperative view after ostectomy to expose root surface for full coverage restorations.

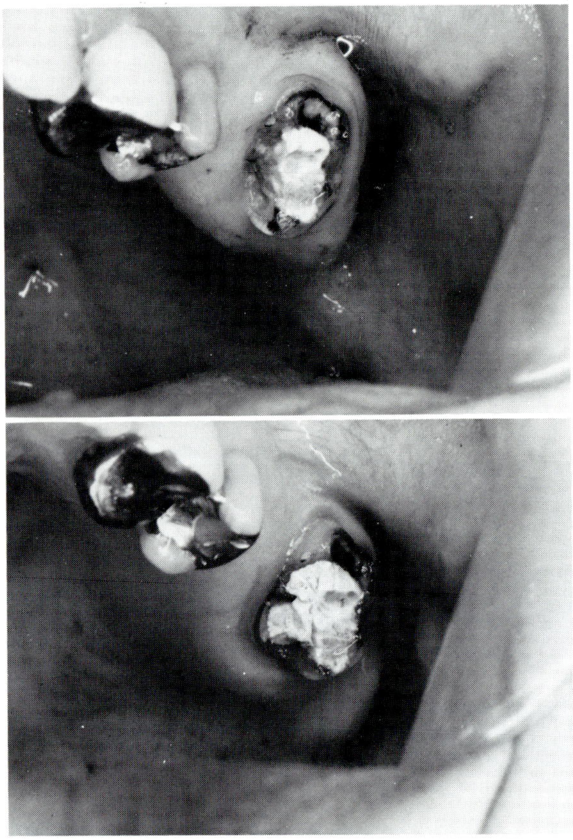

A

B

Fig. 5-53. A, Broken-down crown of upper left second molar. **B,** Postoperative view after ostectomy to expose root surface for full coverage restoration.

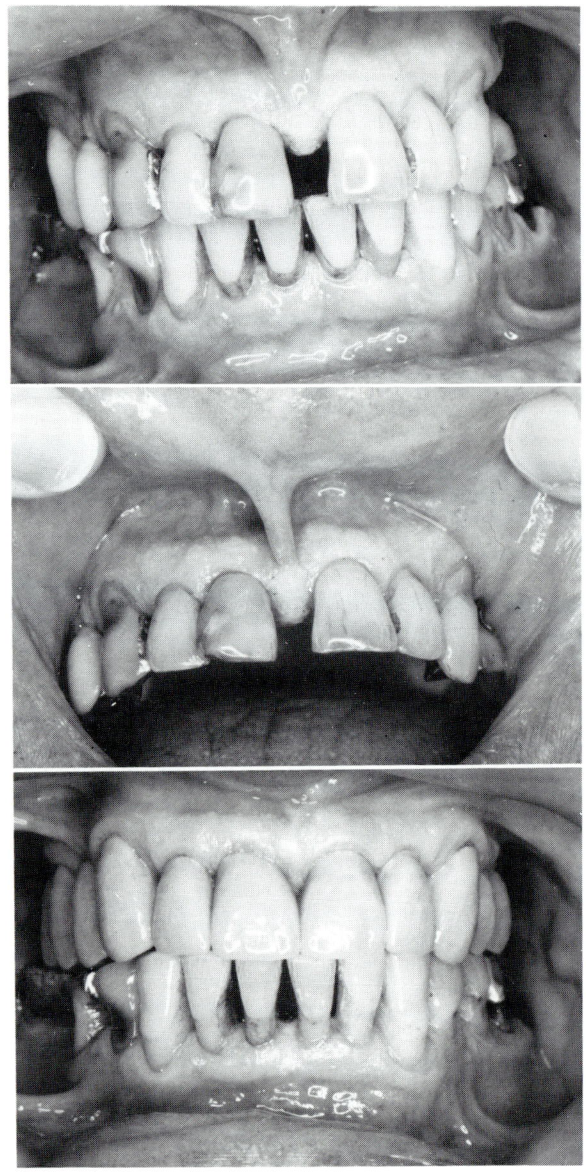

A

B

C

Fig. 5-54. A, Pocket formation about upper incisor teeth involving large frenum and separation of teeth. **B,** Lip extended, illustrating frenum involvement. **C,** Postoperative view after frenectomy and orthodontic movement of incisor teeth.

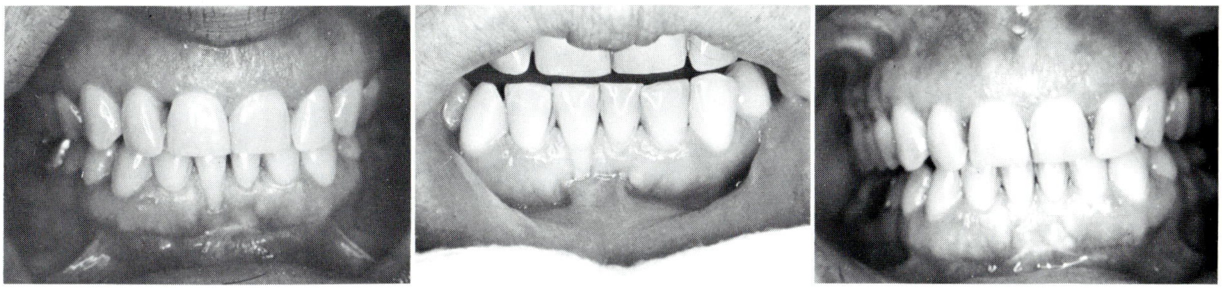

A B C

Fig. 5-55. A, Gingival recession about lower right central incisor tooth caused by improper toothbrushing and broad lower frenum attachment. **B,** Enlargement of frenum in **A. C,** Postoperative view after frenotomy and lowering of attachment of incisive and mental muscles. Attached gingiva now covers previously denuded root of lower right central incisor tooth.

A

B

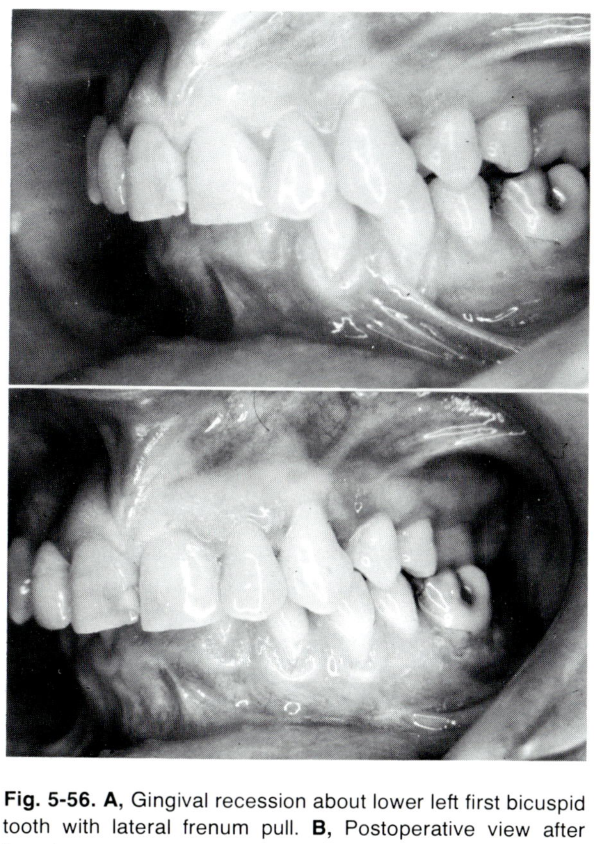

Fig. 5-56. A, Gingival recession about lower left first bicuspid tooth with lateral frenum pull. **B,** Postoperative view after frenotomy.

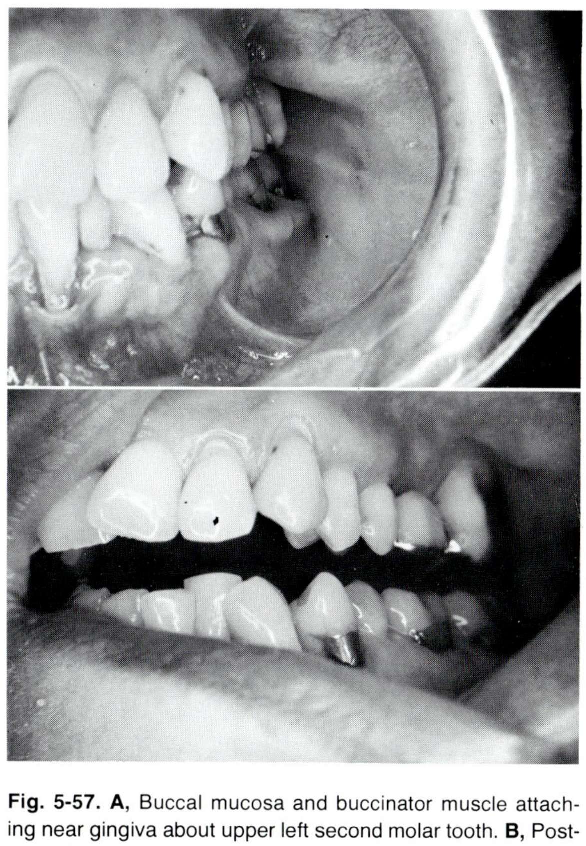

A

B

Fig. 5-57. A, Buccal mucosa and buccinator muscle attaching near gingiva about upper left second molar tooth. **B,** Postoperative view after separation of buccinator muscle attachment and deepening of vestibular fold.

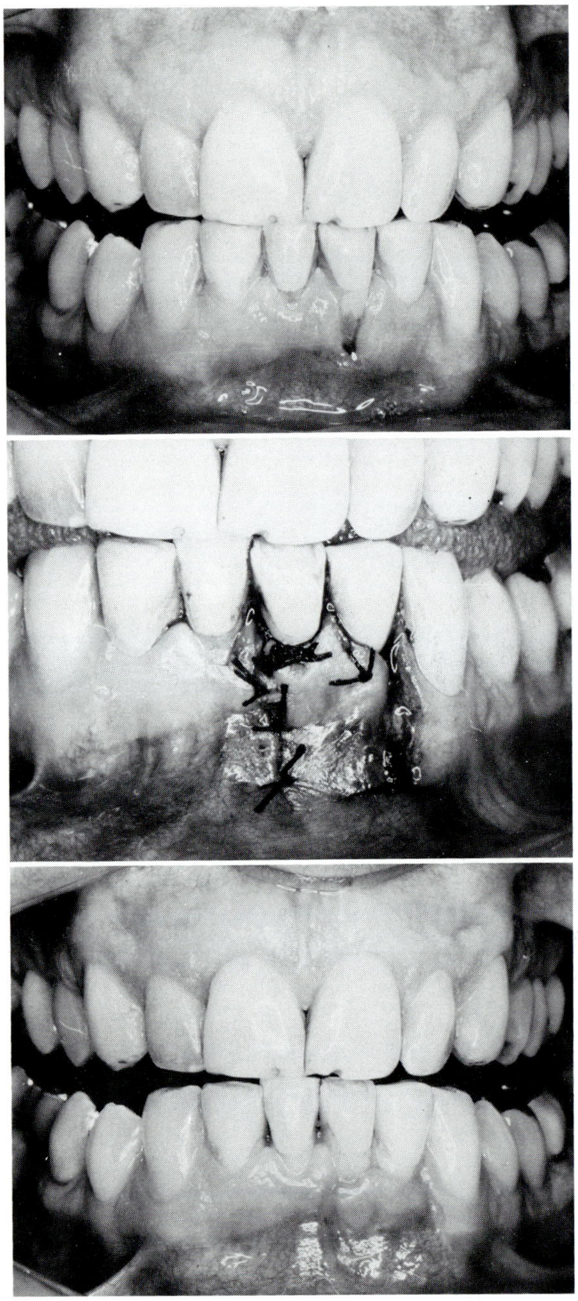

A

B

C

Fig. 5-58. A, Recession of gingiva about lower left central incisor tooth. **B,** Lateral positioned flap or pedicle graft from lower left lateral incisor area. **C,** Postoperative view after pedicle graft. Attached gingiva now present about lower left central incisor tooth.

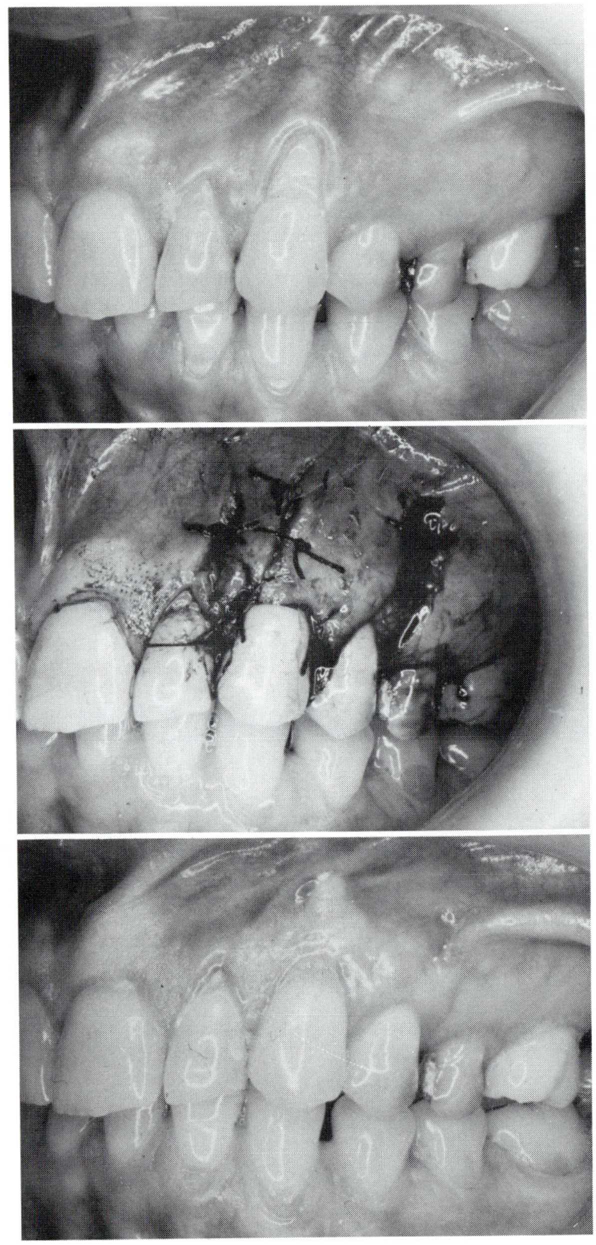

A

B

C

Fig. 5-59. A, Severe gingival recession about upper left cuspid tooth into alveolar mucosa. **B,** Pedicle graft from upper left first bicuspid and lateral incisor areas. **C,** Postoperative view after pedicle graft. New zone of attached gingiva is present about upper left cuspid tooth.

A B C D

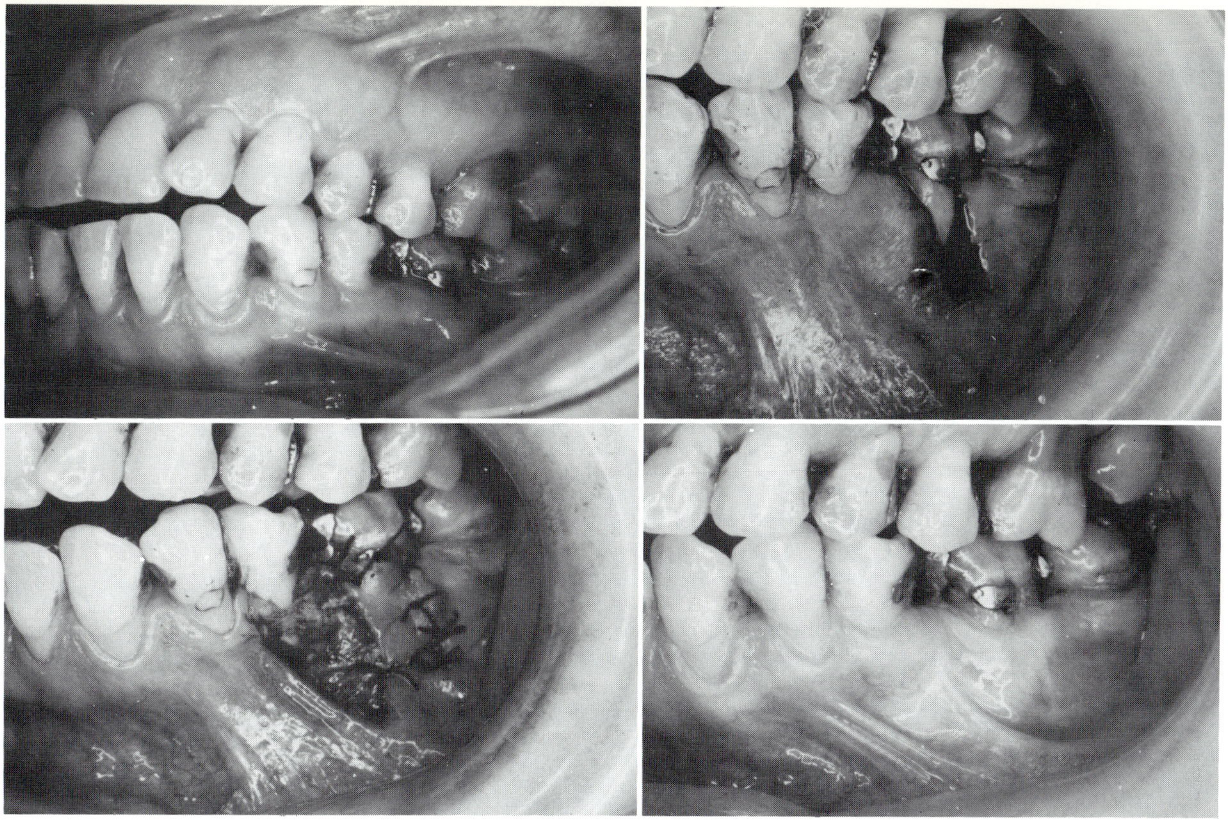

Fig. 5-60. A, Deep pocket formation about lower left first molar tooth extending into alveolar mucosa. **B,** Bone resorption about mesial root of lower left first molar. **C,** Pedicle graft from lower left second bicuspid area. **D,** Postoperative view after pedicle graft. Note eradication of pocket and new zone of attached gingiva about mesial root of lower left first molar tooth.

A B C

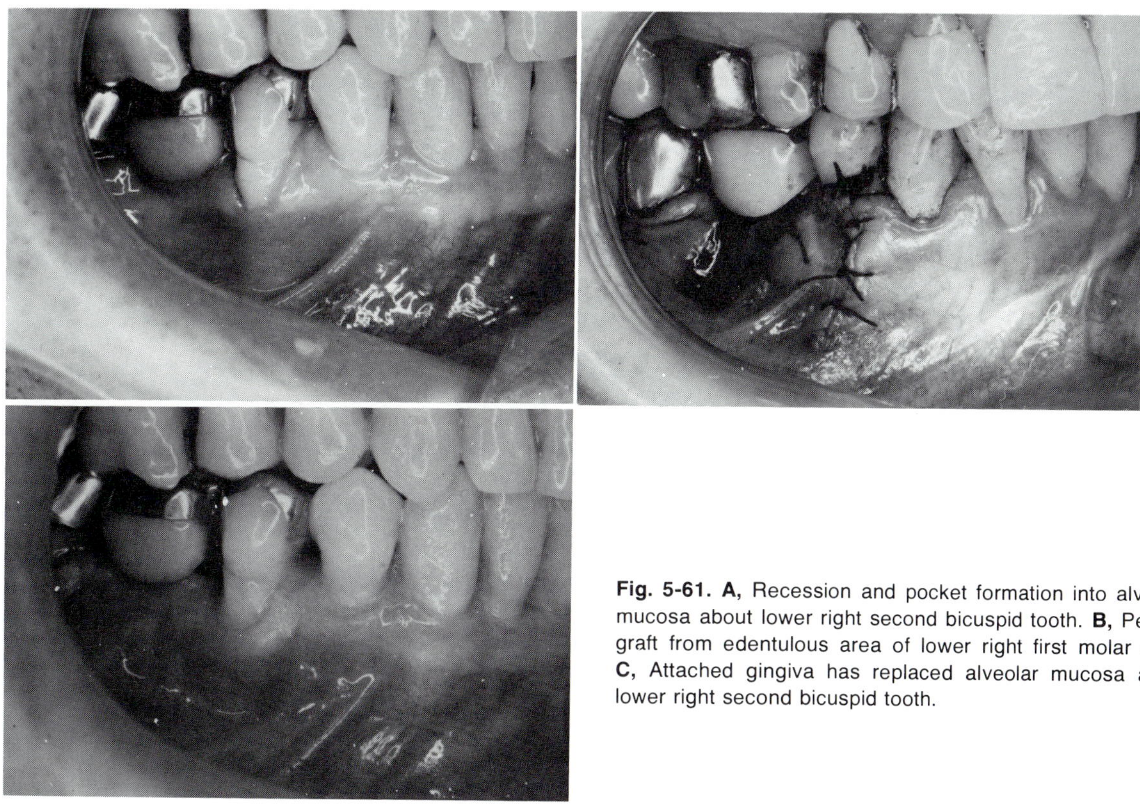

Fig. 5-61. A, Recession and pocket formation into alveolar mucosa about lower right second bicuspid tooth. **B,** Pedicle graft from edentulous area of lower right first molar area. **C,** Attached gingiva has replaced alveolar mucosa about lower right second bicuspid tooth.

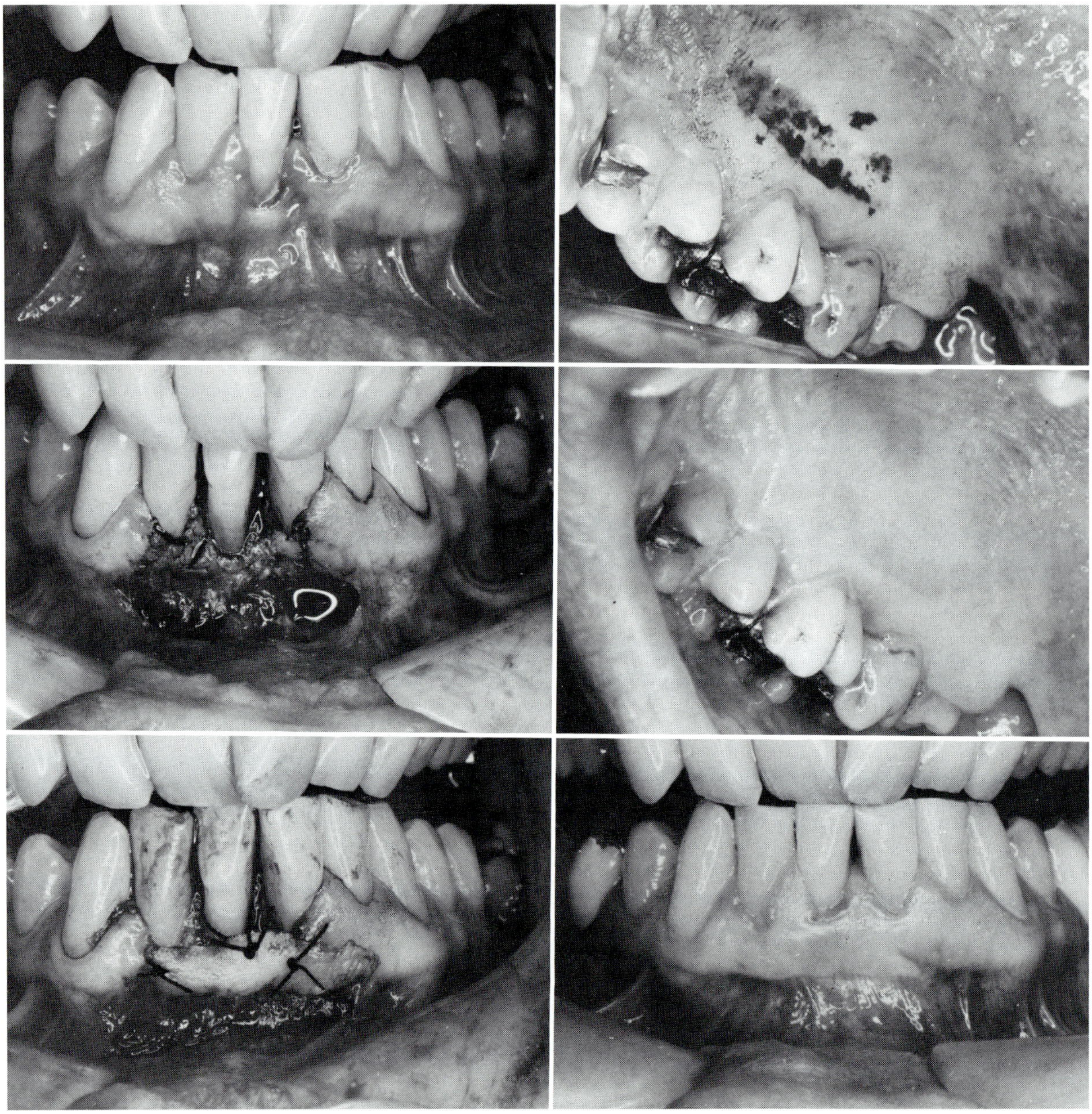

Fig. 5-62. A, Gingival recession and pull of lower labial frenum about lower right central incisor tooth. **B,** Preparation of recipient site for free mucosal graft. **C,** Free mucosal graft sutured in recipient site. **D,** Palatal donor site of graft. **E,** Healed donor site. **F,** Postoperative view after free mucosal graft. Note new attached gingiva about lower right central incisor tooth and elimination of frenum pull.

A

B

C

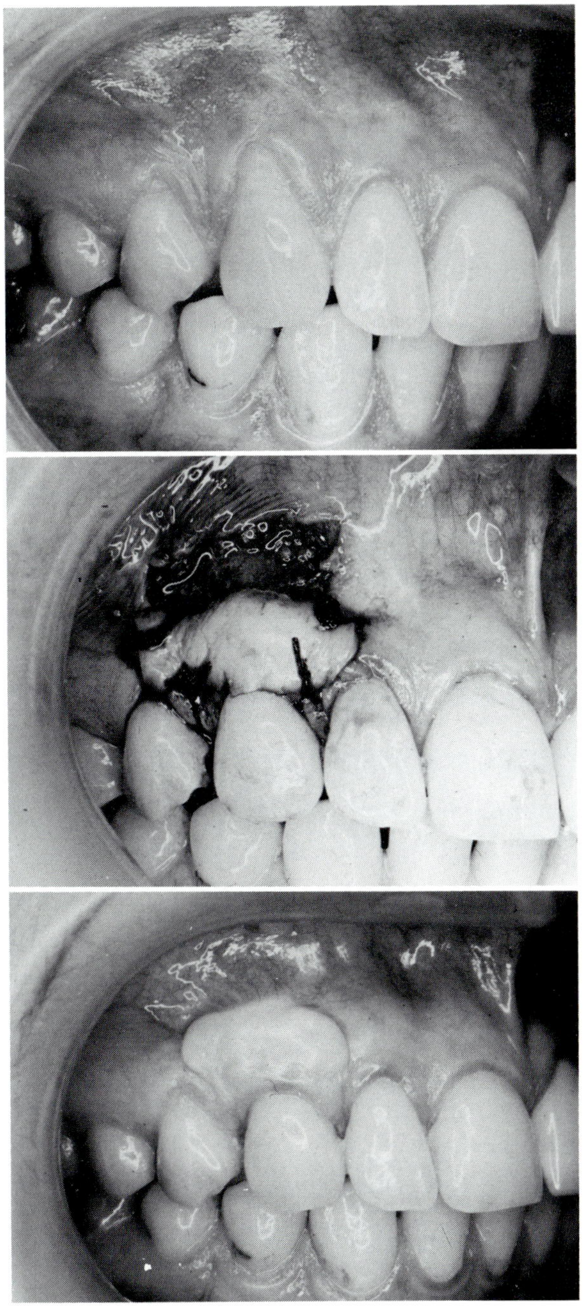

Fig. 5-63. A, Gingival recession about upper right cuspid tooth. **B,** Free mucosal graft from palate sutured in recipient site. **C,** Postoperative view after free mucosal graft. New zone of attached gingiva is present about upper right cuspid tooth with complete coverage of exposed root surface.

A B C

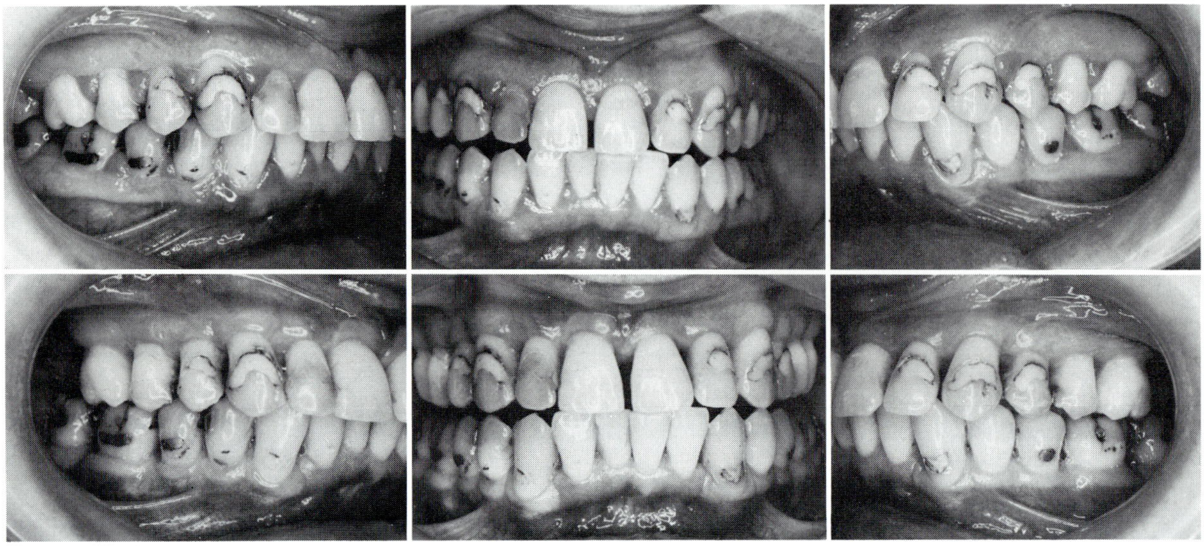

D E F

Fig. 5-64. A to **C,** Periodontitis, moderately advanced. **D** to **F,** Postoperative views after mucoperiosteal flaps with internal or reverse beveled incisions. Elimination of pockets with retention of attached gingiva.

A B C

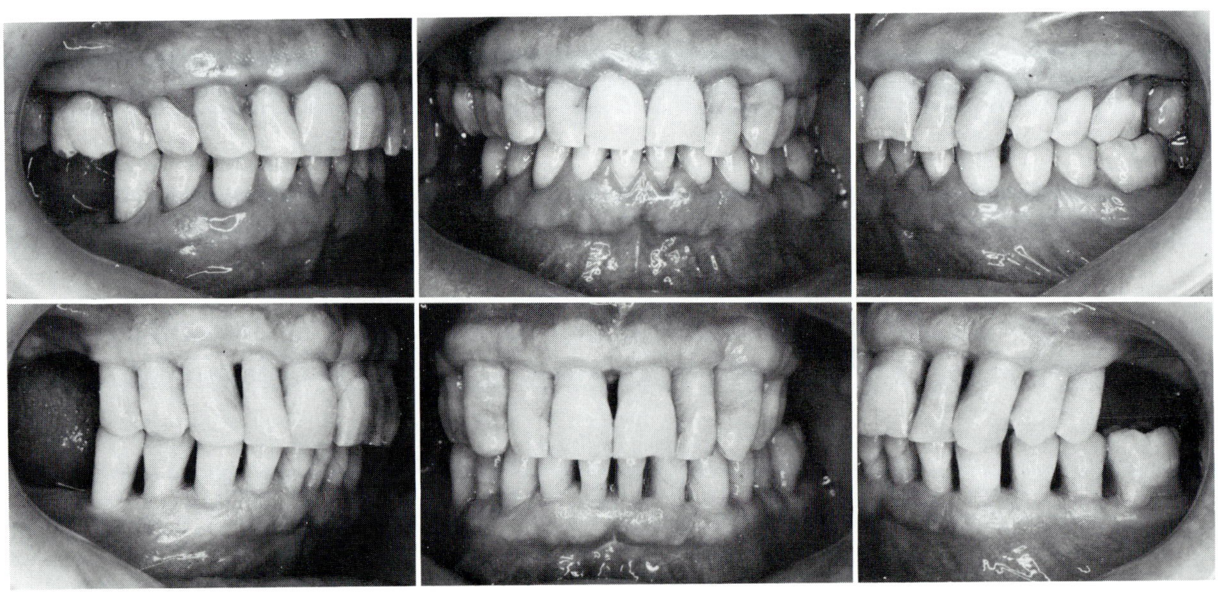

D E F

Fig. 5-65. A to **C,** Periodontitis, well advanced. **D** to **F,** Postoperative view after apically positioned internal beveled flaps. Elimination of pockets with apical positioning of attached gingiva and alveolar mucosa.

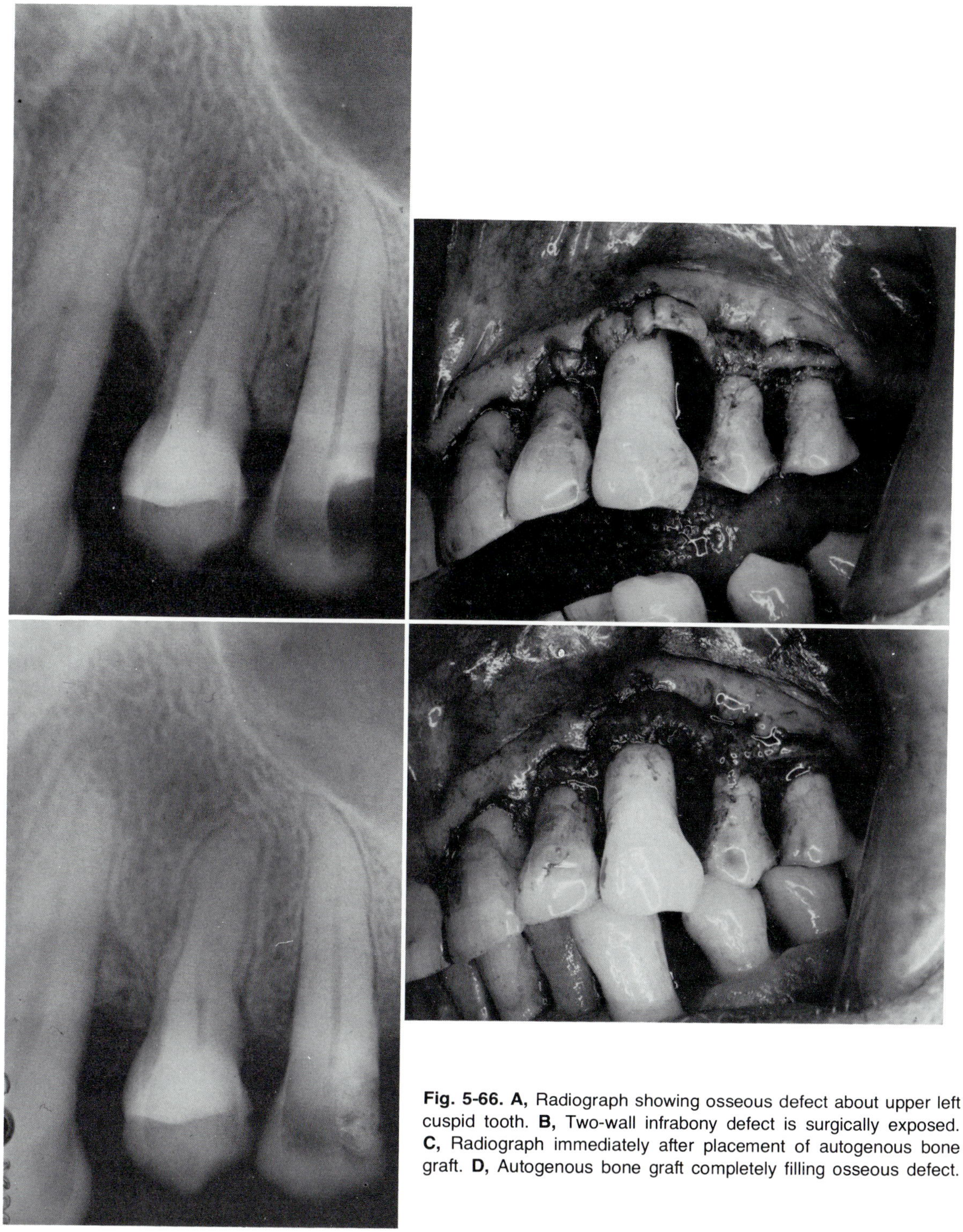

A B C D

Fig. 5-66. A, Radiograph showing osseous defect about upper left cuspid tooth. **B,** Two-wall infrabony defect is surgically exposed. **C,** Radiograph immediately after placement of autogenous bone graft. **D,** Autogenous bone graft completely filling osseous defect.

A 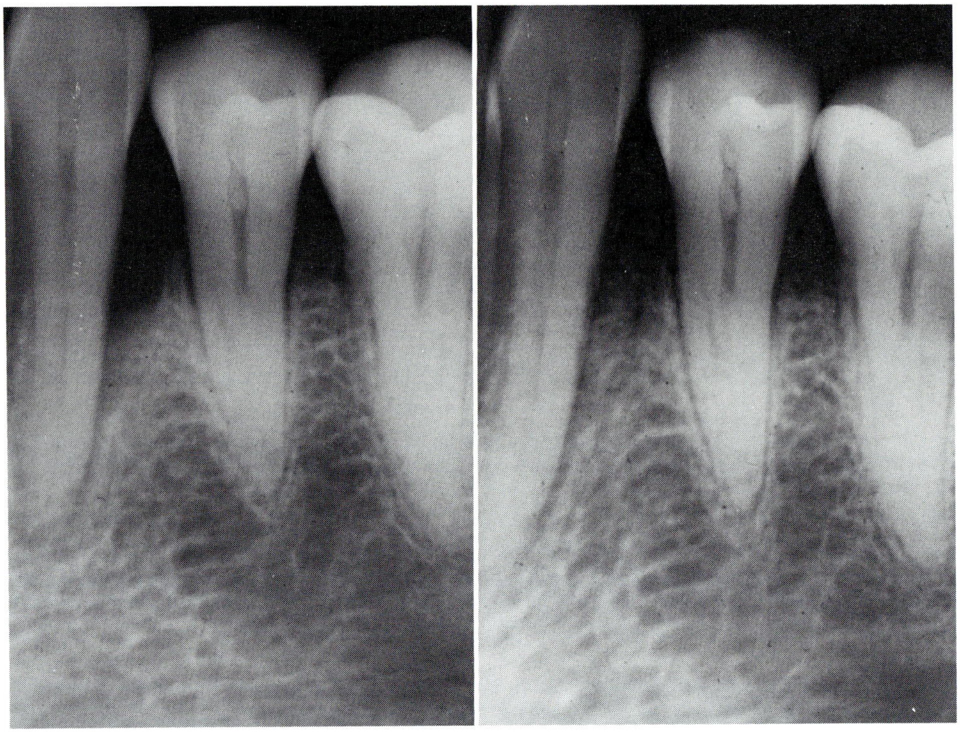 B

Fig. 5-67. A, Osseous defect about distal of lower cuspid. **B,** Postoperative radiograph after autogenous bone graft.

A 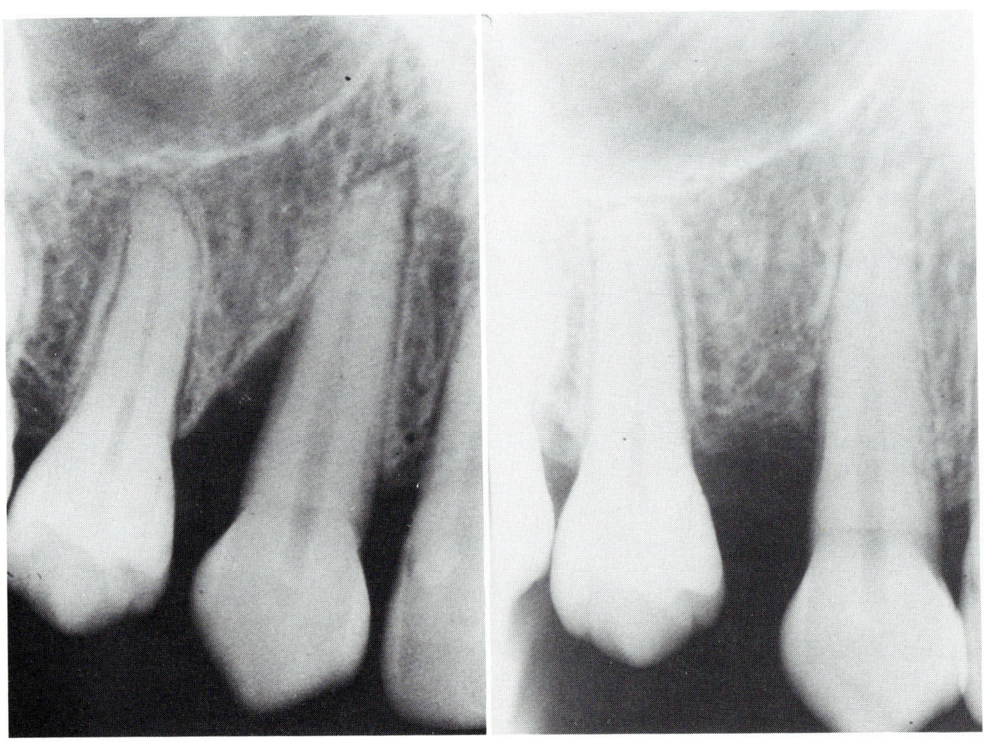 B

Fig. 5-68. A, Osseous defect about distal of upper cuspid. **B,** Postoperative radiograph after autogenous bone graft.

A

B

C

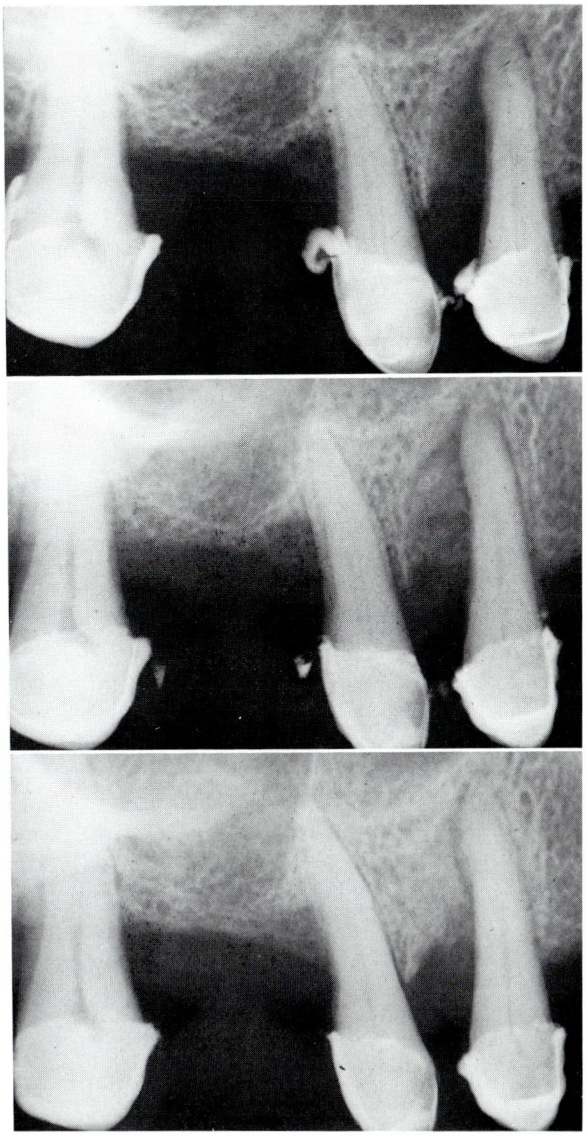

Fig. 5-69. A, Deep two-wall infrabony defect about distal of upper first bicuspid tooth. **B,** Radiograph immediately after placement of autogenous bone graft. **C,** Postoperative radiograph illustrating bone regeneration after 6 month interval.

A

B

C

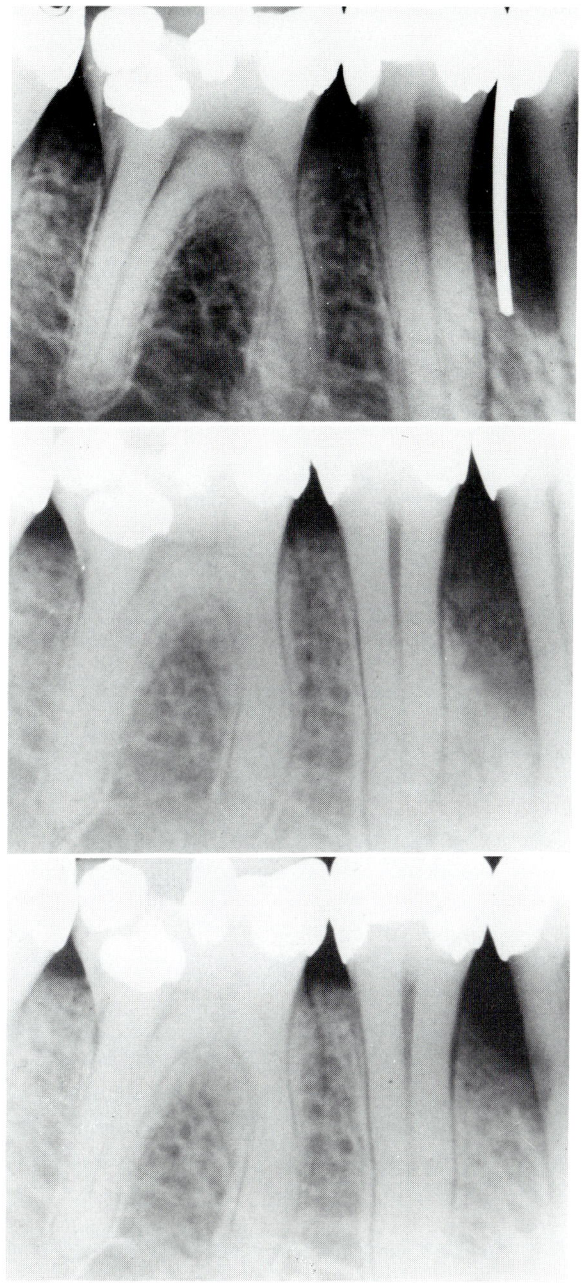

Fig. 5-70. A, Osseous defect about distal of lower first bicuspid tooth. **B,** Radiograph immediately after placement of iliac bone marrow graft. **C,** Postoperative radiograph of iliac bone marrow graft after 1 year.

REFERENCES

1. Bowers, G. M.: A study of the width of the attached gingiva, J. Periodontol. **34:**201, 1963.
2. Fish, S. W.: Etiology and prevention of periodontal breakdown, Dent. Progr. **1(4):**234, 1961.
3. Glickman, I.: Clinical periodontology, Philadelphia, 1964, W. B. Saunders Co.
4. Goldman, H. M., and Cohen, D. W.: Periodontal therapy, ed. 5, St. Louis, 1973, The C. V. Mosby Co.
5. Grant, D., Stern, I. B., and Everett, F. G.: Orban's periodontics, ed. 4, St. Louis, 1972, The C. V. Mosby Co.
6. Provenza, D. V.: Oral histology, Philadelphia, 1964, J. B. Lippincott Co.
7. Sicher, H., and Bhaskar, S. N.: Orban's oral histology and embryology, ed. 7, St. Louis, 1972, The C. V. Mosby Co.

CHAPTER 6

PROSTHETIC-PERIODONTAL INTERRELATIONSHIPS

GENERAL CONSIDERATIONS

The most important task in dentistry is the preservation and maintenance of the natural dentition in health. Restorative dentistry and periodontics are interdependent and interrelated in this particular objective. In other words, restorative dentistry and periodontics should not be practiced as separate and distinct clinical entities, because it is essential that the patient receive a total health service, not a number of individual procedures. The teeth and their supporting structures, because of their intimate functional dependence, should be viewed as a mutually protective team, each contributing to the health of the other.

The periodontal tissues are the ultimate testing ground for the validity of all concepts of occlusal function. In the final analysis the response of the periodontal tissues is the yardstick by which longevity of prosthetics is measured.[1]

Modern periodontic concepts have made possible the retention of many teeth that previously were condemned for extraction, in spite of the fact that the treated dental apparatus is somewhat different than the normal. Reference is made here to new sulcular depths, variations in crown-to-root ratios, embrasure spaces, bifurcation and trifurcation areas, etc. The proper periodontal environment is created before restorative procedures are undertaken.

Concurrent periodontal and pulpal disorders may be related to, or independent of, each other. For example, products of a necrotic pulp may drain through the gingival sulcus or the furcation and produce a periodontal pocket. Infection and inflammation associated with destructive periodontal disease may cause pulpal degeneration. Pain, altered vitality of the pulp, suppuration, periodontal pockets, and radiographic changes may be associated with both disorders.

The close interrelation of periodontal health and correct prosthetic function is of the utmost importance. The functional stimulation provided by the properly designed and executed dental restorations is supportive to the periodontium and is essential for its preservation. Similarly, periodontal health is very necessary for the proper function of the dental restorations. In other words, the periodontal tissues must be restored to health, and the operative and fixed prosthesis must be constructed in a manner that fulfills the necessary biologic concepts for the maintenance of this healthy state.

From the periodontal viewpoint we must end up with an adherent gingival attachment to the tooth that can barely be probed. But how can this phenomenon be accomplished? (See Fig. 6-1.)

To begin with, it can be said that we can see only that which we understand. If we understand the basic sciences and their applications to our problems and

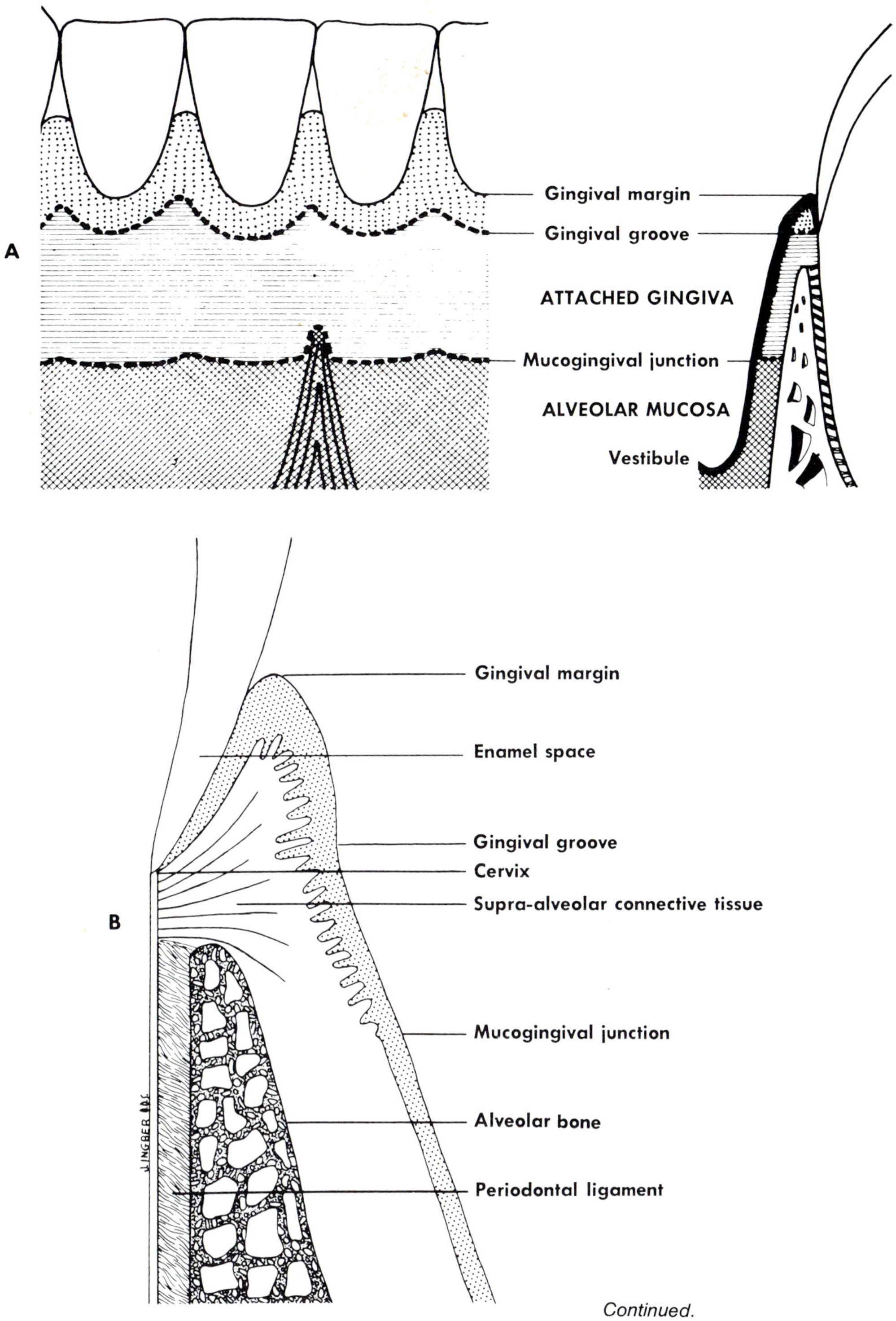

Continued.

Fig. 6-1. A, Anatomic relationships of normal gingiva. **B,** Anatomic relationships of marginal periodontium. **C,** Histologic relationships of marginal gingiva. **D,** *a,* Suprabony pocket on the labial surface. The excision is along the dotted line to remove the marginal epithelium and produce a bevel. The epithelium lining of the pocket is removed later by curettage. *b,* Diagram of an infrabony pocket. An initial incision is made along the dotted line to remove the superficial tissue prior to subgingival curettage. (Adapted from a television course given by Dr. Erwin M. Schaffer; in carefully selected cases, I have had good success with the technique.) (Courtesy Dr. Henry M. Goldman and Dr. D. Walter Cohen.)

C

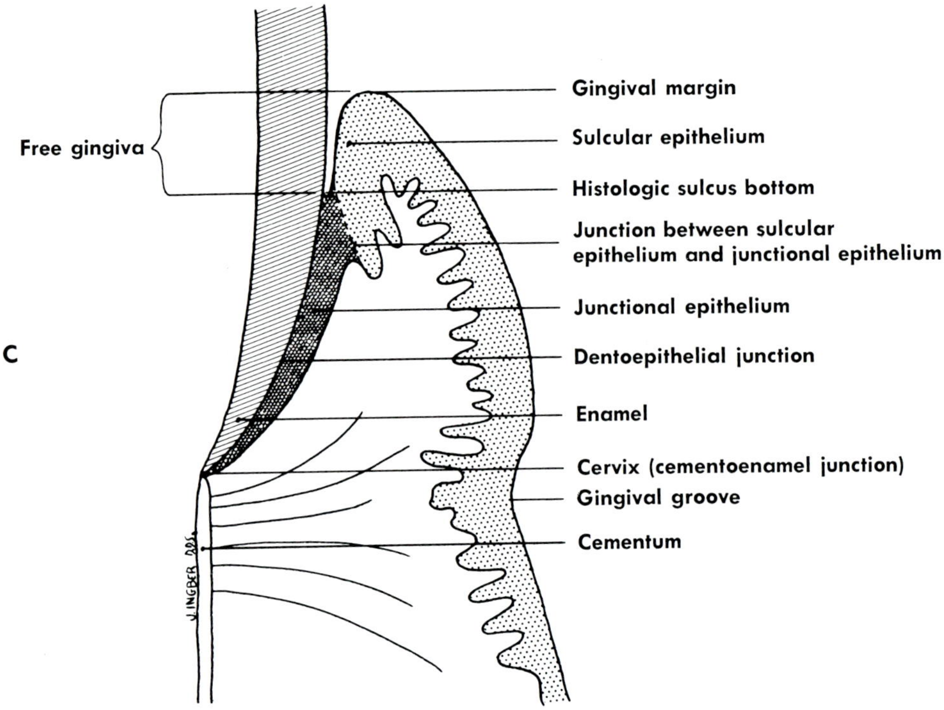

D

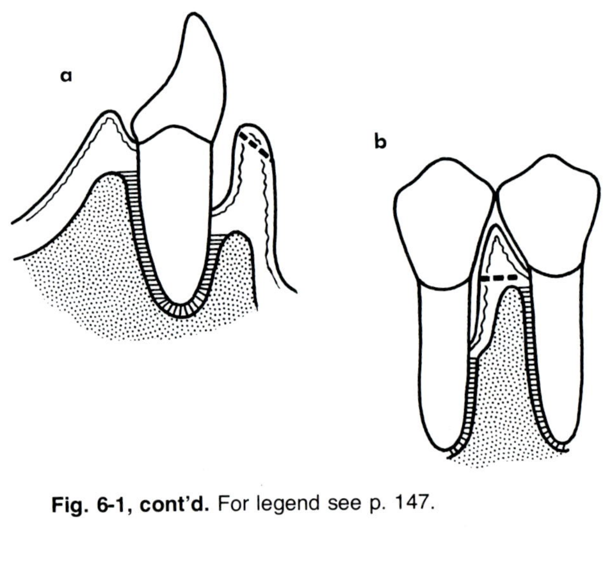

Fig. 6-1, cont'd. For legend see p. 147.

then transfer this biologic knowledge to clinical practice, we can accomplish our work on a biomechanical basis.

The next thing is to know (1) that in gingival disease the attached gingival margin has lost its adherence and is retractile, (2) that the diagnostic signs of gingival disease are changes in the gingival margin, texture value, color value, form value, adherence, and also bleeding and purulent exudate, and (3) that the prime requisites for periodontics is to eradicate the lesion, prevent recurrence, set up an ideal environment, obtain gingival margins that have sharp edges and are curved parabolically to the mesial and to the distal, have mobility of the vestibular fold, since past experiences showed us that the so-called "push-back" operation immobilized the fold, and control or harness mobility.

Goldman[2] refers to the area from the gingival margin to the vestibule as the *gingival wall,* despite the fact that the characteristics are different in the various areas such as the gingiva, attached gingiva, alveolar mucosa, and vestibule. The blood supply to the gingiva comes through the gingival wall.

Before any restorative work is started it is necessary to complete coronal and subgingival scaling, because resolution of inflammation and shrinkage of gingiva may influence the treatment program. It may also become obvious at this time if there is adequate or inadequate attached gingiva, and it will be possible to glean some indications of the patient's ability and motivation to carry out the necessary home care and indications of the rapidity of calculus formation and sordes accumulation.

A review of some of the essentials of a periodontal examination may be in order at this time, especially gingival changes:

1. Color changes. Normal gingiva is pink to coral pink; deviations from normal are reflected as red, magenta, and, in some cases, a very pale pink.

2. Marginal contour. Healthy gingival margin is thin and knife-edged and completely fills interproximal embrasures. Deviations from normal health are reflected in margins that are swollen, edematous, receded, and irregular.

3. Papillary contour. Healthy interdental papillary contours point in an anterior region; in the posterior region they may be flattened or slightly concave. Such papillary contours usually reflect the architecture of the underlying bony structure in health and disease. Papillary contour is also influenced by the interproximal contacts of the teeth.

4. Texture. Under normal circumstances the attached gingiva is textured and stippled. Alveolar mucosa is smoother, loosely attached, dark red in color, reflecting its vascularity and nonkeratinization. Gingival inflammation exhibits attached gingiva as glossy with diminished or total absence of stippling. Normally attached gingiva is firm and tightly adapted to the underlying bone.

5. Sulcus. Healthy gingival sulcus is supposedly "0" mm. in depth. It usually is not so, because the periodontal probe can be introduced at least to some depth. Pocket formation usually reflects swelling, edema, loss of stippling, bleeding, etc.

Other important considerations are tissue tone, adhesion, and the position of tissue in relation to the crown and root of the tooth. Also the arch form, crown form, position of the contact areas, carious lesions, trauma from occlusion, and mobility should be evaluated as etiologic factors.

Mobility is a clinical symptom that must be evaluated very carefully. Practical considerations require us to ask whether the tooth has too great an amount of horizontal or vertical mobility to consider the prognosis favorable, whether it is firm enough to support a fixed or removable restoration that may be required, and whether the pathology accompanying the mobility makes it injurious to the other local structures.

Each tooth in both arches should be checked for mobility patterns, and the clinician has to rely on his visual acuity and subjective judgment. The best assessment of mobility can be made by the use of two mirror handles, placing one handle facially and pushing lingually and the other handle lingually and pushing facially. The mobility pattern is determined in relation to what is considered normal movement for the case under consideration. Teeth slightly more mobile than normal (#1 mobility) can usually be corrected by eliminating the cause; teeth more mobile than this (#2 mobility), but not too excessive, may require fixed splintage for stabilization and reorientation of forces of stress; teeth exhibiting excessive mobility (#3 mobility) usually must be removed because of a poor prognosis. Tooth shape and size, as well as crown-to-root ratio, should be noted, since these are factors often directly related to the presence of mobility in areas of heavy occlusal function.

The *periodontal probe* should be used routinely because of its diagnostic value. It is an important instrument to use in assessing the existing bone form present in periodontal disease. It follows the epithelial attachment around each tooth, which reflects the underlying bone topography.

Six individual measurements are taken for each tooth. They are taken at three different points on both the facial and lingual surfaces of a tooth—at the mesiofacial and mesiolingual line angles, at the distofacial and distolingual line angles, and at the midfacial and midlingual surfaces. Circumferential probing is used to obtain more accurate measurements.

The information obtained by probing, when tied in with roentgenographic studies, observation of the soft and hard tissues of the oral cavity, and cast analysis allows the clinician to treat his patients more definitively. All this is very important in mouth rehabilitation, because an appraisal of the periodontium is necessary to anticipate tissue reactions that may complicate treatment or, in the end, render it useless.

If a surgical phase is indicated it may be necessary, in some instances, to temporarily splint the teeth. Reattachment or "bone-fill" procedures, attached gingiva extensions, root amputations, pocket elimination, gingiva and bone contouring, gingiva and bone reduction to produce greater crown length, etc. can now be carried out.

It is important that the dentist treating periodontal lesions comprehend the exact nature of the process involved. Therapy to obtain a healthy gingiva will not overcome mobility of teeth produced by occlusal trauma. The dentist must evaluate each case and understand the various changes that are occurring. It is necessary to eliminate or control the agents producing the disease process.

The procedures that can be used to obtain a healthy gingiva or to control some of the agents producing the disease process are subgingival curettage, gingivectomy, mucogingival surgery, and osseous surgery.

The technique of subgingival curettage consists of the scaling and planing of the root and the removal of the sulcular lining of the ulcerated tissue. These two parts may be accomplished as one procedure. This procedure is founded on the degree of tissue shrinkage that can result after resolution of inflammation; this is directly dependent upon the character of the tissue and the local environment. In other words, pockets that are relatively shallow in nature and the gingival wall, which consists of soft edematous tissue and whose local environment will not prevent shrinkage, may be treated successfully by curettage.

In the eradication of pockets by shrinkage, it is of the utmost importance that the curettage be thorough and use be made of sharp instruments complemented with a keen sense of touch. The soft tissue side of the pocket has certain characteristics—edema, cellular infiltration, and very little fibrosis. The edema and cellular infiltration are manifestations of inflammation resulting from the calculus and bacterial plaque in the periodontal pocket. The tissue is soft and may vary in color from blue to red. If the tissue is fibrotic, it is firm, making it difficult to induce shrinkage; in this type of situation gingivectomy is the treatment of choice.

The shrinkage, initiated by subgingival curettage, can be increased and maintained by gingival massage. Proper home care by the patient is very important (Fig. 6-1, *D*).

Some of the indications for gingivectomy are:

1. Moderate depth pockets accompanied by long-standing gingival inflammation with fibrosis so that curettage would result in poor architectural form or leave a deepened sulcus
2. Sharply varying levels of gingival margin in adjacent areas
3. Interproximal tissue loss with crater formation instead of the normal papilla
4. Thickened gingival margins
5. A case that presents relatively even horizontal bone loss

Some of the indications for mucogingival surgery are:

1. Abnormal frenum attachment
2. Extremely shallow mucobuccal fold so that there is no room for the normal gingival complex
3. Cases where it is necessary to increase the zone of attached gingiva

Some of the indications for osseous surgery are:

1. Thickened marginal bone due to pattern of destruction by periodontal disease
2. Loss of interproximal septal bone with crater formation
3. Sharply varying levels of bone in adjacent areas
4. One- and two-wall infrabony pockets
5. Bifurcation and trifurcation involvement to produce acceptable contour
6. Sharp angles and ledges of bone

An appropriate waiting period is followed by a reevaluation of the case for bone fill, pocket closure, mobility reduction, clarification of prognosis of doubtful teeth, etc.

The aim of good dentistry is to create optimal functional conditions in order to give the supporting dental tissues the optimal chance of maintenance or recovery under pathologic conditions.

Restorative dentistry at its very best is an irritant to the gingival tissues. The more we can stay away from the attachment apparatus, the more favorable will be the end result.

Healthy interdental papillae exhibit many and varied shapes depending upon (1) the anatomic form of the underlying interdental bone, (2) the proximity of the roots of teeth, allowing for or limiting interdental space, (3) the shape and outline of the interdental space as formed by the proximal surfaces of the teeth, and (4) the alignment or malalignment of the teeth to each other.

The proximal surfaces of crowns must be shaped and contoured to physiologically accept the papillae and not to limit their health (see discussion of coronal contours in Chapter 6).

Therapeutic procedures directed solely to eliminating pocket depth, with failure to give adequate consideration to the causative influences, will only result in the perpetuation of the disease. It is necessary to eliminate all other factors capable of impairing the reparative capacity of the tissues.

The better the functional relation between the maxillary and mandibular teeth in every possible position, the more favorable is the strain on the supporting tissues. The tooth contact mechanism must function in physiologic equilibrium with the periodontal supporting tissues.

Studies of the occlusion includes evaluation of the roentgenograms, casts, the subjective history, and the clinical situation. Because we have pathology to contend with, the role of occlusion is very important and does not allow for the wider area of occlusal tolerance permitted in the presence of high periodontal health.

Teeth that have lost their crest attachment ligaments merit the kindest occlusal treatment possible. This can be in the form of what Harvey Stallard has called "organic occlusion." In such an occlusion the teeth can be used in their three natural groups—rear teeth, corner teeth, and front teeth. All of the occlusal elements should be restored, and they should be so arranged as to suit the lateral border movements and centric relation. Along with organizing the occlusion, it is necessary to organize the disclusion just as fully. By disclusion is meant the taking of the rear or posterior teeth out of occlusion immediately upon the least excursive action either laterally or protrusively.

In other words, the guiding principle is to provide the best centric position attainable, but total freedom from eccentric bicuspid and molar occlusion. To avoid balanced occlusion, the disclusive factors must be consulted at once and utilized. We must fix the occlusal level so that as the condyles are protruded and detruded, the posterior teeth are taken out of gear. If a suitable vertical overlapping of the upper incisors and cuspids can be established, and if the lingual surfaces of these teeth can be given proper concavities, their disclusive actions will correspond to the condylar lateral, protrusive, and opening actions.

Being particular in proper occlusal relations is as much in order in terminal dentitions as in less injured dentitions.

In summation, it can be said that prognosis concerning therapy of periodontal disease should be regarded not only on a tooth-by-tooth basis but on the dentition as an apparatus functioning in health. We must determine the type of pocket present and its extension, the crown-to-root ratio, the root form (square area of root for attachment apparatus), interradicular area involvement, mobility pattern, local environmental factors, tooth position in arch, occlusal factors, etc.

To reiterate, the elimination of the disease process is a primary objective, but it is the maintenance of the dentition in health that constitutes an even more important aspect.

The restoration of proper function, in my opinion, is more difficult to attain than the elimination or control of the tissue lesion. However, we must keep in mind that in attaining good function by means of restorations we do not create or recreate a periodontal lesion, that a healthy gingival margin is established or maintained by means of good adaptive fit and proper contour, and that the periodontium should not be stressed beyond its capacity to adapt.

Histologic structure of the attachment apparatus

I believe that a short résumé of some essential histologic facts in regard to the attachment apparatus, which serves as a suspensory mechanism for the tooth, as a pericementum for the maintenance of the root covering, and as periosteum for the alveolar bone, and which is composed of the cementum, the alveolar housing (alveolar and supporting bone), and the periodontal ligament, is in order at this time because of its importance to a basic understanding of the problems that confront us in treating periodontal disease.

The primary function of the attachment apparatus is to enable the tooth to perform its function by resisting forces that would tend to dislodge the tooth. Three factors operate[3]: (1) the principal fiber apparatus of the periodontal ligament, (2) the shape and size of the root of the tooth, and (3) the fluid content of the periodontal ligament. Churchill[4] indicated that a hydraulic mechanism, operating via the fluid content of the blood of the periodontal ligament, acted as a means for absorbing force on the tooth.

The tooth is attached to the alveolus by numerous bundles of collagenous tissue (principal fibers) arranged in groups, and between the groups is loose connective tissue together with blood vessels, lymph vessels, and nerves. These principal fibers function as the investing and supporting mechanism for the tooth and are called the periodontal ligament.[3]

The *periodontal ligament* is the connective tissue that surrounds the root(s) of the tooth and attaches it to the bony alveolus. It is continuous with the connective tissue of the gingiva. "The gingiva is masticatory mucosa covering the underlying attachment apparatus, and is subdivided into the free and attached gingiva. The *'free gingiva'* is made up of the tissues from the gingival margin to the base of the gingival sulcus, and the *'attached gingiva'* extends from the base of the sulcus to the mucogingival junction. The *'alveolar mucosa'*, which is lining mucosa, is found apical to the mucogingival junction and is continuous with the mucous membrane of the cheek, lip and floor of the oral cavity."*

The functions of the periodontal ligament are (1) formative, (2) supportive, (3) protective, (4) sensory, and (5) nutritive. According to Sicher[5] the *formative function* is fulfilled by the cementoblasts and the osteoblasts, which are essential in building cementum and bone, and by the fibroblasts, which form the fibers of the ligament. In other words, this function is necessary for replacement of tissue—cementum, periodontal ligament, and alveolar bone. The *supportive function* is that of maintaining the relation of the tooth to the surrounding hard and soft tissues—in other words, maintaining and retaining the tooth. By limiting the masticatory movements of the tooth, the periodontal ligament *protects* the tissues at the sites of pressure. This is achieved by connective tissue fibers that comprise the bulk of the ligament. *Functions that are sensory and nutritive* to the cementum and alveolar bone are carried out by the nerves and the blood vessels in the periodontal ligament.

*From Kraus, B. S., Jordan, R. E., and Abrams, Leonard: Dental anatomy and occlusion, Baltimore, 1969, The Williams & Wilkins Co., p. 190.

Amsterdam[6] has pointed out that the periodontal ligament provides the basis for tooth anchorage and is responsible for two basic functions: (1) it acts as a true ligament and limits movement of the hard structures as seen in joints and (2) it functions as double periosteum, laying down cementum on the tooth and bone in the alveolus.

The main tissue elements in the periodontal ligament are the principal fibers, all of which are attached to the cementum. The fiber bundles extend from the cementum to the alveolar wall, across the crest of the interdental septum to the cementum of the adjacent tooth, or into the gingival tissue. "The bundles of collagenous fibers are so arranged that they can be divided into the following ligaments: (1) *gingival ligament*—the fibers of this ligament attach the gingiva to the cementum. The fiber bundles pass outward from the cementum into the free and attached gingiva; (2) *transseptal* (interdental) *ligaments* connect adjacent teeth. The ligaments, but not the single fibers, run from the cementum of one tooth over the crest of the alveolar bone to the cementum of the neighboring tooth (Fig. 6-2); (3) *the alveolodental*

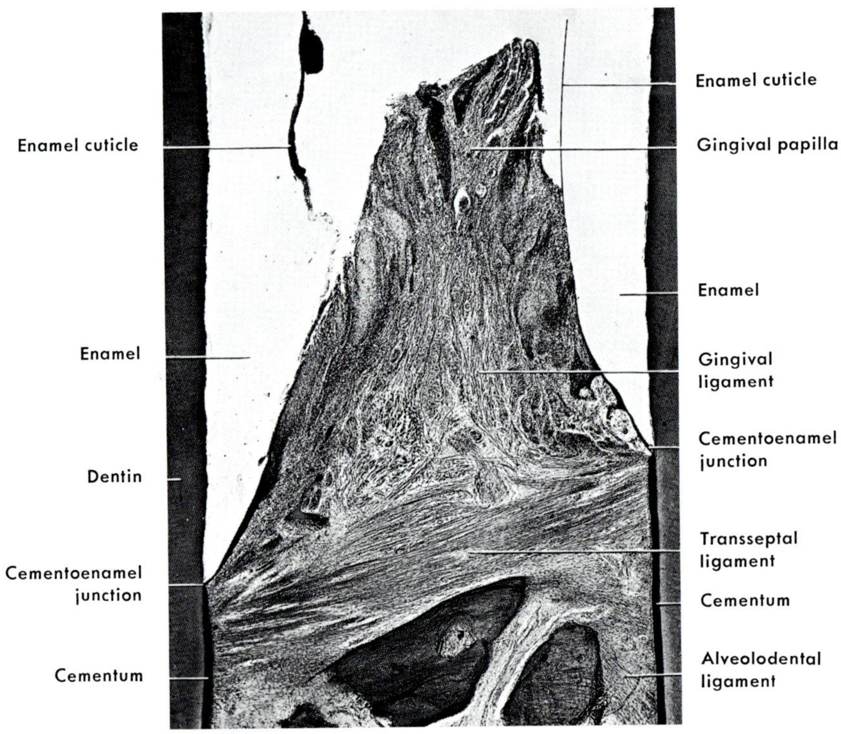

Fig. 6-2. Transseptal ligament connects adjacent teeth. (From Sicher, Harry, and Bhaskar, S. N., editors: Orban's oral histology and embryology, ed. 7, St. Louis, 1972, The C. V. Mosby Co.)

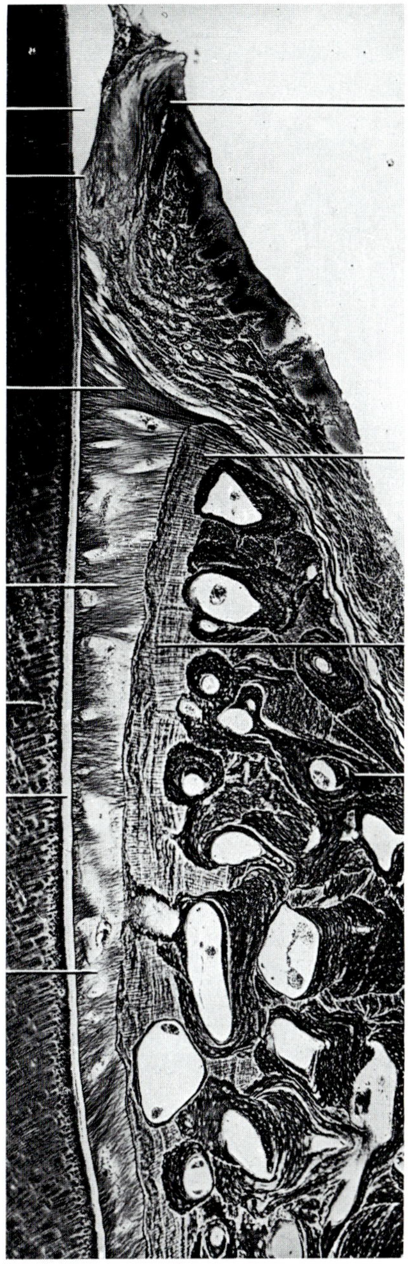

Fig. 6-3. Alveolodental ligament. (From Sicher, Harry, and Bhaskar, S. N., editors: Orban's oral histology and embryology, ed. 7, St. Louis, 1972, The C. V. Mosby Co.)

ligament attaches the tooth to the bone of the alveolus (Fig. 6-3). It consists of five groups of bundles: (a) *alveolar crest group*—the fiber bundles of this group radiate from the crest of the alveolar process and attach themselves to the cervical part of the cementum; (b) *horizontal group*—the bundles run at right angles to the long axis of the tooth, from the cementum to the alveolar bone; (c) *oblique group*—the bundles run obliquely. They are attached in the cementum somewhat apically from their attachment to the bone. These fiber bundles are most numerous and constitute the main support of the tooth against masticatory forces; (d) *apical group*—the bundles are irregularly arranged and radiate from the apical region of the root to the

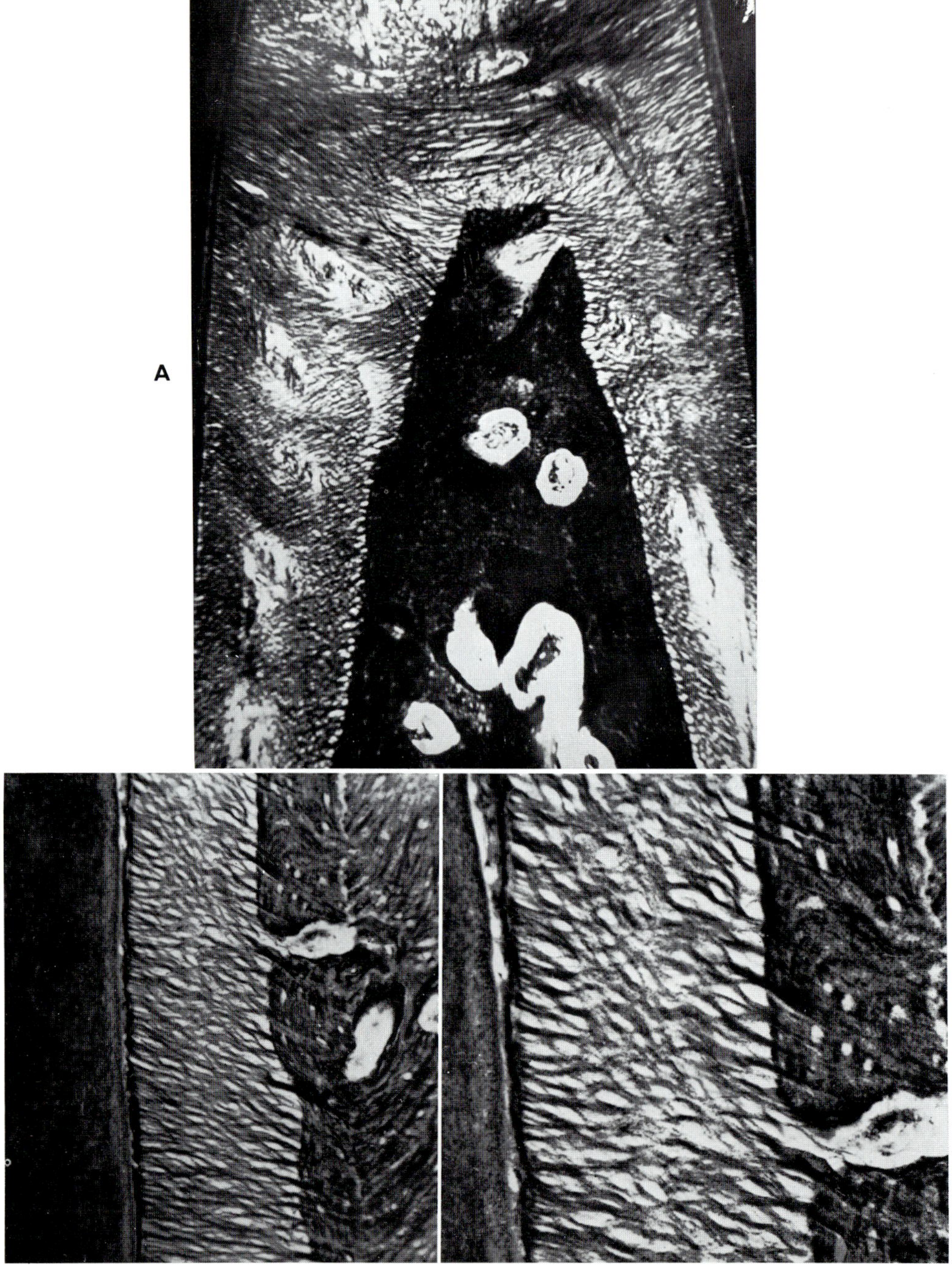

A

B

C

Fig. 6-4. A, Periodontal ligament of premolars of a monkey. Interdental and alveolar bundles of principal fibers may be seen. The fibers are intertwined between cementum and bone in an intermediate plexus. **B,** Periodontal ligament of a rat molar. Note the "braiding" of the periodontal fibers in the intermediate plexus. (Silver impregnation; × 400.) **C,** Higher magnification of an area of **B.** (× 800.) (**C** courtesy Dr. Ino Sciaky.) (From Sicher, Harry, and Bhaskar, S. N., editors: Orban's oral histology and embryology, ed. 7, St. Louis, 1972, The C. V. Mosby Co.)

surrounding bone; (e) *interradicular group*—from the crest of the interradicular septum, bundles extend to the furcation of multi-rooted teeth.

"The principal fibers of the periodontal ligament are white collagenous connective tissue fibers, and they cannot be lengthened. There are no elastic fibers in the periodontal ligament. The apparent elasticity of the periodontal ligament is due to the arrangement of the principal fiber bundles. They follow a wavy course from bone to cementum, thereby allowing slight movements of the tooth during mastication. Near the bone the fibers seem to form larger bundles before their insertion into it. Although the bundles run directly from bone to cementum, the single fibers do not span the entire distance. The bundles are 'spliced or braided' and chemically bound together from shorter fibers in an intermediate plexus midway between cementum and bone (Fig. 6-4). The presence of an intermediate plexus is common to the periodontal ligament of all mammalian teeth because they move occlusomesially by continuous eruption during their functional period. These movements necessitate a continued adaptive readjustment of the suspensory ligament. This rearrangement does not occur by the embedding of new fibers in bone and cementum, as previously assumed, but by the formation of new chemical links in all probability by mucopolysaccharides, between the alveolar and the dental fibers in the intermediate plexus.

"The interdental or transseptal ligaments also consist of fibers that are shorter than the ligaments themselves. In contrast to alveolodental and interdental ligaments, the fibers of the gingival ligament seem to extend directly from the cementum into the gingiva.

"The 'growth movements' or the eruptive movements of the tooth in both vertical and horizontal directions require, of course, continual changes of the supporting tissues, cementum, bone, and suspensory ligaments, i.e. alveolodental, interdental, and gingival ligaments. Therefore, alveolodental and interdental ligaments consist, as do all other ligaments, of fibers that are shorter than the ligament itself. Only by this arrangement, by the physiochemical 'splicing' of shorter fibers to form a ligament, can ligaments adjust to growth in length. In the dental ligaments, however, the adjustive changes are manifold. Some alveolodental fibers have to lengthen, for instance, to allow horizontal tooth movements—'drifting' of the teeth (mesial in man). In a closed dentition with contact wear the interdental ligaments have to shorten. In axial movement the functional arrangement of the alveolodental ligament has to undergo continual changes. All adjustments occur in a middle zone of these ligaments that has been called the *'intermediate plexus.'*

"This plexus, in which the fibers arising in the cementum on one side and in the bone on the other are 'spliced', is characteristic for all mammalian teeth. However, its dimensions are correlated to the speed of eruptive movements.

"The presence of an intermediate plexus and its significance for the rearrangement of fibers of the periodontal ligament make it clear that the continued apposition of cementum serves primarily to maintain the vitality of the cementum."*

SALIENT FACTS

1. Amsterdam[6] has said that the *gingival unit* (free gingiva, attached gingiva, alveolar mucosa) provides a tough collagenous and epithelial covering to the neck of the tooth and the underlying attachment apparatus, which in turn protects these underlying structures from the bacterial flora of the oral environment.

2. Only axial resultant forces transmitted to the periodontium produce true physiologic stimulation of the fiber apparatus. Orban[7] said that the supporting structures of the teeth are built to withstand much force and load if applied in the long axis of the teeth. The fibers of the periodontal ligament are very strong, and the cementum will often tear from the surface of the dentin before the fibers give way. The alveolar bone can withstand much force applied as a pulling force but will yield to resorption if exposed to pressure, even slight pressure. Lateral stress may be more than the tissue can tolerate.

3. *Cementum* is one of the three hard tissues of the tooth. It is the hard bonelike tissue covering the anatomic roots of the teeth. The deposition of cementum is a continuous process in response to stresses and attrition of the teeth.[8] It is associated with the aging process and continuous tooth eruption. It is the least calcified of the hard tissues, and it can be scraped away with a sharp curette. The suspensory fibers of the periodontal ligament are embedded in this tissue.

Cementum does not resorb and form, but grows by apposition of new layers, one upon another. Cemental apposition is slow—changes in function will bear great influence on the activity of cemental growth.[9]

---

*From Sicher, Harry, and Bhaskar, S. N., editors: Orban's oral histology and embryology, ed. 7, St. Louis, 1972, The C. V. Mosby Co.

Cementum piles up over the years and, therefore, the tooth has to erupt to make room for the cementum. This leads to attrition of teeth compensated by mesial drift of teeth. Probably attrition, to a certain degree, is a good thing. We must keep in mind that physiologic eruptive movement of human teeth is characterized by a vertical component in compensation for occlusal wear and a mesial component in compensation for the wear at their contact areas.[10]

Cementoblasts are connective tissue cells found on the surface of cementum. Connective tissue fibers from the periodontal ligament pass between the cementoblasts into the cementum. These fibers are embedded in the cementum and serve as an attachment for the tooth to the surrounding bone. Their embedded portions are known as Sharpey's fibers.

4. *Alveolar bone* is bone that is deposited next to the periodontal ligament and is itself supported by bone. It comprises that portion of the alveolar process which lines the sockets into which the roots of the teeth fit. It is thin, compact bone pierced by many small openings through which blood vessels, lymphatics, and nerve fibers pass, and it is also a very labile structure that responds biologically to the stresses brought to bear upon the teeth. It is referred to roentgenographically as lamina dura and when the tooth is lost the lamina dura disappears.

The bone housing the tooth is dependent upon the function exerted on the tooth to maintain its structure. Between the compact bone making up the alveolus and the external parts of the jaw are numerous *trabeculae* of supporting bone, which are advantageously arranged to take up the stresses that the teeth transmit to the bone surrounding them. The architectural arrangement of the trabeculae and their character are related to the demands of function.

Tissue elements of the alveolar process are no different from those of bone elsewhere. The bone of the alveolus is constantly resorbed and rebuilt. Resorption of bone is brought about by the osteoclasts, and formation of new bone is initiated by the activity of the osteoblasts.

5. Cementum and alveolar bone have different characteristics, the former (cementum) very slow-growing tissue without a resorptive phase, whereas bone is much more active, undergoing resorption and apposition continually (Fig. 6-5).

The periodontal ligament, composed principally

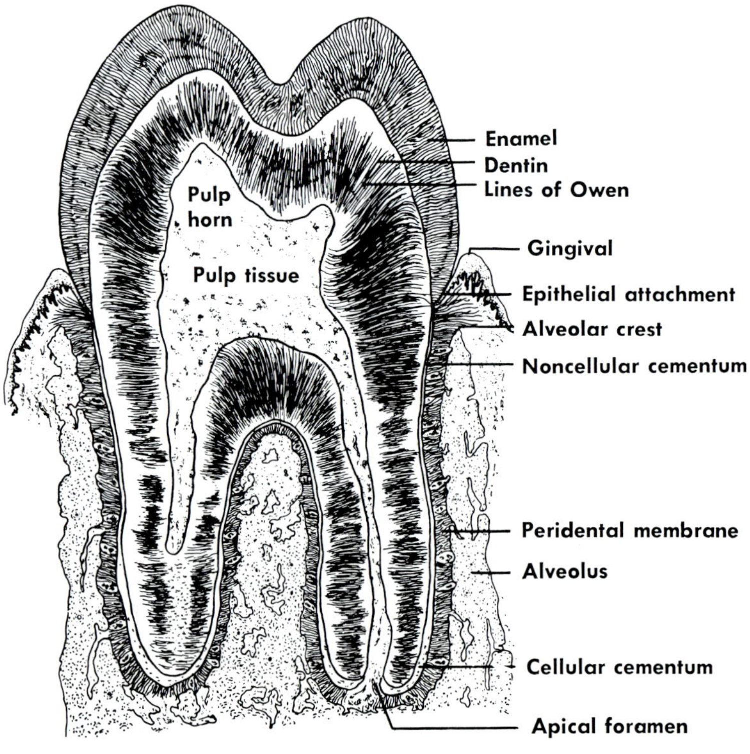

Fig. 6-5. Section of human maxillary molar cut buccolingually to show general relationships of tooth and surrounding tissues. (From Bevelander, Gerrit: Essentials of histology, ed. 6, St. Louis, 1970, The C. V. Mosby Co., p. 163.)

of collagenous connective tissue, is the retaining mechanism for the tooth fibers of the periodontal ligament being embedded in the cementum and the alveolar bone.

Goldman[9] has called attention to the fact that the turnover rate of collagen must be taken into consideration. Collagen has a relatively slow turnover rate. It is most likely that the turnover rate on the cementum side is different from that on the bone side. Since the activity of cementum and bone are not alike, but since they are anchored to one another, there must be a mechanism for independence of these tissues. Or, in other words, this necessitates a junction phenomenon to connect the two sides which is accomplished by the "intermediate plexus." This allows for the faster turnover rate for alveolar bone in contrast to cementum.

6. The function of the gingival fibers is to support the gingiva, keeping it closely adapted to the tooth surface, thus sustaining the gingiva against the forces placed on it during function. It also inhibits apical migration of the epithelial attachment (Fig. 6-6).[3]

If the fiber apparatus breaks down or is destroyed, mobility occurs.

7. Investigators seem to agree that the thickness of the periodontal ligament varies in different individuals, in different teeth in the same person, and in different localities on the same tooth.

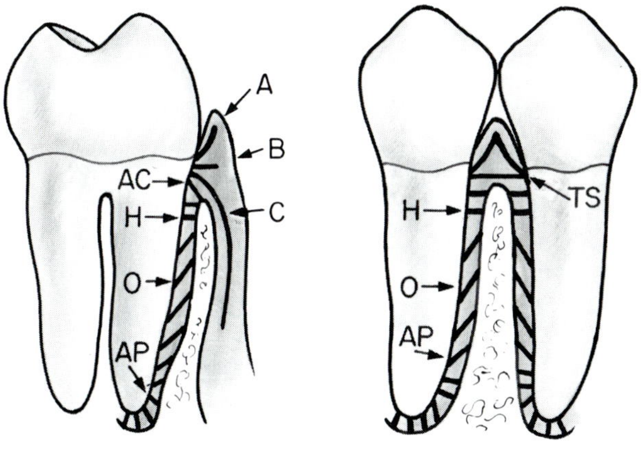

Fig. 6-6. Principal fiber groups of the gingival unit and attachment apparatus. Gingival fibers: group a *(A)*, group b *(B)*, and group c *(C)* are seen in the buccolingual sketch on the left. The transseptal fibers *(TS)* are seen in the mesiodistal sketch on the right. Periodontal ligament fibers: alveolar crest fibers *(AC)*, horizontal fibers *(H)*, oblique fibers *(O)*, and apical fibers *(AP)*. (Adapted from Kraus, B. S., Jordan, R. E., and Abrams, Leonard: Dental anatomy and occlusion, Baltimore, 1969, The Williams & Wilkins Co.)

8 The depth of the healthy gingival sulcus rarely exceeds 2.5 mm.

9. The three structures that have been elaborated upon—the cementum, periodontal ligament, and bone—form a functional unit. Every movement of the tooth is transmitted through the cementum to the fiber apparatus of the periodontal ligament and thus to the bone. A greater or lesser function than usual will lead to corresponding adaptive structural changes.

Orban[5] has pointed out that in loss of function the periodontal ligament becomes narrower, the regular arrangement of the principal fibers is lost. The cementum becomes thicker, but finally aplastic, and does not contain Sharpey's fibers. The alveolar bone also appears aplastic and lacks Sharpey's fibers (Fig. 6-7).

For restorative dentistry the importance is obvious, because the supporting tissues of teeth out of function are unable to carry the load placed upon the tooth by the restoration, be it a crown, bridge, or any appliance in contact with its opponent, be it a tooth, bridge, or denture. This may account for some of the trouble we have with patients attempting to use restorations under these conditions, especially without the elapsing of time so as to allow the supporting tissues to become adapted to the new placement. The tissues must adjust and rearrange in response to new functional demands. Not only is it important to obtain a regeneration of fiber bundles attaching the tooth to the alveolar bone, but it is also of the utmost importance to obtain as ideal a functional relation between the teeth as possible.[5]

All of the material in this section allows for a good understanding of the physiology of the attachment apparatus.

We not only establish an environment that is conducive to the health of the *periodontium* but also to the physiologic function of the muscles, temporomandibular joints, and associated structures. We must not transgress the periodontium, the joint, or the muscles. The aim of good dentistry is to create optimal functional conditions in order to give the supporting dental tissues and associated structures the optimal chance of maintenance or recovery under pathologic conditions.

The theme of this chapter is the stability of teeth in the periodontium and the maintenance of the health of the attachment apparatus. Among other things, it will deal with the biologic implications of

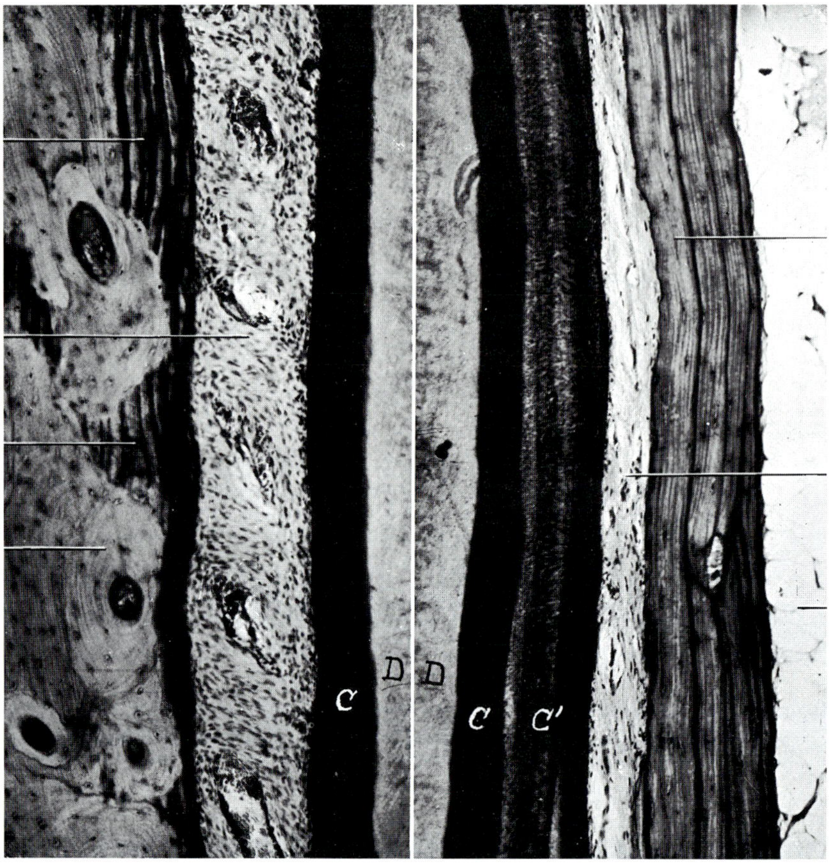

Fig. 6-7. A, Periodontal ligament of a functioning tooth; **B,** periodontal membrane of a nonfunctioning tooth. In the functioning tooth the periodontal ligament is wide and principal fibers are present. Cementum *(C)* is thin. Bundle bone has Sharpey's fibers. In the nonfunctioning tooth the periodontal space is narrow, and no principal fiber bundles are present, cementum is thick (*C* and *C'*). Alveolar bone is lamellated, containing no Sharpey's fibers. *D,* Dentin. (From Sicher, Harry, and Bhaskar, S. N., editors: Orban's oral histology and embryology, ed. 7, St. Louis, 1972, The C. V. Mosby Co.)

occlusal forces in the maintenance of periodontal health. *It will deal with form and function—form as it relates to function.*

Despite the fact that I am thoroughly in accord with the modern concept of periodontics, I might add that complete pocket elimination, as important as it is, comes to naught if stability in function is not attained. Therapeutic procedures directed solely at eliminating pocket depth, with failure to give adequate consideration to the causative influences, will only result in the perpetuation of the disease. It is necessary to eliminate all other factors capable of impairing the reparative capacity of the tissues. In many cases periodontics alone is not enough.

Basic objectives of periodontal prosthesis

Following are the basic objectives of periodontal prosthesis.

1. To reduce lateral stresses
2. To distribute stresses equitably
3. To eliminate areas of food impaction
4. To eliminate premature and/or deflective contacts; to eliminate occlusal traumatism—primary or secondary
5. To direct occlusal stresses of functional forces in the long axes of the teeth with the removal of any conflict between joint and teeth during normal function
6. To correct tooth contours
7. To correct temporomandibular joint conditions

To accomplish these objectives, a number of factors must be taken into consideration.

1. In planning treatment for a debilitated dentition, a major objective is the sequential integration of all technical procedures—periodontal,

surgical, orthodontic, endodontic, and prosthodontic.

2. Therefore, one must be trained not only in prosthodontics, but must develop an overall concept, particularly in periodontics, endodontics, and orthodontics.
3. A careful mounting of the patient's dental casts should be made on an instrument that copies his mandibular movements so that a diagnosis of the functional relations may be made by studying them in conjunction with roentgenograms and all other available data (muscles, joints, systemic factors, and parafunctions).
4. It is of the utmost importance to give certain form to teeth and certain relation of teeth to each other in order to ensure the health of the periodontium. All this, of course, implies an understanding of the normal function of the stomatognathic system.

The oral cavity must be considered as a whole, a tooth being an integral part of a highly organized mechanism that, in the ideal, functions harmoniously and physiologically.

The fundamental requirement of a successful biomechanical result is a harmonius relationship between form and function. Therefore, the object of periodontal prosthesis is, by alteration of the functional relations, to create forms that will reduce stress and distribute forces throughout the entire supporting structures of the mouth. But to achieve this, these tooth forms also must be in harmony with the muscles and temporomandibular joints. We must use every tool at our command and not place our reliance on treatment of local factors alone. We must take intelligent advantage of the tools and knowledge that are available so as not to hamper nature in her struggle to maintain a healthy mouth.

To reduce the forces and stresses by a harmonious relationship between form and function, nature provided us with cusps. Unlike the mandible of the herbivorous animal, the human mandible in all its paths of motion, horizontal or vertical or any combination of the two, describes arcs that demand natural cusp forms to maintain a state of functional equilibrium as a means of avoiding stresses resulting from unequal forces.

Compromises in cusp forms that, by oversimplification, attempt to circumvent the physiologic requirements of healthy supporting structures become pathologic cusp forms, which end by defeating themselves. Nature's response in an effort to achieve functional equilibrium with pathologic cusp forms results in the drifting of teeth, inflamed and thickened gingival tissues, loose partial dentures, etc.

Splinting will prevent teeth from drifting but will not prevent stresses on supporting structures. Splinting is necessary when the functional relations are such that it is impossible to achieve functional stability of individual teeth. However, splinting is not a crutch to be used as a substitute for adequate occlusal forms.

Now we go to the question of the part adaptation plays in condoning our sins of omission. The burden of struggling to adapt to pathologic functional relations creates stresses that, when they exceed physiologic limits, become an intolerable insult, to which nature's response is inflammatory anger. Human beings eventually pay the price for the so-called adaptive capacity. The adaptive capacities are essentially compromises of basic mechanical and biologic laws. When one deviates from the original, the price must be paid eventually in some form such as loss of teeth, function, or joint dysfunction pain syndrome.

It is the lack of adaptation that produces the sick mouth. It would appear then that the objective of restorative treatment is to create a prosthesis adapted to the individual requirements of form and function, to obviate the forces and stresses resulting from lack of adaptation.

A knowledge of the science of occlusion is necessary for the proper correction of the local tooth contact mechanism so that it is capable of functioning in physiologic equilibrium with the periodontal supporting tissues. The better the functional relation between the maxillary and mandibular teeth in every possible position, the more favorable is the strain on the supporting tissues.

"Occlusion in its fullest interpretation includes a knowledge of the anatomy and physiology of the muscles of mastication, the temporomandibular articulation, of jaw-to-jaw relationships, tooth form and position, mandibular movements, vertical dimension, functional and afunctional uses and abuses of teeth, of the periodontal supporting tissues, that is, the periodontal ligament, and, above all else, the alveolar bone and its reaction to the transmission of stresses to it by tooth contacts through muscle power.

"In all studies and treatment of occlusions a differential diagnosis must be made between discrepancies of jaw-to-jaw relationships and tooth-to-tooth positions.

"The determination of correct jaw-to-jaw relationships and tooth-to-tooth positions is based on an understanding of centric relation and centric occlusion.

"A physiologic occlusion implies a balance between occlusal stress and tissue resistance. It may be natural to the individual or it may be acquired through reconstruction.

"*Occlusal* stress is based on: (1) *function,* which may be masticatory or non-masticatory, (2) *force,* which is initiated by the muscle and transmitted by the teeth, and (3) *tissue* resistance, which is represented by the bone and the periodontal ligament.

"It then becomes clear that in order to produce an acquired physiologic occlusion which will balance occlusal stress and tissue resistance, our efforts in equalization must be concerned with the muscles, tooth form, tooth position, jaw relationship and function."*

In other words, the biomechanics in these cases requires a balance between the forces of occlusion and the resistance of the periodontal supporting tissues.[12] An occlusal concept must be correlated intimately with the influencing factors of the temporomandibular articulation and the incisal guidance.

OBTAINING BASIC OBJECTIVES

Now the question arises—how do we attain these goals?

First, a complete examination must be made so that we can arrive at a properly evaluated diagnosis and thereby be able to evolve a total treatment plan. In this way we know what type of case faces us. (1) Is it just a case of bad dental work complicated with some gingival inflammation and a primary occlusal traumatism requiring some curettage, some selective grinding, well-made restorations constructed on an adjustable articulator, and proper home care instructions, or (2) is it a bad, periodontally involved mouth with mobile teeth, migrations, osseous lesions, collapsed posterior bite, etc? The latter is my idea of an example of the indication for procedures referred to as periodontal prosthesis. In these types of cases, after hopeless teeth have been removed, curettage, repositioning of teeth, gross selective grinding (if necessary after tooth movement), osseous and mucogingival surgery, and provisional splinting to help redirect eccentric stresses into direct forces within the long axes of the teeth must be done, and usually in that procedural order. It is in the provisional stage that the case can be evaluated properly as to the possibility of achieving our treatment objectives. If this is possible in the provisional stage, the treatment objectives will carry over to the permanent stage. By creating a different environment the dental mechanism can survive.

Much debate goes on as to partial versus full coverage in tooth preparations used in periodontal prosthesis. In what has been mentioned previously as a case of bad dental work, without serious complication, it really does not matter most of the time which type of preparation is used because there are no problems of crown-to-root ratios, coronal contours, embrasure forms, and unilateral or bilateral splinting.

However, in the second example, a case in need of involved periodontal surgery that will alter the architectural form, the embrasures, and gingival position, only full coverage can be considered. The biomechanics of the case requires full coverage.

It must be kept in mind that the full crown is the most difficult restoration to make properly in our whole repertoire of restorations—because it is almost humanly impossible to reproduce the anatomic contours of a tooth in its entirety, especially in its proper relation to the gingival tissues for maintenance of periodontal health. Intelligent, well-trained, and sincere dentists, being quite aware of what has just been written, would not use full coverage if partial coverage would suffice, but, for the survival of an involved periodontal prosthesis case, full coverage utilized with finesse, understanding, and precision technique is a "must." Full coverage must provide an architectural environment capable of maintaining and preserving the integrity of the supporting structure.

Another important step that we are trying to achieve is an accurate method of transferring records of oral movements to an instrument so that all the work can be done on that instrument.

The accurate recording and transferring of mandibular relations is now attainable, provided certain principles are understood and executed carefully.[13,14]

We must concern ourselves with a *center* that can be easily located and can be useful for our procedures—in other words, a center that will enable us to reproduce the patient's movements on a suitable articulator.[15]

In the evolution of our knowledge of functional harmony the face-bow has come to play a very prominent part. Pioneers in this field—Snow, Gritman, Gysi, and others—recognized the need for a means of orienting the cusps to each other in a rotational relationship that would produce a vertical thrust within the axis of the supporting structures.

---

*From Fox, Lewis: The occlusal factor in periodontal disease, Alpha Omegan **43:**124-133, 1949.

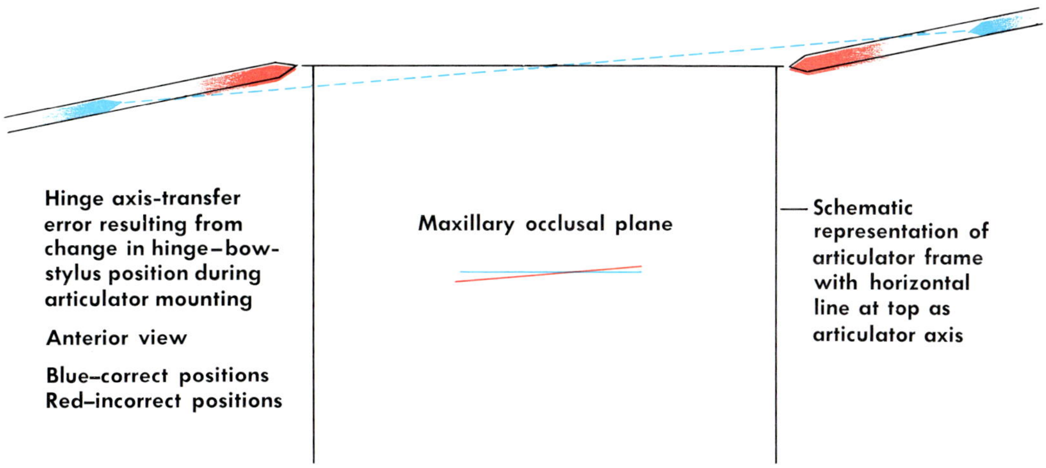

Fig. 6-8. Alteration of position of stylus pins to conform to fixed intercondylar distance of articulator (which usually occurs in a conventional face-bow mounting) can cause axis to be displaced by as much as ½ inch.

The hinge-bow is a precise refinement of the philosophies known and tested for over 60 years. The importance of the hinge axis mounting does not lie alone in the convenience of opening or closing the bite on an articulator. If that were its only objective, we could achieve it by simple repeated remountings with successively thinner bites. The real importance of the hinge axis is the fact that it is the inescapable anatomic center of all rotary movements of the mandible as the teeth make contact with each other, whether it be mastication, swallowing, or bruxism.

A conventional face-bow mounting in which the position of the stylus pins is altered to conform to the fixed intercondylar distance of the articulator can cause the axis to be displaced by as much as ½ inch (Fig. 6-8).

Weinberg[16] pointed out that biologic variables must be considered a source of error in all techniques. Steel instruments are precise and rigid, whereas muscles, ligaments, and bone have a degree of physiologic tolerance. The effect of external stimuli—pain, temperature of waxes, muscle distension, weight of instruments, muscle tone at time of measurement, head position, force exerted by the dentist, the psychic stimuli by the patient or dentist—is another variable factor.

I believe that our ability to treat and save mouths is directly related to our ability to capture and transfer jaw function to the restoration. If we do just that, according to Stuart and Stallard,[17] (1) the cusps will be well geared to the axes of the condyles. Achieving this, the teeth are strengthened and stabilized, and premature wear is kept to a minimum; (2) the directions of the grooves will conform to jaw motions, and the cusps will have grooves to work in and grooves to idle in without colliding (the grooves between cusps are channels in which cusps may travel without collisions); and (3) the timing of the Bennett movement which is expressed in the concavity of the lingual surface of the upper cuspid is dependent upon the lateral condylar movements.

By gearing the cusps to the axes of the condyles, the new restorations are then shaped so that the cusps of the teeth glide by each other without interference, never touching, but shearing the food by reason of the close tolerances created in the carvings of the restorations.

Protection of investing tissues

In many instances patients will come to us with some form of periodontal disease, and they will be told that their present pathologic condition can be arrested or cured. After extensive gingival or subgingival curettage or periodontal surgery, the crown and bridge restorations, as planned, are completed and cemented.

After a while, despite proper toothbrushing, stimulation, etc., these extensive and expensive restorations are surrounded by enlarged, edematous, and inflammatory gingivae. In some instances recession takes place. Why did this happen after so much time and effort had been expended by the dentist and/or periodontist? Why, after our primary objective to cure pathology had been accomplished, has pathology been recreated? Probably we have failed to take into consideration what constitutes correct tooth preparation and impression taking in these cases, the importance of physiologic tooth form as applied to both the temporary coverage and permanent restoration, and the importance of tooth position and function. Tissues that are allowed to become inflamed and distorted architecturally certainly will jeopardize the final result and often will be the cause for failure. It is directly proportional to the correctness of the crown-tissue relationship. The crown must create the maximum opportunity for the maintenance of the health of the free marginal gingiva and the gingival sulcus, and it should not create a gingival problem or further periodontal disease. Existence of systemic disturbances capable of altering the periodontal tissues also will impair the maintenance of a healthy periodontium.

It has been said many times that subgingival extensions of full-coverage margins produce an environment unfavorable to the health of the marginal gingiva, resulting in tissues that are more rolled, more thickened, and more inflammatory in character. Is this the fault of the restoration or the dentist? Can a better understanding of tooth form and function, cavity design, and skillful and careful use of the necessary tools and materials prevent this catastrophe? I think so.

CRITERIA FOR SUCCESS IN PERIODONTAL THERAPY

At this point let us establish the criteria for success in periodontal therapy:

1. One factor is the conversion of a pathologic gingival attachment to health. The gingivae should be firm, pink, and with physiologic architectural form. The sulci should be of a depth within the range of "norm."

2. The tooth should be capable of physiologic function. It should be firm in the socket and should function without tenderness or movement.

3. Roentgenographically, the crestal bone should be cortical in character, and the lamina dura should be intact.

4. The periodontal climate should be conducive to health for maintenance.

5. The oral hygiene program should be satisfactory.

6. The dentition should function as a healthy apparatus.[18]

In periodontal prosthesis we must deal with the restoration of alterations in form as it relates to function. It is essential to master typical preparations and procedures, but it is also advisable to learn the fundamental principles that enable us to introduce change when function dictates deviation.

A healthy periodontium, in which the free gingival margin is in a stable relationship to the tooth, is essential to the success of the restoration. This healthy periodontium must exist prior to the making of the preparation and must be maintained after the restoration has been placed.

In health, the exposed part of the tooth in the mouth is surrounded by a peripheral seal (epithelial attachment) regardless of the gingival level or contour. Our operative and restorative procedures must try to preserve this protective feature.

CLINICAL ANALYSIS OF PERIODONTAL PROBLEMS

Trauma from occlusion

The resistance of the periodontium to occlusal load takes place in the attachment apparatus—cementum, periodontal ligament, and alveolar bone.

Because of the design of this system, vertical forces generally are tolerated better than horizontal forces. The principal and periapical fibers of the periodontal ligament are arranged to withstand the forces best in a vertical direction, parallel to the long axis of the tooth.

It generally is recognized that trauma from occlusion and gingival inflammation represent different types of tissue changes that initially occur in different areas of the periodontium. Gingival inflammation starts in the gingival margin and is caused by local irritation, whereas trauma from occlusion involves the supporting periodontal tissues rather than the gingiva.

Trauma from occlusion is injury in the periodontium produced by occlusal forces. It occurs in several stages—the first is injury, the second is repair, and the third is a change in the morphology of the periodontium if the offending force is chronic. In such a case the periodontium is remodeled to cushion its impact.[1] The periodontal ligament is widened at the expense of the bone, and the tooth becomes loose with its resultant mobility pattern. In other words, the widening of the periodontal ligament space, the loss of lamina dura definition, resorption of the alveolar housing, cemental tears, root resorption, pathologic migration of teeth, etc. reflect degenerative changes as a result of occlusal dysfunction—the adaptive capacity of the masticatory system has been exceeded.

The attachment apparatus has the ability to adapt to and function within a broad range of functional demands. If the stresses are applied to the tooth axially, all the fibers of the periodontal ligament are stretched and, as a group, are very strong and resistant. However, if the stress is not axial but is more or less horizontal, some fibers are stretched and some are compressed. This is transmitted to the bone as pressure and tension.

Unquestionably bone responds more favorably to tension than it does to compression, but it is true that bone, in many instances, has some capacity for resisting and sustaining compressive force. What we must keep uppermost in our minds is that the reaction of bone to force depends upon the degree of its application. If it is slight and intermittent, no resorption of bone occurs. If it is more intense and sustained, it is quite likely that a certain amount of resorption will occur, but if the amount of force is excessive and sustained, it may result in bone resorption, degeneration and necrosis of the periodontal ligament, possible root resorption, and loss of function. This type of injury can bring the root surface into contact with alveolar bone.

In other words, the recognizable lesions of occlusal traumatism are the result of the magnitude, severity, duration, and frequency of the applied force, modified by the repair ability of the host. The most damaging forces are those that are repetitive and those with a horizontal component.

Glickman[1] has said: "The periodontium is built to meet the functional demands of the tooth; support of the tooth is the only reason for its existence. The tooth depends upon the periodontal tissues to keep it in the jaw; the periodontal tissues depend on the functional activity of the tooth to remain healthy."

Sochat and Schwarz[19] aptly express it: "Excessive occlusal forces can cause periodontal disease, but that disease is not gingivitis or periodontitis. When forces exceed the adaptive capacity of the periodontium a lesion develops in any or all of the tissues of the attachment apparatus (cementum, periodontal ligament, alveolar bone). That lesion is called 'occlusal traumatism.'

"Occlusal traumatism is a highly destructive periodontal disease, but it does not cause inflammation or periodontal pockets. It causes degeneration and necrosis of the periodontal ligament, resorption of the alveolar housing and, in some cases, root resorption.

"Occlusal traumatism is multifactorial in its etiology. The common causative ingredients generally found in varying proportions are occlusal interferences and heavy parafunctional activity. It should always be kept in mind that, as with any other disease process or injury, the effects of these etiologic factors are modified by the reparative ability of the host. Like most other biologic systems, the attachment apparatus has the ability to adapt to and function within a broad range of functional demands. Regardless of how the occlusal surfaces of the teeth come together, as long as the host can adapt, no pathology will develop. In other words, 'occlusal interferences' and/or bruxism cannot be equated with disease."*

If trauma occurs and inflammation is present at the same time, the inflammatory reaction might extend into the tissues damaged by trauma.

Pocket formation (gingival irritation and inflammation with destruction of the gingival fibers) is not caused by occlusal trauma. The occlusal trauma lesion is localized in the attachment apparatus (it is a highly destructive noninflammatory change which occurs in any or all of the tissues of the attachment apparatus) and does not influence the gingival fiber apparatus. One must regard the periodontal traumatic lesion and pocket formation as distinct processes. Orban[20] has said that occlusal trauma is always restricted to the intra-alveolar tissues and does not cause changes of the gingiva such as pocket formation, recession, or gingivitis.

In other words (1) trauma is not a primary etiologic factor in producing periodontal disease—it is a severe aggravating factor—and (2) trauma may accentuate pocket depth if it occurs in association with other local irritants. In such instances trauma induces destructive changes in the periodontal ligament, and inflammation in the marginal gingiva, within the confines of the gingival and transseptal fibers, is aggravated and spreads faster and farther into the tissues damaged by trauma. Trauma deflects the pathway of inflammation, and we have on our hands a biomechanical problem.

Primary occlusal traumatism is the result of excessive force in the presence of a normal amount of supporting tissue that will alter the attachment apparatus but will not produce any significant gingival changes or form periodontal pockets.[21] It refers to the degenerative changes which occur as a result of excessive forces. This phenomenon may occur in the presence of marginal inflammatory disease. In the absence of inflammation of the gingival unit, primary occlusal traumatism, according to Ramfjord,[22] is referred to as *pure primary occlusal traumatism* (Fig. 6-9).

---

*From Schwarz, Melvyn S., and Sochat, Paul: Occlusion and periodontal disease, J. S. Calif. Dent. Assoc. **40:**524-526, 1972.

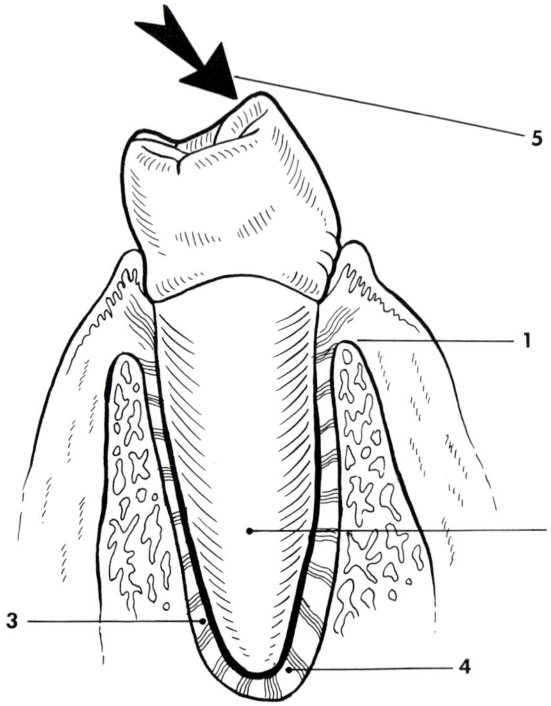

Fig. 6-9. Primary occlusal traumatism. *1,* Height of alveolar bone (normal); *2,* fulcrum point; *3,* area of pressure; *4,* area of tension; *5,* horizontally applied pathologic force. (Redrawn from Amsterdam, M., and Abrams, L.: Periodontal prosthesis. In Goldman, H. M., and Cohen, D. W.: Periodontal therapy, ed. 5, St. Louis, 1973, The C. V. Mosby Co.)

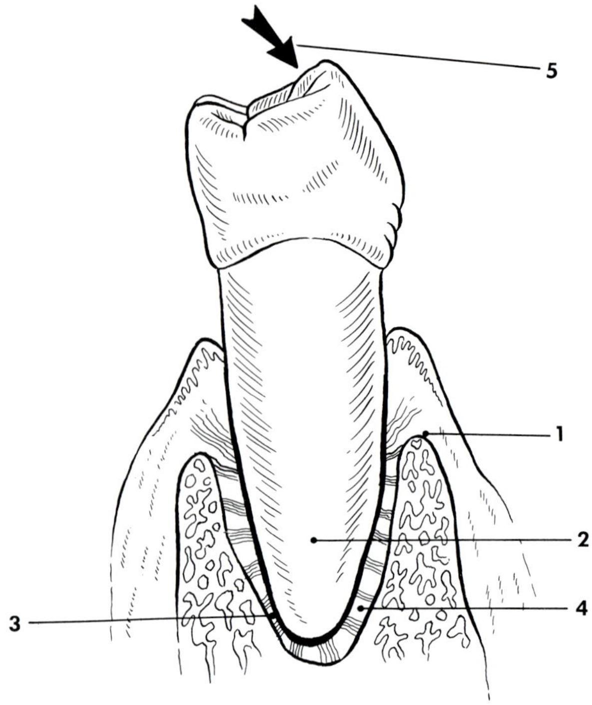

Fig. 6-10. Secondary occlusal traumatism. *1,* Height of alveolar bone (lost due to previous disease); *2,* fulcrum point; *3,* area of pressure; *4,* area of tension; *5,* horizontally applied force during normal function. (Redrawn from Amsterdam, M., and Abrams, L.: Periodontal prosthesis. In Goldman, H. M., and Cohen, D. W.: Periodontal therapy, ed. 5, St. Louis, 1973, The C. V. Mosby Co.)

Signs of healing of primary occlusal traumatism may be clinical or roentgenographic. *Clinical changes* include (1) decrease in tooth mobility, (2) maintenance of migrated tooth in the corrected position, and (3) disappearance of pain or tenderness. *Roentgenographic changes* include (1) thinning of periodontal ligament space (becomes distinct) and (2) lamina dura (alveolar periphery) becoming distinct and intact.

Secondary occlusal traumatism is trauma coupled with gingival inflammation. It creates a summative effect, leading to the loss of supporting structure because of the inflammatory penetration into the periodontal structures, resulting in an apical migration of the epithelial attachment. It refers to the effect on already reduced or weakened periodontal structures by occlusal forces which may or may not be abnormal, but which are excessive for reduced weakened supporting structures. The quantity of the attachment apparatus has been reduced; there is inadequate mechanical resistance of the attachment apparatus. An apical shift in the positioning of the fulcrum of the tooth within its alveolus creates an adverse leverage factor on the remaining alveolar housing of the tooth.[22] This situation, coupled with the presence of parafunctional traumatic influences (grinding and clenching), makes for a most difficult problem. All these factors create an alteration in form and function—a disparity of embrasure forms, crown-tissue relations, and marginal gingiva, a change in the crown-to-root ratio (see Fig. 6-10). This type of condition produces a specific type of periodontal pathology, which is referred to as angular bone destruction.

In secondary occlusal traumatism there is no potential for reversibility. Splinting is the treatment.

Whether injury occurs to normal periodontal structures from abnormal occlusal forces or occurs to already weakened periodontal structures from normal or excessive occlusal forces depends on (1) the resistance and response of the tissues to the forces and (2) those morphologic features of the teeth (crown form, root form, crown-to-root ratio, tooth position), arch form, and supporting structures which resist or modify the forces.

Impairment of tissue resistance may occur from

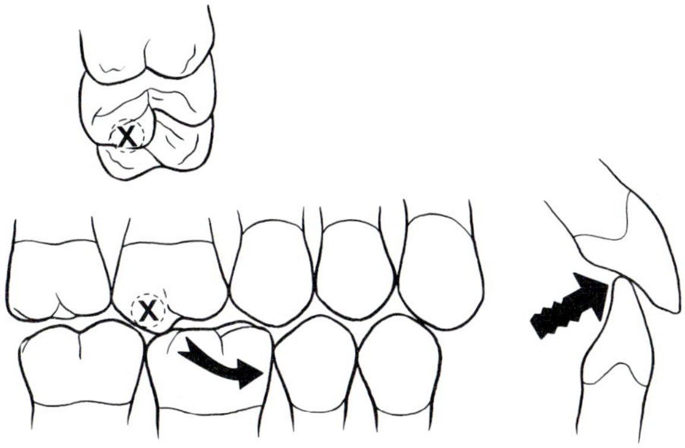

Fig. 6-11. Direct and indirect trauma from occlusion. The centric pathway prematurity *(X)* deflects mandible anteriorly creating indirect trauma and its sequela, fanning or pathologic migration of the maxillary anterior teeth.

alteration of the metabolic activity and structural integrity of the tissues as a result of local or systemic disturbances.

To summarize some important facts, angular bone loss on opposing posterior teeth combined with a mobility pattern and a migration of anterior teeth caused by bone destruction creates a syndrome that points up the existence of direct and indirect trauma from occlusion. Direct trauma is periodontal injury in the area of initial occlusal prematurity. Indirect trauma is injury in areas to which the mandible is deflected by the initial prematurity (Fig. 6-11).

A force is traumatic because the destructive changes it induces exceed the reparative capacity of the tissues. The extent of involvement of the supporting structures in a traumatic situation is dependent upon the interplay of direction, duration, intensity, and frequency of the applied force. The afunctional contacts of teeth produced by clenching and grinding habits also are important factors that require serious consideration.

Excessive forces upon the teeth result in pathologic changes, which are manifested clinically by mobility and/or migration of teeth because of a loss of the attachment apparatus necessary for tooth stability and temporomandibular disturbances, and roentgenographically by a widening of the periodontal ligament space, loss of lamina dura definition, root resorption, and resorption-induced radiolucencies of supporting bone. Cemental tears are in evidence, and it is somewhat common to observe pathologic attritional wear of teeth, cuspal and root fractures, and pulpal changes from a hyperemic pulp to one that has undergone degeneration. Ramfjord[22] has pointed out that a change in the percussion sound (from a sharp sound to a dull one) is the result of the resorption of the lamina dura and increased width and consistency of the periodontal ligament. He noted that an increase in tooth mobility is due to replacement of dense functional periodontal tissues by granulation tissue following a widening of the periodontal ligament space after resorption of the alveolar bone.

It is therefore obvious that occlusal forces not only have influence on tooth structures, but also upon the structures of the periodontium; variations in the functional requirements are met by structural changes within the range of adaptability. Disturbances in this equilibrium can occur if the functional demands are beyond the tissue tolerance and adaptability. The physiologic limits of irritation must always be measured by the resistance values of the individual and his tissues. These resistance values must be computed on the basis of the presence or absence of certain signs and symptoms that are known to be associated with trauma from occlusion. In the absence of the signs and symptoms of periodontal breakdown, we may be justified in accepting health as evidence of repair and adaptation.

The aforementioned facts point up the importance of the creation of optimal functional conditions in order to give to the supporting tissues the optimal chance of maintenance or recovery under pathologic conditions. Avoidance of mesial and distal drifting, distorted lateral stresses, food impaction, and pocket formation cannot be overstressed.

Crown-to-root ratio

The relation of the clinical crowns to the clinical roots of the teeth is of the utmost importance. The crown-to-root ratio is the proportion between the clinical crown and clinical root, and it is important in the resistance against leverages of oral forces. This factor must be kept in mind when considering the problem of loss of supporting tissues, which creates an adverse leverage on the remaining alveolar housing of the teeth, and, if complicated by parafunctional movements, the problem becomes even more exaggerated. The ideal situation would be clinical crown-to-root ratios that are practically equal in proportion. If this is not possible, multiple abutments and splinting of teeth must be instituted to equalize as much as possible the ideal ratio balance.

In the evaluation of crown-to-root ratios the vertical aspect of the teeth is not the only factor to be considered, but also the size, shape, and form of

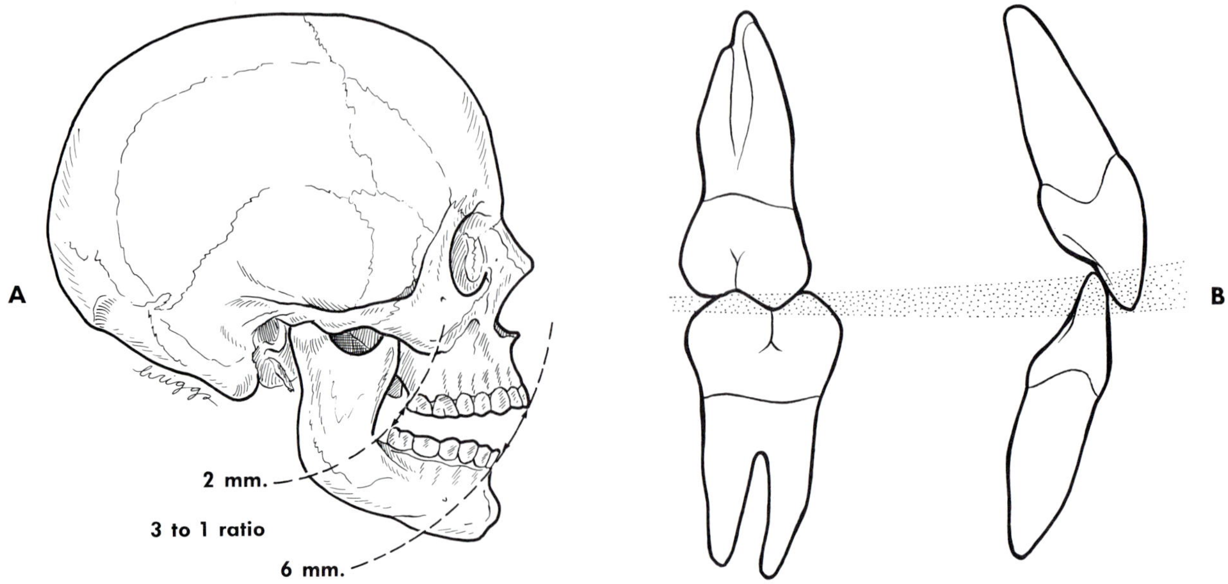

Fig. 6-12. Reduction in clinical crown length. **A,** Relative difference between opening in anterior part of mouth as compared to posterior area. Ratio is approximately 3:1. **B,** Difference between amount of overbite in anterior and posterior areas of mouth is shown as a shaded band. Any decrease in clinical crown length of posterior teeth will have a threefold effect on anterior teeth. (Redrawn from Amsterdam, M., and Abrams, L.: Periodontal prosthesis. In Goldman, H. M., and Cohen, D. W.: Periodontal therapy, ed. 5, St. Louis, 1973, The C. V. Mosby Co.)

the crown as it relates to the size, shape, form, number, and position of the roots. Axial inclination of the tooth and its relation to its housing, as well as the type and amount of remaining bone and the number and distribution of remaining teeth, also must be considered seriously.

Reduction of the clinical crown length of the crown-to-root ratio that shows adverse leverages is a limited procedure, particularly in the posterior teeth, with the exception of extruded teeth and raised cusps on tilted teeth. Bohannan and Abrams[23] have shown that a 1 mm. reduction in posterior height results in a 3 mm. increase in the anterior overbite. Reduction of the height of anterior teeth is feasible, as a rule, allowing for better function and esthetics, but before performing this operation the problems of anterior incisal guidance, esthetics and phonetics, lip line, and the possibility of pulpal involvement should be studied carefully. Intentional or elective vital pulp extirpation is good clinical judgment and practice in many instances.

"Very little reduction can be accomplished on posterior teeth. The main reason for this is found in the mechanics of jaw closure and the relationship of the anterior and posterior parts of the dental arch to the center of mandibular rotation. The nearer the tooth is to the condyle, the shorter will be its arc of closure, and, consequently, the less distance it will travel in the closing movement. Because of this, a 1 mm. closure in the molar region may result in as much as a 3 mm. closure anteriorly (Fig. 6-12). Therefore, any effort to reduce the crown length of posterior teeth generally creates a problem anteriorly. This can lead to an unacceptable situation both esthetically and functionally, the 'open bite' occlusion being an exception. Anterior teeth, on the other hand, can be shortened within esthetic limits to effect a more favorable crown-to-root ratio."*

As previously stated, intentional vital pulp extirpation is good clinical judgment and, in a number of cases, allows for the retention of teeth that would otherwise have to be sacrificed. This fact should be considered seriously when arriving at a total treatment plan. Should abutment teeth be moved into position orthodontically, should they be telescoped, or should intentional pulp extirpation be used? Not only is elective endodontics indicated sometimes in the reduction of crown length to effect a better crown-to-root ratio,

*From Bohannan, Harry M., and Abrams, Leonard: Intentional vital pulp extirpation in periodontal prosthesis, J. Prosthet. Dent. **11**:781-789, 1961.

but also in the establishment of parallelism of clinical crowns and in the reorientation of the plane of occlusion.

Root resection

In some cases of multirooted teeth involved periodontally, the hopelessly diseased part of the tooth can be removed surgically, and the part that can be treated successfully, both periodontally and endodontically, may be retained to serve as an abutment tooth for a fixed prosthesis. The feasibility of this plan hinges on whether the tooth structure that remains is sound with a substantial bony support, is located properly relative to its alveolar housing, and demonstrates an attachment apparatus with a well-defined lamina dura and thin periodontal ligament space as seen roentgenographically.

The periodontic and endodontic procedures must be executed successfully, correct occlusal relations and coronal contours must be established, stabilization must be attained by means of a fixed splint, and oral physiotherapy must be possible of attainment.[24,25]

The operative procedure is to treat the root to be retained endodontically and then to split the tooth, and remove the hopelessly periodontally involved root (or roots) (Fig. 6-13). Stabilization by means of a provisional splint then should be instituted until there is sufficient evidence of periodontal healing, after which a permanent restoration can be constructed and positioned.

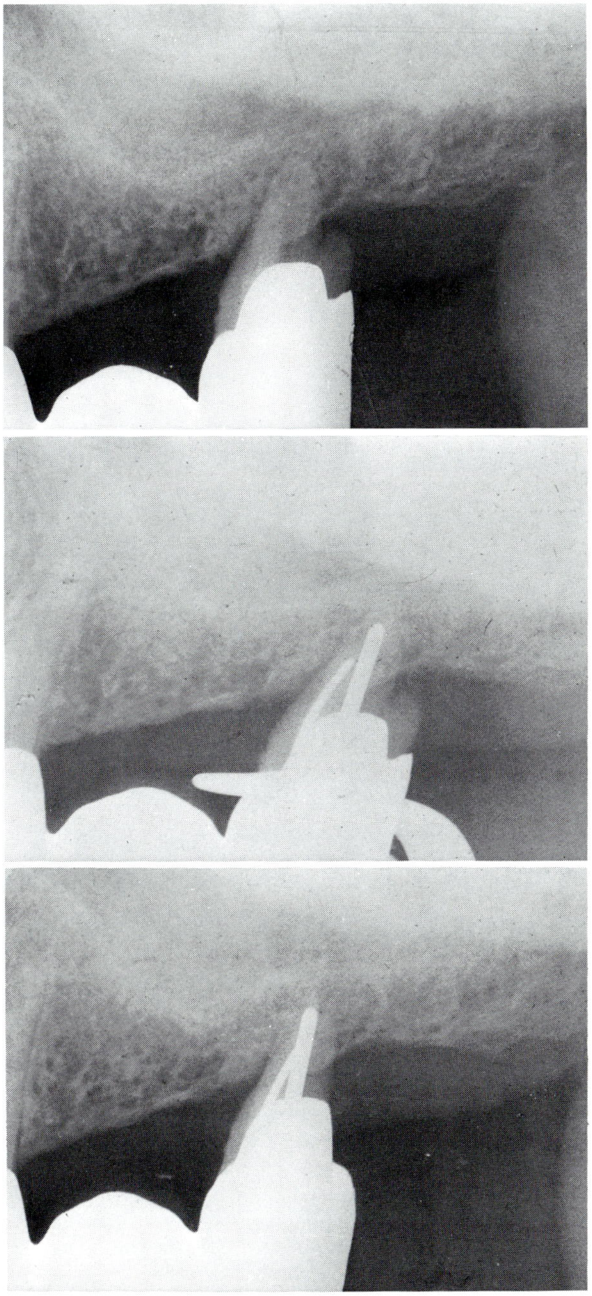

Fig. 6-13. Hopelessly periodontally involved root. Roots to be retained were treated endodontically, and involved root was split and removed.

This therapy of root resection also can be used in cases in which all the canals of a multirooted tooth cannot be treated successfully by endodontic means. After the flap has been loosened and turned back, the root to be resected is severed at the cementoenamel junction with a fissure bur and is removed. The entire crown of the tooth is left in place. Usually double abutments are used in these cases to increase stabilization (Fig. 6-14).

Coronal contours

Crown form and tooth position are important considerations in the etiology of periodontal disease. The restoration of the correct form of a tooth will help regain its function. Crown form plays an important role in the protection of the gingival tissues from the traumatizing effects of many foodstuffs, thereby making it essential for the gingival contours and the occlusal and incisal forms of the restored teeth to be shaped so as to shunt food and protect the marginal gingivae. The importance of the correct contour in the cervical third region of all teeth cannot be over-

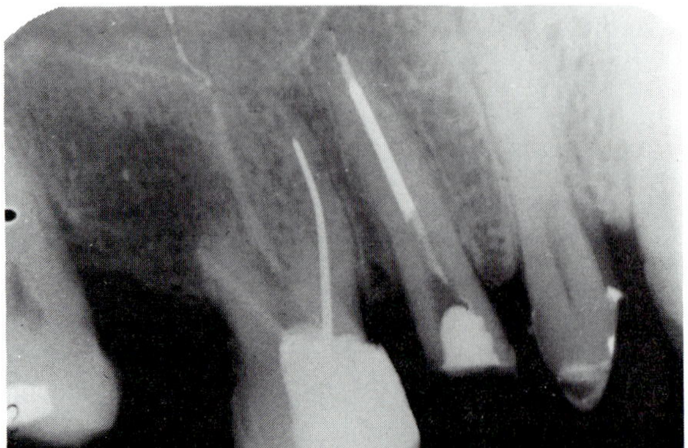

Fig. 6-14. A canal in a multirooted tooth (upper first molar) that could not be treated successfully by endodontic means. Flap was turned back and root resected, leaving entire crown intact. A fixed splint was constructed utilizing two bicuspids and this tooth as abutments to increase stabilization.

A

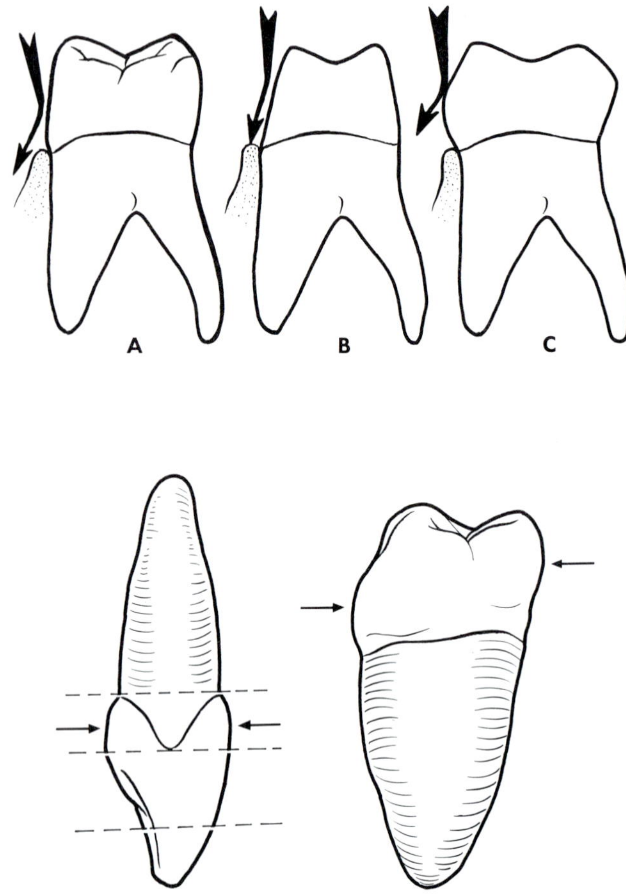

Fig. 6-15. A, Facial and lingual contours (protective). Schematic drawings of curvatures labially, buccally, and lingually. *A,* Normal curvatures as found on mandibular molar. Arrow shows path of food material as it is avalanched over these curvatures during mastication. *B,* Molar with little or no curvature. The gingiva is likely to be stripped or pushed apically through lack of protection and consequent overstimulation. *C,* Molar with curvature in excess of normal. Gingiva will be protected too much and will suffer from lack of proper stimulation. Food material and bacterial cultures may lodge under these curvatures, promoting pathologic disturbance. *D,* Normal cervical curvatures as found on maxillary incisors. The crests of curvature are opposite each other labiolingually. *E,* Curvatures as found on mandibular posterior teeth. Protective curvature is located at cervical third to buccal and at middle third to lingual surface. (Redrawn from Wheeler, R. C.: J. S. Calif. Dent. Assoc. **31**:382, 1963.)

emphasized, because while correct convexities assist in maintaining and protecting the health of the gingivae, an excessive contour in this area causes the investing tissues to lose their tone and also results in the formation of food pockets, causing a chronic inflammation of the gum tissues (Figs. 6-15 and 6-16).

Amsterdam[21] has told us that the basic functional implement of the masticatory organ is the dental unit (Fig. 6-17).

The *dental unit* consists of the *tooth,* the *attachment apparatus,* and the *gingival unit.* The tooth consists of the anatomic crown and the anatomic root; the attachment apparatus is composed of the cemen-

B

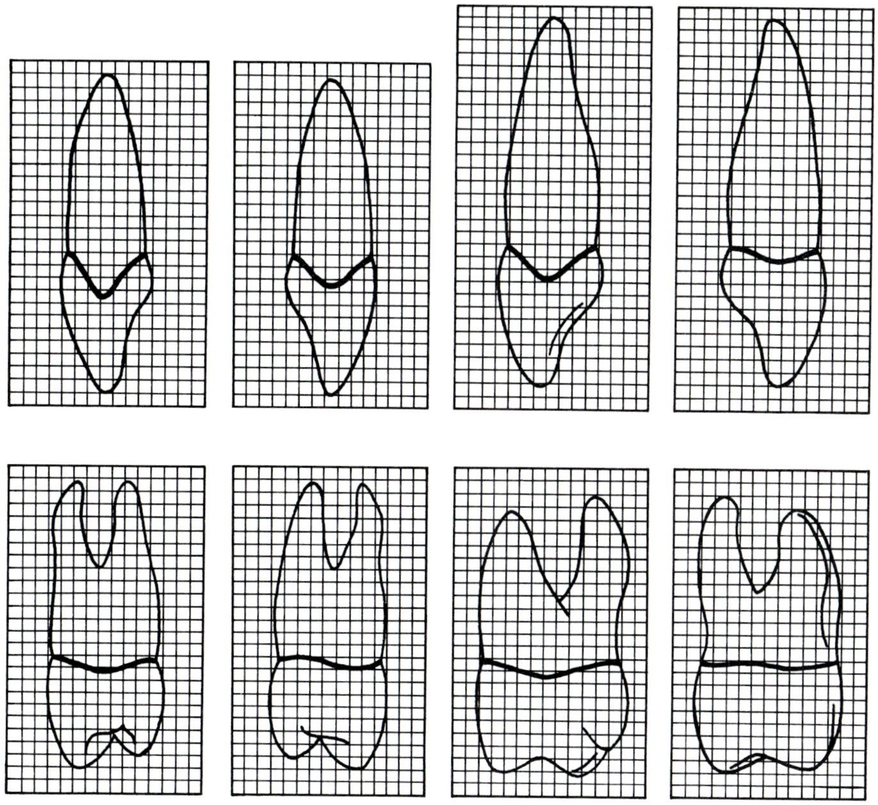

C

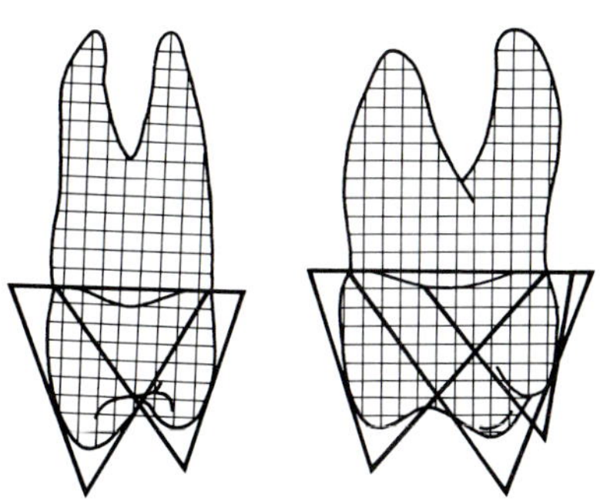

Fig. 6-15, cont'd. B, Graphs of typical forms of maxillary teeth accenting the outlines of cervical lines mesially and distally. **C,** The functional form of the teeth when outlined schematically from the mesial or distal aspects is that of the fusion of two or three cones. Left maxillary premolar; right maxillary first molar. (Redrawn from Wheeler, R. C.: A textbook of dental anatomy and physiology, ed. 4, Philadelphia, 1965, W. B. Saunders Co.)

tum, the alveolar housing, and the periodontal ligament (its primary function is to enable the tooth to perform its function by resisting forces that would tend to dislodge the tooth); and the gingival unit provides a tough collagenous and epithelial covering to the neck of the tooth and the underlying attachment apparatus, which in turn protects these underlying structures from the bacterial flora of the mouth.

Careful examination of the gingival unit shows that its weakest link lies in the sulcular area, the epithelium lining of which is protected from the injurious effects of food retention, impaction, and plaque by the contours and positions of the anatomic or clinical crowns.

The gingival attachment to the tooth is at the cementoenamel junction. The enamel swells out from the cementoenamel junction, forming the cervical

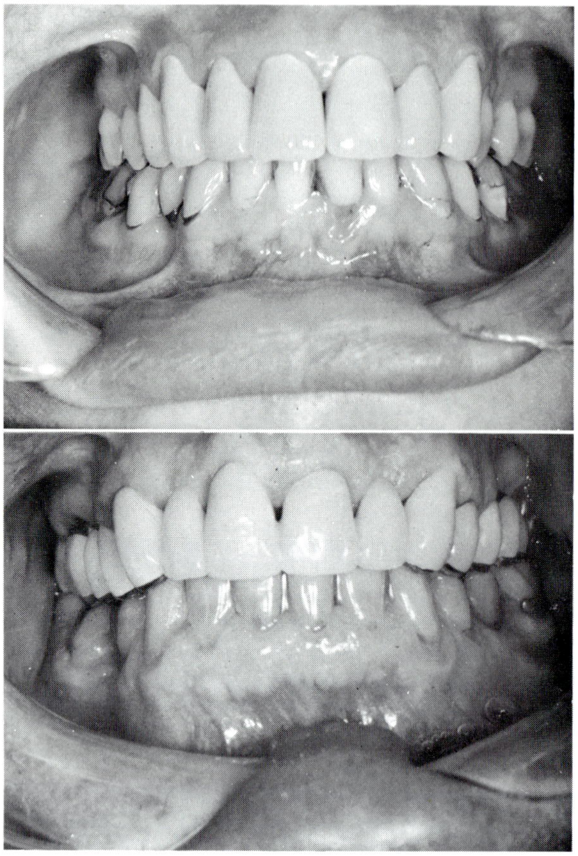

Fig. 6-16. Results of correct coronal form, especially in cervical third area, maintaining and protecting health of gingivae (15 years postoperatively).

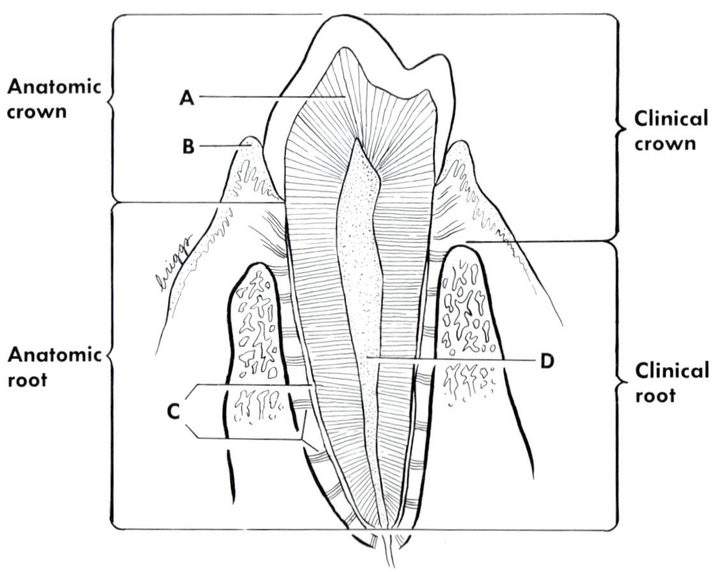

Fig. 6-17. Basic dental unit consists of the tooth *(A)*, gingival unit *(B)*, attachment apparatus *(C)*, and pulp *(D)*. (Redrawn from Amsterdam, M., and Abrams, L.: Periodontal prosthesis. In Goldman, H. M., Schluger, S., Fox, L., and Cohen, D. W.; Periodontal therapy, ed. 3, St. Louis, 1964, The C. V. Mosby Co.)

ridge, the deflective convexity under which the free marginal gingiva rests. Ideally, the cervical ridge and the tip of the free marginal gingiva are of the same width so that the gingival portion of the anatomic crown facially and lingually forms a continuous line with the facial or lingual surface of the tissue, turning the corner mesially and distally to the interproximal papillae. This enamel ridge is the deflecting contour of the tooth that acts to protect the free gingival margin. The surface of the tooth should not extend buccally, lingually, or labially beyond the surface of this tissue; otherwise, the functional stimulation of the tissue by the musculature will be lost.[26]

Tooth crowns have a fairly uniform facial and lingual curvature at the cervical third. The facial and lingual surfaces of the crowns exhibit convex contours of approximately 0.5 mm. at the gingival third, and in mandibular molars it may be as great as 1 mm. on the lingual surface.[27] This convexity is precisely related to the position of the gingival sulcus and directs the passage of food away from the sulcus and onto the more keratinized surface of the attached gingiva. (See Fig. 6-18.) The curvature also should allow sufficient functional stimulation for necessary tissue massage because the gingival tissues are directly dependent upon the functional stimulation of mastication to retain their normal healthy character.

Morris[28] says: "The contour may vary in different mouths, in different parts of the same mouth, or on the same tooth. If such contours do not protect against food impaction but rather permit free muscular flow, the final shapes of those surfaces will range from flat to the most subtle of convexities. These forms are more truly comparable to natural curves and will most likely preserve gingival health. (See Fig. 6-19.)

"The rationale of muscular molding and cleansing, rather than that of food impaction, more adequately explains clinical phenomena and is a more accurate guide for the construction of gingivally tolerated full crowns."*

To reiterate: The importance of establishing a correct anatomic form in the restoration cannot be overemphasized. A basic relation exists between the form of the tooth and its function. Particular attention may well be given to the enamel curvatures on the facial and lingual surfaces of the cervical third of the crown. These natural curvatures have a definite function in that they maintain the desired tension between the tooth and the free gingival margin and per-

*From Morris, Melvin L.: Artificial crown contours and gingival health, J. Prosthet. Dent. **12:**1146-1155, 1962.

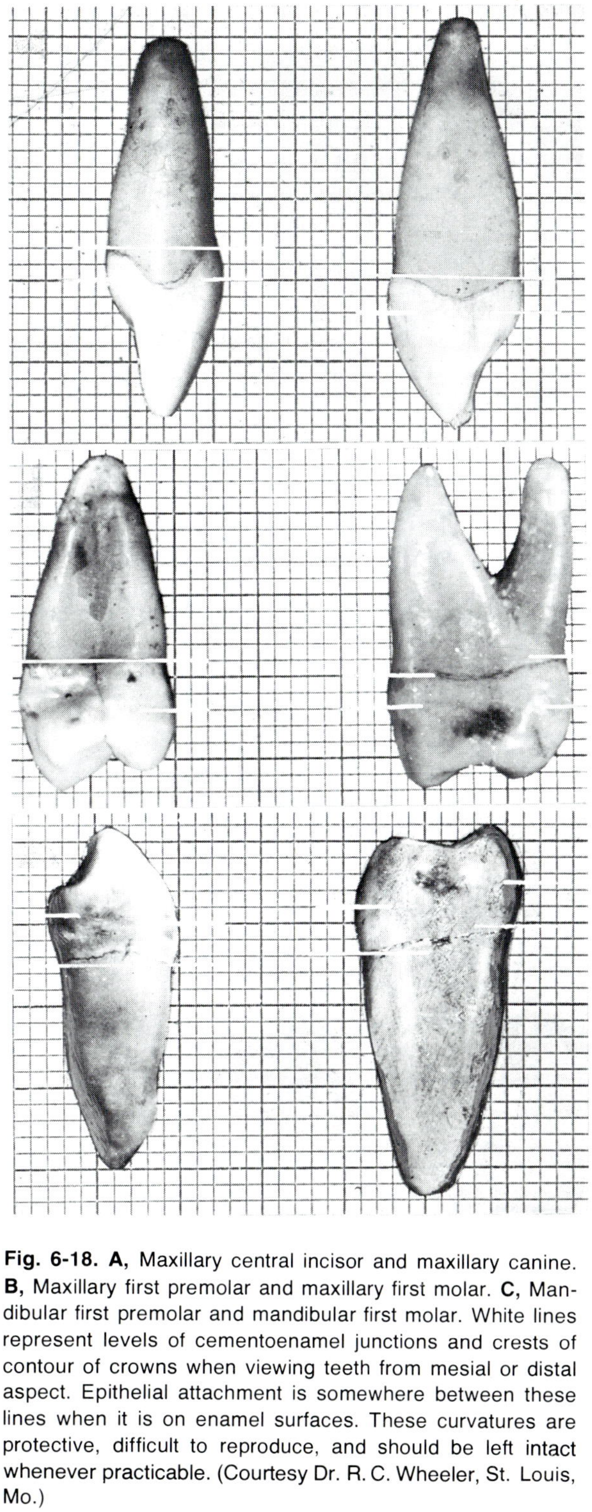

A

B

C

Fig. 6-18. A, Maxillary central incisor and maxillary canine. **B,** Maxillary first premolar and maxillary first molar. **C,** Mandibular first premolar and mandibular first molar. White lines represent levels of cementoenamel junctions and crests of contour of crowns when viewing teeth from mesial or distal aspect. Epithelial attachment is somewhere between these lines when it is on enamel surfaces. These curvatures are protective, difficult to reproduce, and should be left intact whenever practicable. (Courtesy Dr. R. C. Wheeler, St. Louis, Mo.)

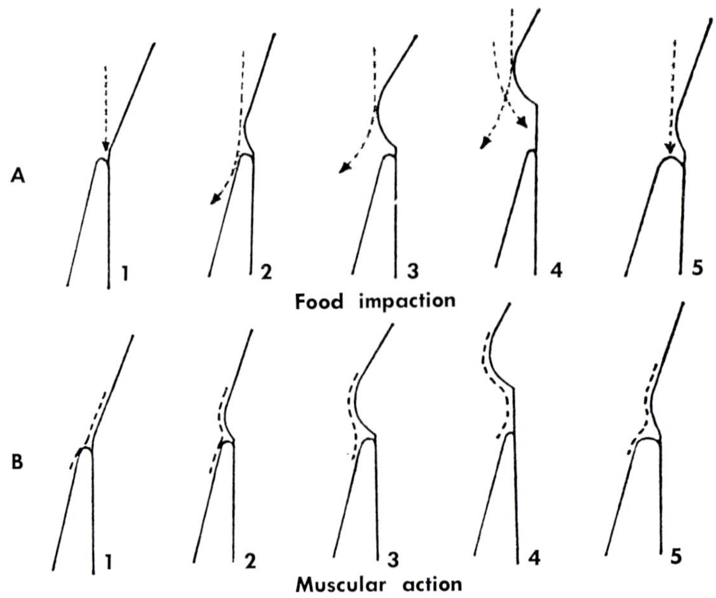

Fig. 6-19. Comparison of identical contour conditions that are interpreted in two different ways. **A,** Food impaction theory regards bulges as protection against impaction of food into buccal and/or lingual crevice. **B,** Muscle action theory pictures a constant cleansing and molding action by muscles and food, which can be impaired when the necessary intimate contact is prevented by a bulge of crown or bone. *1,* No coronal contour: **A,** unhealthy—direct food impaction with no protection; **B,** healthy—most efficient muscular action. *2,* Slight "physiologic" convexity: **A,** healthy—food is deflected to outer surface of gingivae; **B,** healthy—good muscular action. *3,* Thick crown contour: **A,** unhealthy—food is deflected away from gingivae; no stimulation; **B,** unhealthy—muscle contact is prevented by bulge of crown. *4,* Thick crown contour with gingival recession: **A,** unhealthy—bulge is too distant to protect gingivae; **B,** healthy—a distant bulge cannot prevent muscular contact with gingivae. *5,* Thick bone with "physiologic" crown contour: **A,** unhealthy—food can be impacted on wide gingival surface and then toward gingival crevice; **B,** unhealthy—muscular contact is prevented by bulge of bone. (From Morris, M. L.: J. Prosthet. Dent. **12:**1146-1155, 1962.)

mit the necessary frictional stimulation of these tissues in masticating. If the curvature established by restorative measures is less or more than the natural curvature, the restoration will cause irritation and lead to gingival disturbances. Exaggeration of the degree of curvature of the cervical third is a common error in restorative work.

Proper coronal contours and proper tooth alignment lend to an individual and collective self-protection of the masticatory apparatus. When fabricating dental restorations, all factors must be considered to create the best possible environment for tissue health and access to plaque.

Perel[29] has this to say in regard to the problem under consideration: "The placement of a protective contour above the marginal gingiva does not enhance the health of sound gingiva. To the contrary, it may predispose the soft tissue to inflammatory changes. This would occur through the accumulation of debris and the lack of access to the marginal gingiva by food under mastication, by the surrounding musculature, and by oral hygiene appliances. As such, undercontoured axial crown surfaces may be the contours of choice."*

Eissmann, Radke, and Noble[30] have said: "Axial contours must be so related to the gingival architecture, the adjacent and opposing teeth, and to the adjacent musculature to promote continuing gingival health. Restorations must be contoured to function physiologically, i.e. effectively and protectively, and be capable of being kept clean by means of muscular stimulation, food flow patterns, and tooth cleansing devices.

"Protective contours are convexities, such as food deflection prominences which prevent food impaction, and that stimulating contours are concavities, such as sluice-gates and embrasures, which provide ready

---

*From Perel, Morton L.: Periodontal considerations of crown contours, J. Prosthet. Dent. **26**(6):627-630, 1971.

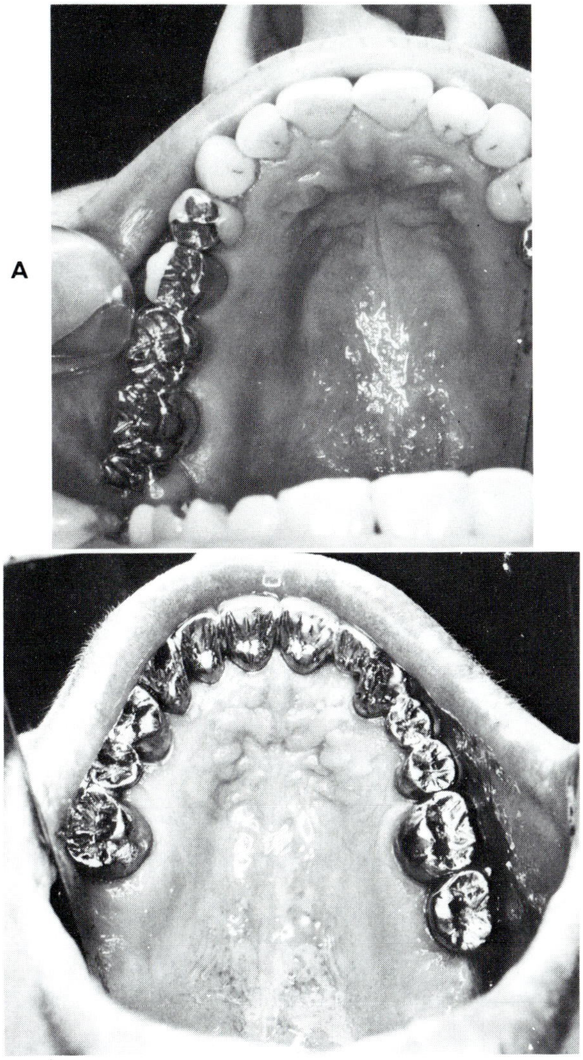

Fig. 6-20. A, Note natural concavities on maxillary incisors below contact areas, exposing gingiva to stimulation necessary for a healthy tissue tone. B, An endeavor was made to accomplish the same principle in the fixed splint—to open access to interproximal embrasures for good hygiene.

access for cleansing of tooth surfaces and for the massaging of gingival tissues.

"Natural concavities are arranged to expose gingiva to stimulation necessary for a healthy tissue tone (Fig. 6-20). As the distance from occlusal table to the free gingival margin increases the necessity for protective convexities decreases, and the accentuation of natural concavities found in tooth forms becomes increasingly important. Because of effects of plaque formation, which outweighs food impaction problems, decrease axial curvatures and decrease them in proportion to the crown length (Fig. 6-21).

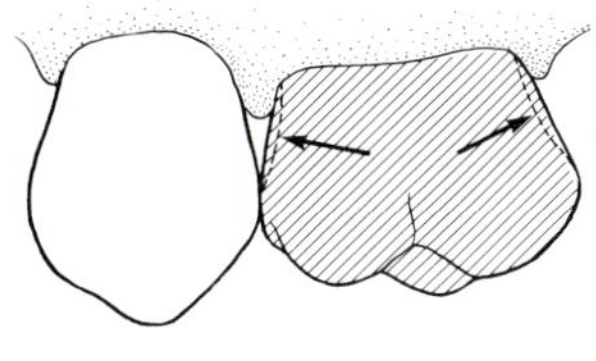

Fig. 6-21. The proximal surfaces of restorations should be flat or slightly concave, giving an obtuse lingual embrasure below the contact area.

"Deflection prominences on facial and lingual surfaces are beneficial in patients with short clinical crowns. They augment muscular adaptation and support."*

Yuodelis, Weaver, and Sapkos[31] have said: "So-called 'protective' convexity not only serves as a food trap, but also prevents massage of the gingival margin. This cervical bulge overprotects the microbial plaque. Plaque buildup begins in, and its retention is greatest in, the cervical region of the tooth gingiva to the height of contour.

"The flatter the contour, the less plaque retained. The explanation for this lies in the accessibility to oral hygiene measures. The authors have never observed teeth with little or no facial or lingual curvature that demonstrated a free gingival margin that had been stripped or pushed apically because of lack of protection and consequent overstimulation."†

My approach to this problem, at the present time, is the creation of a rather subtle deflection ridge—to flatten the facial and lingual contours to a great extent. This not only prevents food impaction but also affords a massaging action to the gingiva. This subtle deflection ridge is precisely related to the position of the gingival sulcus (keeping in mind that the weakest link of the gingival unit lies in the sulcular area) and directs passage of food away from the sulcus and onto the attached gingiva. It allows the restoration to function harmoniously with the surrounding gingival tissues. A great effort is made to have a smooth, gradual transition from the restoration to the tooth structure (Figs. 6-22 and 6-23).

In cases of surgically lengthened clinical crowns, as in that of the normal anatomic crown, the height of coronal contour is to be placed at the cervical third of

*From Eissmann, H. G., Radke, R. A., and Noble, W. H.: Physiologic design criteria for fixed dental restorations, Dent. Clin. N. Am. **15**(3):543-568, July, 1971.

†From Yuodelis, R. A., Weaver, J. D., and Sapkos, S.: Facial and lingual contours of artificial complete crown restorations and their effects on the periodontium, J. Prosthet. Dent. **29**(1):61-66, 1973.

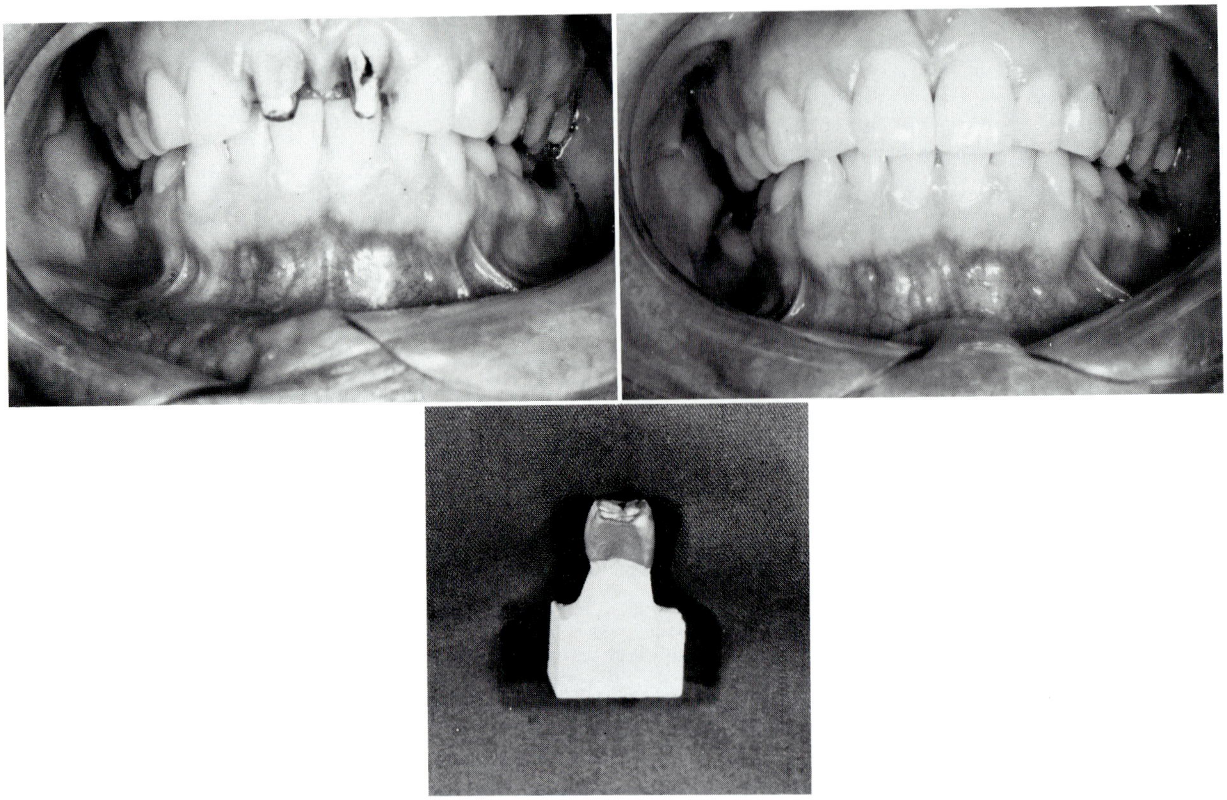

Fig. 6-22. Results of the author's efforts to have a smooth, gradual transition from the restoration to the tooth structure.

the crown. The clinical crown varies markedly with the anatomic crown because of the alveolar and supporting bone loss with resultant apical migration of the epithelial attachment, and the deflecting contours of these teeth are no longer physiologic as a result of the changed tooth–soft tissue relationship. The gingival third of this type of restored teeth, with the apical reposition of the gingival attachment to the tooth and their exposed root surfaces, which may be susceptible to demineralization and decay, must be contoured to imitate true anatomic crown form, making use of double deflecting contours with the most subtle of convexities, if it is to be compatible with the gingiva (Figs. 6-24 to 6-27).

Where furcations have been exposed, the crown and exposed root surfaces should be covered, but care must be taken not to cover the furcation opening with the crown margins (Figs. 6-28 and 6-29). The area should be treated as if it were an interdental papillary region so that adequate oral physiotherapy may be carried out.

When a removable appliance is indicated, it is most essential to design the denture base and connectors so that proper skirting of the gingival and proximal tissues is provided. This prohibition also applies to solder joints.

Restorative dentistry, if not executed properly, can be an etiologic factor in periodontal disease or recreation of this condition after periodontal therapy. Gross to subtle errors in restorations will cause or recreate pathology. A great deal depends on the way in which the tooth is prepared and the restoration is contoured.

Keep in mind that reproduction of the cervical third is almost humanly impossible; so think carefully before destroying all of it in tooth preparations. Also, teeth possess a protective capacity by virtue of their individual coronal contours and collective alignment.[21]

The forms of the facial, lingual or palatal, and interproximal surfaces of the teeth should be modified in periodontal prosthesis to improve their influence on the character of function.

Embrasures

When teeth are in proximal contact, the spaces that widen out from the contact area are known as embrasures. Embrasures protect the gingiva from food impaction and deflect food so as to massage the gingival surface.

Embrasure form is related directly to the coronal form of the proximal areas of adjacent teeth and must be designed in all aspects to protect the interdental papillae and the underlying interproximal bone. These tissues will be influenced greatly by their environment.

Joe H. Smith helped me immeasurably to understand better the role of the interdental topography in periodontal disease which is most essential.

Healthy gingivae may possess either col-shaped or triangular-shaped papillae. The ideal gingival picture is one in which triangular-shaped papillae are found.

Smith[32] has told us that the reason for the col existing as it does is the relationship of the gingival papillae to the contact areas of the adjacent teeth. The most common place for the col-shaped gingiva is between posterior teeth because of the wider tooth contact area. It is common also between anterior teeth, where the contact area extends apically enough to prevent the triangular-shaped papilla from forming. Another area is around crowded teeth, when the roots are close together.

While all col-shaped papillae are not clinically diseased, most diseased papillae are col shaped or cratered to some degree. Stahl[33] demonstrated in histologic sections that the middle part of the col is thin and devoid of the protective substance that covers stratified squamous epithelium and is subject to friction, that is, keratin. The buccal and lingual peaks were covered with keratinized epithelium that became unkeratinized as it approached the middle of the col.

Since bacteria and their enzymes are present in the col and the middle portion of the col is not subject to friction and thereby devoid of keratin, the inflammatory process will start in this vulnerable area. It is necessary to alter the cratered shape of the interdental alveolar crestal bone to obtain an acceptable architectural form that will maintain itself in function and health.

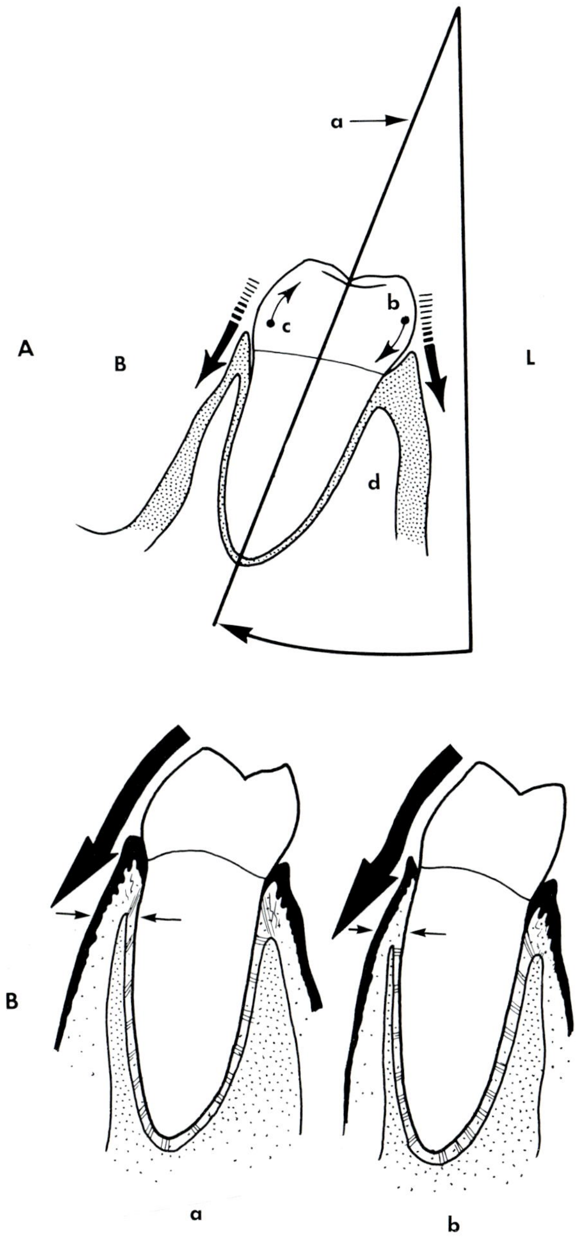

Fig. 6-23. A, The positioning of the axial center *(a)* of the molar is such that the crown is inclined toward the lingual *(L)* and away from the buccal *(B)*. This causes the height of crown contour *(b)* of the lingual to be depressed apically. At the same time the height of crown contour on the buccal *(c)* is elevated coronally. Also note that the increased contour on the lingual surface is apparently well designed to function with the increased thickness of the osseous and soft tissues *(d)* found on the lingual surface of the mandibular molar. **B,** The proper relations between amount of crown contour and the thickness of the periodontal tissues. A severely convex crown form is properly related to the thick tissues. This results in a continuity of crown form and tissue form and creates a sulcular area less likely to accumulate microbial plaque and debris. The desirable objectives of crown form and gingival health are created by having a flatter crown contour properly related to thinner periodontal tissues. (Adapted from Kraus, B. S., Jordan, R. E., and Abrams, Leonard: Dental anatomy and occlusion, Baltimore, 1969, The Williams & Wilkins Co.)

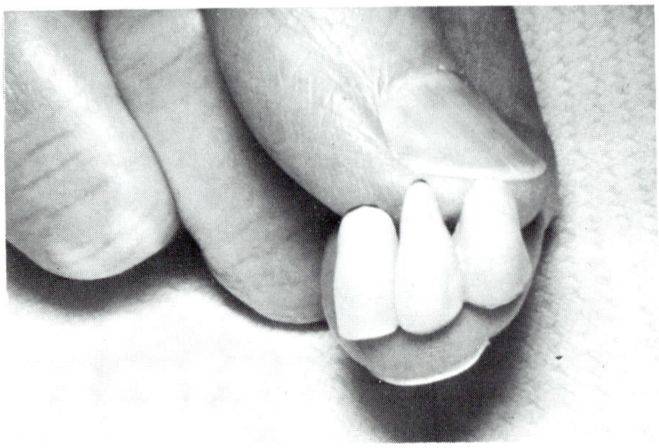

Fig. 6-24

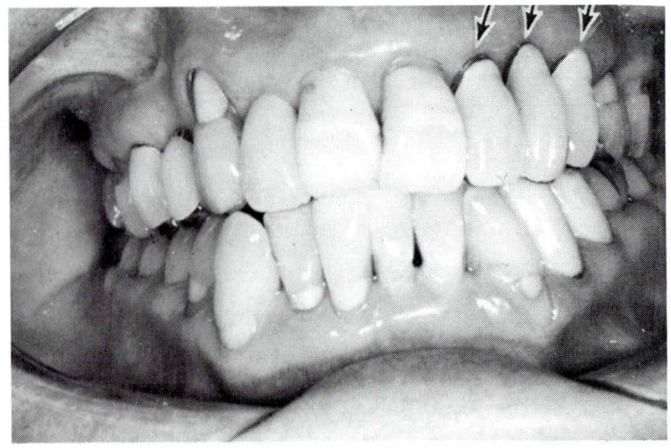

Fig. 6-25

Figs. 6-24 and 6-25. In cases of surgically lengthened clinical crowns, place height of coronal contour at cervical third of crown. If it is to be compatible with the gingiva, contour to imitate true anatomic crown form, making use of double deflecting contours with most subtle of convexities.

Fig. 6-26

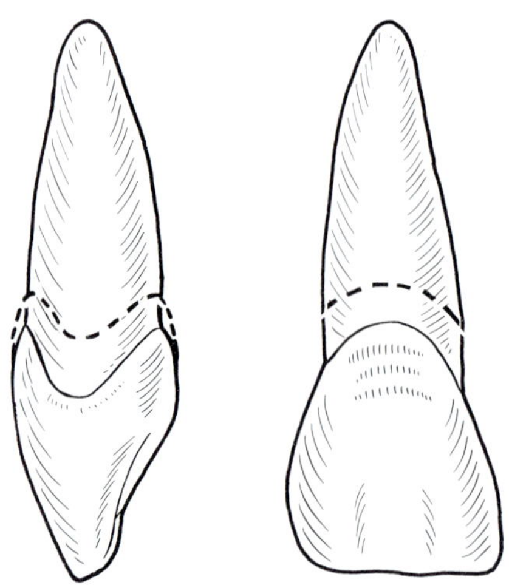

Fig. 6-27

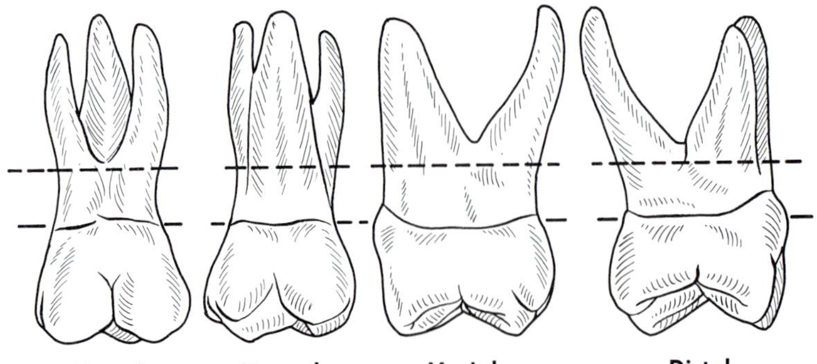

Figs. 6-26 and 6-27. Because of great difficulty of restoring cervical third, some investigators believe that crown form may be extended on root trunk of single-rooted teeth, but no attempt should be made to cover root trunk of multirooted teeth because of complicated form of root trunk. An exception—if caries or erosion demands it. In that case original root form must be reproduced to maintain proper dental hygiene. (Redrawn from Wheeler, R. C.: J. S. Calif. Dent. Assoc. **31**:389, 1963.)

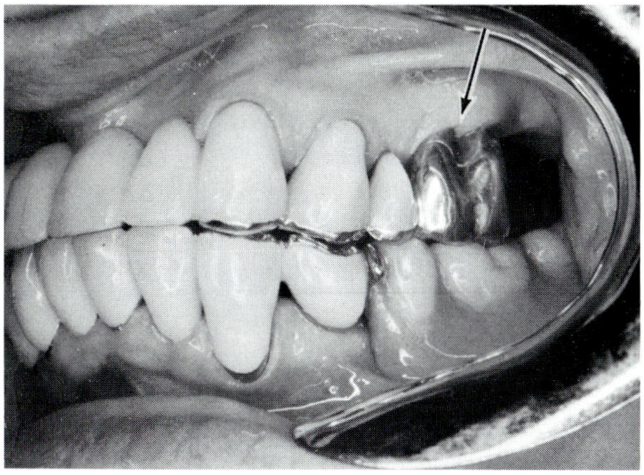

Fig. 6-28

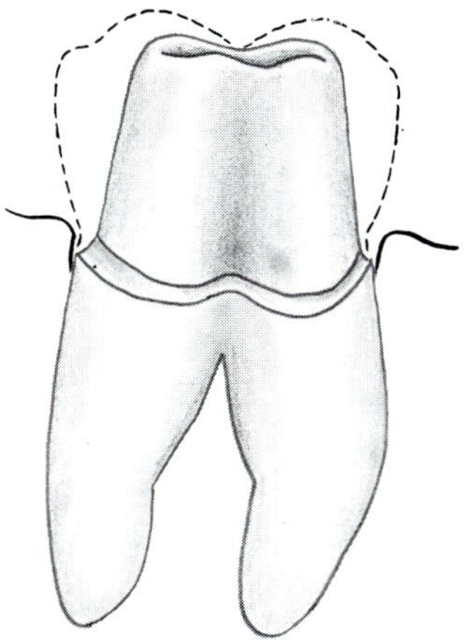

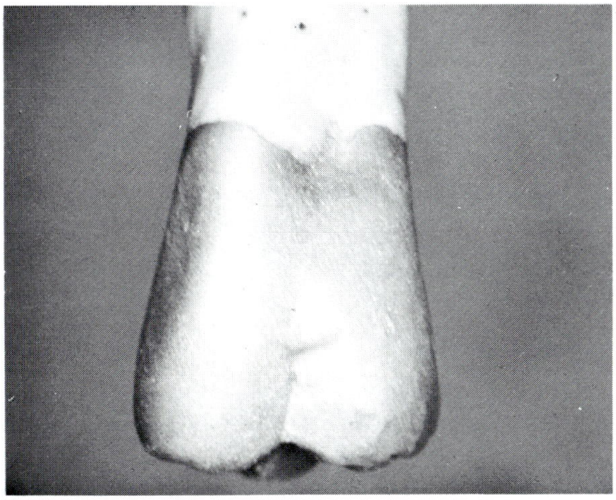

Fig. 6-29

Figs. 6-28 and 6-29. Where furcations have been exposed, crown and exposed root surfaces should be covered, care being taken not to cover furcation opening with crown margins. Adequate oral physiotherapy must be carried out.

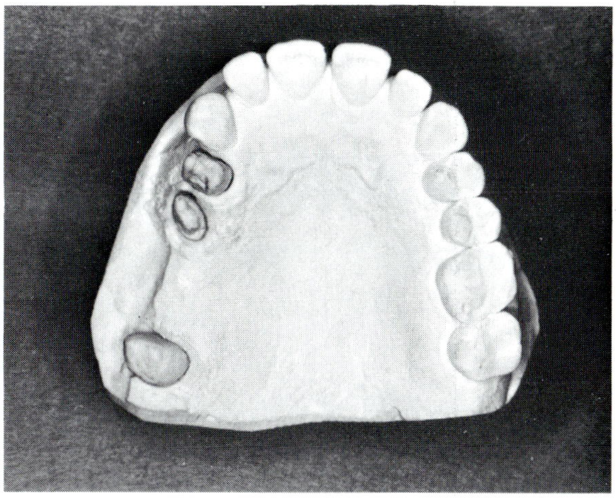

Fig. 6-30

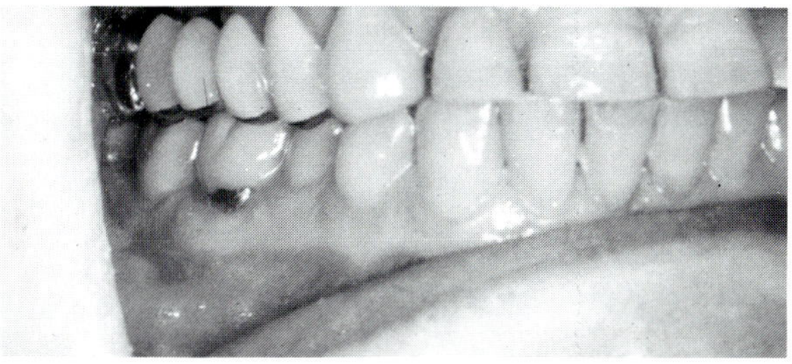

Fig. 6-31

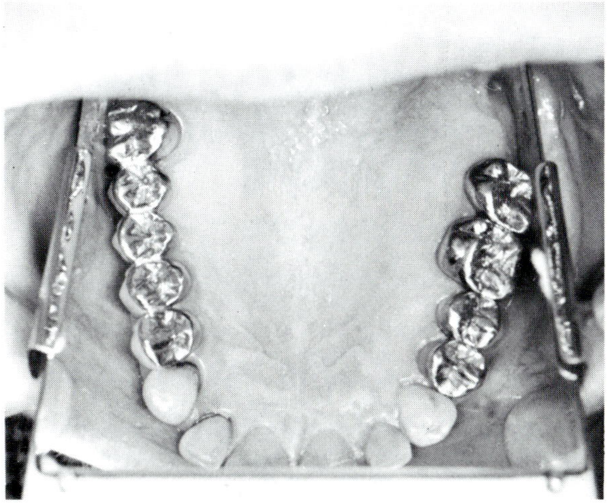

Fig. 6-32

Figs. 6-30 to 6-32. Rotated and tilted teeth may widen, narrow, or even obliterate the embrasures. Crowded or obliterated embrasure may present an insoluble problem necessitating great care in crown form and solder joints to allow for interdental stimulation and lavage.

This enables the overlying gingiva to assume the new shape of the contoured bone, at a distance from the contact area that will permit the necessary cleansing and dental massage. Thus regrowth of the papilla to its original height is prevented, and with conscientious home care the keratinization of the epithelium of the papilla will increase.[32]

Healthy interdental papillae exhibit many and varied shapes depending upon (1) the anatomic form of the underlying interdental bone, (2) the proximity of the roots of teeth allowing for or limiting interdental space, (3) the shape and outline of the interdental space as formed by the proximal surfaces of the teeth, and (4) the alignment or malalignment of the teeth in a jaw to each other.[34]

Anatomic variations of teeth may pose special problems in the shaping of full crowns and pontics. Among these variations are tilted and rotated teeth that distort, widen, narrow, or even obliterate the embrasures. A crowded or obliterated embrasure may present an insoluble problem, necessitating the use of much home care including brushing, interdental stimulation, and lavage. (See Figs. 6-30 to 6-32.)

The interproximal contour and contact point of the restoration will depend upon the size, shape, and height of the papilla. The contact area must be placed correctly and, in many cases of large interdental embrasures, moved gingivally. Keep in mind that the interproximal space should be large enough to accom-

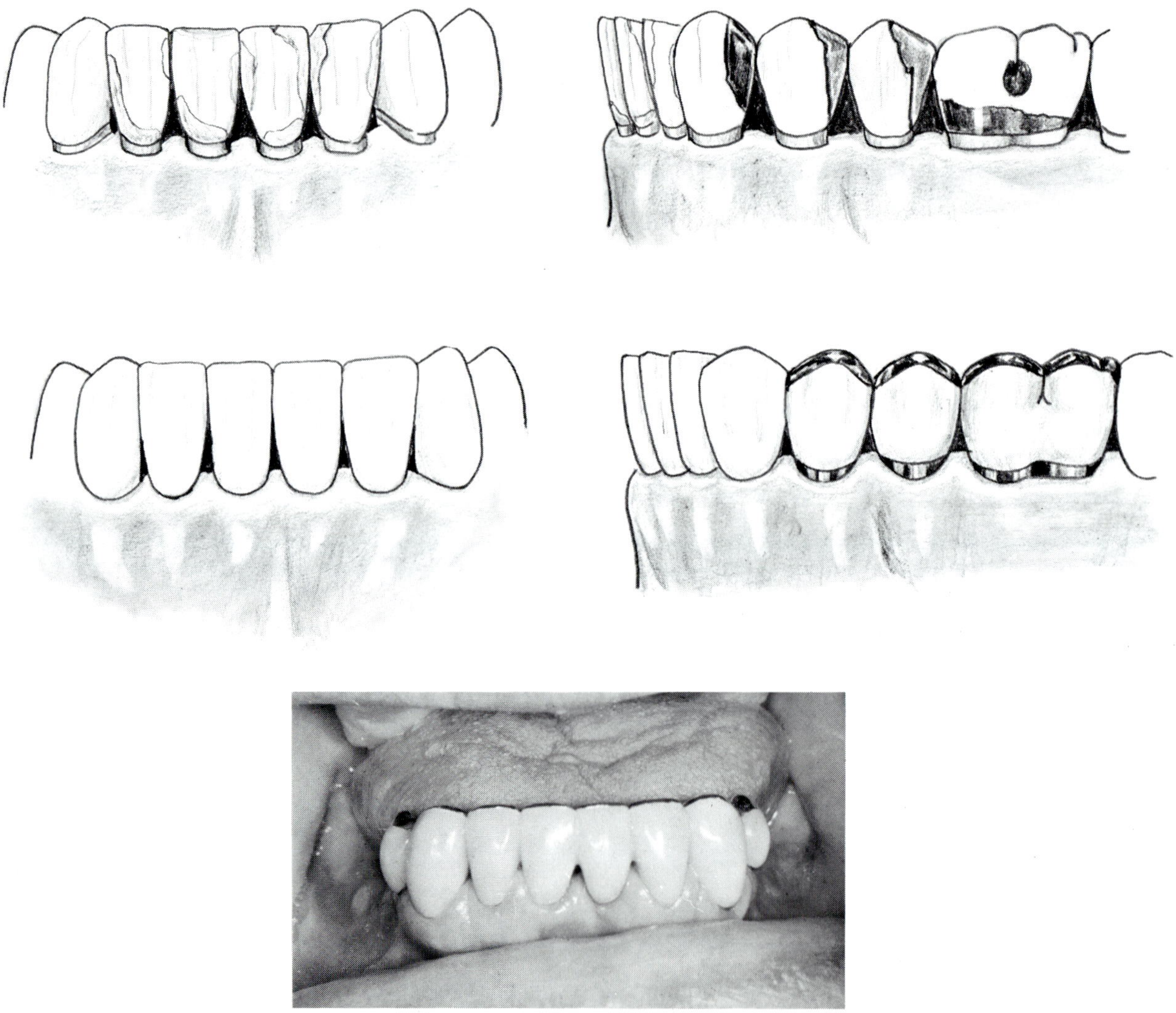

Fig. 6-33. Contact areas must be placed correctly. In cases of large interdental embrasures move gingivally. Keep in mind, however, that interproximal space should be large enough to accommodate papilla without restriction.

modate the papilla without restriction, which also permits proper oral hygiene and tissue stimulation of these interdental tissues. (See Fig. 6-33.)

The proximal surfaces are either flat or, in some instances, concave. "The proximal surfaces of the restorations create the interproximal embrasures that form the canopy that houses the interdental papilla. The roof is created by the very tight and correct positioning of the contact areas of the teeth. The walls are formed by the proximal surfaces of the adjacent teeth. The base is formed by the cementoenamel junctions of the proximal surfaces."*

Correct interproximal embrasures result in a proper arch alignment which possesses a definite continuity of tooth forms. This continuity is expressed as a gradual modification in form from anterior to posterior teeth and demonstrates a continuous alignment of occlusal tables, central fossae, and cusp tips. The ideal would be a fine harmony of tooth form, alignment, arch continuity, and proper architecture and positioning of the gingival tissue.[35]

Proximal surfaces of adjacent teeth should tend to be mirror images of each other, and adjacent marginal ridges should be of equal height, as should be cementoenamel junctions.[21] To reiterate: The proximal surfaces of crowns must be so shaped and contoured so as to physiologically accept the papillae and not limit their health. The mesial and distal marginal ridges of the same tooth tend to converge from the buccal toward the lingual. The facial half of a tooth is wider than the lingual half, therefore lingual embrasures are larger than the buccal embrasures (acute on buccal and obtuse on lingual).

Occlusal and incisal embrasures are formed by adjacent marginal ridges. Careful rounding of these ridges reduces mesiodistal dimension of occlusal tooth surfaces without forming a crevice that would tend to lodge food. This rounded marginal ridge forms an occlusal embrasure, and at the lingual extension of the occlusal embrasure the marginal ridges are interrupted by "sluice grooves." This forms an obtusely broadened embrasure, which helps in the proper pattern of food flow and results in healthy gingiva because of less possibility of plaque retention[30] (Fig. 6-34).

Special attention must be given to all the *transitional line angles* (mesiobuccal, distobuccal, mesiolingual, distolingual) in tooth preparation as well as in the fabrication of the restoration. Amsterdam and Abrams[21,35] have called attention to the fact that "the axial line angle which forms the transition between the flat or concave proximal surface and the convex facial or lingual surface deserves special attention. This angle generally exhibits the same contour as the proximal surface and forms the opening for the residence of the interdental tissue. This axial line angle is referred to as the transitional line angle, and the dentist's or technician's inability to recognize this angle and thereby overcontour it leads to the eviction of the interdental tissue and its subsequent sequelae of gingival deformation"* (Fig. 6-35).

Burch[36] has said that all the transitional line angles of the teeth are straight between the proximal contact point and the cementoenamel junction, with the exception of the lingual line angles (mesiolingual and distolingual) of the maxillary molars, where there may be a slight convexity.

Ideally, the cementoenamel junctions of proximating teeth will be at the same level; crestal bone height will be parallel with the relative heights of the proximal cementoenamel junctions, and the distance between the base of the contact areas and the cementoenamel junction will be the same in adjacent teeth. Sufficient room will be created by these symmetrical walls for the establishment of an adequate interdental gingival papilla with a minimum of col formation.

Ritchey and Orban[37] reported the following in a research project:

1. If approximating tooth surfaces are relatively flat, the septa must of necessity be narrow and the crests more or less pointed. If mesial and distal tooth surfaces are strongly convex, the interdental septa will be wide and the crests flat.

2. In the absence of periodontal disease the configurations of the crests of the interdental alveolar septa are determined by the relative positions of the cementoenamel junctions. The width of the interdental alveolar bone is determined by the tooth form present.

3. In the presence of periodontal disease, alterations in the configuration of the interdental alveolar septa are governed principally by the specific pathologic process.

In other words, Ritchey and Orban[37] and also O'Connor and Biggs[38] have studied the interproximal contour of the alveolar bone, and they found that the normal architecture of the alveolar crest paralleled the

*From Amsterdam, Morton, and Abrams, Leonard: Periodontal prosthesis. In Goldman, Henry M., and Cohen, D. Walter: Periodontal therapy, ed. 5, St. Louis, 1973, The C. V. Mosby Co.

*From Amsterdam, Morton, and Abrams, Leonard: Periodontal prosthesis. In Goldman, Henry M., and Cohen, D. Walter: Periodontal therapy, ed. 5, St. Louis, 1973, The C. V. Mosby Co.

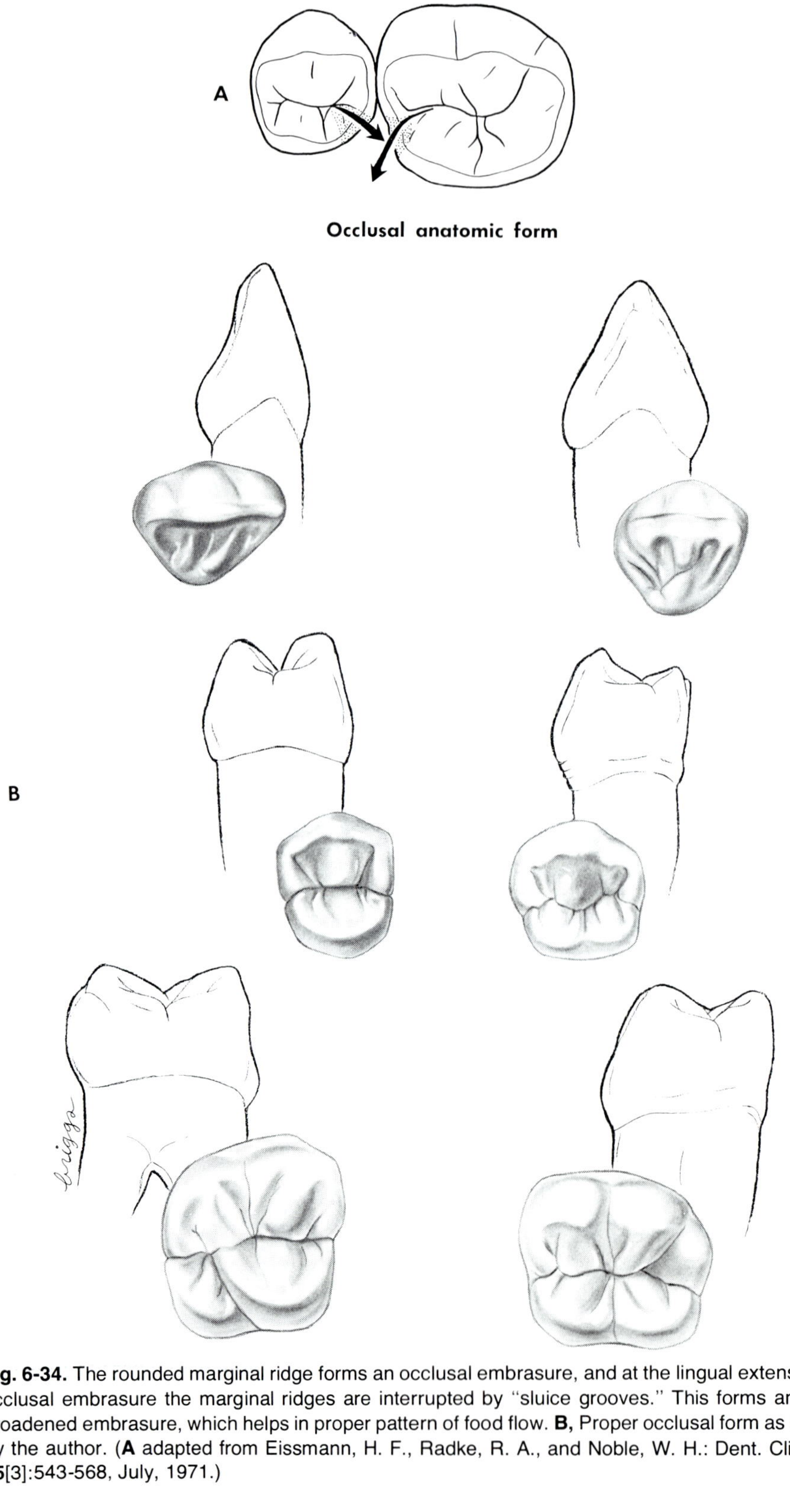

Fig. 6-34. The rounded marginal ridge forms an occlusal embrasure, and at the lingual extension of the occlusal embrasure the marginal ridges are interrupted by "sluice grooves." This forms an obtusely broadened embrasure, which helps in proper pattern of food flow. **B,** Proper occlusal form as visualized by the author. (**A** adapted from Eissmann, H. F., Radke, R. A., and Noble, W. H.: Dent. Clin. N. Am. **15**[3]:543-568, July, 1971.)

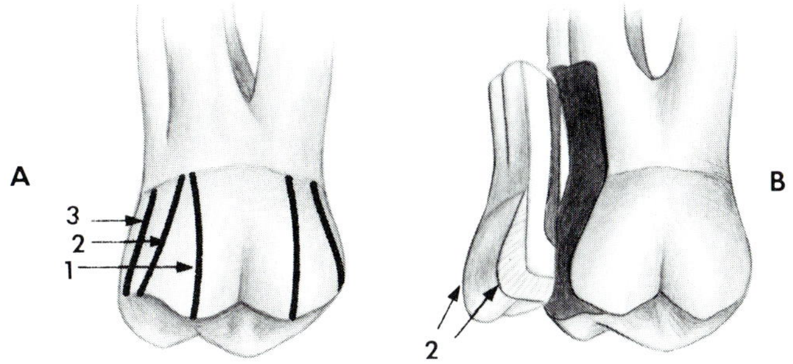

Fig. 6-35. A, Normal coronal contours of tooth can be divided into three areas: *(1)* buccal surface—convex with height of convexity in gingival third of crown; *(2)* transitional line angle—very flat; *(3)* proximal surface—flat and in some instances concave. **B,** Proximal section of tooth from transitional line angle to transitional line angle has been removed to emphasize flattened design of this area. (Adapted from Amsterdam, Morton, and Abrams, Leonard: Periodontal prosthesis. In Goldman, Henry M., and Cohen, D. Walter: Periodontal therapy, ed. 5, St. Louis, 1973, The C. V. Mosby Co.

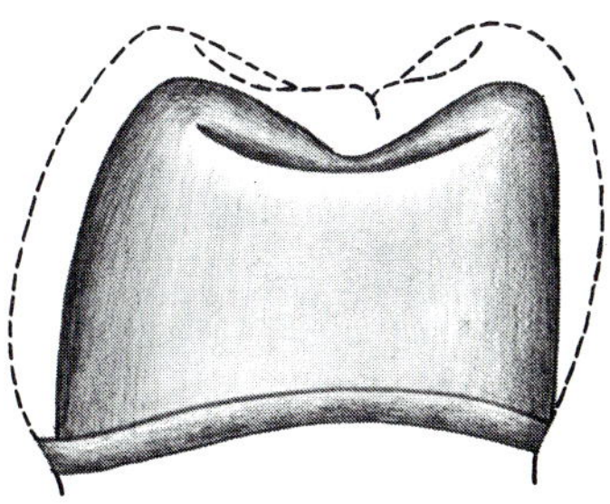

Fig. 6-36. Facial shoulder should be carried into interproximal embrasure in use of veneer crowns. This provides space for casting and veneering material without encroaching on triangular space.

cementoenamel junction of the teeth throughout the mouth. The interproximal areas of the molar regions were predominantly flat, whereas convex interproximal areas were found from the mesial aspect of the second premolar forward as the dominant configuration.

All this information points up most vividly the disastrous results of posterior bite collapse with the drifting and extrusion of molars and bicuspids, giving rise to the development of unlevel marginal ridges and marginal gingiva and altered embrasure forms. For every unlevel marginal ridge there is an unlevel cementoenamel junction, which gives rise to angular crestal bone formation that may lead to alveolar osseous defects such as infrabony pockets since inflammation and occlusal traumatism are part and parcel of this situation.

After periodontal therapy we are confronted many times with unusually long clinical crowns. The embrasure spaces are now long and opened, and buccolingual concavities are found on the mesial and distal surfaces of the maxillary and mandibular canines and maxillary bicuspids. Also the furcations of all molars are exposed. All this necessitates the negotiation of the cemental surface of the root or roots, requiring an excellent knowledge of tooth form to avoid gross to subtle errors in the restoration that would recreate pathology.

The fact that in many instances the enlarged, edematous, inflammatory gingivae are caused by improper cavity design, especially in the interproximal area, must not be overlooked. The facial shoulder should be carried into the interproximal embrasure in the use of veneer crowns. When no shoulder is provided on the proximal surface, the gold framework must be extended into the interproximal space to make room for acrylic resin or porcelain. This added bulk outside the normal contour of the tooth encroaches on the triangular space and leads to a pathologic periodontal condition and also an unesthetic, abnormally shaped crown.[39] In other words, sufficient tooth structure must be removed on the proximal surfaces to allow for the restoration of proper embrasure form. (See Figs. 6-36 and 6-37.)

By all means avoid injury to the tissues through careless use of cutting tools (especially with high-speed equipment), improper handling of the impression material, poor marginal fit of both temporary and permanent restorations, entrapment of tissue between the crown margin and the prepared tooth, retention of excessive cement subgingivally, etc. In tooth preparation, by the careful selection of instruments it is possible to avoid cutting the outer epithelial layer; only the inner crevicular epithelium is touched subgingivally. (See Figs. 6-38 and 6-39.)

The interproximal space is more difficult to maintain than the buccal and lingual tissue. The interproximal space occupied by the papilla must not be violated (Fig. 6-40). All operative and restorative procedures must be done with a minimum of gingival insult.

Margin placement

The question as to where to finish the crown margin—supragingivally or subgingivally—is often asked. Caries, restorations, and cosmetics in many instances indicate subgingivally. If this is the case—how far subgingivally? The acceptable healthy gin-

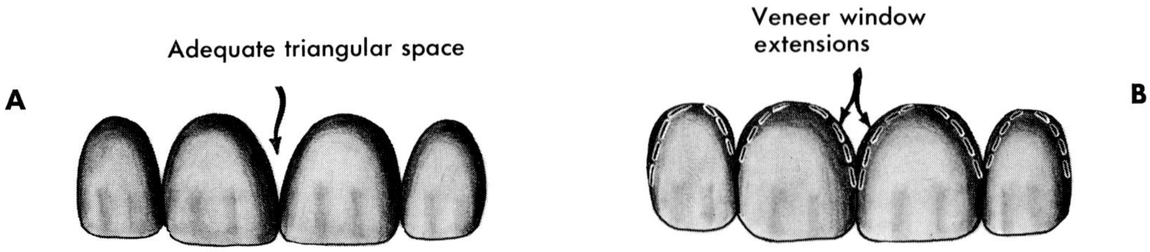

Fig. 6-37. A, A full crown should provide proper interproximal contour for esthetics and adequate space for papillae. **B,** If gold framework is extended into interproximal space, added bulk outside normal contour of tooth encroaches on triangular space. (From Weinberg, L. A.: Atlas of crown and bridge prosthodontics, St. Louis, 1965, The C. V. Mosby Co.)

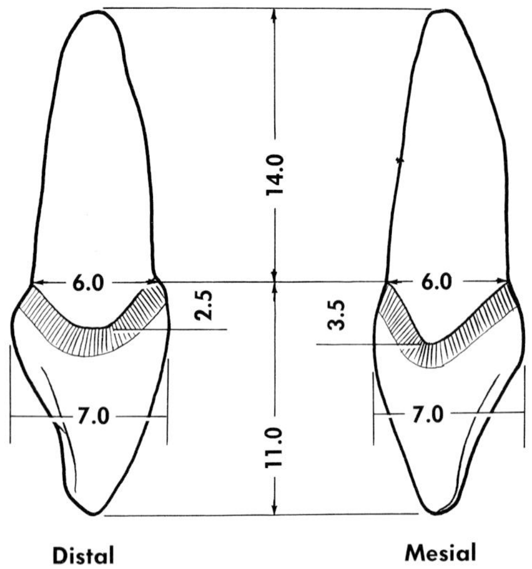

Fig. 6-38. Mesial and distal curvatures of cervical line (cementoenamel junction) on maxillary central incisor demonstrate points of measurement in determining relation between curvature of cervical line mesially and distally. Other points of measurement of crown and root are outlined. The shaded area in form of a band on enamel follows curvature and represents epithelial attachment of gingival tissue to enamel of crown. (Redrawn from Wheeler, R. C.: J. S. Calif. Dent. Assoc. **31**:385, 1963.)

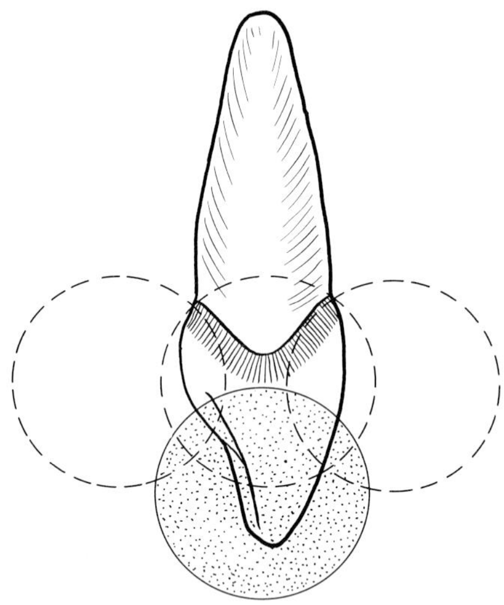

Fig. 6-39. A study of Fig. 6-38 brings to mind the possibility of injury to epithelial attachment if extreme care is not exercised in crown preparation. Ascertain height of attachment. (Suggested by Dr. R. C. Wheeler, St. Louis, Mo.)

gival sulcus is from 1.5 to 2 mm. in depth. The margin of the restoration should finish short of the epithelial attachment, which means that it should not be more than 1 to 1.5 mm. subgingival, depending, of course, upon the depth of the sulcus. This approximate distance is necessary to allow for a "biologic width of connective tissue and epithelial attachments of the gingival unit to the tooth."*[40] If supragingival—how far supragingivally? Whenever possible, it is advantageous to lay the peripheral margins on sound enamel with a definite abrupt bevel and a fair distance above the gingival margin since it not only facilitates accurate marginal adaptation of the gold margin, but also prevents tissue irritation.

Marcum[41] has shown that the ideal area for placement of the margin of a restoration is at the level of the gingival margin.

Caution must be exercised not to go subgingivally into areas where the gingival tissues would not be receptive to this transgression. According to Gordon,[42] these are areas where (1) the band of attached gingiva is very narrow, (2) the gingival margin ends in areolar tissue or the tissue is not keratinized properly, and (3) the anatomic form of the facial alveolar

*From Gargiulo, A. W., Wentz, F. M., and Orban, B.: Dimensions and relations of the dentogingival junction in humans, J. Periodontol. **32**:261-267, 1961.

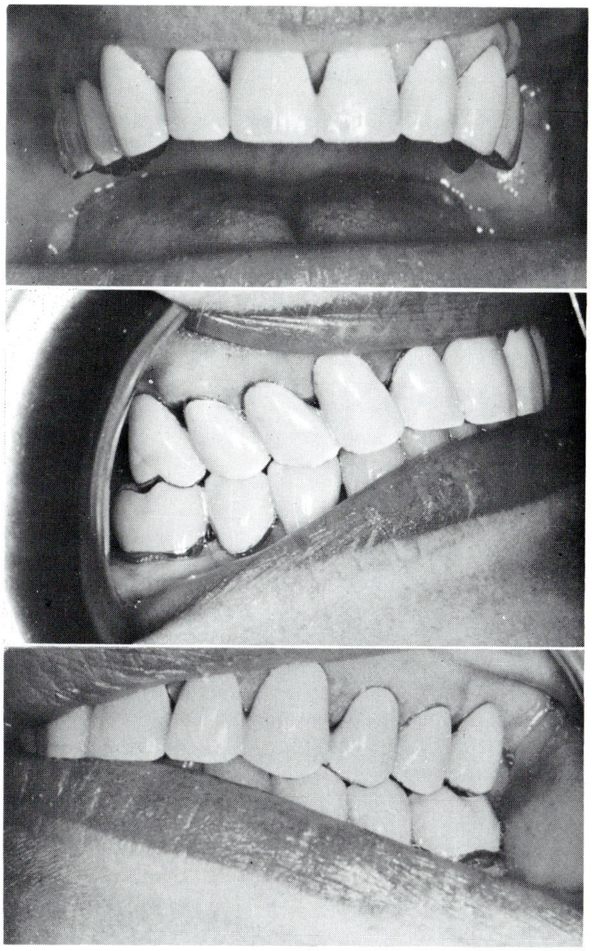

Fig. 6-40. Interproximal spaces occupied by papillae have not been violated. Case at present is of 17 years' standing.

bone and gingival tissue is so thin that the area is not conducive to subgingival extension.

When the outer plate of bone and the gingival tissue are thin, the thickness of the subgingival portion of the crown becomes critical, for if the crown is rendered thick in the facial area, it causes the free marginal gingiva to be distorted, and the response in most instances will be recession or inflammation.[43] Also keep in mind that inadequate thickness or inadequate contour of a restoration subgingivally may cause insufficient support of the gingival unit and subsequent loss of gingival tone.[6] In other words, an adequate amount of tooth structure must be removed to afford a continuous and favorable contour of the restoration—not too thin or too thick. The margin should allow for the smoothest possible transition from the restoration to the tooth structure and, by all means, the surfaces of the restorations should be kept as smooth as possible.

In margins of restorations that are extended subgingivally, the deeper the preparation is extended into the crevice, the greater is the hazard for irritation close to the insertion of the periodontal fibers into the cementum.

"Physiologic contouring must fully afford a massaging action to the gingiva. This action may be transmitted by the gingival tissues, surrounding the tooth like a muscular curtain, to the margin extending into the sulcus approximately two-thirds (1.5 mm.) of its depth. Plaque retention is minimized by tissue movement, tooth movement, and the flushing action of sulcular fluids, provided the restoration is skilfully contoured to form the smoothest possible transition from tooth structure."*

In the biologic approach the margins are placed at any level which will best serve the health of the periodontium.

Waerhaug[2] has said that no structural continuity exists between gingiva and enamel. His research activities indicate that the generally accepted theory concerning the epithelial attachment and its practical implications is open to serious question. It has been suggested that no true attachment exists and that the epithelial cells facing the tooth normally are kept in contact with the enamel surface by adhesion, tissue tonus, and fibers of the free gingiva. Therefore, the term "epithelial cuff" instead of "epithelial attachment" appears more appropriate (Fig. 6-41, *C*).

Recent electron microscopic and radioautographic studies have provided a clearer understanding of the nature of the dentoepithelial interface.[43]

"Toward the end of enamel maturation, the plasmalemma of the ameloblasts in contact with the enamel surface develops *hemidesmosomes*. The space between the cell membrane and the enamel surface is occupied by a *basement lamina* joining the cells to the enamel surface. The hemidesmosomes and the basement lamina are believed to form the attachment apparatus joining the epithelium to the tooth. A similar attachment apparatus is also found between the external surface of the reduced enamel epithelium and the surrounding connective tissue. The basement lamina facing the tooth surface is referred to as the *internal basement lamina,* whereas the basement lamina facing the connective tissue is called the *external basement lamina*. The biologic mechanism that unites epithelial cells to the tooth surface may be

---

*From Eissmann, Harold F., Radke, Ryle A., and Noble, Warden H.: Physiologic design criteria for fixed dental restorations, Dent. Clin. N. Am. **15**(3):543-568, 1971.

A

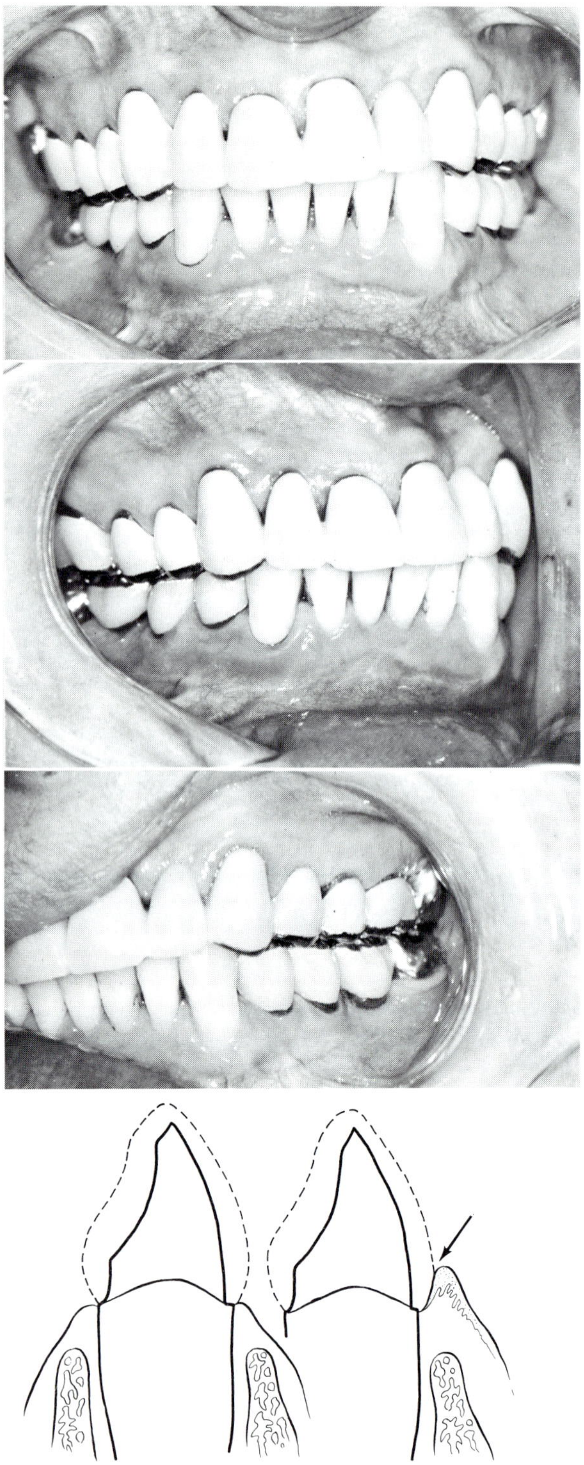

B

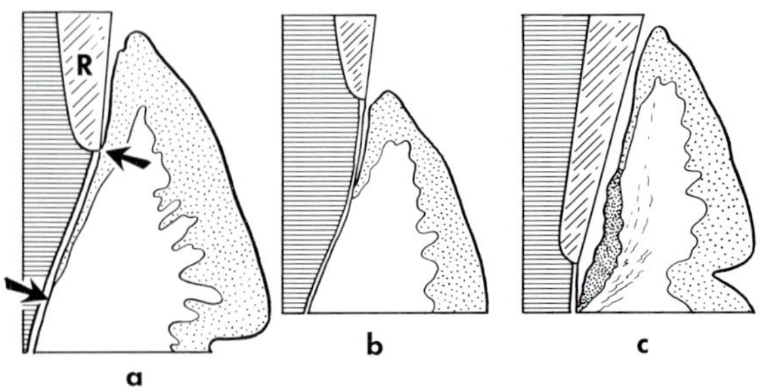

C

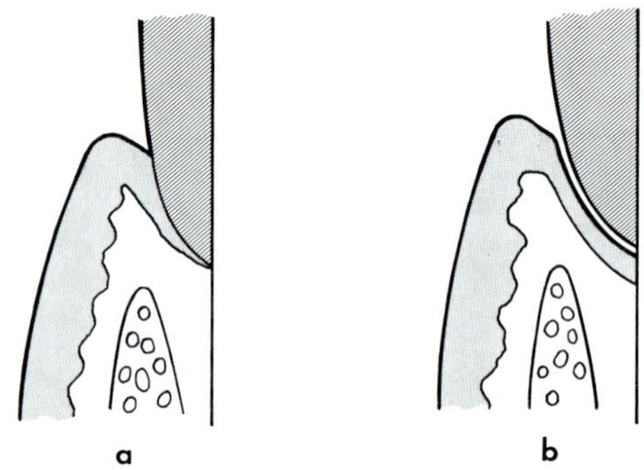

Fig. 6-41. Tooth preparation was started just after epithelization of gingiva had taken place. Supragingival margins were established, which allowed for great accuracy in impression taking and marginal adaptation of cast restoration. As gingival tissues matured, a shallow crevice developed and supragingival margin became subgingival. **B,** *a,* Margin of restoration *(R)* should extend to base of gingival sulcus for gingival fibers to hold margin firmly against restoration. *b,* Incorrect location of margin of restoration at crest of gingival sulcus—a caries-susceptible area. *c,* Incorrect location beyond base of gingival sulcus detaches epithelial attachment and gingival fibers from tooth, causing apical migration and pocket formation. **C,** *a,* Gottlieb's version of true epithelial attachment. *b,* Waerhaug's version that no structural continuity exists between gingiva and enamel—we have instead an "epithelial cuff." (**B** courtesy Dr. Irving Glickman.)

properly described as the epithelial attachment. This term should not be used to describe an epithelium such as the junctional epithelium or reduced enamel epithelium. Its morphologically recognizable components consist of hemidesmosomes and the internal basement lamina."*

After periodontal surgery the sulcular depth is negligible. However, in a short period of time the depth may increase to 1 to 2 mm., which is a usual finding. Knife-edged gingival margins begin to roll slightly. Goldman has described this phenomenon as "creeping reattachment." Therefore, there is the need to wait several months before starting tooth preparation and restorative measures.

Rosen and Gitnick[44] begin tooth preparations, if circumstances permit, just after epithelization of the gingiva has taken place, which is usually 6 to 8 weeks after periodontal surgery. By so doing, a supragingival margin is established, which allows for great accuracy in impression taking (hydrocolloid, rubber base, or silicone) and in marginal adaptation of the cast restoration. Later, as the gingival tissue matures a shallow crevice develops, and the supragingival margin becomes subgingival. Whenever possible, I choose this method, and the end results are most satisfactory. (See Fig. 6-41, *A*.)

PROXIMAL CONTACT AREAS

The purpose of proximal contact areas is to develop tooth stability and arch integrity and to prevent food retention by the contact areas being sufficiently tight. Contact points wear into contact areas; contact areas wear as a result of proximal attrition as one grows older. Eissmann[30] describes it as "physiologic splinting." (See Figs. 6-42 to 6-46.)

PROTECTION TO THE LIP, CHEEK, AND TONGUE SYSTEM

Abrams[35] has called attention to this most important fact. What is meant is (1) the buccal horizontal overlap of the upper posterior teeth, which serves to keep the lip and cheek mucosa away from the cutting surfaces of the mandibular teeth, (2) the lingual horizontal overlap of the lower posterior teeth, which in turn keep the tongue away from the cutting surfaces of the upper teeth, and (3) the distal horizontal overlap of the upper second molar, which also protects the cheek musculature from injury in jaw closure.

*From Goldman, Henry M., and Cohen, D. Walter: Periodontal therapy, ed. 5, Saint Louis, 1973, The C. V. Mosby Co., p. 24.

Parafunctions

TYPES

Parafunctions may be defined as occlusal habits that result in tooth-to-tooth or foreign object–to–tooth contact. They are mandibular movements other than those associated with chewing, swallowing, or speech.

Some pernicious habits such as grinding and clenching may be practiced at night, as evidenced by soreness of teeth or the masticatory muscles in the morning. Patients under emotional stress may even continue these habits during the day when not masticating or swallowing.

Some patients have such habits as biting on fingernails, bobby pins, pipes, thread, or toothpicks, habitually pressing one anterior tooth against another, or tapping on incisal edges of anterior teeth.

Sucking habits or biting on the tongue or lips does not transmit such heavy forces as aforementioned since the intermediate object is softer, but the constant application of these forces still may be enough to cause migration of the teeth.

Observation of the patient's swallowing pattern is important. In normal swallowing the teeth are brought together in centric relation and the tongue is pressed against the palate in the area of the anterior palatine papilla. Incorrect swallowing, in which the tongue places heavy pressure on the anterior teeth or may even be forced between them, is a major cause of open bite. Myofunctional therapy methods may be used to treat these patients.

In bruxism the teeth and supporting structures are involved, and, because of this grinding, they both abrade and exert pressures leading to attrition of teeth and loss of alveolar bone. A type of bruxism, clenching, may produce severe alveolar bone destruction because of the forceful sustained biting pressure (Fig. 6-47).

Bruxism may be initiated by local factors such as cusp interference, mobile teeth, improperly contoured fillings, and "indeed any continuing stimulus to the afferent nerve endings in the periodontal tissues, which normally are associated with the reflex arcs of the rhythmical movements of mastication."*[45] Discrepancies in occlusal contacts, primarily in centric relation–centric occlusion pathways, causing the patient to slip into an acquired relationship, are of prime importance in triggering off the bruxism

*From Walsh, J. P.: The psychogenesis of bruxism, J. Periodontol. **36**:417-420, 1965.

Figs. 6-42 to 6-45. The illustrations in this series (Figs. 6-42 to 6-45) adapted from Wheeler, Russell C.: A textbook of dental anatomy and physiology, ed. 4, Philadelphia, 1965, W. B. Saunders Co.

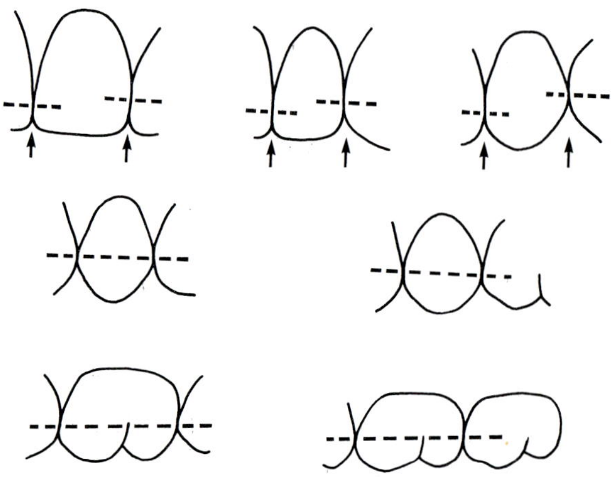

Fig. 6-42. Outline drawings of the maxillary teeth in contact, with dotted lines bisecting the contact areas at the various levels as found normally. Arrows point to embrasure spaces.

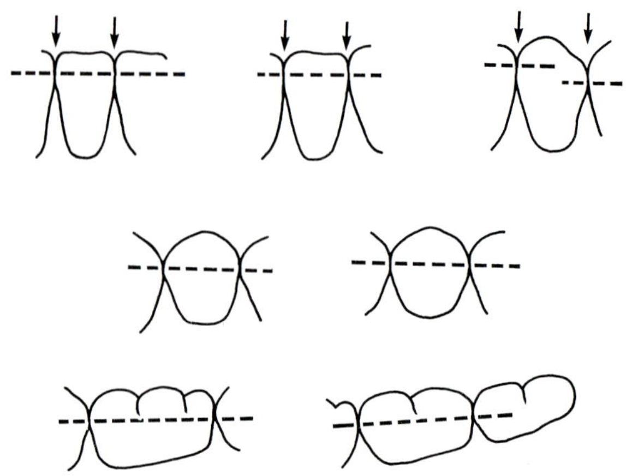

Fig. 6-43. Contact levels found normally on mandibular teeth. Arrows point to embrasure spaces.

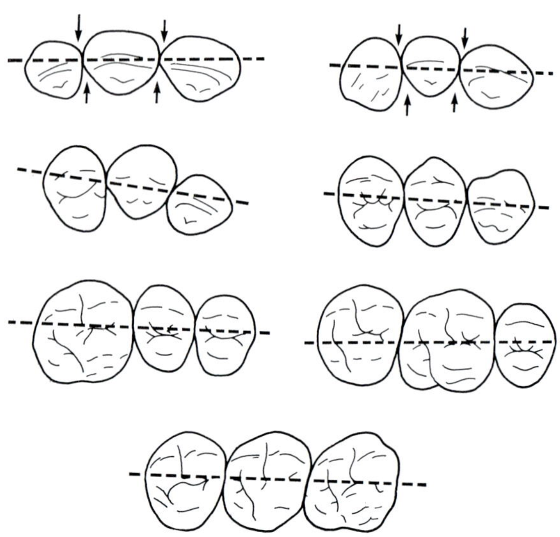

Fig. 6-44. Outline drawings of the maxillary teeth from the incisal and occlusal aspects, with broken lines bisecting the contact areas. These illustrations show the relative positions of the contact areas labiolingually and buccolingually. Arrows point to embrasure spaces.

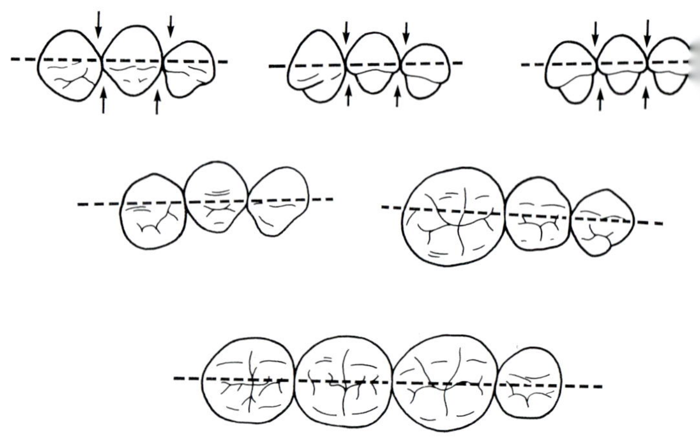

Fig. 6-45. Contact relation of mandibular teeth labiolingually and buccolingually when surveyed from the incisal and occlusal aspects. Arrows point to embrasure spaces.

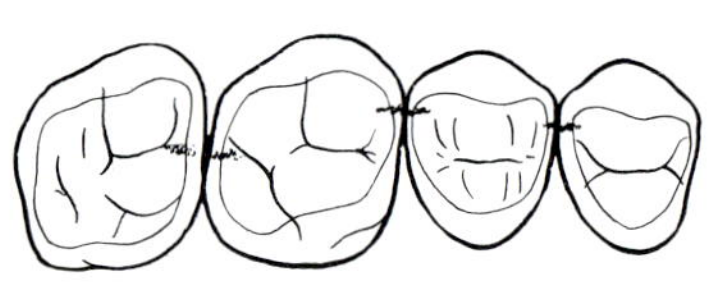

Fig. 6-46. Another view indicating the buccolingual location of the proximal contact areas.

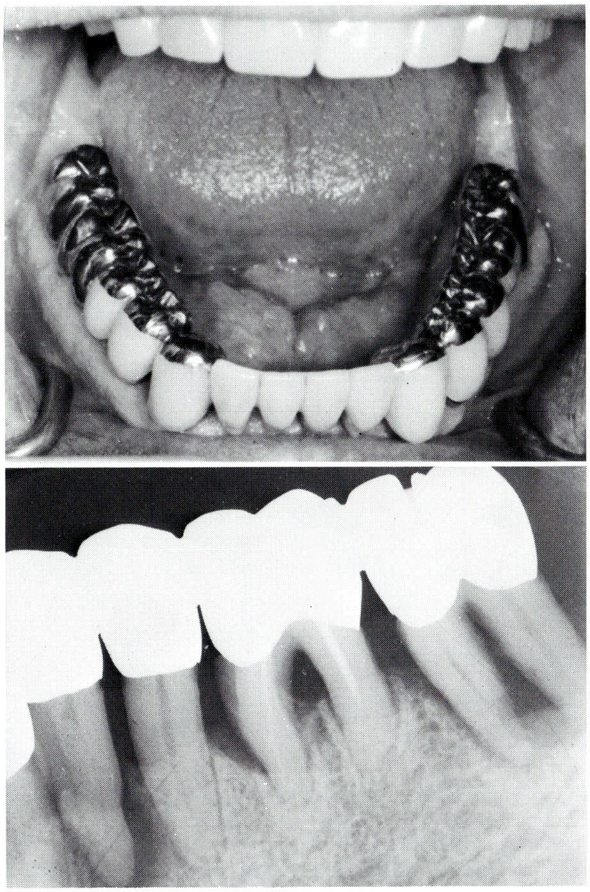

Fig. 6-47. A "bruxer" and "clencher," because of his sustained biting pressure, produced severe alveolar bone destruction in spite of well-established prosthetic-periodontal interrelationships.

habit.[46] Parafunctional tooth contacts are believed to be the initial insult in the origination of the lesion of primary occlusal traumatism.[21]

It is unquestionably true that this action, parafunctional tooth contacts, is complex, being of both local and emotional origin. It is correct to say that local tooth interferences play an important role in the initiation of these destructive habits, thereby requiring a correct centric relation–centric occlusion relationship. In my opinion, after many years of close observation, the most important factor in bruxism is undoubtedly psychologic or emotional tension, which is manifested through the muscular system. Occlusal interferences act as a trigger for bruxism if combined with nervous tension, but objective observation and careful questioning of these patients will bring to the fore that they are the kind of people who either experience disproportionate anger or who do not know how to express rage effectively. They have a need to prevent aggressive tendencies from being manifested, and many of these people have a set, determined, or hostile facial expression.

Fenichel[47] considers that the physical effects of being emotionally "damned up" produce changes in the muscular system, either hypertonic or hypotonic or both alternating. He designates this field as "psychogenic dystonia," examples being grinding and clenching of teeth.

Psychiatrists regard bruxism and clenching as the oral outlet for subconscious aggressions. It may be the result of emotional or psychologic stress. Hostility is turned inward to remove frustrations. In other words, bruxism serves as a safety valve to relieve emotional tension and aggressiveness–it takes out on self the frustrations and tensions which beset his or her personality.

These neurotic habits (bruxism, clenching, clamping, tongue thrusting) are very difficult to eliminate once they become well established, and since these habits, as a rule, do not permit rest periods for tissue repair, they may produce severe periodontal pathology. Bruxism is performed on a subconscious reflex-controlled level.

A clarification of terminology is in order at this time. *Clenching* is very closely related to bruxism. Most of the clenching forces are expended in torquing pressures upon the teeth, which can cause severe periodontal destruction. It can be intermittent or repetitive. *Clamping* is a sustained forceful contact of teeth. It is said that the prime factor in this instance is duration rather than frequency of application of the force. *Tongue thrusting* is a condition in which the muscles of the tongue exert a powerful force when applied with pressure upon the lingual surfaces of the teeth. When the action is habitual, it can result in trauma of the posterior teeth as well as the anterior teeth. The tongue can be observed to occupy spaces between the teeth when the patient swallows or speaks.

The *effects of bruxism* include: (1) abnormal occlusal wear, (2) thickening of the periodontal ligament space, (3) increase of mobility of some or all of the teeth, (4) a flattened, highly glazed wear facet, (5) damage to the attachment apparatus, (6) hypertrophy of the muscle itself because of the increased use of the musculature which characterizes bruxism; this increases the power potential of muscles for greater applied force to the teeth, supporting periodontal structures, and temporomandibular joints, and (7) creation of dysfunctional muscle and temporomandibular joint pain, etc.

"CENTRIC BRUXISM" AND "ECCENTRIC BRUXISM"

Ramfjord[22] designates nonfunctional gnashing and grinding in eccentric excursions as *"eccentric bruxism"* and clenching in centric as *"centric bruxism."*

"Both eccentric and centric bruxism are expressions of an increased muscle tonus. Whether eccentric or centric bruxism dominates depends on the location of the occlusal interferences that act as trigger factors for nonfunctional jaw movements.

"*Eccentric bruxism* usually has eccentric interferences (especially occlusal interferences on balancing side) for trigger factors, while *'centric bruxism'* is more often associated with occlusal instability in the immediate vicinity of centric (a discrepancy between centric relation and centric occlusion or interferences in the retrusive range).

"*Eccentric bruxism* has a dual etiologic background of psychic stress (repressed aggression, emotional tension, anger, fear) and occlusal interference. An interplay of three mechanisms: (1) emotional or nervous tension, (2) pain or discomfort, and (3) occlusal interferences provide the neuromuscular basis for bruxism."*

The mechanics of occlusion in a rehabilitated or a natural dentition requires an expression of harmony in centric and eccentric movements to eliminate muscle strain and the exerted forces of bruxism. Any arrangement of teeth short of this goal must assume the risk of inducing the phenomenon of bruxism.

ACRYLIC RESIN BITE GUARDS

Acrylic resin bite guards, or night guards, are removable splints for the treatment of bruxism and temporomandibular disorders. They are used as a palliative measure in patients who continue to "brux" after correction of occlusal disharmonies and attempts to correct psychogenic factors.

Alginate or hydrocolloid impressions are taken of both arches, and stone casts, as porosity-free as possible, are made. A hinge-bow transfer is made for mounting the upper cast on an adjustable articulator, and two or three centric relation bites are taken for the mounting of the lower cast on the adjustable articulator by the split-cast method.

The casts are surveyed, and a line is drawn approximately 1 mm. gingival to the survey line or height of contour facially and lingually. This line is the borderline of the bite guard.

*From Ramfjord, Sigurd P., and Ash, Major M., Jr.: Occlusion, ed. 2, Philadelphia, 1971, W. B. Saunders Co.

The area that is gingival to the borderline is blocked out with wax. A baseplate wax form is created over all surfaces above the line, the occlusal surface being almost flat. The free-way space must not be encroached upon, and the centric position must be correct.

Cuspal interferences are removed by moving the articulator protrusively and through right and left lateral excursions, after which these wax forms are invested and cured in clear acrylic resin. The cured bite guard or guards then are seated on the casts and adjusted very carefully protrusively, laterally, and for centric position; then they are polished (Fig. 6-48).

By correctly carrying out these procedures the bruxing movements of the mandible are converted to gliding actions over the smooth acrylic surfaces so that the periodontium is protected from injury by eccentric forces.

These acrylic splints are worn at night on one or both jaws, depending upon the mobility patterns and upon the patient's willingness to wear one or two plastic splints (Fig. 6-49). If one is to be worn, it should be placed in the arch exhibiting the greatest mobility pattern. It has splintage value which stabilizes the teeth and prevents occlusal wear.

In some cases we may have to resort to drugs or psychotherapy to achieve muscle relaxation.

PRELIMINARY CORRECTIVE PROCEDURES

Orthodontics

By far the most common reason for the spontaneous movement of teeth in the adult is periodontal disease. In periodontal disease spatial derangements of arch form, induced by drifting, extrusion, and tipping of one or more teeth, frequently are exhibited. We must make use of orthodontics to create a situation that will allow our periodontal and prosthetic treatment procedures to succeed. If extensive tooth movements involving gross repositioning of the root base and fulcrum area of the tooth is indicated, the patient should be referred to a trained orthodontist.[48] However, minor orthodontic tooth movement can play a most important role in the comprehensive treatment plan in periodontal prosthesis and belongs in the realm of the periodontist and prosthodontist. Minor tooth movements can be accomplished with relative ease through the use of removable appliances of various types (Figs. 6-50 and 6-51). Orthodontic treatment should precede periodontal treatment, that is, after initial treatment, consisting of curettage for reduction of inflammation, removal of deposits, etc., but before osseous surgery.

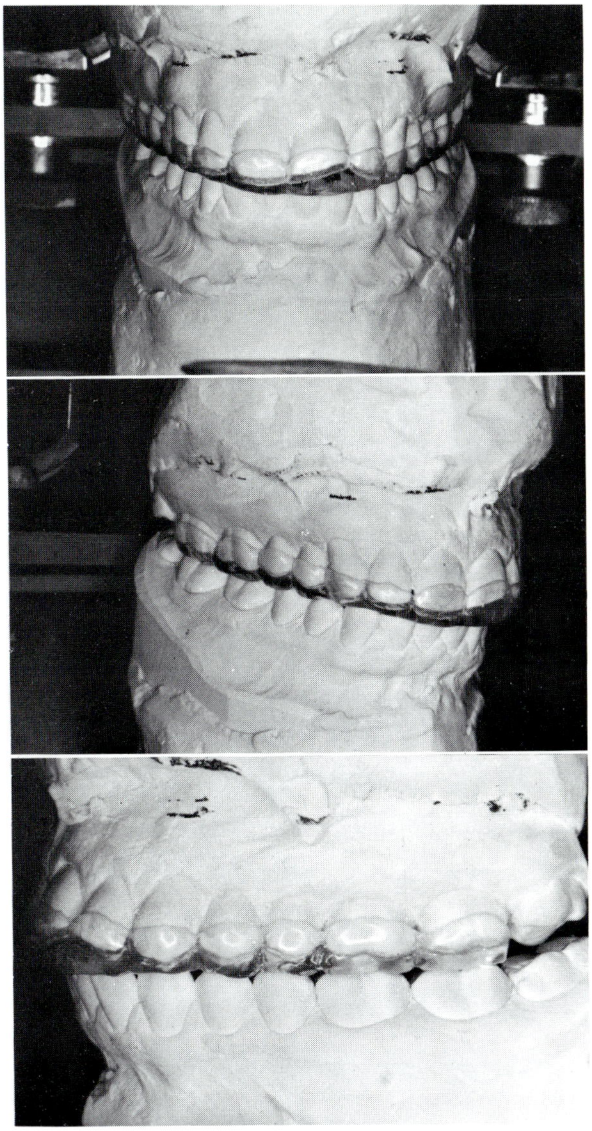

Fig. 6-48. Acrylic resin bite guard on adjustable articulator after construction for adjustments in all mandibular excursions and before being polished.

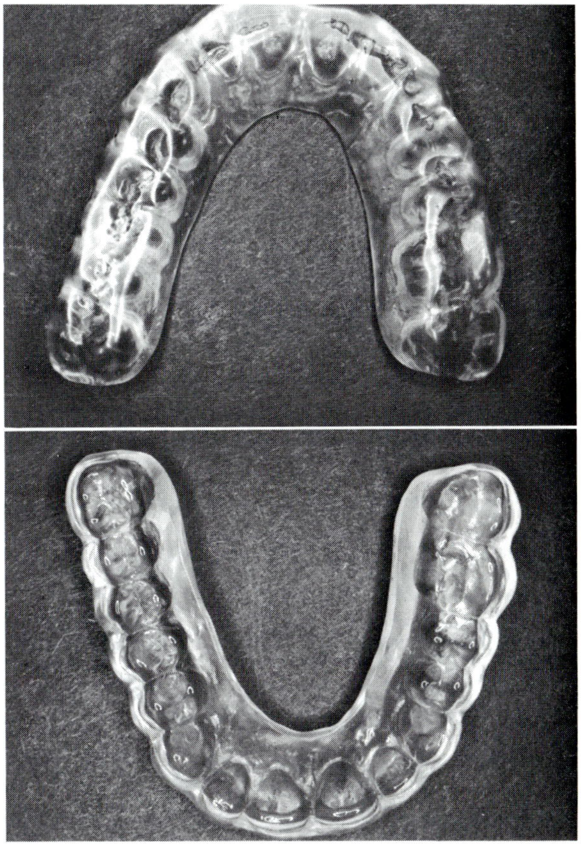

Fig. 6-49. Finished acrylic resin bite-guard splint, which is worn at night.

Malaligned teeth should be moved orthodontically, either for better management of abutments or for better relation to the residual ridges. Many astute students of the subject believe that, barring this possibility, such teeth should be extracted regardless of their periodontal status. Utilization of gross warpage of occlusal tables to compensate for severely malposed and cross-bite situations or otherwise inadequate arch-to-arch relations causes the force recipient areas of the restored teeth to be located poorly with respect to their root support. Existing malpositions of the abutment teeth or purposeful distortion of the restored crown cannot be condoned if the resulting crown-to-root ratio is basically incompatible with the resistance of the periodontium. Tooth preparation is a poor substitute for correct tooth position.

Amsterdam[21] points out that, in our procedural objectives in periodontal prosthesis, teeth that have migrated or tilted as a result of loss of arch continuity, loss of supporting bone, occlusal stress, etc. should be so positioned and axially inclined, if possible, that their roots are located within the confines of their periodontal structures. They should be positioned centrally within their alveolar housing for optimal distribution of force and stress to the remaining root support. Then we have correct distribution of forces over basal bone. In other words, those teeth that have migrated or tilted to unfavorable positions should be realigned so that it is possible to direct forces in a favorable direction by occlusal design. This enables the resultant forces upon the teeth to be transmitted in a more favorable axial direction. Be-

A B C D E F

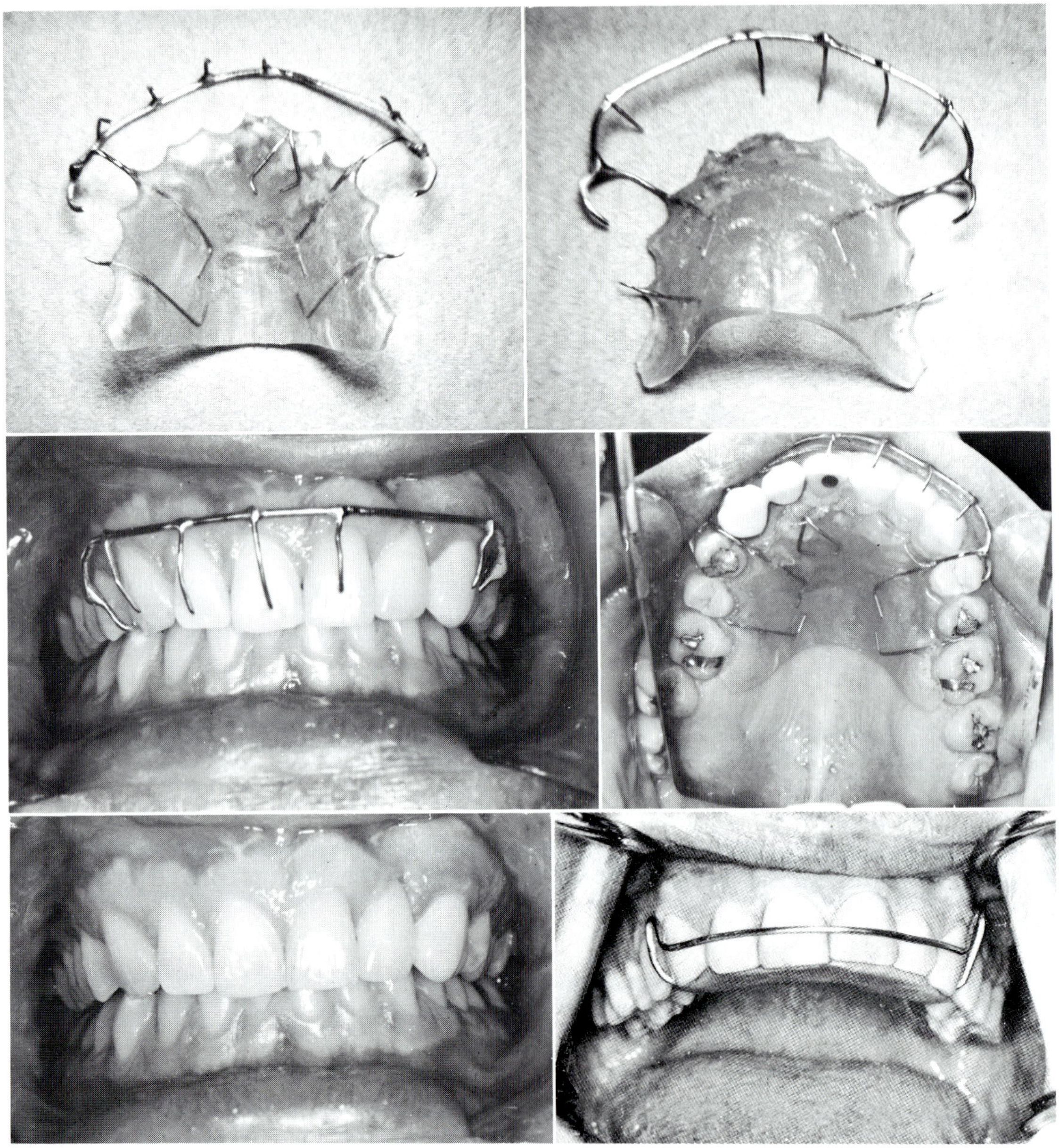

Fig. 6-50. A to **E,** Minor tooth movement can be accomplished by use of removable appliances such as Hawley retainer and its modifications. These illustrations show various views of this type of appliance in and out of mouth and result obtained. **F,** Hawley appliance with a platform area on palatal surface used in a deep overbite case. (**F** from Goldman, H. M., Schluger, S., Fox, L., and Cohen, D. W.: Periodontal therapy, ed. 3, St. Louis, 1964, The C. V. Mosby Co.)

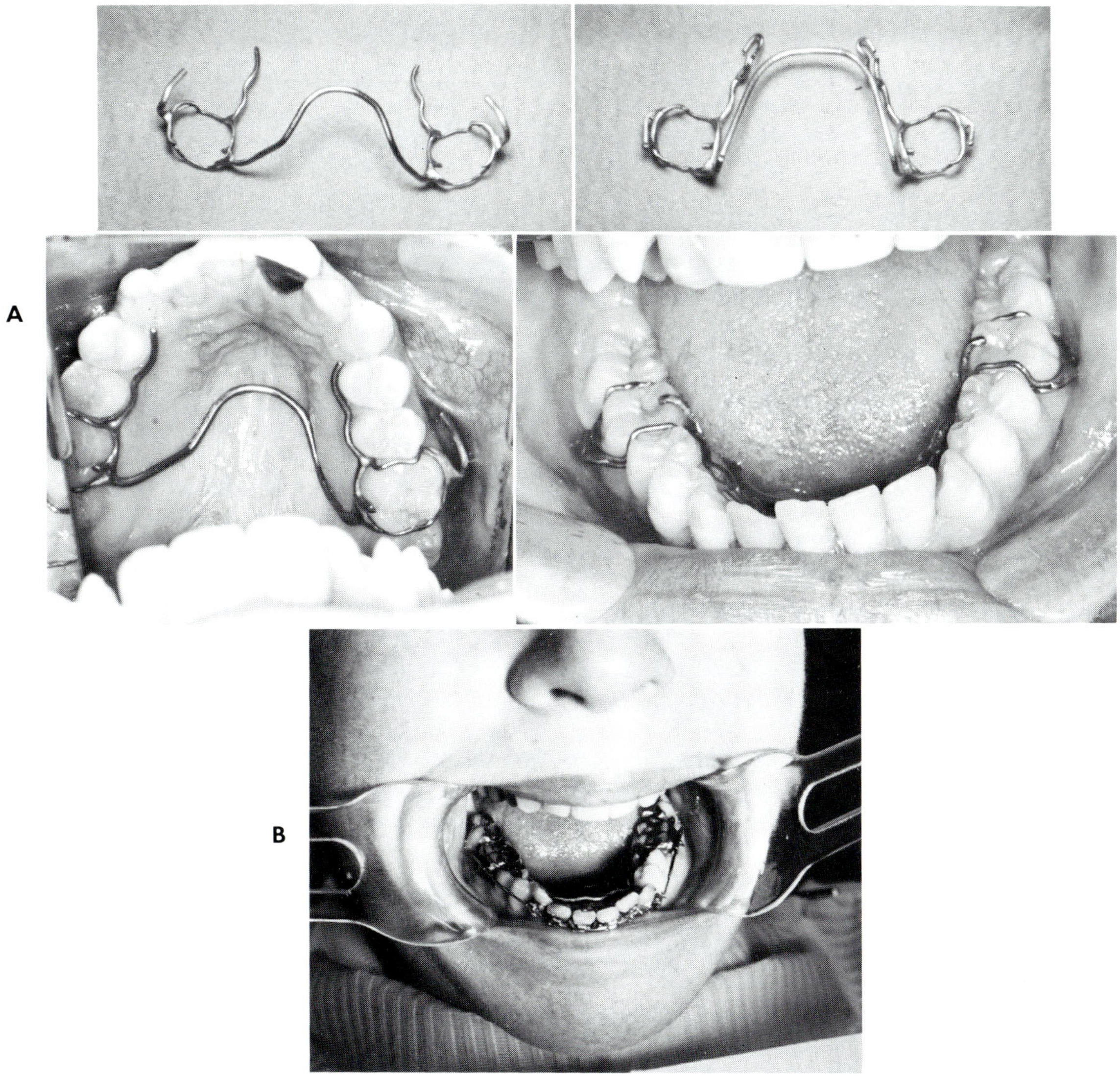

Fig. 6-51. A, These illustrations show Crozat appliance (primary upper appliance and primary lower appliance) in and out of mouth. Orthodontic treatment should precede periodontal treatment. **B,** An adult patient undergoing major orthodontics.

sides providing force control, it also allows for the establishment of proper physiologic tooth form, gingival architecture, embrasure patterns, and esthetics. It also allows us to realign marginal ridges and cementoenamel junctions. Despite all this, there are times when asymmetry of the jaws and malalignment of the teeth in the arch may require a compromise of ideal objectives.

Before considering any technologic procedures, let us consider in more detail some basics, some objectives, and other factors involved in tooth movement.[5]

"Orthodontic tooth movement depends upon bone resorption and bone formation stimulated by properly regulated pressure and tension. These stimuli are transmitted through the medium of the periodontal ligament. If the movement of teeth is within physiologic limits (which may vary with the individual), the initial compression of the periodontal ligament on the pressure side is compensated for by bone resorption, whereas the stretch of the bundles of the periodontal ligament on the tension side is balanced by bone apposition. The presence of an intermediate plexus (see discussion of histologic structure of the attachment apparatus earlier in this chapter) in the alveodental and interdental ligaments allows a rather speedy adjustment after orthodontic movements. The absence of an intermediate plexus in the gingival fiber bundles prolongs such a readjustment, and may be responsible for the relapse, for instance, after rotation of a tooth."*

Orthodontic movements may be of value for the periodontal patient, if it will accomplish one or more of the following: (1) a more harmonious relationship between the adjacent teeth in each jaw and between the teeth in opposing jaws, (2) facilitate restorative procedures, and (3) increase the value of the teeth to the patient by improving their appearance.

Important factors in tooth movements to be considered are: (1) *bone support*—amount and type of bone to be dealt with, (2) *space*—there must be sufficient space available into which the tooth can be moved, (3) *force of pressure*—this must be controlled within acceptable limits of the patient's bone physiology, (4) *type of movement*—in minor tooth movement, teeth are not actually moved but tipped (Do not tip a tooth out of its axial alignment. Bodily movement of the entire tooth requires more exacting appliances or banding.), (5) *understanding of levers, leverage,* and *bone physiology,* (6) *types of appliances for minor tooth movement,* including fixed (wire ligatures, rubber dam elastics, etc.) and removable (Hawley, Crozat, etc.), and (7) *retention and stabilization*—after the teeth have been relocated, it is very important to support them in the new position during the time it takes to rebuild the bone.

So, for the patient in need of mouth rehabilitation, tooth movement can be a major therapeutic tool in many cases. It can be used to gain, for example, better relationships of the anterior teeth in order to obtain posterior disclusion. It can also make possible more ideal restorative procedures, establish proper space for pontics, prevent overcontoured restorations, close open contacts, make it easier to parallel abutment teeth, establish maintainable embrasures, and, by a reordering of the gingival environment, make plaque control more attainable.

The restorative dentist should, as a rule, use simple limited orthodontic appliances for his purposes and for relatively short periods of treatment time. Removable appliances can accomplish the desired results in a considerable proportion of cases. After the teeth are moved orthodontically into proper position, one should observe carefully whether roentgenographic evidence shows apparent improvement in the bone contiguous to the periodontal pocket.

In summation, it can be said that indications for orthodontic treatment in adult patients are functional and/or esthetic. *Functional indications* are (1) occlusal disharmonies associated with functional disorders (cross-bite relations, tipping and migration of premolars and molars, etc.), (2) extreme vertical and/or horizontal overlap causing an unfavorable load on the teeth and/or the gingivae, (3) crowding of teeth, and (4) cases where orthodontic treatment facilitates prosthetic treatment. *Esthetic indications* usually comprise malocclusions which cause emotional or psychological disturbances and, in turn, involve important social aspects.[49]

Ross[50] has shown that teeth will move into more favorable positions and the periodontium will become healthier as the interocclusal relations improve between the maxillary and mandibular teeth. All the movements occur without the use of orthodontic appliances, merely as a result of periodontal therapy. The therapy includes reshaping of the teeth by grinding, scaling, curettage, home care, and, at times, periodontal surgery. This he refers to as *reactive positioning*.

"Reactive positioning refers to the movement of a malposed tooth into a new position after the blocking or moving forces have been partially or completely removed. The blocking and moving forces that produce malpositioning may be adjacent or opposing teeth; muscular forces such as tongue pressure and lip pressure; and the pressure from foreign objects used in such habits as fingernail biting, pencil biting, and the use of toothpicks.

"The response of the tooth in the new position also depends upon the distribution and amount of periodontal support around the malposed tooth, the potential of the periodontium for healing, and the type of function to which the tooth is subjected in the new position.

"The teeth are usually reshaped over several visits. This permits the malposed teeth to move a small distance after each appointment of grinding. If pockets are present, pocket eradication and elimination of dense granulation tissue will complement the grinding in producing movement and tightening of the teeth."*

---

*From Sicher, Harry, and Bhaskar, S. N. editors: Orban's oral histology and embryology, ed. 7, St. Louis, 1972, The C. V. Mosby Co.

*From Ross, Ira F.: Reactive positioning and improved gingival architecture, J. Periodontol. **34:**444-446, 1963.

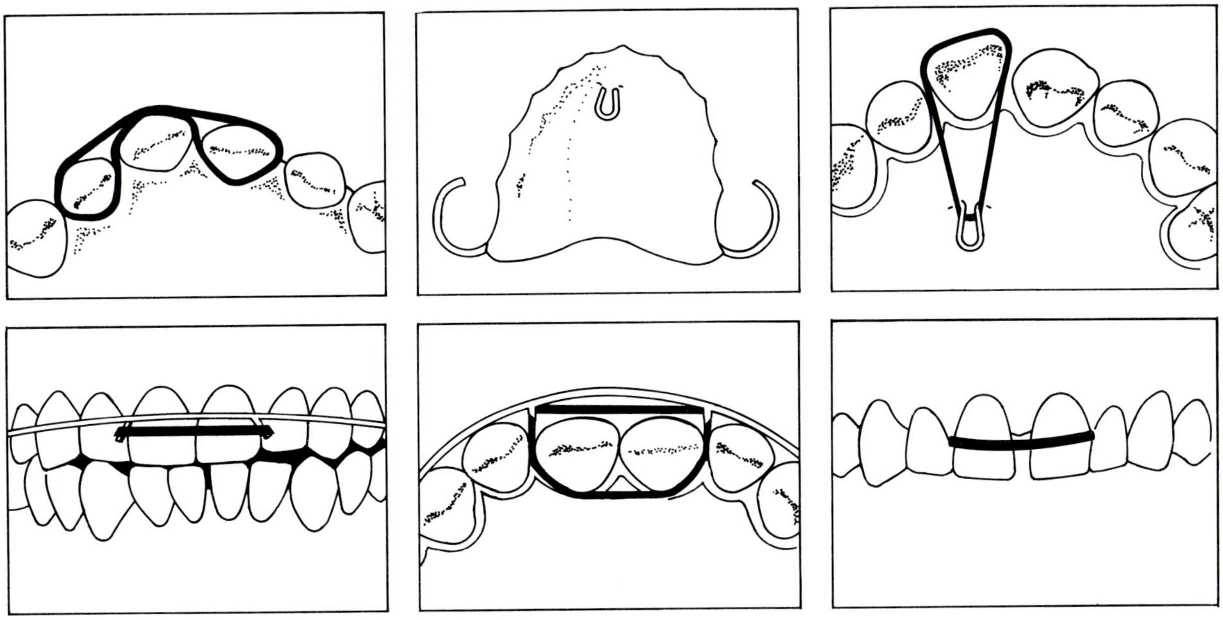

Fig. 6-52. Minor tooth movement with rubber dam elastics. One or more teeth can be moved lingually, labially, mesially, or distally, supplying the required anchorage by the use of an acrylic-wire appliance or labial arch wire.

A Hawley retainer and rubber dam or latex elastics can be used effectively to create the movement of malaligned and tilted teeth to proper position.[51]

Arch wires, clasp arms, finger springs, hooks for rubber or wire ligatures, reciprocal bracing, bite planes, and many other special appliances can be adapted to the removable prosthesis during the treatment period (Fig. 6-52).

Certain basic concepts of tooth movement must be kept in mind, and it must be understood what types of movement of teeth must be accomplished. The three basic procedures involved are (1) rotation of teeth, (2) facial or lingual movement, and (3) mesial or distal movement.

Alteration of the position of the fulcrum area of the tooth should be done only by a trained orthodontist. Instead, a tipping action against the fulcrum is employed because usually a coronal migration has taken place with little alteration of the position of the apex of the root. Therefore, the rationale of treatment is to correctly position the coronal portion of the tooth by tipping or working against the fulcrum area.[48]

The bite plate is used extensively as a prerestorative treatment. It is a relatively simple appliance made of acrylic resin of horseshoe design, having arrow type clasps that are usually placed in the bicuspid and molar interdental buccal embrasures near the cervical region and a labial arch wire contacting the six upper anterior teeth. On the anterior palatal surface a flat bite wall is made, extending from cuspid to cuspid. The flat plane meets the incisal edges of the lower six anterior teeth at an angle of 90 degrees so that only a vertical force is exerted on them. If the incisal edges of the lower teeth are very uneven, level them so that uniform contact is made against the bite wall. Also, be sure to avoid depression in the bite wall so as not to interfere with the free movement of the mandible. Do not encroach too much upon the freeway space.[52]

Cases exhibiting the following may be helped with this type of appliance or one similar to it.

1. Cases exhibiting deep overbite that may affect the successful treatment of periodontal disease and subsequent restorative treatment may be helped by a combination of tooth movements, including the intrusion of lower anterior teeth and extrusion of posterior teeth.

2. Upper anterior teeth can be moved lingually to place them in a more desirable position over the basal bone so that stresses upon them will result in the least amount of trauma to the supporting mechanism, with resultant decreases in food impaction areas and an improved esthetic appearance.

3. Teeth may be moved facially into a more favorable position, while moving others lingually and intruding or extruding others.

Many other cases and uses of this appliance can be cited. Elongation of posterior teeth with alveolar bone to fill a defect is certainly much desired with the use of the Hawley retainer. We also move tooth to bone or bone to tooth.

Grassline ligature also can be used to bring teeth together. This type of ligature is used as the moving force, and stainless steel wire can be used as the anchor. The grassline ligature should be changed weekly.

Provisional splinting can provide anchorage for an orthodontic appliance from which the necessary force can be exerted.

Treatment should be accomplished as simply and rapidly as possible. After realignment of the teeth a period of stabilization should follow, wherein the teeth are maintained in their corrected position. Splinting in many instances provides permanent retention for the teeth that have been moved.

With a knowledge of the physiology of the involved tissues, a few basic techniques, and the application of the necessary materials, minor orthodontic tooth movement can be executed successfully, leading to the successful completion of the subsequent periodontal and prosthodontic procedures and their maximum longevity.

MAJOR ORTHODONTICS*

Few textbooks or reference periodicals describing the rearrangement of teeth in the adult dentition, either as an aid to restorative dentistry, as a substitute for restoration, or as a replacement, were published prior to 20 years ago. With the enhancement of techniques of both restorative dentistry and orthodontics, the adult patient has profited greatly by a cooperative effort between these important fields of dentistry.

As all publications concerning the etiology of malposed teeth and jaws declare, the prime cause of all malocclusions is heredity, closely followed by premature tooth loss. It is probably as common for the parent of an orthodontic patient to realize the personal need for either or both orthodontic and restorative dental care as it is for the restorative dentist to require the aid of orthodontics in the realization of a better end result to a problem in his restorative practice. In some instances either branch of the profession, that is, either orthodontics or restorative dentistry, may be alone the answer to a problem.

*Contributed by Earl E. Shepard, Professor and Chairman, Department of Orthodontics, Washington University School of Dental Medicine, St. Louis, Mo.

The following cases and illustrations will show orthodontic procedures in preparation for restorative procedures.

CASE 1

Uprighting of abutment teeth was desirable and was accomplished with a removable acrylic and wire space opener as originally described by Dr. Herrick of Iowa (Case 1-1 to 1-7).

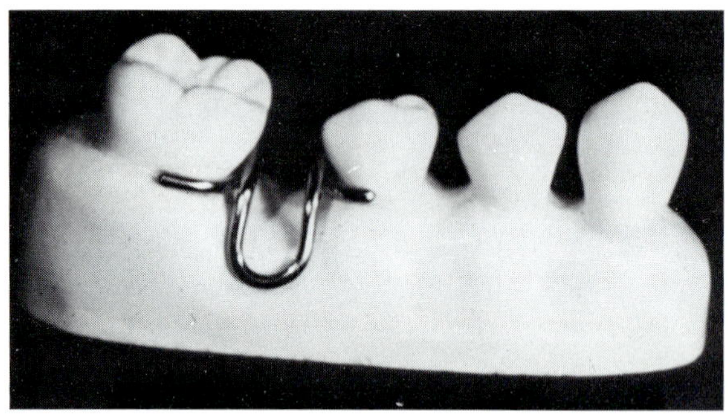

Case 1-1

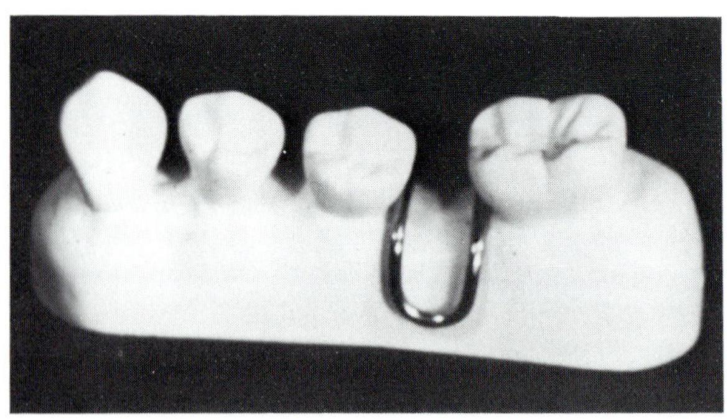

Case 1-2

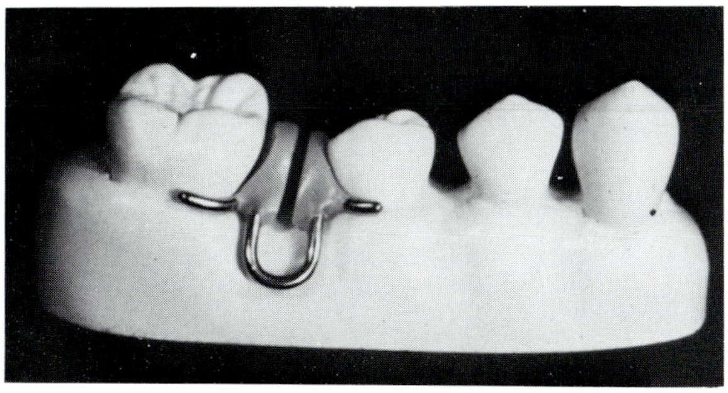

Case 1-3

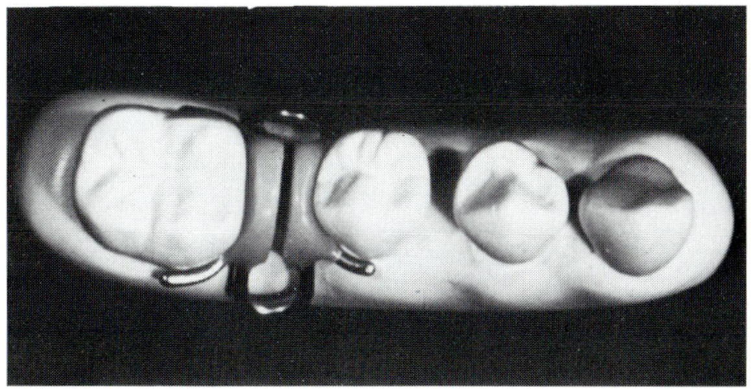

Case 1-4

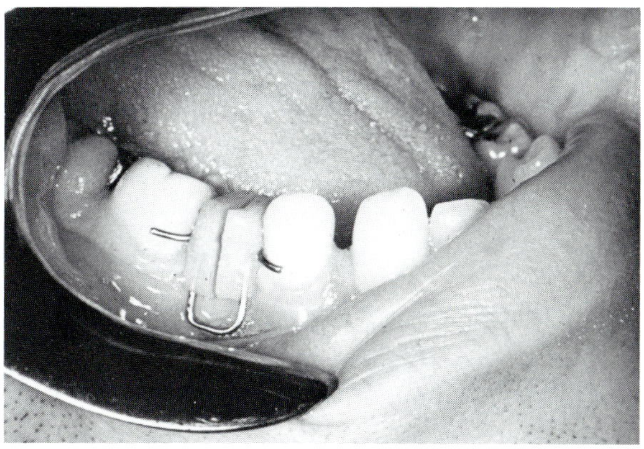

Case 1-5

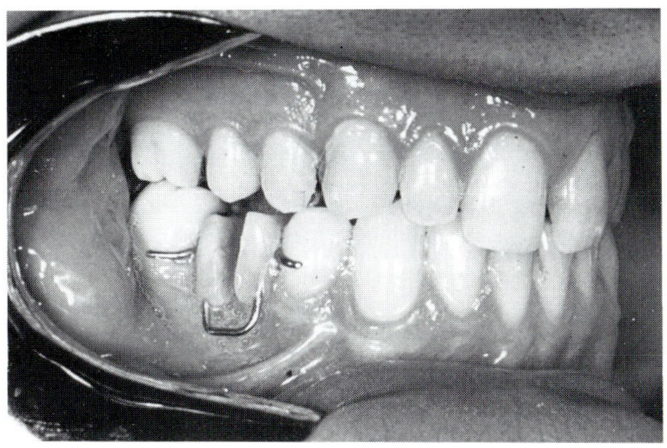

Case 1-6

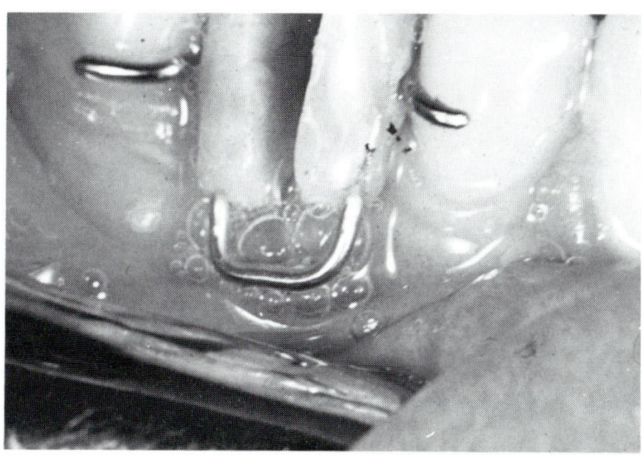

Case 1-7

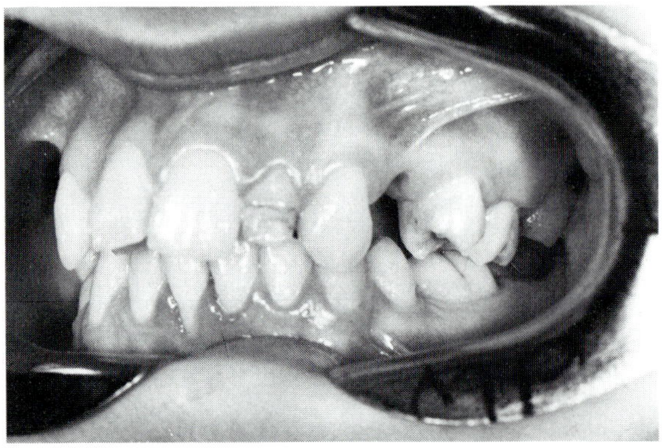

Case 2-1

CASE 2

A young adult had torsiverted and malaligned maxillary anterior teeth, a hypoplastic left lateral incisor, as well as a completely buccoverted left maxillary second premolar. The right and left maxillary first premolars were extracted, and a banded light wire appliance was employed to align the anterior teeth (Case 2-1 to 2-5). These illustrations reveal an improved tooth alignment as well as vertical dimension.

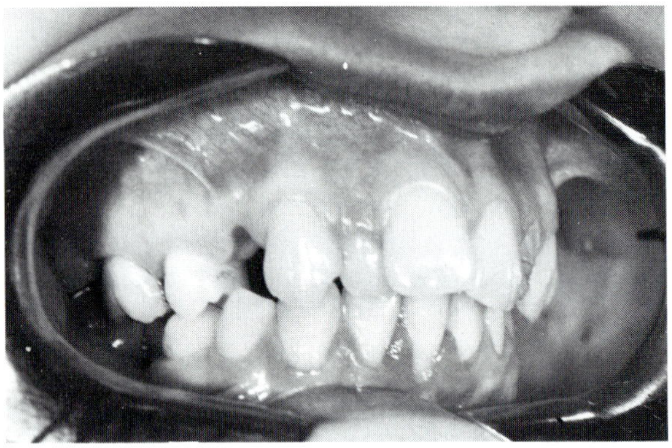

Case 2-2

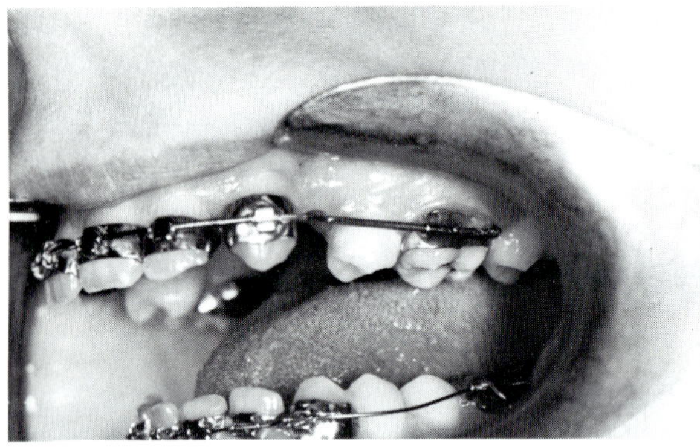

Case 2-3

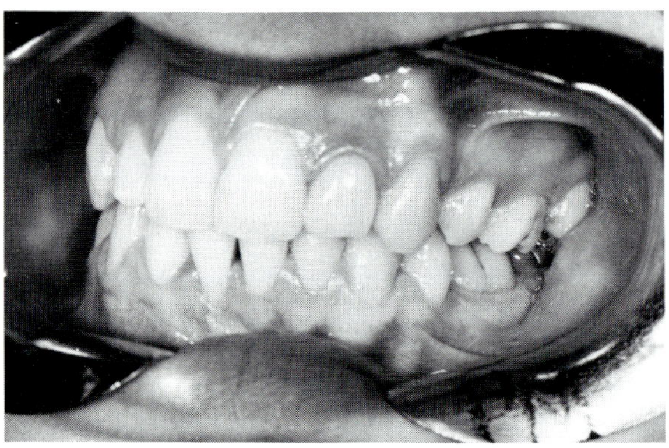

Case 2-4

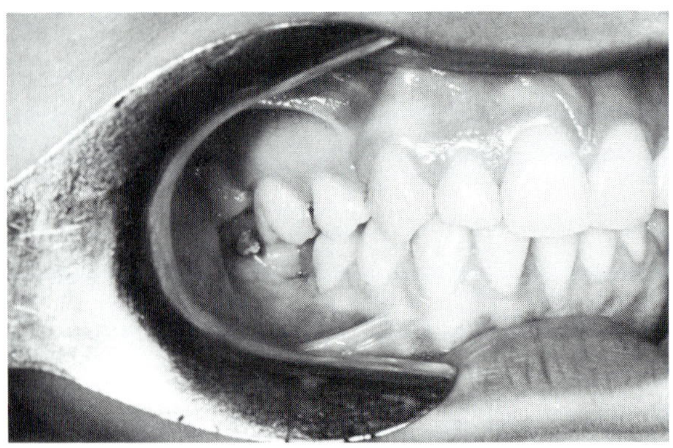

Case 2-5

CASE 3

A young woman presented herself with a rather unsightly left maxillary central incisor dowel crown restoration and wearing a palatal denture carrying a labially posed right maxillary central incisor. The right mandibular central and lateral incisors were in labioversion, making it impossible to correctly align a replacement tooth.

A modified mandibular Hawley appliance was utilized to move the labioverted teeth lingually. Proper alignment of the mandibular incisors permitted a properly aligned replacement (Case 3-1 to 3-3).

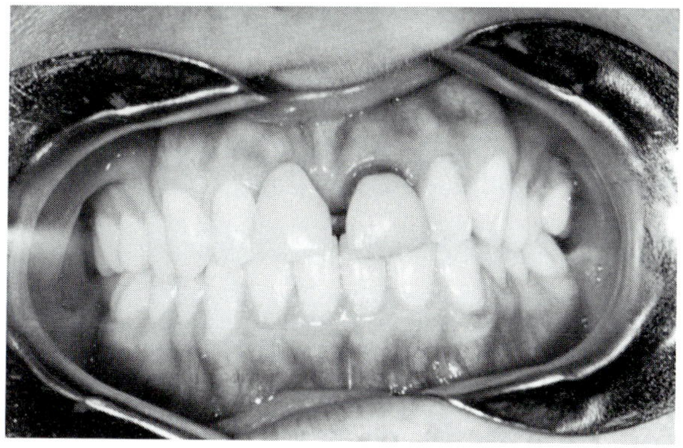

Case 3-1

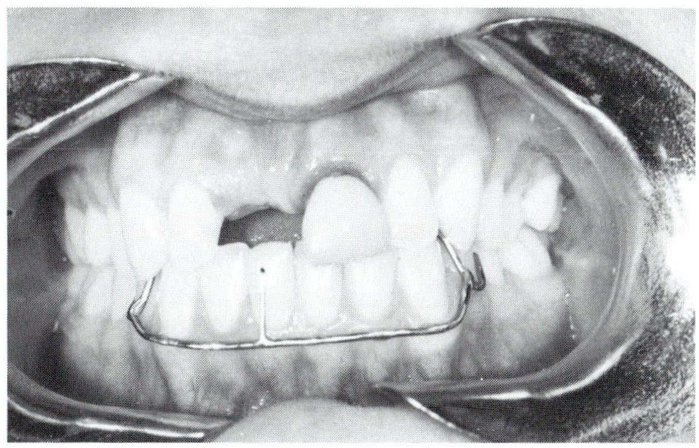

Case 3-2

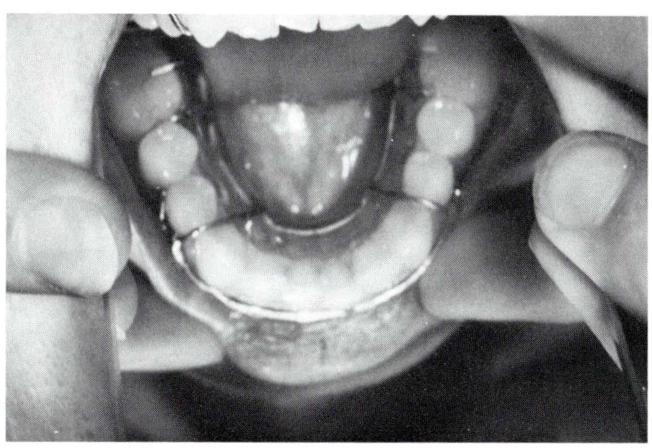

Case 3-3

CASE 4

A young woman presented herself with prematurely lost right mandibular lateral incisor and first permanent molar as well as maxillary lateral incisors. The vertical dimension is drastically closed. The patient related that, because of their extremely malposed positions, the aforementioned incisors were extracted some years previously.

A light (twin) wire appliance was utilized with anchorage supplied from the banded molar teeth, incisors, and canines and intrusive tension was directed to the anterior teeth.

After some 28 months of orthodontic therapy, the vertical dimension decidedly improved. The remaining maxillary central incisors were extracted and mouth rehabilitation undertaken (Case 4-1 to 4-5). (Mandibular retaining appliance is in place in some illustrations.)

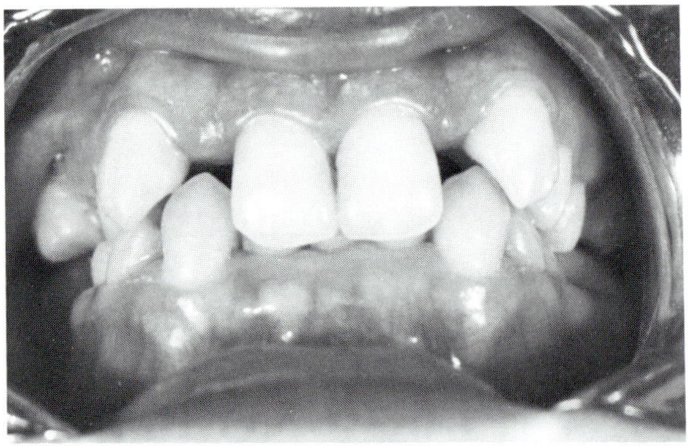

Case 4-1

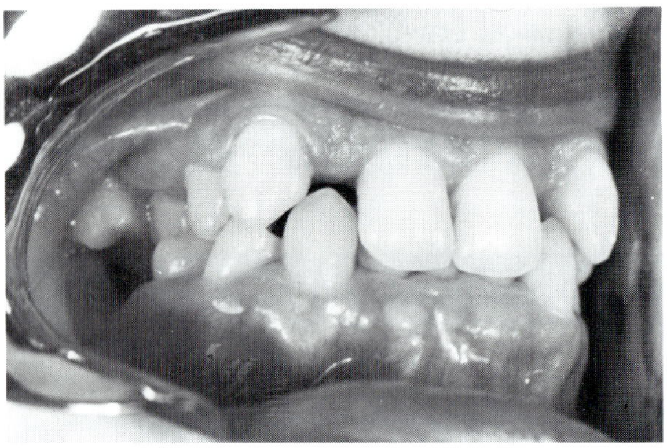

Case 4-2

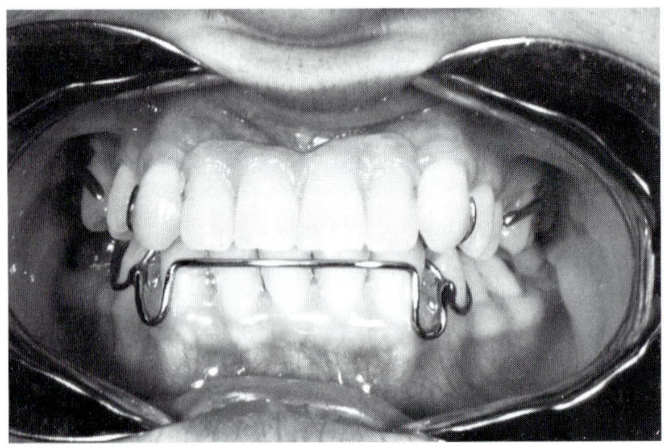

Case 4-3

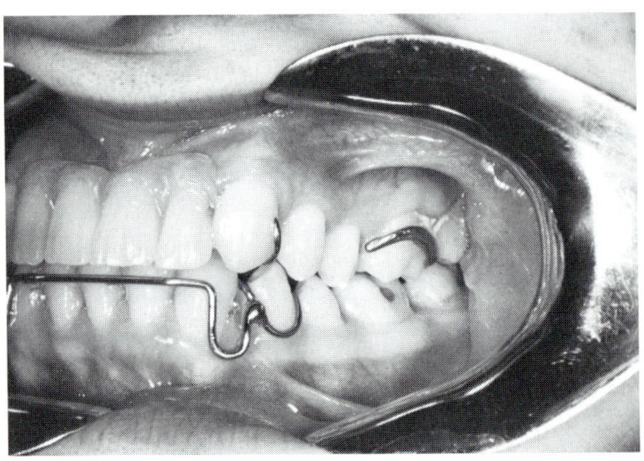

Case 4-4

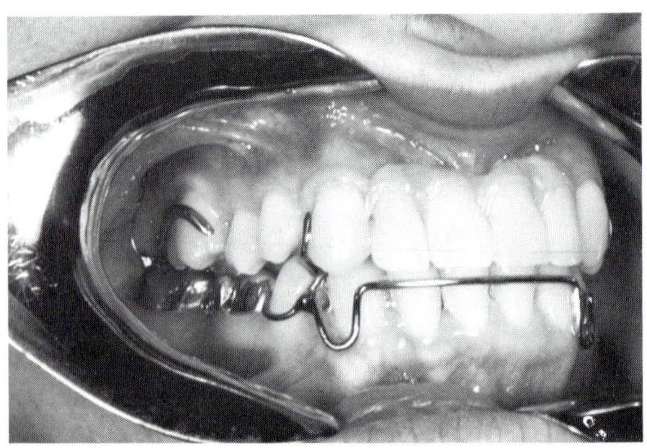

Case 4-5

CASE 5

A young man 21 years of age was referred for possible rearrangement of the anterior teeth so that an ill-fitting bridge could be replaced.

The bridge pontics were removed, and a Hawley high labial type removal appliance was constructed which carried acrylic teeth replacing the right maxillary central and lateral incisors. As the overjet was improved by means of the vertical springs of the removable appliance, the acrylic pontics were likewise reduced labially by grinding and polishing.

Note the improvement in the overjet, and the new restorative replacements (Case 5-1 to 5-9).

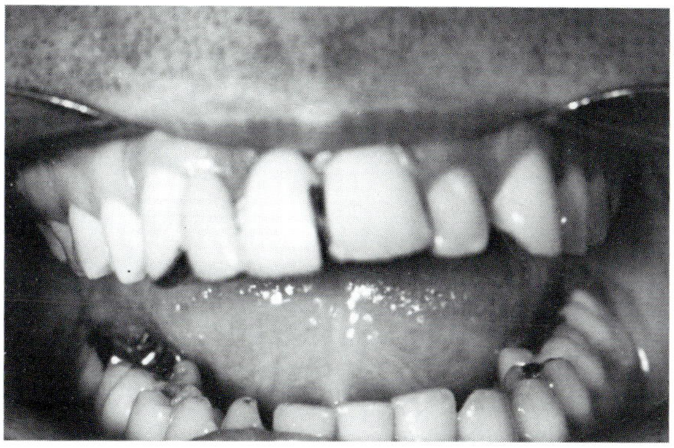

Case 5-1

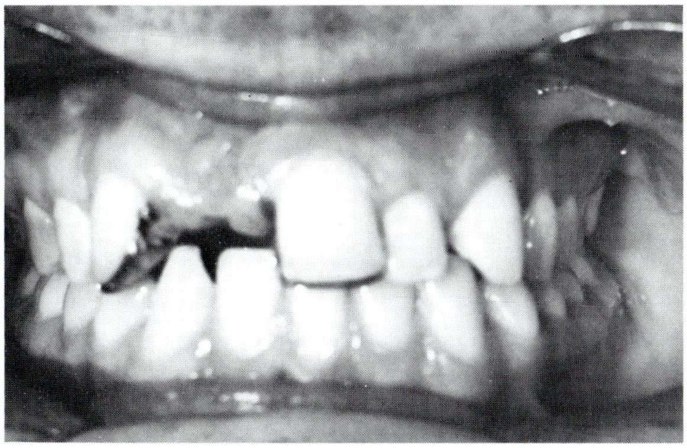

Case 5-2

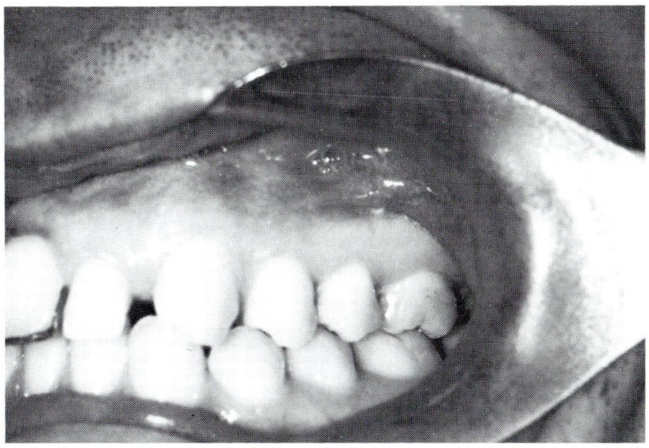

Case 5-3

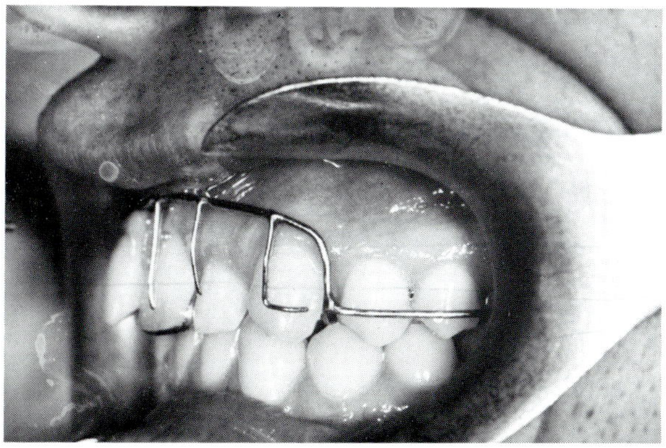

Case 5-4

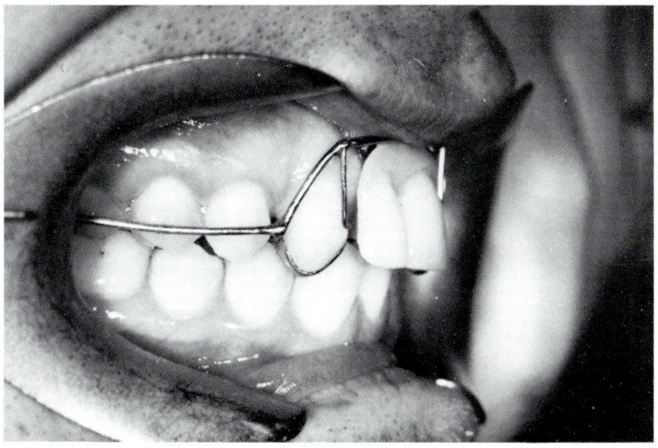

Case 5-5

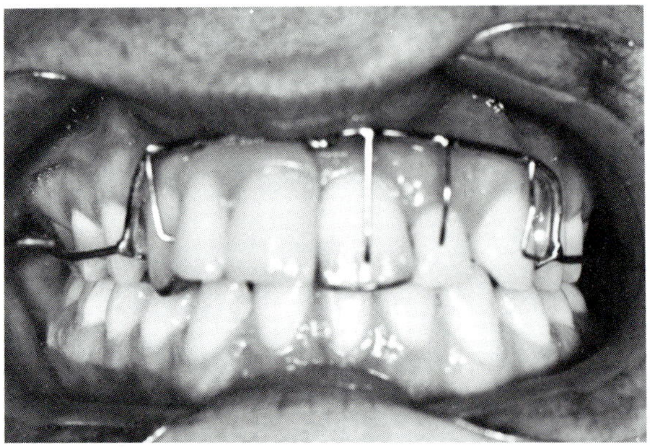

Case 5-6

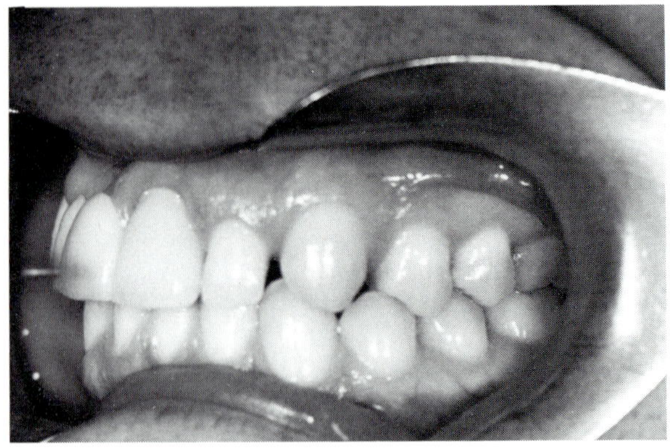

Case 5-7

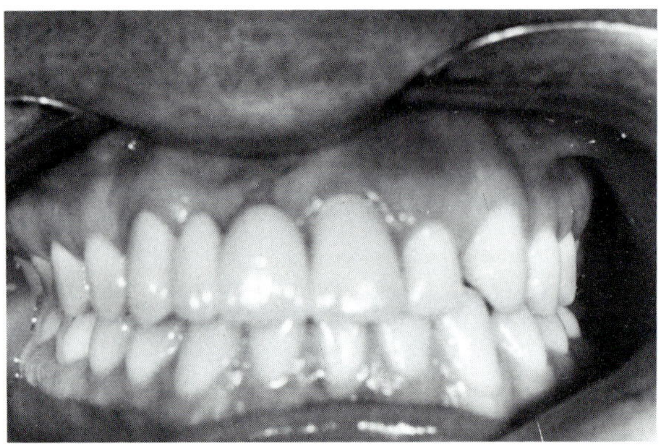

Case 5-8

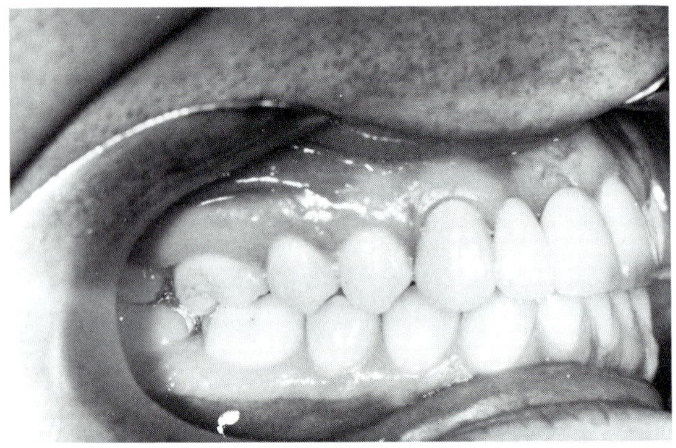

Case 5-9

Selective grinding

An important consideration in an analysis of occlusion is the functional contact relationships between the maxillary and mandibular teeth. The sound effect of a patient tapping his teeth together in centric occlusion should be noted, possibly with the aid of a stethoscope. Stable tooth contact with balanced muscle activity will elicit a sharp, well-defined sound; an unstable occlusion will give various and uneven sound effects.

The recognition and correction of occlusal interferences in the natural dentition are facilitated by an understanding of the physiology of mandibular movements rather than by mastery of a regimented series of grinding rules.[53]

The teeth that receive the impact of a slide from centric relation to centric occlusion often are exposed to a much stronger and more traumatic force than the posterior tooth with the premature contacts (see Fig. 6-11).[22]

Disharmony between centric relation and centric occlusion is a factor that causes improper wear and loss of the supporting structures of the teeth.

We want to establish a centric occlusion that is associated with a true centric relation, that is, the terminal hinge relation of the mandible.

If reshaping of the surfaces of the teeth is indicated, we should remember that the general anatomy of each tooth should be retained so that, when reshaped, the function of each tooth will be improved and the life and health of its supporting structures lengthened because of the relief of abnormal stress.

Occlusal adjustment by means of selective grinding is an operation of limited value in mouth rehabilitation. The displacement of the mandible anteriorly in patients in need of periodontal prosthesis is usually of a half cusp width or greater, and it is very doubtful that selective grinding can achieve a matching of the cuspal elements of the mandibular to the maxillary teeth. Proper intercuspation in these instances can be accomplished only by procedures used in periodontal prosthesis.

Never do preventive occlusal adjustment. Avoid the grinding of prematurities if clinical and roentgenographic evidence show no pathologic disorder and no joint symptoms. In these cases the patient has developed a protective proprioceptive reflex and, by all means, do not disturb it.

CONTRAINDICATIONS

Selective grinding cannot be used for the following conditions:

1. Large displacement of the mandible anteriorly or laterally
2. Deep overbites
3. Closed bites
4. Flat, heavily abraded occlusal surfaces
5. Severe amounts of alveolar bone resorption
6. Excessive mobility of teeth
7. Numerous open contact areas, migrated teeth
8. Numerous edentulous areas

OBJECTIVES

Following are some important objectives in selective grinding:

1. Leveling of extruded teeth
2. Reduction of prematurities in the path of closure from physiologic rest to swallowing contact
3. Enhancement of optimum holding contacts of teeth in centric position
4. Establishment of proper occlusal plane
5. Bringing occlusal forces into direction of long axes of teeth; directing forces closer to center of occlusal table within range of root form and closer to the center of the tooth
6. Reduction in size of contact surfaces
7. Reduction in wedging effect in teeth
8. Elimination of balancing contacts
9. Adjustment of clinical crown to clinical root ratio
10. Incisive group function
11. Leveling of marginal ridges and reduction of plunger cusps
12. Improvement of the occlusal and interproximal embrasures—reduction of effects of functional irritation
13. Retaining of sharpness of cusps and establishment of smooth gliding planes
14. Narrowing of buccolingual diameter to improve form and function in relation to the gingival tissues
15. Reduction of lateral thrusts—buccolingually and mesiodistally
16. Reduction of interferences in the incisal guidance relationships

TECHNIQUE

Complete analysis of the articulation and occlusion of the dentition is not possible, in my opinion, without properly mounting the casts of the case on an adjustable articulator. A written list of the adjustments made on the casts is made for the purpose of reproducing the cuts made on the casts to the actual teeth or restorations when work is started on the patient.

Upper and lower alginate, hydrocolloid, or rubber base impressions are taken for the construction of accurate study casts for mounting on an adjustable articulator so that they are on the same axis as the teeth of the patient.

The hinge axis of the mandible is determined either approximately by palpation, by an average measurement, or by a hinge axis determination. Full registrations would more than compensate for the time required to take them (Chapter 17), but axis-mounted casts will suffice.

A hinge-bow transfer for mounting the upper study cast on the adjustable articulator is made, followed by two or more correctly registered centric relation bites for mounting the lower study cast on the articulator by the Lauritzen split-cast method.

A determination of the premature contacts and interferences is the next order of business, but before this procedure is undertaken the basic principles and rules for grinding must be established.

Lauritzen[54] has called our attention to the fact that *basic principles* are absolute and inviolate, whereas *rules* are not absolute and may be violated, provided basic principles are adhered to. All rules (except the rule MU-DL) are based on a normal buccolingual relation of the occlusion; thus they do not apply for teeth in crossbite relation.

CORRECTION OF CENTRIC OCCLUSION

"*Basic principle:* Maintain the cusps as far as possible because they are prerequisites for harmonizing the excursive motions.

"*Rule: MU-DL.* When the occlusion has to be repositioned to a more distal position, trim mesial inclines of upper cusps (the tips of the cusps are moved more distally) and distal inclines of lower cusps (the tips of the cusps are moved more mesially).

"*General cusps to be trimmed:* Buccal lowers and lingual uppers."*

CORRECTIONS OF EXCURSIVE MOVEMENTS (AFTER CENTRIC OCCLUSION HAS BEEN ESTABLISHED)

"*Basic principle:* Never take teeth out of centric occlusion.

"*Protrusion—Rule: BU-LL.* Buccal upper cusps (trim their distal inclines) and lingual lower cusps (trim their mesial inclines). In anterior region trim labially of lower anteriors and lingually of upper anteriors.

"*Lateral excursion:*

"*Working side—Rule: BU-LL.* Buccal upper cusps (trim their inner inclines) and lower lingual cusps (inner inclines).

"*Balancing side—Rule: LU or BL.* Select either lingual upper cusps (inner distal inclines) *or buccal lower cusps* (inner mesial inclines). Never trim both cusps."*

Premature contacts and interferences are determined with the use of typewriter ribbon† on the mounted stone casts. The plaster teeth are trimmed with a knife, following the rules of grinding, and then a grinding list is made before proceeding to chairside operations.

Grinding in the mouth is done with small stones (small inverted cone stones or diamond points), using typewriter ribbon, wax strips (as suggested by Dr. Bernard Jankelson‡), and thin carbon paper. Carbon paper is the least desirable medium to use for this purpose since it marks everything and is not definitive enough. The occlusal indicator wax is good. With the adhesive side against the tooth the wax should be pressed well in place over the occlusal, buccal, and lingual surfaces of the area. The patient should be asked to wet the occlusal indicator wax with his tongue and his mandible is guided into the closure until the wax is thinned or penetrated. The point of penetration is easily located with an explorer point; a mark is made through the point of penetration with a waterproof pencil. The wax strip is removed and the pencilled areas ground with small inverted cone stones.

*From Lauritzen, Arne: Lecture notes, Post-Graduate Study Groups, 1953, 1961.

†Madame Butterfly Brand, No. 10 inking, ¾ inch, manufactured by Miller-Bryant-Pierce, Aurora, Ill.

‡Occlusal indicator wax, Kerr Mfg. Co., Detroit, Mich.

In grinding one must never leave a flat plane or surface. All articulating surfaces are rounded or parabolic because all jaw movements are rotary. Equal contact can be maintained only by rounded surfaces.

The decision as to where grinding is to be performed is based on the procedures of establishing an articulation.[13] A clear understanding of these procedures will reveal the shortcomings of selective grinding as a treatment, and it also will prevent the grinding away of the wrong surfaces.

Always remember that the centric contact is the most important contact and the one that must be preserved (Figs. 6-53 and 6-54).

At this time, I wish to outline the procedures I use daily in my practice of dentistry,* applying the basic principles and rules of grinding.

As an example, sometimes a patient presents with a lower tipped molar which is distal to the upper molars. In a case like this, in testing incisal relations, (1) if any premolars or molars contact, remove tooth structure from buccal cusps of the upper teeth and lingual cusps of the lower teeth and (2) make a groove in the distal of the lower tipped molar for the upper cusp to pass through.

In testing cuspid relations in the lateral excursion in the tip-to-tip contact, if any posterior cusps interfere or make simultaneous contact on the idling or balancing side, make a groove in the upper teeth for the lower cusps to pass through, and make a groove in the lower teeth for the upper cusps to pass through. Follow the rules of grinding: grooves are sloped toward the mesial from the markings on the upper teeth and distally from the markings on the lower teeth.

In testing relations on the working side and if any interferences between bicuspids or molars appear in the tip-to-tip relation, remove tooth structure from the buccal cusps of the upper teeth and lingual cusps of the lower teeth.

After removal of any bicuspid and molar interferences in the tip-to-tip cuspid relation (on both the working and idling or balancing sides), test the occlusion nearer centric relation, that is, just a little inside the tip-to-tip cuspid relation. Again, remove any interferences as previously executed and keep testing "successive stations" nearer and nearer centric relation, eliminating interferences until centric relation closure is reached.

Repeat the same procedure for the opposite lateral movement beginning with the tip-to-tip cuspid

*As suggested by Charles E. Stuart, Ventura, Calif.

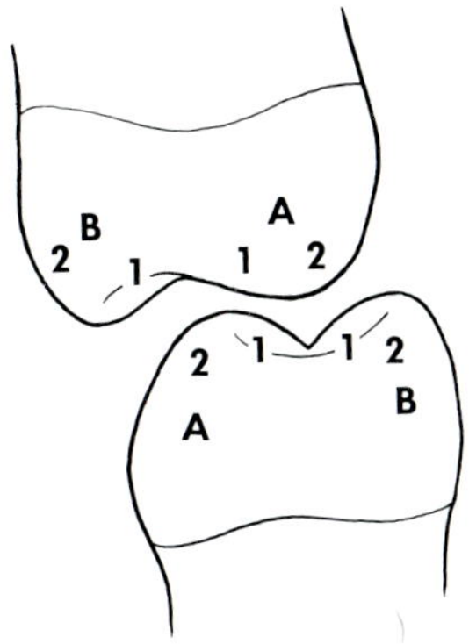

Fig. 6-53. A, Centric cusps. Maxillary lingual cusps and mandibular buccal cusps. The primary stop to vertical closure. **B,** BU-LL cusps. Buccal upper cusps and lingual lower cusps. *1,* Inner inclines: Cuspal inclines of the teeth facing toward the central groove. *2,* Outer inclines: Cuspal inclines of the teeth facing away from the central groove.

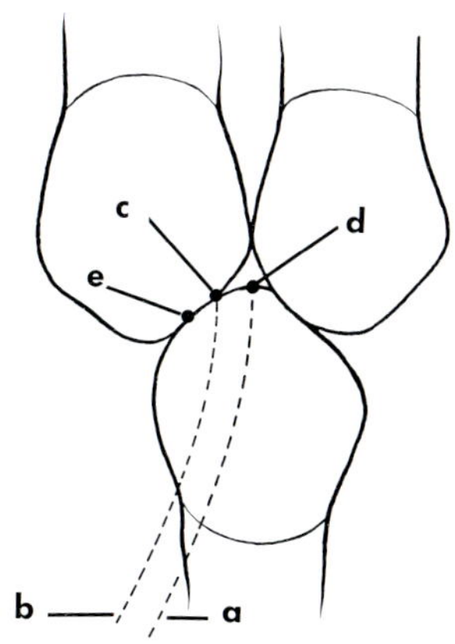

Fig. 6-54. Two maxillary bicuspids in occlusal contact with a mandibular bicuspid at the most closed position. Arc *a-d* is the acquired path of closure programmed by the occlusal condition. Arc *b-c* is the path of closure about the terminal hinge axis until first occlusal contact is made on a deflecting incline at point *e* and then the mandible is propelled forward to point *d,* the most closed position. (Courtesy Niles F. Guichet.)

relation, and gradually working nearer and nearer centric relation.

In testing lateral excursions, slight hand pressure is applied on the idling or balancing side toward the working side so that the total side shift or Bennett movement is secured.

The centric position is adjusted last. Tip the patient's head back, and have him close his jaw lightly in its rearmost position. With the marking material positioned between the teeth have the patient close from the first contact to full intercuspation. Interferences are removed from the mesial slopes of the upper teeth and the distal slopes of the lower teeth. Next, deepen the fossae to give the centric related intercuspation slightly more closure than the patient had in the former forward intercuspation.

Finally, make certain that the patient's intercuspation has even pressure on both sides and that the premolars close simultaneously with the molars. We want mesiodistal as well as bilateral equal closure. We now have maximum intercuspation—the jaw is in a rearmost, midmost, and uppermost position.

We must test the eccentric relations first, as outlined above, to make sure that our centric position contacts are not destroyed in the eccentric excursions. Or, in other words, the eccentric relations have been consulted before the centric relation intercuspation can be made. *The eccentric contacts are relieved, and then the centric relation intercuspation is made* (Fig. 6-55).

Also, during the "remount" procedure with the gold restorations, the interferences in eccentric relations are corrected before those of the centric position. This sequence, as previously stated, helps to prevent overreduction of a casting in centric relation. The amount of correction necessary in gold restorations, as a rule, is usually slight compared with initial adjustments required for correction of gross interferences.

Before dismissing a patient, restore anatomic detail and polish all cut surfaces. Make sure the patient is comfortable and has a negative occlusal perception.

Overbite and overjet

The following definitions are those of Ross.[55]

Incisal guidance is the path on the lingual surfaces of maxillary teeth along which the incisal edges, or labial surfaces, or both, of the mandibular incisor teeth glide. This path directs the movement of the mandible from intercuspal position to protrusive position. Relation between the maxillary and mandibular anterior teeth also effects the movement of the mandible in its lateral excursions. Incisal guidance is the result of four factors: (1) overbite, (2) overjet, (3) length and amount of contact between maxillary and mandibular anterior teeth, and (4) position of contact on the maxillary and mandibular anterior teeth.[55]

Overbite refers to the vertical distance between the incisal edge of the longest maxillary anterior tooth and the longest mandibular anterior tooth in intercuspal position (Fig. 6-56).

Overjet refers to the horizontal distance between

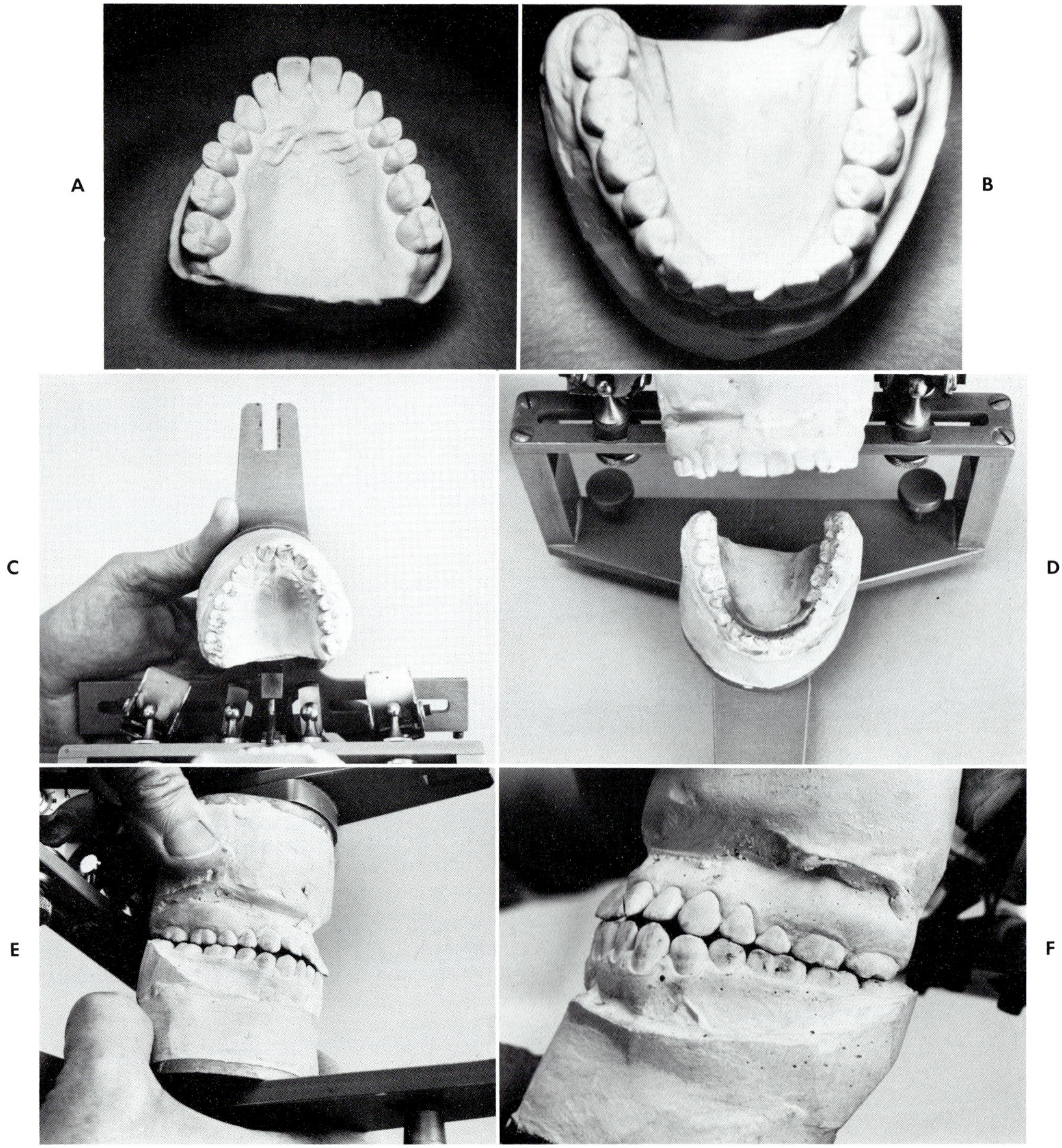

Fig. 6-55. A to **F,** A case from practice applying the basic principles and rules of grinding as described in the text.

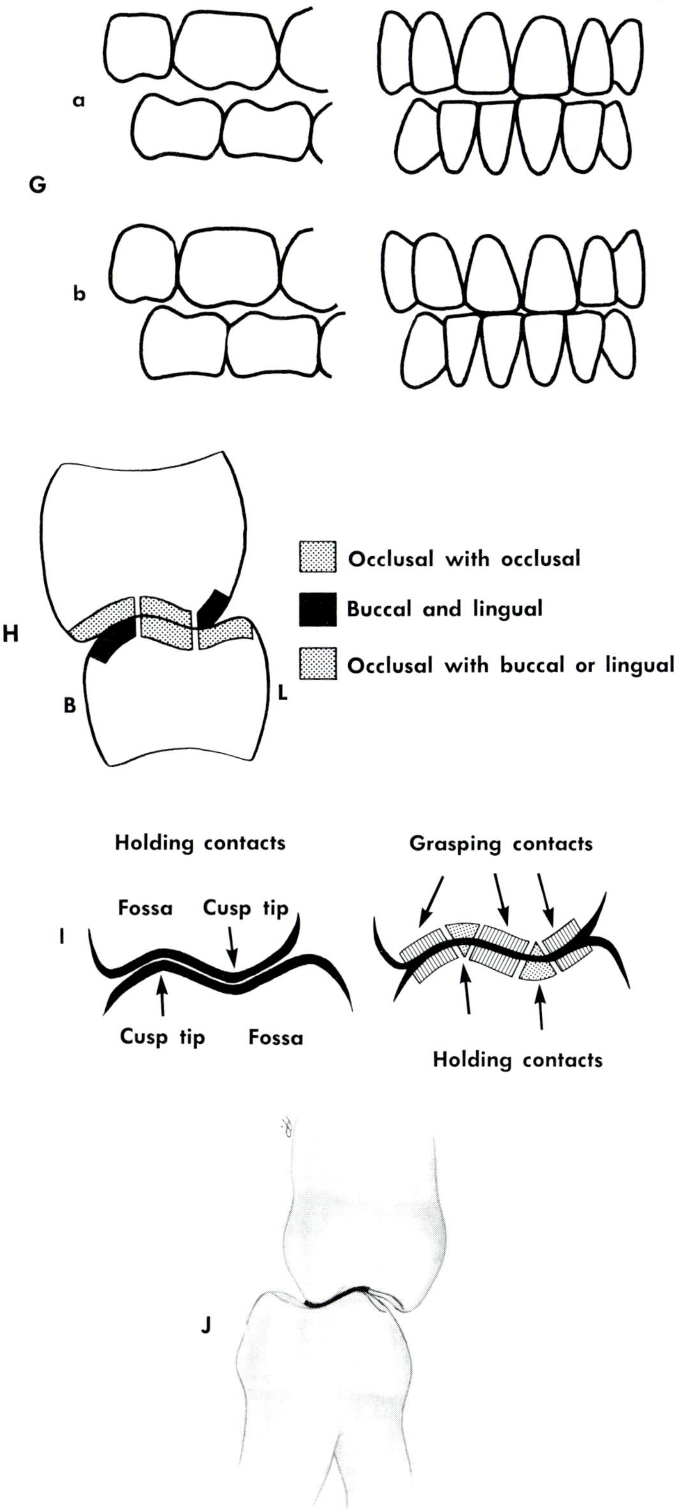

Fig. 6-55, cont'd. G, Protrusive glide and anterior prematurities. *a,* Concept of balance in terms of distribution of force and stress as represented by group function or at least central incisors (posterior contact not necessary). **H,** Surfaces to be reduced in selective grinding; **I,** holding and grasping contacts; **J,** the shaded area between the upper and lower teeth indicates the area of potential contact in centric occlusion. Inner aspect of the upper lingual cusps and inner aspect of lower buccal cusps as well as a small amount of the outer aspect of lower buccal cusps and upper lingual cusps have potential for contact. (**J** courtesy Morton Amsterdam.)

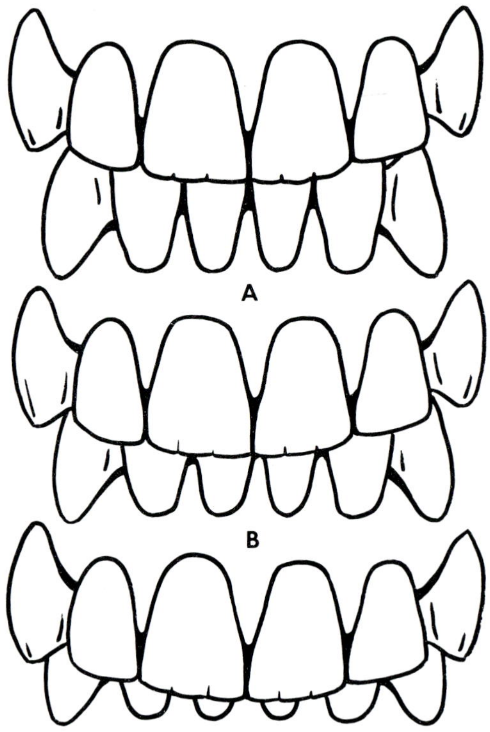

Fig. 6-56. Different degrees of overbite. **A,** Slight overbite. **B,** Moderate overbite. **C,** Marked overbite. There is more rigid control and more chance for bone loss with the deep overbite than with the shallow overbite (if the overjet is minimal). If the overjet is moderate or marked, the degree of overbite is less important. (From Ross, Ira F.: Occlusion—a concept for the clinician, St. Louis, 1970, The C. V. Mosby Co.)

the most anterior part of the labial surface of the mandibular anterior teeth and the closest point on the lingual surface of the maxillary anterior teeth in intercuspal position. The greater the overjet, the more freedom in moving the mandible forward and laterally, and the less injury to the anterior teeth during these movements (Fig. 6-57).

The amount of overjet and the length, amount, and position of contact between the anterior teeth seem to be more important in determining whether there will be trauma from occlusion around the anterior teeth. The amount of overbite seems less important.[55]

Ramfjord[22] calls attention to the fact that a traumatic and unstable occlusion is seen where there is an inadequate overjet related to a deep overbite in a patient with bruxism. The maxillary anterior teeth are moved labially, resulting in a loss of the centric stops of the mandibular incisors. With a loss of centric stops there is a subsequent extrusion of the mandibular incisors and the development of interferences in lateral and protrusive excursions of the mandible.

Temporomandibular joint dysfunction

The temporomandibular joint is a complex mechanism that has a precise manner of function, and the problem of temporomandibular joint disorders is a complex one which has to do with occlusal disharmonies, lack of eccentric mobility, and psychological factors.

Some are of the opinion that occlusion is the major etiologic factor (it is true that the occlusion of the teeth must be arranged to harmonize with the normal function of the joint, and if this harmony fails to exist, the temporomandibular joints will suffer proportionately); others say that psychologic and muscle factors are of the greatest etiologic importance. It is also true that there is a significant relationship of psychologic factors to nonorganic temporomandibular joint dysfunction, and that tension produces muscle fatigue and spasm which can be the underlying or key factor in temporomandibular joint disorders (derangements and pain).

To begin with, a complete clinical examination following a good medical and dental history, correlated with a cognizance of the possibility of psychogenic factors, especially the centering of the psychic stress in the region of the temporomandibular joint, is of the utmost importance. Stethoscopic examination can be of some help in revealing crepitation and clicking in the joints (Fig. 6-58).

The *pain dysfunction syndrome* of Laskin[56] appeals to my thinking and experience. Pain, muscle tenderness, clicking, or alteration of mandibular movement are cardinal symptoms of the temporomandibular joint pain dysfunction syndrome. Muscle spasms caused by tensional habits of the individual are probably due to the fact that these individuals cannot accept their deep-seated dependency needs, whereas with a physical pain symptom it permits them to be dependent on others for care which consciously they believe to be factual. Unquestionably, one cannot discount occlusion as a factor, but muscle spasm is probably the primary cause in most pain symptomatology of the temporomandibular joint. The occlusal and psychologic factors operate, as a rule, together and produce the pain dysfunction syndrome (PDS).

Lerman[57] has said that "the activity of certain motor units is increased disproportionately. If these motor units maintain physiologic adequacy and can

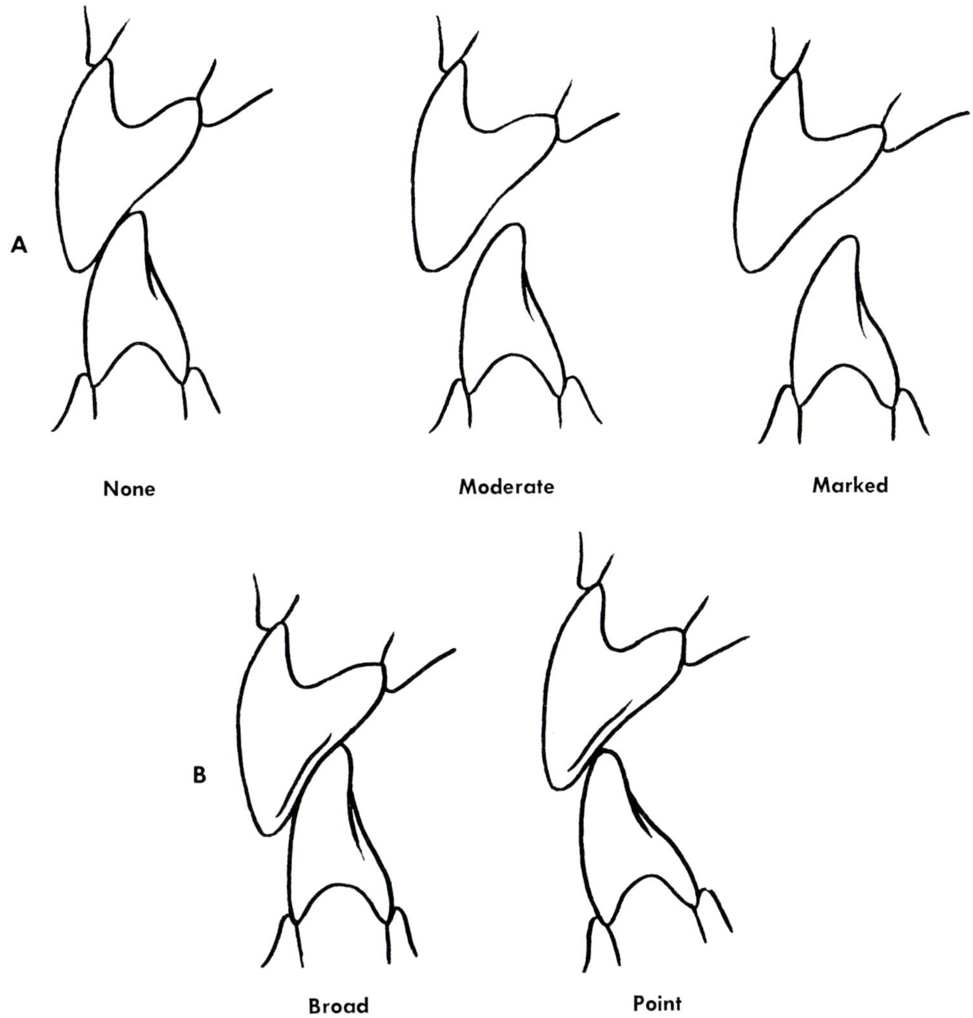

Fig. 6-57. A, Different amounts of overjet. With no overjet, the mandible is restricted in horizontal and vertical mandibular movements. There is a good possibility of mobility of the anterior teeth and anterior bone loss. With moderate and marked overjet, the mandible has greater freedom in horizontal and vertical movements. There is less chance of mobility of the anterior teeth and anterior bone loss. **B,** Different amounts of contact between anterior teeth. Both sets of teeth have the same overjet relation. There is more rigid control and more chance of increased mobility and bone loss with broad contact. There is more freedom and less chance of destruction with point contact. (From Ross, Ira F.: Occlusion—a concept for the clinician, St. Louis, 1970, The C. V. Mosby Co.)

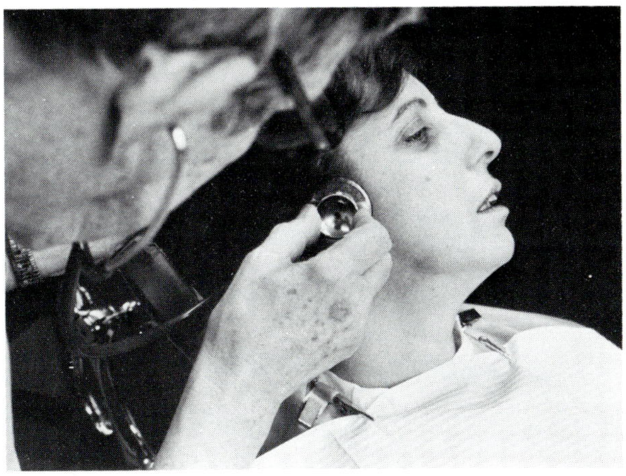

Fig. 6-58. The use of the stethoscope in temporomandibular joint examination.

satisfy accommodative responses Pain Dysfunction Syndrome does not develop, and patient remains asymptomatic. When they cannot, however, the affected motor units become progressively more incoordinated, finally going into spasm.''*

Tension resulting from interfering cusps can encourage clenching and gnashing. ''Irregular occlusion of the teeth can be considered a type of trigger that causes discomfort in referred areas when an individual is under stress. This results in heightened tension and perpetuates the cycle.''†

Occlusal malfunction can be responsible for subjective and objective symptoms in the temporomandibular joint complex. When occlusal discrepancies are responsible for abnormal muscle function, the most frequent offenders are cuspal interferences in the centric relation pathway and interferences on the balancing side in lateral mandibular glide. When this happens, a painful syndrome ensues.

Dawson[58] is of the opinion that even though emotional stress can be a contributory factor, it does not cause the problem. If the occlusion is perfected to the point that there is no muscle tenderness to palpation, the syndrome will disappear or cease to exist. If pressure exerted on the mandible causes pain or tenderness at either joint region, the condyle is being held by muscle, and it is not in the terminal hinge position. What happens is that the prolonged contraction of the external pterygoid muscle is required to position the mandible anterior to its ligament-braced terminal axis.[59]

The pterygoid muscles, because they are involved with deviation of the mandible, must be examined for tenderness to palpation (Fig. 6-59). Tenderness on palpation is usually indicative of abnormal function. Also observe the temporalis muscle for possible trouble. In fact, palpate the entire side of the head and neck for soreness, and also any muscle that can be reached intraorally.

Another factor that should be seriously considered in the temporomandibular dysfunction problem is the ''myofascial pain dysfunction syndrome (MPD).'' Freese and Scheman[60] tell us that it is of muscle origin, and the pain is due to spasms of the muscles of mastication. Myofascial pain is the term applied to those pain syndromes originating in myofascial structures. ''A myofascial trigger area is a small, circumscribed, very hypersensitive area in myofascial tissues from which impulses arise to bombard the central nervous system and produce referred pain. It is a physical sign, not a symptom, and the patient is usually unaware of it'' (Fig. 6-60).* Myofascial trigger areas can be activated by any motion that stretches the structure containing the trigger area—needling (administration of a local anesthetic), opening the mouth for long periods of time (long dental sessions), intense heat or cold, etc.

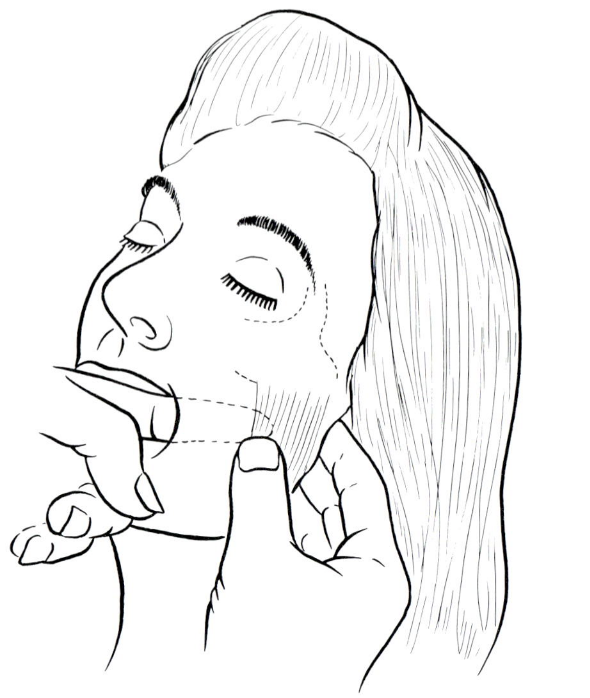

Fig. 6-59. Palpating the origin of the internal pterygoid muscle. The right hand encompasses the superficial portion of the masseter.

Shore[61] has called attention to the fact that if the external pterygoid muscle moves incoordinately, the condyle does not remain in its normal place in the center of the disk, but rides on its thickened outer edge. When the jaw opens fully, the disk snaps into place, producing the click that is felt and heard. If this clicking is allowed to persist, muscle spasm, limitation of motion, and pain often result (Fig. 6-61).

Still another factor that merits consideration is the apparent scientific proof that Moffett[62] has re-

*From Lerman, Martin D.: A unifying concept of the TMJ pain-dysfunction syndrome, J.A.D.A. **86**(4):833-841, 1973.

†From Laskin, D. M.: Etiology of the pain dysfunction syndrome, J.A.D.A. **79:**147, July 1969.

*From Freese, Arthur S., and Scheman, Paul: Management of temporomandibular joint problems, St. Louis, 1962, The C. V. Mosby Co., p. 115.

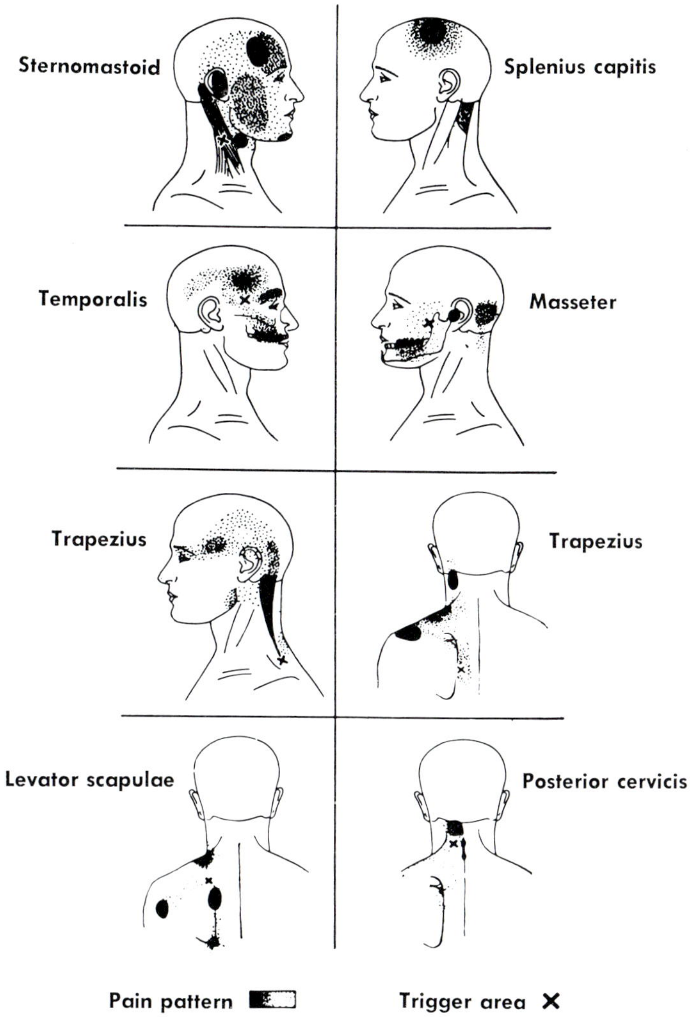

Fig. 6-60. Zones of reference in the head and neck. Solid black areas indicate "essential zones" and the stippled areas indicate "spillover zones"; the heavier the stippling, the more frequent this area is a zone of reference. (From Travell, J., and Rinzler, S. H.: Postgrad. Med. **11**:425-427, 1952. In Freese, A. S., and Scheman, P.: Management of temporomandibular joint problems, St. Louis, 1962, The C. V. Mosby Co.)

ported, which shows that remodeling of the bones of the temporomandibular joint may occur and, if so, we would have an alteration of the maxillomandibular relations.

Treatment of temporomandibular joint dysfunction calls for concomitant therapy of three major structures—temporomandibular joint, musculature, and teeth.

Patients with acute exacerbated pain must be given symptomatic relief before any correction of occlusal disharmony is undertaken, because during acute pain, trismus, and limitation of mandibular movement is not the right time to perform this procedure. At this time it is impossible to determine proper centric relation, because we are dealing with an unstable temporomandibular joint that should not be used as a foundation for occlusal therapy. The patient's terminal hinge position must be accurately determined in order to help him. The terminal hinge axis moves in its skull relations as the temporomandibular joint becomes more stable. Dyer[63] defines a stable temporomandibular joint as a "pain-free joint from which accurately taken maxillomandibular records may be duplicated over a period of several years without changes in the border movements of the mandible."

In other words, treatment should combine psy-

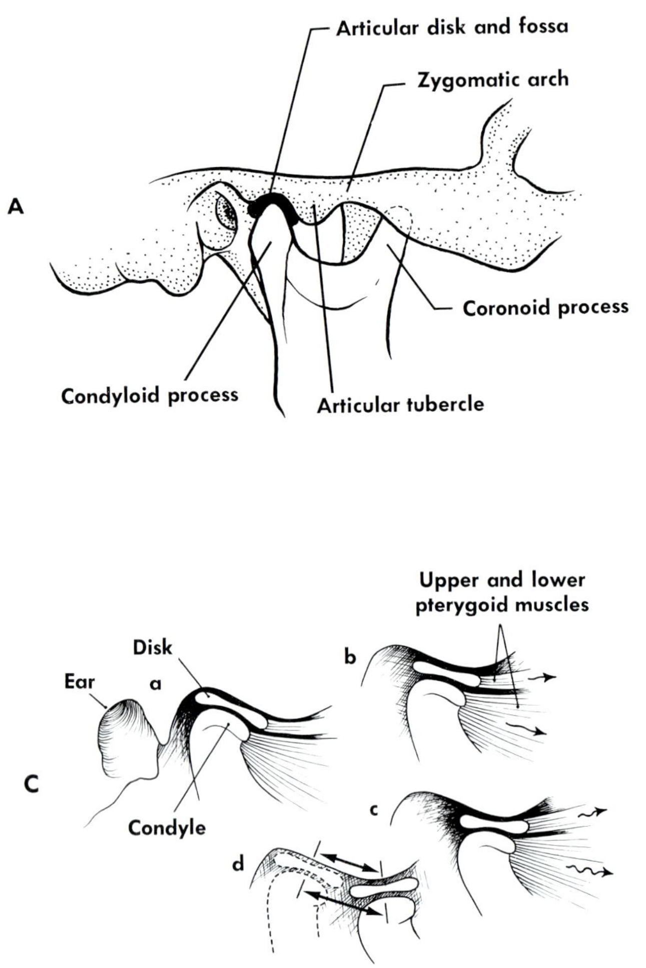

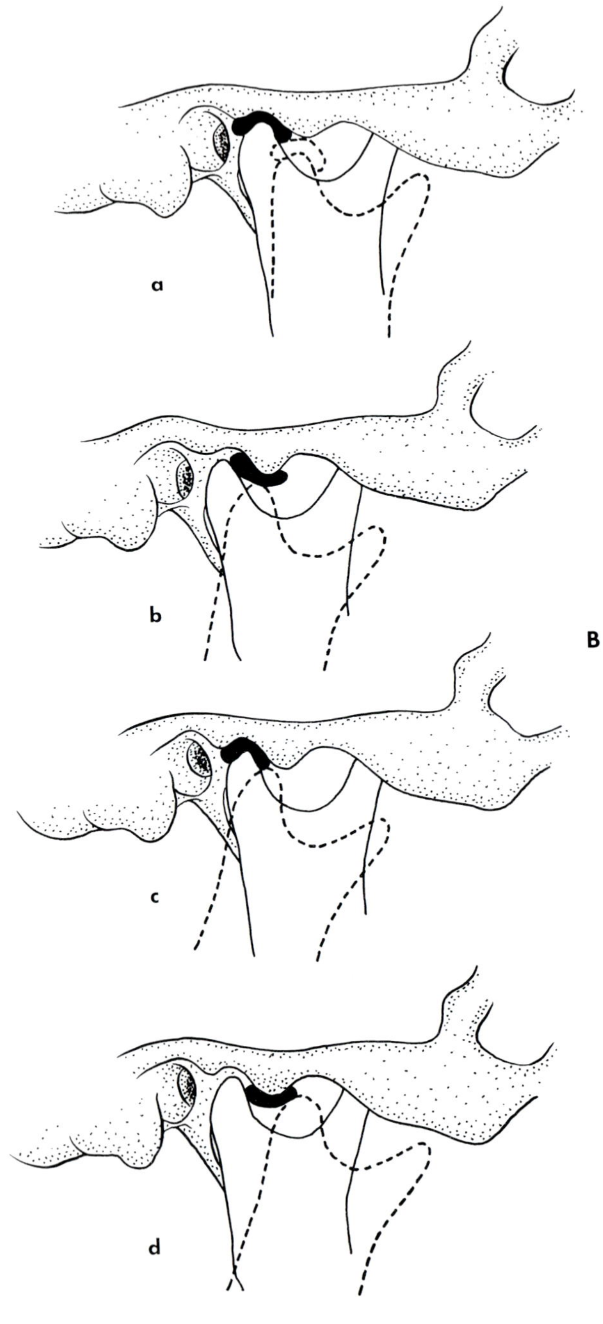

Fig. 6-61. If the external pterygoid muscle moves incoordinately, the condyle does not remain in its normal place in the center of the disk—it rides on the thickened outer edge of the disk. There is a sound upon opening and another when the condyle returns to the closed position. Persistent clicking leads, as a rule, to muscle spasm, limitation of motion, and pain.

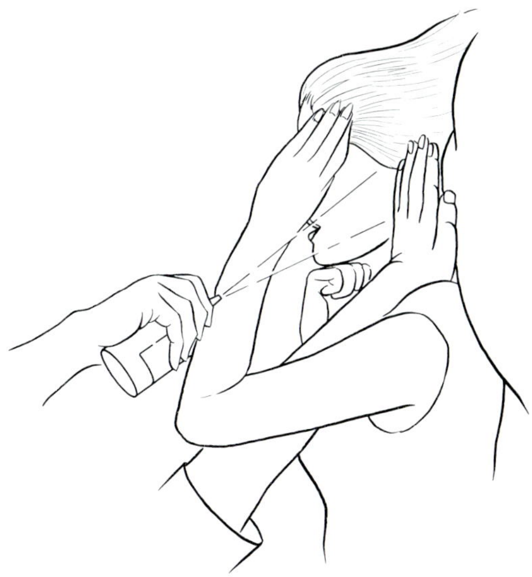

Fig. 6-62. Application of ethyl chloride spray. Spray areas of skin overlying the temporomandibular joint and the masseter and temporal muscles at a distance of about 2 feet from the face.

chologic and physiologic modalities. Pain and tension must be controlled and spasm eliminated. Intra-articular injection is indicated in some cases of an acutely tender temporomandibular joint. An effective agent for injecting into the joint is prednisolone butylacetate (Hydeltra T.B.A.), and a good result usually can be expected.

Adjuvant therapy such as moist heat, analgesics, muscle relaxants, tranquilizers for tension, ethyl chloride spray (blocks out myofascial trigger mechanism), direct injection of procaine hydrochloride into the muscles, and intramuscular injection of vitamin B_{12} to aid in the restoration of general body nutrition is also part of the treatment[64] (Fig. 6-62).

Temporary occlusal splints or bite planes are usually effective in relieving temporomandibular joint dysfunction. It is thought that the relief comes from the simple expedient of changing the old neuromuscular pathways (elimination of the disturbing input upon the neuromuscular mechanism from occlusal interferences) by allowing freedom for eccentric movements. It facilitates muscle relaxation and decreases the dysfunctional muscle forces. We are trying to stop the cycling effect of continued painful use of masticatory muscles. The idea is to restrict all masticatory function within painless limits.

By adjusting the occlusal splint or maxillary orthopedic appliance on an adjustable articulator before positioning in the patient's mouth, and by continuous adjustments after placement to keep up with changes that take place in the temporomandibular joint over a period of time, we endeavor to attain (1) a coincidence of centric relation and centric occlusion, (2) a cusp-to-fossa relationship, whereby the buccal cusps of the lower teeth are seated into a definite fossa in the upper acrylic appliance, (3) cuspid protection or working side contact through a lateral range of approximately 1 mm., and (4) no idling or balancing side contacts. (See Figs. 6-48 and 6-49).

Dyer[63, 65] has said that the mandible must be supported during all testing of translatory movements (right and left lateral and protrusive). The condyles must be held in initimate contact with the meniscus and articular eminence—and if this is not done a subluxation of the condyles can occur. "The dentist must firmly support and guide the lateral movements of the mandible in order to secure the maximum degree of pivot and lateral shift, and support should be given to the posterior angles of the mandible during protrusive test excursion."*

Attention should be given to any deviate swallowing habits, because if the habit is not corrected the orthopedic appliance will be of little benefit in the effort to stabilize the temporomandibular joint.[63]

We must also keep in mind that psychologic factors, according to Lerman,[57] lead to an overall increase in masticatory muscle activity, whereas occlusal factors increase muscle activity selectively. Some individuals are psychologically predisposed to magnify the stress-generating potentials of their life situation, which can result in increased bruxism and clenching activity. In some cases of this type, I resort to psychotherapy to help in functional procedures.

When symptoms have been reasonably relieved, selective grinding or restorative measures or both are carried out to correct the occlusal disharmony, which can produce functional temporomandibular joint disease. In other words, the occlusal correction, by whatever means deemed necessary, should be muscle oriented, aimed at restoring the mandible to its neuromuscular position, and elimination of all interferences which cause muscle incoordination.

Habit training for temporomandibular joint pain

1. Suppress yawns with the palm of your hand.
2. Eliminate thick sandwiches or any wide opening while eating (such as whole apples, corn on the cob, etc.).

*From Dyer, E. H.: Personal communication.

Habit training for temporomandibular joint pain—cont'd

3. Avoid all hard or tough foods.
4. Avoid gum chewing.
5. Do *not* test your jaw by determining how wide you can open or how much you can move the lower jaw forward or to the right or left sides.
6. Do not clench your teeth tightly together.
7. Do not crack ice with your teeth.
8. Avoid holding small objects between your teeth, such as pins, pencils, toothpicks, pipes, etc.
9. Do not attempt to cut thread with your teeth or bite your fingernails.
10. Do not sleep with the side of your face on a pillow with your hand under the pillow, which may push the jaw toward the opposite side.
11. Eliminate habits of opening the mouth wide, such as in laughing, attempting to open your eustachian tubes when coming down from high altitudes (airplanes, mountain driving) or *any* extensive movements of the jaw you may have acquired in various expressions of emotion.
12. If you have been told that you "grind" your teeth while asleep, try to learn to sleep on your back and without any pillows.
13. Avoid any long dental appointments.
14. To repeat—do *not* try to test your jaw by trying to open it wide or making any extensive forward or sideward movements.

Neurophysiologic point of view

The following are some observations made by Jerge[66]:

"A strictly mechanical approach to the study of the kinesiology of the mandible based on morphology of the temporomandibular joints or the functional relationships of teeth disregards the very complex nervous system mechanism which is superimposed on this mechanical system.

"The tooth as a whole has an array of receptors around it which can receive information about pressure stimulation from any direction."*

In both horizontal and vertical lesions of bone in periodontal disease, the loss of periodontal ligament support means sensory deprivation as well as loss of mechanical support. In the case of the deeply penetrating vertical lesions of bone (which suggests a disorganized periodontal ligament in that area and that the sensory mechanism of the tooth is impaired) the tooth develops a "blind side" (Fig. 6-63). Such a tooth, deprived of its innervation on one side, cannot relate to the nervous system any information about pressure impinging on it from the side of the lesion. Sensory impulses from periodontal ligament receptors exert some control over the jaw musculature, which in turn moves the mandible. Ultimately, as the infrabony lesion becomes more circumferential, the tooth becomes more a "passive" structure in the dental arch. It is unable to influence mandibular movements via trigeminal reflexes.

The tooth that has no sensory nerve supply will be buffeted about by the forces which impinge upon it, and it has no ability to influence the direction or magnitude of these forces. The sensory neurons of the periodontal ligament are essential components of the reflex arcs which control mandibular muscles and ultimately the force exerted on the dentition by muscular contraction.

"The extent to which the teeth have healthy periodontal ligaments and nerve supplies, and the extent to which the dentition as a whole relays coordinated information, determines the extent to which mandibular movement is coordinated with all the parts of the dentition. It is often coordinated only in relation to some or most of the parts."*

The impairment of this nervous mechanism by the lesions of periodontal disease is a factor to note.

Temporary coverage

Temporary restorations used during mouth rehabilitation have to be fitted well. If not, displacement of teeth, faulty occlusal pathways, and disturbed temporomandibular joint function during this critical period may jeopardize the final result.

Gingival and pulpal inflammation can be controlled by using acrylic resin coverage for teeth and a soft periodontal dressing for tissues.

Inadequate, immediate, temporary measures will create marked periodontal disturbances. Overextended temporary crowns present a problem. Detachment of the gingival fibers for a short period of time is unlikely to produce permanent damage, but after

*From Jerge, Charles R.: Comments on the innervation of the teeth, Dent. Clin. N. Am., pp. 117-127, March, 1965.

*From Jerge, Charles R.: Comments on the innervation of the teeth, Dent. Clin. N. Am., pp. 117-127, March, 1965.

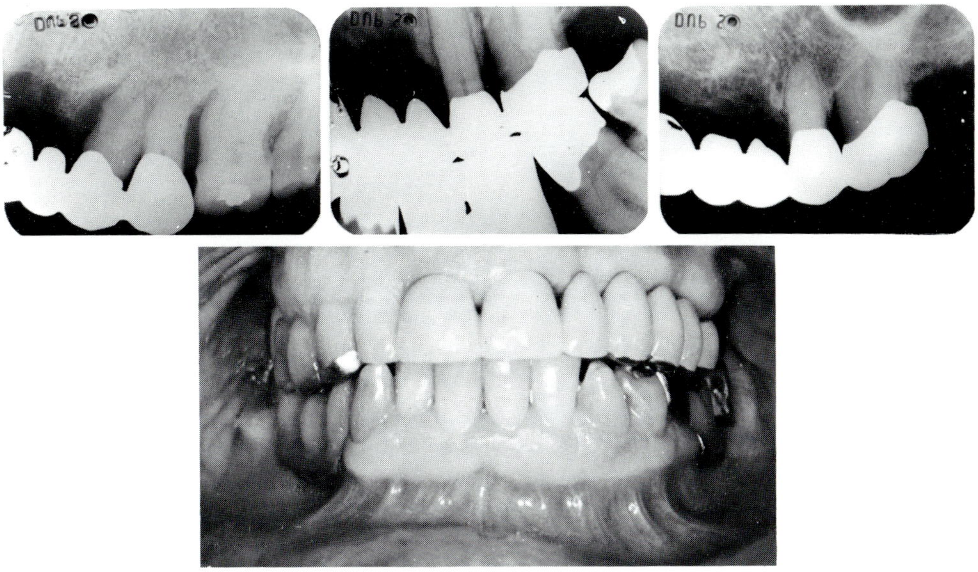

Fig. 6-63. Because of deeply penetrating bone lesion, which suggested development of a "blind side," the first bicuspid was removed. Establishment of proper occlusal relations and making use of bilateral splintage in upper arch seems to indicate that healing is taking place.

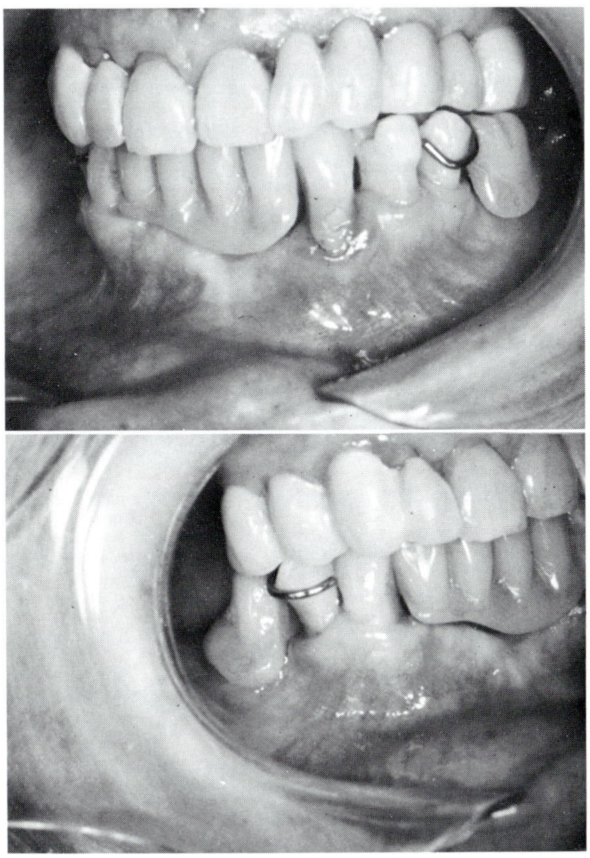

Fig. 6-64. Overextended and poorly contoured temporary crowns and pontics creating marked periodontal disturbances in upper arch.

approximately 1 month such crowns introduce the risk of gingival recession. (See Fig. 6-64.)

The temporary restoration must foster the healing of the gingival tissue and must create an environmental relationship that will keep the tissue healthy and unchanged during the period from the preparation of the tooth to the placement of the completed restoration.

The marginal fit of the temporary restoration should simulate, as much as possible, that of the finished restoration. Margins should be knife-edge, well adapted, and cover the entire prepared surface of the tooth to afford maximum protection to the preparation while offering minimal irritation to the soft tissue environment. Good contours and correct embrasure form also should be developed. (See Fig. 6-65.)

Temporary coverage also can be useful for the establishment of prognosis of questionable teeth as it affects the final treatment plan.

Therapeutic splinting

PRINCIPLE

Splinting is a biologic procedure. Individual tooth movement is not obliterated by splints and fixed appliances as some have thought. On the contrary, it is directed so that the entire periodontal ligament is stimulated fairly uniformly.

Since a splint distributes the supporting force of the tooth more uniformly, there will not be as much

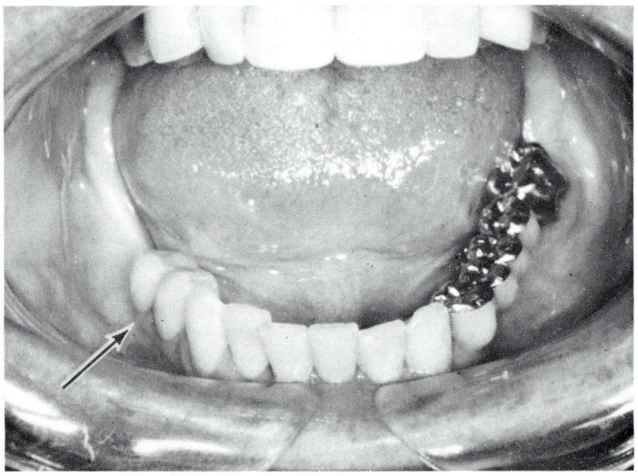

Fig. 6-65. Development of good contours, correct embrasure form, and marginal fit offers maximum protection to preparation and minimal irritation to soft tissue environment (arrow).

movement by any one part of the tooth's supporting periodontal ligament as there had been prior to splinting. Therefore, the tooth will appear tighter after splinting.

In other words, a rigid fixed splint does not cause a partial degeneration and atrophy of the periodontal structures from lack of functional stimuli.

Only axial resultant forces transmitted to the periodontium produce true physiologic stimulation of the fiber apparatus. The oblique fibers of the ligament are stimulated and oriented to resist the axial forces. Lateral forces, however, are resisted by the coronal and apical fibers; the orientation and strength of these fibers are not sufficient to adequately resist and dissipate these lateral forces, especially when there is a loss of supporting bone and periodontal ligament.

The principle of splinting teeth in either unilateral or cross-arch relation is a necessary adjunct to the treatment of periodontally involved teeth. It minimizes the effects of loss of support; it is necessary to establish posterior support for which there is a great need.

Splinting transforms several single-rooted teeth into a new multirooted tooth. Splinting of two single-rooted teeth not only alters the center of rotation about their root surfaces, but also allows the teeth incorporated into the splint to function as a multirooted dental unit. An increase in total root area creates a more favorable crown-to-root ratio. It is the procedure to employ when teeth must withstand forces beyond their physiologic limit; it offsets adverse factors with which we are faced. (See Fig. 6-66.)

PURPOSE

The purpose of the splint should be to distribute and direct the functional and afunctional forces, to bring them within the tolerance of the remaining supporting tissues, and to eliminate any mobility that may be present. Or we may say that it is a reorientation of the forces and stresses that come into play in the dental apparatus in such a way that the teeth are brought within the range of the adaptive capacity of the periodontal tissues. Fixation provides mechanical advantage and simultaneously restricts excessive tooth movements.

The primary purposes of splinting are as follows[18]:

1. Stabilization. Under stabilization we increase the resistance patterns to mesial, buccal, lingual, and distal vectors of force: (a) root area of resistance is increased and (b) reciprocal antagonism to force patterns is provided. Actually, under pure stabilization procedures the force may remain the same as before splinting, but the resistance is increased.

2. Reorientation of force and stress. Because of splinting, the unit area of resistance to force and stress is increased. The direction of force is altered, the total force may be the same, but the point of stress may be altered—its terminal direction may be rerouted.

The secondary purposes of splinting are (1) improvement of form and function of the teeth, (2) modification of occlusal contact patterns, (3) adjustment of jaw relations, and (4) improvement of masticatory efficiency.

Splinting of teeth will radically change the periodontal distribution of impacts from occlusal forces. However, splints require a great deal of accuracy with regard to occlusal relations, because after insertion of the splint there is not adaptive movement of the teeth to accommodate various occlusal discrepancies.

Unilateral splinting[21] is the joining of two or more teeth in one plane of an arch segment. In this type of splint the resistance is primarily against mesiodistal force action. The only buccolingual resistance is that afforded a weakened abutment by its firm neighbors (Fig. 6-67).

As long as the patterns of mobility of two adjacent teeth are not identical, splinting two such teeth together will provide some stabilization. A concomitant of stabilization is a certain amount of bone healing.

Bilateral splinting,[21] or cross-arch splinting, involves the inclusion of teeth on two or more segments of an arch up to and including the entire arch. In this type of splint action the resistance to force is in all directions, and weakened or mobile teeth actually

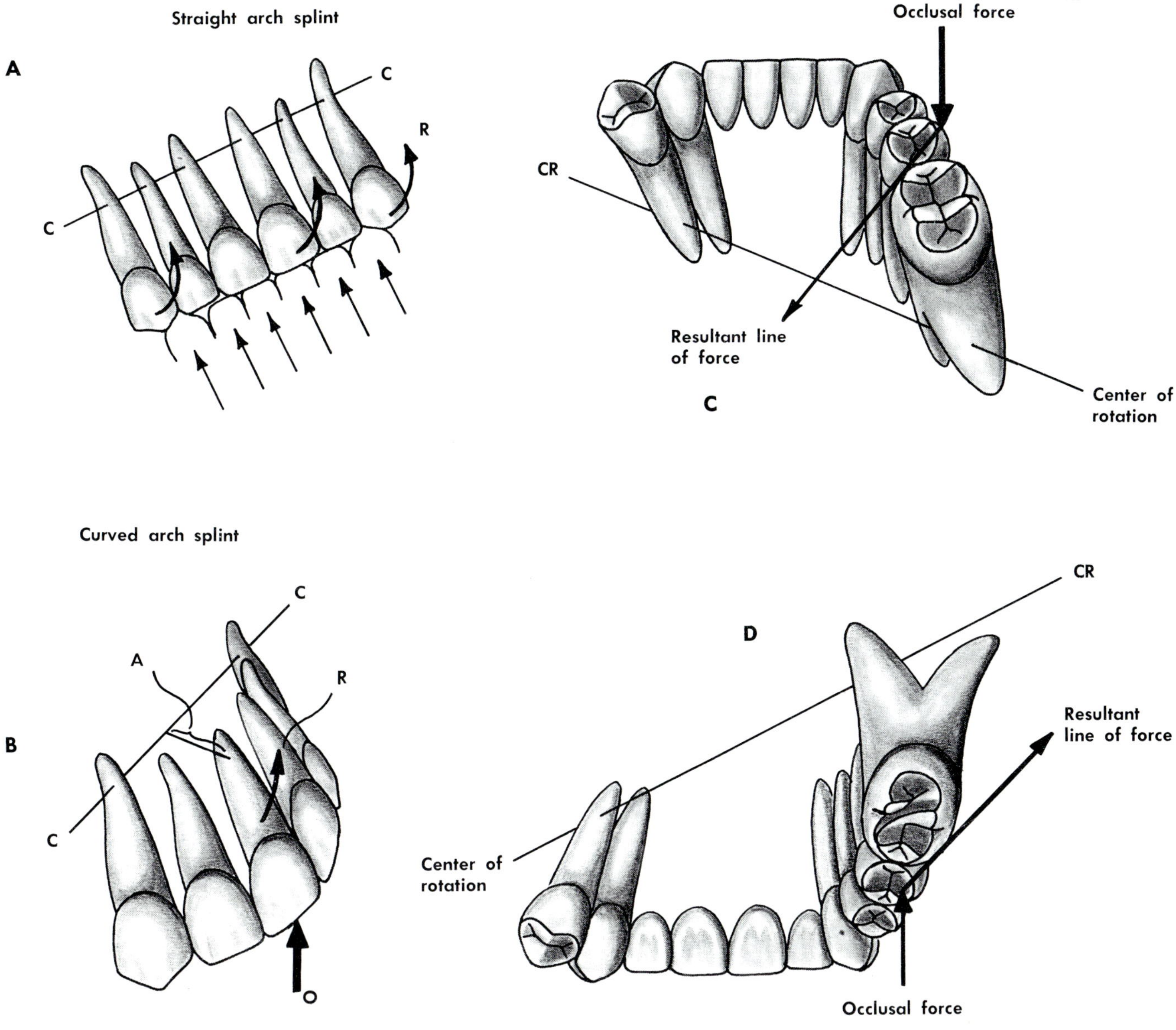

Fig. 6-66. A, Simultaneous occlusal pressure on a straight arch splint can cause whole splint to rotate; *R,* about the center of rotation; CC, passing through the area of apical third of teeth. Force on each tooth in splint is quite similar to that created by occlusal pressure on unsplinted tooth. **B,** Anterior curved arch splint. Because of curve in arch, central and lateral incisors would be *A,* anterior, to CC, center of rotation. This causes a change in *R,* the direction of force, which is now more apical than the tipping, which occurs when teeth are arranged in straight arch splint. **C,** In a mandibular curved arch splint occlusal force on buccal slope of posterior tooth produces lingual resultant of force. This resultant may pass through or near center of rotation, causing little or no torque. **D,** In a maxillary curved arch splint of similar design center of rotation, *CR,* usually passes near the apical third of terminal abutments. Occlusal force on upper buccal cusp incline produces a resultant line of force which is buccal in direction, while center of rotation is lingual to tooth. This results in a great deal of torque. (Courtesy Dr. L.A. Weinberg, New York, N.Y.)

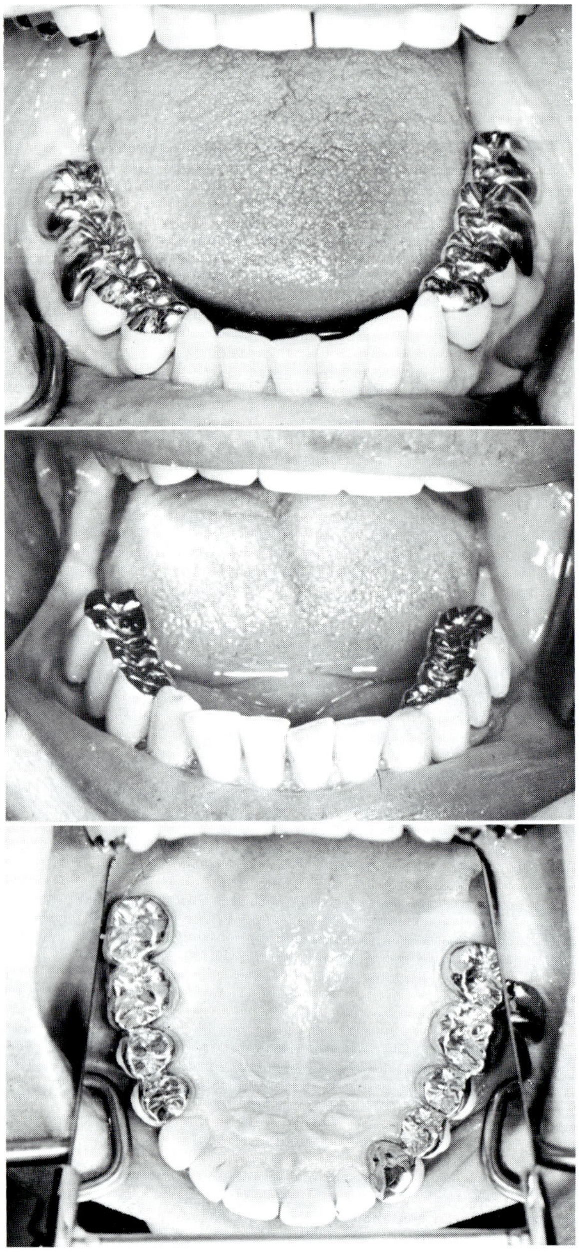

Fig. 6-67. Cases in which unilateral splinting was used to provide some stabilization and bone healing.

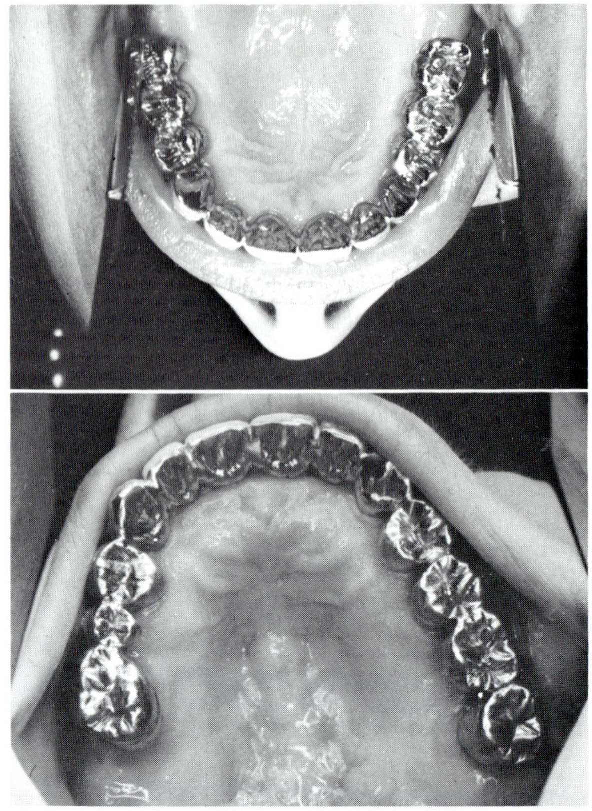

Fig. 6-68. Cases in which bilateral or cross-arch splinting was used to offer as much resistance as possible to force in all directions.

can give support to other mobile abutments. (See Fig. 6-68.)

The greatest effect is achieved from cross-arch stabilization; with such a tying together of teeth, forces, whether functional or otherwise, will be distributed among all the teeth in the arch. Because forces of occlusion are multidirectional, the ideal splint for reducing buccolingual mobility patterns is one that takes advantage of turning the dental arch; it provides maximum resistance against the multidirectional forces that occur in the mouth. Although the distribution may not be equal, it may suffice to make the load tolerable for the periodontium. (See Fig. 6-69.)

Such a distribution of abutments produces the "so-called 'tripod effect,' which means that a tipping force will act as a well tolerated intrusive force upon one or more of the abutments."* In other words, in splinting anterior teeth include a tooth distal to each cuspid (this prevents faciolingual and anteroposterior tipping movements and prevents excessive lateral forces), and when splinting the posterior segment extend the splint anteriorly beyond the cuspid to include at least the lateral incisor, but better still the lateral and central incisors (this prevents faciolingual movement of the splint) (Fig. 6-70).

---

*From Ramfjord, Sigurd P., and Ash, Major M., Jr.: Occlusion, ed. 2, Philadelphia, 1971, W. B. Saunders Co.

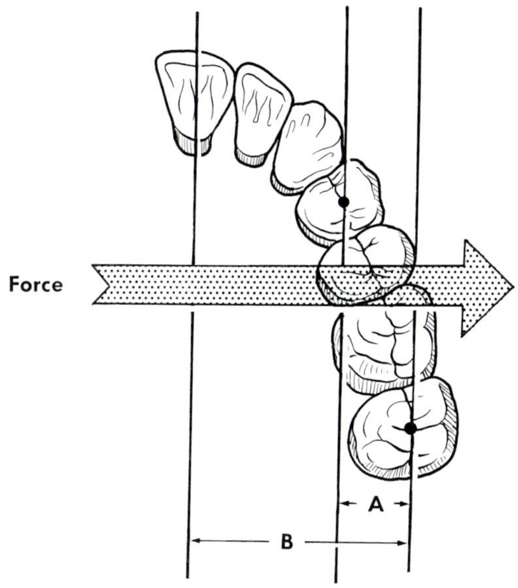

Fig. 6-69. Resistance to buccolingual force is relatively poor when splint runs from first bicuspid to second molar because of small distance, *A,* in buccolingual direction between second molar and first bicuspid. When splint is extended to central incisor, effective buccolingual distance is increased to *B,* which is much greater than *A,* and therefore provides superior resistance to force in lateral (buccolingual) direction. (Redrawn from Simring, Marvin, and Thaller, Jack L.: J.A.D.A. **53:**429-434, 1956.)

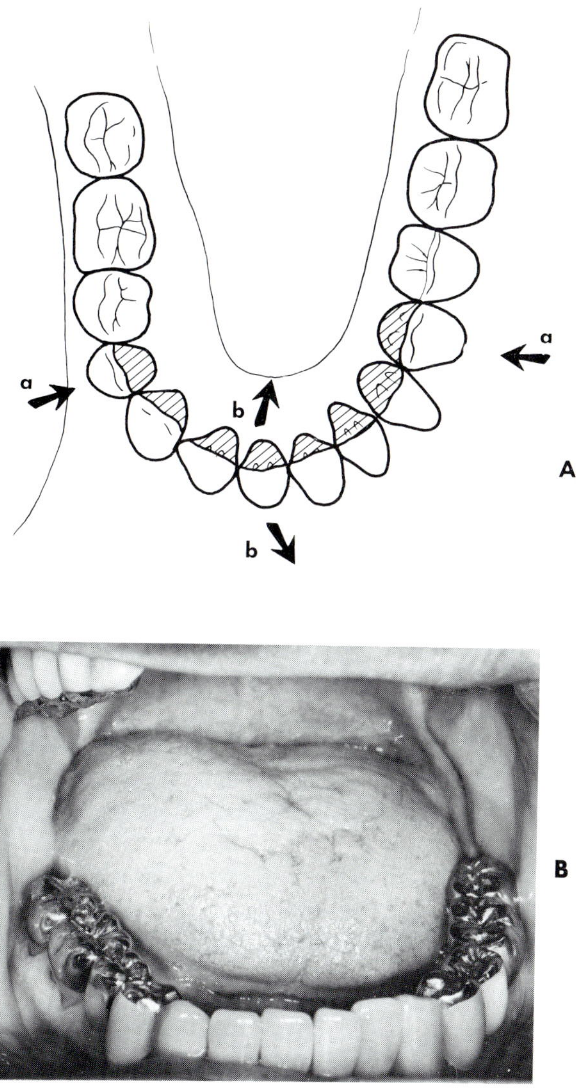

Fig. 6-70. A, In splinting anterior teeth include a tooth distal to each cuspid. This provides superior resistance to force in lateral (faciolingual) direction and anteroposterior tipping. **B,** Case from practice. Anterior splint using cuspid, first bicuspid (right and left) as abutments.

Integrating the advantages of cross-arch splinting and vertical endodontic endosseous splinting is biologically and physiologically sound and beneficial.

Keep in mind that (1) when only one tooth in a splint is traumatized, the periodontium of all the splinted teeth suffers (Fig. 6-71), (2) a sufficient number of firm teeth should be included in the splint, if possible, (3) the slight compression of the mandible of about 0.5 mm. in wide opening of the jaw does not seem to affect splints on the teeth,[67] (4) if roots are too close together, it is impossible to achieve periodontal health in the interproximal areas after splinting, (5) there is a tendency for teeth that are rather loose to move slightly from the pressure of cementation at the time of the seating of the splint (examine periodically for cement "wash-outs"), (6) it is always important to provide sufficient overjet with a deep overbite so that the patient can do unrestricted lateral excursions (to prevent a broken splint, splint movement, muscle or temporomandibular joint pain, etc.).

In selected cases it may be possible to achieve bilateral splint action by means of a removable palatal strap, instead of the customary anterior fixed splints. This permits bilateral stabilization of the posterior segments in the absence of anterior tooth restoration. The palatal strap can be removed when stabilization takes place, and the "female attachments" can be filled in.

TYPES

TEMPORARY OR PROVISIONAL SPLINTS

Provisional, or "healing," splints are employed for a limited period of time (1) to aid healing by

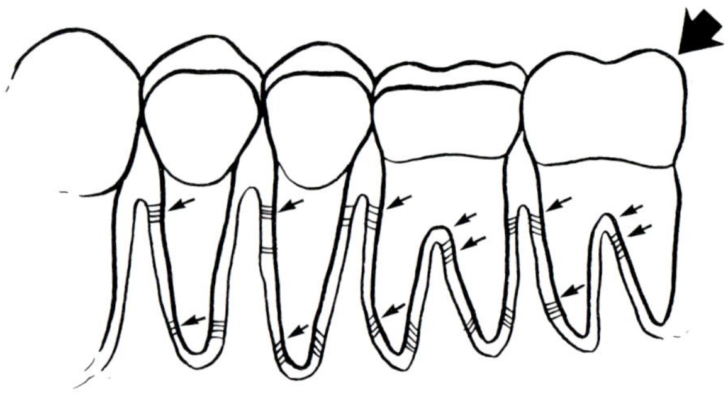

Fig. 6-71. Premature contact on one tooth in splint injures periodontium of all splinted teeth. Direction of transmitted injurious force is indicated by large arrow. (Redrawn from Stein, R. Sheldon: Perio-therapy guidelines, Dent. Times, October, 1964.)

limiting the mobility of the healing tissues, (2) to immobilize and relieve the periodontium about to undergo periodontal surgery, and (3) to assist in determining the prognosis of questionable teeth. Can changes in the attachment apparatus caused by occlusal traumatism be corrected and the teeth be stabilized in function by these means of periodontal surgery and stabilization and reorientation of force and stress? Will the periodontal ligament space remain abnormally wide, and will the teeth remain mobile? Even though the provisional splint has been cemented with zinc oxide—eugenol cement for a minimum of 2 months, has pulpal repair taken place? Will bite guards be necessary to overcome or minimize habit patterns—or can these habits be overcome? Is the patient cooperative in home care?

Above all, remember this: provisional splints tell us if the case will be a success or a failure.

PERMANENT SPLINTS

Permanent splints serve as constant adjuncts to the maintenance of periodontal health. They are employed when the periodontal support has been lost so that ordinary physiologic forces may not become injurious. The square area of attachment apparatus in relation to span and function must be "shored up." Complete fixation will secure the necessary stability.

TELESCOPIC SPLINTING

Telescoping is the process of fitting a full coverage primary casting, or coping, to a prepared tooth and then placing a secondary casting, or superstructure, over the primary casting.[68] It is not necessary to parallel the tooth preparations, but the copings must be paralleled. The tooth preparation is made along the direction of the inclination of the tooth without jeopardizing the pulp when teeth are tilted and it is difficult to obtain parallelism of preparations.

The telescopic principle of splinting, as explained and demonstrated to me by Morris Feder about 15 years ago, has been of inestimable assistance in the handling of many cases requiring periodontal prosthesis. Frictional irritation of the dentin during removal and reseating of the permanent splint, opening and spreading of margins caused by repeated removals of the splint with the reverse hammer, etc., "wash-outs" and ensuing caries, and even complete destruction of the coronal portion caused in great part by lack of parallelism of abutment teeth and improper occlusal relations, but also by the fact that temporary cement lacks the rigidity and durability to meet conditions of stress and flexure to which long multiunit restorations are subjected, etc., have been some of the drawbacks to the one-piece bilateral splint. It must be remembered, too, that permanent cementation of this type of splint is quite a task to accomplish, and, even if this is possible, the problem of removal after permanent cementation can be done only with almost complete mutilation of the splint. In patients requiring periodontal prosthesis, removal of the splints at times for alleviation of symptoms or for repair to individual teeth or tissues is not only probable, but also very possible in many cases of recent date or of many years' standing.

Primary casting or coping

FABRICATION OF COPING

This coping affords tooth protection because it is permanently cemented, thereby avoiding some of the bad effects of the one-piece, temporarily cemented splint as previously mentioned. However, for the prepared tooth to be protected from sensitivity and caries the primary coping must be constructed and fitted properly.

These copings are constructed with parallel vertical walls to ensure accurate seating of the superstructure and to prevent movement of the teeth to conform to the prosthesis. This coping is critical since it must fit the tooth accurately and must create a receptive condition for the superstructure (Fig. 6-72).[69,70]

A shoulder is made around the gingival margin of the coping. On proximal surfaces the shoulder is coronal to the gingival papilla, which is protected by the contour and position of the shoulder and the solder joints. On the lingual surface the shoulder is coronal to the gingival margin, and this holds true for the

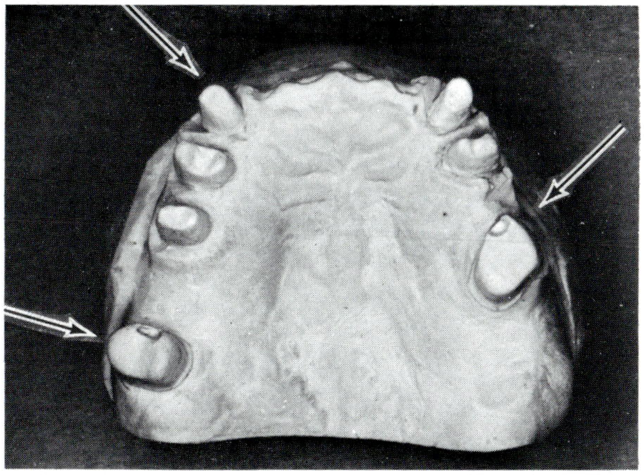

Fig. 6-72. Copings (arrows) constructed to aid in parallelism. Cervical third area must be properly contoured and marginal fit must be accurate.

facial surface, with the possible exception of the upper anterior teeth where the margin extends to, or slightly under, the gingiva.

In other words, the shoulder in the coping is supragingival on the lingual and interproximal surfaces, and in some instances on the facial surface a chamfer which blends with the interproximal shoulder is developed. A shallow groove is made around the coping at the junction of the vertical walls and the shoulder to obtain better interlocking (Fig. 6-73). Because of the parallel walls of the copings and the slight groove in the shoulder, likelihood of rotation of the superstructure on the copings is prevented and retention is provided.

The primary copings are waxed as thin as possible, the cast, with waxed dies, is positioned on the surveyor table, and the surveyor, with appropriate tools, is used to obtain the correct taper of the waxed copings for adjacent parallelism. Marginal limits should be established and the correct anatomic form should exist at the cervical third so that the recreation of pathology is avoided.

The wax patterns are then sprued, invested, and cast. After the castings are recovered and placed on their respective dies in the "working cast," they are rechecked on the surveyor for possible undercuts, parallelism, and correct amount of taper, and any corrections are made by drilling with the proper bur or stone, which is aligned in the handpiece holder attached to the surveyor.

Recheck the anatomic contour of the finished castings at the important cervical third area, finish the margins with great care, and polish this area very

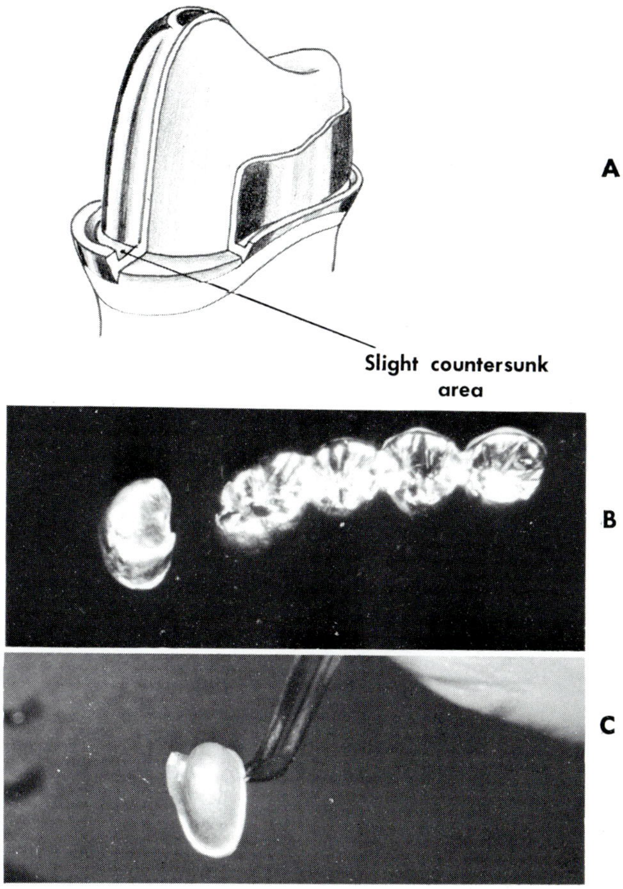

Fig. 6-73. A, A shoulder is made around gingival margin of coping. A shallow groove is made around coping at junction of vertical walls and shoulder to obtain better interlocking. **B,** A fixed splint requiring use of a coping for proper seating of bridge to prevent movement of teeth to conform to prosthesis. **C,** Proper development of proximal surface to avoid impingement on interdental papilla and still obtain good solder joint.

thoroughly. Copings are left as individual units, splinting being provided by the superstructure. However, the soldering of adjacent copings allows for additional support for mobile teeth. (See Fig. 6-74.)

The copings are then seated on their respective tooth preparations and checked out for marginal fit and gingival contour, after which hinge-bow transfer, centric relation bites, and overall plaster impressions are taken for construction of casts and mounting on an adjustable articulator for the construction of the superstructure.

The superstructure is constructed in sections, making use of the principle of "cross-linkage" (Fig. 6-75). By cross-linkage of abutments over soldered copings, a bilateral splint can be divided into two or

A

B

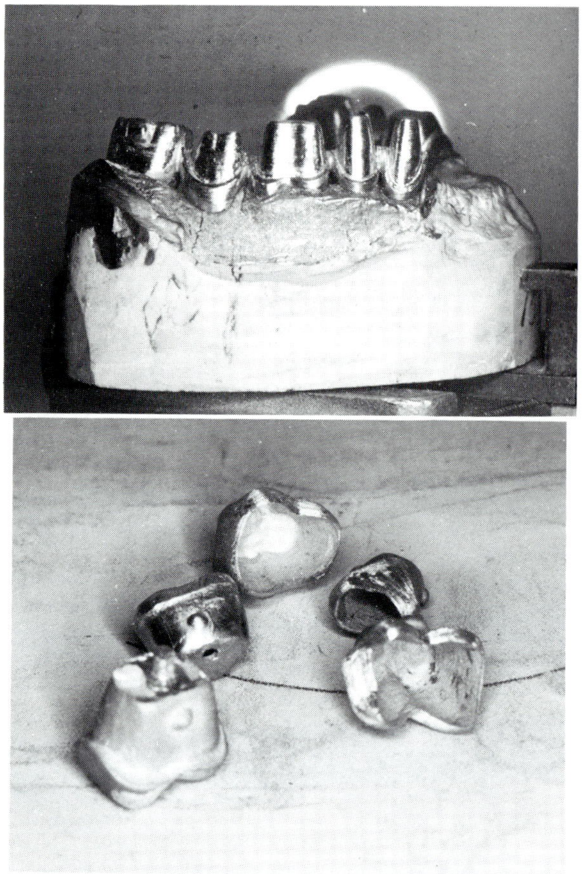

Fig. 6-74. A, Copings being milled for paralleling of walls and development of shoulder. Note proper positioning of solder joints to avoid crowding out of interdental papillae. **B,** A series of copings. (**A** courtesy Morris Feder, Philadelphia, Pa.)

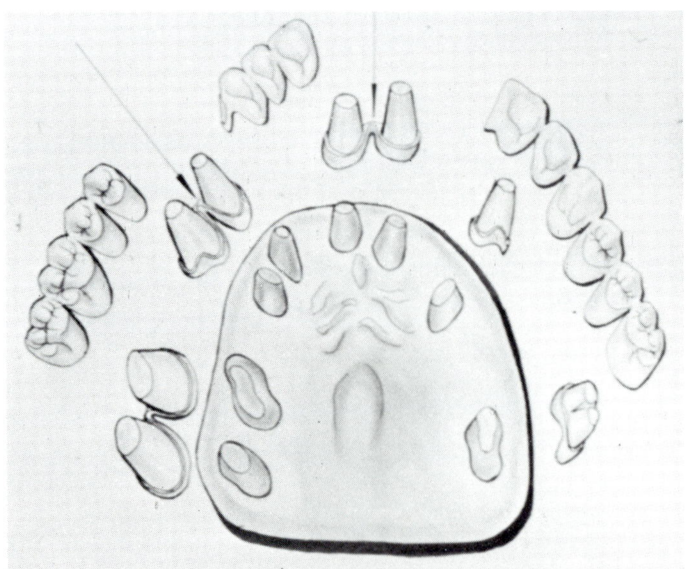

Fig. 6-75. Principle of cross-linkage. A bilateral splint divided into several small units and still retaining advantages of fixed splinting around arch. (Courtesy Morris Feder, Philadelphia, Pa.)

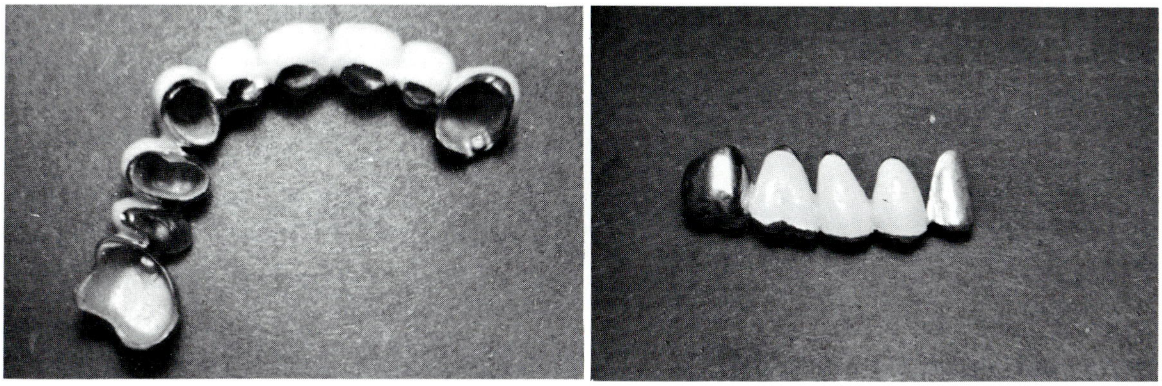

Fig. 6-76. Entire arch was splinted with two components in which a solderless joint was used to unite sections.

three small units and still retain the advantages of fixed splinting around the arch. "Three separate overlays effectively unite the entire arch by overlapping the copings that are soldered where the sections of the superstructure are not soldered."* The path of insertion of these sections are developed in the laboratory on the "working cast."

This type of splinting permits stabilization when teeth are in malposition and not parallel, provides effective resistance to occlusal forces in all directions, and allows for any section of the splint to be removed for repair and maintenance, such as renovation of veneer facings, creation of pontics if and when it becomes necessary (extraction site is permitted to heal and then the superstructural crown is modified into a pontic by reshaping it and processing acrylic into it), in endodontic therapy, etc.

Sectional splints

As previously mentioned, it is difficult and hazardous to cement full arch splints in one piece, regardless of whether partial or full coverage retainers are used. Therefore, the entire arch should be splinted with two or three components in the splint (as pointed out in section on telescopic splinting) where a solderless joint can be used to unite the components (Fig. 6-76). Use also can be made of a semirigid joint provided by a key and key-way, or a semiprecision or precision attachment in cases requiring the union of components of a splint, in which the support is adequate and the mobility of the teeth is not marked (Fig. 6-77).

*From Prichard, John, and Feder, Morris: A modern adaptation of the telescopic principle in periodontal prosthesis, J. Periodontol. **33:**360-364, 1962.

Semirigid or precision attachment connections between various parts of the splint rank next to fixed rigid splints in stability and controlled stress distribution. These connections should, if possible, be made deep, parallel, and as rigid as possible. Interlocking joints provide the desired splinting effect, and positive assurance should be given that abutment castings are fully seated upon cementation.

Some very capable dentists feel that in full arch splinting, when indicated, there should be a stressbreaker behind each cuspid so that the anterior teeth may be used without disturbing the posterior teeth and the posterior teeth can be used without pumping and rocking the anterior teeth.

Cementation

The primary copings are cemented with permanent cement as individual or coupled units, but not before the superstructure has been completed and the whole case has been fitted and checked out for all necessary periodontal and restorative conditions. This is accomplished by seating the case (copings and superstructure) with zinc oxide powder (Moyco) and petroleum jelly for at least a period of 2 weeks. If on removal of copings and superstructure this paste is white and intact in all castings and gingival tissues appear healthy, the cementation of the primary copings with a permanent type of cement (oxyphosphate of zinc cement, E.B.A., Caulk's Zebacem) can be done (see discussion on cementation in Chapter 12).

The superstructure is cemented with a zinc oxide–eugenol temporary cement.

Ample vertical space for better retention of the primary copings and space for two castings, as well as ample tooth reduction facially to accommodate two castings and veneering material, must be con-

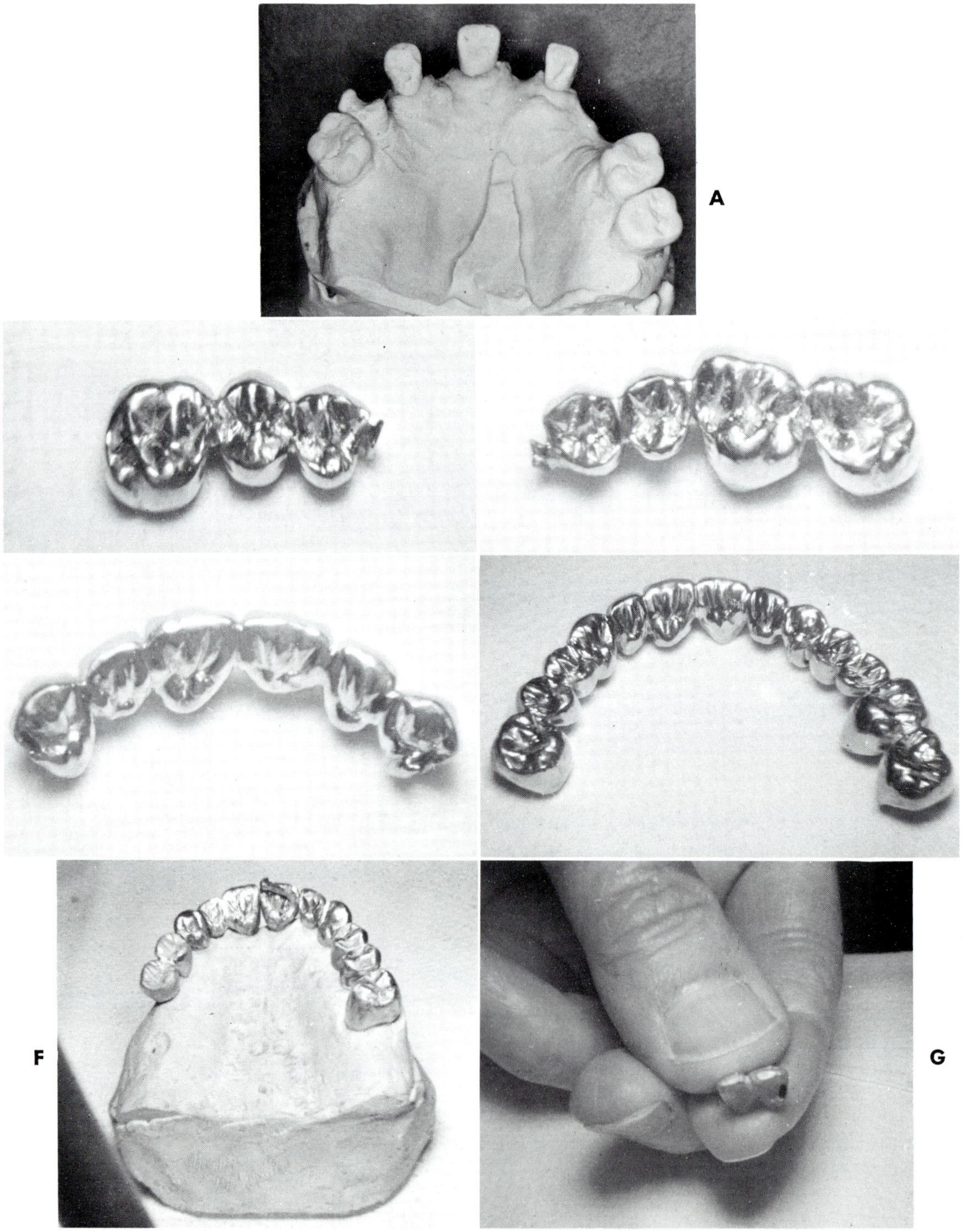

A B C D E F G

Fig. 6-77. A to **E,** Semirigid joints provided by precision attachments. **F** to **I,** A key and key-way.

H

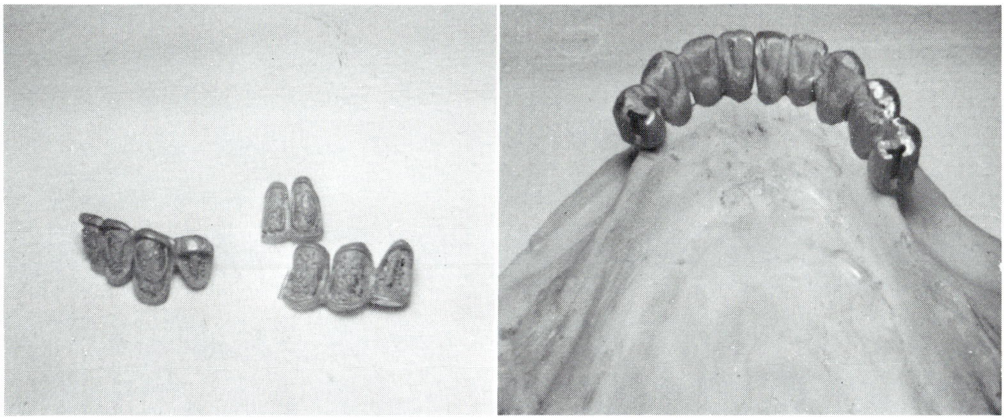

I

Fig. 6-77, cont'd. For legend see opposite page.

sidered seriously. This requirement presents a problem with patients with short teeth or with crowded, small, lower anterior teeth.

Splinting of any nature creates a problem of maintaining good oral hygiene. The most thorough practice of oral physiotherapy must be utilized by the patient, with constant appraisal by the dentist.

Thorough clinical and roentgenographic examinations are necessary for a continual evaluation of the situation and its progress and prognosis.

If all of this—diagnosis and treatment planning, treatment procedures, postoperative care—is done thoroughly, the patient can and does in many, many instances retain his teeth for a number of years, making it worthy of the expenditure of time, energy, worry, and money involved in these cases of periodontal prosthesis.

In summation let us remember that, in splinting, the stabilization and fixation of mobile teeth occur. The teeth act together in such a way that they support one another and distribute and redirect forces among themselves. The shape of the dental arch, the position of the teeth within the arch, and the quality and amount of remaining alveolar bone are other important factors influencing the effectiveness of this procedure, which also includes the mobility patterns of the teeth, crown-to-root ratio, shape and size of the roots of the teeth, length of the edentulous space, and occlusal requirements. Buccolingual, mesiodistal, vertical, and rotational movements can be counteracted.

Splinting should not be visualized as complete elimination of functional movements because, even though in the most rigid of splints we have eliminated forces in the horizontal direction, we still have not eliminated forces in the direction of the long axes of the teeth. The functional stimuli that are exerted in the long axes are enough to keep the supporting tissues in good functional condition, and splinting does not stop functional stimulation.

But by all means keep foremost in your mind that, although the concept of splinting is a very important adjunct in therapy, its advantages should not be abused nor should its presence be substituted for proper occlusal relations. This principle of splinting should be combined, for maximum benefits, with altered coronal surfaces, and the teeth should be in functional harmony with the mandibular movements.

Jerge[66] has told us that splinting teeth imposes a totally unnatural condition on the sensory mechanism of the teeth. Under ordinary conditions periodontal ligament receptors of one tooth are not excited by pressure on another tooth 3 or 4 cm. away or by one on the opposite side of the dental arch. The need of more research along these lines is certainly urgent.

Promiscuous use of splinting is not recommended. If mobile teeth can be retained in proper position and function without splinting, in spite of the excessive loss of supporting bone, well and good, but in cases categorized as in need of periodontal prosthesis, which I have seen and treated, this is not possible. The entire dental mechanism has been interfered with, and experience has taught us that the dental mechanism can survive in a different environment. Both full coverage and splinting are indicated in these cases.

Therapy must be focused on measures that will aid in the recovery to health of the periodontal tissues and in the minimizing of the overall loss of support as it affects function on the teeth.

RESTORATIVE PROCEDURES

Acrylic resin masks

VALUE OF MASKS

The removal of gingival tissues and alveolar bone, with its aftermath of exposed roots, lengthened clinical crowns, and enlarged interproximal embrasures, in the treatment of periodontal disease can leave, in many instances, unsightly oral structures, especially in the upper anterior region, from upper right second bicuspid to upper left second bicuspid. Besides the difficulty in the maintenance of proper mouth hygiene, the problem of esthetics, which is of such psychologic importance to the patient, cannot be taken lightly.

The solution to this problem is an acrylic resin mask, which is not difficult to construct and which serves the following purposes: (1) provides good esthetic effect and psychologic comfort, (2) gives the lengthened clinical crown a more normal appearance by covering the exposed roots, (3) prevents tendency of upper lip from being caught in the concavity produced by the abnormally long incisors, (4) prevents excessive accumulation of foodstuffs in the enlarged interproximal embrasures, and (5) can be inserted and removed with little effort and is easily cleaned.[71]

TECHNIQUE OF CONSTRUCTION

1. After a thorough prophylaxis, take an alginate impression of the upper arch, being sure to obtain an accurate reproduction of the labial and buccal gingival tissues, especially in the area of the right second bicuspid to the left second bicuspid. Pour a stone cast (Fig. 6-78, *A*).

2. Make an acrylic palatal core that extends slightly into the interproximal embrasures from the lingual side to prevent the impression material from entering the embrasures from the labial and buccal sides too deeply when the final impression is made.

3. An acrylic resin impression tray is made (Fig. 6-78, *B*) for the labial and buccal surfaces. This is the tray that will give us a detailed impression of the teeth, the interproximal embrasures, and gingival tissues. Both the palatal core and impression tray are made of cold-cure acrylic resin.

4. With the palatal core in position, a proper mix of alginate impression material is placed in the specially constructed acrylic resin tray, and an impression is taken, positioning the tray facially. Examination of the completed impression should record in exact detail the labial and buccal surfaces of the teeth, including the incisal and occlusal edges from right

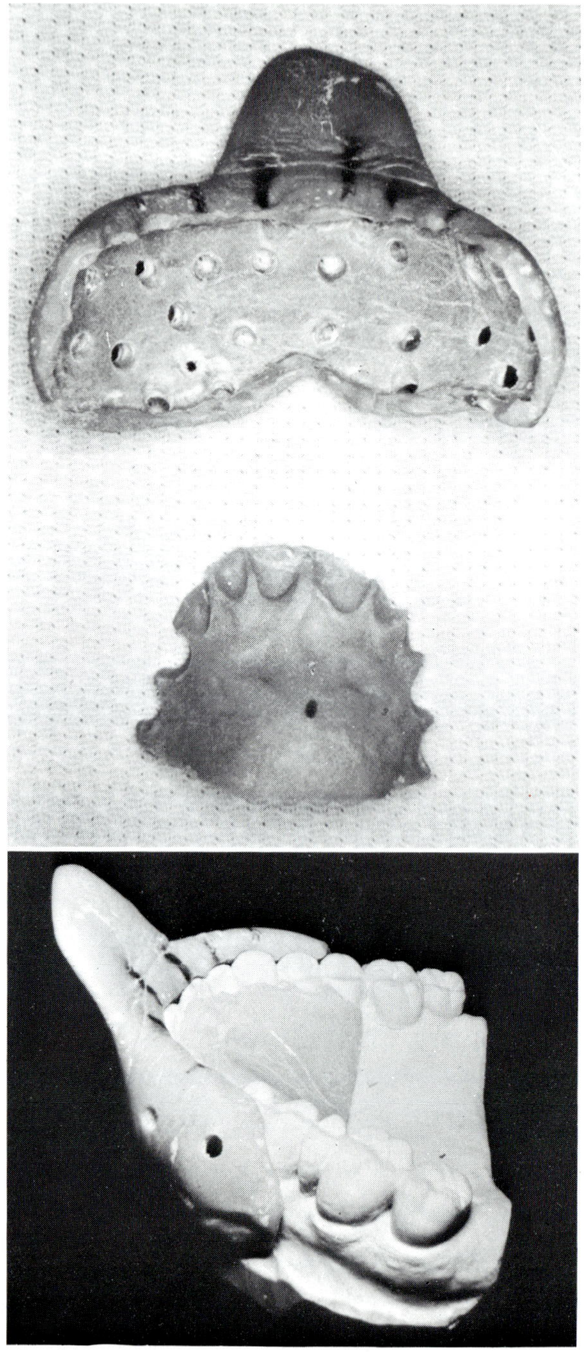

A

B

Fig. 6-78. Construction of an acrylic resin mask. **A,** A stone cast, which has been made from good alginate impression, is used to make palatal core, which extends slightly into interproximal embrasures from lingual side to prevent impression material from entering embrasures from labial and buccal surface too deeply when final impression is made. **B,** A facially positioned acrylic resin impression tray is made also.

A

B

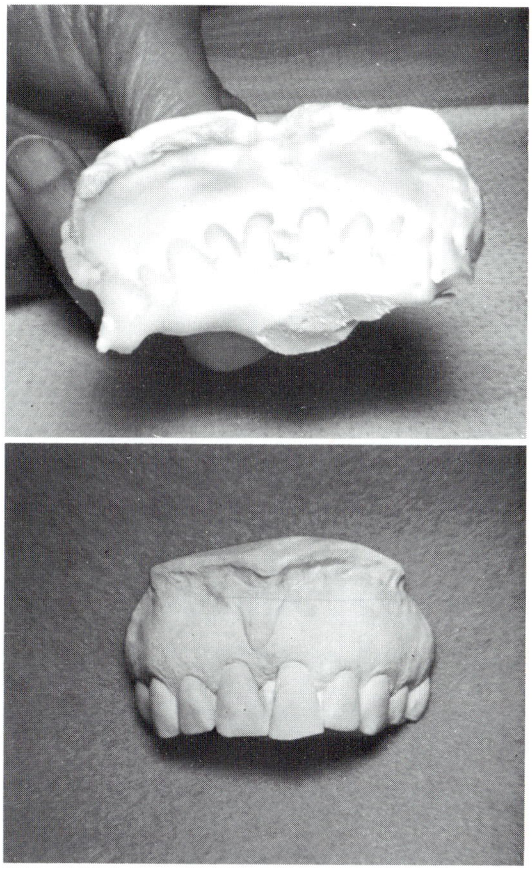

Fig. 6-79. A, Alginate impression taken in specially constructed tray (be sure palatal core is in position). **B,** An accurate stone cast made from impression.

A

B

C

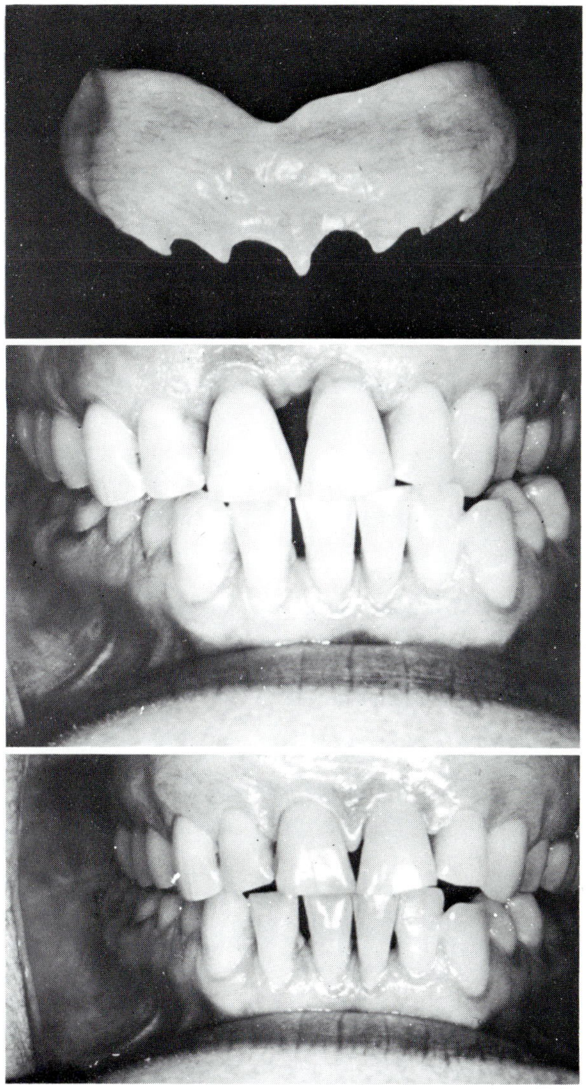

Fig. 6-81. A, Completed mask—projections of mask slip into embrasures and hold it in place. **B** and **C,** Preoperative and postoperative photographs of case.

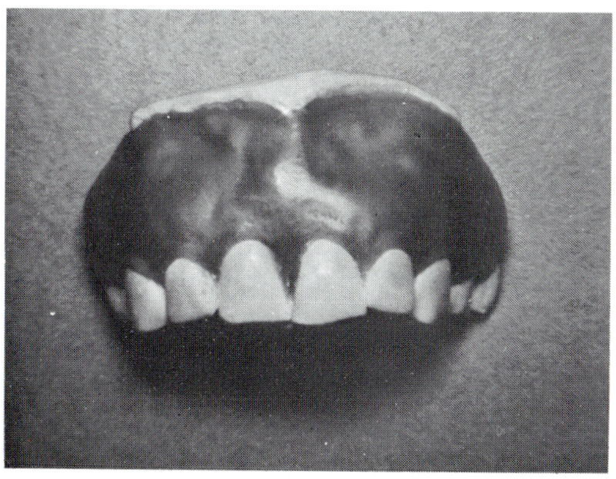

Fig. 6-80. Acrylic resin mask waxed and carved.

second bicuspid to left second bicuspid, the interproximal embrasures, labial and buccal gingival tissues, and frenum. An accurate stone cast is made from this impression (Fig. 6-79).

5. The acrylic resin mask is waxed and carved (Fig. 6-80) and processed in heat-cured acrylic resin, after which it is refitted on a duplicate cast, stippled, and thoroughly polished.

The projections of the plastic mask into the embrasures hold the appliance in position without the aid of any other form of retention (Fig. 6-81).

Pontics

BASIC REQUIREMENTS OF PONTIC DESIGN

A pontic not only restores a missing tooth, but also maintains oral function in a physiologic and esthetic manner. The pontic must be of proper mechanical and cosmetic design, and must also be acceptable to the biologic environment in which it functions. It should provide comfort and support to the adjacent tissues.

Pontic form is very important. It must include in the topographic anatomy of the restoration the basic convexities, concavities, cusp form, and groove outlines. In other words, proper contour and form of the entire pontic must be developed. Its contour and form must ensure proper sanitation and stimulation of the mucosa. Conformation of the gingival contacting area of the pontic must not deny access of stimulation to the underlying gingival tissue because this tissue must be subjected to stimulation to have its health maintained. This is provided by the contact of food, tongue, cheek, and oral hygiene aids if embrasures are incorporated properly for the passage of this food and the mechanical stimulation of the edentulous mucosa.

Stein[72] has the following to say as to the basic requirements that must be met in the design of pontics:

1. Pontics must restore the proper degree of function. The functional relationships of the cusps is the most critical consideration in the design of the occlusal surface of pontics. Because of the fact that the cusps should be in harmony with the functional pattern of the entire dentition, the necessity for the proper recording and transferring of mandibular relations becomes more obvious. It is to obviate the need to narrow or limit the coronal width, that is, make it arbitrarily two thirds or less of the faciolingual occlusal width even when the periodontal support and the resultant leverage to the roots are not ideal. Reduction in occlusal width would come at the expense of centric contact, which, by all means, should not be sacrificed. The fixed splint should be constructed anatomically and physiologically correct, thereby allowing for a meticulous distribution and direction of stress to all the roots of the teeth and to the residual ridges.

2. The secondary functional demands of esthetics, phonetics, and the protective role of food deflection must be satisfied by the conformation of the faciolingual surfaces.

3. Specific posterior pontic design (Fig. 6-82):

"A correctly designed posterior pontic should have the following characteristics:

a. "All surfaces should be convex, smooth, and properly finished.
b. "Contact with the buccal contiguous slope should be minimal (pinpoint) and pressure-free (modified ridge lap).
c. "The occlusal table must be in functional harmony with the occlusion of all of the teeth.
d. "The buccal and lingual shunting mechanisms should conform to those of the adjacent teeth.
e. "The over-all length buccal surface should be

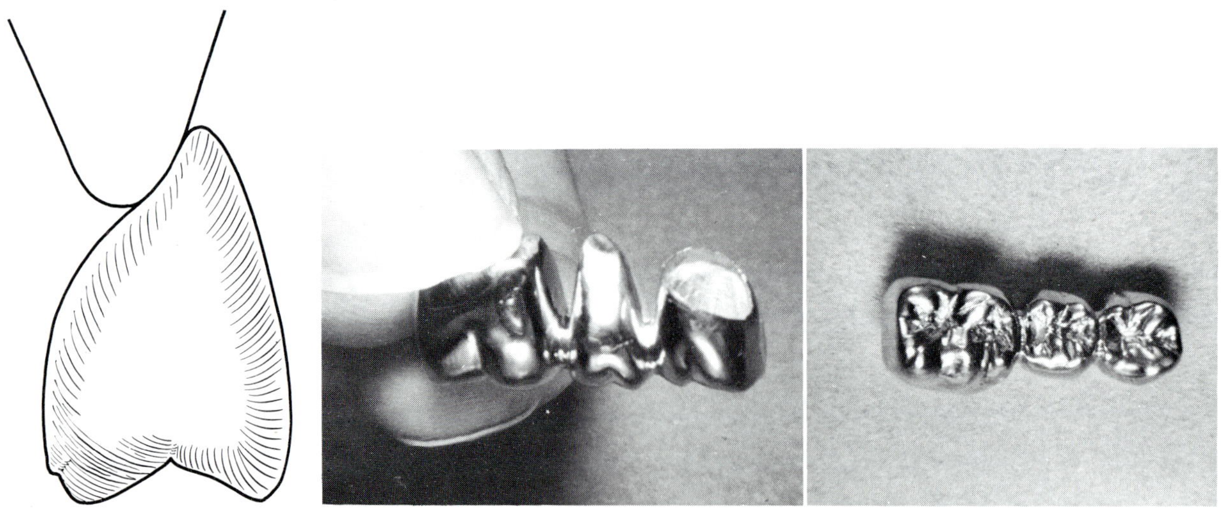

A B C

Fig. 6-82. A, Modified ridge-lap type of pontic. **B** and **C,** Properly developed posterior pontic—lingual and modified ridge-lap view and occlusal view.

equal to that of the adjacent abutments or pontics."*

4. Specific anterior pontic design:

"A correctly designed anterior pontic should have the following characteristics:

a. "All surfaces should be convex, smooth, and properly finished.
b. "Contact with the labial mucosa should be minimal (pinpoint) and pressure free (lap facing). Esthetics may require a long area of contact to prevent the 'black space' appearance if the residual ridge is excessively resorbed.
c. "The lingual contour should be in harmony with adjacent teeth or pontics."*

The design of the pontic is the important factor in preventing inflammatory reactions beneath pontics, provided that, in addition to design, all surfaces are properly polished so that surface smoothness is attained. Pontics should have minimal contact with the ridge and should cover as little of the ridge as possible within the demands of esthetics and comfort. Where multiple pontics are to be placed, use ridge-lap type instead of bullet-nose pontics because there is less food retention. The ridge-lap type of pontic follows the facial contour of the ridge to the crest, where it joins the lingual surface. The lingual surface of the pontic should follow the normal tooth form for a distance of approximately half of its occlusogingival length and then should taper in a convex line to meet the facial portion at the crest of the ridge.

Hirshberg[73] has come to the conclusion, after considerable study and observation, that ridge-lap pontics were less desirable than spheroid or modified spheroid pontics in maintaining mucosal health since inflammation developed beneath them. In other words, the oral mucosa is more likely to remain healthy under spheroid or modified spheroid pontics than under ridge-lap pontics—"a deflective protective convexity over the lingual half of the alveolar crest appeared to decrease the amount of plaque accumulation"* (Fig. 6-83).

Eissmann[30] says that the sanitary contoured pontic could well serve as a standard concept for pontic design and be termed the "physiologically contoured" pontic. Its form offers the most favorable balance between comfort, support, and hygiene, and it could be related to various ridge conditions (average resorption; broad, blunted ridge; excessive resorption) (Fig. 6-84).

Never relieve the cast to get better pontic adaptation. It may result in pressure atrophy of the underlying ridge as well as periodontal breakdown on the teeth adjacent to the edentulous areas.

Inflammation from periodontal pockets into the adjacent edentulous mucosa is another important factor to be taken into consideration. This inflammation can extend for varying distances into this area, making it necessary to eliminate the inflammatory processes of both the diseased gingiva and the edentulous mucosa. When this treatment has been carried out, it will reestablish the healthy contour of

*From Stein, R. Sheldon: Pontic-residual ridge relationship: a research report, J. Prosthet. Dent. **16**:251-285, 1966.

*From Hirshberg, Saul M.: The relationship of oral hygiene to embrasure and pontic design—a preliminary study, J. Prosthet. Dent. **27**(1):26-38, 1972.

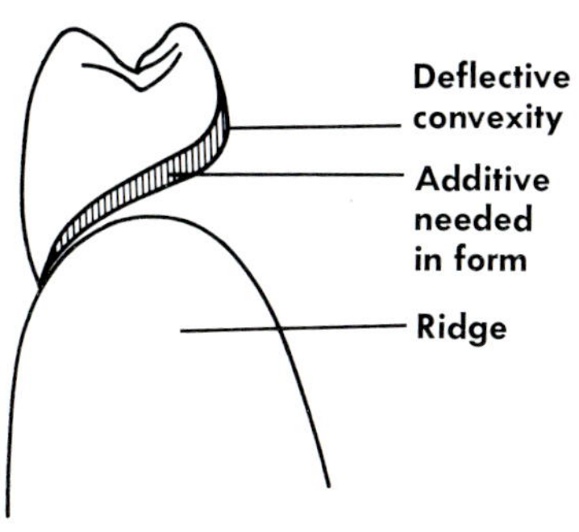

Fig. 6-83. A spheroid or modified spheroid pontic. (Redrawn from Hirshberg, Saul M.: J. Prosthet. Dent. **27**[1]:26-38, Jan. 1972.)

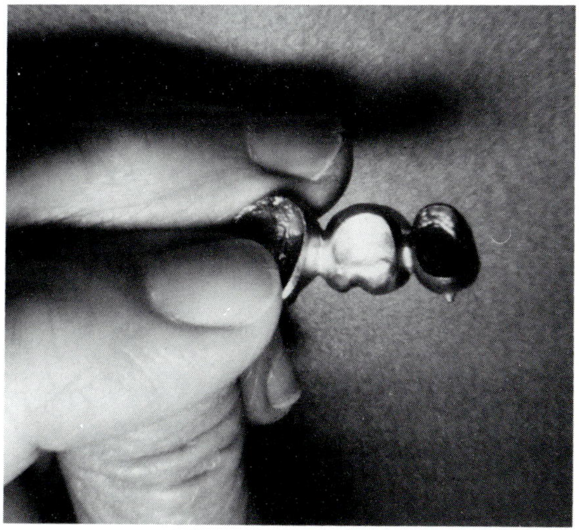

Fig. 6-84. A pontic form offering a balance between support, comfort, and hygiene.

the gingiva and adjacent mucosa. In other words, periodontal treatment should not be limited to only the elimination of periodontal pockets and the restoration of gingival health. It should also create the gingival-mucosal environment that is necessary for the proper function of fixed and removal partial prostheses.[72] In other words, edentulous mucosa must be treated so that it is smooth and attached firmly to the bone. If the tissue were fibrotic and peaked at distal and mesial papillary margins of the abutment teeth, the pontic would have to be radically modified to fit the available space, but by recontouring the edentulous mucosa and eliminating the peaked papillae, the pontic design can fulfill the requirements of function, esthetics, and oral hygiene.

SANITARY TYPE PONTIC

The sanitary type pontic reduces the risk of periodontal involvement. It consists of a cast occlusal surface, the undersurface of which is rounded or convex faciolingually. Food passes under this surface, cleansing the surface of the mucosa and gingiva. The rounded undersurface of the pontic and surrounding tissues also can be cleansed by rubbing it with a folded dental napkin. Because of esthetics, its use should be limited to the posterior region of the mouth.

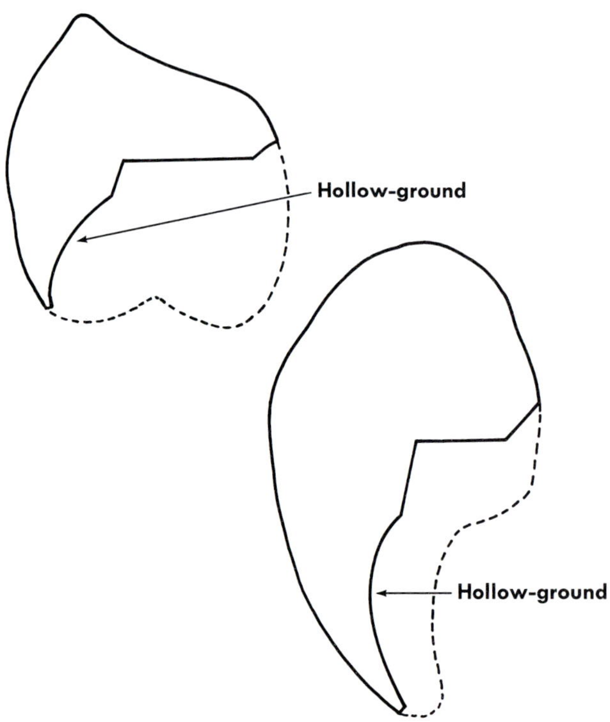

Fig. 6-85. Cross sections of hollow-ground facings showing bulk of metal with minimum display of gold.

PORCELAIN VENEERS

Porcelain is resistant to abrasion, dimensionally stable, and insoluble in oral fluids. It is biologically acceptable.

The elastic limit of porcelain is so low that fractures occur from extremely small shearing and impact forces.

A porcelain facing in combination with a gold backing creates the best pontic from a biomechanical standpoint. The porcelain must be in an area where there is neither tension nor compression. An optimal biomechanical design is our objective; facings break because basic principles of good design are violated. It is necessary to have sufficient gold to rigidly resist occlusal forces. Incisal and occlusal edges must be treated correctly. The gold backing must have sufficient bulk, distribution, strength, hardness, and correct shape to resist distortion in function, and all this is possible without an undue display of gold (Fig. 6-85). A properly formed backing prevents shearing forces

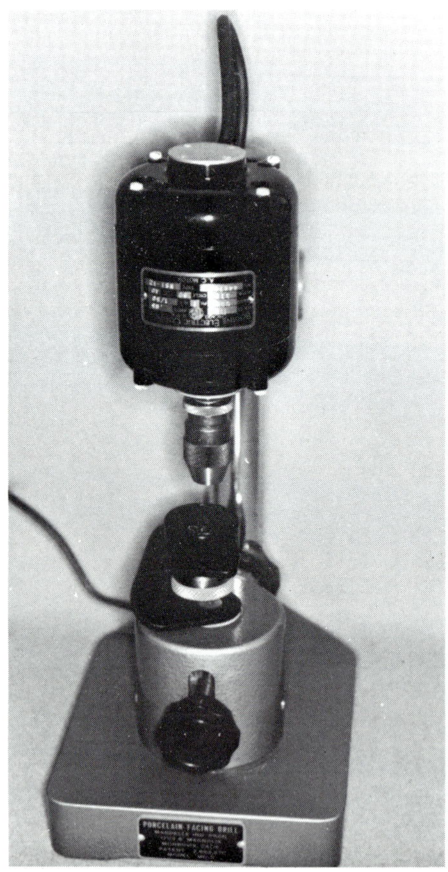

Fig. 6-86. Special drill press used in fabrication of reverse pin facing.

from being transmitted to the facing and thus eliminates failures caused by breakage. Use a gold that is sufficiently hard, such as a type 3 or 4 gold.

REVERSE PIN FACING

The reverse pin facing is fabricated from a porcelain denture tooth by means of a special porcelain drill press (Fig. 6-86).[74,75]

Since this type of facing is inserted into the backing from a horizontal direction, it can be modified on all six surfaces. Excellent design and esthetics can be obtained when using this type of facing. Many molds and shades are available. Porcelain can be added to the ridge-lap surface.[76]

Retention is secured over the entire lingual surface of the facing instead of by one or two pins that have

A

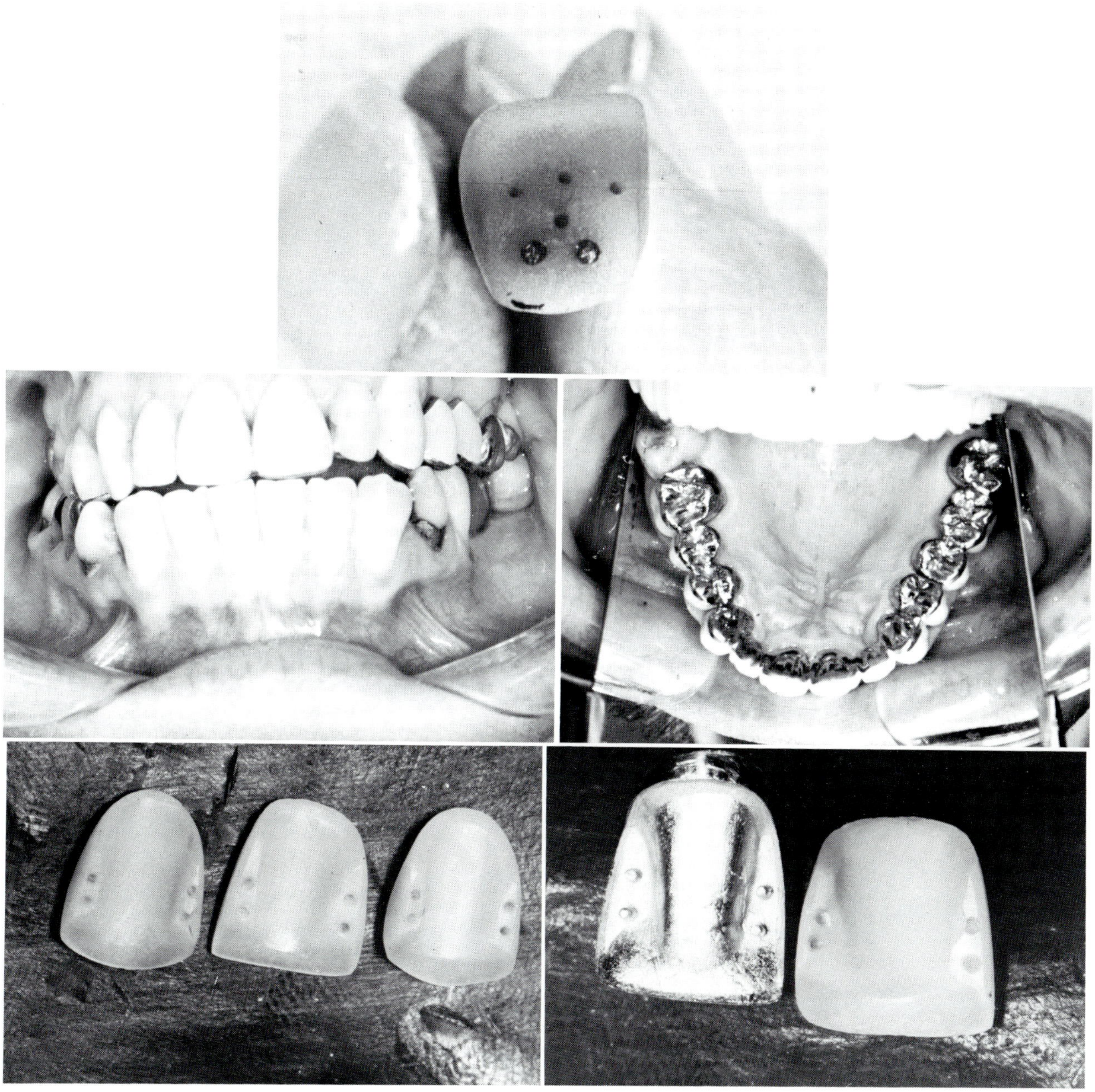

B

Fig. 6-87. A, Retention is secured over entire lingual surface of facing for pontic. Perlon pins are inserted into prepared holes (which are cut at an angle), wax-up completed, and casting made. This method is excellent for both pontics and veneer facings for crowns. **B,** Preparation of reverse pin facings for veneer crowns.

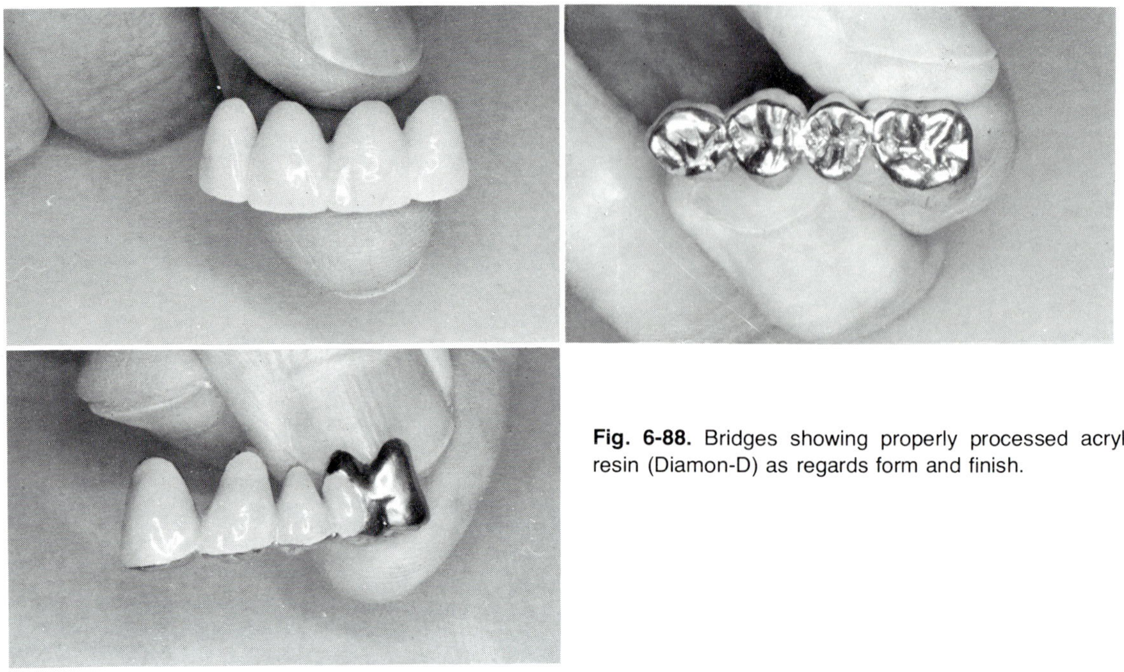

Fig. 6-88. Bridges showing properly processed acrylic resin (Diamon-D) as regards form and finish.

porcelain fused to them, which allows for more chance of creating lines of fracture (Fig. 6-87).

ACRYLIC RESIN VENEERS

Acrylic resin falls short in its ability to resist wear and abrasion and is not tolerated as well by the soft tissues as is porcelain. However, many periodontal prosthesis cases require the use of the best type of acrylic resins because of length of spans, mobility patterns, torque, etc., and the telescopic principle of splinting, which allows for ease of renovation of facings, is the answer to this big problem (Fig. 6-88).

FUNDAMENTAL PRINCIPLES FOR CANTILEVERED PONTICS

A pontic no wider mesiodistally than the average bicuspid may be cantilevered off the end of a multiunit bridge to prevent extrusion of opposing teeth (Fig. 6-89). Proper contour of such terminal pontics is most important because of the absence of protection from a proximal tooth, which increases the risk of food accumulation under the pontic. It is preferable for the cantilevered pontic to fit against the mucosa of the alveolar ridge—it is fairly easy to keep clean and comfortable to the tongue.

A minimum of two abutment teeth (if a cuspid or first molar can be one of the abutments so much the better) should be used to support the pontic. The exception is a winged lateral from a cuspid or a small space from a molar. (See Fig. 6-90.) Some prosthodontists are of the opinion that one or two pontics between the abutment teeth are preferable because this will increase the lever arm support (Fig. 6-91).

PROSTHETIC-PERIODONTAL TREATMENT PLANNING

Procedural integration

In many instances the nature of the procedures dealing with the treatment of deeply involved debilitated dentitions calls for a coordinated teamwork approach as regards the prosthodontist, periodontist, oral surgeon, orthodontist, and endodontist. Careful planning is of the utmost importance, and the prosthodontist, who should have an overall concept of these specialties, must assume the full responsibility of the supervision of the treatment and outcome of the case. This necessitates not only a logical sequence of treatment, but also a complete agreement of the procedural plan by all specialists that are involved in the case.

The ability to correlate diagnosis, pathology, and etiology to therapy is of paramount importance. An oral examination, medical history, complete series of roentgenograms, evaluation of psychogenic factors, and properly oriented study casts on an adjustable articulator are indispensable aids for a competent diagnosis and treatment plan. Correction of any nutritional deficiencies and other general health disturbances is undertaken with the assistance of the physician.

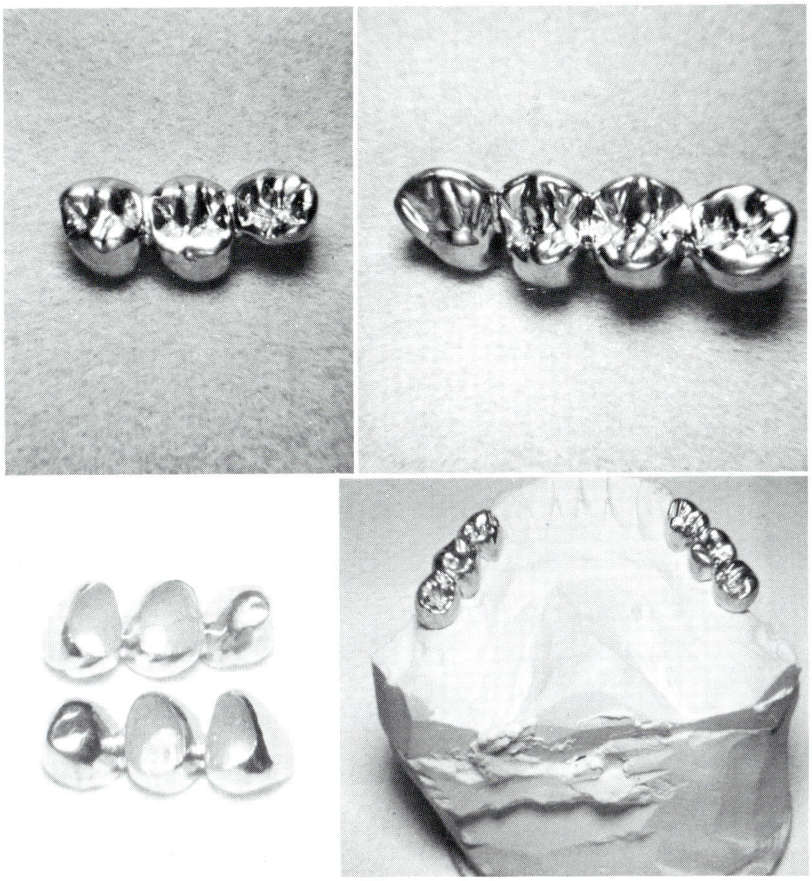

Fig. 6-89. Cantilevered pontics. Pontic is no wider mesiodistally than average bicuspid. Good contour is necessary, and in these cases cantilevered pontic should fit against mucosa of alveolar ridge since it is fairly easy to keep clean. It also will be comfortable to tongue.

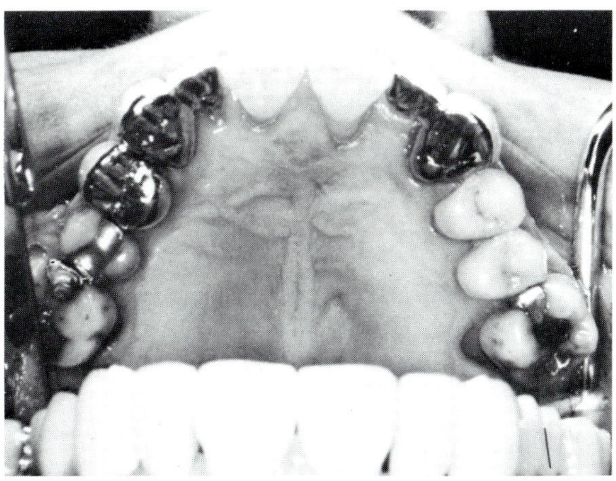

Fig. 6-90. Minimum of two abutment teeth should be used to support cantilevered pontic with exception of a winged lateral from a cuspid or very small space.

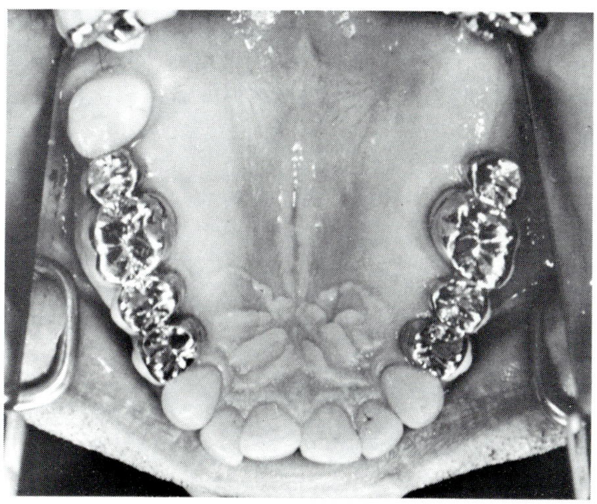

Fig. 6-91. One or two pontics between abutment teeth are preferable since this will increase lever arm support.

Carefully timed restorative and periodontal procedures can augment each other to provide superior treatment. A working plan following the outline below may be formulated[18]:

1. Scaling and/or curettage
2. Minor orthodontic movement
3. Occlusal adjustment of gross occlusal interferences
4. Temporary fixed splints
5. Periodontal surgery
6. Periodontal prosthesis
7. Bite guards (if indicated) for minimizing habit patterns
8. Oral hygiene program
9. Maintenance care

The dentition is to be restored to as nearly normal position and function as possible by construction of all restorations and replacements that may be required, giving careful consideration to the impaired supporting tissues of each tooth as well as the entire dentition.

Initial treatment

It is necessary to prepare the mouth for restorative procedures by creating the proper periodontal environment.

Initial periodontal therapy consists of a thorough scaling and/or curettage. All gross calcareous accumulations are removed, and as thorough a job as possible is done with root debridement of these deposits. Diseased cementum is removed, and curettage of the tissue side of the pocket is accomplished so that an environment that will promote healing is obtained. This is followed by a polishing of the tooth surfaces and the institution of physiotherapy. In some instances diastemas have closed after this initial treatment.

Although in involved cases this treatment may be only of a marginal nature, it is an important procedure because it reduces inflammation and allows for a better evaluation of the problem at hand. It, in conjunction with the roentgenograms and study casts, tells us if surgical procedures are necessary to fully eradicate any residual periodontal involvement. Probing of pockets and interradicular areas allows us to determine which teeth are hopelessly involved and are to be condemned to extraction, which can be treated by advanced periodontal methods, which may need root resection and endodontics, and whether elective endodontics can help us with the problems of parallelism, crown-to-root ratio, etc. Also, much can be learned about the patient's healing capacity, indications of rapidity of calculus formation and sordes accumulation, and his ability and motivation to carry out necessary home care. Another important factor to consider is that a field debrided of local irritants such as coronal and root calcareous deposits gives us an environment that allows for better and quicker healing after surgery, be it periodontal or removal of teeth.

Minor orthodontic corrections

Teeth that present a deficient axial relationship to basal bone, not allowing for correct distribution of forces over basal bone or poor contact relationships to adjacent teeth, should be corrected by orthodontic means before instituting any further periodontal therapy. Teeth must be positioned correctly to basal bone.

As previously stated (see discussion on orthodontics), when mass anchorage is required for proper alignment of the teeth, the patient should be treated by a trained orthodontist, but, when a tipping movement will suffice, malposed teeth often may be treated successfully by using a Hawley retainer or some modification of it, a Crozat appliance, grassline or steel wire ligatures, or rubber dam elastics.

Selective tooth grinding

Next in procedural sequence is selective tooth grinding for the relief of gross occlusal disharmonies. If orthodontic aids have not been used or are limited in their possibilities, the extent and nature of occlusal adjustment, which was indicated prior to tooth preparation, is directly related to tooth position. Extruded and drifted teeth must be corrected.

Temporary acrylic resin splints

Temporary acrylic resin splints are constructed in advance of the contemplated periodontal surgery.

Impressions (alginate, hydrocolloid, rubber base) are taken for the construction of casts, as are a hinge-bow transfer for correct orientation of the upper cast on the adjustable articulator and centric relation bites for the mounting of the lower cast by the split-cast method. The stone teeth on the casts are prepared (with burs and stones) for the construction of temporary acrylic resin splint "shells," which will be rebased upon completion of tooth preparations (Chapter 9).

This type of appliance (temporary splint) is necessary in many instances before advanced periodontal therapy for elimination of architectural deformities of the periodontium is started because it stabilizes mobile teeth and affords an immediate opportunity to improve the functional tooth relations of the dentition by changing the direction and distribution of stress on the teeth. It can serve also as a matrix for holding a surgical pack following periodontal surgery.

Osseous resection also can be used, at the time of surgery, to lengthen clinical crowns so that better retention is provided for the retainers, but only if a favorable crown-to-root ratio will still obtain.

Preliminary tooth preparations

In cases of advanced periodontal disease the full coverage preparation and restoration is the one of choice because of the many requirements it is able to fulfill. Despite the importance of tooth structure conservation, the preservation of the supporting structures of the teeth is of prime importance. With changed embrasures, architectural form, and gingival position, only full coverage can be considered.

However, in cases exhibiting mild or moderately advanced periodontal involvement, showing facial and lingual contours that are intact and physiologic and not in need of bilateral splinting, indications and contraindications for the use of full coverage restorations have to be considered. In my opinion these are not the type of cases designated in the category of periodontal prosthesis (a widespread devastating generalized loss of the supporting periodontal structures accompanied by extensive pocket depth and varying degrees of mobility patterns calling for restorative treatment as an adjunct to periodontal therapy), but this is a matter of personal opinion, and I do not care to leave the impression that all patients in need of mouth rehabilitation call for the use of full coverage.

The teeth should be carefully prepared, ending the preparation just short of the gingival line. Retentive preparations should be made (Chapter 8). The preparation of the final marginal finish line and other necessary preparation alterations will be made after complete periodontal healing and before impressions for the final restorations are made.

Treatment of preprepared acrylic resin "shell" splints

Preprepared acrylic resin "shell" splints, made from preoperative casts (Chapter 9), are fitted, and any necessary adjustments for complete seating and occlusion are made prior to the rebasing procedure.

Make a mix of acrylic resin, place this material, when ready, into the splint, and reseat the splint, having the patient close in centric closure—on a piece of tinfoil if there is an opposing acrylic splint—to prevent the surplus acrylic resin material from uniting the two splints. Press the facial and lingual excess material in a gingival direction, molding it to the prepared tooth surfaces with moistened fingers. As the material begins to set adapt it more densely subgingivally and interproximally to the prepared teeth with a flat-bladed instrument, which is coated with splint lube to assure accurate registration of the marginal areas. Keep moving the splint up and down on the prepared teeth during the setting of the rebase material to break away from any undercut areas, especially in areas beyond the preparations. After complete set has taken place remove the splint and contour it very carefully, not only coronally but interproximally as well for correct anatomic form.

Reestablishment of correct coronal form will help in gingival protection. Crown-to-root ratio can be improved, and reduction of the incisal guide angle will tend to decrease the horizontal overloading of the anterior teeth. The splints also provide necessary rigidity for mobile teeth and seem to help in maintaining the organizing blood clot intact for optimum healing after surgery. Carelessly constructed temporary splints, however, will not promote proper healing of the tissues.

The acrylic resin splints are then cemented with a zinc oxide–eugenol temporary cement.

A word of caution is in order at this point. It is the prosthodontist's obligation to periodically inspect and maintain the fit and function of the splints during the various phases of treatment for protection of the periodontium and pulp. This holds true during the surgical healing phase, after the placement of a new set of splints or additional revamping of the old ones after periodontal healing (the finalized provisional splints), and in many instances after placement of the permanent splints.

After cementation of the temporary splints the patient returns to the periodontist for final periodontal treatment by surgical means, soft tissue and osseous. During this phase of the treatment the periodontist can remove the splints, facilitating his approach to inaccessible areas. A reorientation of the mucogingival tissue may have to be resolved for maintenance of periodontal health.

Finalized preparation

With the supporting structures completely healed, the preparations are refined and extended, impressions are made, and restorations are completed. The general rule is that preparations should not be finalized until the gingiva is healthy and its position on the root has been established.

The way in which the tooth is prepared and the restoration contoured is important. Sufficient tooth substance must be removed, and shoulder and chamfer preparations must be executed properly to allow for a

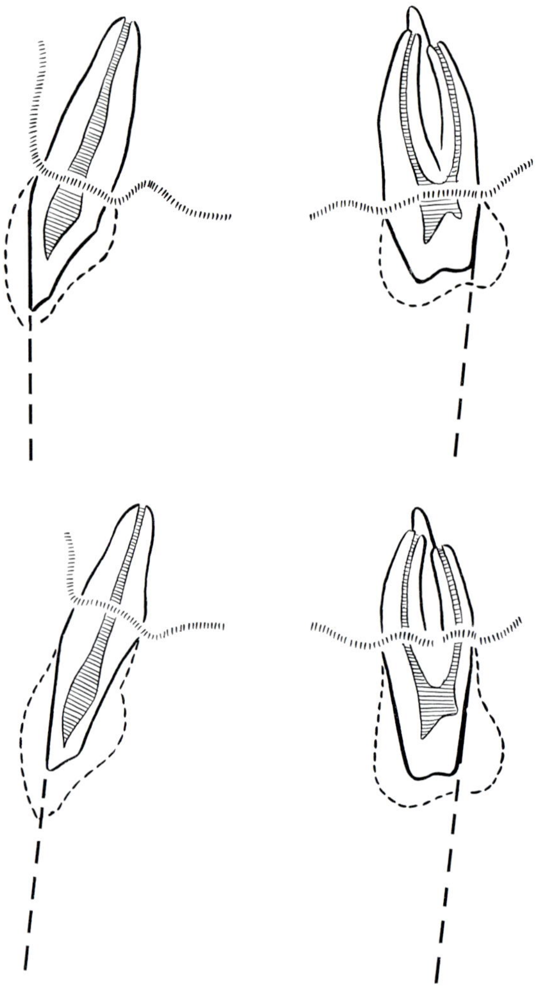

A

B

Fig. 6-92. A, In cases that do not have lengthened clinical crowns because of periodontal surgery, paralleling of anterior abutment tooth, even with its labial inclination, to posterior second molar abutment tooth can be done with comparative ease and safety. The distoproximal slice may have to be angulated slightly. **B,** Same situation with lengthened clinical crowns requires acutely angulated distoproximal slices of maxillary molars so that they are in same parallel plane with prepared labial surface of maxillary anterior quadrant of teeth.

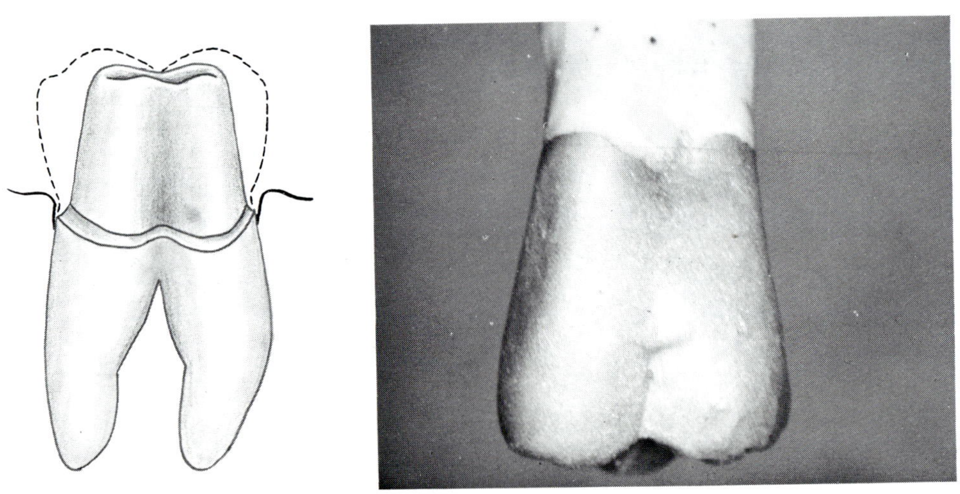

Fig. 6-93. "Barrel-out" preparations in furcations.

correct replacement with the restoration. Particular care must be taken at the proximal line angles, where the width of the shoulder or chamfer is often inadequate and where added bulk in the restoration is needed to achieve a desirable esthetic effect, at the same time avoiding a displacement or crowding of the interdental papilla. In other words, sufficient space for the restorative material is created by an adequate preparation, and thus it is possible to carve ideal contours.

Distoproximal slices of maxillary molars must be angulated acutely so that they are in the same parallel plane with the prepared labial surface of the maxillary anterior quadrant of teeth (Fig. 6-92). It is necessary to "barrel-out" preparations in furcations (Fig. 6-93).

"Principles of parallelism must be adhered to when anterior and posterior teeth are to be included in the same bridge. At times, even after orthodontic aid in repositioning of abutment teeth, parallelism is impossible because of the direction of the root areas. Telescopic copings and crowns may be used as an aid in paralleling and in seating and interlocking sections of fixed bridges. Teeth prepared for the reception of a telescopic crown must sometimes be tapered slightly more than a normal preparation. (See Fig. 6-94.)

"When preparations extend onto root surfaces or end at the cemento-enamel junction and the areas almost touch the corresponding area of the adjacent tooth, it is necessary to try to chamfer up to that area of contact. This is done to provide space for internal bulk, to give marginal strength to the crown, better gingival esthetics to the veneer, and provide interproximal embrasure space for the tissue to be located in health."*

---

*From Minker, Jules S.: Simplified full coverage preparations, Dent. Clin. N. Am., pp. 369, 371-372, July, 1965.

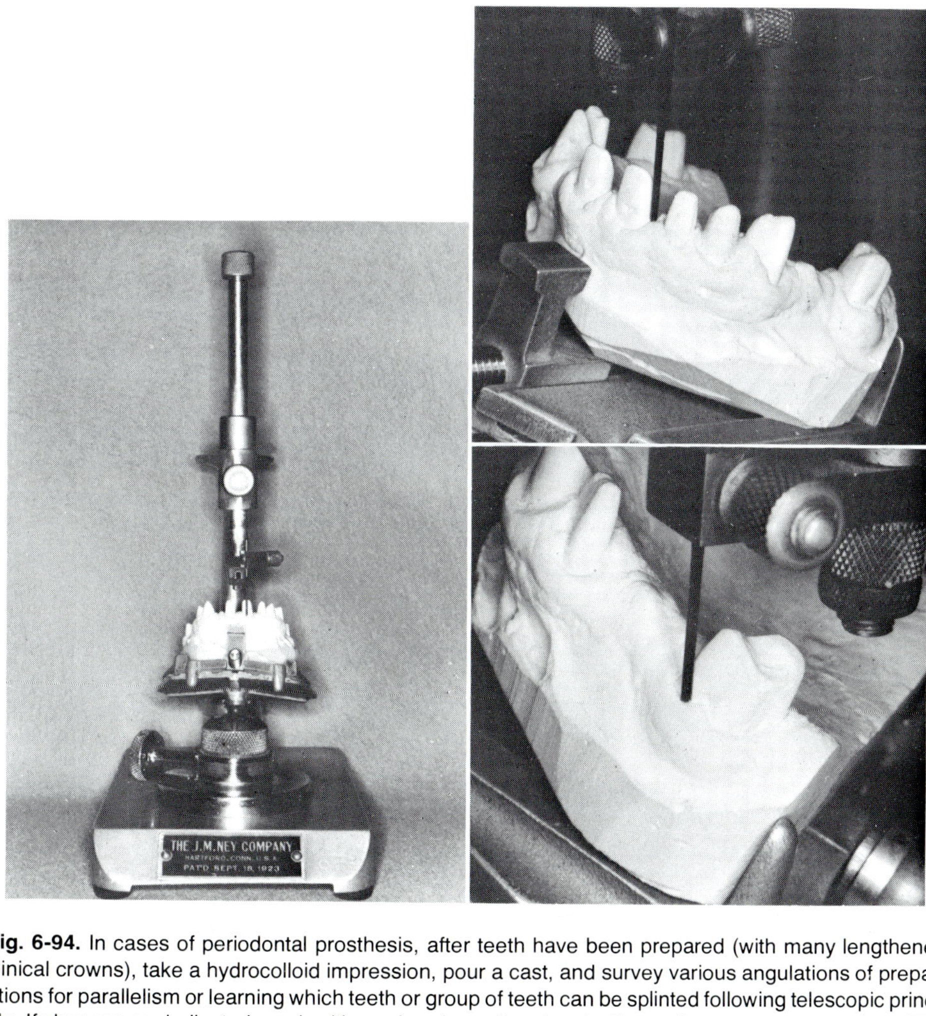

Fig. 6-94. In cases of periodontal prosthesis, after teeth have been prepared (with many lengthened clinical crowns), take a hydrocolloid impression, pour a cast, and survey various angulations of preparations for parallelism or learning which teeth or group of teeth can be splinted following telescopic principle. If changes are indicated, mark with a colored pencil and make these changes on preparations. The small amount of time necessary to make this survey pays good dividends.

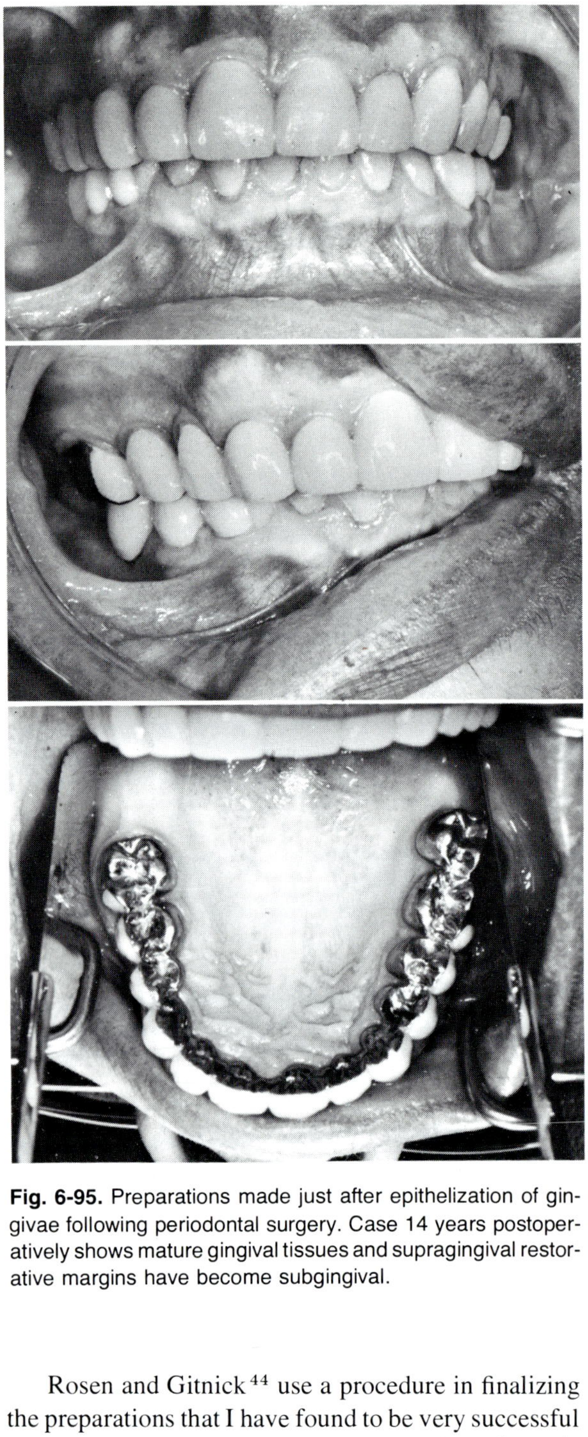

Fig. 6-95. Preparations made just after epithelization of gingivae following periodontal surgery. Case 14 years postoperatively shows mature gingival tissues and supragingival restorative margins have become subgingival.

Rosen and Gitnick[44] use a procedure in finalizing the preparations that I have found to be very successful in my cases. The preparations are made just after epithelization of the gingiva has taken place, which is usually in 6 to 8 weeks after completion of the periodontal surgery. Since no gingival sulcus exists during early stages of maturation, a subgingival margin cannot be established. Visibility and access in the cervical region are best before the complete maturation of the gingival tissues, which takes place in approximately 3 months. At this particular time "the tissue matures, connective tissue is laid down, the surface becomes stippled and keratinized and a shallow knife-edged gingival sulcus develops."* As the gingival tissues mature, a shallow crevice develops and the supragingival restorative margin becomes one that is subgingival (Fig. 6-95).

In endodontically treated teeth a cast post or an endo-post with cast gold cores is constructed and cemented with oxyphosphate of zinc cement. These postanchorage cast gold cores are made parallel to the adjacent preparations by making use of the surveyor.

Provisional and permanent restorations

After finalization of tooth preparations, full upper and lower hydrocolloid impressions (since no subgingival margins exist), a hinge-bow transfer, and centric relation bites are taken for the construction of the working casts and for the proper orientation of these casts on an adjustable articulator. At this stage we can construct well-made provisional splints (gold-acrylic veneer), provided we feel our objectives such as assurance of the retention of repositioned teeth, roentgenographic evidence indicating a return of a physiologic width of the periodontal ligament and definitely defined lamina dura and trabeculae of bone, proper keratinization of the periodontal tissues, firm and stippled gingival tissues with good color and contour, reduction of mobility, and clarification of prognosis on doubtful teeth have now been achieved. Biologic crown form, rigidity for stabilization of mobile teeth, improved functional tooth relations to promote the completion of the healing of traumatic lesions, and a more conducive environment for the reorganization and stabilization of the surrounding bone around the orthodontically moved teeth must be given prime consideration. The case must be solved and evaluated properly in the provisional stage, and all procedures must be executed with the utmost care and thought so that all can benefit from present-day knowledge.

A change in the vertical dimension of occlusion may be necessary occasionally because of the collapse of the dental apparatus, especially posterior bite collapse.

Any increase in an existing vertical dimension of occlusion must be made with extreme prudence. If you

*From Rosen, H., and Gitnick, P. J.: Integrating restorative procedures into the treatment of periodontal disease, J. Prosthet. Dent. **14:**343-354, 1964.

A

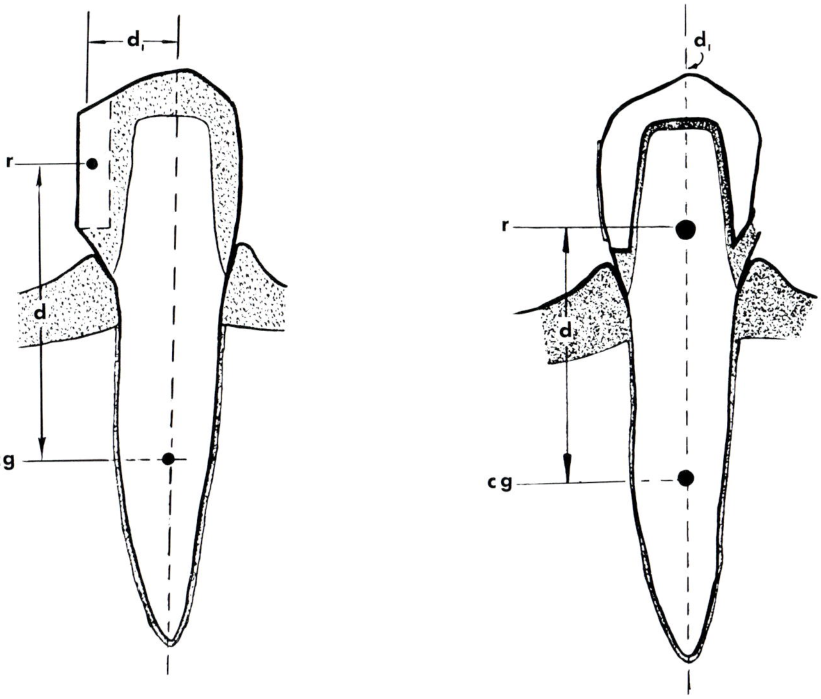

B

C

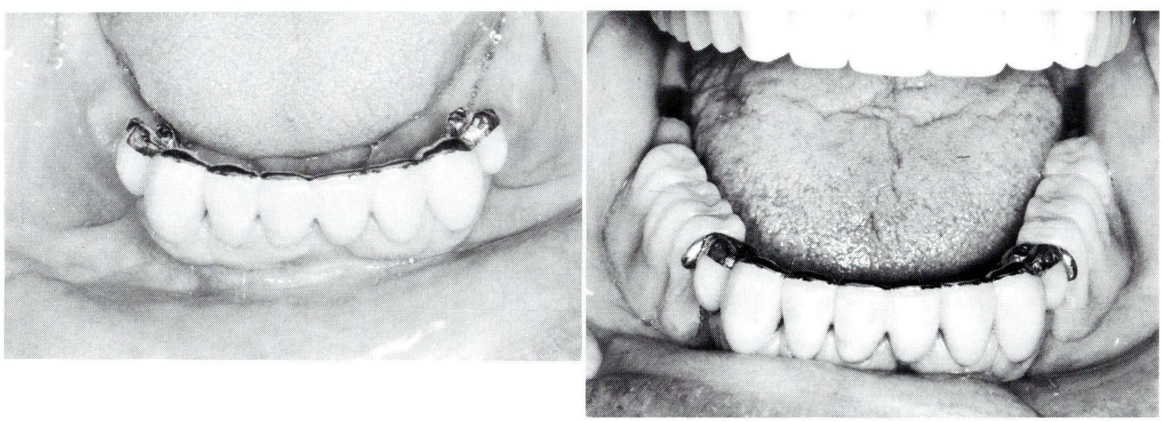

D

Fig. 6-96. A, Location of stress-receiving area in abutment tooth for removable partial denture prosthesis, utilizing key and keyway prefabricated precision attachment. *cg,* Center of gravity or fulcrum point of the root support—hypothetical ideal location for resistance to force by root housing. *r,* Point of force transmission by denture retainer. d_1, Distance from axial center of root to retainer. *d,* Distance from retainer transmitting site to center of gravity of root support. **B,** Location of stress-receiving area in abutment tooth for removable partial denture prosthesis, utilizing telescopic crown retainers. Note reduction in dimension of d_1 and *d* as compared to **A.** *Cg,* Center of gravity or fulcrum point of root support—hypothetical ideal location for resistance to force by root housing. *r,* Point of force transmission by denture retainer. d_1, Distance from axial center of root to retainer. *d,* Distance from retainer transmitting site to center of gravity of root support. **C,** to **D,** If a removable appliance is indicated, make use of internal precision attachment or telescopic partial denture. Case in which internal precision attachment was used is shown. (**A** and **B** from Abrams, Leonard, and Feder, Morris: Alpha Omega **55:**123-136, 1962.)

wish to avoid trouble, do not impinge upon the interocclusal space. Skurnik[78] says that "this position is an anatomic and functional entity differing greatly among individuals. . . . Some individuals require more and others less of this arbitrary space [2 to 3 mm.] for optimum efficiency in mastication, speech, esthetics, and neuromuscular adaptation."*

When we are satisfied that our objectives have been achieved, which may take some time in certain cases, we are ready for the completion of the case. In some cases in which gold-acrylic veneer restorations have been used, these restorations can be used as the permanent ones. In some instances a completely new permanent case has to be made. The procedures followed in the construction of these cases at this stage is thoroughly covered by a step-by-step procedure of a practical case in Chapter 17.

Removable partial dentures

If a removable appliance is indicated, only the internal precision attachment or telescopic partial denture should be used (Fig. 6-96). Since the center of rotation of a tooth carrying an attachment is much closer, compared to a circumferential clasp, to the actual center, functional stress is resolved into a vertical intrusive force. Without circumferential pressure, supporting structures are under stress only during function. The insertion and removal are limited to one exact path, which places no stress on abutment teeth during these operations.

Cementation

The permanent case is cemented temporarily with Moyco powder and petroleum jelly, be it a telescopic case with copings and superstructure or otherwise constructed, for a minimum of 2 weeks. On removal of castings, if a "wash-out" has taken place, rest assured that the same will be true of permanent cementation. This is caused by torquing due to a lack of parallelism or an occlusal factor. If, however, on removal of the castings (crowns, copings, superstructures) the powder has a pure white color, one can proceed to "hard cement" the case; for telescopic restorations the copings are cemented permanently (oxyphosphate of zinc cement, E.B.A., Caulk's Zebacem), and the superstructures are cemented temporarily with Moyco zinc oxide–eugenol cement.

Remove all excess cement with great care, using a sickle-shaped explorer or worn curettes, to ensure against gingival irritation. Traces of temporary cement adhering to the surfaces of the acrylic veneers and natural teeth may be removed with Orange solvent.

If indicated, a bite guard or guards can be constructed for minimizing habit patterns (see discussion on parafunctions).

Home care

The final phase of any mouth rehabilitation case is adequate instruction for home care—suitable toothbrushing, flossing, interdental stimulation, and use of the Water Pik.

The dentist must observe how and what the patient does with this important assignment—his ability and motivation to carry out home care. Without real motivation for a systematic regimen of toothbrushing and gingival stimulation, the case, regardless how well executed, will "go down the drain."

The periodic recall system must be instituted and carried out by all means.

Oral physiotherapy

Proper instruction and supervision of oral care at home are as important as any service we render our patient in mouth rehabilitation. We must make a supreme effort to motivate the patient to conscientiously perform the necessary cleansing procedures, which must be maintained properly. However, without cooperation of the patient in this respect all other therapy seems unwarranted.

Recurrence of periodontal disease and caries at the margins of restorations may well be evident if properly instituted care is not taken to ensure routine massage of supporting tissues and the thorough cleansing of all the surfaces of the teeth. A caries-susceptible patient must understand the plaque concept of incipient caries and how to cope with it. *Let us reiterate—home care is most essential.*

Colbern,[79] in summarizing Arnim's[80] lecture, has this to say:

"Dr. Arnim states that dental plaque is one of the causes of the most common dental diseases, dental caries and periodontal disease. The microcosm is located between the teeth, in the gingival crevice, in pits and fissures, and all habitually unclean areas. The microcosm is a composite of the dental plaque or zooglea (slime-layer), the bacteria, food, and the products of metabolism. The zoogleal (living glue) gel forms a semipermeable layer under which the bacterial colonies can multiply to cause disease. *In the carious lesion,* the bacteria form the acid to dissolve the teeth in areas where the microcosm is not removed from

---

*From Skurnik, Harry R.: Treatment planning for occlusal rehabilitation, J. Prosthet. Dent. **9:**988-1000, 1959.

the habitually unclean areas of the tooth surface. *In the periodontal lesion,* the microcosm is located in the gingival crevice and the end products of protein degradation produce gingival inflammation which causes the breakdown of the circular and other connective tissue fibers in the gingivae at the neck of the tooth. This causes the gingivae to lose its purse string-like adaptation to the tooth and the gingivae becomes flabby, irritated, and swollen. Upon further progress of this situation, the microcosms in the crevice causes calculus to be formed in the pocket, the pocket becomes deeper due to the continuing inflammation, the bony support is destroyed, the tooth becomes loose and is finally lost. The problem, as Dr. Arnim sees it, is then to control the microcosm effectively so that the disease does not have a chance to occur. Once the microcosm is removed it takes 24 to 48 hours for the microcosm to grow back in quantity, and the longer the microcosm is present, the harder it is to remove."*

A strong bundle of circular fibers inhabits the tip of the free gingival margin. The bundle is soon lost when inflammation occurs—with the presence of disease, the circular band fibers disintegrate rapidly and soon lose their identity. It rebuilds when injurious agents are removed.[81]

Arnim is largely responsible for innovations in methodology, implementation, and techniques of patient motivation, leading to a more realistic and effective approach to oral physiotherapy.[82]

Adequate oral hygiene includes the correct instrumentation of toothbrushes, stimulators, floss, irrigating devices, and other oral hygiene aids in such a manner that they do not irritate the periodontal tissues.

The aids advocated by Arnim are (1) disclosing wafers, (2) soft nylon toothbrush, (3) unwaxed dental floss, and (4) water spray.

1. Disclosing wafers. This type of wafer is used to measure tooth cleanliness. It consists of a water-soluble vegetable dye compounded into a flavored tablet (a palatable food color tablet of F.D.C. red No. 3 [Erythrocin]). It stains the dental plaque red so that it is visible and can be removed. It does not color the teeth or restorations if they are free of plaque. The cervical and interproximal areas exhibit the heaviest staining pattern. Since the common denominator of the causes of dental diseases is plaque, it is readily seen that if it can be removed promptly, the disease cannot exist. At recall visit, the teeth should be restained, and, using a large hand mirror, the patient should be shown the bacteria on his teeth that are associated with inflamed gingiva.

The patient should use a disclosing wafer daily until he becomes very proficient in the cleansing of the teeth, after which once a week will probably be sufficient to act as a check-up on his oral physiotherapy efficiency.

2. Toothbrush. The primary objective of brushing the teeth is removal of coronal accretions such as food debris, soft deposits, bacterial clumps, and stains. Regular removal of adherent microorganisms from the surfaces of the teeth and the prevention of calculus formation in the cervical regions are of particular importance in avoiding cariogenic activity and periodontal pathosis.

An Oral B30 or Oral B40 soft nylon toothbrush or a Butler toothbrush with rounded bristles are my choices. The toothbrush removes dental plaque from three surfaces of the tooth—facial or cheek or lip side, lingual or tongue side, and occlusal or biting surface. The procedural steps for correct use of the toothbrush are as follows:

a. The brush is placed with the side of the bristles flat against the attached gingiva and the handle parallel to the occlusal surfaces; the side of the bristles is pressed firmly against the gums.
b. The brush is moved along the attached gingiva to the marginal gingiva.
c. As the brush moves onto the tooth surfaces, it is rotated slightly to about 45 degrees, and the stroke is continued until the entire facial or lingual surface has been passed over with the brush.
d. The occlusal surfaces are scrubbed with a rotary and a forward and backward movement of the bristle points. Brushing of the tongue is advocated in many cases.[83]

Brushing alone, no matter how carefully performed, does not provide a completely satisfactory method of interproximal cleaning. Interproximal tissues, particularly gingival sulci and "col" areas, cannot be cleaned satisfactorily.

3. Dental floss. Interproximal surfaces are relatively inaccessible to the toothbrush; retention of disclosing stain after careful toothbrushing is proof of this fact. A thin, unwaxed floss should be used regularly for consistently effective results in these areas. Removal of stained microorganisms is attained also.

Unwaxed dental tape is easily passed through the contact areas with a gentle "sawing motion" so that

*From Colbern, Robert: Effective oral hygiene for full mouth rehabilitation, Second International Congress of Gnathology, San Diego, Calif., 1965.

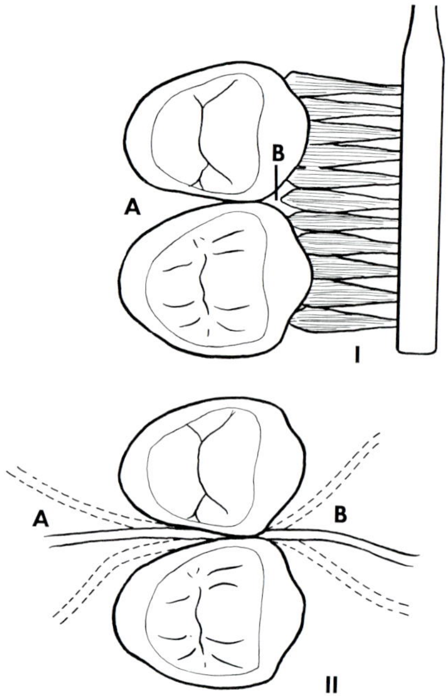

Fig. 6-97. *I,* Occlusal view showing limitation of toothbrush cleaning interproximally (note areas *A* and *B*). Both proximal tooth surfaces and interproximal epithelium are not cleaned and stimulated. *II,* Supplemental use of dental floss, properly executed, will clean and stimulate tooth surfaces and gingival margins.

it does not suddenly snap through the contact area and traumatize the gingiva. The tape is moved in a buccolingual and up and down "sawing motion" direction through the contact areas to the gingival margin on the mesial side of the tooth first, and then the distal surface. Colbern[79] says that the pressure of the tape against the tooth causes the filaments of the tape to separate, forming a number of individual cutting edges which remove the debris. One should floss before brushing, because it clears the interproximal areas and permits better brush penetration (Fig. 6-97).

4. Water spray. Cohen and Bohannan[82] have told us that the gingival sulcus and the interdental col usually harbor bacteria and debris, and the toothbrush and floss fail to reach the depths of these areas consistently.

Forced irrigation removes the dental plaque from the crevice between the tooth and the gum, it being necessary to pass the water spray (Water Pik*) around each tooth and between the teeth, under pontics, and into "female" attachments in precision removal partial dentures, to thoroughly flush and cleanse these areas.

*Aqua Tec Corp., Denver, Colo.

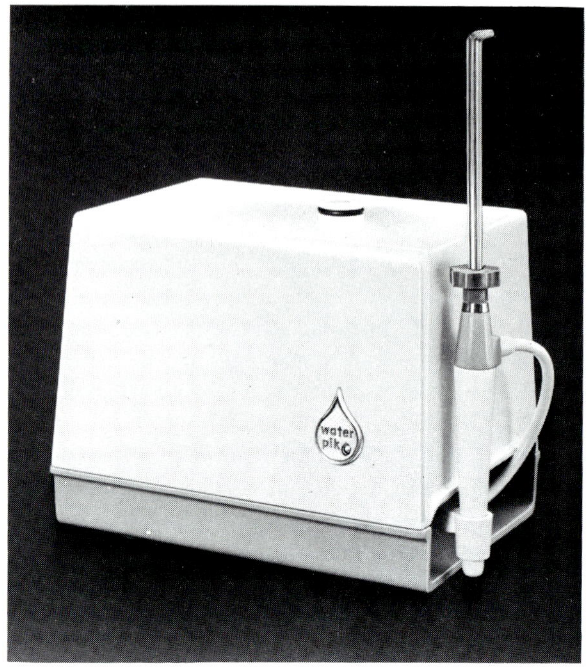

Fig. 6-98. Water Pik for forced irrigation to remove dental plaque from crevice between tooth and gum.

This type of appliance should be an integral part of daily oral physiotherapy, and it is excellent for use in compromised results when some residual depth remains and in cases where pocket elimination is contraindicated. The water spray has proved to be the answer to the elimination of subgingival microcosm.

The Water Pik (Fig. 6-98) produces a gentle intermittent compression of the gingival tissues, twenty times each second, as evidenced by momentary blanching at the height of the pulse. It thoroughly irrigates the gingival sulcus by lifting the free gingival margin and flushing out the crevice. Deep periodontal pockets are irrigated thoroughly with cyclic surges of water pressure.

Using controls, Cantor and Stahl[84] studied the effect of a water pressure device on human gingival cols. Tissue specimens of gingival papillae showed that the device did not affect the degree of keratinization in the col after 1 month's use. However, a statistically significant reduction in inflammation occurred in the col and adjacent area of crevicular epithelium. Some harmful effects can accrue when water pressure irrigating devices are used with too much force. Set at medium or slightly lower in some cases.

I firmly believe, in spite of the fact that some

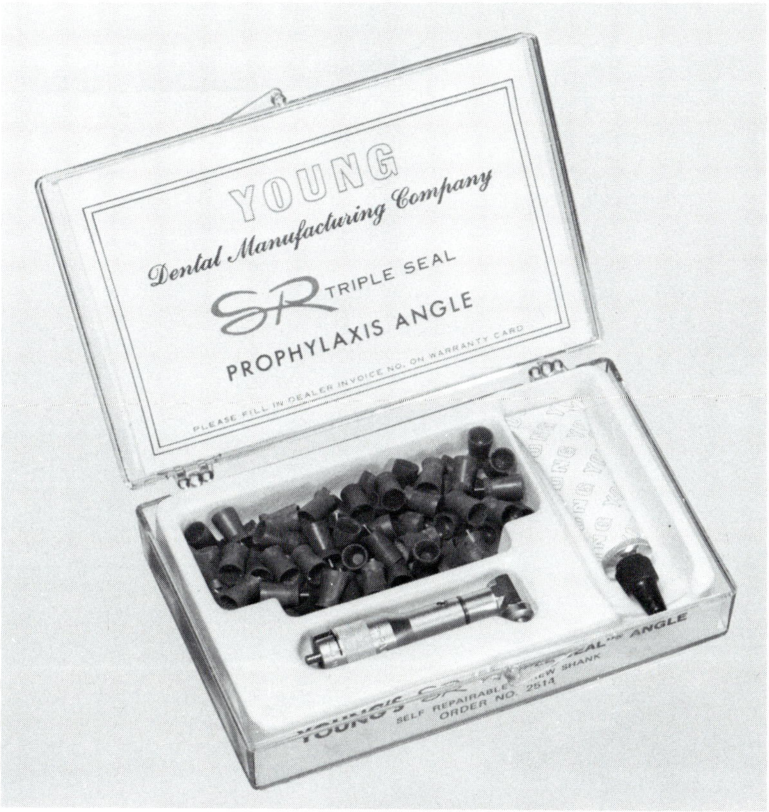

Fig. 6-99. I like and use the Young prophylaxis angle and accessories. (Courtesy Young Dental Mfg. Co., St. Louis, Mo.)

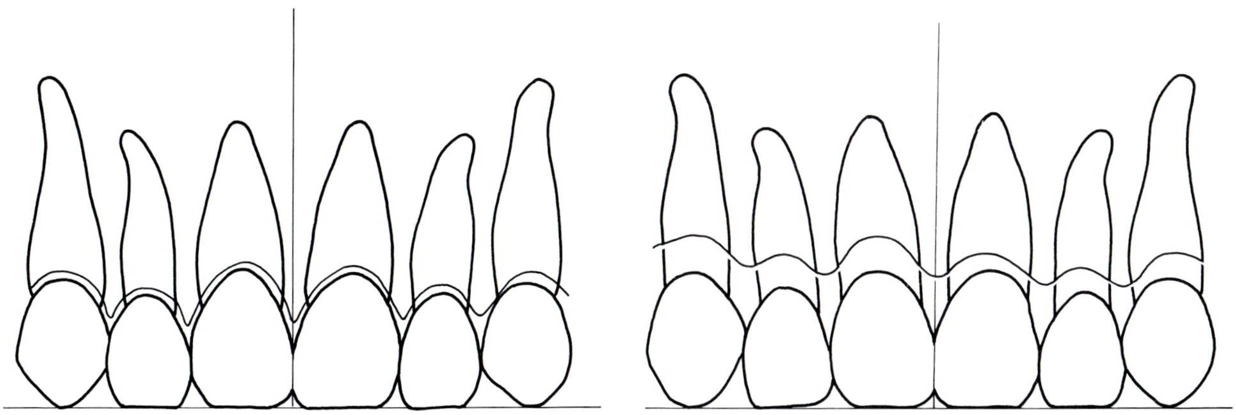

Continued.

Fig. 6-100. Schematic drawings showing development of biomechanical restoration beginning with **A,** condition as presented by the patient, **B,** after periodontal surgery, **C,** preparations, keeping in mind parallelism, elective endodontics, crown-to-root ratio, etc., **D,** teeth before preparation *(A),* after preparation *(C),* and biomechanical restoration *(B),* and **E,** biomechanical restoration. (Redrawn from illustrations courtesy Morris Feder, Philadelphia, Pa.)

C

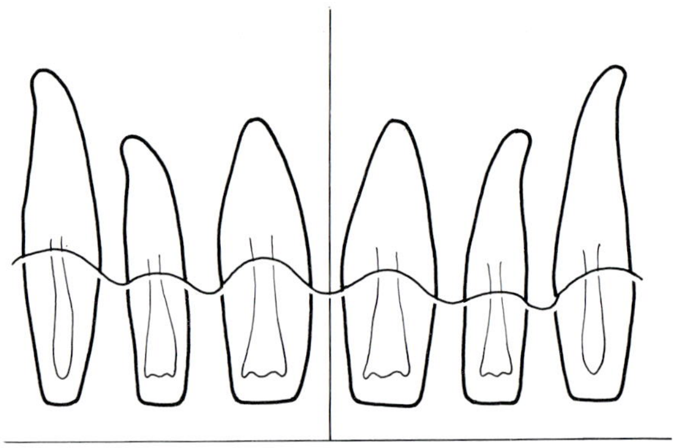

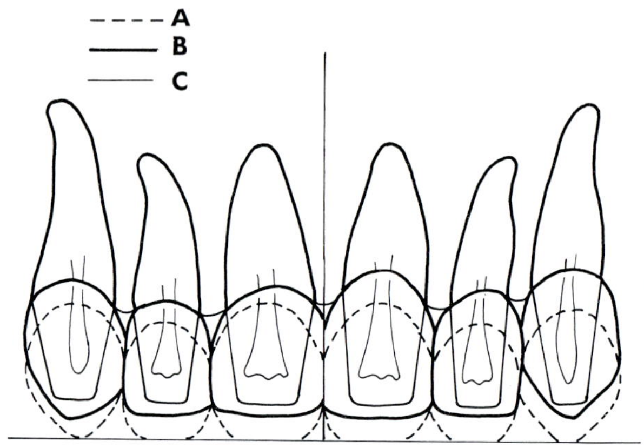

D

E

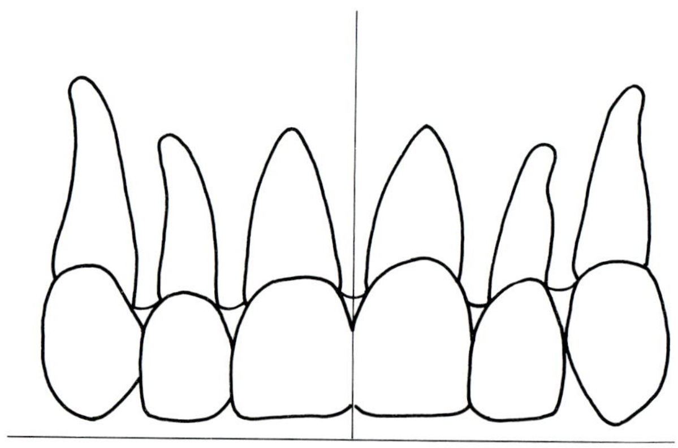

Fig. 6-100, cont'd. For legend see p. 241.

periodontists disagree with me, that the water spray, properly regulated, has been of great help in maintaining many severe cases in a good state of health.

INTERDENTAL STIMULATORS

Interdental stimulation (rubber tip, Stim-u-dents, round toothpicks) is imperative, Most gingival problems start interproximally where the toothbrush cannot reach.

Insert the stimulator interproximally until it is wedged tightly, and then massage the tissues with a pumping motion, up and down and in and out several times. At first this procedure may be painful and produce hemorrhage. However, by so stimulating the swollen pathologic tissues, it allows them to repair themselves and return to a state of normalcy. The tenderness and hemorrhaging will disappear.

Friction applied to the interproximal spaces will

serve to prevent or decrease the severity of gingival disease. Friction applied to healthy epithelium will produce keratin formation, and properly keratinized epithelium does not bleed under moderate pressure.

Intrasulcular brushing, cleansing of the interdental sulcus with dental tape, stimulators, irrigating device, and good restorative dentistry provide the best means of ensuring the health of the interdental tissue.

Bodkins (zon dental bridge cleaners*) are used to pass the dental floss beneath the pontics of a bridge so that it can be kept clean; pipecleaners are handy for cleansing of furcations.

Dentifrices have polishing qualities and detergent action but are of no therapeutic value to the periodontium. Use one with as little abrasiveness as possible. After debridement of crown and roots of teeth use a fluoride-containing tooth paste for prophylaxis (Fig. 6-99).

The use—the "why" and "how"—of the disclosing tablet, toothbrush, unwaxed floss, interdental stimulators, water spray, bodkins, and other aids is the basic information to be communicated to the patient. He must clean his teeth frequently to prevent accumulation of adherent masses that cause dental disease. The gingival tissues must assume and maintain a normal healthy tone, color, and form.

Good dentistry is of little value unless the patient controls recurrent caries and periodontal disease in his mouth.

The maintenance phase is the basic aspect of complete treatment. The patient's oral hygiene program must be supervised very carefully, and the interest of both the patient and the dentist must be sustained.

*Johnson & Johnson, New Brunswick, N. J.

Concluding remarks

The preservation of the integrity of the individual dental unit is of the utmost importance—it is part of a self-protecting mechanism.

The function and future life of the restoration depend upon the preservation of the epithelial attachment and the normal form of the crown—physiologic form and function.

When splinting is necessary, additional stability is obtained by the correct posterosuperior position of the mandible.

In periodontal prosthesis we can modify the anterior guidance and the vertical dimension, working within the limits of the established free-way space. It is also possible to establish favorable or acceptable esthetic, phonetic, and masticatory patterns.

This method of treatment, periodontal prosthesis, should not be used as an excuse to justify poor occlusal relations. All of the occlusal elements should be restored, and they should be arranged to suit the lateral border movements and centric relation.

If not executed properly, restorative dentistry can be an etiologic factor in periodontal disease or recreation of this condition after periodontal therapy. Gross to subtle errors in restorations can be responsible for pocket formation and loss of alveolar bone. A great deal is dependent on the way in which the tooth is prepared and the restoration is contoured.

The patient must have, on completion of the mouth rehabilitation, a negative occlusal perception.

Caution is necessary to prevent the definition of the "normal" to exclude individuals with an abnormal dental biomechanism in appearance, which may be functioning in a good physiologic state (Figs. 6-100 to 6-102).

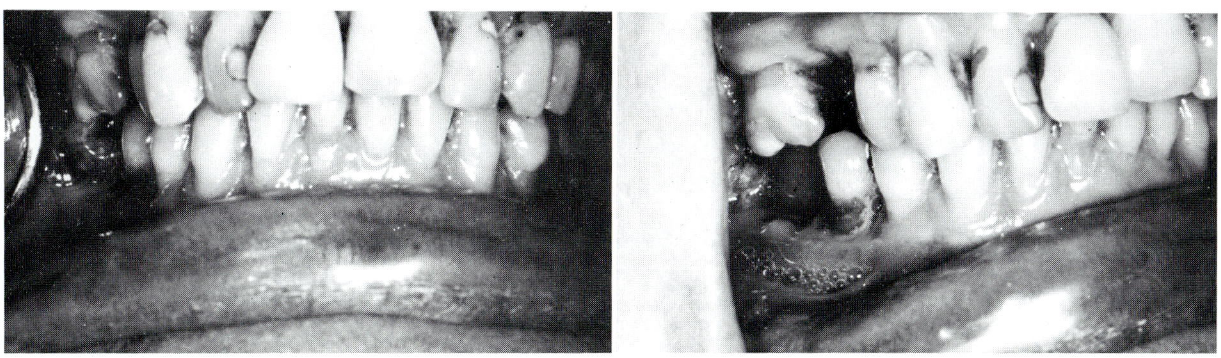

Continued.

Fig. 6-101. Illustrations of cases (preoperative and postoperative) that were referred for correction of coronal form and splinting. They were considered terminal cases, but clinical study and observation were desired to evaluate procedures in relation to gingival health.

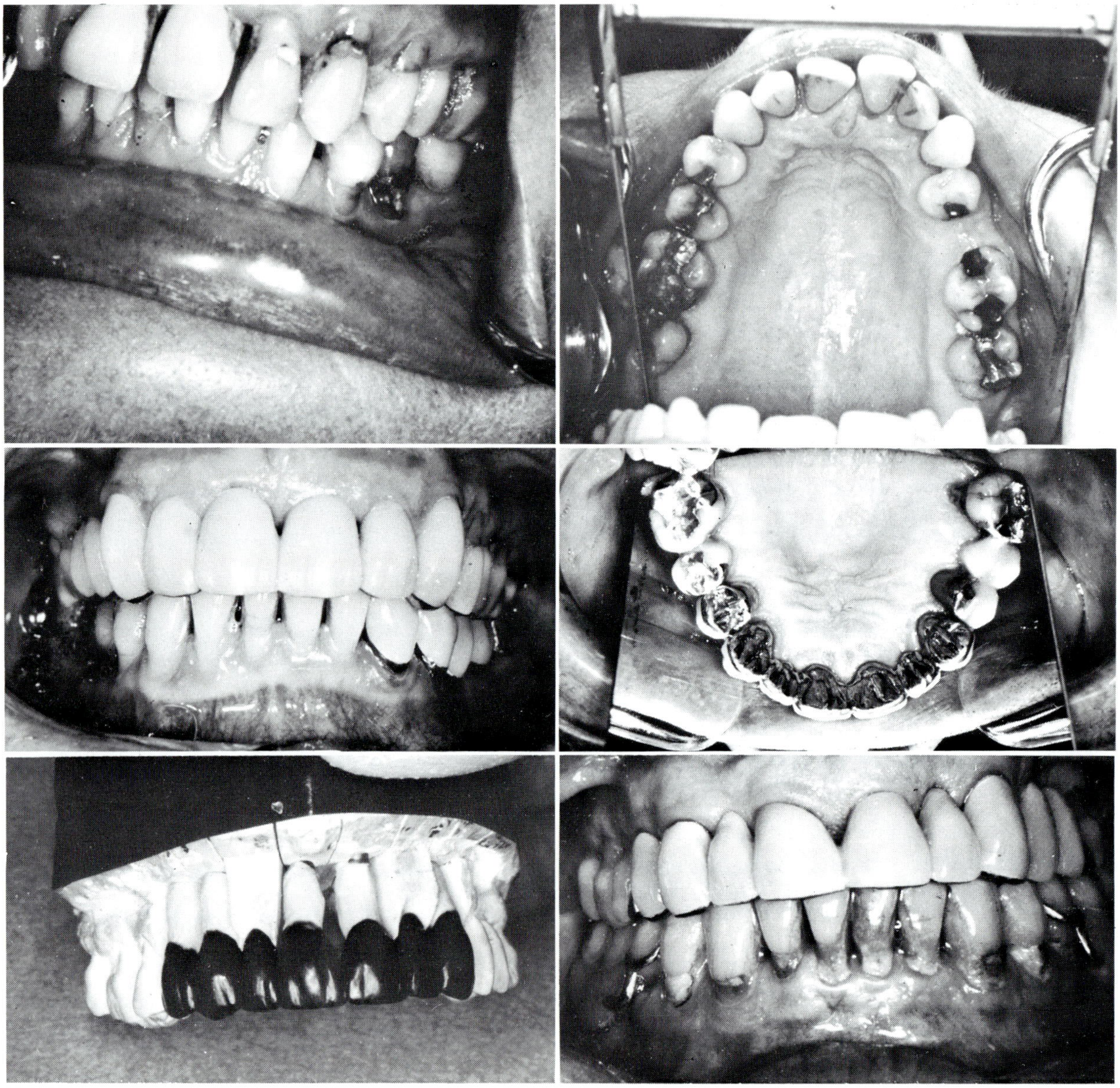

Fig. 6-101, cont'd. For legend see p. 243.

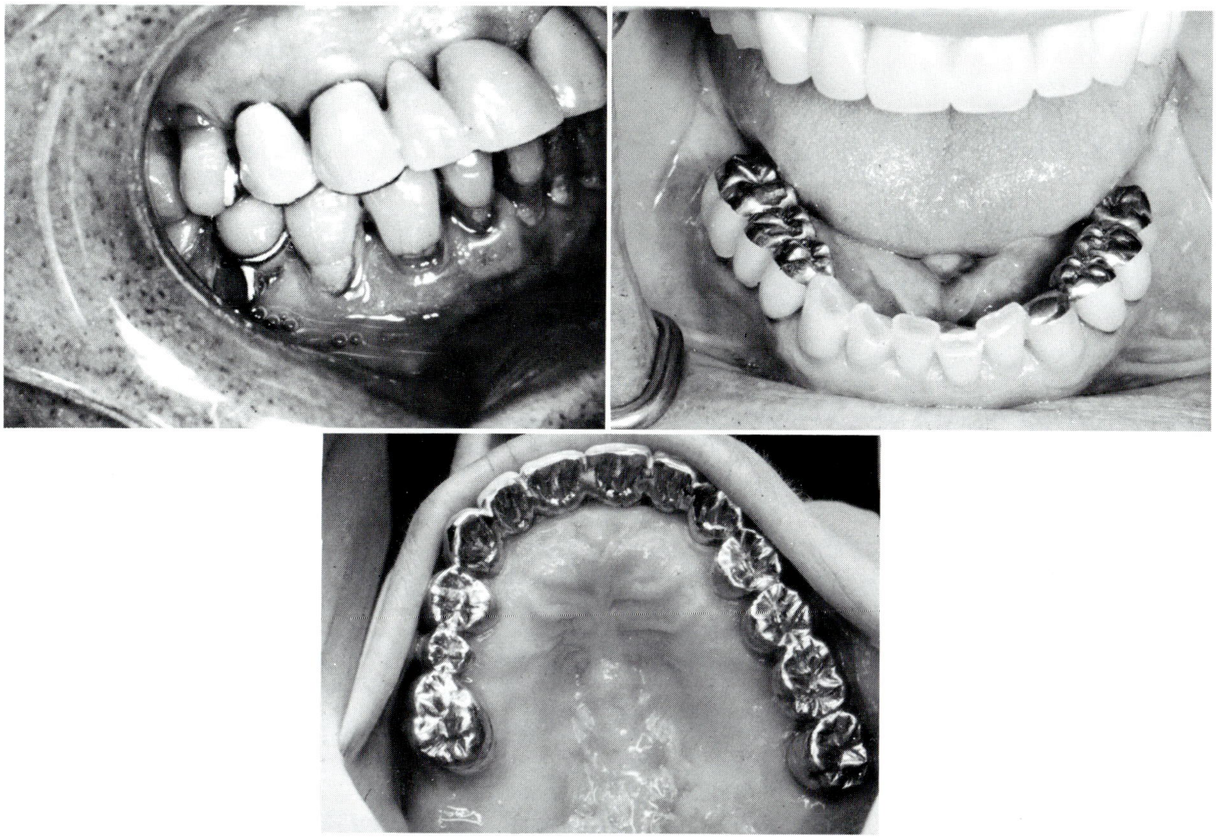

Fig. 6-101, cont'd. For legend see p. 243.

A B C

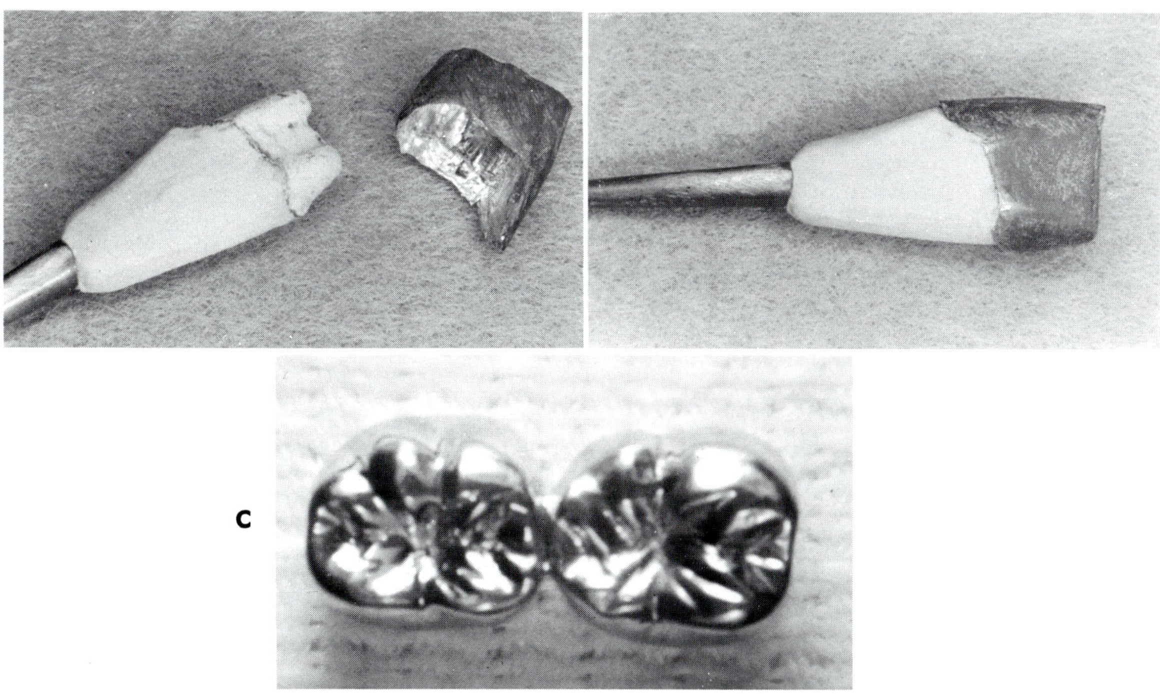

Fig. 6-102. A and **B,** Stone die and DuraLay coping for purposes of "transfer" when taking impression for working cast. **C,** Two-tooth splint showing correct positioning of soldered contact area—anatomically and vertically.

REFERENCES

1. Glickman, Irving: Lecture notes, Mid-Atlantic States Conference on Dentistry, Buck Hill Falls, Pa., 1964.
2. Goldman, Henry M.: Lecture notes, Post-Graduate Course in Periodontics, Boston University, School of Graduate Dentistry, Boston, 1970.
3. Kraus, B. S., Jordan, R. E., and Abrams, Leonard: Dental anatomy and occlusion, Baltimore, 1969, The Williams & Wilkins Co.
4. Churchill, H. R.: Meyer's normal histology and histogenesis of the human teeth and associated parts, Philadelphia, 1935, J. B. Lippincott Co., p. 142.
5. Sicher, Harry, and Bhaskar, S. N., editors; Orban's oral histology and embryology, ed. 7, St. Louis, 1972, The C. V. Mosby Co.
6. Amsterdam, Morton, and Abrams, Leonard: In Goldman, Henry M., and Cohen, D. Walter: Periodontal therapy, ed. 5, St. Louis, 1973, The C. V. Mosby Co.
7. Orban, Balint, and Wentz, Frank M.: Periodontal membrane; cementum; alveolar bone, J. S. Calif. Dent. Assoc. **23**(11):37-40, 1955.
8. Gottlieb, B.: Biology of cementum, J. Periodontol. **13:**13, 1942; Aisenberg, M. S.: Histology and physiology of the supporting structures, J.A.D.A. **44:**628, 1952.
9. Goldman, Henry M.: Histologic structure of the attachment apparatus, Alpha Omegan **50:**102-106, Sept. 1957.
10. Sicher, Harry: Personal communication.
11. Fox, Lewis: The occlusal factor in periodontal disease, Alpha Omegan **43:**124-133, 1949.
12. Fox, Lewis: Operative dentistry in the atomic age, Alpha Omegan **51:**75-79, 1958.
13. Lucia, Victor O: Modern gnathological concepts, St. Louis, 1961, The C. V. Mosby Co.
14. Granger, Ernest R.: Practical procedures in oral rehabilitation, Philadelphia, 1962, J. B. Lippincott Co.
15. Lucia, Victor O.: A technique for recording centric relation, J. Prosthet. Dent. **14:**492-505, 1964.
16. Weinberg, Lawrence A.: Physiologic objectives of reconstruction techniques, J. Prosthet. Dent. **10:**711-723, 1960.
17. Stuart, Charles E., and Stallard, Harvey: Principles involved in restoring occlusion to natural teeth, J. Prosthet. Dent. **10:** 304-313, 1960.
18. Goldman, Henry M.: Lecture notes, Mid-Atlantic States Conference on Dentistry, Skytop, Pa., 1956.
19. Schwarz, Melvyn S., and Sochat, Paul: Occlusion and periodontal disease, J. S. Calif. Dent. Assoc. **40:**524-526, 1972.
20. Orban, Balint: Personal communication.
21. Amsterdam, Morton, and Abrams, Leonard: Periodontal prosthesis. In Goldman, Henry M., Schluger, Saul, Fox, Lewis, and Cohen, D. Walter: Periodontal therapy, ed. 3, St. Louis, 1964, The C. V. Mosby Co., pp. 762-813.
22. Ramfjord, Sigurd P., and Ash, Major M., Jr.: Occlusion, ed. 2, Philadelphia, 1971, W. B. Saunders Co.
23. Bohannan, Harry M., and Abrams, Leonard: Intentional vital pulp extirpation in periodontal prosthesis, J. Prosthet. Dent. **11:**781-789, 1961.
24. Amsterdam, Morton, and Rossman, Samuel R.: Techniques of hemisection of multirooted teeth, Alpha Omegan **53:**4-15, 1960.
25. Lloyd, Ralph S., and Baer, Paul N.: Periodontal therapy by root resection, J. Prosthet. Dent. **10:**362-365, 1960.
26. Wagman, Sydney S.: Tissue management for full cast veneer crowns, J. Prosthet. Dent. **15:**106-117, 1965.
27. Wheeler, Russell C.: Complete crown form and the periodontium, J. Prosthet. Dent. **11:**722-734, 1961.
28. Morris, Melvin L.: Artificial crown contours and gingival health, J. Prosthet. Dent. **12:**1146-1155, 1962.
29. Perel, Morton L.: Periodontal considerations of crown contours, J. Prosthet. Dent. **26**(6):627-630, 1971.
30. Eissmann, H. F., Radke, R. A., and Noble, W. H.: Physiologic design criteria for fixed dental restorations, Dent. Clin. N. Am. **15**(3):543-568, July, 1971.
31. Yuodelis, R. A., Weaver, J. D., and Sapkos, S.: Facial and lingual contours of artificial complete crown restorations and their effects on the periodontium, J. Prosthet. Dent. **29**(1): 61-66, 1973.
32. Smith, Joe H.: The interdental gingival topography and its role in periodontal disease, Tex. Dent. J. **82:**20-25, 1964.
33. Stahl, S. S.: Morphology and healing pattern of human interdental gingiva, J.A.D.A. **67:**48, 1963.
34. Kohl, J. T., and Zander, H. A.: Morphology of interdental gingival tissues, Oral Surg. **14:**287-295, 1961.
35. Abrams, Leonard: The self-protective features of the dentition. In Kraus, B. S., Jordan, R. E., and Abrams, Leonard: Dental anatomy and occlusion, Baltimore, 1969, The Williams & Wilkins Co.
36. Burch, James G.: Ten rules for developing crown contours in restorations, Dent. Clin. N. Am. **15**(3):611-618, July, 1971.
37. Ritchey, Beryl, and Orban, Balint: The crests of the interdental alveolar septa, J. Periodontol. **24:**75-87, 1953.
38. O'Connor, T. W., and Biggs, N. L.: Interproximal bony contours, J. Periodontol. **35:**326, 1964.
39. Weinberg, Lawrence A.: Esthetics and the gingivae in full coverage, J. Prosthet. Dent. **10:**737-744, 1960.
40. Gargiulo, A. W., Wentz, F. M., and Orban, B.: Dimensions and relations of the dentogingival junction in humans, J. Periodontol. **32:**261-267, 1961.
41. Marcum, J. S.: The effect of crown margin depth upon gingival tissue, J. Prosthet. Dent. **17:**479-487, 1967.
42. Gordon, Irving: The danger zone—use and abuse of full coverage, Alpha Omegan **54:**126-131, 1961.
43. Goldman, Henry M., and Cohen, D. Walter: Periodontal therapy, ed. 4, St. Louis, 1968, The C. V. Mosby Co., p. 26.
44. Rosen, H., and Gitnick, P. J.: Integrating restorative procedures into the treatment of periodontal disease, J. Prosthet. Dent. **14:**343-354, 1964.
45. Walsh, J. P.: The psychogenesis of bruxism, J. Periodontol. **36:**417-420, 1965.
46. Beaudreau, David E.: The role of the posterior fixed bridge in occlusion, Dent. Clin. N. Am. pp. 13-24, March, 1965.
47. Fenichel, Otto: The psychoanalytic theory of neurosis, New York, 1945, W. W. Norton & Co., Inc.
48. Rhoads, John E.: Repositioning of malposed teeth prior to oral rehabilitation, J. S. Calif. Dent. Assoc. **31:**346-354, 1963.
49. Posselt, Ulf: Personal communication.
50. Ross, Ira F.: Reactive positioning and improved gingival architecture, J. Periodontol. **34:**444-446, 1963.
51. Sternlicht, Harold C.: Tooth movement in periodontal disease, J. S. Calif. Dent. Assoc. **27:**324-332, 1959.
52. Tylman, Stanley D.: The use of the bite plate as a prerestorative measure, J. Can. Dent. Assoc. **23:**134-140, 1957.
53. Christensen, Gordon J., and Lundeen, Harry C.: Restorative dentistry in general practice. In Morris, Alvin L., and Bohannan, Harry C.: The dental specialties in general practice, Philadelphia, 1969, W. B. Saunders Co., pp. 513-568.

54. Lauritzen, Arne: Lecture notes, Post-Graduate Study Groups, 1953, 1961.
55. Ross, Ira F.: Occlusion—a concept for the clinician, St. Louis, 1970, The C. V. Mosby Co., pp. 19-22.
56. Laskin, D. M.: Etiology of the pain dysfunction syndrome, J.A.D.A. **79:**147-153, July, 1969.
57. Lerman, Martin D.: A unifying concept of the TMJ pain-dysfunction syndrome, J.A.D.A. **86** (4):833-841, 1973.
58. Dawson, Peter E.: Temporomandibular joint pain-dysfunction problems can be solved, J. Prosthet. Dent. **29**(1):100-112, 1973.
59. Ramfjord, S. P.: Dysfunctional temporomandibular joint and muscle pain, J. Prosthet. Dent. **11:**353-373, 1961.
60. Freese, Arthur S., and Scheman, Paul: Management of temporomandibular joint problems, St. Louis, 1962, The C. V. Mosby Co.
61. Shore, Nathan Allen: Muscle exercise to prevent clicking in the temporo-mandibular joint, Dent. Dig. **67**(4):166-167, April, 1961.
62. Moffett, B., Jr., Johnson, L., McCabe, J., and Askey, H.: Articular remodeling in the adult human TMJ, Am. J. Anat. **115:**119-130, 1964.
63. Dyer, E. H.: Importance of a stable maxillomandibular relation, J. Prosthet. Dent. **30**(3):241-251, 1973.
64. Shore, Nathan Allen: Temporomandibular joint dysfunctions, J. Prosthet. Dent. **10:**366-373, 1960.
65. Dyer, E. H.: Personal communication.
66. Jerge, Charles R.: Comments on the innervation of the teeth, Dent. Clin. N. Am., pp. 117-127, March, 1965.
67. Burch, James G.: Lecture notes, International Academy of Gnathology Seminar, San Diego, Calif., 1971.
68. Gordon, Theodore: Telescope reconstruction—an approach to oral rehabilitation, J.A.D.A. **72:**97-105, 1966.
69. Abrams, Leonard, and Feder, Morris: Periodontal considerations for removable prosthesis, Alpha Omegan **55:**123-136, 1962.
70. Prichard, J. F., and Feder, Morris: A modern adaptation of the telescopic principle in periodontal prosthesis, J. Periodontol. **33:**360-364, 1962.
71. Schweitzer, Jerome M.: Esthetics and hygiene after extensive periodontal treatment, J. Prosthet. Dent. **10:**284-287, 1960.
72. Stein, R. Sheldon: Pontic-residual ridge relationship, a research report, J. Prosthet. Dent. **16:**251-285, 1966.
73. Hirshberg, Saul M.: The relationship of oral hygiene to embrasure and pontic design—a preliminary study, J. Prosthet. Dent. **27**(1):26-38, 1972.
74. Shooshan, E. D.: The reverse pin-porcelain facing, J. Prosthet. Dent. **9:**284-301, 1959.
75. Shooshan, E. D.: A pin-ledge casting technique; its application in periodontal splinting, Dent. Clin. N. Am., pp. 189-206, March, 1960.
76. Staffanou, Robert S., and Thayer, Keith E.: Reverse pin-porcelain veneer and pontic technique, J. Prosthet. Dent. **12:**1138-1145, 1962.
77. Minker, Jules S.: Simplified full coverage preparations, Dent. Clin. N. Am., pp. 371-372, July, 1965.
78. Skurnik, Harry R.: Treatment planning for occlusal rehabilitation, J. Prosthet. Dent. **9:**988-1000, 1959.
79. Colbern, Robert: Effective oral hygiene for full mouth rehabilitation, Second International Congress of Gnathology, San Diego, Calif., 1965.
80. Arnim, S. S.: Microcosms of human mouth, J. Tenn. Dent. Assoc. **39:**3-28, 1959.
81. Arnim, S. S., and Hagerman, D. A.: The connective tissue fibers of the marginal gingiva, J.A.D.A. **47:**271-281, 1953.
82. Cohen, D. Walter, and Bohannan, Harry M.: Current periodontal therapy. In Goldman, Henry M., Forrest, Stephen P., Byrd, D. Lamar, and McDonald, Ralph E.: Current therapy in dentistry, vol. 1, St. Louis, 1964, The C. V. Mosby Co., pp. 60-67.
83. Mesrobian, Armen Z.: Simplified oral physiotherapy or gingival home care, J.A.D.A. **63:**98-99, 1961.
84. Cantor, M. T., and Stahl, S. S.: Interdental col tissue responses to the use of a water pressure cleansing device, J. Periodontol. **40:**292, 1969.

CHAPTER 7

ESSENTIAL AND FUNDAMENTAL FACTORS INVOLVED IN CROWN AND BRIDGE PROSTHODONTICS

A consideration of the many phases of crown and bridge prosthodontics as we see it today demands of the dentist more exacting attention to the biologic, physiologic, engineering, mechanical, and esthetic phases of construction. The fixed partial denture, properly planned and skillfully constructed, affords a health and preventive service that is not comparable to any other type of replacement. It requires great precision and the most ardent attention to fine detail; we must design our appliances to conform to physical and engineering principles, as well as to biologic requirements.

By the biologic requirement we mean the condition of the abutment teeth, the pulps of these teeth, the hard and soft investing tissues, and the design of the appliance in order to be conducive to the health of those tissues. We must keep in mind that fine workmanship and accurate technique are very important, but if the end result only fills a space and fails to conform to the biologic requisites of the mouth, then the efforts for the most part are usually expended in vain. Do not permit any portion of a fixed or removable prosthesis to rest on interproximal embrasure area. This applies to solder joints, pontic areas, retainers, connectors, and denture bases.

By the physiologic requirement we mean that the appliance should be constructed with those anatomic details characteristic of natural teeth in order to restore lost efficiency, which includes functional occlusion. We must consider the question of how teeth function as a completely integrated unit.

In other words, the planning of the restoration should entail the consideration of the foundation upon which it is to be supported, the teeth to be employed as abutments, the importance of the intermaxillary relationship, harmony and balance of occlusion, the mechanical and engineering principles essential to good construction, comprehensive knowledge of the properties of the materials involved, and the problem of esthetics.[1] The biomechanical aspects must be interrelated harmoniously and, if this is accomplished, the oral tissues will accept the restorations biologically. The oral cavity must be considered as a whole, a tooth being an integral part of a highly organized mechanism which in the ideal functions harmoniously and physiologically.

The fundamental requirement to maintaining a successful result is a harmonious relationship between form and function. The object of restorative dentistry is, by alteration of the functional relations, to create forms which will reduce stress and distribute forces throughout the entire supporting structures of the mouth. But to achieve this, these tooth forms must likewise be harmonious with the functional relations of the muscles and temporomandibular joints. We must use every tool at our command and not place our reliance on treatment of local factors alone.

And so, to create the architecture which will achieve a harmony of *form* and *function,* we must know how to take intelligent advantage of the tools and knowledge that are available. It would appear then that the objective of restorative treatment is to create prosthetic appliances which are adapted to the individual requirements of form and function, so as to obviate the forces and stresses resulting from lack of adaptation.

Splinting is necessary where the functional relations are such that it is impossible to achieve functional stability of individual teeth. It will prevent teeth from drifting but will not prevent stresses on supporting structures. It should not be used as a crutch to substitute for adequate occlusal forms but should be used as an adjunct in the creation of a physiologic environment.

Requirements for success of a fixed partial denture include:

1. A thorough examination, which must include the proper selection of the most desirable type or method of replacing missing teeth. The prime purpose of any fixed partial denture is to preserve the remaining teeth. This should receive the greatest consideration. The purposes of restoration of masticatory function, phonetics, and improvement of esthetics become secondary with relative values according to the individual requirements.

2. A favorable occlusion or a condition in which this important factor can be obtained. We must note the discrepancies of jaw-to-jaw relationships and tooth-to-tooth positions. This determination of correct jaw-to-jaw relationships and tooth-to-tooth positions is based on an understanding of centric relation and centric occlusion. We are seeking a balance between occlusal stress and tissue resistance—it may be natural to the individual or it may be acquired through restorative measures.

3. Careful selection and designing of retainers. An ideal retainer is (a) one that requires the least amount of destruction to the abutment tooth, (b) one that least destroys the outline form of the tooth, (c) one that has the least amount of marginal line, (d) one that can be finished about its periphery with great accuracy and its margins positioned so as to be less susceptible to caries or recurrence of caries, (e) one that will be so rigid (have structural adequacy) that it will withstand the requisite load without distortion or deformation or opening of margins when subjected to functional stresses, (f) one that will have frictional adaptation and protect the tooth against its fracture, (g) one that least destroys the cervical marginal ridge, (h) one whose preparation can be made without trauma to the pulp or surrounding tissues, (i) one that is an accurate complement to the lost tooth structure, (j) one that is readily cleansable, and (k) one that fulfills the requirements of esthetics.

Myers[2] has aptly pointed out that displacing stresses concentrate at the junction between the restoration and the tooth at the cement lute, and that the weak point in a bridge is the cement lute.

"Dental cements are not adherent, and do not bond to the retainer or to the tooth. Cements hold a bridge in place by mechanical locking. If stresses in the cement lute are too high, the cement will break and the bridge will become loose.

"Dental cements have high compressive strengths, but low tensile and shear strength. Therefore, it is important to design bridge retainers in a way that transmits the functional forces to the cement lute as compressive forces and not tensile or shear forces. This can be accomplished by having the axial walls of retainer preparations as near parallel as possible and as long as the tooth will allow" (Figs. 7-1 and 7-2).*

4. Incorporating into the restoration those anatomic details characteristic of natural teeth (axial and occlusal surfaces). Occlusal anatomy has an indirect influence on the loads transmitted to the teeth. Normal occlusal surfaces are curved, ridged, and tuberculated. The triangular ridges, tubercular in form, produce many of the points of occlusal contact. Nature placed at each side of the ridge a supplemental groove to permit escape of the bolus and reduce leverage. Ridges and grooves increase the sharpness and shearing action of teeth and reduce friction between opposing surfaces by keeping the contacting area to a minimum, thereby reducing the load transmitted to the abutment teeth (Fig. 7-3).

---

*From Myers, George E.: Textbook of crown and bridge prosthodontics, St. Louis, 1969, The C. V. Mosby Co., pp. 11-13.

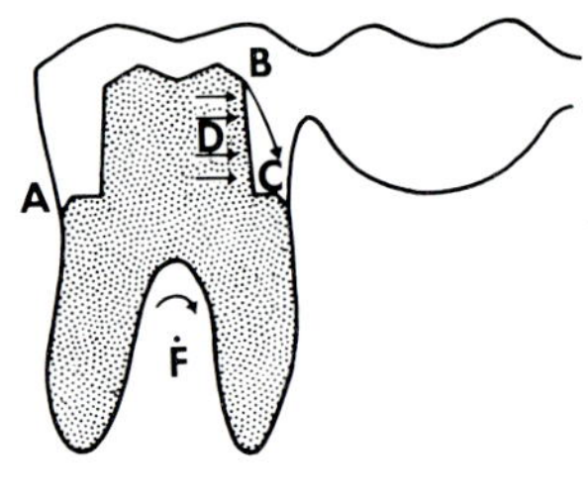

Fig. 7-1. Effect of a mesial tilting force on molar abutment and the retainer of a bridge with long axial walls and minimum taper. For the tooth to move out of the retainer about point *A,* point *B* would have to move through the retainer on arc *BC.* Cement along the mesial axial wall is subjected to compression. *F,* Natural rotation point of tooth; *D,* compressive force against cement. (Redrawn from Myers, George E.: Textbook of crown and bridge prosthodontics, St. Louis, 1969, The C. V. Mosby Co.)

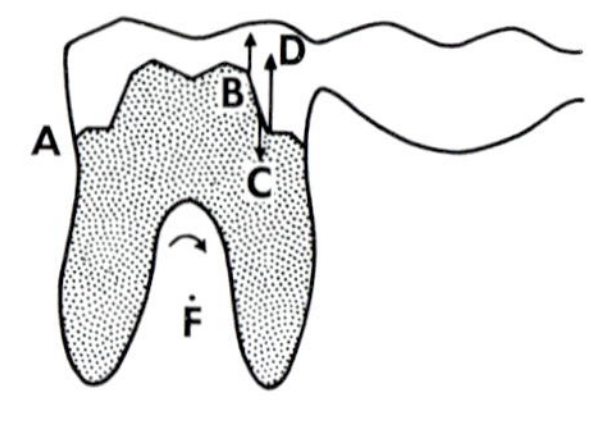

Fig. 7-2. Effect of a mesial tilting force on molar abutment and the retainer of a bridge with short axial walls and a greater degree of taper. For the tooth to move out of the retainer about point *A,* point *B* would move along the arc *BC,* which does not pass through the retainer. The cement on the mesial axial wall is subjected to shear. *F,* Natural rotation point of tooth; *D,* tensile and shear forces against cement. (Redrawn from Myers, George E.: Textbook of crown and bridge prosthodontics, St. Louis, 1969, The C. V. Mosby Co.)

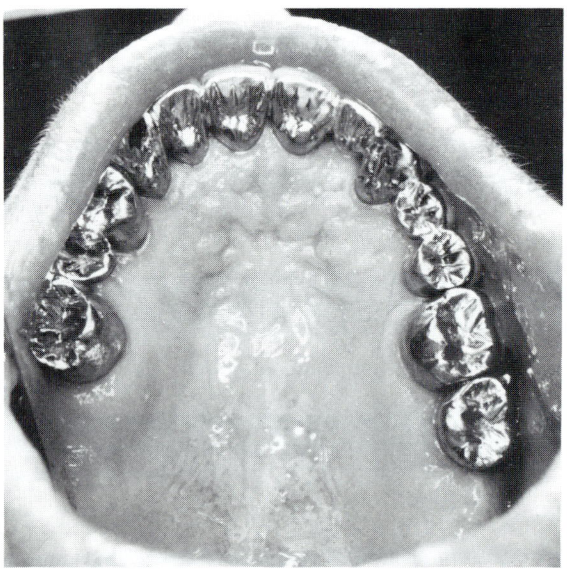

Fig. 7-3. Occlusal anatomy has an indirect influence on the loads transmitted to the teeth. Normal occlusal surfaces are curved, ridged, and tuberculated.

5. Adequate consideration of the biologic, physiologic, mechanical, engineering, and esthetic factors in order that our appliances conform to the laws of nature, which we know to be unchangeable.

Failures, therefore, in fixed partial denture construction can be avoided, to a considerable extent, by the proper selection of dental materials for the case at hand, correct abutment preparations, avoidance of faulty fabrication of the appliance by being well versed in good technical procedures, and application of the basic laws of mechanics and engineering in the construction of these appliances.

Reynolds[3] has said that lack of sufficient rigidity in a fixed prosthesis is a frequent cause of failure. Rigidity is obtained by the use of the proper materials arranged in the correct shape, form, and thickness in regard to the forces acting upon them. Flexure can cause damage to the abutments and may result in loosening of the retainers and fatigue of the metal.

Also of importance is a consideration of the stresses of occlusion, keeping in mind the fact that vertical stresses need not greatly concern us because these stresses are more favorable due to the histologic structure of the periodontal ligament. But the lateral stresses present a different problem and must be kept within biologic limits. Fixed partial dentures transmit forces through their abutments to the periodontium.

Consideration must also be given to:

1. The alignment of the abutment teeth (do they occupy their normal positions in the arch?).

2. The physical aspect of the tooth itself as to size and shape of the crown (is it long, medium, or short; is it well formed, bell-shaped, etc.?), as well as the number of roots and their shape, length (short or tapered roots can create a problem), alignment, and bone height or level.

3. The ratio of the bone support to the length of the tooth. Periodontal support may be determined by the application of a rule, Ante's law,[4] which states that "in fixed bridgework the combined pericemental area of the abutment teeth should be equal to or greater in pericemental area than the tooth or teeth to be replaced."*

---

*From Ante, I. H.: The fundamental principles of abutments, Mich. Dent. Soc. Bull. **8:**14, 1926.

4. Crown-to-root ratio. A crown-to-root ratio of 1:2 in linear measurement is considered ideal, and a crown-to-root ratio of 1:1 in linear measurement is probably an absolute minimum, providing use is made of multiple abutments applying the principle of splintage. This gives us some assurance that the occlusal load transmitted to the abutment teeth can be tolerated within their factor of safety, which includes their reserve capacity, and determination can be made of the load-bearing ability of the abutment teeth.

Other factors to be considered are:

1. Length of span to be replaced (is it a long or short span?). The longer the span and the greater the stresses and strains or torques on the abutment teeth, the more consideration must be given to the crown-to-root ratio and splintage.

2. Contact and alignment of adjacent teeth.

3. The long axis relationship. Keep forces, if possible, directed along the long axis of the tooth, and keep in mind that the maximum deviation from parallel can be no more than 25 to 30 degrees.

4. The structure of the supporting bone such as thickness, pattern, and density. The trabeculae should be uniform, both in their size and distribution, and, if they are, the bone can withstand the load of proper function. The functional demands placed upon the supporting structures must not exceed the metabolic activity of the bone for that particular patient. Glickman[5] has pointed out that each patient has a bone factor (the response of alveolar bone to local etiologic agents in periodontal disease is governed by interrelated systemic influences), and the bone factor for each

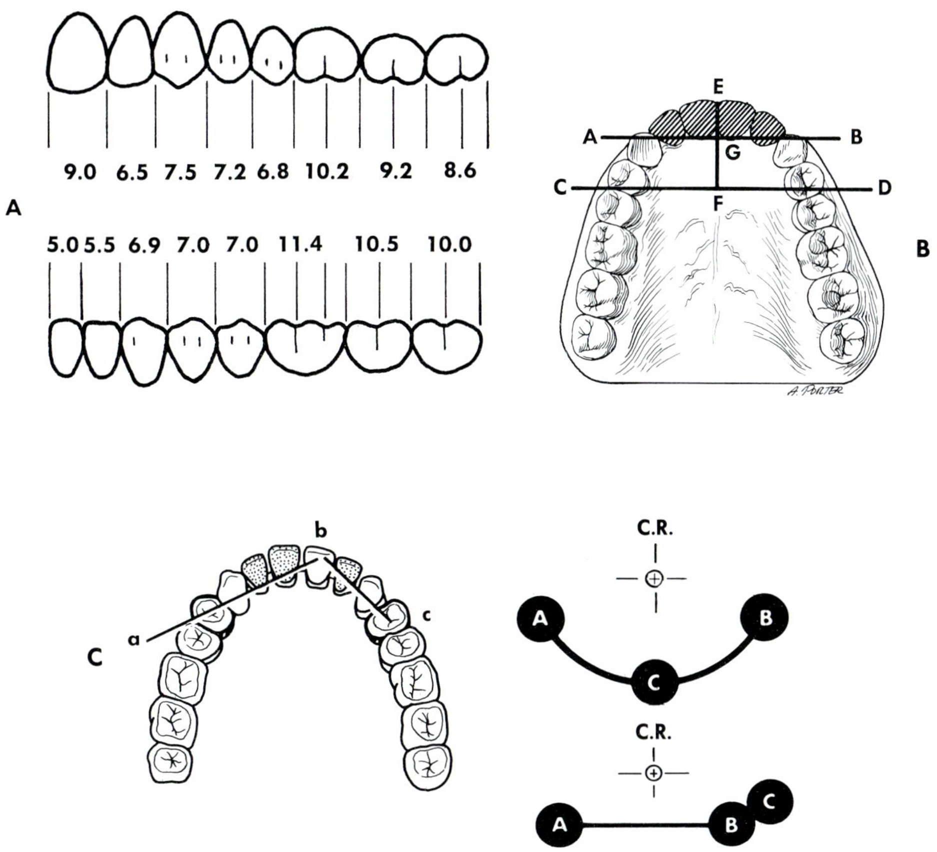

Fig. 7-4. A, A knowledge of the mesiodistal width of average natural teeth is important in selection of abutment and pontic design. **B,** Line *AB* is the fulcrum line around which the fixed partial denture tends to rotate; line *CD* is the distal extent of the abutments; line *EG* is the lever arm; line *GF* is the counterbalancing arm. Line *GF* should equal or exceed line *EG* in all fixed partial denture situations. **C,** The greatest leverage occurs when four maxillary incisors are replaced in a narrow tapered arch. The presence of a single incisor will considerably shorten the lever arm. (**A** and **C** courtesy J. Marvin Reynolds; **B** adapted from Reynolds, J. Marvin: J. Prosthet. Dent. **19**[5]:483-488, May, 1968.)

patient must be evaluated and classified before placement of fixed restorations.

5. Arch form. "Restorations involving anterior teeth are shaped in the form of an arc. When forces are applied to the pontics, a rotational effect occurs on the abutments and a vertical force is exerted on the terminal ends of the fixed partial denture. The counterbalancing force supplied by the abutments should equal or exceed that of the pontics as indicated by the length of the lever arm. The lever arm is determined by drawing a perpendicular line from the fulcrum line to the point on the pontics farthest from this line. The fulcrum is a line joining the abutments adjacent to the edentulous space at the proximo-occlusal angles of the preparation (Fig. 7-4). The greatest leverage occurs when four maxillary incisors are replaced in a narrow tapered arch. The presence of a single incisor will considerably shorten the lever arm. A long lever arm can be equalized by using additional abutments."*

6. Pontics. The first consideration in designing a pontic is strength; the second is anatomic form that will function in mastication and provide surfaces that are easily cleansable; and the third is esthetics. The normal mucosa over a ridge is firm and unyielding; it is attached to the underlying bone by a dense fibrous tissue. The tissue-contacting surface of the pontic should be convex in form, smooth, make minimal contact, be free of pressure, and be confined within the area of the immovable mucosa of the ridge (if extended into the movable border tissue inflammation and irritation will result). The occlusal surface of the pontics should harmonize with the buccolingual dimension of the natural teeth and recreate the normal buccal and lingual form to the height of contour. Reducing the width of pontics does not materially reduce the forces transmitted to abutments.[3] Narrowing the pontic somewhat in its lingual half widens the lingual embrasures from the contact areas and is considered good practice. Advantage should be taken of the hollow-grinding principle, which greatly reduces facing fracture, because these failures are usually due to stresses of mastication being carried indirectly through an inadequate gold reinforcement that is insufficiently rigid to resist bending. In the anterior part of the mouth, interproximal exaggeration cannot be carried out as much as in the posterior regions because of esthetic considerations, but one cannot overlook the fact that adequate embrasures between pontics and abutments, as well as between adjacent pontics, are very important. Correctly shaped, they allow flushing action and do not retain food particles.

*From Reynolds, J. Marvin: Abutment selection for fixed prosthodontics, J. Prosthet. Dent. **19**(5):486, 1968.

Faust[1] has called attention to the importance of noting and recording pertinent midline information. In the case of the cuspid-to-cuspid fixed partial denture, through drifting or maladjustment of teeth and because of the importance of a correct esthetic placement of the midline, it will often be found that one of the laterals will have to be smaller than the other in order to get it into the space. This is exactly the condition that often is found in nature, and it is very conducive to naturalness of appearance. Far too many of our cuspid-to-cuspid restorations disregard proper midline placement and the natural irregularity of teeth as to position, size, and shade, with the result that our restorations are often very unesthetic.

Another essential in the considerations of important factors in the construction of fixed partial dentures is the *health of the dental pulp*. Normal pulps atrophy gradually and the dentin becomes more consolidated as the age of the patient advances. This makes possible the employment of fixed restorations in older teeth where a younger pulp would be less suitable. This does not rule out the necessity of always making certain of the pulp's size, position, and degree of calcification by x-ray diagnosis and the pulp's response to diagnostic stimuli. For this purpose of diagnosis the thermal change induced by a pointed piece of ice is the one preferred. The response of a normal pulp disappears immediately, while the response of a degenerating pulp lingers upon removal of the stimulus.

ENGINEERING PRINCIPLES*

The construction of a fixed partial denture must follow definite laws of mechanics and their subdivisions of kinematics, dynamics, kinetics, and statics. It is impossible to guess at the forces to which such a structure is exposed (strains, stresses, torque, equilibrium), and therefore one must make use of principles of mechanics acceptable to engineering practice. The fixed partial denture provides the most stable foundation to vertical and horizontal loading and stresses the periodontium most favorably through tension. Teeth which are periodontal risks should not be used at less

*As a teacher and clinician, I have taught and applied in practice the principles of mechanics acceptable to engineering practice to avoid failures of dental restorations. I have drawn extensively in this section, with permission, from the excellent research work of R. C. Brumfield and E. S. Smyd.

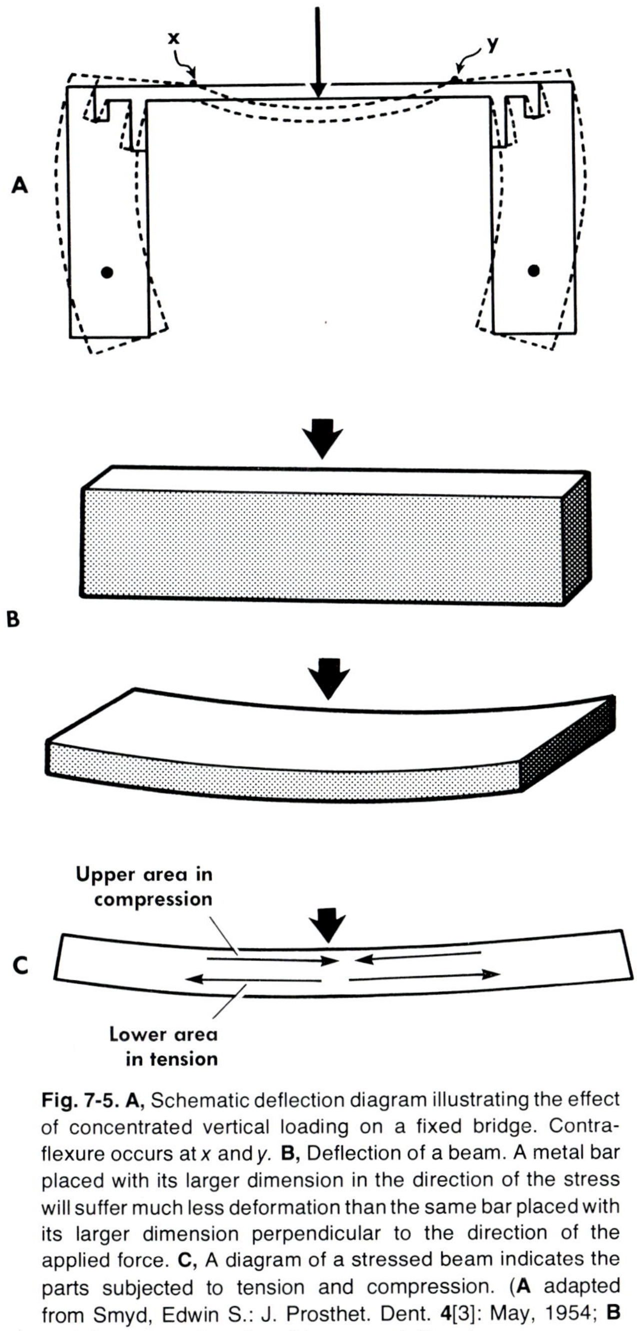

Fig. 7-5. A, Schematic deflection diagram illustrating the effect of concentrated vertical loading on a fixed bridge. Contraflexure occurs at *x* and *y*. **B,** Deflection of a beam. A metal bar placed with its larger dimension in the direction of the stress will suffer much less deformation than the same bar placed with its larger dimension perpendicular to the direction of the applied force. **C,** A diagram of a stressed beam indicates the parts subjected to tension and compression. (**A** adapted from Smyd, Edwin S.: J. Prosthet. Dent. **4**[3]: May, 1954; **B** and **C** courtesy American Thermocraft Corp.)

than their maximal capacity to take tensile stress.

According to Brumfield[6]: "The principles governing the load-carrying capacities of dental bridges are those of beams, for all such bridges are beams. A beam is any structural member which changes curvature under load. When occlusal loads come upon the dental bridge, it deflects slightly under the influence of those loads, and so changes curvature" (Fig. 7-5).*

If a fixed partial denture is to be a satisfactory beam, (1) it must not be too long (too long a span) for the number of retainers, (2) the retainers must have adequate retention, and (3) lateral occlusal forces, which produce torquing of abutment teeth, should not be excessive in order to avoid displacement of the restoration from its abutments.

If a long span bridge must be used, keep in mind that the strength of a long span bridge is not as great as a short span bridge because it will carry a greater load. Every auxiliary device possible to strengthen it must be employed. This includes the use of a partial denture gold (type 4) for its construction, which will increase the load-carrying capacity of the bridge. At least the use of a type 4 gold for the pontics is in order, because bending stresses are greater near the middle of the bridge than near the end supports (Fig. 7-6). Tough metals like partial denture gold alloys take stress in tension well, so a crown is a rigid structure, even though its walls may be thin, providing a type 4 gold alloy is used.[7]

"All this points out one of the important principles governing the deflection strength of dental bridges—the greater the yield strength of the metal used in a bridge, the greater the load-carrying capacity of the bridge or, in other words, the higher the yield strength the greater the biting stresses a metal can withstand. Assuming identical design, the load-carrying capacity is proportional to the yield strength. That is, the load-carrying capacity of a type 4 alloy of 80,000 p.s.i. yield strength is twice that of a type 3 alloy of 40,000 p.s.i. yield strength. Another important principle is that a shorter span bridge will deflect less than a longer span bridge or, we can say, a three-unit bridge will deflect only half as much as a six-unit bridge. The connection between these two principles is obvious. For example, if you design a three-unit bridge with a specific section thickness and use a type 3 alloy, you can use the same section thickness for a six-unit bridge, provided you use a type 4 alloy. Thus, both bridges

*From Brumfield, R. C.: Load capacities of posterior dental bridges, J. Prosthet. Dent. **4**(4):530, 1954.

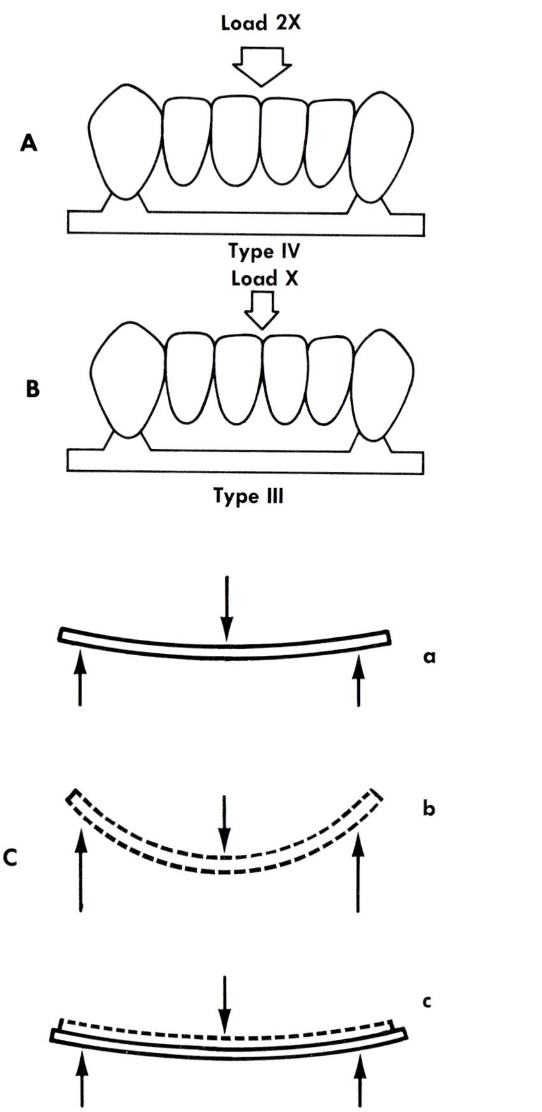

Fig. 7-6. Type 4 gold, **A,** has twice the load-carrying capacity of the type 3 gold, **B,** and is more ideally suited for long span bridges. **C,** Schematics demonstrate the strengthening influence of a material with high moduli of elasticity. *a,* "Stiff" material like steel or type 3 gold alloy will deflect little to a given load; *b,* tooth structure with low moduli of elasticity will deflect greatly to the same load; *c,* the deflection of a composite of tooth structure and type 3 gold alloy will deflect about as much as the type 3 alloy itself. Most of the stress is borne by the metal. (**A** and **B** courtesy J. F. Jelenko & Co., Inc.; **C** adapted from Smyd, Edwin S.: J. Prosthet. Dent. **11**[1]:95-111, Jan.-Feb., 1961.)

will be structurally similar as regards load carrying capacity.''*[8]

If the estimated load-carrying capacity of a particular bridge is equal to or greater than the biting pressures for the teeth replaced by pontics,† the bridge may be considered entirely satisfactory as a load-carrying device. The load-carrying capacity of fixed restorations varies directly with the proportional limit (the greatest stress that a material will sustain without a deviation from the law of proportionality of stress to strain) of the metal used in its construction. Yield strength may be taken as synonymous with proportional limit for design purposes.

Soldered joints should be made as thin with as great a strength as possible, and as deep occlusogingivally as is permissible so as to show strengths comparable to those of the pontics by partaking of the strength characteristics of the metal portion of the bulky pontics which they join. At the same time the need for interproximal stimulation and cleansing should be considered. It is necessary to get sound, gas-oxide-free joints between the parts. This also gives the joint strength to bear occlusal loads. Where bending moments are large, joints should be located as far as possible from the center of the bridge span.

In summation, in regard to factors related to load-carrying capacities of dental bridges it can be said[9]: ''There are three factors that are of determinative influence on the load-carrying capacity of the dental bridge: (a) the loads that are to come upon the bridge, both as to intensity and as to character (static, impact, concentrated, etc.); (b) the form and shape of the structure that receives the loads; the load placing, and the consequent stresses induced within the structure; (c) the ability of the material from which the structure is built to withstand the stresses induced within it. These three factors are not related to each other.''‡

Smyd[10, 10a] defines *torque* as a force acting through a moment arm or lever which produces rotation about a given point or axis. Torque deforms or stresses the body on which it acts, and the deformation

*From Tuccillo, Joseph J.: Load carrying capacities of dental alloys, Thermotrol Technician **24**(2):4, 1970.

†See Table 40-1, Biting forces of human teeth and recommended design loads, in Tylman, S. D.: Theory and practice of crown and fixed partial prosthodontics (bridge), ed. 6, St. Louis, 1970, The C. V. Mosby Co.

‡From Tylman, S. D.: Theory and practice of crown and fixed partial prosthodontics (bridge), ed. 6, St. Louis, 1970, The C. V. Mosby Co., p. 911. (Structural investigation and design of dental restorations [bridges]; relationship of structural design to biologic acceptance.)

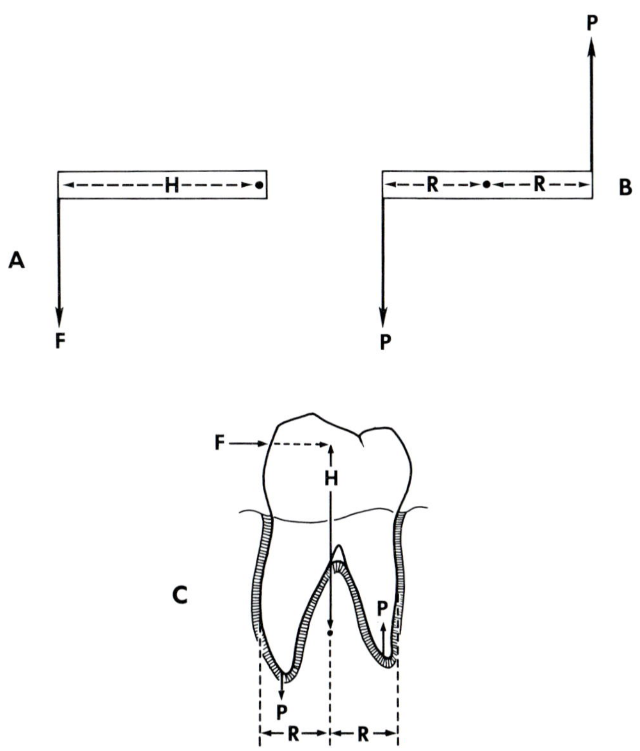

Fig. 7-7. **A,** Simple illustration of torque. **B,** Torque through action of a couple. **C,** The torque of the applied force *F* is resisted by the torque of the couple in the investing structures. At equilibrium, FH = P · 2R. (Adapted from Smyd, Edwin S.: J. Prosthet. Dent. **11**[1]:Jan.-Feb., 1961.)

may be compressive, tensile, a combination of these two, or torsional. Torque and bending are largely responsible for many prosthetic failures. It is one of the most harmful stresses to which abutment teeth may be subjected.

"A *couple* is a pair of equal paralleled forces acting in opposite directions, but not on the same point. A couple also produces torque, and by definition the measure of a couple is one of forces times the perpendicular distance between them, or P · 2R" (Fig. 7-7).*

"All bodies, however rigid or massive they may be, are beyond question deformed by the application of force. It does not matter how small the forces may be, the deformations are necessarily present. Mastication gives rise to forces which produce deformations of compression, tension, shear, deflection (bending), elongation, and torsion of highly significant magnitude in the investing tissues, the teeth, and the restorations."†[11]

A consideration of stress and of the three basic types of stresses is in order at this time. Stress is the internal reaction to the external force and is equal in intensity and opposite in direction to the applied external force. The three basic types of stresses are (1) tension, (2) compression, and (3) shear. "*Tension* re-

*From Smyd, Edwin S.: The role of torque, torsion, and bending in prosthodontic failures, J. Prosthet. Dent. **11**(1):95-111, 1961; also Smyd, Edwin S.: Role of mechanical stress in dentistry, New York J. Dent. **28**:227-235, 1958.

†From Smyd, Edwin S.: Dental engineering, J. Dent. Res. **27**: 649, 1948.

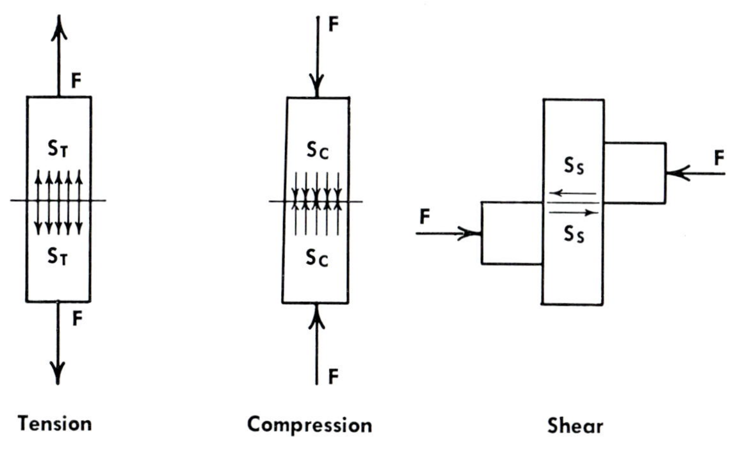

Fig. 7-8. The three basic types of stresses. (From Peyton, F. A., and Craig, R. G.: Restorative dental materials, ed. 4, St. Louis, 1971, The C. V. Mosby Co.)

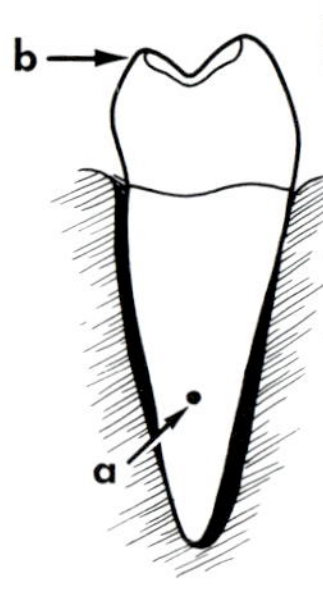

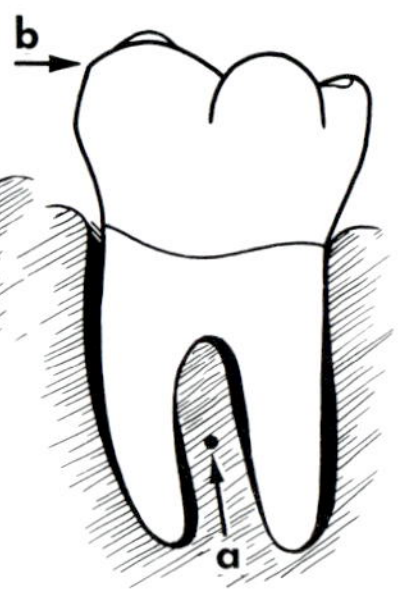

Fig. 7-9 Fig. 7-10

Fig. 7-9. A single-rooted tooth rotates to transverse force on the center *a* in the apical third of the root of the tooth.
Fig. 7-10. The lower molar rotates to transverse force *b* about a center *a* in the radicular bone. Translation of the roots occurs. (Figs. 7-9 and 7-10 adapted from Smyd, Edwin S.: J. Prosthet. Dent. **11**[1]:Jan.-Feb., 1961.)

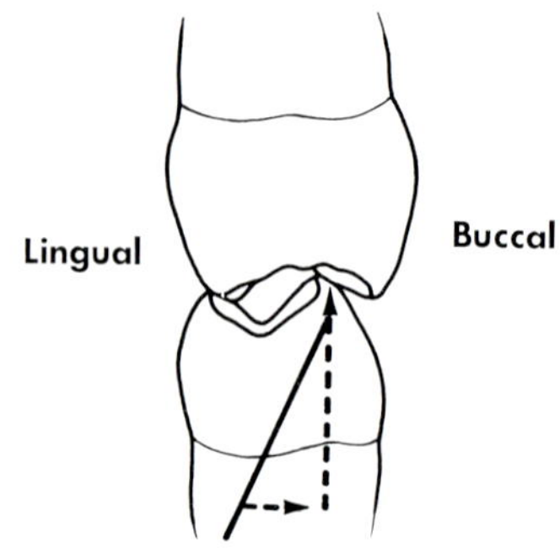

Fig. 7-11. Vector analysis of forces acting when the lower posterior teeth are in contact with the uppers and the mandible moves from "working" bite to centric relation.

sults in a body when it is subjected to two sets of forces which are directed away from each other in the same straight line; *compression* results when the body is subjected to two sets of forces in the same straight line and directed toward each other; *shear* is the result of two sets of forces being directed toward each other, but not in the same straight line'' (Fig. 7-8).*[12]

A single-rooted tooth is under mechanical disadvantage to take horizontal loading. Single-rooted teeth describe rotational movements when subjected to lateral forces, and an axis of rotation is established somewhere near the apical third of the root of the tooth (Fig. 7-9).[10]

The multirooted teeth are better able to take horizontal loading if the force is directed across the roots. Multirooted teeth also turn on axes in the apical third of the roots, but if the transverse force is directed across the roots, one root moves down under the force and the root nearer the point of application of the force moves up. Rotation occurs about a point in the bone septum between the two roots (Figs. 7-10 and 7-11).

The periodontium and bone take tensile stress well, much better than they take compression. If compression is sustained by the tooth and its investing structures, we have a condition known as osteoclasia. Osteogenesis takes place on the tension side. In the resolution of restorative problems, we should maximize tensile stress and minimize compressive stress in the investing structures of the teeth.

''Fixation of abutments reduces tooth movements, places more periodontal fibers in tensile stress through increasing the orbits of tooth rotations, gains mechanical advantage and simultaneously reduces stress in the fibers and bone. Fixation reduces the stress in the periodontal ligament through leverage.

''Torsion of individual teeth occurs frequently in mastication, and it is much more significant when its effects are increased through leverage. A good example is a fixed partial denture between an upper cuspid and the first molar. The patient bites into a crust of bread that is very resistant to mastication, and the crust is compressed against the occlusal surface of the first bicuspid pontic and the lingual incline of the cuspid abutment. Three things occur: (1) the cuspid is depressed more deeply in its socket than the molar because the load is concentrated over the cuspid; (2) bending of the fixed partial denture occurs in the region of the bicuspid; and (3) the cuspid is moved laterally. The molar resists the lateral displacement so there is both bending and twisting of the metal framework. The same thing occurs in all posterior fixed partial dentures during eccentric mastication'' (Fig. 7-12).*

An ideal bridge is one in which, when seated, there is a condition of equilibrium.

Equilibrium is a state in which all forces balance not only as to translative tendency but also to their rotative tendency.

Reed[13] has said that the two kinds of motion, translation and rotation, are the first principles of kinematics and may be expressed as follows. *Pure translation* is a change in position or bodily movement of an object without change in direction of any of the axes or lines

*From Peyton, F. A., and Craig, R. G.: Restorative dental materials, ed. 4, St. Louis, 1971, The C. V. Mosby Co., p. 61.

*From Smyd, Edwin S.: The role of torque, torsion and bending in prosthodontic failures, J. Prosthet. Dent. **11**(1):95-111, 1961.

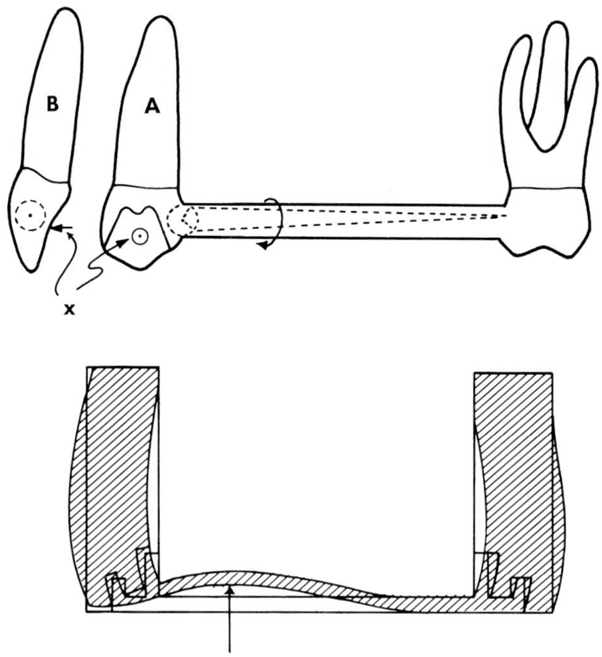

Fig. 7-12. When concentrated loading occurs on the fixed partial denture in the cuspid–first bicuspid region, both bending and torsion occur simultaneously. *B* is a side view of *A*. Transverse force is applied at *x*. (Redrawn from Smyd, Edwin S.: J. Prosthet. Dent. **11**[1]:Jan.-Feb., 1961.)

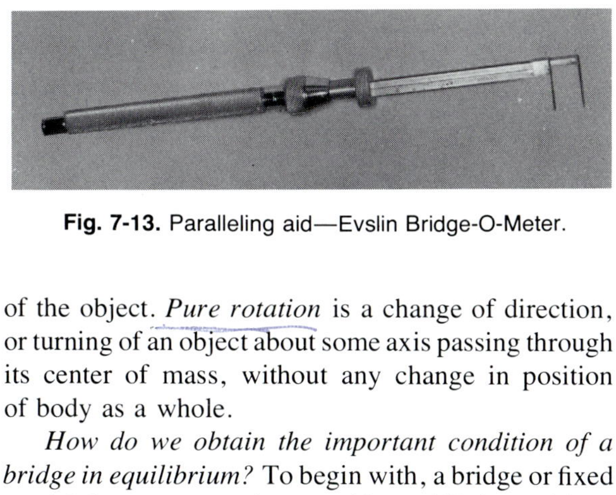

Fig. 7-13. Paralleling aid—Evslin Bridge-O-Meter.

of the object. *Pure rotation* is a change of direction, or turning of an object about some axis passing through its center of mass, without any change in position of body as a whole.

How do we obtain the important condition of a bridge in equilibrium? To begin with, a bridge or fixed partial denture cannot be seated in equilibrium without harmful stresses resulting unless (1) the walls of the abutment preparations are parallel or converge 2 degrees and not over 5 degrees (which enhances functional retention), and (2) the walls of the abutment teeth are surveyed with an instrument so adjusted as to ascertain the amount of inclination of the teeth and the amount of tooth structure which must be cut (this can be determined in the mouth and on study casts) to obtain this parallelism. After the teeth are prepared, a further check must be made to see if what we had in mind has been accomplished. This also includes any grooves, wells, pits, pinholes, etc. (Fig. 7-13). In other words, to have a fixed partial denture in equilibrium we must be able to insert it without undue stress in any direction. The bridge should go to place with no resistance other than the frictional resistance natural to two closely adapted surfaces. If the appliance goes to place with a "snap" it is not in equilibrium. It is true that nature may, at times, adjust to this torsion, but since one of the fundamental laws of mechanics has been violated some damage will result (periodontal ligament, bone absorption).

It is my opinion that it would serve us well to conform to the precept that equilibrium, the elimination of torsion, and the neutralizing of stresses are paramount to success; and in the surety of proper tapers, surface coverage, correct placement of grooves, pins, wells, etc. we greatly increase retention. So, use a mechanical guide, as a rule, and keep in mind that dependence on visual guidance to detect mechanical imperfections can create problems.

The desired property of a casting is rigidity, which is obtained by the use of the proper material, properly shaped and disposed in the correct manner with respect to the direction of the load. Jones[14] has called attention to the fact that the I-beam, the angle iron, the channel iron, and others are structural shapes giving the greatest strength with the least material and are rigid because of their shapes. These also must be used correctly with respect to the direction of the load.

Dental cement, as previously stated in this chapter, can take great stress in compression—6,000 to 12,000 p.s.i. The security of the bond may be questioned if the bond is subjected to shear or diagonal tension. Dental cement acts as a bond not through adhesion, but rather as a keying mechanism between the irregularity and roughness of the restoration on the one side and the irregularity and roughness of the tooth on the other side.[10]

"The strength of the cement bond is determined by the following factors: (1) the strength of the cement in compression, tension, and shear; (2) the number and size of the interlocking keys; (3) the areas of the bond between opposing walls; (4) the taper of the cavity preparation; (5) the tolerance or closeness of fit between the casting and the tooth; and (6) coupling. The most important of these factors controlled by the dentist is coupling.

"The deficiency of the cement bond in shear and diagonal tension may be made up by some form of male-female engagement or coupling. Either *internal* *engagement* with a pin or dowel or extension of the dovetail into a groove in the buccal and lingual tooth structure (the casting furnishes the male and the tooth structure the female part of the coupling) or *external engagement* (the crown is the female and the tooth structure the male component) is used. Since dislodging forces acting on an abutment casting are not usually coaxial with the draft of the prepared tooth, mechanical coupling between the metal of the casting and the tooth may be employed to resist torque. Cement under the mechanically coupled parts is thus in compressive stress, the best possible way to load dental cement."*

In other words, the dowel and the crown provide the most effective coupling between the retainer and the tooth. Both the dowel and the crown present a continuously opposing surface to the tooth and, when prepared with little taper, both provide good mechanical coupling. The coupling should be such that the deflection and torsion set up in the prosthetic structure place the cement under the retainers in compressive stress. We must not depend upon cement to take the stress in shear or diagonal tension except in direct axial traction. If you feel that the prosthetic structure will subject the cement bond to great shear stress, be sure that the retainers are full cast veneers or at least well-designed and executed three-quarter crowns.

The life of a fixed bridge may be considered as a continual contest between load and abutments. A successful bridge is one in which the balance is always in favor of the abutments. First consideration should be the abutments available—how many are there? Next, what is the character of the bone in which they are supported? What vertical length do the abutments have? How much is extraosseous, how much intraosseous? In a case of horizontal atrophy in an older patient with hard supporting bone evident in the roentgenogram, the apparent excessive extraosseous length may not be a serious deterrent.

The load to which a bridge is subjected is governed by the opposing forces. Obviously, those forces which would be exerted through the medium of an opposing full denture would be markedly less than forces which would be exerted by sound, natural opposing teeth. Broad, flat occlusal surfaces greatly increase the load during the masticatory process, whereas anatomically carved occlusal surfaces properly articulated with opposing normal anatomic forms minimize the vertical pressures required in mastication, and only after complete contact of the opposing dentition is the full load exerted.

Leverage exerted upon a bridge is a very important consideration. Deviation of the fixed partial denture restoration from a straight line between the two primary abutments is an important cause of leverage occasionally overlooked.[15]

Salient facts

1. Abutment castings that support a prosthetic level through either fixation or precision attachment must be rigid and retentive through coupling.
2. Attachment castings share in the kinematics of the structures they support.
3. The dowel and the crown provide the most effective coupling between the attachment casting and the tooth.
4. Since attachment castings share in the bending of the pontic(s), the great danger of failure in dental restorations lies in thin sections of attachment castings.
5. The cavity preparation should conform to engineering principles so that structural demands upon the physical properties of the tooth and the restorative materials shall be properly met.
6. Cavity preparation should be, if possible, relatively shallow but extensive. Have square cut seats.
7. While a certain amount of "pitch" in the cavity walls is essential, it is easy to destroy resistance form by too much taper.
8. "All other things remaining equal, a two-tooth bridge will bend eight times as much as a one-tooth span, and a three-tooth span will bend twenty-seven times as much. We should take advantage of this fact.

"We want the metal parts of our bridge to be as thick occlusogingivally as possible, especially for long span bridges, to keep bending of the bridge span down so that the abutment castings will not be wrenched loose from the teeth; we want our abutment castings stiff so that they will not crumble the cement binding them to the teeth.

"Pontics should have as much metal from the occlusal to the gingival surface as the circumstances warrant. To accept less makes the pontic springy, which bends and twists the abutment castings excessively, especially in long sections.

"The deflection of the pontic on concentrated loading tends to thrust the teeth apart, and the dovetails are raised out of their seats in the teeth (Fig. 7-14).

"The only part of the bridge assembly which places cement under compression is the cervical floor

*From Smyd, Edwin S.: The role of torque, torsion, and bending in prosthodontic failures, J. Prosthet. Dent. **11**(1):95-111, 1961.

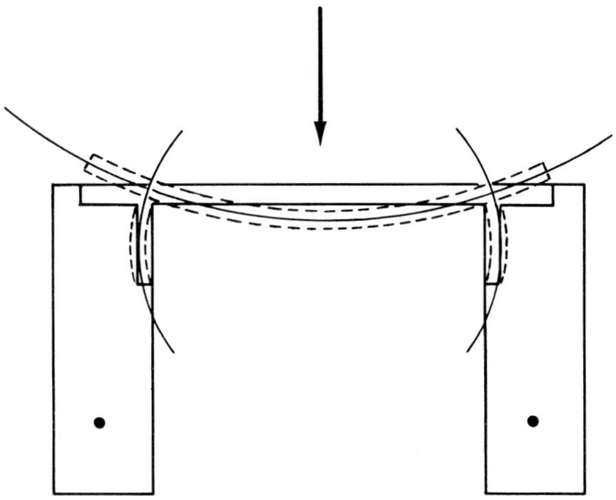

Fig. 7-14. Deflection diagram of a fixed bridge. (Courtesy Edwin S. Smyd.)

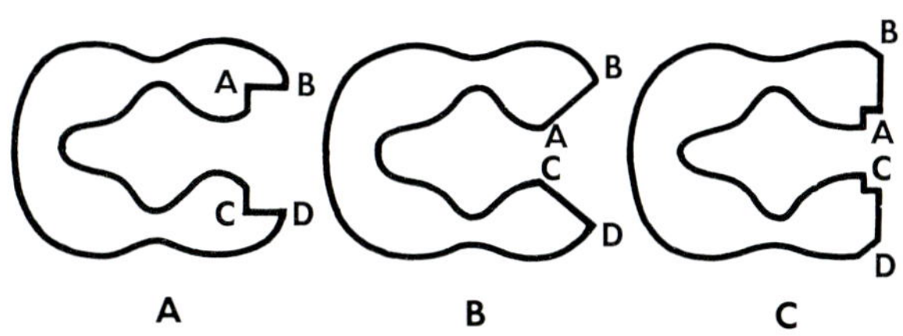

Fig. 7-15. The more nearly the proximal flange is cut as a box with parallel and opposing walls the stronger the bond, **A.** Black's box preparation, **B,** is nearer the ideal than the slice preparation, **C.** (Adapted from Smyd, Edwin S.: J. Prosthet. Dent. **2**[5]:Sept., 1952.)

of each abutment casting. These considerations establish as sound and reasonable the preparation of cavities with large flat cervical floors, and with provision for a thick proximal flange"*[16] (Fig. 7-15).

RETENTION

Preparations must provide amply for the mechanical retention of the fixed partial denture retainers. The displacing forces that a bridge transmits to the retainers are greater than those that fall on a single restoration, and therefore the retainers must have adequate strength to resist deformation under functional stresses. Consideration of the pontic, which acts as a lever, is also important, because we get a magnification of the occlusal forces transmitted to the retainers and abutment teeth.

Retention is obtained by close adaptation to nearly parallel walls, the variation from absolute parallel being sufficient only to permit the withdrawal of the pattern and the subsequent seating of the restoration. A retentive surface involves quantity as well as the degree of parallelism between walls. We must take into consideration not only that retention can also be increased, and more adequate strength obtained in our retainers, by the use of proximal boxes and grooves, locked grooves, bevels, occlusal keyways, pits, wells, pins, etc., but we must also evaluate the potential strength of the remaining bulk of tooth structure and the objective to increase the overall approximating surface area of tooth to casting so as to increase the quantity of cement which will effectively resist shearing. This is not the increasing of bulk cement, but rather increasing the effective number of square millimeters which can be effectively used and, especially, the necessity to increase the effective cementing surface when involved with short teeth. Of course, all this involves a projection of the probable forces to which the retainer and abutment tooth will be subjected, a determination of where the cleavage may occur, and the application of good design principles, forethought, and imagination.

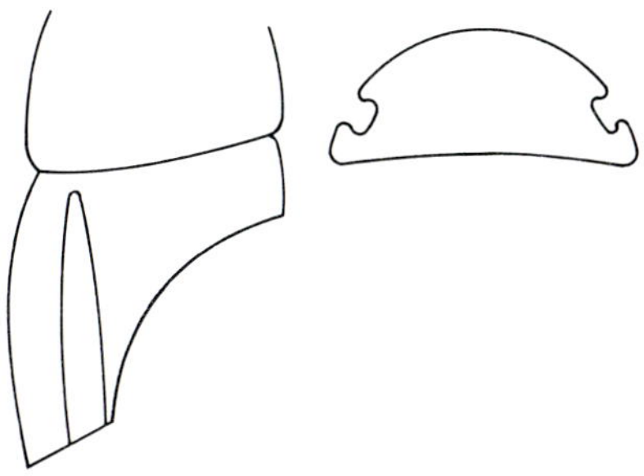

Fig. 7-16. Locked groove or oval groove is superior to the V shaped or round grooves. Retention is increased against lifting forces and also forces acting in a lingual direction.

Attention has been called to the use of grooves for additional retention of retainers. The locked groove or oval groove is superior to the V-shaped or round grooves (Fig. 7-16), because retention is tremendously increased against lifting forces and forces acting in a lingual direction, especially in reference to a three-quarter crown. In this type of preparation (three-quarter crown) the V-shaped groove is made with a No. 700 or No. 701 tapered cross-cut fissure bur, which does not add much retention against lifting forces in a vertical direction but which does prevent dislodgment in a lingual direction, providing the retainer is sturdy and will not spread mesiodistally. Probably in teeth of normal or longer crown length this type of

---

*From Smyd, Edwin S.: Mechanics of dental structures, J. Prosthet. Dent. **2**(5):668-692, 1952.

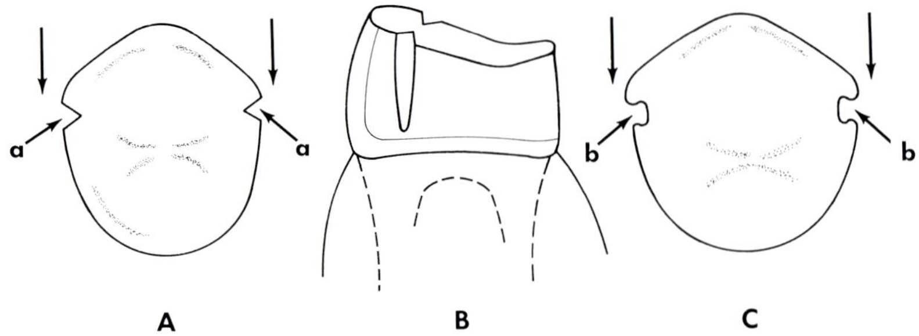

Fig. 7-17. A, These grooves have not added much to retention against lifting forces in a vertical direction, but they do prevent a dislodgment of the attachment in a lingual direction, providing attachment does not spread mesiodistally. **B,** In posterior teeth of normal or better crown length, this type of groove (V) usually has sufficient retention factors to carry properly constructed bridges. But in short crown teeth, retention is frequently inadequate against vertical lifting forces and the attachment can loosen. **C,** With the oval form groove retention is increased tremendously.

groove may be satisfactory, but in short crown teeth I believe it is inadequate. By making the oval or locked groove, which is made by first cutting the grooves in the usual manner with a No. 701 cross-cut taper fissure bur, then changing to a No. 700 cross-cut taper fissure bur, and moving this bur (No. 700) buccally and then lingually in cutting, the retention is increased tremendously. The resultant flanges on the casting made for this preparation become, in effect, like posts in canals and (1) increase the retention against lifting, vertical forces and (2) help the retainer resist spreading forces because the mesial and distal side walls of the retainer cannot move outward unless the tooth structure which forms the lip of the oval groove breaks away (Fig. 7-17), a condition that rarely occurs. I use the locked or oval groove in all three-quarter crown preparations, in full crown preparations where the crown of the tooth is short, and in many atypical inlay preparations.

Attention must also be called to the fact that besides retention of the retainers to the abutment teeth, there is another form of retention in fixed partial denture construction. That is retention of the abutment teeth themselves in the jaws. (A thorough coverage of the principles of splintage, the indications for the use of multiple retainers, etc. can be found in Chapter 6.)

Another essential in the retention of fixed partial dentures has to do with tooth form and function or tooth anatomy and physiology. The form and size of facial, lingual, and occlusal surfaces of retainers and pontics are of great importance. The buccolingual width of the working surface must not be too great (it should be approximately 60% of the distance from the buccal to the lingual wall at the widest part of the tooth), because the rocking forces are thereby increased detrimentally (Fig. 7-18). Our tooth form must

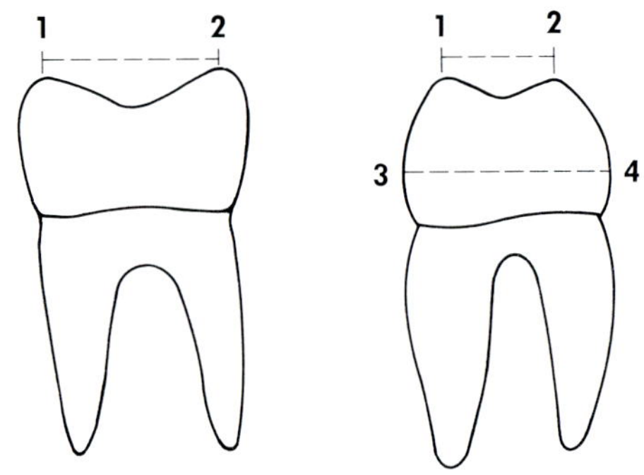

Fig. 7-18. The buccolingual width of the working surface must not be too great to avoid increased rocking forces.

be in accordance with nature's plan so as to overcome any resultant stress, or as much as possible.

The following are some of the important factors in influencing retention of fixed partial dentures: (1) correct tooth selection, design, and preparation to accept the proper retainers, (2) accurate construction and fit of the retainers, (3) adequate root support of abutment teeth, (4) correct tooth form and function, and (5) adequate strength of gold alloy used so as to have retainers that resist deformation under functional stresses.

Lorey and Myers[17] have made an excellent study of the retentive qualities of bridge retainers, and their findings can be substantiated clinically by many cases completed by me and kept under very close observation as to their retention (not considering any recurrent caries or accidental blows) over a span of many years.

Their tests were made by cementing the retainers on test dies and applying tensional forces in the line of draw of the preparation. The force required to break the cement seal and loosen the castings gave a value representing the retention of the casting. Each restoration was also tested in this manner before cementation to the die. Bureau of Standards dies gave the highest values obtained in the study because of large surface area and uniform taper of the preparation.

The findings of Lorey and Myers are very interesting and important to the clinician. For example, in some instances, the looser fitting castings gave higher values after cementation than those obtained from tight castings. They concluded that (1) there is no support for seeking excessively tight castings clinically as a criterion for good retention. In all probability the tight casting reduces the thickness of the cement lute below the optimum in some areas and reduces the retention value, whereas (2) the well-fitting casting which seats readily probably provides a more uniform space for the cement lute, and thereby higher retention values are obtained.

They also found that the addition of the cingulum pin to anterior three-quarter crowns increased retention, that pinledge restorations need not only pins but also ledges and recesses, which contribute considerably to the retentive values of the restoration, and that the full crown gave the maximum retentive value of all types of retainers. Retentive values increased with increased surface area of the preparation.

Another important finding was that the retention values of uncemented castings gave no indication of the retention values obtained after cementation.

Retainers

There are certain basic and fundamental principles upon which mechanical techniques are founded, and these principles continue to be applicable even though methods may change. Maximum of care and attention to details in making retainers on the abutment teeth is most essential.

Partial veneer crowns and full veneer crowns are the favored types of retainers for the majority of fixed partial dentures. The crown type retainers completely or partially surround the abutment teeth and tend to strengthen them.

A well-designed and accurately constructed partial veneer retainer offers ample strength and retention. Facial margins of partial veneer crowns may be placed where they are practically invisible.

To meet the stress of occlusion, do we prepare steps, etc. at right angles to the applied force? Likewise, in deciding on our retainers do we determine the type to be used by the fact that a more tense frictional grip is secured in a long, well-formed tooth than in a short tooth or short bell-shaped crown? Another factor in dislodging retainers is our failure to reestablish normal occlusion, thereby subjecting the retainers to an abnormal stress or strain. A study of occluding surfaces shows abutment teeth in abnormal occlusion many times, and it has been pointed out that a pathologic occlusion may often be prevented, or in early life corrected, by orthodontic treatment, or in later life by selective grinding of tooth surfaces or by occlusal reconstruction. We must also keep in mind that the stronger the forces of mastication, the greater the need for heavier occlusal protection; retainers of fixed partial dentures that are opposed by removable partial or full dentures are, as a rule, subjected to less strain than in the case of natural teeth; patients who show a small cuspid rise and long gliding contacts with the opposing teeth need more occlusal protection than those with a greater cuspid rise.[2]

As to the question of partial versus full coverage, what we must keep in mind is to make a proper analysis of each case. The indiscriminate use of full coverage for all teeth is to be avoided.

Amsterdam[18] has aptly said that when the clinical crown and the anatomic crown are practically the same, general dentistry is most efficient and periodontal therapy is rather simple. Use of partial coverage (onlays, partial veneer crowns, etc.) are ideal because guides for coronal contours are present, embrasure forms are preestablished, and adequate amounts of attached gingiva and adequate vestibular depth are present. In other words, keeping in mind the concept of the individual dental unit and maintenance of arch integrity; proper cavity preparations, including some occlusal adjustment by selective grinding, scaling, and, in some cases, subgingival curettage; proper technical procedures as to impression taking, casting, soldering, and cementation; minor orthodontic therapy (if indicated); and a good home care program offer the best potential for a good therapeutic result.

However, if the clinical crown and the anatomic crown are dissimilar, it is imperative to make use of full coverage. We are confronted with mobile teeth in need of splinting for mechanical retention and reshaping of coronal forms, for restoration of the relation of the clinical crown to its surrounding tissues, for covering and protecting exposed root structure, for esthetics, etc. However, this type of coverage, in spite of some of its disadvantages, cannot be abused (and it is being abused) as to treatment planning and mechanical execution. The potential of full coverage and splintage offers an excellent means of treating a complexity of problems faced in advanced restorative dentistry.

Types of abutment preparations

The types of abutment preparations include the inlay type and its various modifications, the overlay or veneer type, and a combination of the two. The typical mesio-occlusal (M.O.) or disto-occlusal (D.O.) inlays as retainers will usually end in failure unless advantage is taken of additional retention such as the Hoffer tripod principle, the Knapp slice-lock, or the methods advocated by Kyprie and the selection of teeth with proper length. The onlay, in some cases, offers greater possibilities depending on the degree of occlusal spread, additional retention possibilities, and the length of the axial walls.

The veneer type is represented by the three-quarter crown, the full crown, the pinledge, and half-crown (mesial version of the veneer crown).

In using the three-quarter crown as a fixed bridge retainer it is important to select the square type of tooth in the anterior region, and in the posterior region a bicuspid or molar of sufficient length.

The three-quarter crown, when used in carefully selected cases and avoiding extensively decayed teeth that do not permit the laying of retentive grooves in sound dentin, offers maximum retention with a minimum sacrifice of tooth structure. Its retention depends upon the staple formed by the mesial and distal converging grooves, which are laid just beneath the labial plate of the enamel and extend well toward the cementoenamel junction to give a firm lock about the cingulum, and a pin in the region of the cingulum. It is necessary, in this type of retainer, to have a sufficient thickness of metal at the linguoincisal portion of the tooth (to avoid opening of the margin because of work hardening of the gold alloy) and to avoid too tapering a preparation and a too soft gold alloy (Fig. 7-19).

The pinledge, the type in which the dowels are cast instead of using metal wire, is preferred. The dowel holes must be slightly larger so as to be able to get a good impression of the walls (by means of a hydrocolloid syringe), but the retention is much greater. One must be cautious in its preparation because of possible pulp involvement, but this type of retention (tripodism) is one of the best mechanical retentive forces that we have for use in the mouth. However, in using this type of retainer keep in mind the length of the span, the masticatory forces involved, and the amount of torque, torsion, and bending it will be subjected to in function and nonfunctional usage.

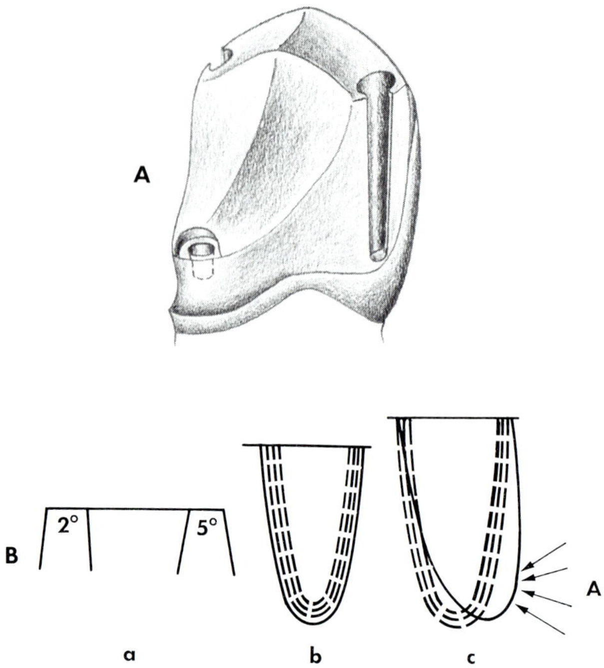

Fig. 7-19. A, Preparation of an anterior three-quarter crown. **B,** Ideal taper of walls of preparation should be between 2 and 5 degrees *(a)*. If grooves are parallel the bridge can be seated in a state of equilibrium *(b)*. However, if a groove is out of parallel a force would be exerted at *A* which would cause torsion *(c)*. (**B** adapted from Reed, Ray R.: Northwest Dent., Oct., 1943.)

Selberg's modification of using two dowel wells, one at the junction of the enamel and dentin near the incisal and the other in the cingulum area, and a proximal box or locked (oval) groove will offer a tremendous amount of resistance to displacement.

A number of failures have occurred with this type of retainer because of margins that "open up." Resistance can be increased to this by grooving adjacent to the margin for increased bulk, and by keeping the margin away from the area of stress in occlusion (Fig. 7-20).

The full gold veneer crown and *the porcelain or plastic veneer crown* fulfill all the mechanical requirements needed in a retainer, and they are the most retentive of all the retainers that we have at our command. They fulfill our needs as a retainer not only in well-formed and well-positioned teeth but in cases of extremely short or extensively decayed teeth and in those cases where gingival decay is prevalent. On bell-shaped teeth, the buccal and lingual margins need only extend slightly below the height of contour. The preparation should not be made too conical so as to have adequate retention (Fig. 7-21).

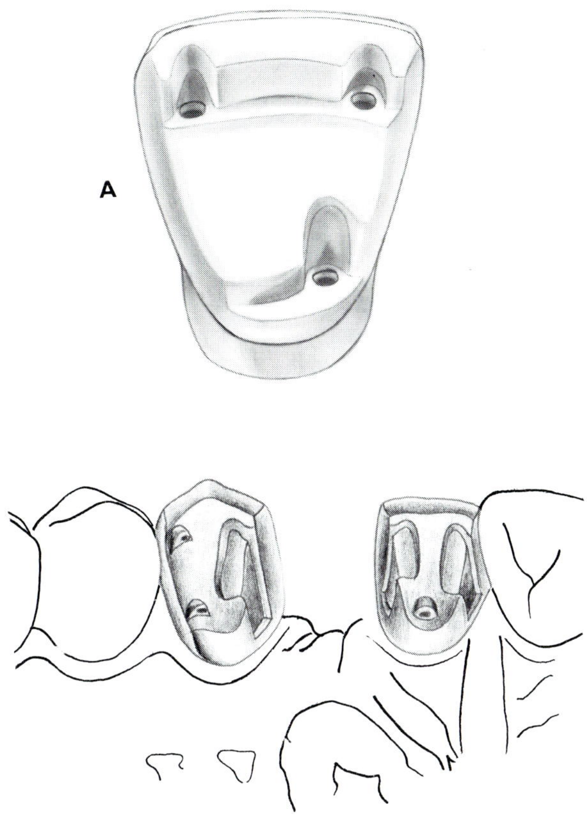

Fig. 7-20. A, Pinledge preparation—linguoincisal view. **B,** Modification of the pinledge preparation. (**A** from Sturdevant, C. M., Barton, R. E., Brauer, J. C., and Harrison, M. L.: The art and science of operative dentistry, New York, 1968, McGraw-Hill Book Co.)

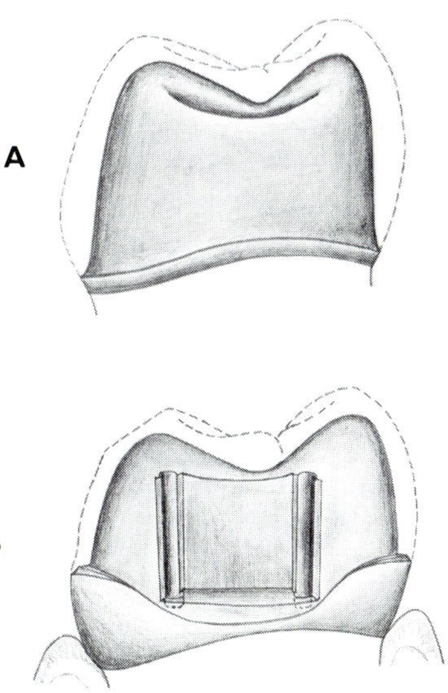

Fig. 7-21. A, The full gold veneer crown preparation (chamfer marginal finish line). **B,** The modified onlay preparation. This is also appropriate for bell-shaped teeth.

It is believed that at this time the following pertinent statements regarding full coverage are in order. This will be repeated again at the appropriate time because of its importance.

"Clinical evidence clearly demonstrates that subgingival extensions of full coverage margins produce an environment unfavorable to the health of the marginal gingiva. In the area adjacent to full coverage, it is difficult to maintain marginal gingiva which are thin and acceptably contoured for physiologic function and food flow.

"In contrast to the maintenance of healthy gingiva around enamel and cementum of natural tooth substance, the gingival tissues around full coverage seem to be more thickened, more rolled, and generally more inflammatory in character.

"Even with the most careful techniques of tooth preparation and tissue handling during preparation of tooth, impression taking, temporization, and final cementation, the full coverage extended subgingivally limits the opportunity for the marginal gingiva to achieve maximum patterns of health.

"This is not an indictment of full coverage. There has, however, been a tendency to utilize this procedure without definitive indication. Where indicated and demanded in the therapeutics of restorative dentistry, it can be utilized to advantage. Where full coverage is therapeutically utilized with finesse and understanding and precision technique, it offers much in many clinical circumstances."*

The half-crown or *the mesial version of the veneer crown* is usually for teeth that are tilted mesially. The surfaces covered are the mesial half of the buccal and lingual surfaces and the mesial surface and the mesial half of the occlusal surface, with an extension to the distal sulcus. The grooves are located on the buccal, mesial, and lingual surfaces, respectively. We must bear in mind that all grooves must be parallel to one another, particularly as their number increases in the one preparation. Where the abutment teeth are tipped or when it is not advisable to extend the preparation into the distal aspect of the tooth, the grooves can be positioned in a direction parallel to the anterior abutment. This type of preparation allows for the restoration of the mesial cusps of the tipped molar to the established occlusal plane, thereby also restoring functional occlusion (Fig. 7-22).

There are many other preparation possibilities (combinations of the various types) depending on one's ingenuity and ability.

*From Fox, Lewis: Letters to the editor, Dent. Times **3:**6, 1961.

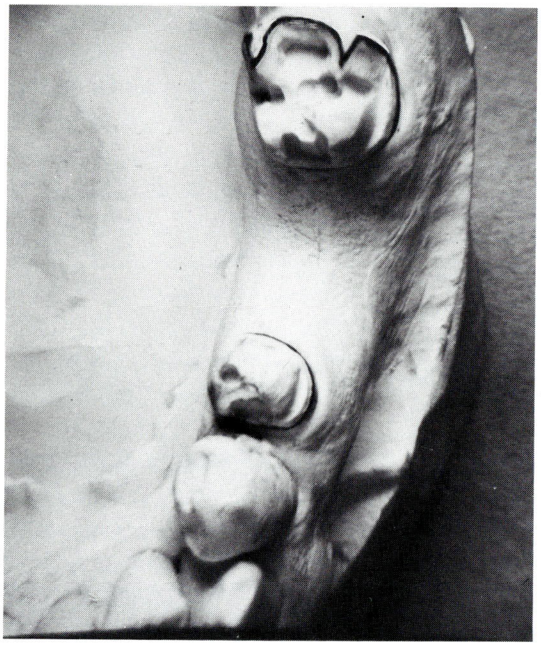

Fig. 7-22. A modified half-crown preparation (molar).

Whenever possible, it is advantageous to lay the peripheral margins on sound enamel with a definite abrupt bevel and slightly above the gingival margin, since this not only facilitates accurate marginal adaptation of the gold but prevents gingival tissue irritation. Always keep margins away from all stressful situations; avoid placing margins of retainers within the range of functional glide paths. Never end a preparation where an opposing cusp may rub over the margin of the restoration. If this is done it will enhance the likelihood of burnishing and curling the margin of gold, and enamel rods in this area are also more likely to break down. Create the lowest total length of margin possible and practical which is in accord with the needs of the restoration for durability first and esthetics second. Preserve, whenever possible, those areas which have good contour, are kept well cleansed by the patient, and cannot be improved upon by the restoration. This means there may not always be a need to bury the margin in the gingival crevice. Evaluate the situation and place the margin either above or below any area where debris is likely to accumulate.

The abutment preparations should always be protected between sittings by means of temporary inlays or crowns constructed from a "quick-cure" acrylic. These are used to maintain the proper mesiodistal relation, prevent sensitive cavities, maintain proper relation of occluding teeth, and prevent chipping of delicate margins. These temporary restorations are cemented with a zinc oxide–eugenol mixture which gives an antiseptic and anodyne effect. (Also refer to Chapter 8 for technical procedures.)

Proper reduction of vertical walls and occlusal surfaces of teeth to be used as abutments in fixed partial denture construction is of the utmost importance. The reduction of the occlusal surface by 2 mm. should be a clearance of 2 mm. created with all pathways of movement (lateral, protrusive) considered and allowed for, in addition to centric clearance. Greater efficiency of function requires greater care in design. We must endeavor to avoid the possibility of a patient wearing through a casting or the possibility of grinding through a casting while adjusting it or of grinding a casting into a mutilated nonentity.

Welter[19] has classified some of the most probable causes of, or reasons for, grinding of castings (other than ill fit). They are:

1. There was unrecognized Bennett shift (hence not allowed for).
2. There was an upward displacement of the condyle and teeth as the teeth left centric position.
3. The "bite" had been opened on the articulator without corresponding compensation having been made on the horizontal condylar inclination settings or through incorrect lateral bites, resulting in a higher setting than the patient has.
4. An incorrect "centric bite" had been used.
5. An incorrect vertical center of rotation (intercondylar distance) caused improper ridge placement (both position and direction), cusp placement, groove depth, cusp height, and cusp angle.
6. Half models (quadrant impressions) had been used which make the proper positioning of abutments relative to the opposing model difficult, if not impossible. They are less stable or secure when placed in the "bite" and mounted. Half models subtract the opposite side of the arch from the use of the technician, thus eliminating the use of any help in guiding the models over one another and at least taking advantage of any obvious facet or visible patterns present in the mouth.

The areas usually requiring compensatory grinding are a result of:

1. Bennett shift—grooving toward the buccal and/or lingual to allow the opposing cusp additional room to escape laterally from centric position.

2. Sagittal displacement (immediate upward or gradual upward movement)—the inner inclines of the upper buccal cusps and/or the deepening and widening of the escape route from centric position, to allow room for the lower buccal cusps to travel without interference toward the buccal and the upper lingual cusp to escape toward the lingual of the lower tooth which it opposes.
3. Horizontal condylar inclination too high on the articulator—balancing contacts, for example, from centric position distobuccally on the inner aspect of the slopes of the lower buccal cusps to allow room for the upper lingual cusp to pass. Protrusive contacts also will require some relief.
4. Incorrect centric relation—cusp shortening or fossa deepening and generally trying to get it to fit into the opposing tooth. All lateral excursions must also be checked.
5. Incorrect intercondylar distance—cusp ridges, cusp height. You will generally be cutting new grooves, probably through cusps.
6. Half models—anywhere and everywhere in an amount depending on your good luck.
7. Combinations of the previous six—start over.

TOOTH FORM AND FUNCTION (TOOTH ANATOMY AND PHYSIOLOGY)

A thorough knowledge of detailed dental anatomy and physiology is of the utmost importance, because it requires a great deal of knowledge and skill to restore each and every minute detail of anatomic form to a tooth so as to allow it to function properly and at the same time to preserve the supporting tissues and create a negative occlusal perception. Unless we are willing to unite all the elements—the teeth which are the working surfaces of the chewing mechanism, the maxilla and the mandible, the temporomandibular joints, the muscles and ligaments controlling the movements of the mandible, the neuromuscular complex, the supporting tissues, tongue, lips, cheeks, etc.—which compose the dental mechanism into one unit, it is impossible to reach a correct understanding of tooth function. We must endeavor to get correct relation of the teeth in arches, because correct detailed tooth form with incorrect mandibular relation creates problems. Until each tooth is properly supported by, and associated with, its fellows in a normal way, tooth function cannot properly take place. Then, and only then, can the significance of tooth form be comprehended. Then the value of each groove, ridge, cusp, etc. becomes apparent, and the functioning of the masticatory elements is more fully understood.

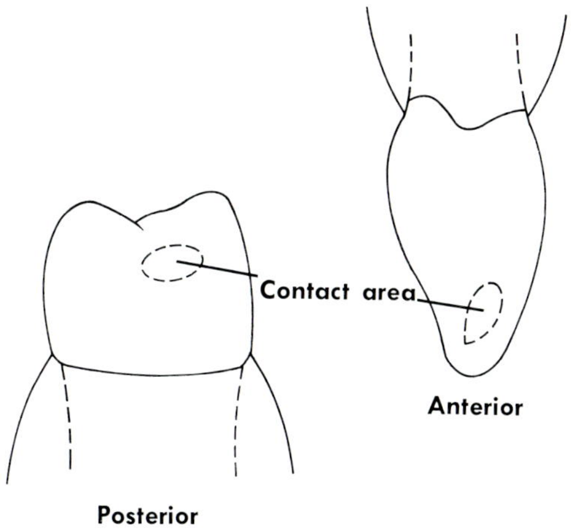

Fig. 7-23. Anterior restoration contact area is placed to the facial and incisal, and posterior restoration contact area is placed in most instances to the facial and occlusal.

Serious consideration must be given to the facial, lingual, occlusal, and proximal surfaces so as to end up with a contour that will fulfill the proper form, function, and esthetic needs, and that will not create periodontal disease or a malocclusion.

The anatomy of the mesial and distal portion of a tooth involves four important embrasures: the occlusal, gingival, facial, and lingual. To begin with, the proximal surfaces must be shaped to either flat or concave below the contact area on its approach to the cementoenamel junction. The occlusal, facial, and lingual embrasures must be so contoured as to direct the bolus of food away from the soft tissues, but at the same time permitting proper massage of these tissues. The gingival embrasure must be contoured so as not to allow impingement of interdental papilla and also allow for good oral hygiene. (For a detailed discussion and illustrations of coronal contours refer to Chapter 6.)

Contact areas

The anterior restoration contact area is placed to the facial and incisal, and in posterior restorations to the facial and occlusal (Fig. 7-23). Dental floss must "snap" through these contact areas without undue pressure. If the contact area has a "plus" contact, the teeth in the arch may all be shifted to a degree that may cause some malocclusion. If the contact area has a "minus" contact, food impaction will result not only in patient discomfort but also in possible recurrent decay and periodontal disease.

Occlusal surfaces

The occlusal surface must have proper anatomic form, which means the restoration of all cusps, fossae, grooves, and ridges in such a way so as to function properly with its counterpart in the opposing arch. Excessive occlusal contact can cause pulpal involvement, periodontal disturbances, etc., whereas no occlusal contact may cause opposing tooth to drift out of the proper occlusal plane, which may cause malocclusion and loss of chewing efficiency.

Occlusal surfaces are practically 50% to 60% as wide as the crown through its greatest diameter buccolingually. A detailed study and very close observation of occlusal surfaces of teeth will show many important and interesting facets. Reynolds[20] calls attention to the fact that the occlusal surface of a tooth has cusp tips, marginal ridges, triangular ridges, supplemental ridges, developmental grooves, supplemental grooves, and fossae—the elements of occlusion. "The following facts are observed in the occlusal elements: (1) definite cusps, ridges, and grooves exist on molars and premolars; (2) the buccolingual width of the occlusal table is about the same on molars as that on premolars; (3) each cusp has a primary ridge with a smaller supplementary ridge on each side; (4) each primary ridge is at least twice as wide as each supplementary ridge; (5) the primary and supplementary ridges are biconvex; (6) the lingual surfaces of anterior teeth have a definite concave surface incisogingivally; and (7) the incisal edges of anterior teeth are rounded. The elements of occlusion are common to all teeth, but they are more defined in some than they are in others."*

All natural mesial or distal marginal ridges, with very few exceptions, are broken by spillways, permitting escape of food over the ridge and into the wide (obtuse) lingual embrasure. This performs a very definite function in that it limits the field of susceptibility to caries and periodontal disease, decreases the occlusal load or stress, and gives tone to the large fibrous gum tissue forming the base of the lingual embrasure, which in turn is supported by a heavy mass of bone. Without spillways, nature's scheme is defeated.[21] Nature has wisely provided for food escape with embrasures, supplemental grooves, spillways, etc., which makes trapping impossible. We must have sluiceways and contact areas, escapeways on lingual (mesially and distally) which opens up lingual embrasure form; in other words, we must shape the occlusal surface to biomechanical needs (Fig. 7-24). If our restorations are so made to fill the fossae or if the marginal ridges are made too high or sharp instead of rounded and continuous, the escapeways are closed and the food cannot escape when teeth are clenched. Teeth may become lame, and septal tissue will hypertrophy and bleed.

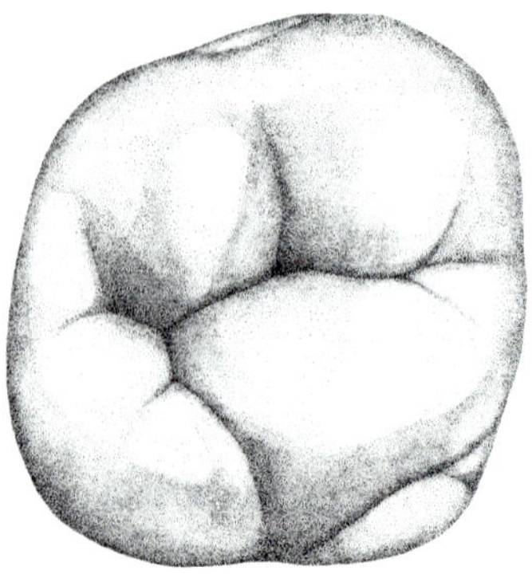

Fig. 7-24. Occlusal surface must have proper anatomic form—cusps, fossae, grooves, ridges, supplemental grooves, embrasures, spillways.

As to the question of decreasing the occlusal load or stress, Prime,[21] some years ago, called attention to the fact that the lingual cusps, by being smaller or narrower mesiodistally than the buccal cusps, create the wide lingual embrasures. The lingual cusps receive the greater part of the load, and because they are smaller they diminish the stresses and leverages to the periodontium.

Prime[21] also observed that (1) the narrowing of the tubercle on the mesial of the first bicuspid compensates for the narrow distal surface of the cuspid, with which it forms a most efficient contact area (Fig. 7-25) and (2) in unworn teeth, as a rule, the stresses fall very near the long axes as illustrated by parallel lines; while on worn teeth, the stresses are not only much greater in degree but are spread over wider and more dangerous areas, within the parallel lines (Fig. 7-26). Reduction of occlusal contact points of two convexities to flat surfaces will multiply our leverages greatly.

It would be appropriate to say that we should not omit spillways or gateways; we should keep occlusal surfaces convex so as to produce occlusal contact points and not flat surfaces, so that food can escape more easily; we should make lingual embrasures obtuse; we should not have too wide or overly wide occlusal surfaces, etc.

Occlusal disharmony is often present in the cases requiring replacement of teeth, and such disharmony should be corrected before the bridge is made. Post-

---

*From Reynolds, J. Marvin: Occlusal wear facets, J. Prosthet. Dent. **24**(4):371, 1970.

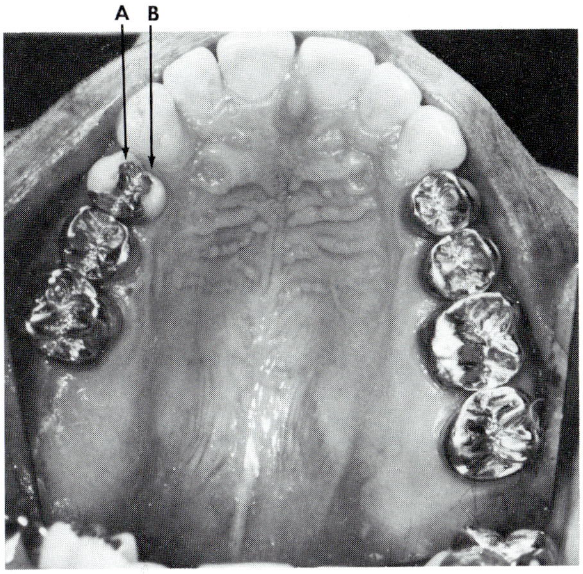

Fig. 7-25. Note the narrowing of the tubercle *(B)* on the mesial of the first bicuspid to compensate for the narrow distal surface of the cuspid *(A)*, with which it forms a most efficient contact area.

poning adjustment until after the bridge is in position may result in impairment of the bridge.

Interference of the cusps, broad occlusal contacts, and the overloading of abutment teeth often subject these teeth to stresses beyond the limits of biologic safety.

The teeth can readily be divided into cutting surfaces, or points, and planes on which these surfaces or points function. Sharpness of cutting cusps minimizes the essential application of force in function. By proper selective grinding procedures (refer to Chapter 6) undesirable guiding tooth inclines may be reduced while cusp sharpness is retained. The same cusps definitely maintain the maxillomandibular relation.

When we have interfering convex surfaces and we wish to reduce them, we must reduce the surfaces by grinding away and around the spot and carrying the whole surface down without creating a broad occlusal surface or, what is worse, a concavity. The idea is to create occlusal forms meeting at contact points, at the same time keeping them as near in line with the long axis of the tooth or teeth as the conditions will permit.

In a full coverage crown, have the line of force generated during mastication directed from the cusp tip to a point within the confines of the root. In posterior teeth being restored with full coverage crowns, make certain modifications such as reducing the

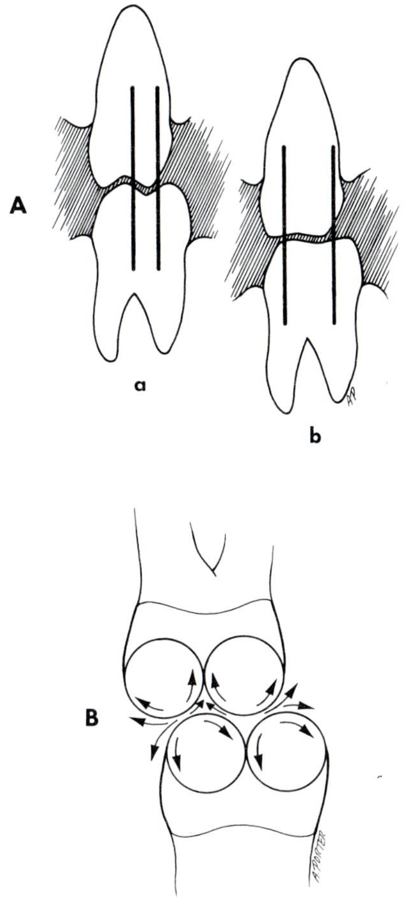

Fig. 7-26. A, Stresses of occlusion in unworn teeth fall very near the long axes (note parallel lines *a*), and on worn teeth stresses are spread over wider and more dangerous areas (note parallel lines *b*). B, Circles representing balls that will touch at small contact points similar to the manner in which unworn teeth occlude. Arrows illustrate escape of food in all directions from the contacting points.

facial-lingual dimension from cusp tip to cusp tip so as to fulfill the above-mentioned specification. This modification will somewhat reduce the force to the attachment apparatus and will thereby provide some protection to it. The occlusal table, in other words, must be located, if possible, over the root support, and it should be approximately half of the overall buccolingual width of the tooth. This permits forces to be transmitted axially where they are best withstood (Fig. 7-27).

Teeth should be given form characteristics to compensate for their inclination in the arch. Keep in mind that at least portions of the buccal surfaces of the lower teeth and lingual surfaces of the upper teeth are really part of the occlusal scheme (act as occlusal surfaces), and that no tooth functions alone.

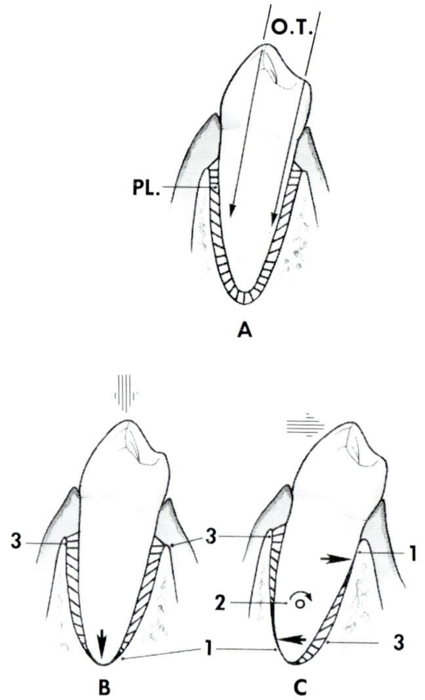

Fig. 7-27. Protection of the attachment apparatus. **A,** Diagrammatic representation of a tooth and its periodontium. The occlusal table *(O. T.)* is located over the root support and is about half of the overall buccolingual width of the tooth. This permits forces to be transmitted axially where they are best withstood. **B,** When vertical force (large arrow) is applied to the tooth the zone of crush *(1)* is minimized and the zone of stretch *(3)* or resistance is increased. Therefore, vertical forces are best withstood. **C,** When horizontal force (large arrow) is applied to the tooth, a fulcrum *(2)* is created about which the root rotates within the alveolus causing an increased zone of crush *(1)* or destruction and a decreased zone of stretch *(3)* or resistance. Horizontal forces are not tolerated as well as vertical forces. (Adapted from Kraus, B. S., Jordan, R. E., and Abrams, Leonard: Dental anatomy and occlusion, Baltimore, 1969, The Williams & Wilkins Co.)

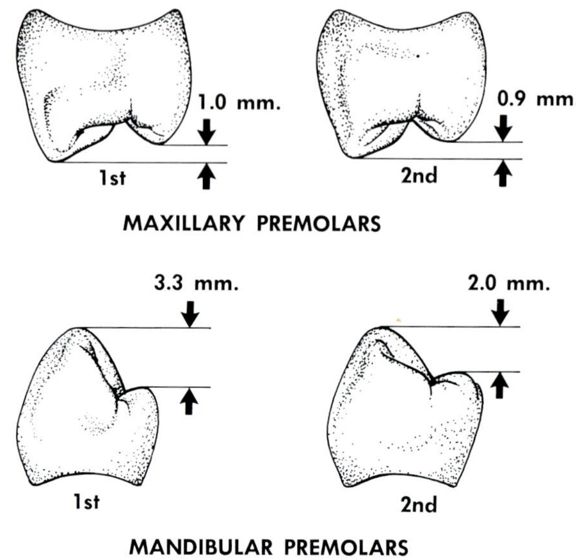

Fig. 7-28. The buccal cusps of premolars are longer than the lingual cusps by the amounts shown. (From Shillingburg, H. T., Jr., Kaplan, M. J., and Grace, C. S.: J. S. Calif. Dent. Assoc. **40**[9]:Sept., 1972.)

Shillingburg, Kaplan, and Grace[22] have reported a very significant fact, which is that "the buccal cusps of maxillary and mandibular premolars were found to be significantly longer than the respective lingual cusps. The difference amounts to 1.0 mm. in first premolars and 0.9 mm. in second premolars in the maxillary arch; and 3.3 mm. for first premolars and 2.0 mm. for second premolars in the mandibular arch" (Fig. 7-28).*

Our occlusal surface designs and physiologic contouring of restorations must be harmonious with biomechanical requirements so as to function harmoniously with the oral environment. Lack of attention to these requirements and basic details will cause damage to the oral mechanism and be a distinct disservice to the patient.

BROKEN-STRESS BRIDGE

In my opinion, the broken-stress or semifixed bridge should only be considered when complete fixation of the abutment teeth may prove hazardous, because an attempt to parallel a badly tipped abutment tooth with one in normal position will often result in loss of retention and dangerously deep preparations. Also, in a five-tooth fixed partial denture (abutment teeth, for example, being upper cuspid, second bicuspid, second molar), it is of the utmost importance to consider the placement of a keyway on the distal surface of the middle abutment because (1) the movement of the nonrigid connector is enough to prevent the middle abutment from serving as a fulcrum (the excessive force transmitted to the terminal retainers as a result of the middle abutment's fulcrumlike position can cause the weaker retainer to loosen), (2) most posterior teeth tilt mesially when subject to occlusal forces, and (3) because of this fact, any mesial move-

*From Shillingburg, H. T., Jr., Kaplan, M. J., and Grace, C. S.: Tooth dimensions—a comparative study, J. S. Calif. Dent. Assoc. **40**(9):830-839, 1972.

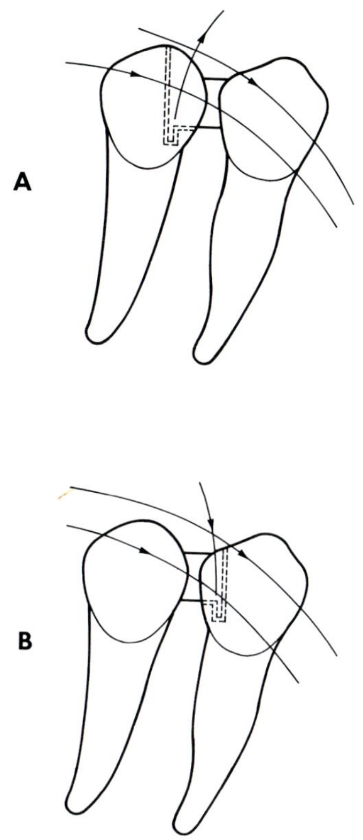

Fig. 7-29. A, The dislodging effect of mesial drift upon the key between two abutment teeth when the keyway is placed in the mesial of the distal attachment. **B,** The resultant force when the key and keyway are placed on the distal surface of the mesial attachment. The mesial drift tends to pull the key down into the keyway progressively tighter and tighter.

ment tends to seat the key into the keyway more solidly, whereas placement of the keyway on the mesial side causes the key to become unseated during its mesial movements, which can create a pathologic mobility to develop in the cuspid abutment and thereby cause the failure of the cuspid retainer (Fig. 7-29).

Whenever we must use the broken-stress bridge it must be executed with precision, because it should only be used as a means of convenience of positioning the bridge with the least amount of tooth destruction.

In the average broken-stress bridge the secondary abutment retainer, which receives the lug or male component, is usually of a simple inlay type (a disto-occlusal inlay), and the lug must be free so that the primary abutment may function independently of the secondary. If little tolerance occurs in the lug the secondary abutment casting may come loose. When it is desired to limit movement at the secondary abutment, as with a precision lug, the secondary abutment should be prepared with as much retention as possible —the severity of loading at the secondary abutment will then approximate that at the primary abutment.[10]

A nonrigid joint is used by some dentists in those cases where one of the abutment teeth has greater mobility than the others, but the coupling of a second sound abutment tooth approximating the weaker abutment tooth would be better clinical judgment (Fig. 7-30).

The important phases of crown and bridge prosthodontics dealing with (1) abutment preparations (Chapter 8), (2) impressions (Chapter 9), (3) waxing and casting (Chapter 10), (4) soldering (Chapter 11), and (5) cementation (Chapter 12) are discussed and illustrated in the indicated chapters of this book.

Pin retention methods to retain appliances have been perfected in recent years. Some of the current uses of pin retention will be discussed in this section in the light of reinforcement of restorations against future troubles, and also as aids in "trouble-shooting" when necessary. I believe it has been of immeasurable assistance in my extensive execution of crown and bridge prosthodontic procedures.

Replacement of acrylic facings with pins, solderless joints (utilization of pins to create rigid joints between crown and bridge units without the use of solder), replacement of a retainer that went "sour," and restoration of its continuity with the fixed prosthesis are examples of aids in "trouble-shooting" which are of the utmost importance.

Courtade[23] has said that the ideal pin attached to a cast restoration is made from a wrought wire that is threaded, serrated, or knurled and that has a square end that has been beveled.

Measuring devices have an important place in the armamentarium for pin usage. A dial micrometer,* which is a gauge that will read to 0.00025 inch, is important for checking diameters of twist drills, impression pins, and pins to be used in the final casting. Also, the Dial-A-Pin-Cutter† which cuts wire with a square end makes use of the shear principle suggested by Moffa. No bur or distortion of any practical significance has been noted with the use of this tool. One squeeze of the pliers will cut a pin accurately to the desired length, and it will have a smooth end. Any number of pins of equal length can be cut by using this device (Fig. 7-31).[23]

Venting and cross-pinning of full crowns must be taken very seriously in the process of cementation.

*Techni-Tool, Silverman's, Philadelphia, Pa.

†Dial-A-Pin-Cutter, Whaldent, Inc., Brooklyn, N. Y.

"Experimentation has shown that the minimum space between inner occlusal surface of the casting and occlusal surface of the prepared tooth was 20 to 25 microns. As a rule, when non-vented full crowns are cemented with oxyphosphate of zinc cement, the occlusal cement thickness may be as much as 250 microns (0.025 mm.). Venting allows for the escape of excess cement, thereby permitting full seating at the gingival margin; prevents occlusal elevation and, therefore, disturbance of established occlusal relationship, and minimizes post-operative sensitivity by eliminating pressure of cement fluids on dentinal tubules. (Refer to Chapter 12 for techniques of venting full crowns.)

"Cross pinning and venting can be accomplished in one operation. A contra angle twist drill (0.028 inch) is slowly rotated at 500 r.p.m. through the vent hole before cementation, with the crown in place on the tooth, to the depth of about 1 mm. Therefore, when the crown is cemented the gold threaded pin of proper length and diameter serves not only as a closure for the vent hole, but also as a 'cross pin'. Caution must be exercised in making sure that the threaded pin is not turned beyond the first tooth contact, be-

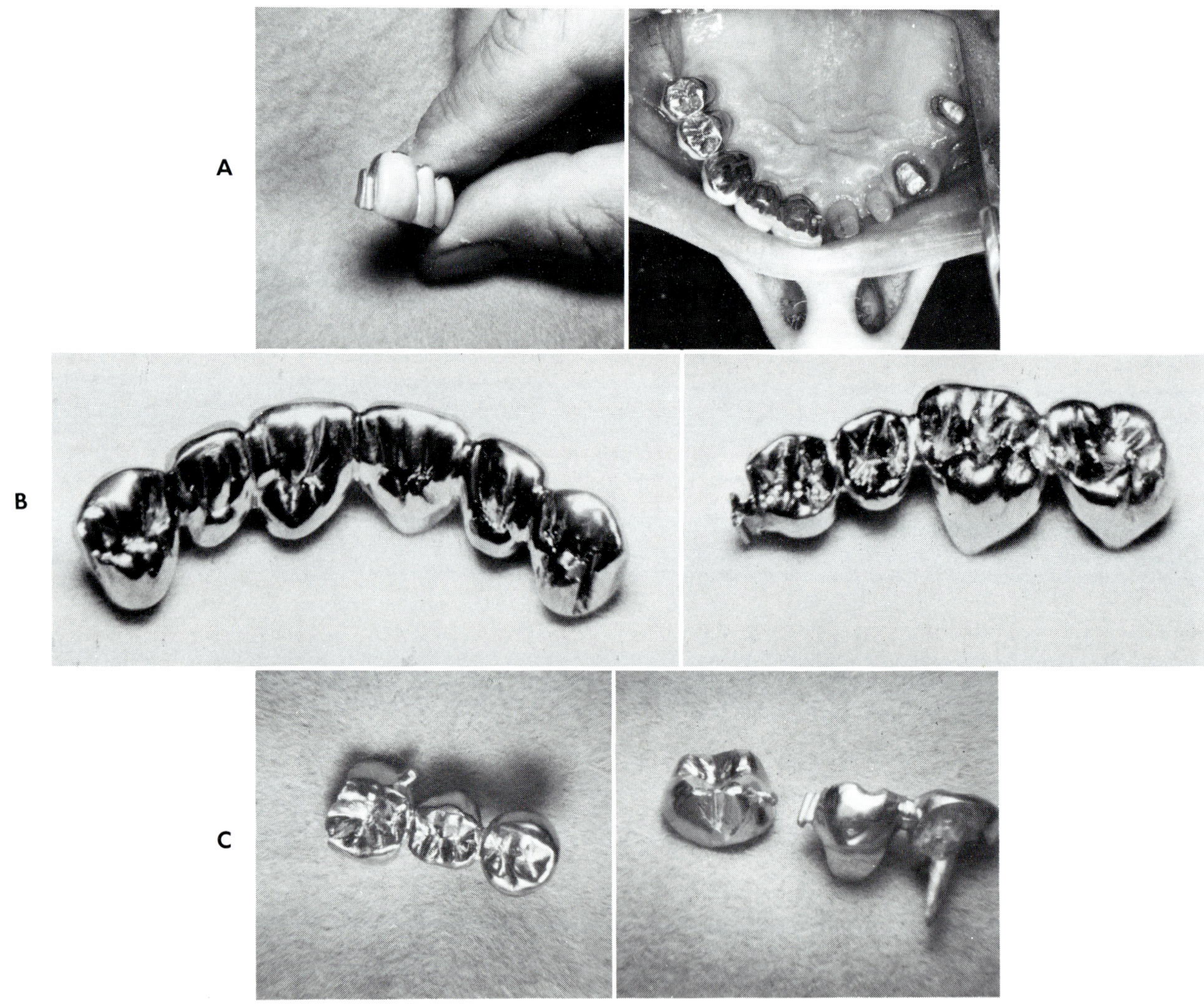

Fig. 7-30. Use of the nonrigid joint. **A,** The "hand-made" type. **B,** Use of the internal precision attachment. **C,** Use of the P-D. (Ideally, the nonrigid joint should be placed into the distal of the mesial retainer. However, this case has been in service for 10 years.) **D,** The J. M. Ney "plastic forms" (Ney Broken-Stress Connectors—the Ney Mortice Rest, the Ney Mini-Rest, and the Ney MS attachment.) **E,** The J. F. Jelenko Tele-Seal/Pontic-Seal.

D

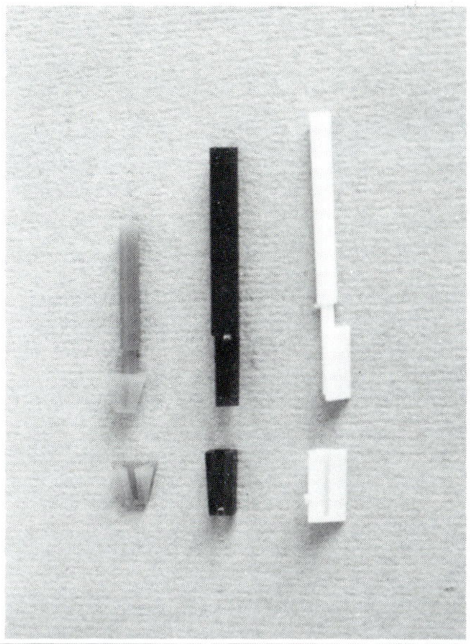

E

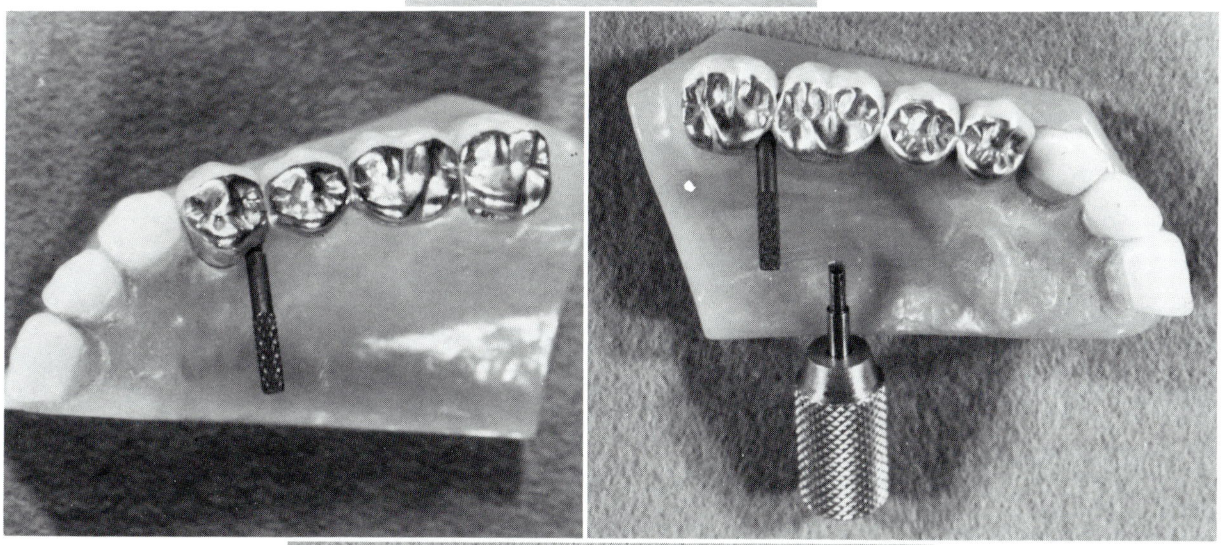

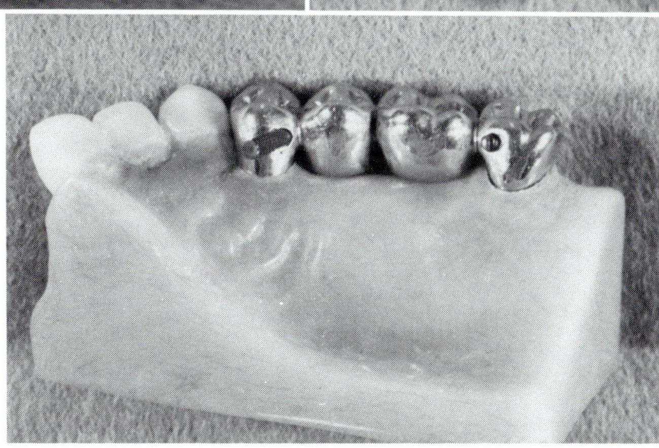

Fig. 7-30, cont'd. For legend see opposite page.

A

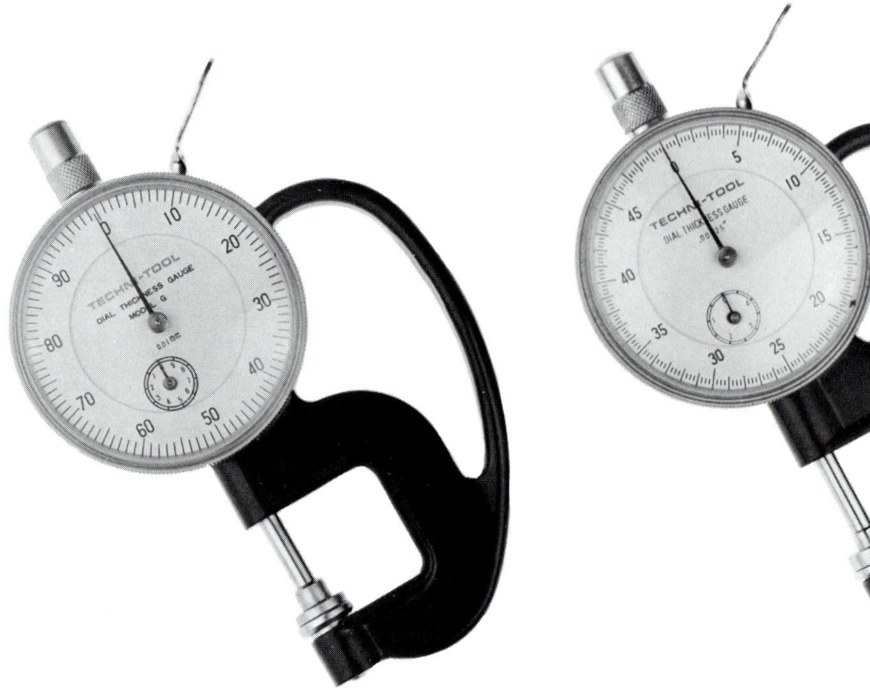

Fig. 7-31. A, Techni-Tool dial micrometers are accurate measuring instruments. One most commonly used in United States is on the right. It measures to 0.00025 inch. Type G, on the left, measures to 0.01 mm. **B,** Dial-A-Pin Cutter is recommended for cutting precious metal pin stock. Pin is cut with no bur or increase in diameter. Regular wire cutter from hardware store may be used when end of cut pin or post will be embedded in pattern but not in precise channel. **C,** Top, Lactona Logo depth gauge. Bottom, Whaledent Omni-Depth guide. These are useful for measuring depth of pin channels and posthole preparations. They are read in millimeters. (From Courtade, G. L.: J. Prosthet. Dent. **16:**748, 1966.)

cause excessive turning of the screw may elevate the crown from its seated position.''*[24]

SELF-SHEARING PIN

Pins should be selected that will require the least modification after their installation.

''The self-shearing pin† which measures 5 mm when installed fulfills the above mentioned requirement most frequently. The twist drill bit is 5 mm. long, and by permitting the drill bit to enter the tooth to one-half its length, a channel of the ideal depth is produced. This allows 2 to 3 mm. of the pin to extend above the tooth structure for retention of the restorative material. This type of pin is simple, convenient and efficient to use.

''The pin is installed after the 0.027 mm. channel is lined with copal varnish. The reduction-gear, contra-angle handpiece with its direct drive chuck is utilized in installing the pin. The flat end of the pin is placed into the slot of the chuck and positioned over the channel. The engine is operated at low speed (500 r.p.m.) in a clockwise direction. The pin will thread into the dentin and, upon reaching the base of the pin channel, will shear off at the predetermined 5 mm. level (Fig. 7-32).[25] The threads on the pins provide excellent retention for the restorative material which is condensed around them. The pins may be bent with a bending tool.* Various types of pins can be used'' (Fig. 7-33).†

Moffa, Razzano, and Folio[26] have concluded from a research study based on the Ca^{45} radioauto-

---

*From Courtade, Gerard L.: Pin pointers. II. Venting and cross pinning, J. Prosthet. Dent. **16**(5):978-980, 1966. I wish to express my appreciation to Dr. Gerard L. Courtade for the numerous technical procedures and hints given to me in regard to the use of self-threading pins and tools in many personal communications.

†Whaldent, Inc., Brooklyn, N. Y.

---

*Whaldent, Inc., Brooklyn, N. Y.

†From Courtade, Gerard L.: Pin Pointers. III. Self-threading pins, J. Prosthet. Dent. **20**(4):335-338, 1968.

B

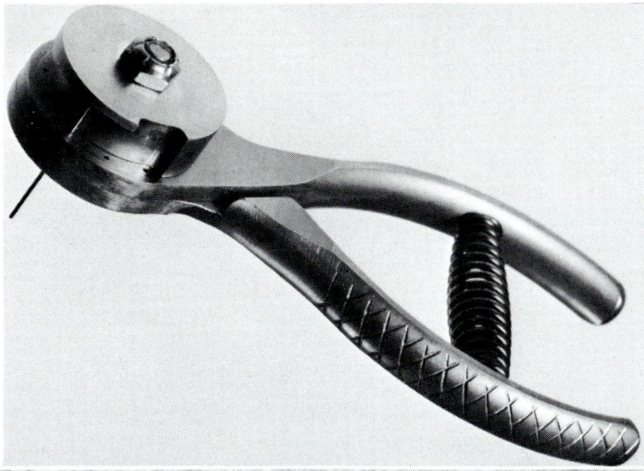

C

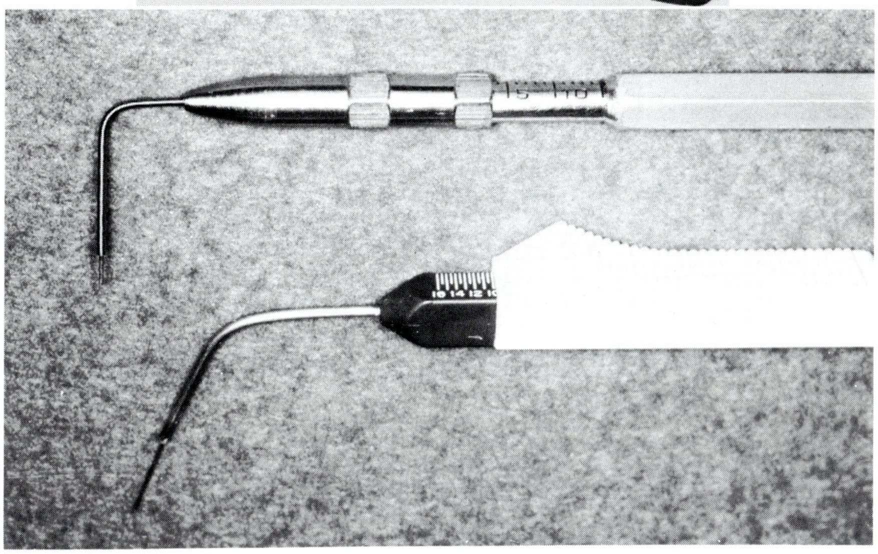

Fig. 7-31, cont'd. For legend see opposite page.

graphic technique, and upon the tensile testing procedures, that:

1. "All pin-retaining devices exhibited microleakage which increased as a function of time.
2. "Cemented pins demonstrated the least initial leakage, but showed the greatest deterioration as a function of time.
3. "Cavity varnish virtually eliminated the leakage associated with the friction-locked and the self-threading pin types and decreased the leakage of the cemented pin types.
4. "Cavity varnish decreased the retention of the cemented pin type by 46 per cent.
5. "Cavity varnish had no significant effect on the retention of friction-locked and self-threading pin types.
6. "When used in conjunction with cavity varnish, self-threading pins were eight times more retentive than cemented pins."*

In another study[27] the conclusions reached were (1) the cemented pins are the least retentive (1×), (2) the friction-locked pins are intermediate in retention (2× to 3×), and (3) the self-threading pins are the most retentive of the three types tested (5× to 6×).

I have used a solderless joint, when indicated, with great success for repairing broken solder joints, closing interproximal contacts between adjoining restorations, splinting of adjoining restorations, and adding additional or repaired retainers to an existing

*From Moffa, J. P., Razzano, M. R., and Folio, J.: Influence of cavity varnish on microleakage and retention of various pin-retaining devices, J. Prosthet. Dent. **20**(6):541-551, 1968.

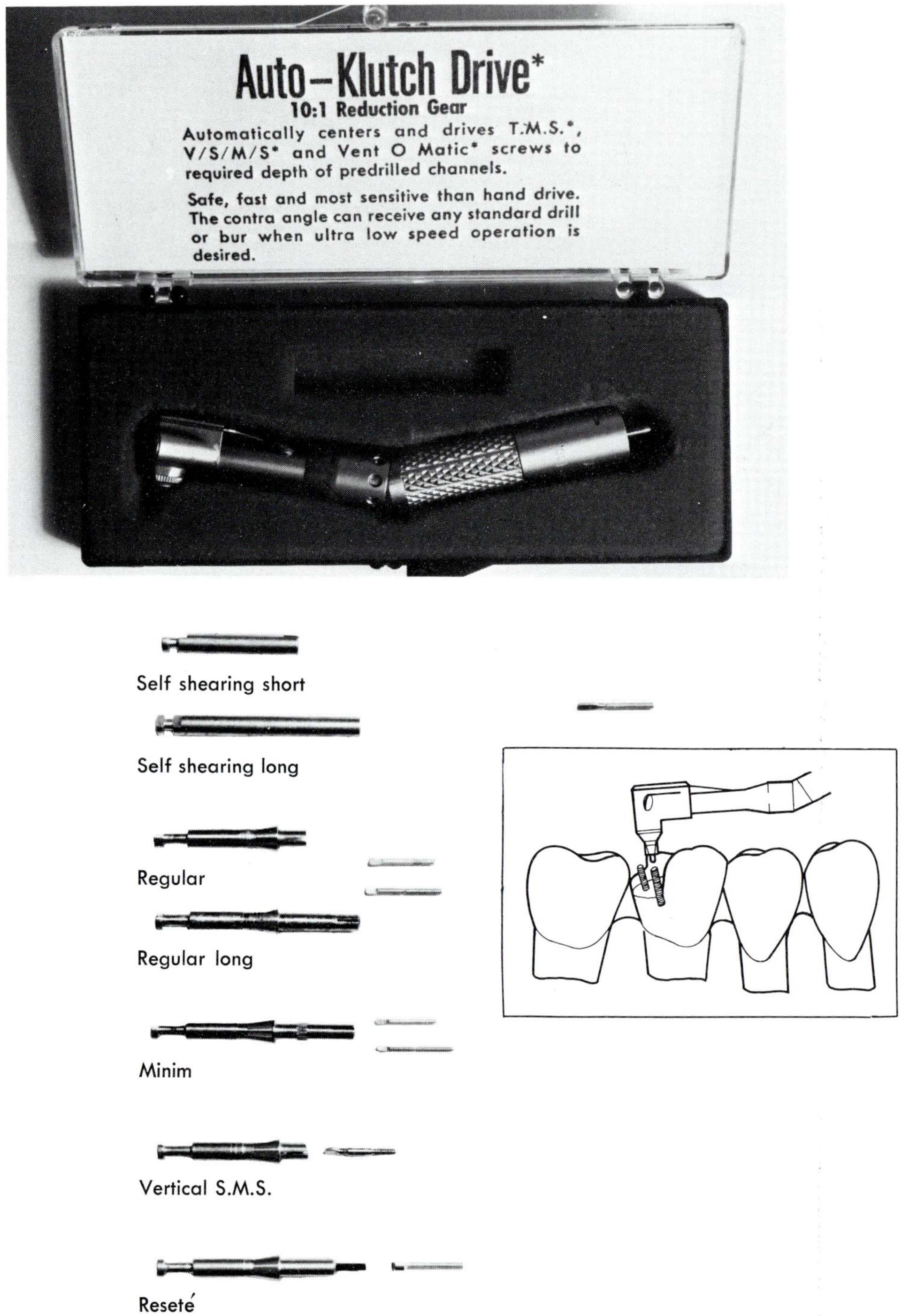

Fig. 7-32. Auto-Klutch installation of a drive contra-angle and a self-shearing pin.

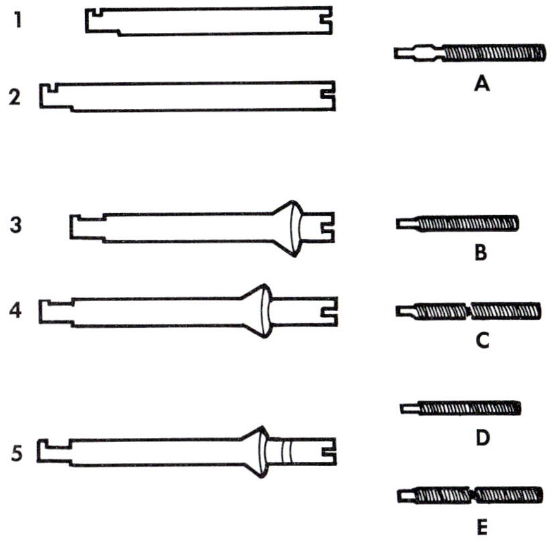

Fig. 7-33. The various types of pins. **A,** A self-shearing pin with short *(1)* and long *(2)* direct-drive chucks; **B,** a regular full-length self-threading pin; **C,** a twin-stage pin (for a 0.027 inch drill) to be employed with short *(3)* and long *(4)* slip drive chucks; **D,** a miniature pin; **E,** a twin-stage pin (for 0.021 inch drill) to be employed with slip-drive chucks *(5)*. (From Courtade, G. L.: J. Prosthet. Dent. **20**[4]:335-338, 1968.)

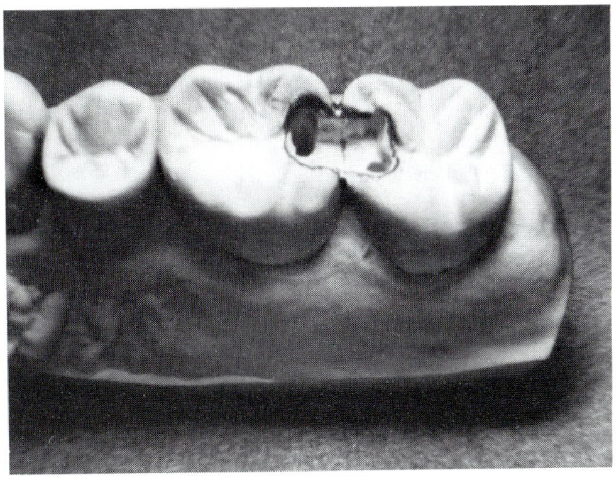

Fig. 7-34. The use of a solderless joint to prevent extrusion of upper second molar after loss of lower second molar.

fixed prosthesis. A channel is prepared in the occlusal surface of adjoining restorations or the lingual surface of anterior teeth to a depth of 1 to 2 mm. and a width (faciolingually) of 2 to 3 mm., using a No. 171 friction grip carbide bur. The proximating ends of the channels of the adjoining restorations are finished with a small slice, the occlusal or lingual surface of the channel is terminated in a dovetail, and the occlusal or lingual surface is beveled for fine marginal adaptation. The next step is the drilling of the pinholes, which can be accomplished, for example in posterior teeth, by creating these parallel pinholes (one buccal and one lingual on each casting) in line with the axial wall of the preparation or just inside of the axial wall of the preparation and a little away from the buccal and lingual walls, with a No. 170 or No. 171 carbide bur to a depth of approximately 3 mm. Increasing the diameter and length of the pins and using, if possible, threaded pins instead of smooth cylindrical pins will increase the retention of the cemented castings. My impression material of choice is hydrocolloid, and the impression is taken after the interproximal area below the preparations in the restorations is ''blocked out'' with a soft wax, thereby avoiding the tearing of the impression (Fig. 7-34).

Another method of preparing the pinholes is to start them with a No. $^1/_2$ round bur run at high speed, followed with a 0.27 twist drill (and then with a 0.028 twist drill) run at slow speed with a reduction-gear, contra-angle handpiece (low speed with high torque) to the depth of approximately 3 mm. (confirmed with an Omni-depth measuring gauge*). When cutting into gold with a twist drill, use a lubricant, a drop of oil at the site of drilling or periphery wax on drill, and a slow pumping motion, which is needed to remove gold shavings. To prevent bending and fracturing of the twist drill use a continuous rotation in the ''down'' as well as the ''up'' motion of the twist drill. When paralleling one pinhole to the other, you can use a steel indicator rod (Jelenko No. 7)† and the ''eye.'' After the preparations have been completed, plastic-headed pins are positioned in the pinholes (be sure that the ''head'' will not hit the impression tray), and a hydrocolloid impression is taken and poured up in die stone. (Refer to Chapter 11 for waxing and casting.)

Another method of repairing and modifying cemented fixed prostheses, which makes use of nonparallel pin bolts (the ''bolt inlay'') as advocated by Weiss,[28] is worthy of careful consideration and study (Figs. 7-35 and 7-36).

The advantages of intracoronal threaded pin retention are many. Standard depth (3 mm.) pinholes may be placed wherever sound dentin remains. Since the holes need not be parallel, they may diverge to avoid pulp exposure. The entire prosthetic appliance is not dependent upon cement for retention, but rather it

*Whaldent, Inc., Brooklyn, N. Y.

†J. F. Jelenko & Co., Inc., New Rochelle, N. Y.

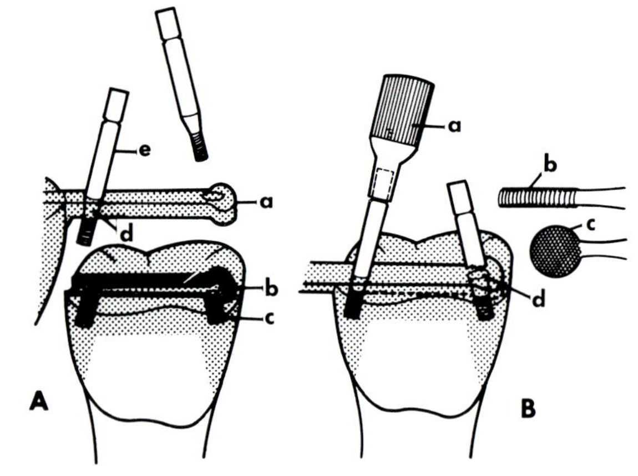

Fig. 7-35. A, The bolt inlay. *a,* The inlay to be bolted. *b,* The occlusal channel prepared in the existing gold casting; *c,* A nonparalleled pinhole. *d,* The tapered part of the pin is inserted in the tapered opening provided in the inlay. *e,* The pin bolt. **B,** The assembly. *a,* The wrench used to screw pins into position. *b,* A cross-cut fissure bur used first at high speed to cut off the pin. *c,* A round diamond stone used to smooth the cut end. *d,* The cut end of the pin. (Redrawn from Weiss, A. B.: J. Prosthet. Dent. **23**[3]:296-309, 1970.)

obtains most of its retentive property from the wedging contact of steel threads against the dentin (Fig. 7-37).*[29]

IMPLANTS

I am, and have been for a long time, an advocate of the use of the endosseous implant, providing proper judgment is used in the selection of the case and the proper technique is followed in its execution. All this requires knowledge, interest, and skills. Proper diagnosis of the anatomic landmarks (sinus, mandibular canal, etc.) is mandatory. The area of the mental foramen and the superior border of the mandibular canal, for example, must be "cleared." A good end result can benefit our patients esthetically, psychologically, and physically.

The implant, which is designed to complement the natural forces operating in the health and welfare of the jaws, is put into bone. The implant is accepted by the tissues in which it has been set and is tightly bound there, providing a tenacious abutment to which a temporary or permanent prosthesis may be attached.[30] It has more resistance to lateral stress because there is more metal-to-bone contact; the rather large openings in the body allow for better growth of

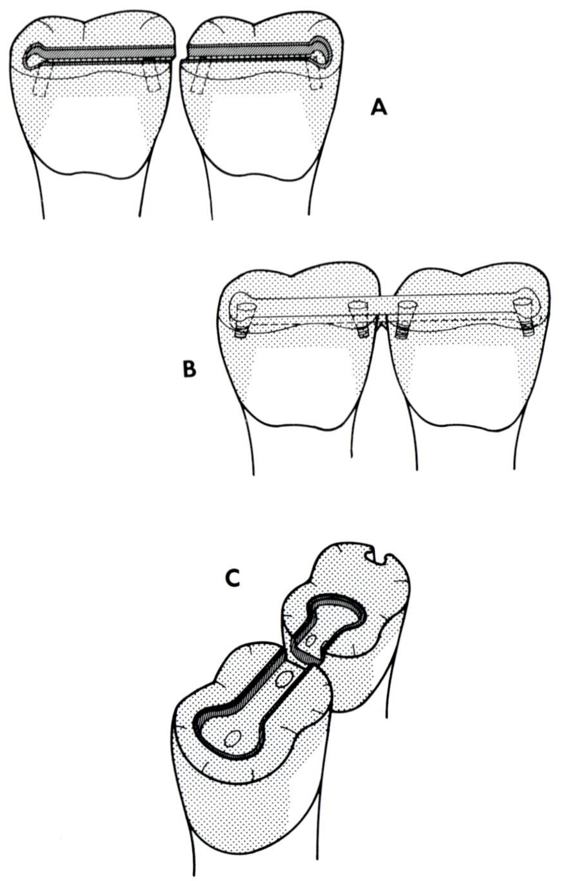

Fig. 7-36. A, The design of the bolt inlay for repairing a broken solder joint or joining approximating restorations for periodontal stabilization. This figure shows the preparations. **B,** Here the bolt inlay is in place. **C,** The design of the bolt inlay is modified when two restorations are to be joined where a precision attachment or deep box is in the proximal surface. (Redrawn from Weiss, A. B.: J. Prosthet. Dent. **23**[3]:296-309, 1970.)

the bone and fibrous tissue through them, and very little bone is surgically removed when placing the implant. It can be custom designed as well as reshaped for a particular bone site (Fig. 7-38).

Linkow[30] has said that an endosseous implant technique cannot be performed on all patients. Because the implant must be set in alveolar bone, those patients with extensive bone resorption are not suitable candidates, but they may be candidates for a subperiosteal implant. In other words, for good results and greater longevity we desire alveolar bone that is high, wide, and dense; but implants can be utilized, at times, when a narrow buccolingual ridge exists and when the ridges are shallow. Patients with severe systemic disease (uncontrolled diabetes, etc.)

---

*I recommend highly Courtade, G. L., and Timmermans, J. J.: Pins in restorative dentistry, St. Louis, 1971, The C. V. Mosby Co.

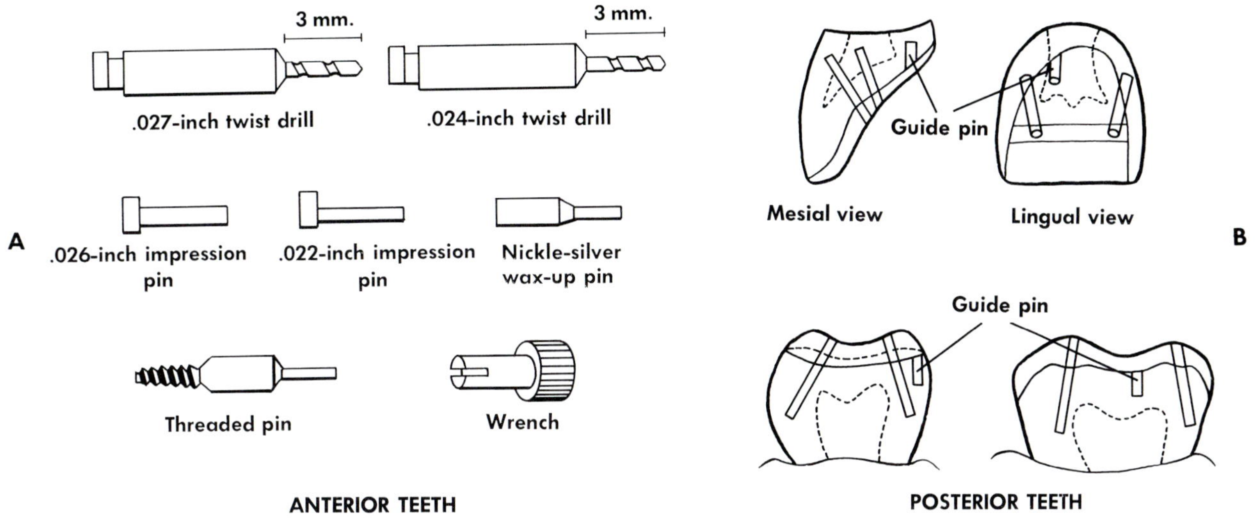

Fig. 7-37. A, The armamentarium. **B,** The direction of the nonparallel pins. (Adapted from Timmermans, J. J., and Courtade, G. L.: J. Prosthet. Dent. **19**[4]:381-392, 1968.)

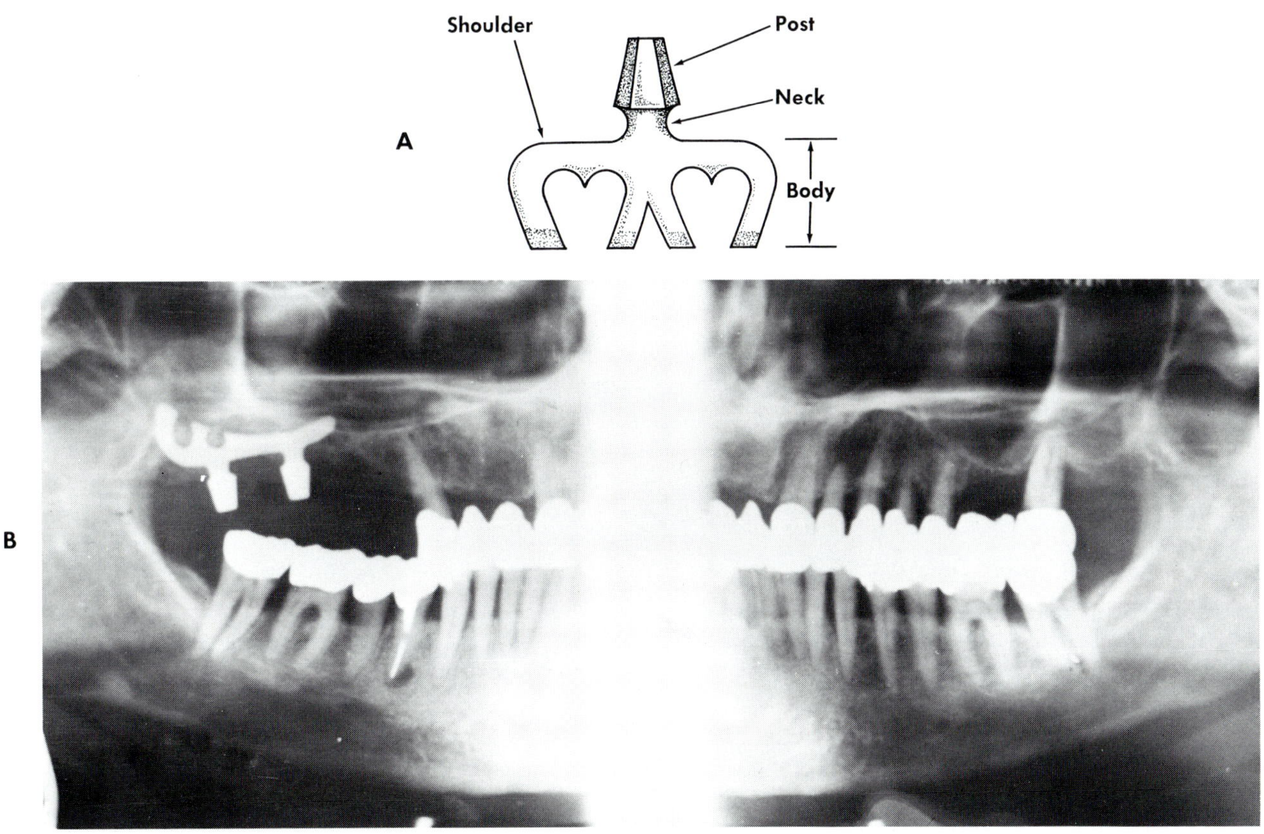

Fig. 7-38. A, A blade implant. **B,** Roentgenogram of a blade implant.

cannot be candidates for any kind of implant intervention.

It is true that oral implantology, its philosophy and techniques, seems somewhat radical to some members of the dental profession. It is also true that at this time insufficient information exists regarding the causes for failures as well as the reasons for successes of implants. Submission of well-controlled objective clinical research is of the utmost importance. Granting that more refined and better means of performing this operation may come along in the future, there is still no question in my mind that what we have today is very valuable and useful, and that is the reason I am involved in its use in the clinical practice of dentistry. A new technique must be carefully judged and evaluated in terms of its inherent merits.

The best reference, in my opinion, for a complete understanding of oral implantology, its philosophy, techniques, and case histories, is *Theories and Techniques of Oral Implantology*, by Leonard I. Linkow.[30]

Bite-opening dangers

Bite-opening is a misnomer in mouth rehabilitation procedures, in my opinion, because it really is not what we have in mind. *Bite-restoring* is a better way of expressing our objective. Why? To begin with, "bite-opening" presupposes the ability to permanently increase the distance between the mandible and the maxilla, which in turn means that the muscles which close the jaw would have to be lengthened (which cannot happen) and, by so doing, a corresponding shortening of the muscles which open the jaw would be necessary. Since muscles work in groups or pairs, there would be a point at which the mandible would be out of muscular control. Considered from a practical and scientific viewpoint, all this is out of the question. Keep in mind that muscle is always the dominant tissue. What really happens under such conditions are changes in the tissues which can be changed, e.g., in the alveolar bone, the dental periosteum, or the true bone of the mandible or maxilla.

"Bite-restoring" means that the bite is opened only to the limit of tolerance of the muscles, etc. which govern the mandible. Vertical dimension increase should not be beyond that which the muscles, supporting bone, and root length permit. The ratio of root length and clinical crown should be within the norm—the clinical crown should not be elongated. We must recognize the fact that the structure and function of the oral cavity impose limits which cannot be exceeded without doing harm.

PORCELAIN-FUSED-TO-METAL RESTORATIONS

Porcelain-fused-to-metal restorations show high physical properties (especially rigidity and impact strength) and can, if properly understood and handled, yield composite structures unexcelled in esthetics, strength, and permanence. With dental porcelains we can also obtain abrasion and stain resistance, which are so desirable.

As a dental restorative material, porcelain has two advantages over other materials: color and tissue compatibility. The combination of porcelain and metal fused together is stronger than procelain alone. The bond appears to be adhesive in nature, with the union occurring by van der Waal's forces and by primary, or chemical, bonds as well.[31] Failure or fracture will, as a rule, occur in the porcelain rather than at the porcelain-metal interface.

All porcelains are generally finely ground ceramic with pigments added for color and shade. Tuccillo[32] has said that the ceramic, when mixed with water, forms a paste with sufficient green strength to be applied to a gold alloy substructure in layers. By vibrating this paste (after applying to the gold alloy substructure) the particles settle and pack together and the excess water is removed (this phenomenon is referred to as condensation). This is then fused at an elevated temperature to form a hard, strong, insoluble (in oral fluids) ceramic body with desirable esthetic qualities in the mouth. The better the condensation, the less shrinkage during firing. Two factors that contribute to condensation are the size and shape of the particles of porcelain powder. Voids that exist between the particles after condensation are subsequently filled during firing and result in shrinkage of the porcelain body. The less water present after condensation, the less shrinkage during firing.

Low and medium temperature porcelains (those generally used in porcelain-fused-to-metal restorations) are those that mature in the temperature range of 1,600° to 2,300°F. These porcelains are glass powders that have been ground from matured or fired porcelain, and are commonly referred to as "frits." On subsequent firing, the particles of "frit" fuse together. The firing temperature depends upon the original composition of the glass, which must be controlled for reproducible maturing temperatures and expansion coefficients.

The amount of firing shrinkage can be as great as 45% volumetrically (12% to 15% linearly).

Porosity in porcelain consists of bubbles or voids caused by trapping of air during fusion. These bubbles, as may be expected, reduce the translucence and strength of the porcelain, and there are more of them with larger size particles of porcelain powder than with smaller size particles. *Porosity can be reduced in a number of ways besides using properly sized particle sizes:*

1. Firing in a vacuum removes the air before it is trapped.
2. Hydrogen or some other diffusible gas is substituted for the ordinary furnace atmospheres. During fusion such gases diffuse out of the porcelain or dissolve in the porcelain.
3. Cooling the fused porcelain under pressure, thus compressing the air bubbles.
4. Therefore, the best method is the use of vacuum.

Vacuum firing can increase the impact strength of porcelain by as much as 48%. This increase is, of course, due to the decrease in the number and size of the air voids.

Many different materials are used to create a porcelain-fused-to-metal restoration. The ultimate in esthetics and strength can be obtained only if each and every material involved conforms to the highest standards of metallurgic and ceramic achievement. It is of the utmost importance that the porcelain be kept at a minimum thickness compatible with good esthetics. Relatively thin porcelain, of uniform thickness and supported by rigid metal, is strong.

Some investigators think that the best way to protect porcelain is not by interposing a gold section between the porcelain and the biting force, as is done with plastic veneers, but by placing gold under the porcelain so that the porcelain is sandwiched in between supporting gold and opposing dentition. It is said that the forces acting upon the porcelain will be mainly compressive and, because porcelain enjoys good compressive strength, a durable restoration is assured. I am certainly in accord with the principle of allowing as much porcelain "wraparound" as possible, but I think one must not overlook occlusal and incisal contacts with opposing teeth. Occlusal contacts can be made with greater precision on metal surfaces than on porcelain surfaces, and there will likely be less wear on the opposing teeth. In most instances, I place occlusal contacts for posterior teeth on metal, and for anterior teeth on metal if the contact can be kept well away from the porcelain-metal junction, because contact at or very near that junction could lead to metal flow and subsequent fracture of the porcelain. In other words, bring the porcelain around the incisal and as far toward the lingual cervical as is feasible.

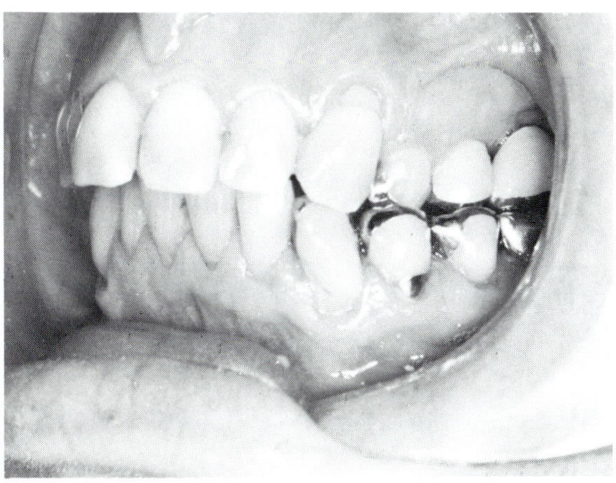

Fig. 7-39. Because of a cross-bite situation distal to the first bicuspid, I used a heavy metal occlusal tip on the second bicuspid porcelain veneer crown.

However, it must be stated that there is rarely a strong indication for prescribing a porcelain veneer but, in special situations (especially in mouth rehabilitation cases), they must be used (Fig. 7-39).

Sigmund Katz[33] has said: "The strength of a porcelain-to-metal construct is the algebraic sum of the strengths of its individual components. If the materials are acting in concert, higher strengths are achieved for the combination than for either individual component. If the materials are acting in opposition, then lower strengths are achieved for the combination. The thermal expansions of the components which have been fused together determine whether the strengths of the components shall act in concert to oppose applied stresses, or shall act in opposition to each other and so vitiate their combined ability to oppose externally applied stresses.

"Porcelain fused to metal is at its maximum strength for the condition of zero internal stress, i.e., when the thermal expansions of the porcelain and the metal are identical. If this condition is not possible (and it will later be shown that it is not obtainable in practice) then the porcelain will be strongest for the condition of minimum stress. Minimum stress can be achieved only when the thermal expansions of porcelain and metal are within the design parameters set by the manufacturer of the porcelain.

"The relationships between the thermal expansions of the porcelain and the metal are somewhat more complex than we would first imagine. For example, we say that the porcelain must always be in compression, and we say this as though the state of compression does something beneficial to the porcelain. This is not so. What is really meant is that the porcelain *must never be in tension.* (Porcelain is weak in tension and strong in compression). The logic is as follows:

"If the metal contracts more than the porcelain on cooling to room temperature, then we say that the porcelain achieves a condition of circumferential compression. True enough, but the only way to arrive at this state is at the cost of developing a radial tension across the porcelain-metal interface. There is no way to place the porcelain in circumferential compression without placing it at the same time in radial tension. This may explain why a small amount of compression is tolerable while a somewhat larger amount of compression results in failure. Even though the porcelain is in circumferential compression, failure has occurred through radial tension. In other words, regardless of the amount of thermal expansion mismatch, porcelain failure is always due to tension, whether circumferential or radial.

"We therefore design our porcelain and metal to develop a small amount of circumferential compression in porcelain, just to be certain that no circumferential tension will be generated as a result of subsequent firing history" (Fig. 7-40).*

*From Katz, Sigmund: Factors affecting the strength of dental prostheses fabricated from porcelain fused to metal, Thermocraft Techn. Bull. **2**(3):1-3, 1968.

The mechanical properties of an air-fired porcelain and a vacuum-fired porcelain are similar; however, vacuum firing does introduce a vital translucence that is not as readily attained in an air-fired porcelain. In other words, a benefit of vacuum firing of porcelain is an increase in vitality due to the increased translucency. There is also some control of the shade through variation of the amount of applied vacuum. Higher vacuum intensifies the shade, and lower vacuum lightens the shade. Vacuum firing also provides an extremely dense porcelain which can be polished to a glazed finish after spot-grinding in some instances, but keep in mind that vacuum firing cannot be a substitute for a poor condensing technique, and porcelains which condense poorly are hazardous whether fired by vacuum or air. To sum up, vacuum firing gives (1) increased translucency, (2) additional shade control, (3) increased density, (4) increased strength, (5) fewer gas blow-ups, and (6) superior esthetics. Use of a vacuum allows for the escape of small air bubbles that are normally trapped in an air-fired porcelain, and the elimination of these small air bubbles confers greater translucence. However, the use of a vacuum-fired porcelain demands careful degassing of the metal prior to application of porcelain. Otherwise, gases adsorbed on the metal will be released, thereby forming very large bubbles at the porcelain-metal interface which can interfere with the bond.[34]

The success of porcelain-fused-to-metal restorations depends on a number of factors. A few of the

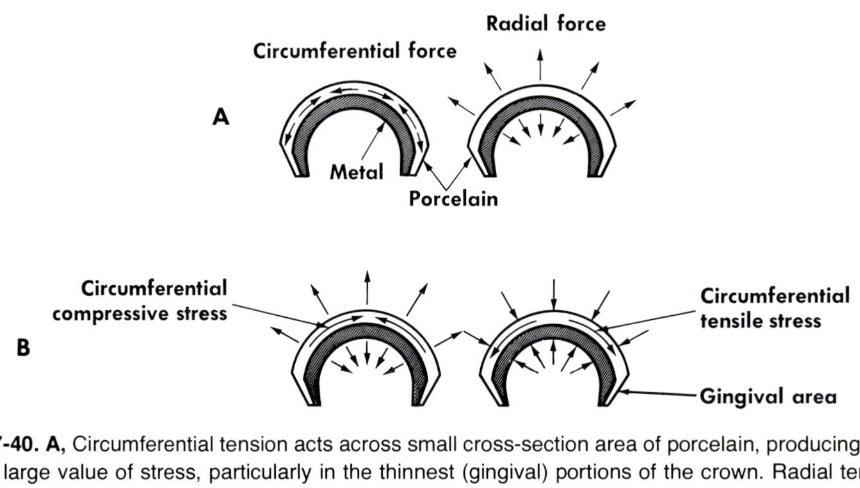

Fig. 7-40. A, Circumferential tension acts across small cross-section area of porcelain, producing relatively large value of stress, particularly in the thinnest (gingival) portions of the crown. Radial tension applied over total area of porcelain-metal interface produces relatively low value of stress (force/unit of area). **B,** If metal shrinks more than porcelain, then porcelain is placed in circumferential compression and the porcelain-metal interface is placed in radial tension. If porcelain shrinks more than metal, then the porcelain-metal interface is placed in radial compression, but porcelain is in circumferential tension. (Adapted from Thermocraft Technical Bulletin **2**[3]:Oct., 1968.)

important ones are (1) matched coefficients of expansion, (2) chemical bond, (3) a good Brinell hardness of the alloy, and (4) sag resistance.

1. Coefficient of expansion or coefficient of thermal expansion is the most important property for both the gold and the porcelain. The coefficient of expansion is the percentage change in length when a material is heated from room temperature to higher temperatures. Therefore it is the most critical property in designing a ceramic-to-metal combination, and it must be adjusted as close as possible between gold and porcelain, with a slight edge being given to the gold. Gold, therefore, should have a slightly higher coefficient of expansion.

To reduce interfacial stresses between the porcelain and metal, their coefficients of expansion should be matched or compatible. The bond between these two materials depends upon this important factor of matched coefficients of expansion. The greater the disparity between the coefficients of expansion of the two materials, the greater the interfacial stress will be; hence, the greater the probability of bond rupture.

As the porcelain-metal combination cools, the metal contracts faster than the porcelain and pulls it together. This leaves the porcelain in compression where it is strongest. If the gold alloy shrinks less on cooling, after firing the porcelain, the porcelain will be in tension, where it is weakest, resulting in crazing of the porcelain surface. Ceramics are strong in resistance to forces that try to shorten their length and otherwise compress them.

Accurate control checks must be made by the manufacturers of these materials to maintain them in a precise ratio to each other.

2. It is also necessary to have a chemical bonding. Oxides contribute to a chemical bond between the alloy and the porcelain. The oxide formation must not affect the color of the porcelain. The main bond is chemical and only slightly mechanical. The mechanical bond results from the gripping of the many grooves in the surface of the metal by the porcelain.

If either of these two all-important factors—matched coefficients of expansion and chemical bonding—is not present in the porcelain-gold pair, then the full strength of the bond will not be developed.

The porcelain and gold must be made for each other to expand and contract compatibly and provide an inseparable bond.

3. It has been found that the ceramic gold alloy actually becomes stronger during the porcelain bake. The full strength potential of the gold is developed.

4. Sag resistance is the ability to withstand sag, creep, or deformation at high temperatures. The importance of sag resistance is primarily its effect on accurate fit of the restoration, not before but after baking on the porcelain. This development also has resulted in higher hardness and greater strength.[35]

In general, I have discussed a few important criteria—the necessary relationship between the thermal expansions of the porcelain and the gold casting to which it is fused, and also the achievement of the necessary optic properties for satisfactory esthetics (which is very important to satisfy a criterion).

But, some years ago, my attention was called to the fact that for maximum reliability, the porcelain must have three additional properties: (1) high strength, measured by transverse rupture modules, (2) high resistance to thermal shock, and (3) the ability to be annealed.[36]

The strength of a porcelain is measured by its ability to resist external forces without breaking. However, resistance to external forces may be sharply reduced by the presence of internal stresses, and it is literally impossible to produce bridgework of the type under discussion without these internal stresses. Therefore, the stronger the porcelain, the greater the ability to resist both internal and external stresses.

High resistance to thermal shock is a property which is of primary interest to the ceramist. Low resistance to thermal shock may make it troublesome to produce the case, since it will check frequently during processing. Sometimes it will pop, with small pieces of porcelain flying from the bridge. Thermal shock failure in the mouth is probably rare, since the temperature differences involved in processing are very much greater than can occur in the oral cavity.

As to the question of the ability of the porcelain to be annealed so as to be able to relieve internal stresses that develop and weaken the porcelain, it can be said that the effectiveness of the treatment will increase impact resistance and also provide a smoothness, ease, and safety in the grinding of the porcelain.

Shelby[37] has aptly listed the requirements for porcelain-fused-to-metal restorations: (1) accurate preparations and impressions, (2) accurate abutment and pontic castings, (3) accurate soldering and ease of soldering, (4) rigidity of the metal framework, thereby obtaining adequate strength of the final restoration, (5) good esthetics, and (6) tissue tolerance.

Before considering the above-mentioned requirements in more detail, a few words about "glazed porcelain" are in order. Glazed porcelain most closely resembles the natural tooth structure—you can have glazed porcelain on the ridge area (glazed porcelain is kind to mouth tissues), it will not erode, it can be used on a "biting" surface, it is not porous and is therefore impervious to mouth fluids, it will not change color.

Certain design principles and precautions in tooth preparation and coping and framework design must be followed when porcelain-fused-to-metal is used in restorative dentistry.

Preparation design

We must involve ourselves in these particular types of restorations with a few changes or adaptations in the conventional preparation procedures for full coverage, not only for maximum strength but also for restoration of function and correct esthetic values.

Crown retention, abutment parallelism, and "no undercuts" in the preparation are most essential. Also, removal of sufficient tooth structure incisally or occlusally (2 mm.) and circumferentially (1.5 to 2 mm.) is necessary to allow the construction of a metal coping (0.33 to 0.5 mm.) of sufficient strength and rigidity and at the same time to fabricate a porcelain restoration of correct anatomic contours (coronal and embrasures) and color. A slight bevel on the shoulder preparation is indicated because a perfect butt joint between metal coping and a square shoulder is difficult to attain. The end result is usually a cement line which eventually washes out, leading to plaque formation and its sequelae, decay and gingival irritation.

In other words, we must always keep in mind not only definitive retentive form and marginal outline, but also proper tooth form and function.

Since room must be created to accommodate a small subgingival metal collar (which must not be covered with porcelain to avoid overcontouring) and without creating undue pressure upon the delicate gingival tissues, we must be very cautious in our technical approach so as not to damage the marginal fibers of the periodontium (Fig. 7-41).

Clinical evidence clearly demonstrates that subgingival extension of full coverage margins produces an environment unfavorable to the health of the marginal gingiva. In the area adjacent to full coverage, it is difficult to maintain marginal gingiva which are thin and acceptably contoured for physiologic function and food flow. In contrast to the maintenance of healthy gingiva around enamel and cementum of natural tooth substance, the gingival tissues around full coverage seem to be more thickened, more rolled, and generally more inflammatory in character.

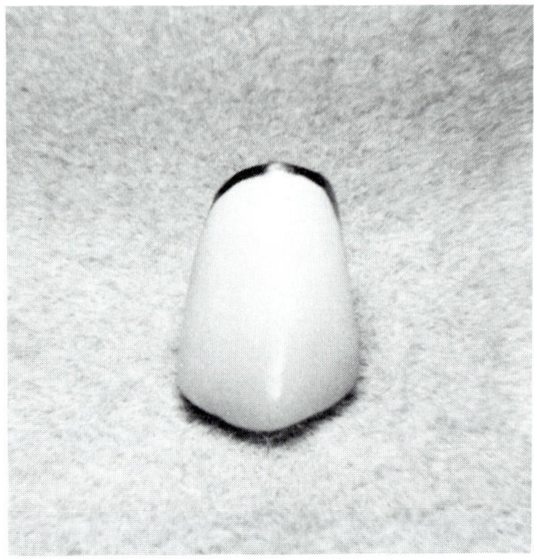

Fig. 7-41. A small subgingival metal collar not covered by porcelain to avoid overcontouring and thereby not damaging the marginal fibers of the periodontium.

A normal healthy condition of the gingival tissues around a porcelain crown, even if not exactly what we desire, can be helped by preparatory measures that will avoid irritating the tissues unduly, by constructing a restoration that is an accurate complement to the prepared tooth, and by making one that has a tooth form that is an accurate anatomic reproduction of the natural tooth.

In this same vein let us ask ourselves the question —where should we terminate the preparation for a full crown? I believe, considering the information mentioned above, that no matter how deep the gingival crevice is, the preparation should extend very slightly into that crevice. To recommend extending the margin of the preparation up to or just short of the epithelial attachment is impractical and misleading, and often results in severe tissue laceration.

There are some teeth where it is impossible to prepare a shoulder because of the anatomy, the condition, and the position of the tooth. Shoulderless or finishing line preparations are the answer. It is imperative that on such a shoulderless preparation, the gold collar be exhibited in the area where insufficient tooth structure was removed.

We should also keep in mind that in a shoulder preparation we have allowance for a wedge-shaped or triangular piece of metal lying in the gingivoaxial line angle of the preparation which will give added strength in this area (Fig. 7-42).

Also, as reported by Shillingburg, Hobo, and Fisher,[38,39] the beveled shoulder has been found to afford some protection against distortion during porce-

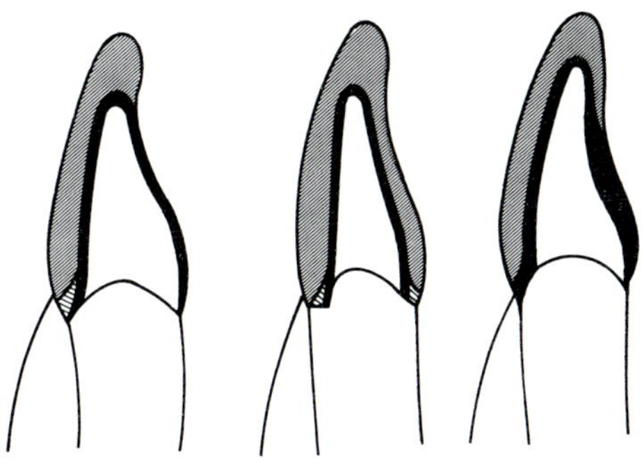

Fig. 7-42. Possibilities of metal-porcelain distribution on anterior restorations. **A,** Chamfer preparation. Gingival margin of restoration should have a wedge-shaped fillet of metal for rigidity when it can be concealed in the gingival sulcus. **B,** Shoulder preparation. This must be reinforced for rigidity, etc. with a wedge-shaped fillet of metal at gingival area. Display of gold at gingival area not necessary. **C,** Shoulderless preparation. Gold collar will be exhibited but usually not noticeable from a speaking distance. (Adapted from Hoffman, E. G.: Dent. Clin. N. Am., March, 1965.)

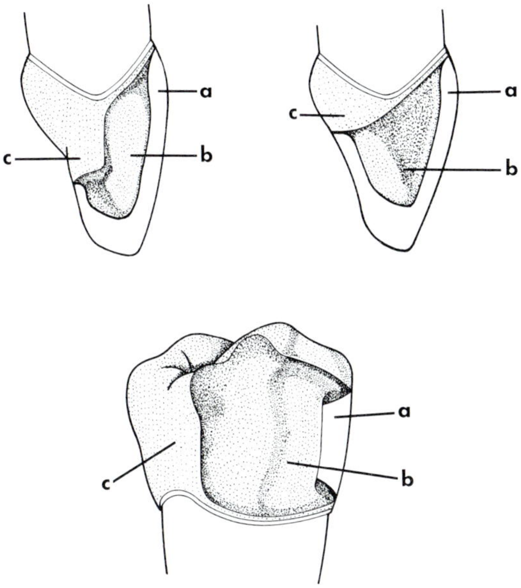

Fig. 7-43. Ceramic crowns with high and low porcelain-metal junctions which will allow for occlusal contacts on metal (high) and occlusal contacts on porcelain (low). *a,* Porcelain; *b,* coping covered by porcelain; *c,* unveneered metal. (Adapted from Hobo, S., and Shillingburg, H. T., Jr.: J. Prosthet. Dent. **30**[1]:28-36, July, 1973.)

lain firing. They are also of the opinion, with which I am in full accord, that the proximal contacts for anterior teeth should be in porcelain, because the appearance of the finished case is improved by not having metal contacts darkening the adjacent teeth, and that the proximal contacts and occlusal surfaces in areas of occlusal contact with opposing teeth on posterior teeth should be in metal, except for the mesial surface of maxillary bicuspids, where the proximal contact and mesial marginal ridge may be done in porcelain if occlusion permits (Fig. 7-43).

SOME IMPORTANT STEPS IN THE PREPARATION

Incisal reduction is made to a depth of 2 mm. and in a plane at right angles to the direction of the force induced by the opposing occlusion (and hollow ground). This allows for 0.5 mm. thickness of metal underlying the porcelain, and the remaining 1.5 mm. of space makes it possible to build an incisal edge on the restoration which has pleasing optic qualities and normal labiolingual thickness. The incisal corners are rounded off or notched to prevent the necessity for metal extending too far into the incisal corners of the restoration.[39]

In the reduction of the facial surface remove enough tooth structure (somewhat deeper axial reduction) to ensure adequate thickness of metal and porcelain while preserving integrity of the pulp. This can be accomplished by preparing in two planes, which gives us maximum esthetics with unnecessary tooth structure destruction (Fig. 7-44). A shoulder of 0.7 mm. width (which is minimal) to 1.5 mm. or, if possible, in some cases 2 mm. is what must be considered. The shoulder should be carried around the proximal angles into the embrasures, usually to a point beneath or slightly lingual to the center of the contact area. At this point we have created what has been referred to as "mesial and distal 'wings,'" and from here the remainder of the proximal surfaces and the lingual surface are prepared using a chamfer finishing line. The lingual surface rarely requires a shoulder preparation as long as sufficient tooth structure is removed to permit adequate thickness for the metal and porcelain at the incisal and middle thirds.

Posterior occlusal surface reduction should be at least 2 mm. and should follow occlusal contour or the primary planes of the occlusal surface. The shoulder is carried around the proximal angles into the embrasures, usually to a point beneath or slightly lingual to the center of the contact area. A chamfer finish line is used for the remainder of the proximal surfaces and the lingual. The facial finish line for

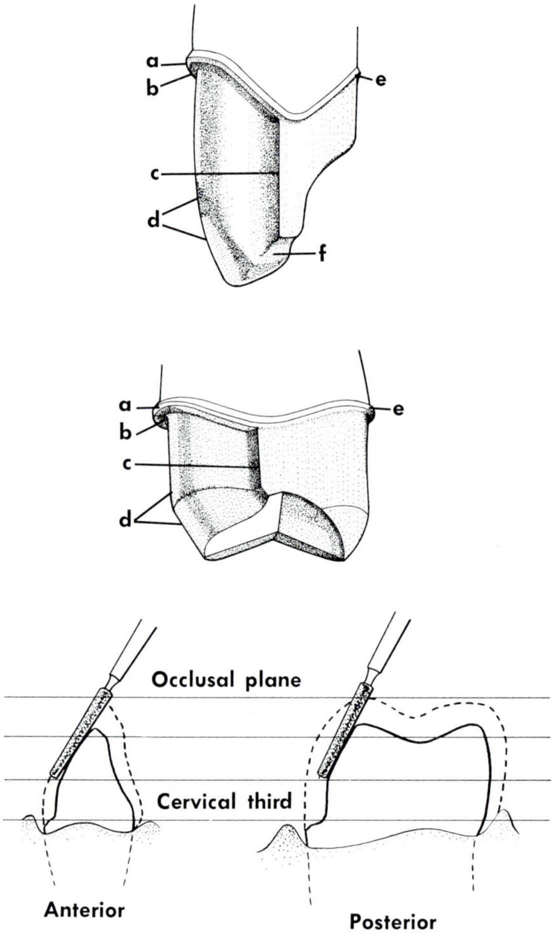

Fig. 7-44. Preparation of an anterior and posterior tooth by preparing in two planes for maximum esthetics and unnecessary tooth structure destruction. *a,* The bevel; *b,* the shoulder; *c,* the proximal "wing" where heavy facial reduction ends; *d,* facial reduction accomplished in two planes; *e,* lingual chamfer; *f,* notches in incisal corners on anterior preparation. (Courtesy Sumiya Hobo and Herbert T. Shillingburg, Jr.)

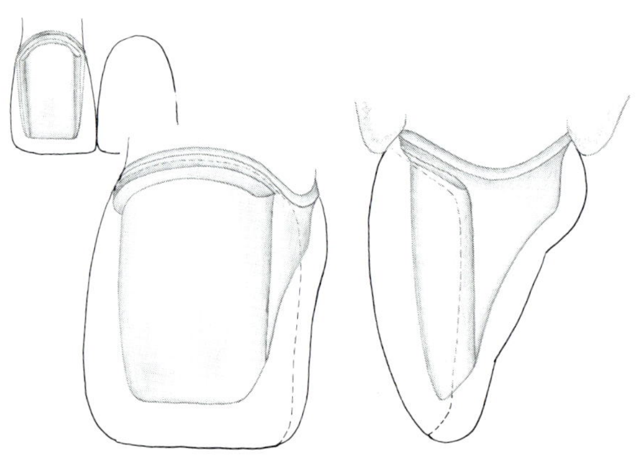

Fig. 7-45. Beveled-shoulder marginal finish line gradually fades into chamfer finish line as it approaches lingual surface.

anterior and posterior teeth is a shoulder with a slight bevel (0.2 mm. or less). Be sure to round slightly all axioincisal and axio-occlusal angles (Fig. 7-45).

The reduction of the occlusal surface by 2 mm. (in our preparations) should be a clearance of 2 mm. created with all pathways of eccentric movement (lateral and protrusive) considered, observed, duly noted, and allowed for, in addition to centric position clearance. Greater efficiency of function requires greater care in design. To wear through a casting is unfortunate, displeasing, and troublesome, and to grind through while adjusting is bad.

Keep the proximal walls of preparations as parallel as possible (2 to 5 degrees to the perpendicular) to gain adequate retention, and in some cases (short preparations, tapering preparations, caries involvement, etc.) a posthole in the cingulum area for additional retention is indicated.

Esthetic recontouring of the gingiva may be necessary to make the teeth appear uniform in length. A high gingival papilla between pontic area and abutment tooth will weaken the metal framework and precipitate breakage of the finished restoration. Cut the papilla with an electric scalpel.

Some dentists are of the opinion that a sliding fit with a chamfered shoulder produces a more intimate and accurate joint and greatly aids retention. However, in my opinion, this type of finishing line does not allow for the use of sufficient bulk of metal for support (and it does not afford protection against distortion during porcelain firing) or enough bulk of porcelain to attain color matching in the gingival third of the veneer unless the restoration is overcontoured in this area. This overcontouring has a deleterious effect on the marginal gingiva and also gives the tooth a bulky appearance, especially when it is carried interproximally.

Do not polish the preparation highly. A slightly textured surface aids cementation.

Periodontally involved teeth where the preparation will finish well down on the root structure are not likely candidates for shoulder preparations and necessitate (with some upper anterior exceptions) a display of a small band of gold supragingivally.

So, summing up it can be said:

1. To achieve harmony it is necessary to remain within the confines of the form and contour of the original tooth.
2. To produce the requisite color and translucence a certain bulk of porcelain is necessary.
3. A good ceramic crown has excellent esthetic characteristics of form and color and promotes

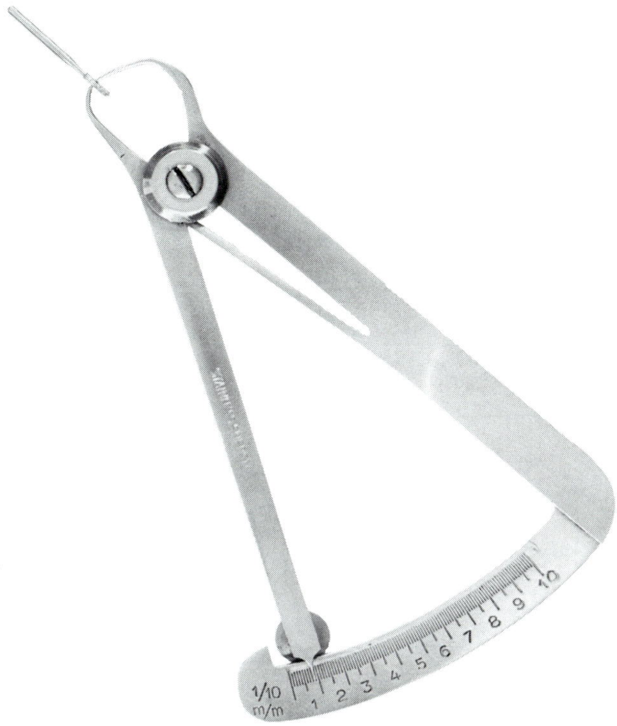

Fig. 7-46. Caliper used to check metal casting thickness and for measurement of diamond stones for depth control in tooth structure removal.

physiologic health of the tissues. Glazed porcelain makes it easier to maintain gingival health since the lack of porosity discourages formation of plaque or calculus.

Berman[40] has described, and I have used exclusively for the last 4 years, a procedure that has improved cutting efficiency over other methods for bulk removal of tooth structure by means of depth control by the instrument itself. This is described in detail and with illustrations in Chapter 8 in the section on full coverage.

In concluding this phase of the porcelain-fused-to-gold section, preparation design, I believe, after many years of experience with this type of restoration, that probably the greatest single cause of failure is inadequate tooth preparation. There is no substitute for sufficient tooth structure removal that can make it possible to satisfy the esthetic and functional demands of the patient. Metal structure, opaquing, shade control, and coronal form are all governed by the tooth preparation. One or more of these factors must usually be sacrificed if the abutment teeth are not properly prepared. For example, if the metal understructure is made so that the facing that is to accept the porcelain is less than 0.4 to 0.5 mm. in thickness, the chances for a successful restoration are minimal. It is important to check metal thickness with an accurate caliper (Fig. 7-46). If the casting is made too thin to avoid overcontouring, the porcelain-gold restoration will distort during "try-in" or cementation or under occlusal stresses and the porcelain will pop off. If, on the other hand, the proper bulk of metal structure is used, the case will be overcontoured, with its deleterious sequelae. Keep in mind, therefore, that the fundamental geometry of the case contributes to good end results. Major considerations in creating this geometry are not only adequate tooth structure removal but also parallelism of the abutment preparations. Lack of parallelism will cause a torquelike force to be exerted on the metal substructure so that it may flex and cause breakage of the porcelain veneer. This may occur at the time of insertion, or at a later time, especially if some small extra masticatory force is applied. If one carries out the above-mentioned precautions, the finished restoration will go to place with finger pressure, sometimes hard finger pressure. The fit should be "passive."

Impressions, temporary coverage, and transfers

The impression is now taken with either one of the elastic impression materials (hydrocolloid, elasticon, or citricon) or a copper tube with modeling compound.

The next step, before dismissal of the patient, is the temporary coverage of the prepared tooth. (For detailed discussion and illustrations of impression taking and temporary coverage refer to Chapter 9).

At a subsequent visit of the patient, a highly important consideration is the need for accurately transferring the dies (if copper or silver plated dies are used) before the construction of the metal structure.

TRANSFERS

1. Extreme accuracy for proper seating and alignment of copper or silver plated dies is possible if cast metal transfers are constructed which fit the dies accurately. A labioincisal or bucco-occlusal opening of the metal transfer assures exact seating on the abutment tooth.
2. A buccal (or lingual) "lug" or a labioincisal or bucco-occlusal "lip" is of great assistance when taking a plaster impression or an acrylic matrix (rebased with a zinc oxide eugenol paste)—alginate "overall" impression (Fig. 7-47).

This accuracy of transfer with well-prepared paral-

A

B

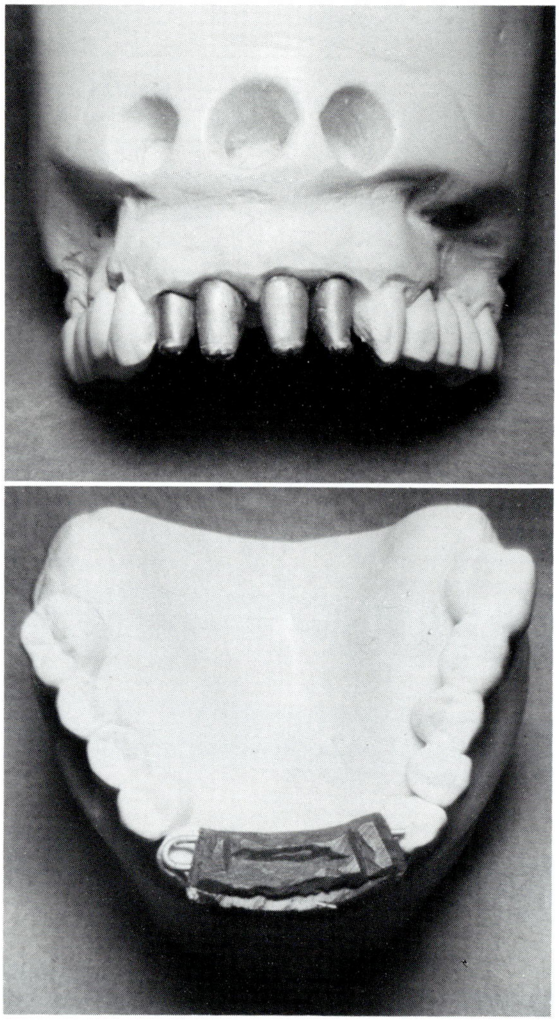

Fig. 7-47. A, Copings with labioincisal "lips" on prepared teeth. **B,** Reinforced modeling compound matrix fitted over incisal "lips," rebased with Kerr's Temp-Bond, and overall alginate impression taken for accurate positioning of the copper-plated dies.

lel abutment teeth creates the base for a well-fitting restoration.*

*I wish to express my deep appreciation, and I feel it applies also to the profession at large, to the pioneer work of J. Johnston, R. Dykema, R. Phillips, G. Mumford, E. Hoffman, L. Weinberg, J. Shell, J. Nielsen, J. Tuccillo, G. Ryge, W. J. O'Brien, A. F. Kelley, Denton Smith, G. Straussberg, S. Katz, G. Katz, M. Kuwata, the research and development staffs of the J. M. Ney Co., J. F. Jelenko Co., American Thermocraft Corp., J. Aderer Co., the Williams Co., the Whip-Mix Corp., Ceramco, Inc., and probably a few other individuals that I cannot call to mind at this time for their basic research and technical application of their findings in the important field of porcelain-fused-to-metal restorations.

Metal structure

Most investigators agree that it is desirable to have the most rigid framework possible to prevent flexing and subsequent porcelain fracture.

Properly designed gold alloy copings and pontics provide the greatest gold strength consistent with maximum porcelain support and esthetics. Coping design is of such importance that it can effect success or failure of the restoration. If there is any deformation of the metal coping, either during initial seating of the restoration or later when it is subjected to occlusal forces, the brittle, inflexible porcelain may fracture. So we are confronted with two interrelated factors—the alloy used and the structural design.

To prevent deformation, the metal structure must exhibit great rigidity and torque-resisting qualities, and its design must ensure an optimum bulk of the proper alloy. Or, put this way, rigidity may be attained, according to Mumford,[34] by (1) using a metal with a high modulus of elasticity and high proportional limit combined with a thicker than normal cross-sectional area, (2) changing the geometry of the cross section, and (3) reducing the load by the use of short spans (two or three tooth sections).

It would be remiss in considering good structural design not to review the causes of failures in porcelain-fused-to-metal restorations. Most failures are the result of excessive stress from various origins. Important stress factors that result in failures are: (1) differences in the coefficient of thermal expansion between the metal and the porcelain, (2) sharp edges or corners at the interface of the metal and the porcelain, and (3) deformation of the cast structure under the porcelain. This type of deformation is usually the result of the metal structure being too thin, resulting in it being distorted by the contraction of the porcelain (shrinkage of the porcelain during fusing). Stresses will also increase as the span increases. The questions that must come to mind are: (1) What is the position of the structural span in relation to the arch? (2) Is it a linear structure (anterior or posterior unit) or a curvilinear structure (both anterior and posterior units)? Structural considerations are quite different when dealing with linear or curvilinear construction.[41]

The span of the fixed partial denture (linear construction) should be limited in size, and the complete arch splint (curvilinear construction) should be broken into segments, if possible, by means of precision attachments or telescopic crowns. This use of segments also keeps dimensional changes during heating and cooling in the baking process to a minimum. If a precision attachment is used the metal boxing should be so prepared so as to allow at least 1.5 mm. metal thickness between male attachment and porcelain to absorb internal stress.

If, however, conditions dictate (position of remaining teeth in the arch, mobility patterns, etc.) that the complete arch splint must be constructed as one unit, an excellent technical suggestion as to how to avoid warpage in this type of long span bridge was given by Purcell.[42] The question that was asked frequently of him was —what causes a long span bridge to no longer fit after it has been subjected to several firings in the porcelain furnace? By long span bridge we are considering complete splints of ten to fourteen units in length. In most cases, the technician is aware that a horseshoe-shaped casting would have a tendency when cast to want to straighten. Consequently, most technicians will attach an 8 gauge wax rod or connector between the two free ends, or from second molar across the arch to second molar. The unit is held together as one piece while it is being cast. This connection should remain in place while porcelain is being fabricated, thus eliminating the possibility of having the posterior segments no longer fit properly on the prepared teeth. Through the addition of this bar, the problem of a misfitting casting after porcelain has been fabricated is usually eliminated.

After soldering the various sections of a complete arch splint into one unit, as discussed and illustrated in Chapter 11, I now also solder a connector from the last retainer on one side across the arch to the last retainer on the other side to avoid warpage of the splint during fabrication of the porcelain veneer.

However, it is found that if the splint is not properly supported that it can, and often does, change with subsequent heats during the firing process of porcelain, and that the splint could change ever so slightly, even though a sag-resistant factor is built into the gold alloy. As a result, the casting will not fit properly after multiple firings.

Castings must be adequately supported to prevent warpage or torque, or both, which can exist particularly with long span bridges. A custom saggar tray should be fabricated for the long span bridge or splint so that it is adequately supported during the firing procedures. This means support on the retainers as well as the pontics. The pontic support areas on the tray should be dusted with powdered silex so that the porcelain will not stick. Such custom trays should be used even though bridge units are not cast as one piece, but rather are cast as one, two, or three multiples and soldered together before the porcelain fabrication has been completed (Fig. 7-48).

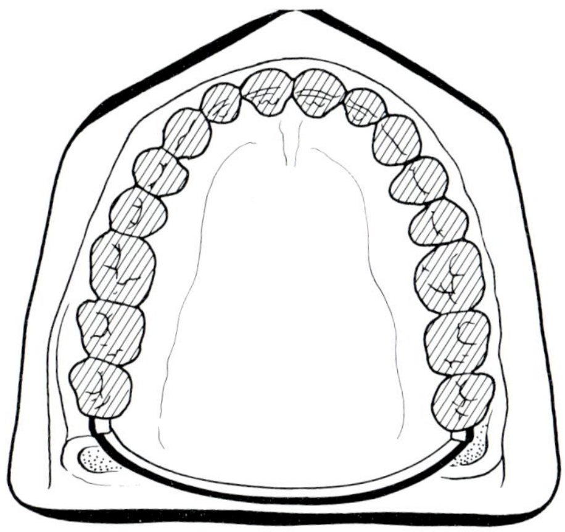

Fig. 7-48. A connector is soldered from the last retainer on one side across the arch to the last retainer on the other side to avoid warpage of the splint during fabrication of the porcelain veneer.

Weinberg[43] has aptly said that there are two principles relating to metal structure rigidity that should be made clear in relation to dental restorations. The first is that the individual castings should always be as rigid or more rigid than the solder joints connecting them. Due to the limitation of space, the solder joint can only have a certain maximum rigidity. Therefore, it should be the weakest link in a fixed partial prosthesis. The rigidity of the solder joint should be the minimum factor in construction. By the addition of the high lingual shoulder and the elongated proximal connecting strut, the substructure coping is now more rigid than the solder joint (Fig. 7-49). Engineering techniques, such as prestressing, could be used to increase the rigidity of assembled dental castings.

Another method of increasing the rigidity of the substructure framework utilizes the engineering principle of corrugation. The principle is extremely simple in that by merely changing the shape of a given material its strength is increased. The modified substructure configuration utilizes the corrugation principle. The rigid lingual shoulder is confluent with the proximal connecting struts which join at the incisal surface. This forms a continuous rigid bar of metal in a corrugated shape. The resultant substructure frame is stronger than if the same thickness of metal were arranged in a straight line at the gingival.

In our discussion of the importance of structural design to obtain a rigid framework, mention was also made that the proper alloy should be used. It is my opinion, which has been formulated by actual usage over a period of years, that ceramic golds with super

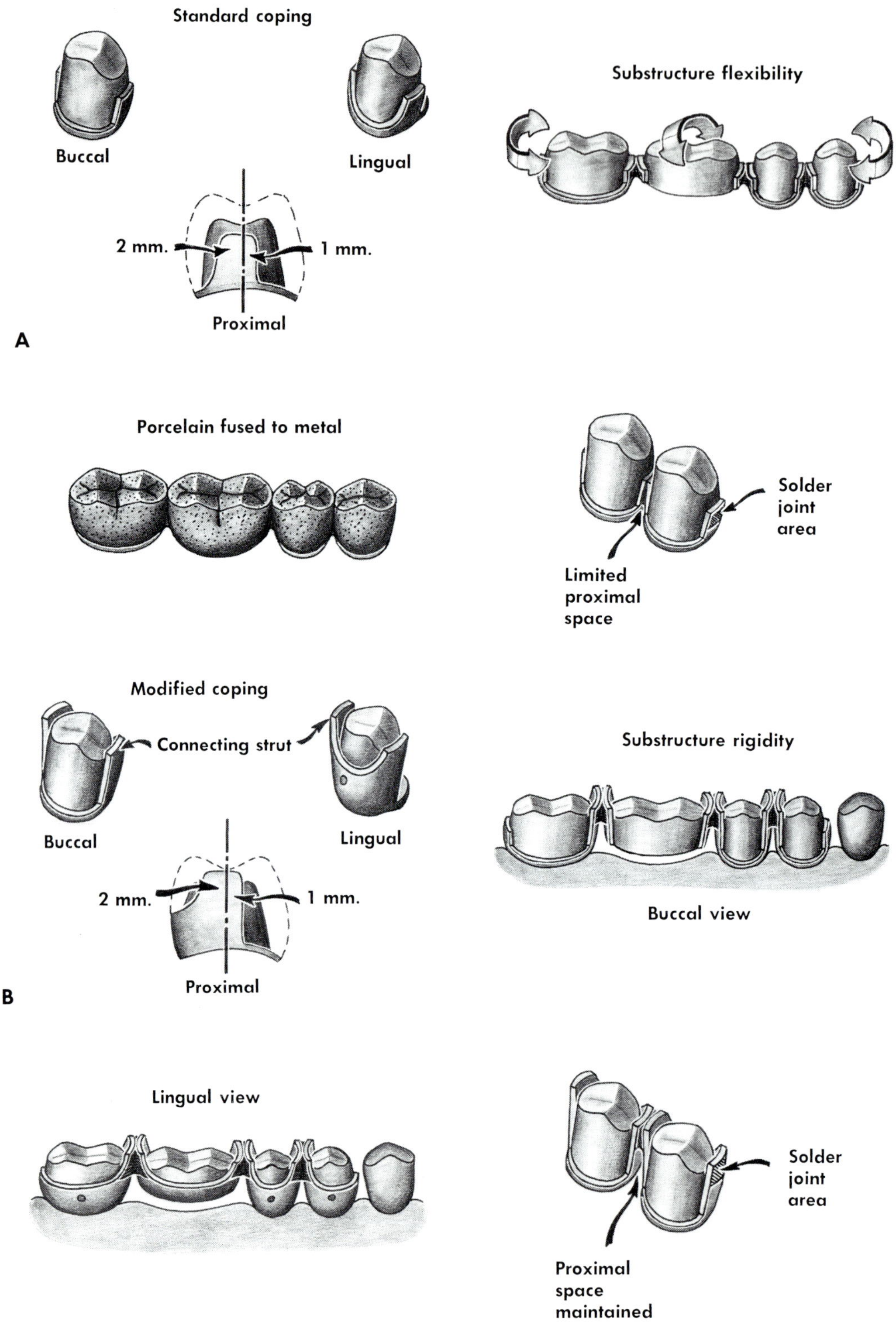

Fig. 7-49. A, Standard coping. **B,** Modified coping (utilizes the engineering principle of corrugation) as used by Kornfeld. **C,** The pontic. **D,** Completed view. **E,** Application of the principle in a practical case. (**D** courtesy Lawrence A. Weinberg.)

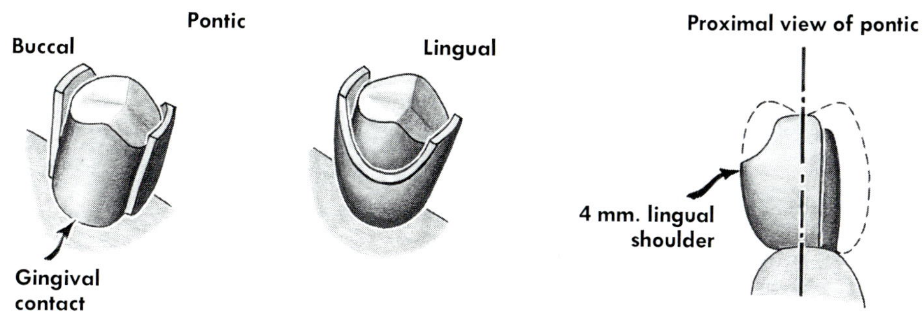

C

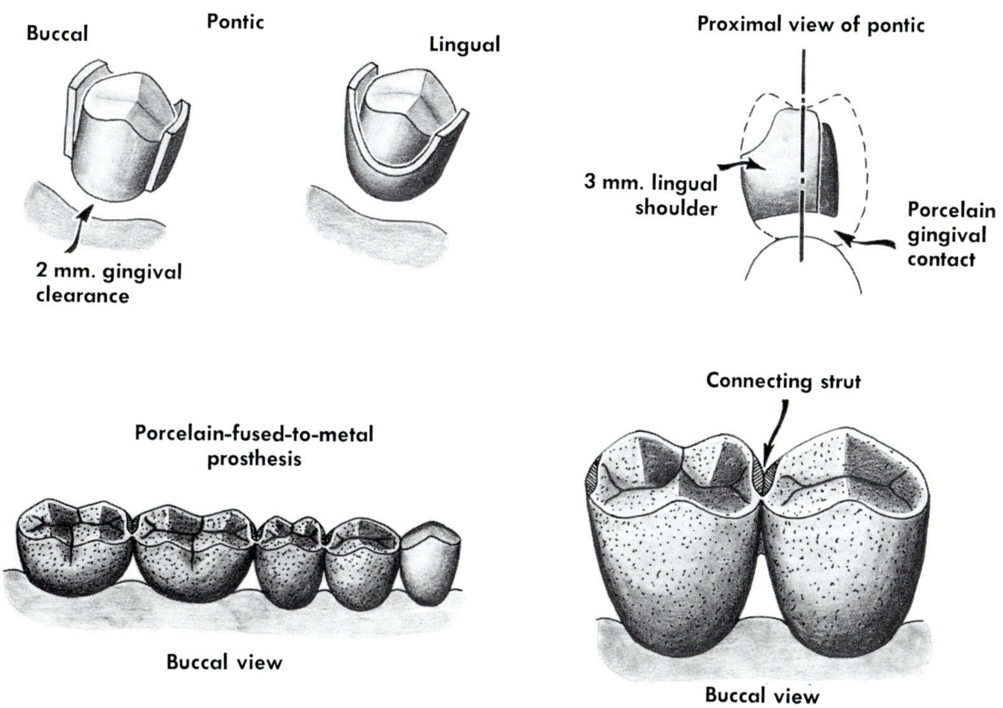

D

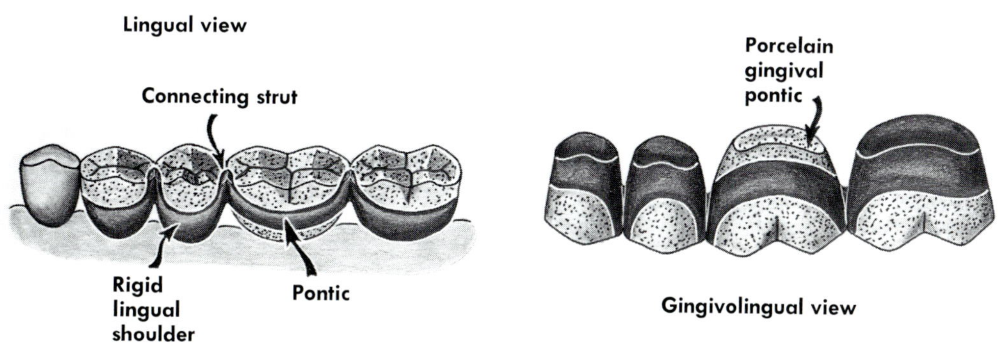

Fig. 7-49, cont'd. For legend see opposite page.

E

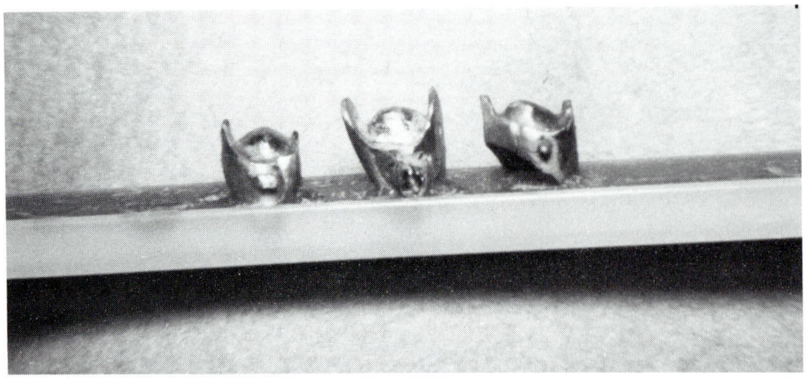

Fig. 7-49, cont'd. For legend see p. 288.

micrograin are the proper types to be used in ceramic restorations.

Super micrograin is a metallurgic process that produces an extremely fine-grained casting in golds for use with porcelain. Super micrograin is locked into the alloy. This means that no matter how many times it is remelted or how many furnace firing cycles a casting is subjected to, its super micrograin size will not change. Its tensile strength, hardness, and handling properties will remain the same regardless of the technique used in the dental laboratory. It retains the structural integrity of the restoration. We can obtain strong, dense castings which are safer for thin, delicate margins. These margins can be finished with no flaking or chipping. It grinds smoothly without drag or well-up of metal. Its elongation allows for good burnishing of the margins, but it is also important to know that all marginal adaptation must be done before the casting or bridge is fired for degassing. Full hardness of the metal is developed during the slow cooling after degassing, which means that it would be more difficult to burnish the margins. A high luster finish can be given to the restoration. We not only have an increased yield strength, which means that more pressure is required to cause any flexing of the metal, but we have the working advantages of castability (eliminates the problem of critical casting temperatures), grindability, burnishability, and polishability. Micrograin solder joints are stronger.[44,45]

Tuccillo[46] has recently checked out the compositional losses that occur when we melt, remelt, remelt, and remelt again without the addition of new metal at each melt. He chose the porcelain gold alloys because they generally contain a small but highly significant amount of base metals that control metal strength and adhesive bonding to the porcelain. He found that there is a threshold value of hardening elements, and by remelting without the addition of new metal with a gas/oxygen torch two or three times we get dangerously close to the threshold value. If the metal is overheated with a gas/oxygen torch (temperatures up to about 2,800° F. are possible, and this is 500° F. above the recommended casting temperature) the threshold value can be reached after two remelts. *Therefore, when melting porcelain gold alloys by gas/oxygen torch do not overheat and add at least 50% new metal.*

Spruing, investing, casting, soldering, and cementation (in regard to the construction of "ceramic" restorations) are discussed and illustrated in detail in Chapters 10 through 12. (Chapter 12 includes finishing and polishing of the casting.)

SALIENT FACTS (DESIGN AND PREPARATION OF THE CASTING, SOME PORCELAIN CONSIDERATIONS)

Porcelain coverage should not terminate at the incisal or bucco-occlusal edges, as it does in conventional veneering, but should be carried onto the lingual or occlusal surfaces (as a hand grips a ball), with the possible exception of the lower posterior teeth in some cases.

An anterior porcelain veneered gold crown is built with a porcelain incisal edge "unprotected" by overlying metal. This is a mechanical necessity and is esthetically better. In my experience it seems that, even though all precautions have been taken in design of the wax pattern and preparation of the casting, the preponderance of incisal fractures has taken place in those veneers where an attempt was made to protect the incisal edge with metal. Not only is translucency interfered with, but pressure exerted on the metal by opposing teeth can deflect the metal and impose a flexing force on the porcelain.

In other words, the incisal edge should be reproduced in porcelain. The areas on the lingual surface making contacts in centric position and the beginnings of the eccentric movements preferably should be metal (contacts should not take place at the porcelain-metal junction—allow a safety margin of at least 2 mm.), since this permits some subsequent occlusal adjustment without the formation of a rough porcelain surface.

In upper posterior crowns or pontics, the porcelain is extended over the occlusal edge and including the occlusal third of the lingual incline of the buccal cusp.

The occlusal surfaces of lower posterior crowns or pontics are left unveneered unless the absolute in esthetics is demanded by the patient. Covering the entire occlusal surface of these posterior teeth with porcelain often leads to inaccurate occlusal contacts, the possibility of excessive wear on opposing teeth, etc. However, if full porcelain occlusals are indicated, the copings should have occlusal planes which are not flat, but rather correspond to the ultimate porcelain contours (Fig. 7-50).

Design of wax pattern

FORMING THE WINDOW

1. The window should be extended sufficiently interproximally. This window may end in a vertical line through the contact area for a single crown. When units are to be soldered together the window margin will have to curve labially as it approaches the contact area to allow a large enough area for the soldered union. *Always consider* (a) the extensions of the area to be veneered with porcelain, (b) the bulk of metal for rigidity, and (c) placement of occlusal contacts.

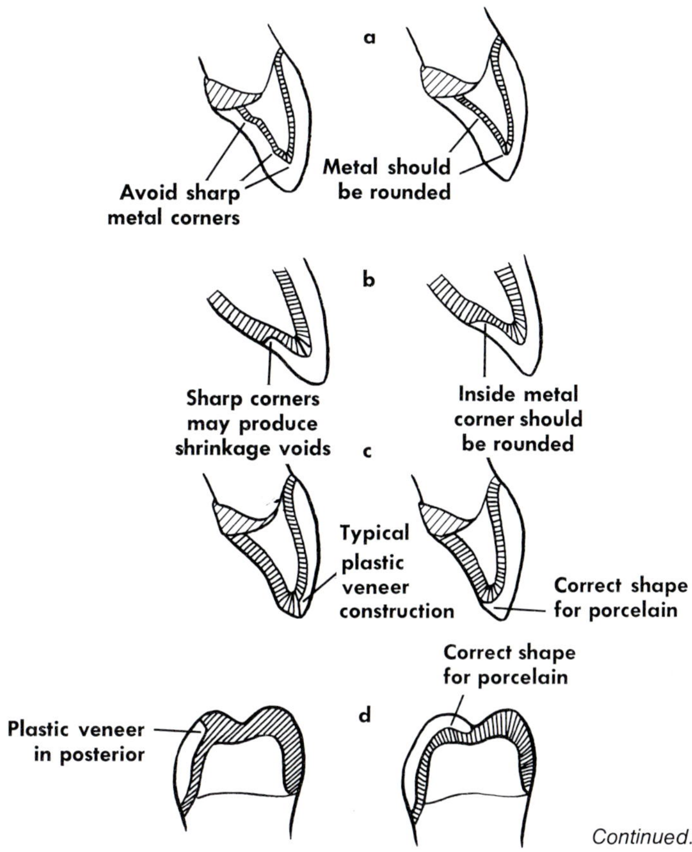

Continued.

Fig. 7-50. Principles to be observed in the designing of the wax pattern, the preparation of the casting, and occlusal factors. Avoid sharp metal corners, shrinkage voids, comparison of plastic and porcelain on anteriors and posteriors, correct shape for posterior porcelain restorations, the lingual surfaces of anteriors and posteriors. (Redrawn courtesy American Thermocraft Corp.)

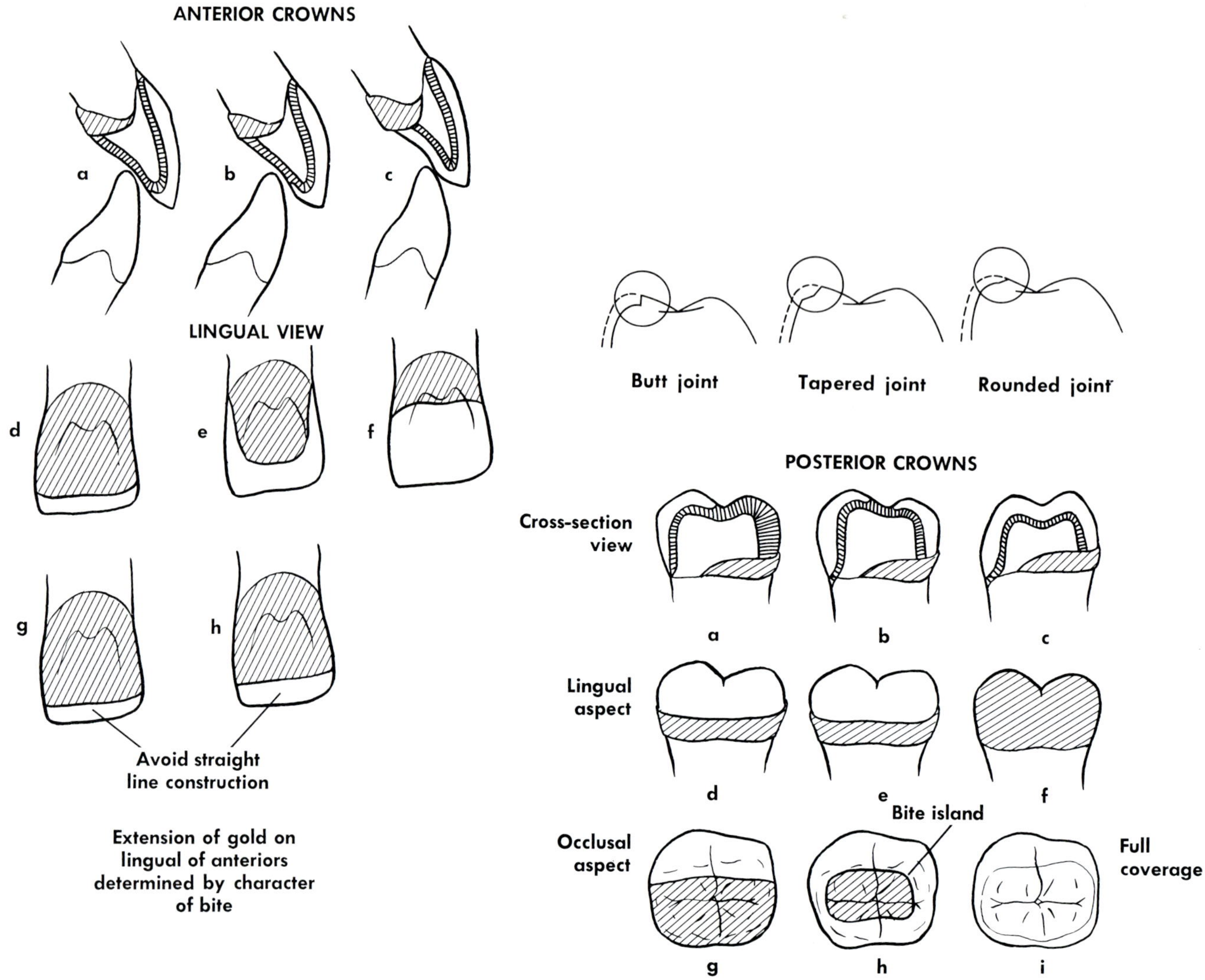

Fig. 7-50, cont'd. For legend see p. 291.

2. The ultimate form of the window should be one exhibiting flowing curves with a convex form (avoid boxings and concavities). By having even-flowing curves, sharp points, corners, or angles on the porcelain-bearing surfaces (which might have a "chisel" effect under pressure) are eliminated. Even-flowing convex contours are best for the veneering area because they distribute stress the best, which means that the possibility of stress concentration which may initiate fracture in the porcelain is minimized. Or it could be said that convex curves may assist in creating a prestressing effect which could increase the apparent strength of the porcelain when subject to tension.

The only concavity will be at the faciogingival angle. Here the sharp angle in the crown preparation (shoulder) should not be reproduced on the surface to be veneered. Neither should the junctions of the facial and incisal or occlusal areas be left sharp—they should be gently rounded (Fig. 7-51).

3. In the design of the wax pattern it is very important to avoid excessive porcelain bulk. It should be never more than approximately 1 to 1½ mm. facially. Strength is achieved by building up the metal understructure to match the tooth contour and baking the porcelain to the metal as evenly as possible. Bulk of porcelain does not result in strength.

4. The thickness of the facial surface of the casting should be approximately the equivalent of a piece of 26 gauge wax (which gives a 0.5 mm. thickness of gold). Some investigators are of the opinion that a 0.3 mm.

thickness of metal after it has been dressed down for the firing of porcelain for single crowns and a 0.4 mm. thickness for retainers would meet specifications.

5. The walls of castings in fixed bridges or splints should not have any "undercuts," because if fracture occurs it is sometimes possible to reshape casting slightly to receive modified porcelain jacket crowns.

6. Mechanical retention is contraindicated. Hoffman[47] has called attention to the fact that mechanical retention of fingers of porcelain seeping into the metal (metal is microscopically porous) makes for an extremely strong bond.

7. The metal structure should be designed so that occlusal contact will not occur at a line of junction of porcelain and gold. It should be at least 2 mm. away from this junction. If not, the contact will result in an eventual burnishing of the metal and flaking of the porcelain.

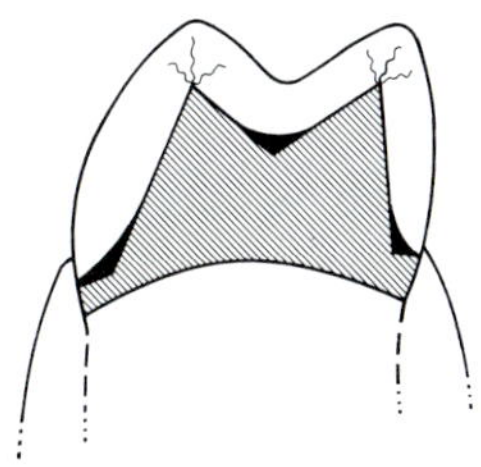

Fig. 7-51. Black areas represent voids that would occur because of sharp angulations instead of the ball shape as porcelain tends to become spheroid on fusing. Crazed lines over sharp projections cause cracking of porcelain under stress. (Courtesy Edward J. Hoffman.)

8. The outer junction of porcelain to metal should be at a right angle to avoid burnishing of the metal and subsequent fracture of the porcelain.

9. The metal substructure for a pontic must be much more rigid for porcelain than for acrylic. Flexion of the substructure must be controlled.

10. In some instances, the metal copings which fit during the "try-in" session apparently do not fit as well after the porcelain has been added. If shrinkage of the porcelain is the primary reason for marginal distortion, increasing the bulk of metal in the right places will minimize this distortion. Tuccillo and Nielson[48] found permanent deformation in porcelain-metal strips as a result of interfacial stress following firing. Shillingburg, Hobo, and Fisher[38] have pointed out that the labial margin where the thickness of metal is limited by esthetic demands is the part that seems to be most subject to distortion. If possible, a small facial collar positioned subgingivally would be advantageous (it is inconspicuous and does not encroach on the space required for porcelain veneering), as would a bulk of metal, if possible, on proximal and lingual surfaces. A lingual collar of metal will add rigidity and should be approximately 3 mm. wide incisogingivally or occlusogingivally (Fig. 7-52).

11. Where the occluding contact is near the cingulum or when little space exists, the metal on the lingual surface must extend past the point of tooth contact in centric occlusion to accommodate eccentric slides during mastication.[49]

12. The straight-line termination of gold and porcelain is to be avoided. The porcelain may extend

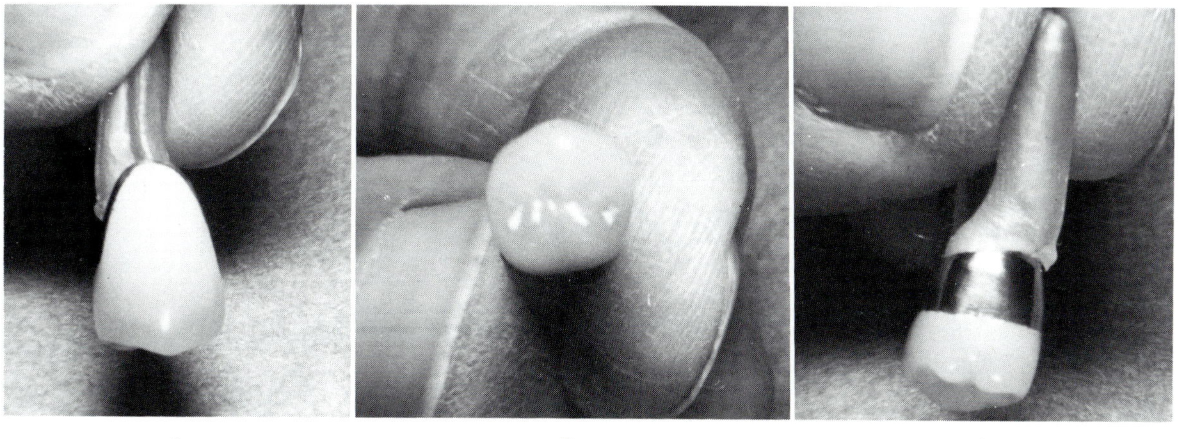

A B C

Fig. 7-52. A bicuspid full coverage porcelain gold crown showing a small facial collar which was positioned subgingivally and the proper bulk of metal on the proximal and lingual. **A,** Facial view; **B,** occlusal view; **C,** lingual view.

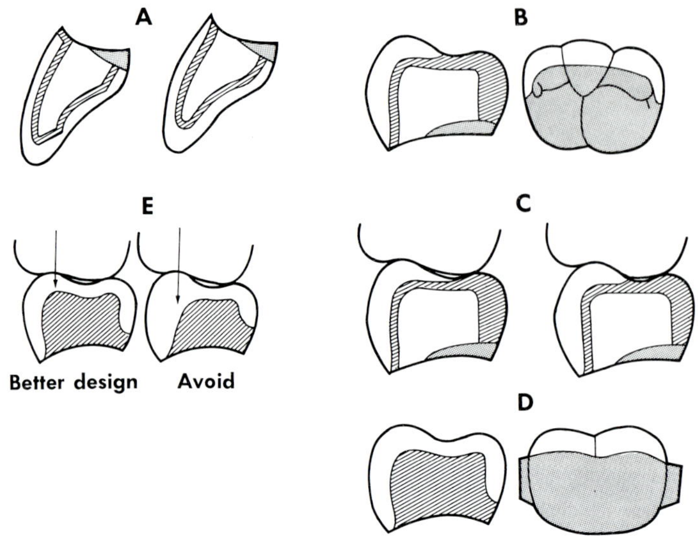

Fig. 7-53. In summation: **A,** avoid sharp corners; **B,** porcelain should fit around casting—over incisal and buccal cusps, and extend around onto proximal surfaces; **C,** avoid feather edges where loads are applied; **D,** design pontics to be similar to the abutments; and, **E,** avoid shearing by backing up porcelain with metal.

around the mesial and distal surfaces of the restoration.

13. The completed framework of a fixed partial denture or splint should be able to go to place completely with no strain or binding with finger pressure—if need be, hard finger pressure. The framework must be rigid so that it cannot bend and cause the porcelain to fracture. We must avoid internal stress against the metal.

14. It is a good idea that the margins of the castings not be made of a knife-edged character until the restoration is ready for final cementation. If so made (knife-edged), they could be damaged during laboratory handling.

15. In summation, a few points to keep firmly in mind when considering the design of the casting are: (a) avoid sharp corners (Fig. 7-53, *A*), (b) carry the porcelain over incisal and buccal cusps, and extend porcelain around onto the proximal surfaces (Fig. 7-53, *B*), (c) avoid feather edges where loads are applied (Fig. 7-53, *C*), (d) avoid straight lines behind incisal tips of porcelain (Fig. 7-53, *D*), and (e) design pontics to be similar to the retainers, and avoid shearing by backing up porcelain with metal (Fig. 7-53,*E*). In other words, the pontic should follow the design of corresponding single units with porcelain tissue contact (if space permits). It is necessary to provide for an equal thickness of porcelain on all units (retainers and pontics).

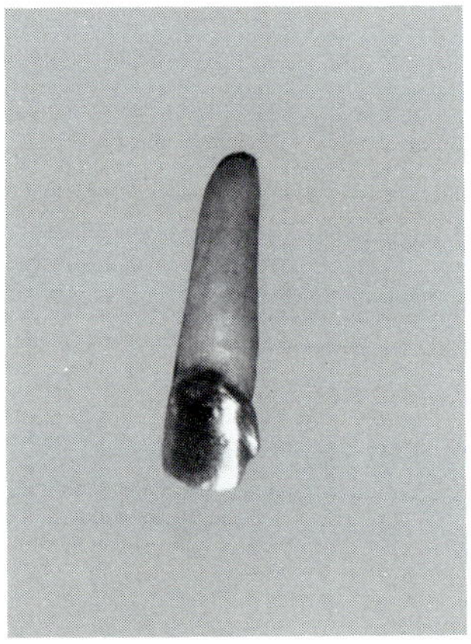

Fig. 7-54. A properly finished ceramic coping.

Preparation of casting

A few salient facts in regard to the "preparation of the casting" will be listed. (For a more detailed discussion refer to Chapter 10.)

1. After completion of the casting process sandblast the casting, or place it into hydrofluoric acid, or both.

2. Finish the casting, by using disks, stones, rubber wheels, etc., to the desired shape or form as previously outlined. Avoid grinding wheels or separating disks made of silicon carbide (green or black color) (Fig. 7-54).

3. Clean in the ultrasonic cleaner.

4. Rinse in ultrasonic cleaner in clear tap water (minimum of 2 minutes).

5. Burn out metal casting (degas) for insurance against contamination and gassing. Prefire from 1,200° to 1,800° F. at the rate of 100° per minute, and hold at 1,800° F. for 10 minutes. Higher temperatures may be used with caution. Cool under glass.

6. Handle casting only with clean instruments. Never touch metal surface with fingers after degassing—this will leave an undesirable oil film on the casting.

The use of vacuum-fired porcelain demands that careful degassing of the metal be carried out prior to the application of the porcelain. To eliminate adsorbed gases the casting is heated in the furnace (as just described); otherwise the gases adsorbed on the metal will be released, forming very large bubbles at the porcelain-metal interface. These bubbles can be large enough to distort the surface contour of the restoration, and at the same time the bond is destroyed.

In the bond between "ceramic" gold alloys and porcelain there is apparently a combination of "wetting adhesion" and "chemical adhesion" with very little "mechanical adhesion." The bond of porcelain and gold will be three times the strength of the porcelain.

Shell and Nielsen's[50] study of the bond between gold alloys and porcelain can be summed up this way:

1. The dental porcelain–to–dental gold bond, if properly made, was primarily one of the interatomic bonding.

2. The total bond had a shear resistance of about 10,000 to 13,000 p.s.i.

3. About one third of this resistance appeared to be due to van der Waals' forces of wetting (which is similar to the force that causes adhesion of frost to automobile windshields).

4. Two thirds of this resistance appeared to be due to chemical bonding, perhaps a mixture of ionic, covalent, and metallic bonding.

5. A mechanical bond did not play an important role in the bond strength proper. Roughening per se did not add to the shear resistance at the bond. The mechanical effect at best could give a bond only half the tensile strength of the porcelain.

Mumford[34] sums up Ryge and O'Brien's experiments on this subject: "Wetting bonds alone provide us with more than adequate strength, and our main concern then becomes that of eliminating some of the factors that produce stress at the interface."*

*From Mumford, George: The porcelain fused to metal restoration, Dent. Clin. N. Am., pp. 241-249, March, 1965.

The careful tailoring of both the porcelain and the gold alloys by the manufacturer to compatible coefficients of expansion allows them to make a strong physical bond. There may be some chemical bonding by a combination of an oxide of the alloy with some ingredients in the opaque layer of porcelain. By either mechanism, the bond of the porcelain to the metal is stronger than the shearing strength of the porcelain. Porcelain alone has poor impact strength.

Some porcelain considerations

Gold alloys can often be improved in physical properties by suitable heat treatment, but very often technicians fail to take advantage of such heat treating because a special operation is required. With standard casting golds a practical partial heat treatment may be effected by cooling for various lengths of time in the casting flask before quenching. An increase in physical properties is also obtained by slow cooling after a soldering operation, but maximum heat treatment requires a furnace treatment.

With most of the "ceramic" gold alloys no special heat treating operation is required because this alloy attains maximum hardness and strength by slow cooling to room temperature from 1,800° to 1,900° F. This is exactly the treatment usually accorded the restoration during the porcelain firing operation.

Only when porcelain is fused completely and properly does it attain all of its physical properties. Porcelain that appears dead or granular or lacks natural glaze is soft, friable, and undependable.

Overfired porcelain (when fired to glass) is under severe tension or stress and seeks to relieve this stress by shearing away from the inner face or by checking.

Underfired porcelain is equally as bad, since the bond is not created (oxides have not bonded).

It is essential that the first opaque bake be taken to a "shine" but not a complete gloss. If this is not done, the bond between the porcelain and the gold will not be as strong even though the gingival bake made subsequently is taken to the correct temperature.

Proper baking means the building of the veneer almost completely to contour and fusing this to a very high biscuit on the first bake. The second bake, if necessary, can be used to make only small additions for better contour. Slow baking or repeated cooling resulting from too frequent furnace opening produces a dull, crystallized porcelain with opaque colors. Repeated firing to a high temperature eventually fuses the porcelain all the way through to give a washed-out, translucent appearance.

Fused porcelain veneer should be comparatively

even in thickness to provide the greatest strength and uniformity of shade (unsupported porcelain, even in bulk, is weaker than a uniform layer). The shade translucency of porcelain varies with the thickness, thus unequal thickness makes good esthetics impossible technically. The shade of the veneer only improves with thickness up to a certain point. Pontics must have the same metal outline as adjacent retainers to obtain uniformity of shade.

When porcelain carving is completed, the case is biscuit fired and returned to the dentist (by resident or nonresident technician) where fit, occlusion, and contour are checked, it is ground to desired shape, and other corrections to be made are indicated by the dentist.

In other words, the role of the dentist in determining the final individualization and coloration of the completed single and multiple-unit restorations in order to satisfy the esthetic demands of the patient is very important. The surface of the biscuit bake is ground both on the model and in the oral cavity to develop the elements of form necessary for a harmonious esthetic result. The color is examined with a moistened surface and the form, color, etc. are compared with adjacent teeth. The surface is then smoothed with rubber polishing wheels used wet, and the porcelain veneer restoration is cleaned in an ultrasonic cleaner. Some technicians, before glazing restorations, pumice them with a wet rag wheel and wet pumice powder. This treatment creates a dull matte finish. A pumiced surface produces a smooth natural appearance and requires a somewhat lower (25° to 50° F.) temperature to finish. This lower temperature makes it easier to achieve a uniform glaze and helps to preserve the fine details of carving that tend to be fused out under higher heat.

Some porcelain is taken from the slab and rubbed or vibrated into the matte surface to cover any slight imperfections or surface irregularities. The excess porcelain is brushed off. At this point additional stain may be applied. Then the case is ready for glazing. Little shrinkage or running should occur in the final bake.

The crown or bridge is now placed in the furnace and brought to glazing temperature. For glazing, the porcelain is heated rapidly to its fusing point and then immediately removed from the furnace. This allows the outer surface to cool rapidly and produces a surface skin on the porcelain as the material attempts to fuse to a sphere. This skin produces a prestressing effect and binds the material tightly around the underlying metal.

The degree of gloss depends on the temperature, the rapidity with which the temperature is reached, the time held at this temperature, and the number of previous firings. It must be emphasized that the difference in temperature between the attainment of the desired degree of glaze and overfusion is quite small. Accurate calibration of the furnace is essential, and frequent visual inspection of the restoration should be made as an added safety factor.

If porcelain work is done in your own laboratory, be sure to check the pyrometer of the porcelain furnace periodically to ensure that the inside muffle temperature is being accurately recorded.

Saggars (made with muffle cement) used for checking pyrometers should not be used again for porcelain. The silver check (1,762° F.) gives off silver oxide, which is a mustard color and which will discolor porcelain. Testing saggars should be made the same height as the saggars which hold the porcelain during firing to ensure accurate calibration. Overfiring of the porcelain seriously affects the strength characteristics of the porcelain. Shade and translucency can also be affected.

In the final individualizing of the "ceramic" restoration, instruments found very useful in these procedures are the Sintered* diamond instruments or the Shofu† porcelain adjustment kit, which are used in making fine incisal or occlusal adjustments. The porcelain kit also contains wheels that are good for polishing cut surfaces after cementation.

I am of the opinion that the dentist should do the reshaping, staining, and glazing of his "ceramic" restorations. To accomplish the "glazing" aspect correctly, the dentist would have to know the thermal history of the restoration. By thermal history or thermal life we mean the amount of firing it can receive before it reaches the glass phase. The coefficient of linear thermal expansion of the glaze must be exactly right for the porcelain being used.

Waltke[51] has the following to say about "glazing":

"By definition, the term 'to glaze' means to give a vitreous (glassy) surface or coating to a ceramic. This can be done in two ways: by the application of a surface substance or by fusion of the body surface. This definition includes the two principal techniques in use to produce glazed surfaces on porcelain crowns and bridges. The first procedure is called a *superficial or applied glaze,* while the latter is referred to as a

*Ceramco, Inc., Long Island City, N. Y.
†Shofu Dental Corp., Menlo Park, Calif.

natural glaze. In either case, the purpose of the glaze is to produce a smooth, durable, and impermeable coating of glass on the surface of the unit. We must produce a layer of glass on the surface of a porcelain (crystalline) body without turning the body itself into glass.

"The correct procedure to follow is to give it a natural glaze. This is accomplished quite simply by cleaning the case thoroughly, preheating it at 1200° F. and firing it rapidly (at a rate of 90°-100° increase per minute) until a glazed condition is observed. The temperature at which the glaze will occur will be dependent on several factors, namely the degree of glaze that is desired, and more importantly, the thermal history of the restoration. If the crown or bridge has been fired rapidly only once or twice, it will glaze at a higher temperature than a restoration that has had three, four, or five bakes, even though they may have been rapid. In any case, the glaze should occur at the fusing point of the porcelain or considerably below it.

"A superficial glaze can be a life saver in some cases. Imagine a full upper or lower reconstruction case that has taken five or six firings to complete. If the dentist grinds the face of one of the units for one reason or another (recontouring purposes, etc.), and if the ceramist tries to produce a natural glaze on the ground unit he runs the risk of ruining the case in two ways: first, he may get too high a glaze on the rest of the case and, second, he may push porcelain out of coefficient tolerance with the metal. Superficial glaze on the ground unit is the answer.

"A case that's had a corrective bake with 1600° porcelain should be glazed with a low temperature superficial glaze. A porcelain jacket crown that needs to be reglazed after its matrix has been stripped may easily be glazed in the same manner without loss of its dimensional accuracy. The two main advantages of the low temperature glazing technic then, may be summed up as follows: it helps the ceramist to glaze porcelain without losing dimensional accuracy, and it also allows him to glaze porcelain without getting it out of coefficient tolerance with the metal substrate."*

Most ceramists prefer to make additions to the glaze bake with a 50/50 mixture of 1,600° and 1,800° F. air-fired porcelain because they require no further smoothing or polishing.

A few of the troubles that can occur when working with porcelain are:

*From Waltke, Robert: Glazing, Ceramco Technigraph **4**(1): Aug., 1972.

1. Bubbling at the gold-opaque interface, which is usually due to unclean metal or small holes on the surface of the casting which is to receive the porcelain.
2. Bubbles or voids of the porcelain due mostly to a poor condensation technique or to a too quick application of heat.
3. Checks or cracks in the porcelain due to overglazing or not understanding the problem of glazing.
4. Small particles of porcelain finding themselves inside the casting and fusing during the baking process. This will destroy the fit unless carefully removed with a Sintered diamond instrument such as No. C-8.*
5. Not observing close enough that the metal structure in the "try-in" phase sprung over slight "undercuts" in the preparation, which will set up stress in the unyielding porcelain which in turn can cause breakage of the porcelain.

Color and shade

In the present era, not only is the restoration of function of great importance but, in many instances, the problem of tooth shade and color is a dimension just as important. The patient desires a prosthesis that has a vital, natural appearance. In esthetic considerations we must deal with (1) form, (2) surface characteristics, and (3) color. This calls for the application of basic color principles, which in turn calls for the use of a common color nomenclature or language. In other words, since many times no proper shade guide can be found to match the particular tooth under consideration, the use of stains and a working knowledge of color principles (hue, chroma, and value) can help us out of this dilemma. Hue, chroma, and value allow us to properly evaluate the characteristics of a colored object. Color, in conjunction with form and contour, plays a major role in the acceptability of the restoration.

Shade guides with an opaque metal backing similar to that of a finished veneer are valuable assets in shade selection. Light reflections from the opaque surface on the "ceramic" metal make the shade matching in a porcelain-fused-to-metal veneer an entirely different problem than that found in the selection of a color match in a straight porcelain jacket crown. Opaques are selected to match the basic color of the tooth and, if done correctly, the reduced thickness of overlying

*Ceramco, Inc., Long Island City, N. Y.

translucent porcelain is not obvious. I have added a small amount of pink to the formula being used, because I believe that makes most body colors more lifelike.

To begin with let us consider the following: (1) what is color? (2) how do we see color? (3) light source variable, (4) selecting a light source for shade matching, and (5) daylight.*

WHAT IS COLOR?

In *Principles of Color Technology,* Billmeyer and Saltzman[52] define color as the result of the physical modification of *light* by *colorants* as observed by the human *eye* and interpreted by the *brain.*

The four preceding nouns describe the complex nature of color; *light* is physical, *colorants* are chemical, the *eye* physiologic, and the *brain,* of course, psychologic. Actually, the eye as a receptor interfaced with the brain as an interpreter is psychophysical in nature. This definition of color is indicative of the variables inherent in seeking and controlling color.

HOW DO WE SEE COLOR?

The entire process originates with the light source, hence the statement "color is light." A light source, whether a phase of natural daylight or an artificial source, emits radiant energy within the visible spectrum, which lies within the wavelengths 380 to 750 nm in the electromagnetic spectrum. White light or north sky daylight contains all of these wavelengths in a nearly equivalent distribution of energy. However, many artificial sources and some phases of natural daylight do not.

LIGHT SOURCE VARIABLES

Light is where color begins. It is obvious that without light there is no color.

Let us consider several light sources and how they act as variables in the way we see color. *Incandescent light,* which is commonly used in the home and in most operatory lamps, emits a great deal of energy in the red-yellow area of the spectrum and very little in the blue area. Therefore, if we illuminate samples of red, yellow, and blue under the incandescent source, we will see that the red and yellow are quite strong or highly saturated, while the blue is weak and lacking in saturation. Under a *cool-white fluorescent source,* however, which is high in blue-green energy and low in red energy, we note that the red is desaturated, the yellow less saturated than under the tungsten or incandescent source, and the blue quite strong and highly saturated. We should note that cool-white fluorescent lamps are used commonly in stores and offices, and when they are used for color selection, they can cause the wrong tie to be selected for a suit, as well as the wrong shade to be selected for a tooth. There are fluorescent tubes manufactured, however, which have full color content and render color much more accurately than the cool-white type. It is unfortunate that all fluorescent sources emit peaks of energy caused by the mercury gases used in stimulating the phosphors. These peaks of energy occur at several points across the spectrum and can cause color distortion when used for critical shade matching.

If we view these same red, yellow, and blue samples under complete color-content daylight illumination, we note that each color is rendered accurately and highly saturated. We can see how light sources act as variables in the color-viewing process by our examination of physical standards; further evidence is provided by the spectral energy distribution curves of these light sources.

SELECTING A LIGHT SOURCE FOR SHADE MATCHING

What qualities are desirable in an ideal light source for shade matching?

1. The light should have complete color content. As we have seen, if a tooth, natural or artificial, has a subtle reddish pigmentation and the light source—for example, a cool-white fluorescent fixture—emits very little red energy, the reddish pigmentation will either be severely attenuated or not evident at all.

2. This full-color content light source should have enough intensity to overcome the influence of ambient room light and excite slight as well as dominant pigmentation in the tooth. The light source should not, however, be so intense that slight color differences are overcome or washed out.

3. The source should be comfortable to the eye, allowing the eye to perceive color accurately and comfortably.

4. The light should be standard—unchanging in quality and quantity from day to night or season to season and, for purposes of color communication, unchanging from place to place.

A color temperature scale exists and is commonly used to index color of light sources in *degrees Kelvin,* which is equivalent to degrees centigrade plus 273.

DAYLIGHT

While some phases of natural daylight have the basic qualities which are desirable for color evaluation

*This material courtesy The J. M. Ney Co., Hartford, Conn.

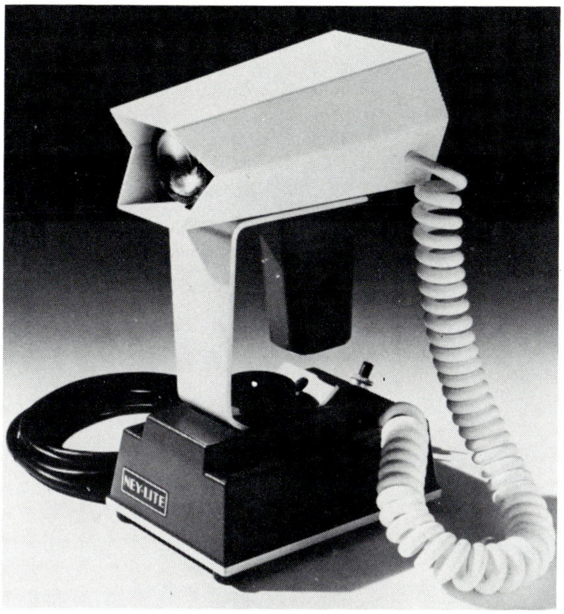

Fig. 7-55. The Ney-Lite.

—i.e., full color content, adequate intensity, and compatibility with the eye—daylight is changing almost constantly in both quality and quantity. The color temperatures of daylight can vary from 1,000° K. during a dusty sunset to a much higher degree Kelvin in a blue sky. The spectral energy distribution likewise can change from a high concentration of blue energy in the north sky at midday to almost entirely red-orange at sunset with practically no blue energy evident.

Due to the obvious vagaries in daylight, dyers, artists, colorists, and people dependent upon daylight for accurate color rendition and reproduction have preferred a phase of daylight described as a slightly overcast north sky at midday.

None of the existing operatory lamps or office luminaries incorporates all of the qualities which we have discussed as being desirable in a standard shade matching lamp. While a few have complete color content, distorting mercury emission lines are in evidence. Some lamps are rated by Kelvin temperature but have unequal distributions of energy. I am using, as an important aid along with a better and broader knowledge of the dimensions of color or color language, the ''Ney-Lite''* (Fig. 7-55), which utilizes the output of a continuous spectrum tungsten halogen source corrected to the spectral energy distribution of preferred daylight at 6,000° K. by a Corning Daylight Filter. The lamp emits an intensity of 400 footcandles, which helps in the exclusion of the undesirable influx of ambient office light, and illuminates the oral cavity with a 2 × 4 inch controlled viewing field. It seems to give a light source that is the next thing to natural daylight and allows one to detect subtle differences in color. It can be useful in making accurate, effective color communication possible.

*The J. M. Ney Co., Hartford, Conn.

Lighting standardization utilizing a technically correct source can assist the dental profession in producing natural, esthetically pleasing restorations with minimal cost and delay.

Sproull[53, 53a] has, and is, making a very important contribution to the problem of color matching in dentistry. In his opinion: ''The Munsell Color Order System is recommended as the system of choice for dentists who wish to gain a working knowledge of color. Once the dimensions of color (Hue, Value, and Chroma) become familiar terms, dentists will have the color language and the necessary tools to approach color matching problems in a logical manner. It is possible to arrange color in a manner that makes this three-dimensional enigma understandable.''*

Hue, the first dimension, is the easiest to understand, and in Munsell's[54] words: ''It is that quality by which we distinguish one color family from another, as red from yellow, green from blue or purple.''†

Value and chroma are more difficult to understand and are often confused with one another. Special attention must be focused on these dimensions.

''*Value* is that quality by which we distinguish a light color from a dark color.''† The *value* of a color is determined by which gray on the value scale it matches in lightness/darkness. The black of the value scale is assigned a value of 0, the white a value of 10. ''Low'' values refer to dark colors, ''high'' values to light colors.

''*Chroma* is that quality by which we distinguish a strong color from a weak one; the departure of a color sensation from that of white or gray; the intensity of a distinctive Hue; color intensity.''† Chroma describes the *amount* of hue in a color. Chroma indicates the purity or saturation of the color, or conversely, its freedom from dilution.

*From Sproull, Robert C.: Color matching in dentistry. Part I. The three-dimensional nature of color, J. Prosthet. Dent. **29**(4):416-423, 1973; Part II. Practical applications of the organization of color, J. Prosthet. Dent. **29**(5):556-566, 1973.

†From Munsell, A. H.: A color notation, ed. 11, Baltimore, 1961, Munsell Color Co., Inc.

MODIFICATION OF A CHOSEN SHADE

''An approach that should be used by a dentist-ceramist team conversant with color language is to specify a shade 69, but with a modification of one or more of the dimensions of color, e.g., a shade 69 but raise the Value. This approach can be effective but is, of course, subject to error.

''The dentist should choose the shade as above, and then modify the color match with porcelain stains while the patient is seated in the office and available for constant reference.''* Value that is too low and/or chroma too strong are situations which frequently are impossible to adjust.

*From Sproull, Robert C.: Color matching in dentistry. Part I. The three-dimensional nature of color, J. Prosthet. Dent. **29**(4):416-423, 1973; Part II. Practical applications of the organization of color, J. Prosthet. Dent. **29**(5):556-566, 1973.

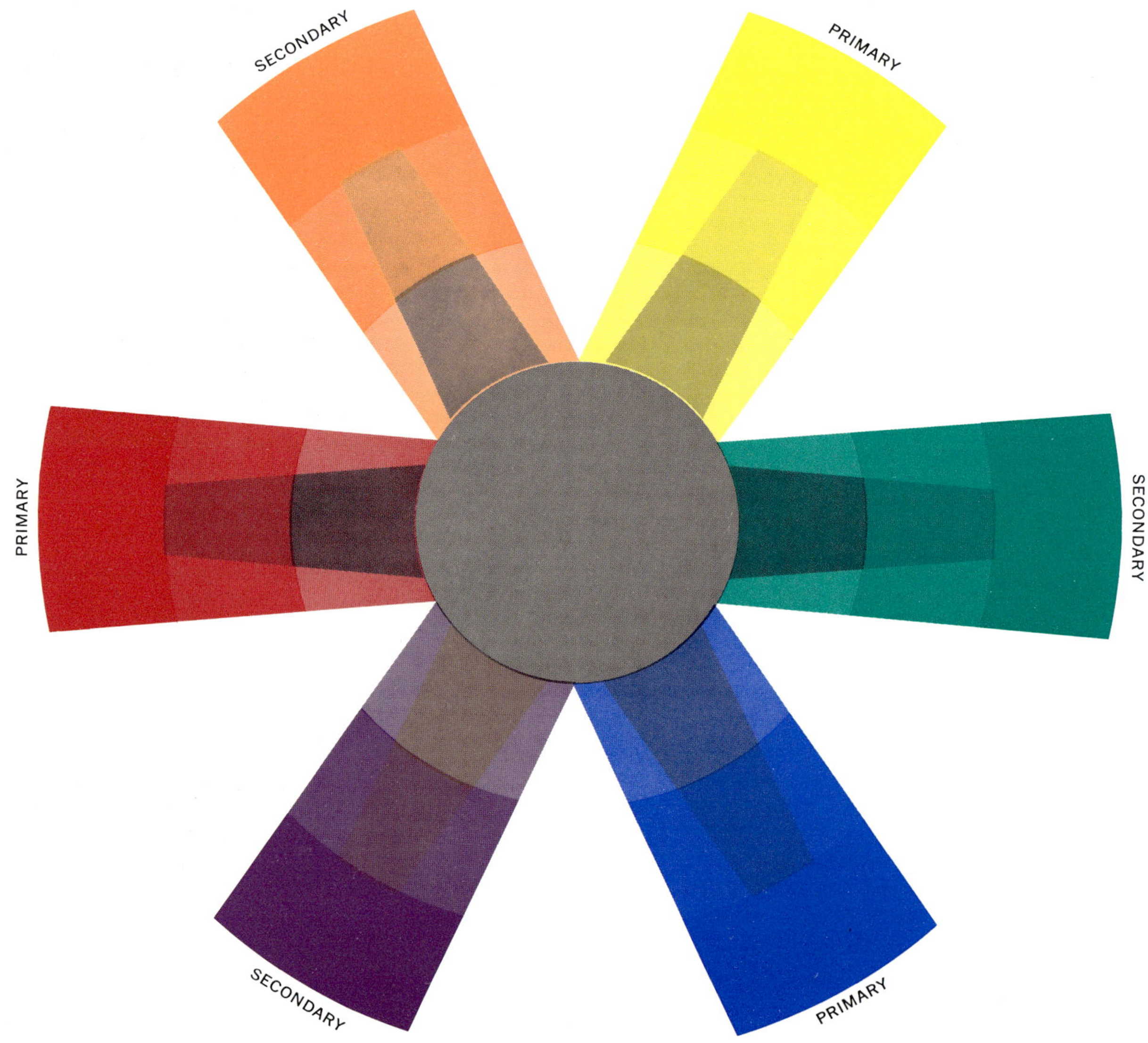

Fig. 7-56. The color wheel. Primary hues are blended to create secondary hues. The complementary hues opposite each other have a neutralizing effect when intermixed. If complementary hues of unequal chroma are blended, the dominant hue is lowered in value (grayer). If complementary hues of equal chroma and volume are blended, a neutral gray is created. (Courtesy Ceramco, Inc., Long Island, N. Y.)

Some authors, in discussing the subject of dimensions of color, will refer to them as hue, brilliance, and saturation while others, as just quoted, use hue, value, and chroma.

The importance of complementary colors cannot be overlooked. Complementary colors are those hues which are directly opposite each other on the color wheel (Fig. 7-56).

It has been said that a knowledge of the effect of complementary hues upon each other is the key to precise shade control in dental ceramics. Shade adjustment does not consist of merely adding a hue (or overaccentuation of hues) that is lacking. It often involves neutralizing an apparent excess of chroma in a given hue or adjusting value.

HOW TO MATCH A SHADE

1. Seat the patient with head erect at the dentist's eye level. Never "tip" the patient back in the chair while the shade is being taken since this will place the light source in the wrong direction.

2. The dentist should stand between the patient and the light source. The best light source is northern exposure with a slightly overcast sky, preferably at noon. This type of light has completely balanced color content. But, as a rule, normal office lighting is not color balanced. You may have, for example, high red, low blue, or high blue, low red color content, etc. present. What you see is the result of the particular light reflected. Can you detect subtle differences in color? Therefore, once again the emphasis must be placed on an understanding of the dimensions of color (a common terminology understood by the dentist and ceramist) and the use of any good aid, such as a "Ney-Lite." Also, if a restoration, in the "biscuit bake" or finished state, is mismatched, it will be necessary to determine which hues dominate the shade and whether the correction involves a change of hue or a change in chroma or in value. Or it may be necessary to change two or even all three of these characteristics. Do you want the shade to be a little lighter, do you want more white added (to increase brilliance), or do you want less yellow (which will reduce its yellow saturation)? It has been said that a dental shade guide has very few colors, but it has these few colors in a range of Hues, Brilliances, and Saturations.

3. Make color observations as quickly as possible so that receptors in the eye for the specific colors do not tire and thereby lose ability for color differentiation.

4. To select a color dimension that will look equally well in bright daylight and under artificial light may necessitate a compromise on shade.

Creating illusions of tooth size by varying tooth form*

1. If a tooth appears too short and broad to match the natural tooth or to fit into the patient's overall facial appearance, eliminate as many horizontal lines, edges, and characteristics as possible and accentuate all vertical aspects.

2. If a tooth appears too long and narrow to match

*This material courtesy J. F. Jelenko & Co., New Rochelle, N. Y.

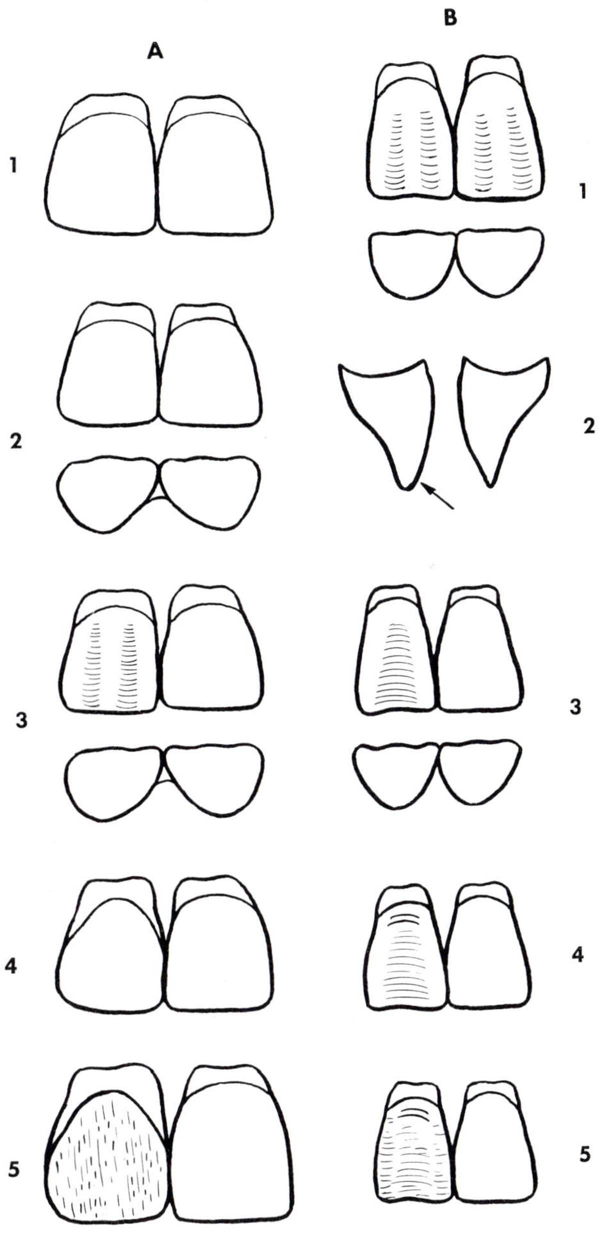

Fig. 7-57. Creating illusions of tooth size by varying tooth form. **A,** Short and broad; **B,** long and narrow. (See text.)

Purple blue	Blue	Blue green	Green	Green yellow	Yellow	Yellow red	Red

Fig. 7-58. The illustrations in this series (Figs. 7-58 to 7-65) courtesy The J. M. Ney Co., Hartford, Conn.

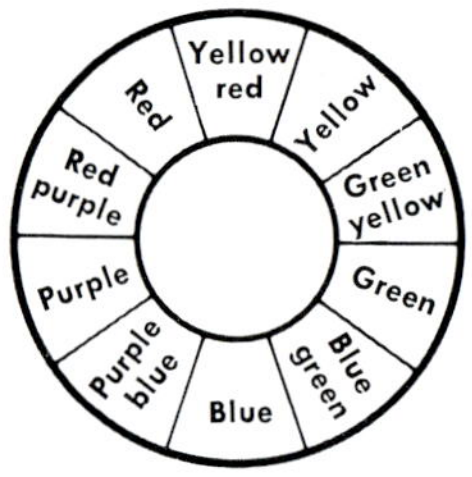

Fig. 7-59

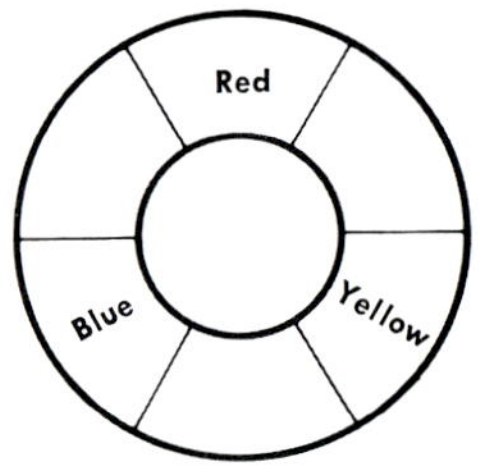

Fig. 7-60

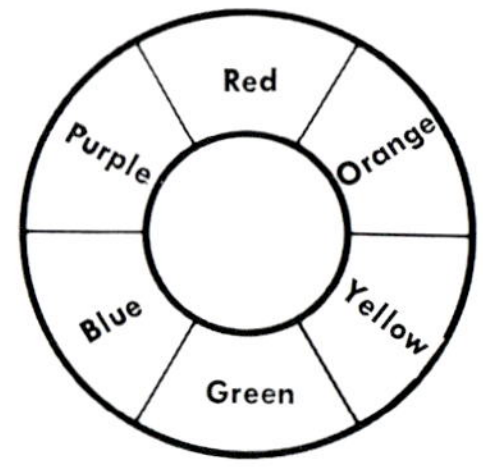

Fig. 7-61

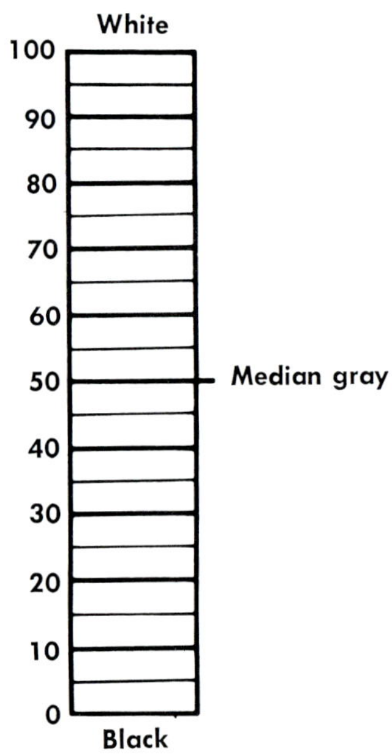

Fig. 7-62

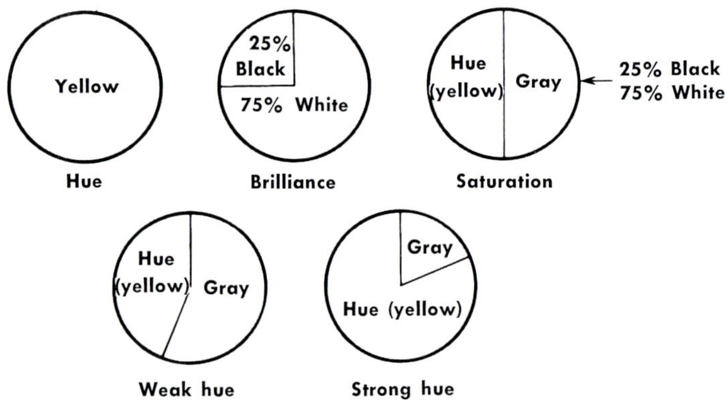

Fig. 7-63

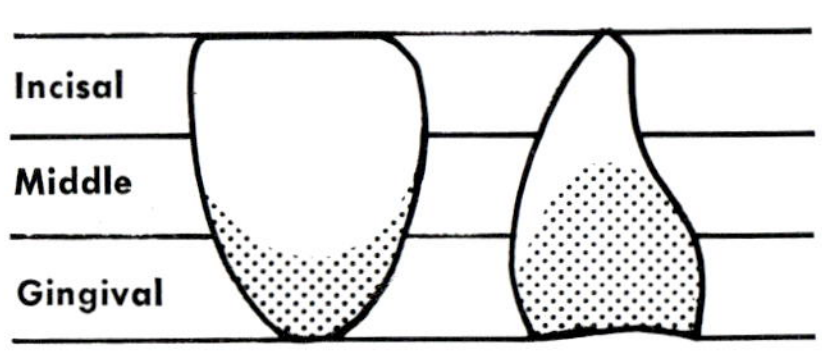

Fig. 7-64

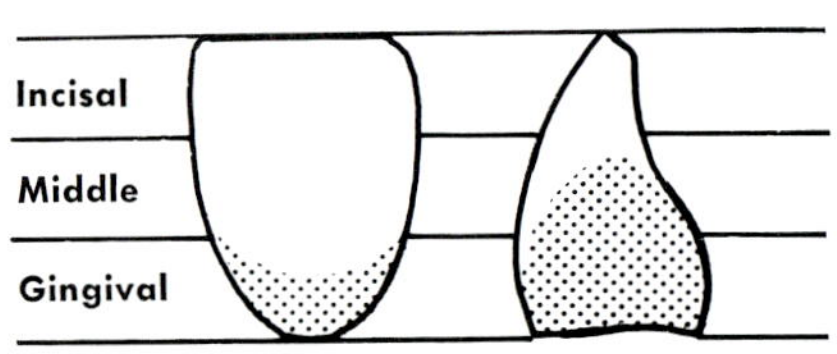

Fig. 7-65

the natural tooth or to fit into the patient's overall facial appearance, eliminate as many vertical lines, edges, and characteristics as possible and accentuate all horizontal aspects.[56]

The formation of vertical highlights tends to create an illusion of greater length, and horizontal highlights creates an illusion of width. Stains, and the way they are applied, can also create illusions of tooth size (Fig. 7-57).

I am of the opinion that, at this time, a more detailed discussion of the dimensions of color is in order. The study of the fundamental principles of light and color, as previously stated, and how these principles are manipulated for practical application resolves itself into a fascinating science.

The dimensions of color*

When working with dental porcelains or plastic materials many technicians have had the experience of having a gray cast spoil the shade they were trying to make. Every color in nature, unless it is pure black or pure white, has gray in it. Unless he clearly understands the role that gray plays in the formulation of colors the technician is sure to have trouble with it from time to time.

Many years ago Doctor E. Bruce Clark described color as a sensation and called attention to the fact that it had three dimensions,—hue, brilliance, and saturation. If all three of the dimensions of color were better understood by the technician he would find it less difficult to produce satisfactory tooth shades in either ceramics or plastics.

The sensations observed when viewing a color may be red or yellow or green; it may be light or dark; it may be strong or weak. The first is the dimension of hue which is the color itself, such as red, yellow, green, or any other color. As the dimension of hue is studied it will be found that most colors are related in some way to the solar spectrum. By allowing sunlight or a beam of artificial light to pass through a glass prism and projecting the beam on a white surface, an array of color can be seen. These are the spectrum colors. They are blue, green, yellow, and red. When these colors are viewed in their proper order in the spectrum, additional colors can be seen (Fig. 7-58).

Starting at the left of the spectrum and moving to the right, a purple blue (violet) color is observed. Continuing to the right it changes to pure blue, then to blue green, to pure green, to green yellow, then to pure yellow, to yellow red and ends with pure red. Pure purple, while not found in the spectrum, can be created by joining the ends of the spectrum to form a circle. The joining of red with blue will result in purple (Fig. 7-59).

These colors represent the entire field of hue and are called chromatic colors. Black and white and any combination of black and white, which will be a gray, have no hue and are called achromatic colors. All colors are made from combinations of the colors of the spectrum and black and white. The spectral colors are blue, green, yellow, and red. Blue and yellow, when combined, will result in green. Green can therefore be eliminated and the remaining colors—blue, yellow, and red—become the primary colors. It is possible to make all colors from combinations of the primary colors and black and white (Fig. 7-60).

When each primary color is mixed with the adjacent color in the circle, secondary colors will be produced. Red mixed with yellow will produce orange; yellow mixed with blue will produce green; and blue mixed with red will produce purple (Fig. 7-61).

When these colors are examined in the color circle it can be seen that there is a secondary color opposite each primary color and vice versa. These opposite colors are said to be complementary colors and when mixed together will produce a color without hue which will be a neutral color, such as white, black, or gray.

Going back to the color circle (Fig. 7-61) which now has six colors, and again mixing adjacent colors, six additional colors can be produced. Adjacent colors can be mixed again and again, producing any number of different colors. Teeth have yellow hues, and these yellows can be distinguished from each other only by the small amount of red or green that can be seen in each of them.

It is important that the technician understand the dimension of hue. He should know the primary and secondary colors, the complementary colors, and the results to be expected when mixing them. *For example: if a green yellow is added to a red yellow in an attempt to strengthen the hue, the result will be a failure because green is a complementary color to red and the hue produced will be a gray yellow.*

The second dimension of color is the sensation of lightness or darkness, and is called brilliance. All colors contain certain amounts of black and white. The more white a color contains, the more brilliant it appears. If all colors have some black and some white in them, and they must have, for no color can be darker than black or lighter than white, all colors then have gray in them because black mixed with white will result in gray. Equal amounts of black and white will

*This material courtesy The J. M. Ney Co., Hartford, Conn.

produce neutral gray. This means then that all tooth shades have a certain amount of gray in them. The quality of the gray as it ranges from black to white will control the lightness or darkness of a tooth shade and give it the dimension of brilliance.

The dimension of brilliance is often confused with the third dimension of color, saturation, which will be discussed later. For example; a green color is observed with other colors that are somber, and the green is referred to as a brilliant color. This may be incorrect. Any color lighter than the green would be more brilliant. It will help to remember that white is the most brilliant color possible and black represents a complete absence of brilliance.

Brilliance is the result of the proportion of black to white in a given color. Saturation is the result of the proportion of hue to the amount of black and white, or gray in color. The range of brilliance in a color can be represented by a scale of neutral grays, starting with pure black as zero and ascending through the dark grays to median gray and on through the light grays to pure white (Fig. 7-62).

Sometimes the technician attempts to darken a tooth shade by adding gray. He will not be successful if the gray he uses is higher on the brilliance scale than the color he is attempting to darken. For example; if the color has a brilliance which is below that of median gray, and a gray which is above median gray is used, the result will be an increase in brilliance which will lighten the color rather than darken it.

The third dimension of color, saturation, is probably the least understood, although it is said to be the most important in matching tooth color. It has been said that a color cannot be darker than black or lighter than white. Its lightness or darkness is controlled by the ratio of the white to black it contains. If this ratio is 25% black to 75% white then the resulting gray will have a value of 75 on the brilliance scale. If this gray is then added to a hue of say yellow, and the yellow had a brilliance of 75, saturation would be the ratio of the yellow to the gray. If 30% yellow, or hue, is mixed with 70% of this gray, the saturation would be weak. If the yellow, or hue, is increased to 90% and the same gray reduced to 10%, then the saturation would be strong. The brilliance would remain the same 75. The hue, or color, can be made weaker or stronger (saturation) without making it lighter or darker. Saturation increases as the amount of gray in a hue, or color, decreases. Brilliance increases as the amount of white *to* black in the gray increases (Fig. 7-63). Many mistakes in shading are made by confusing weak, or low saturation with light colors. A color must have hue, and the stronger the hue appears in a color the more saturated it is said to be. It is important then that the technician understands and can recognize the dimensions of color, hue, brilliance, and saturation, and learns how to control them.

An example of a common mistake in the construction of restorations is when the tooth has gingival and incisal colors that are strong in contrast. If the usual technic of overlaying the gingival color with incisal color is used (Fig. 7-64), the result may be a green yellow in the middle third.

The reason that this may occur is that the gingival color is usually a strong yellow, high in saturation, and the incisal color is a neutral gray. Laying the incisal color over the yellow gingival color will produce a green yellow hue in the middle third, which will spoil the shade. This is the result of the incisal gray color absorbing strongly in the yellow part of the spectrum and reflecting some blue. Where the blue combines with the gingival yellow the hue will be green yellow in that area.

To overcome this a blend color should be used. This can be made by first mixing a sample of equal parts of the gingival and incisal colors. The sample will have the correct brilliance and saturation but will have a green yellow hue. This can be corrected by the addition of a red yellow of the same brilliance and saturation. This blend color can then be used to make the middle third of the shade (Fig. 7-65). Not using a blend color when it is indicated usually results in a mismatch of color even though the gingival and incisal shades were correctly selected.

We have seen that color is a complex interaction of light source, object, and observer and therefore not an exact science, since it is subjective, not objective. The knowledge and tools to control color do exist, however, and have been proved. By utilizing this available technology, the dental profession can bring to esthetic restorations the same technical excellence which it has exhibited in functional restorations.

Properties of veneers—porcelain and resin

The strength of the bond which develops when porcelain is baked against a compatible gold alloy is enormously greater than the almost negligible bond strength of a resin to gold. The difference is responsible for the variations in design of the two types of veneer restorations.

Gold colored alloys with a slight pinkish hue are available to improve the esthetic qualities of resin restorations. This type of alloy is often a definite improvement over many of the regular crown and bridge alloys, which have a slightly grayish color. However, because of their low resistance to abrasion, their high percentage of flow, and their continued dimensional change after polymerization, the use of resins for veneer crowns and some pontics as permanent restorations is not recommended. Exceptions to this recommendation would be in the case of some elderly patients, for economic reasons, in periodontally involved teeth (weak and mobile) requiring extensive splinting, and in some posterior pontics. When resins are used in these situations, I use Thermo-JEL* or Pyroplast,† because these products give a plastic which is much harder, denser, and more resistant to wear, and which clinically seems to possess far greater dimensional stability. (For a more detailed discussion of this type of resin refer to Chapter 17.)

It might be stated that both the porcelain veneers and the resin veneers have some inherent advantages and disadvantages.

The principal advantages of the porcelain-fused-to-metal restoration are: (1) its powerful bond to the metal without necessitating mechanical retention, (2) its greater strength and hardness for resisting wear, and (3) its good esthetics. Its greatest disadvantages are: (1) its tendency to fracture, especially when incorrectly designed, and (2) the difficulty of repairing this type of restoration.

The principal advantages of the resin veneers are (1) ease of fabrication, (2) low curing temperature, and (3) ease of repair. Its greatest disadvantages are: (1) low hardness strength, (2) low wear resistance, (3) lack of bond between the resin and the metal (at most the bond would be very small), (4) its porosity (will absorb mouth fluids and change color), (5) seepage at the acrylic-metal seal, (6) inferior esthetics with gold-acrylic compared with that which can be achieved with porcelain-bonded-to-gold, and (7) its allergic effect on some people.

Requirements for a successful porcelain-fused-to-metal restoration include: (1) harmonious occlusion, (2) good tooth preparation, (3) perfect marginal fit of casting(s), (4) correct coronal form (retainers and pontics) which will allow for embrasures that permit proper tissue stimulation, and (5) correct ridge adaptation of pontics.

A word of caution: Do not promise the patient the impossible (especially as to longevity) in cases involving weak or mobile teeth, long spans, closed bite, cross-bite, etc., because of breakage of porcelain can occur at the time of cementation or breakage of porcelain and complete failure of the case can occur after some service in the mouth.

A series of illustrations relative to the design of the metal supporting structure is given in Figs. 7-66 to 7-102.

Semiprecious alloys for porcelain-fused-to-metal restorations

Semiprecious alloys used for ceramic restorations contain approximately 44% gold, whereas the regular alloys contain about 75% gold. In these types of alloys it is believed that the copper content should be one and one half times more than silver (which apparently causes corrosion); e.g. if the silver content is 20, the copper content must be 30. Increased additions of palladium (a platinum group metal), silver, and certain base metals made it possible to reduce the gold content and thereby lower the cost per unit.

The lower density of this type of alloy has advantages, but it requires special technique considerations which will now be discussed:

1. Because it has a slightly higher melting range, it is more resistant to "sag" when firing porcelain on substructures. It also allows for more thermal stability of the porcelain firing temperature.

2. The lower density means less weight per given span, and less weight means less stress on the restorations during firing and therefore less tendency to "sag."

3. The higher strength of this type of alloy allows for slightly thinner sections to be employed.

4. Because the lower density metals are lighter per given volume of metal, it becomes necessary to compensate for this change in the casting procedure to avoid incomplete castings or miscasts.

The casting pressure is determined by three factors when using a centrifugal casting machine: (1) acceleration, (2) length of the centrifugal arm, and (3) weight of the metal being used. Since the length of the centrifugal arm is a fixed factor, it becomes necessary to increase the acceleration by increasing the turns—a half turn if spring is of the heavy duty type and new, or one (or one and a half) turns if spring is old. The use of larger buttons of metal (increasing the total weight of the metal cast) usually results in overheated and abused metal. Use a smaller button (25% less than the regular ceramic alloy) and add new metal to the button (about 50%), and use heavier gauge wax sprues (10 gauge for copings, 8 gauge for pontics and heavier copings) of about ⅜ inch in length.

Text continued on p. 318.

*Caulk Co., Milford, Del.

†Williams Gold Refining Co., Inc., Buffalo, N. Y.

Figs. 7-66 to 7-103. The illustrations in this series (Figs. 7-66 to 7-103) courtesy The J. M. Ney Co., Hartford, Conn.

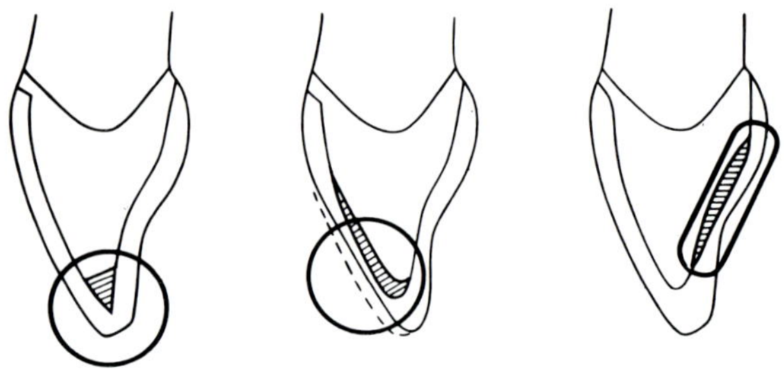

A B C

Fig. 7-66. A, Shows inadequate incisal preparation (less than 1.5 mm.). Hashed area indicates the necessary additional preparation. **B,** If the incisolabial hashed area shown is not reduced, an overcontoured crown having poor color and esthetics results. **C,** On lingual surface reduce as shown by hashed area. This allows for proper design for a tooth-to-tooth relationship.

A

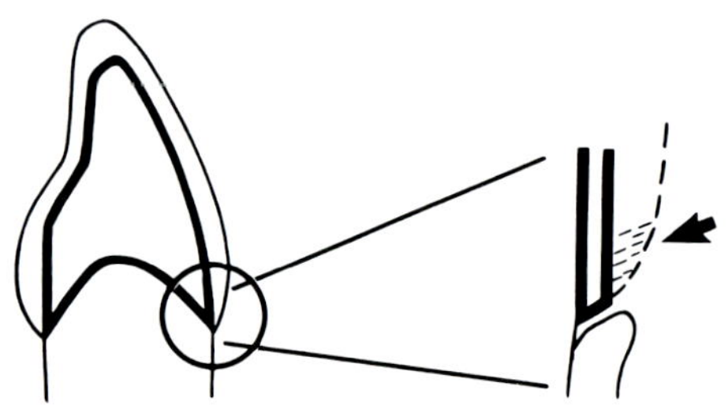

B

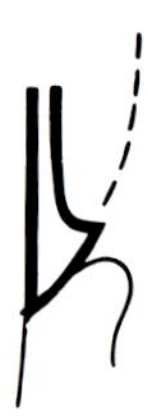

Fig. 7-67. A, A "knife-edge" type of margin preparation. This results in overcontouring and sometimes the opaque shows through the porcelain. **B,** Better contour and thickness. For good color a metal collar on the labial may be utilized. Not the most desirable design for anterior teeth.

A

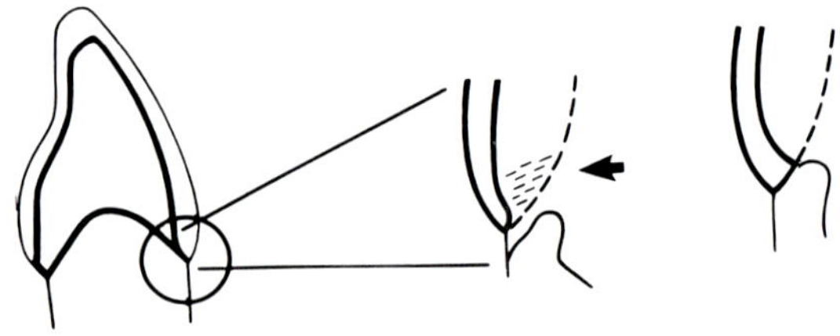

B

Fig. 7-68. A, A chamfered margin. Porcelain fused to the marginal edge can also result in overcontouring and/or opaque showing through. **B,** A metal collar will provide restoration with good contour, and better color can be produced in this area.

A

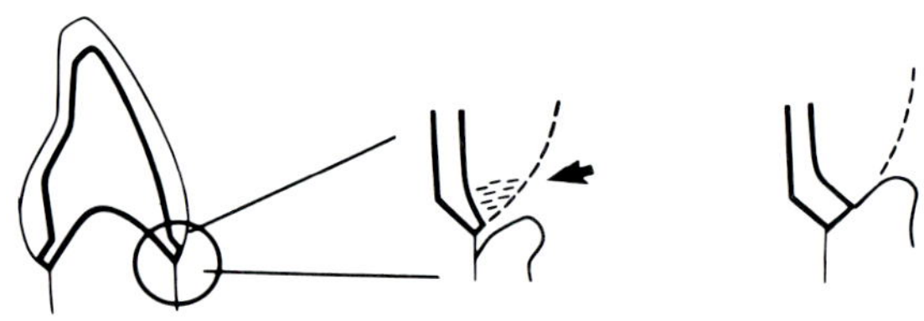

B

C

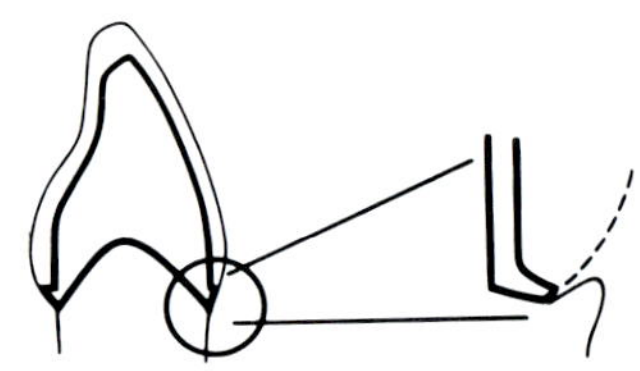

Fig. 7-69. A, The beveled shoulder preparation more closely approaches the amount of reduction necessary for adequate room for metal and porcelain. In **A,** we see the problem of overcontour and color can still result. **B,** A fine labial collar of gold allows for creation of a restoration having proper contour and ample thickness of porcelain to obtain good color. **C,** The shoulder margin provides the ideal amount of room to produce a porcelain-fused-to-gold restoration with good gingival contour and color.

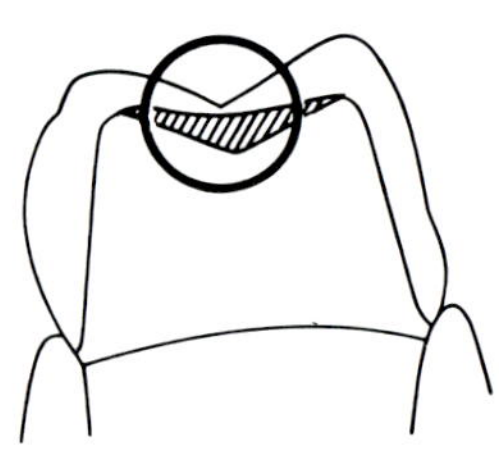

Fig. 7-70. Occlusal surface of a posterior tooth must be reduced a minimum of 2 mm. Be sure to reduce central fossa area sufficiently (see hashed area).

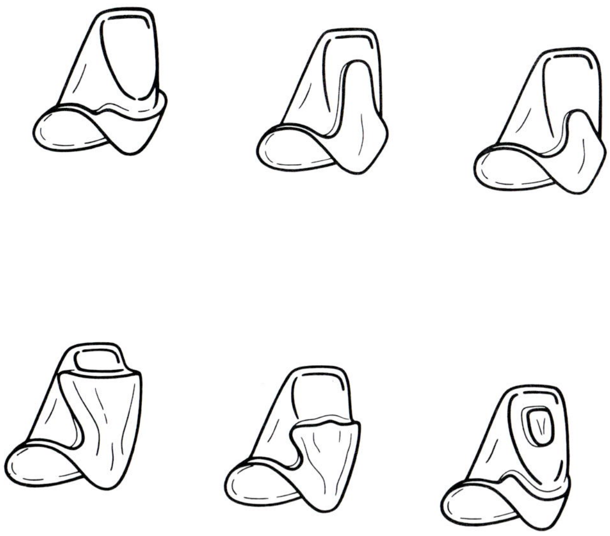

Fig. 7-71

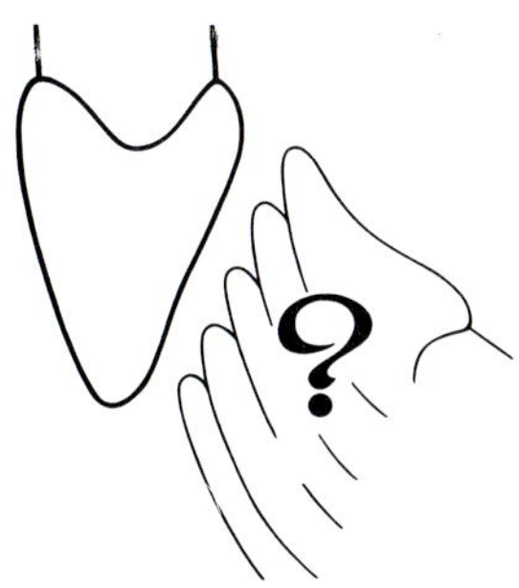

Fig. 7-72

Figs. 7-71 and 7-72. The design for anterior restorations can vary considerably. It is controlled by many factors which include the maxillary and mandibular relationship and the "travel" paths of the involved teeth in all excursions, the main determining factor being that the travel path of the antagonizing tooth not pass over the porcelain and metal junction.

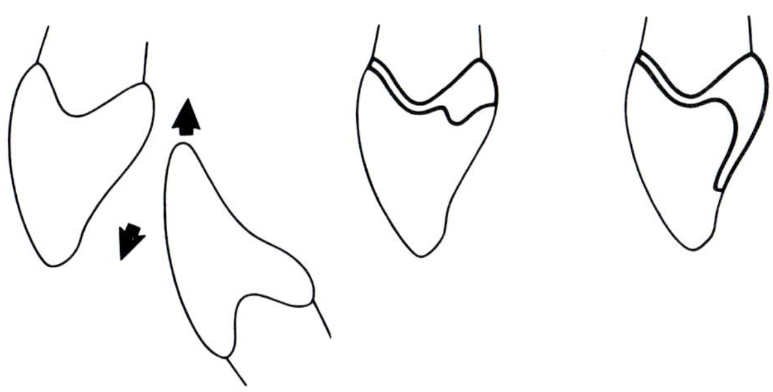

Fig. 7-73. Where no contact or travel paths are present, the restoration can be designed according to the operator's individual preference.

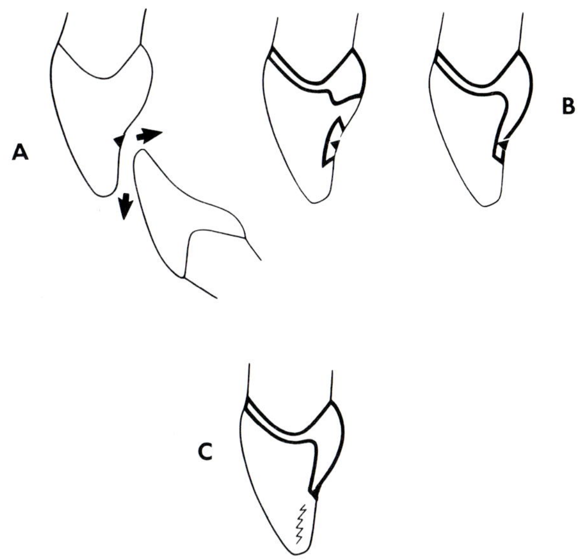

Fig. 7-74. Anteriors having only point contact and no travel path can be designed as illustrated in **A** and **B.** The restoration could also have full coverage of porcelain. In any case the terminating edge of metal should not coincide with the contacting point, **C,** since the possibility of fracture is increased. Where stresses are placed on this junction of porcelain and metal, a distortion of the metal could occur eventually resulting in checking, cracking, or shearing of the porcelain away from the crown.

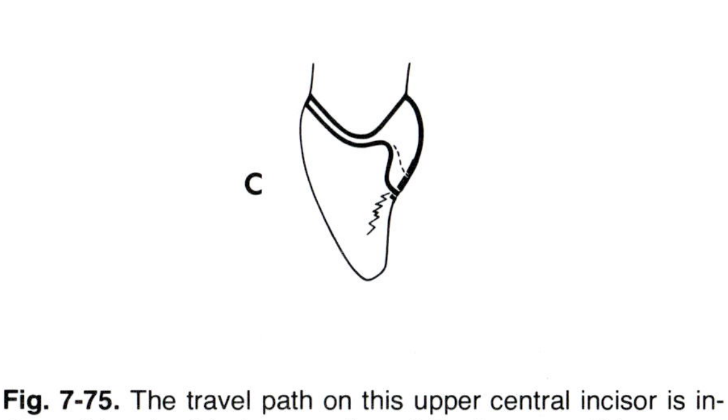

Fig. 7-75. The travel path on this upper central incisor is indicated by the black area. **A** and **B** show possible proper metal structure design. **C** indicates that when the metal is terminated within this travel path or too closely beyond (0.5 mm.), the possibility of fracture is increased.

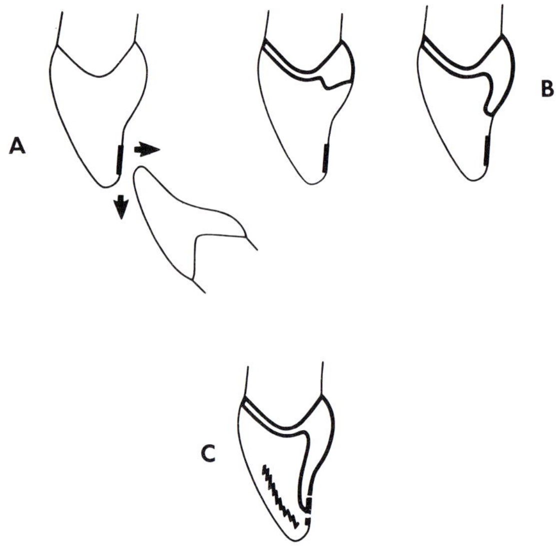

Fig. 7-76. A high or incisal third travel path, as indicated by the black area, necessitates a structure with its metal terminating closer to the gingival and away from any antagonizing tooth contact (see **A** and **B**). **C** illustrates the fracture or shear possibility when this junction of porcelain and metal is within the "travel" area.

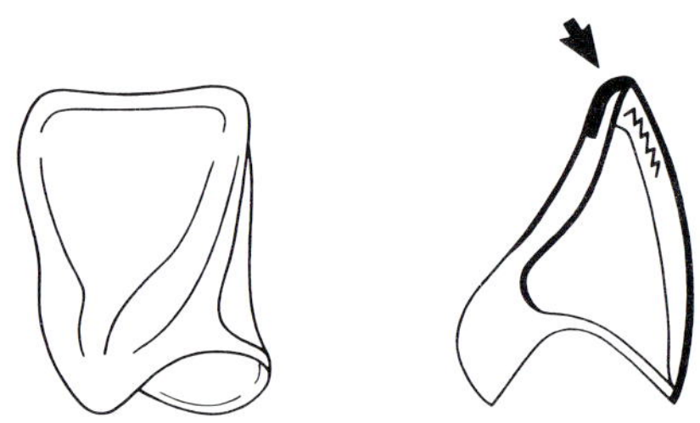

Fig. 7-77. It is strongly recommended that this type of design not be used for anterior or posterior teeth. Even where no travel path is present, normal usage of the crown involving any incisal stresses could result in shearing off of the labial porcelain.

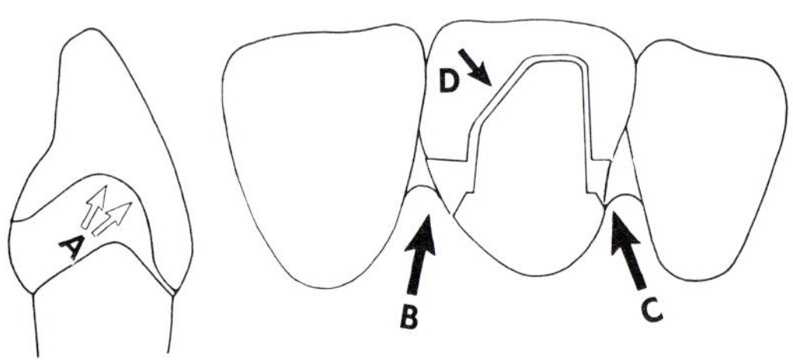

Fig. 7-78. The incisogingival and labiolingual placement of the collar of metal on this type of restoration is extremely important. In those cases where the supporting metal structure is designed with the collar too high or too far labially (as shown by arrows *A*) it limits one's creative ability by the position of this finish line. The esthetic results are determined by its position. Arrow *B* indicates an interproximal overcontour caused by too heavy and too high a collar. Arrow *C* shows a resultant undercontoured situation by too thin a metal collar. Arrow *D* illustrates the metal following the incisal contour of a fractured central incisor, resulting in a bulk of porcelain in one area which could produce checking.

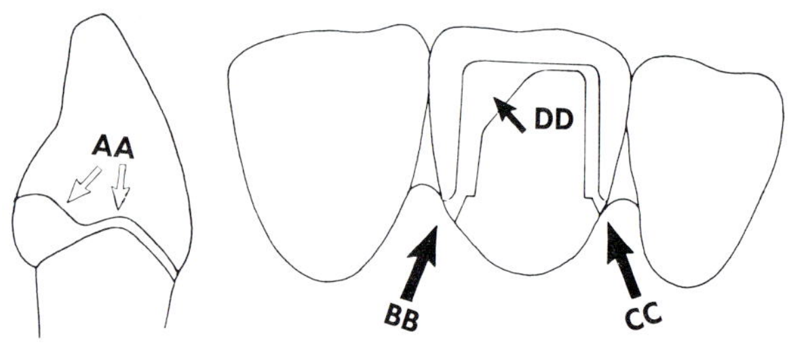

Fig. 7-79. The interproximal area should be free of as much metal as possible, which will allow the ceramist to properly contour the porcelain in these areas. Doing so eliminates the possibility of the metal causing a "graying out" of the gingival interproximal tissue. The double letters *(AA, BB, CC, DD)* show the metal contour corrections necessary in these areas.

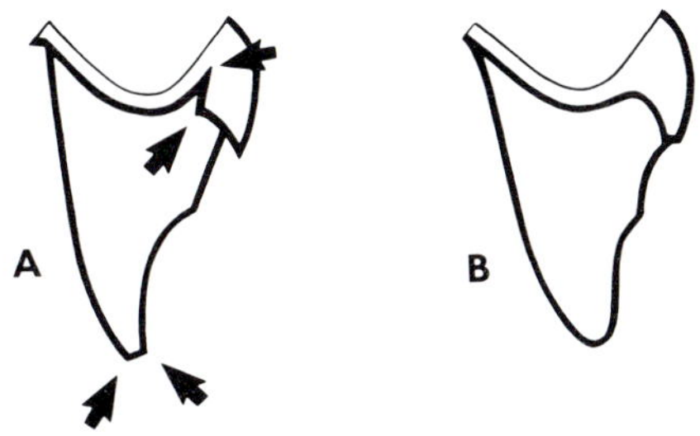

Fig. 7-80. The arrows in **A** point to sharp negative and positive angles which, if not corrected, will result in stress areas and produce checking and/or fracture of the completed case. **B** shows the same restoration with all of these angles contoured properly.

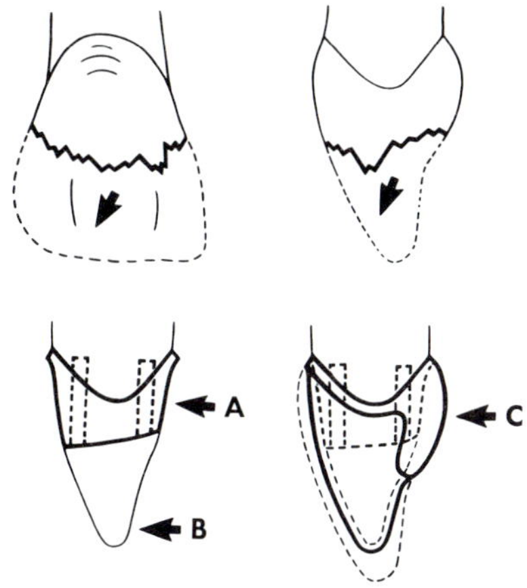

Fig. 7-81. *A* shows remaining portion of the tooth is prepared. The dotted lines indicate Ney parallel pin placement. *B* shows the gold pin core is in position on the prepared tooth. *C* shows a restoration made over the above structure will have adequate retentive qualities *(A, B)*.

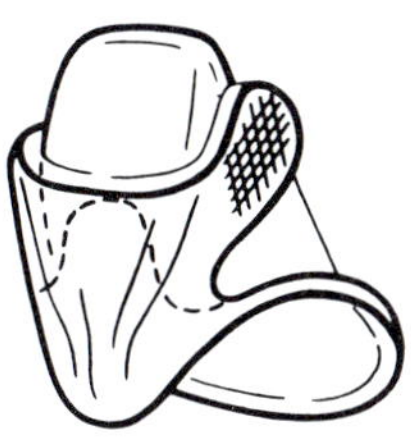

Fig. 7-82. The design requirement for multiple units varies from that used on single units. When an anterior restoration is to be used as an abutment, the design should be similar to that indicated by the hashed area. The dotted line would be the design contour for a single restoration.

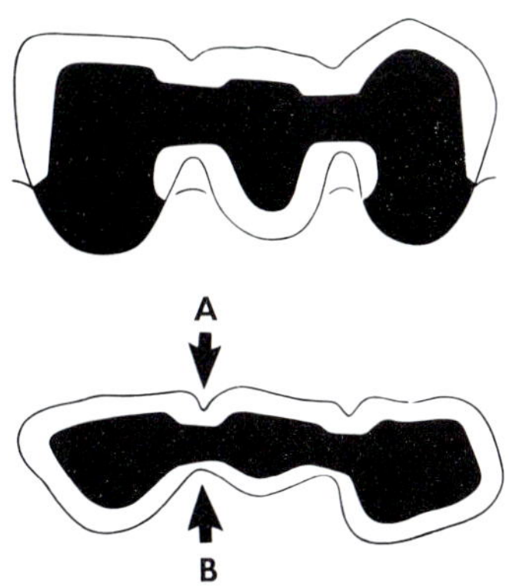

Fig. 7-83. The waxing of the framework should be such as to ensure an even and adequate thickness of porcelain. Interproximal areas should not be waxed in a V shape but rather with a relatively broad and flat contour (3 mm. wide) (arrow *A*) to provide sufficient room to create deep and natural appearing interdental contours. In most instances, any compromise will have to be made on the lingual interproximal area (arrow *B*) to increase the thickness of metal in the connecting area of the frame as a means of providing the necessary strength and rigidity. Breakages at cast connector or solder joint usually not metal failure, but design failure.

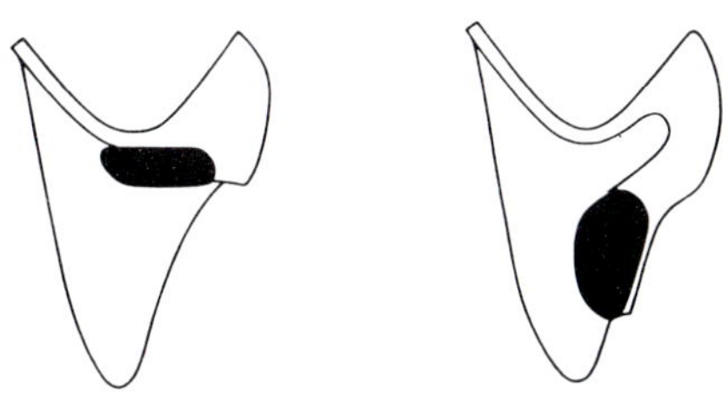

Fig. 7-84. A connector between units, regardless of whether cast or soldered, should be thicker in the incisogingival direction than it is in the labiolingual dimension.

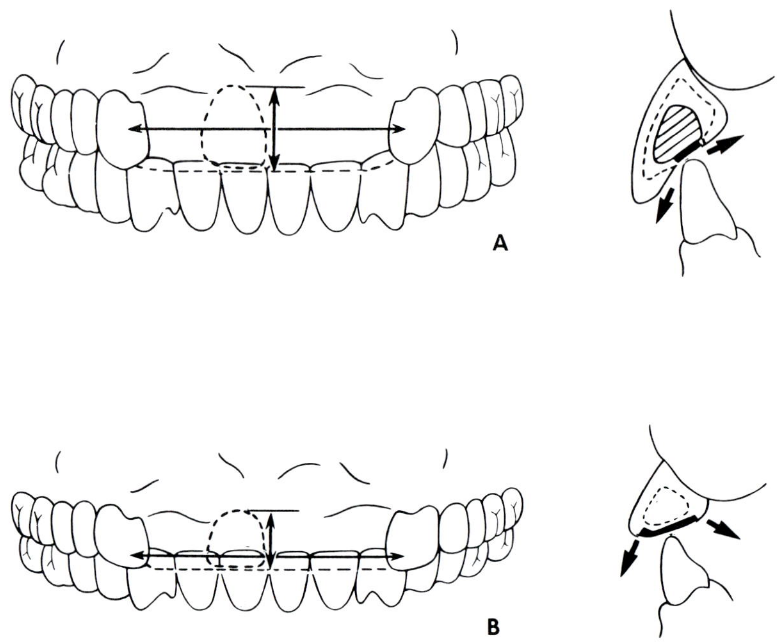

Fig. 7-85. There are situations that contraindicate the construction of a fixed prosthesis using porcelain fused to metal. **A,** Anterior bridge offers no obvious problem—there is enough incisogingival height, connectors can be designed to properly support the case, and good esthetics can be attained. **B,** There is minimal incisogingival room, and span, in relation to this height, is quite long. Compare the cross section of the frames and travel paths in **A** and **B.** Recommendation in case such as shown in **B** would be not to use porcelain fused to metal as a material of choice.

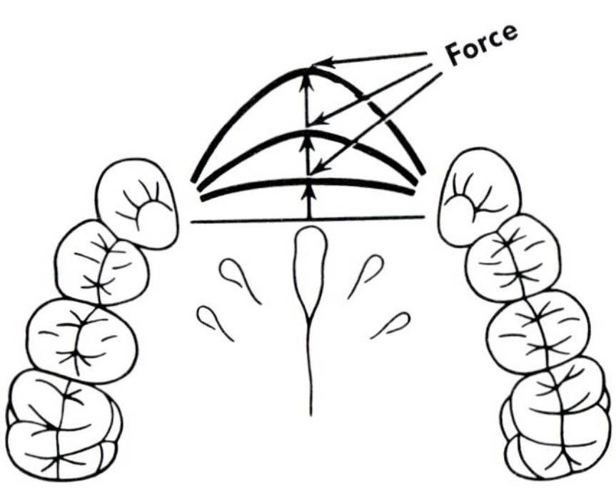

Fig. 7-86. Arch form is another consideration. This figure illustrates three of the possible arch forms. The longer the span, the greater the need for rigidity in the metal substructure.

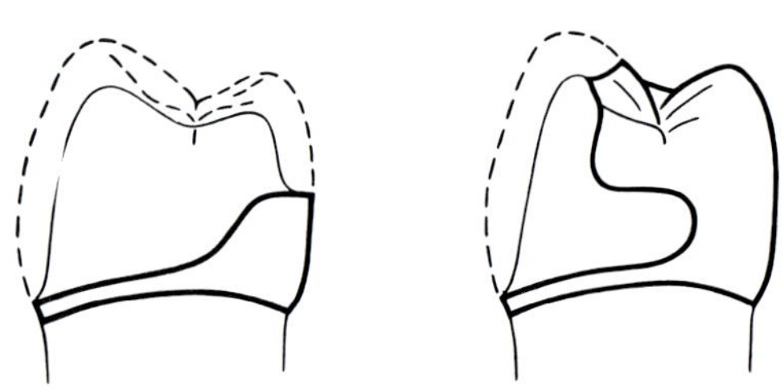

Fig. 7-87. The design selected for use on posterior teeth is also determined by amount of reduction, tooth-to-tooth relationship, and their paths of travel. Here we show correct design for full coverage of porcelain on the left, and on the right correct design for metal occlusion.

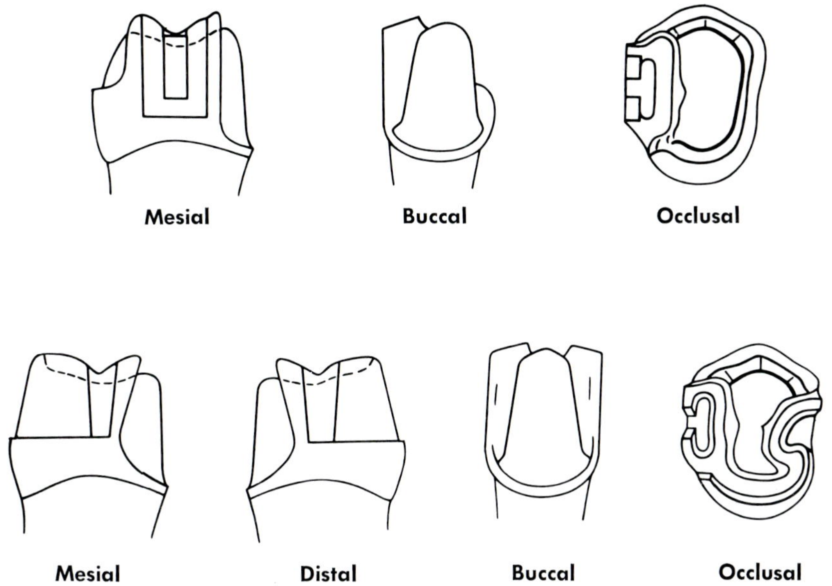

Fig. 7-88. Upper three illustrations show various views where a precision attachment is used. The lower four sketches show a double milled lock with lingual metal shoulder. The occlusal view shows the island of metal surrounding the milled areas to afford protection for the porcelain once it has been applied.

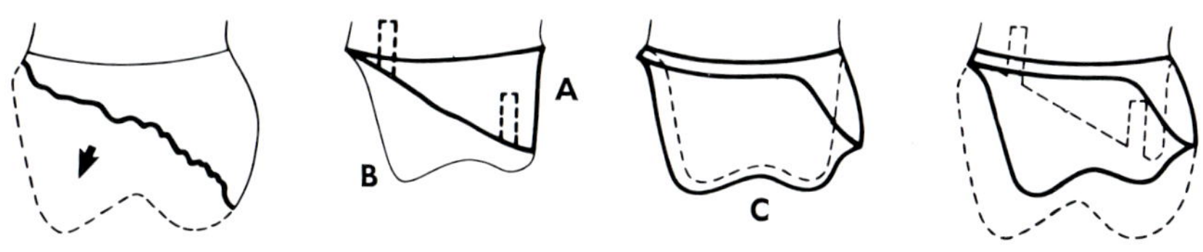

Fig. 7-89. *A* illustrates the preparation, *B* the completed pin core in position on the tooth, and *C* the ceramic coping casting prepared for receiving the porcelain. As an alternate method the retentive parallel pins could be incorporated as an integral part of the ceramic casting.

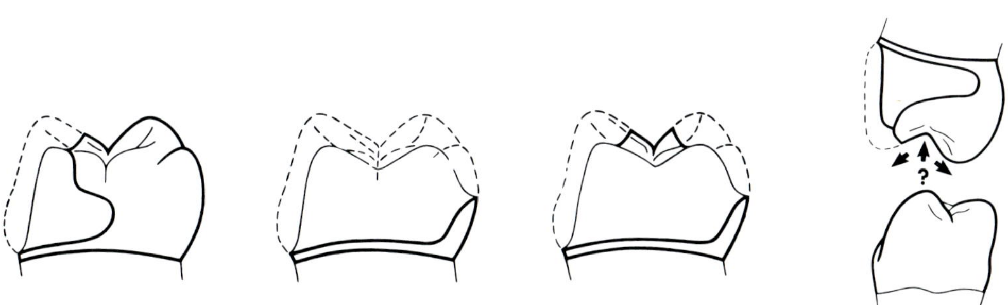

Fig. 7-90. Designs for restoring molars utilizing metal occlusion, full coverage of porcelain, and "island" or "strike" areas. Which of these designs is the most correct again depends on where the antagonizing tooth makes contact and what the travel path of the contacting cusp (or cusps) is.

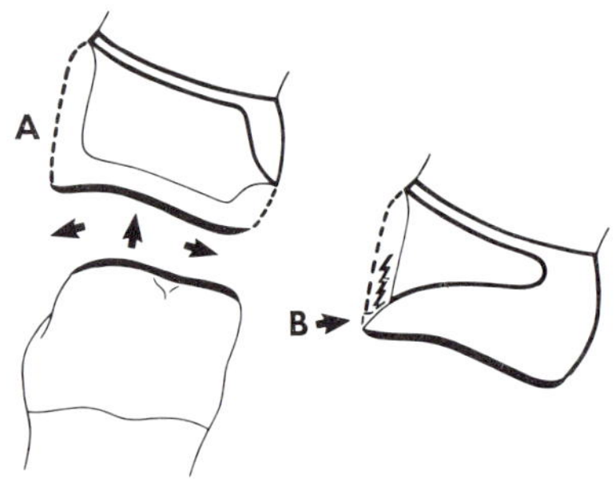

Fig. 7-91. Flat occlusal surface with intimate contact with opposing teeth not only in centric relation but in all excursions. The travel path is indicated by the heavy black line on the occlusal of these drawings. *A* would be the design of choice if adequate occlusal reduction has been made. If a metal occlusion is requested and the metal portion of the restoration is made with a sharp occlusobuccal margin, fracture can be expected. To prevent this, a heavier (2 mm.) occlusobuccal margin *(B)* must be used to prevent any occlusal stresses on the metal from being transferred to the porcelain veneer preventing it from shearing off. Minimal occlusal reduction limits design choice to metal occlusion only.

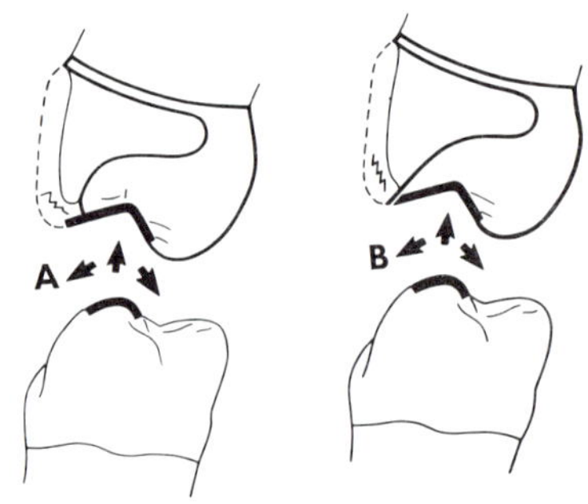

Fig. 7-92. The importance of observing travel paths and their effect on probable fracturing of the porcelain. *A,* Occlusobuccal margin was terminated within the travel path, resulting in fracture of the veneer. *B,* Occlusobuccal margin was extended 0.5 mm. beyond the travel path and, again, resulted in a fractured veneer. The metal is too thin at the porcelain-metal junction, permitting the stresses to be transferred to the porcelain.

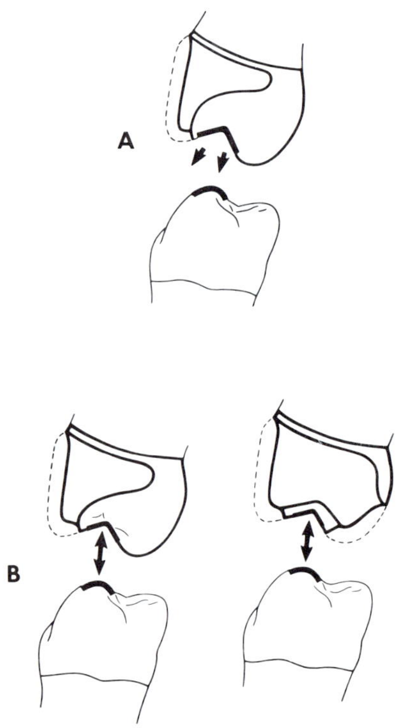

Fig. 7-93. A, Where an occlusal reduction is adequate (2 mm) and occlusal contact occurs in the central fossa with average travel distance, a metal frame can be successfully designed. Notice the metal preparation interproximally to allow freedom of contour of the porcelain for maximum esthetics. **B** indicates the correct design for a metal occlusion and metal strike design. The porcelain-metal margins terminate well away from the end of the travel paths, and the interproximal metal has been eliminated as much as possible.

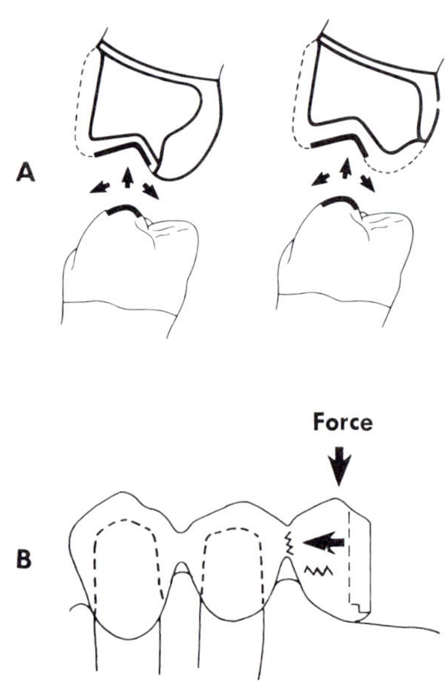

Fig. 7-94. A, The correct designs for full and partial porcelain coverage. It is necessary to keep the junction of porcelain and metal away from occlusal travel paths and to keep interproximals clear. **B,** When occlusal forces are applied on the cantilevered section and adequate strength and rigidity are not provided by properly designing the connector, checking of the porcelain or even breaking off of the cantilevered pontic could occur.

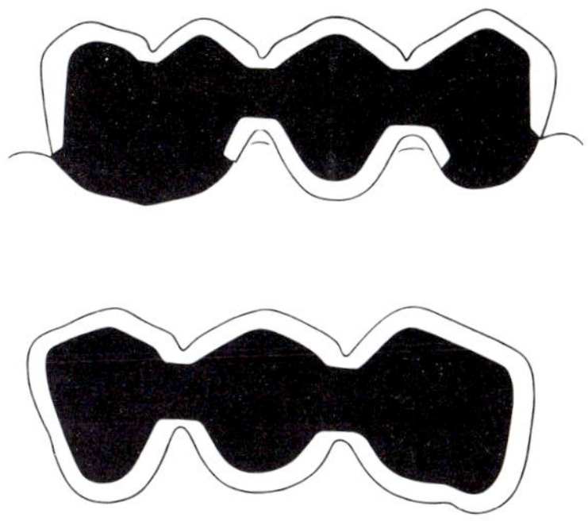

Fig. 7-95. The thickness of the porcelain application should be even to control color. Too thick or uneven application of porcelain in any given area on the restoration could result in checking or cracking after completion of the splint or bridge.

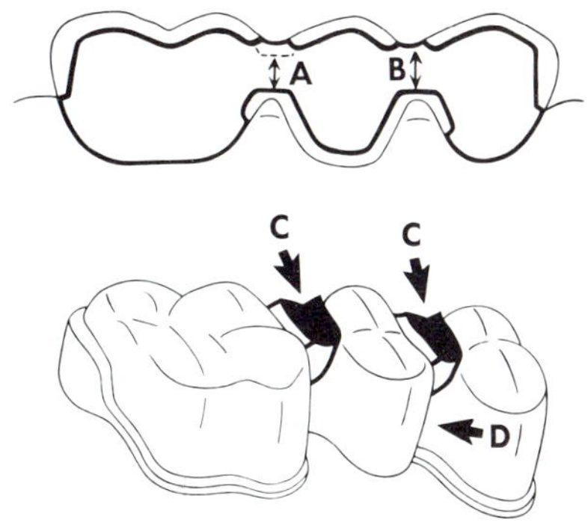

Fig. 7-97. Usually the design for Fig. 7-95, *C,* is shown by arrow *A,* which would lack sufficient strength and be flexible, causing checking, cracking, and shearing of the fused porcelain. By redesigning the connector (arrow *B*) and exposing a small amount of metal on the occlusal surface, sufficient strength and rigidity are gained to allow for the fabrication of a successful case. Arrow *C* shows the amount of metal that will be exposed on the occlusal surface. Contouring of interproximal areas is possible of attainment (arrow *D*).

Connectors—posterior

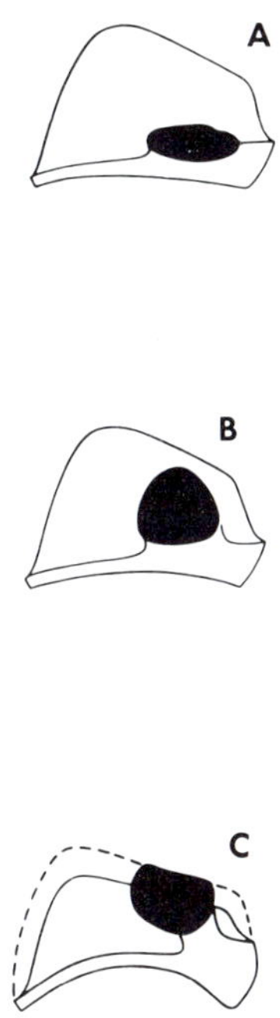

Fig. 7-96. Posterior connections between units (soldered or cast) should be designed with their greater dimension in an occlusogingival direction to obtain the maximum strength and rigidity with a minimal amount of metal. In **A,** the connection will be weak and flexible; **B** shows the correct design. **C,** A solution to provide a properly designed connection on a case where the occlusogingival space is minimal.

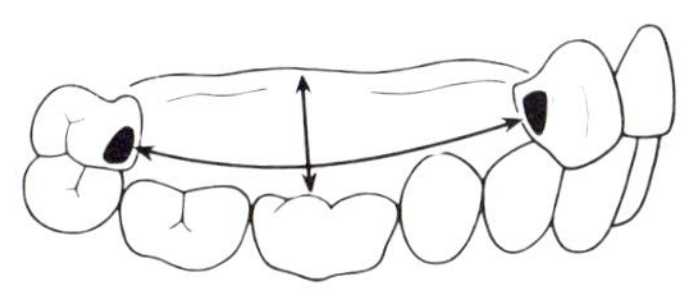

Fig. 7-98. Considerations that determine the success or failure of posterior bridges are length of span, occlusogingival space available, and number of abutments in relation to length of span. Top illustration (a relatively long span) fulfills requirements for a successful restoration.

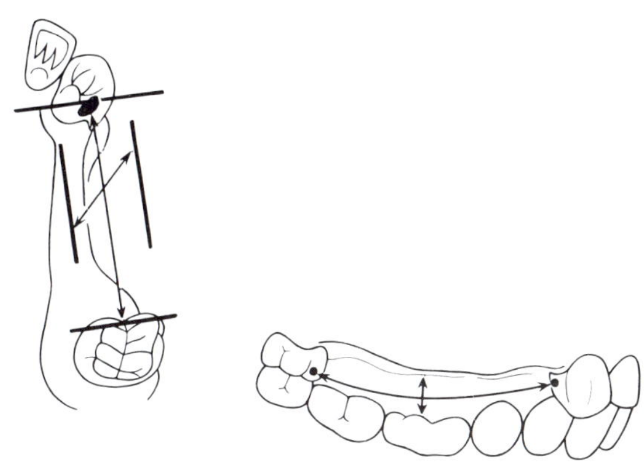

Fig. 7-99. A somewhat similar case but the span is too long in relation to occlusogingival length of abutments, connection areas are too small to provide adequate strength and rigidity, and an irregular occlusal plane on the lower teeth would add to these problems.

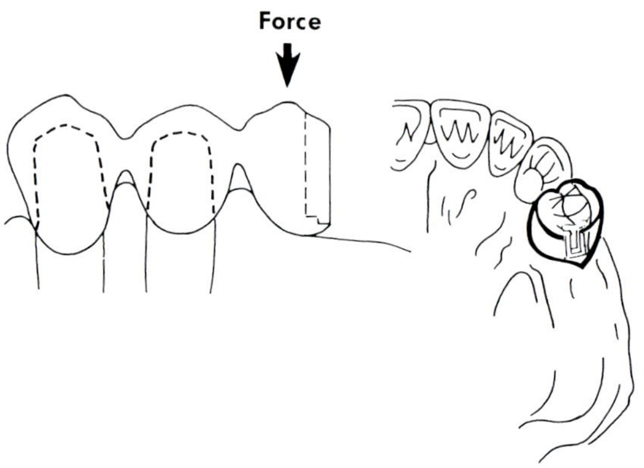

Fig. 7-100. In a case where a cantilevered bicuspid with a precision attachment to retain a removable partial denture is made, be sure adequate strength and rigidity is provided by properly designing the connector to absorb applied occlusal forces.

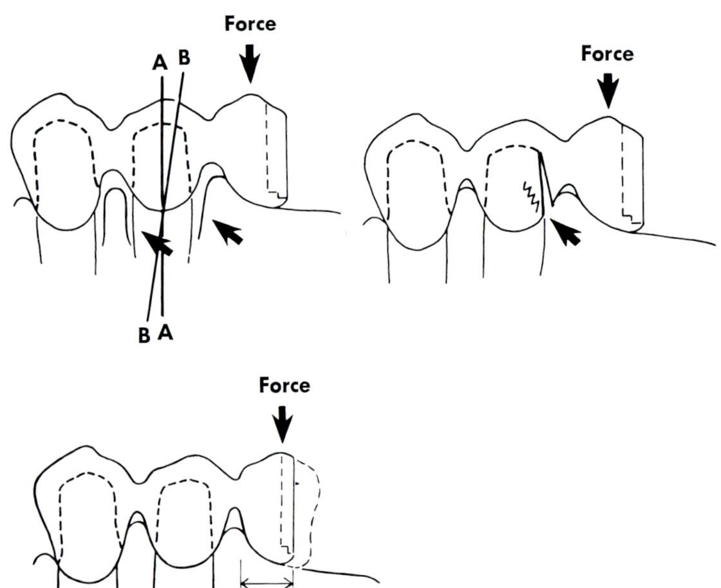

Fig. 7-101. Where the connector does provide enough rigidity and strength to prevent checking or breakage, the forces applied to the pontic are relayed to the abutment tooth's long axis, resulting in possible breakdown of the investing tissues and/or the opening or warping of gingival margins on the retainer castings and/or cracking of the porcelain on these retainers. Where esthetics permits, eliminate the distal half of the pontic (bottom drawing) and, by so doing the stresses placed on the pontic are reduced—in effect we have shortened the arm of the lever and reduced by a considerable amount the stresses on this portion of the restoration.

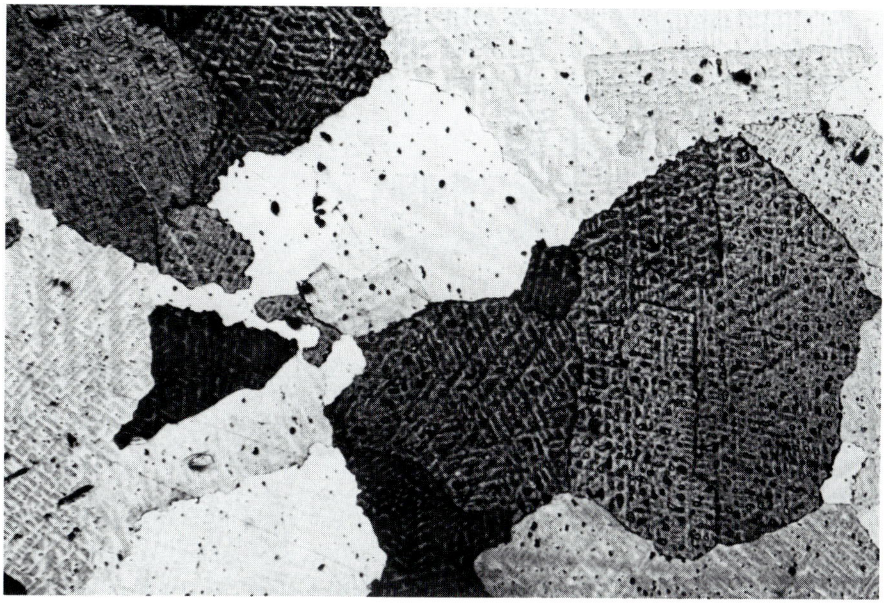

Fig. 7-102. Ceramic gold without super micrograin. Unretouched photomicrograph (30X) shows coarse grain, marked dendritic structure.

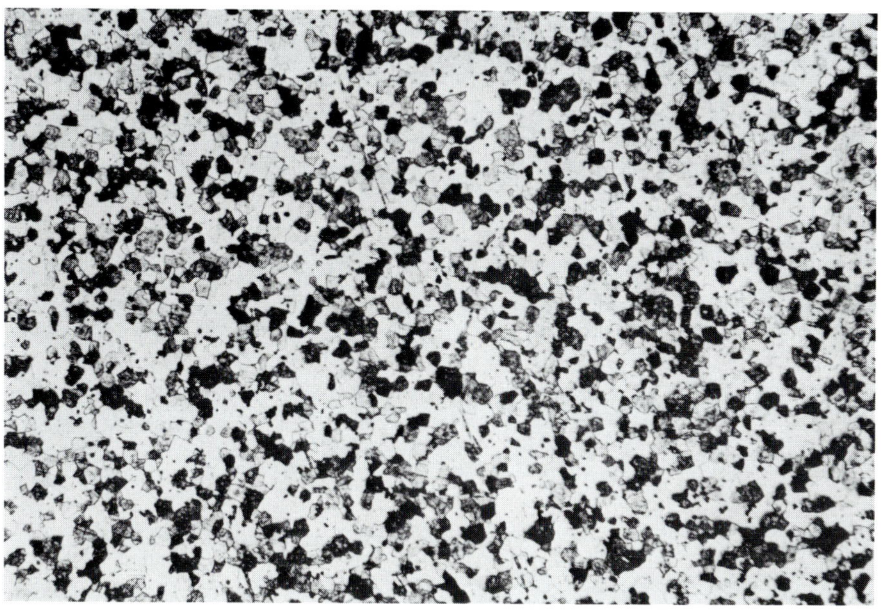

Fig. 7-103. Ceramic gold with super micrograin. Unretouched photomicrograph (30X) shows extremely fine equiaxed grains, total lack of dendritic structure, and absence of porosity.

Figs. 7-104 to 7-111. A series of difficult and interesting cases making use of gold and porcelain.

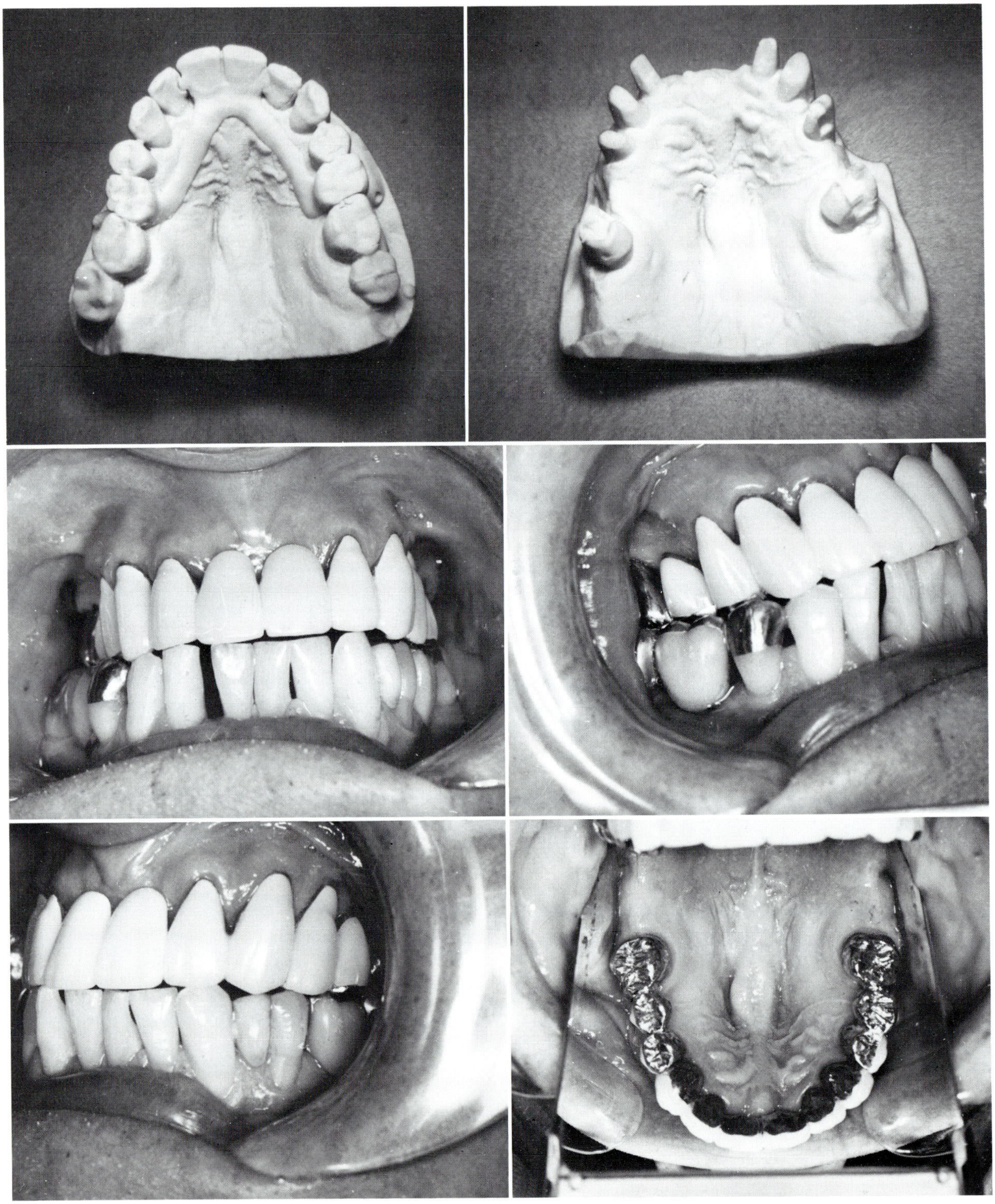

Fig. 7-104. Combination of cross-bite and some end-to-end preoperatively to completion of upper arch.

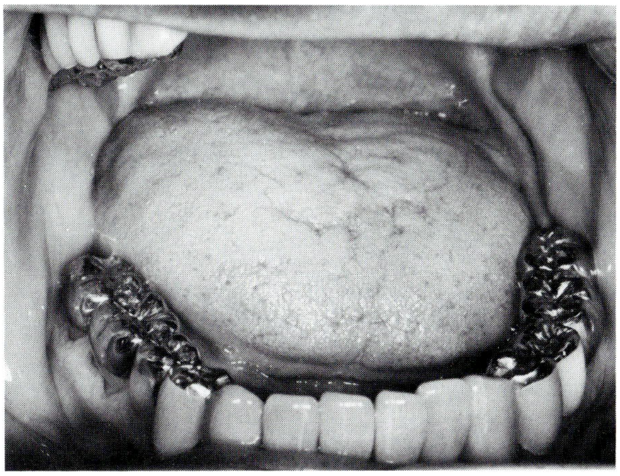

Fig. 7-105. Splint using the right and left cuspids and right and first bicuspids as abutments.

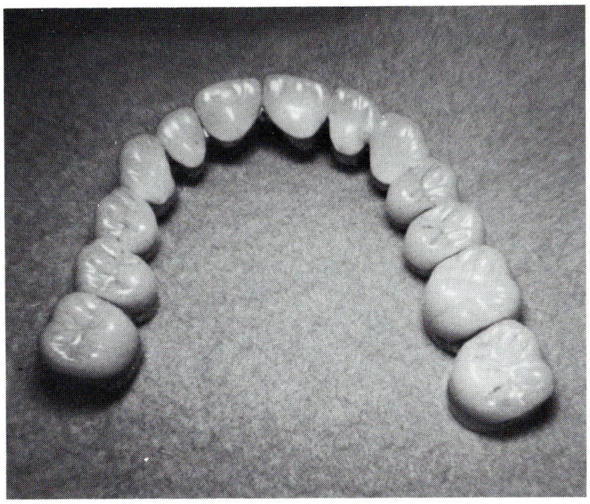

Fig. 7-106. Complete full upper arch splint baked in sections and furnace soldered (see Chapter 11).

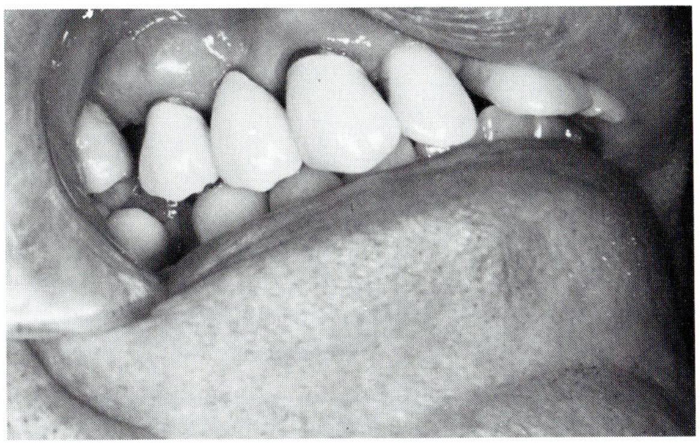

Fig. 7-107. Bridge including cuspid and both bicuspids. Difficulty was buccal alignment without too much overcontouring for periodontal health.

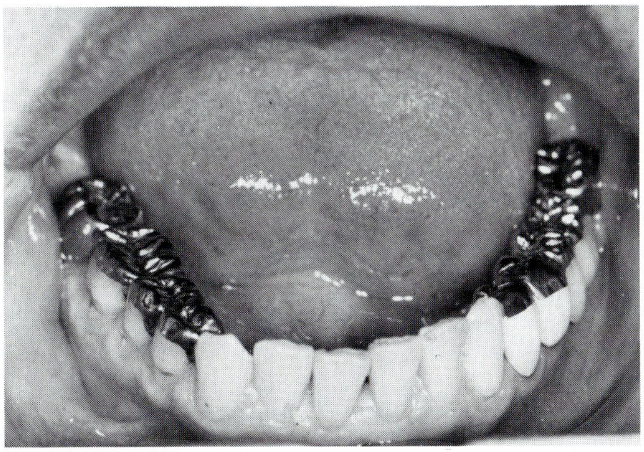

Fig. 7-108. Need for strong gold occlusal protection on left side.

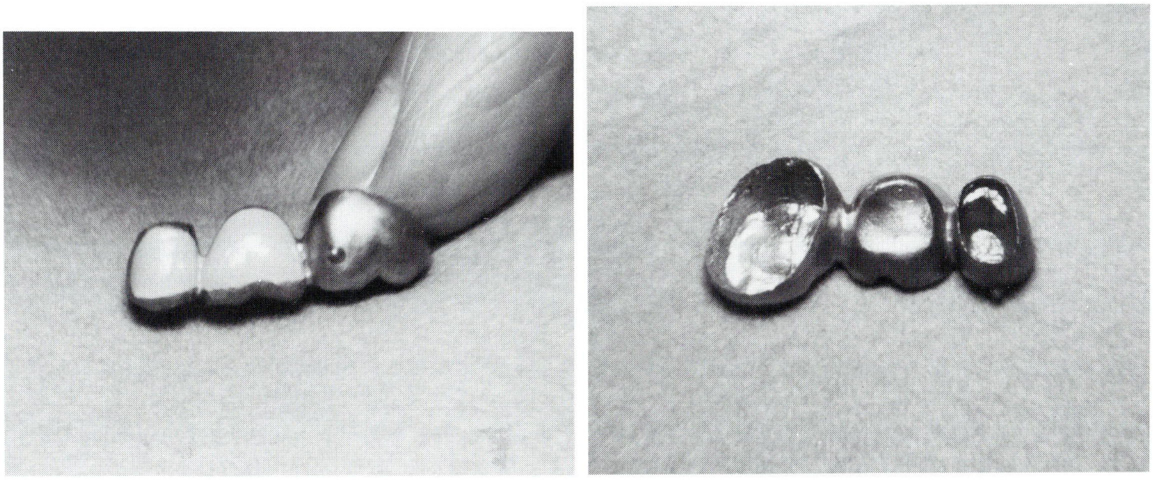

Fig. 7-109. Need for occlusal protection in a cross-bite case.

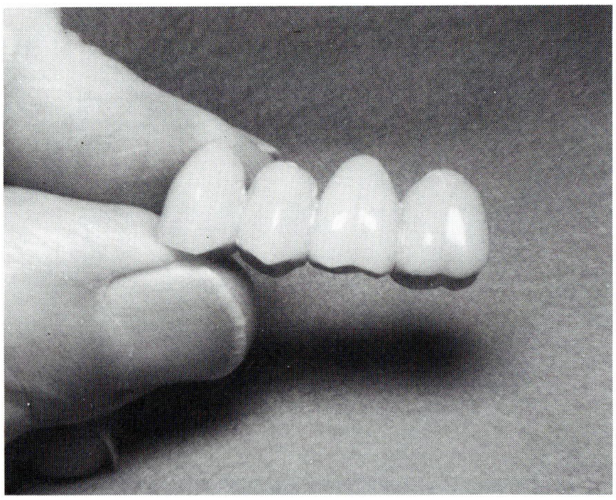

Fig. 7-110. A four-tooth bridge with porcelain enveloping part of the occlusal surfaces.

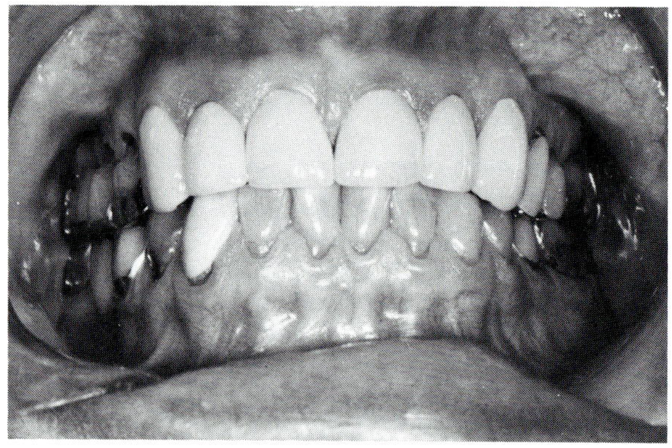

Fig. 7-111. After completion of upper anterior porcelain-fused-to-gold restorations, patient expressed a desire to do the same for many of her posterior teeth.

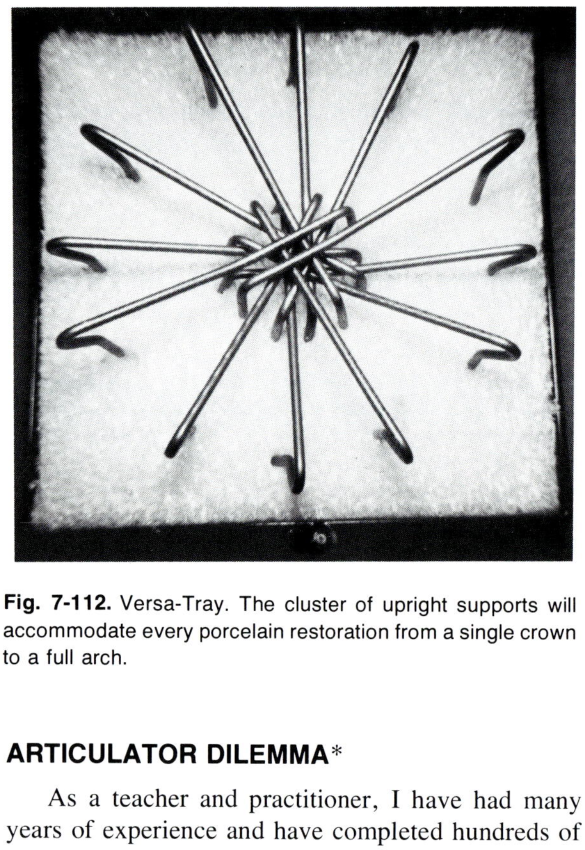

Fig. 7-112. Versa-Tray. The cluster of upright supports will accommodate every porcelain restoration from a single crown to a full arch.

ARTICULATOR DILEMMA*

As a teacher and practitioner, I have had many years of experience and have completed hundreds of cases during this time, having successes and failures with all types of articulators and techniques. I am cognizant of the fact that we have in our midst some exceptionally trained and skillful dentists who can obtain exceptional end results with the use of any type of articulator as an aid in their procedures in full mouth rehabilitation. But my extensive observation has found this to be the exception (a small percentage) and not the rule. So, a consideration of acceptable semiadjustable and fully adjustable articulators, and their limitations, is in order.

To begin with, what constitutes the essential requirements of a functional articulator?

In view of the importance of the coordinated functions of anatomy, physiology, and geometrics and their relation to prosthetic technique, it is mandatory that an articulator have certain characteristics which enable it to accept and maintain various functions.

Of primary importance in this regard is the characteristic of having the condyle spheres situated on the lower member of an articulator and the fossae on the upper member. This arrangement ensures that all rotation (axial centers of rotation) becomes the sole function of the lower member and the product of the rotations expressed as intercondylar distance, while all translatory functions—i.e. Bennett, protrusive, lateral protrusive with curvilinear paths and the working component—can be attributed to the upper member of the analog. Since registrations of protrusive and lateral excursions are necessarily taken while the jaw is in an open position, an articulator is set for these excursions in the same open position. If the condyle path is on the lower member, as the upper member is closed into centric relation, the angle formed by an extension of the condyle path and the articulation plane will be decreased since the maxillary cast will be lowered, while the condylar angulation remains as previously set. The articulation plane is determined by corresponding points on the upper dentition that are used on the lower dentition to determine plane of occlusion.[57] If, on the other hand, the condyle path is situated on

*With the assistance of A. J. De Pietro.

the upper member of an articulator, once set, it and, of necessity, the angle formed remain constant to the maxillary cast in opening and closing movements of all excursions. Plane of reference and fully adjustable side-shift controls are on the upper member.

As important in this regard is the fixed position of the condyle spheres on the lower member of an articulator—that is, fixed to a determined intercondylar distance for an individual case. If such condition is not present on an articulator, when a Bennett and horizontal tilt adjustment is made, the magnitude and direction of the axis of rotation will not remain constant to that of centric relation in eccentric closures. With the condyle spheres fixed on the lower member of an articulator, the relationship of the axis to the fossa remains constant, and the arc of closure remains constant in centric and all eccentric closures. The hinge axis or transverse axis mounting becomes much more practical, since it can be utilized to establish vertical dimension without any alteration in the arc of closure and a definite relation to the settings of the condyle.

An articulator must be capable of accepting a hinge axis or transverse axis mounting and maintaining the true relationship dictated by it. Any movement of the face-bow, either in relation to itself or to the upper member of an articulator, will negate a true hinge axis or transverse axis mounting.

An articulator should have provision to adjust intercondylar distance both medially and laterally (adjustable intercenter distance), since this dimension, in correlation with the Bennett adjustment, determines horizontal radii (intercondylar distance determines the gross horizontal arc while Bennett movement imparts the subtle variations along the arc), and is a necessary factor in the duplication of a given path of a cusp tip. Without the intercondylar distance adjustment, increase or decrease of horizontal radii would be confined within the limitations afforded by the Bennett adjustment acting alone, making nearly impossible duplication of a given path of a cusp tip.

It must be remembered that an articulator must be so constructed that when the intercondylar distance is adjusted, the axis is not distorted in any way, so that the magnitude and direction of the axis remain constant to that of centric in all eccentric closures.

An articulator should have provision for a Bennett adjustment since this movement controlling the rotating centers of the horizontal, vertical, and sagittal axes, increases the magnitude of the functional envelope of motion. This is absolutely a necessary factor in the duplication of a given path of a cusp tip on working and balancing sides.

In close correlation with the Bennett movement is an adjustment that rotates the condyle path about the sagittal axis. This adjustment we shall call "horizontal tilt." As the condyle sphere on the working side rotates about the sagittal axis, the degree and magnitude of drop of the condyle sphere on the balancing side is controlled by the horizontal tilt adjustment in correlation with the Bennett adjustment. Without this feature incorporated into an articulator, duplication of a given balancing cusp height is nearly impossible.

Another essential feature of the condylar assembly of an articulator is, of course, the condyle path. In this regard, the construction of an articulator should permit the changing of the condyle path to that of the specific curvature dictated by the patient, if the normal functional movements of the patient are to be simulated. The use of a straight condyle path, set at an angle determined by a single protrusive registration, can be accurate in the protrusive excursion only at that point at which it was set, since the intermediate movement of the condyle sphere along the path from centric relation to that single point follows a straight line. In only very rare cases will a patient present a straight condylar path. In pantographic registrations the problem of selecting the correct path is a relatively simple one, since the registrations scribed on the lateral plates dictate the correct radius paths to be used.

The working component of the fossae must be so constructed as to be free and capable of independent settings and yet combine in such a manner with the Bennett, lateral, and protrusive settings to function as a smooth continuous structure.[58] The working component must be capable of a setting about the vertical axial center so that the translation of the spherical element can be directed anterior or posterior to this center. It must permit rotation about the sagittal axial center so that translation of the element can be directed inferior or superior to this axial center. All surfaces of the fossae that control translatory angulations must be constructed of a material that will permit subtle adjustments to the angulation by the addition to or removal of portions of the walls that support the spherical structure.

An articulator should have an incisal table that is capable of a limited rotation about the frontal axis and the capability of being locked in a determined position. This adjustment is necessary to accommodate the amount of overbite dictated by anterior guidance, in synchronization with the straight protrusive movement dictated by the condyle path.

An incisal table should have lateral incisal guide planes, capable of limited rotation about the sagittal axis, and the capability of being locked in a determined position. This adjustment is necessary to accommodate the amount of overbite dictated by the canine in synchronization with the lateral excursive movement dictated by the condyle path. In addition, the lateral incisal guide planes should present a slightly curved surface, since the function of the canine guidance is a curved function.

An incisal table should contain the means whereby the point on which the incisal guide pin rests in centric position has the capability of being raised or lowered and locked in a determined position. This point, or adjustable pin, we will call the incisal overbite adjustment pin. A custom-built plastic incisal table can also be used (refer to Chapter 17).

Functionally, an articulator should be sturdy and exact in construction, simple but efficient in mechanics of operation, and capable of maintaining constants and duplicating desired movements. It should accept pantographic registrations and, by all means, maintain centric relation. It should be a teaching aid to the student and a capable tool for the prosthodontist.

In other words, the purpose of an articulator in fixed partial denture prosthodontics is to transfer the effective mandibular movements of a patient to the laboratory bench. An articulator should be capable of adjusting for those essential elements of the determinants of mandibular movement which are of clinical importance. The accuracy of the simulation of the jaw movement controls the accuracy of the fabricated prosthesis. It allows for more accurate occlusal relationships of the restorations and should require but minor adjustments after installation of the case.[59]

Inadequate understanding of the patient's individual functional movements may result in restorations which cause periodontal breakdown of the remaining teeth, temporomandibular joint disorders, or muscle spasm. So the question resolves itself into one which asks: Can we obtain an end result which will not cause periodontal disease or temporomandibular disorders with the correct use of a semiadjustable articulator, or must we use a fully adjustable articulator? In some instances a compromise treatment must be instituted. To compromise one must be able to evaluate findings, consider all the factors involved, and execute the best treatment possible under the circumstances. A simplified procedure which only considers the ease of operation and time involved, but ignores essential requirements, is certainly not practical from the standpoint of the patient. The patient must be made aware of the fact of where and why the compromise is being made. I am in accord with the use of any suitable articulator that can attain the proper goals within reasonable limits of time consumption (an important commodity) and reasonable expertise. But we know that there is a wide gap between those techniques that are too compromising and those that are absolutely uncompromising, that the quality of results do differ, and that a person sees only what he knows. There are no quick solutions, and even our desire for this does not change the fact. A dentist who understands mandibular motion and normal joint function may do an acceptable job of what we refer to as a compromise treatment procedure.

Let us digress for a moment from our discussion of types of articulators and define what we have in mind when we use the word "occlusion," some important characteristics that the patient should exhibit, and the criteria used in the evaluation of the occlusion of the patient.

To begin with, I am of the opinion that occlusion is the common denominator of all dental practice. Celenza[60] has aptly said: "Occlusion is the meeting ground, the coordinator, the hub of the dental wheel for both the basic and clinical sciences."* Fox[61] has said: "Occlusion in its fullest interpretation includes a knowledge of the anatomy and physiology of the muscles of mastication, the temporo-mandibular articulation, jaw to jaw relationships, tooth form and position, mandibular movements, vertical dimension, functional and afunctional uses and abuses of teeth, the periodontal supporting tissues, namely, the periodontal ligament and, above all else the alveolar bone and its reaction to the transmission of stresses to it by tooth contacts through muscle power."†

Amsterdam[62] is of the opinion that the characteristics a patient would exhibit in what may be referred to as a normal occlusion are the following: "(1) the occlusion of the teeth are in maximum contact when the jaws are in centric relation, (2) the teeth are apart when the mandible assumes its rest position, allowing for sufficient free-way space, (3) the cuspal relations of the teeth are such as to allow the mandible to move to and from centric without restraint. There is a coordinated anterior and posterior overbite and overjet relationship, (4) the 'Bennett' movement is a noninterfering factor, (5) the inclination of the roots are in a correct mesial, distal, buccal, and lingual axial direction, (6) there are good proximal contacting relationships of the teeth, (7) the crown-to-root ratio is favorable in all aspects, and (8) the coronal forms of the teeth are such as to provide maximum protection to the investing structures."‡

*From Celenza, Frank: Personal communication.

†From Fox, Lewis: The occlusal factor in periodontal disease, Alpha Omegan **43:**124-133, 1949.

‡From Amsterdam, Morton: Personal communication.

In other words, in evaluating the occlusion of a patient, the dentist must use the primary objectives of function, esthetics, and phonetics as his criteria. There must be (1) good esthetics, phonetics, and periodontal health, (2) freedom from subjective and objective temporomandibular joint symptoms, (3) an absence of retrogade wear patterns of the teeth, (4) the ability to chew adequately, and (5) a negative occlusal perception.

Many dentists are of the opinion that if one could obtain a stable centric occlusion which is coincident with centric relation, it could be said that they could obtain an acceptable result with a simple hinge articulator or, at most, a semiadjustable articulator. But, in spite of the fact that a coincidence of centric occlusion and centric relation is an important basic of our objectives, we must keep in mind that patients have to be capable of reaching their maximum closure comfortably from many positions of the mandible without tooth interference. Therefore, we must understand mandibular motion, how to measure it, and how to duplicate it on an articulator. In other words, centric position may have no deflective or interceptive occlusal contacts, but the eccentric positions may be uncontrolled. And it is possible for these uncontrolled eccentric positions to trigger parafunctional or periodontal insult.

The question that comes to mind is whether these eccentric movements, especially in the so-called involved cases, can be recorded satisfactorily by the use of positional wax records or check-bites on a semiadjustable articulator. Keep in mind that the amount of mandibular side shift tends to increase as the occlusion becomes more mutilated. In my experiences, the final result, when placed in the mouth, did not match the projected results as worked out on the semiadjustable articulator. Error produced by the use of this type of instrument may result in need for more than minimal eccentric occlusal adjustments or uncontrolled amounts of disocclusion. Occlusal forms that at first offered good efficiency become obliterated.

It must be admitted, in all fairness, that a semiadjustable articulator has its place in a general practice of dentistry, but we must understand the criteria of an optimum occlusion. In other words, what are we seeking to accomplish? The dentist has in mind (1) the construction of new occlusal surfaces designed for efficient functioning, and for a distribution of the masticatory loads in keeping with the demands of health, (2) occlusal surfaces which give a point and line contact by means of sharp cusps, well-defined convex ridges, and food-escape grooves that run buccally, lingually, and to the embrasures (occlusal surfaces with all ridges convex not only are efficient masticatory surfaces, but also tend to limit destructive lateral stresses; properly coordinated, these surfaces glide smoothly instead of locking in function), (3) maintenance of healthy periodontal tissues, and (4) preservation of osseous structures.

Guichet's[63] interpretation of the criteria of an optimum occlusion is as follows:

1. *Vertical stress*—incorporates in the occlusion those factors which have to do with the *reduction* of vertical stress.
2. *Horizontal stress*—provides for maximum intercuspation of the teeth with the condyles in centric relation, and provides for horizontal movement of the mandible from the centric related intercuspal position, until those teeth *most* capable of bearing the horizontal load come into function (Fig. 7-113).

In some cases all of these criteria can be satisfied with the use of a semiadjustable articulator, providing we understand the limitations of this type of analog. Keep in mind that adjustments in the mouth can be minimized, many times, in the working and lateral protrusive range by decreasing the angle of the triangular ridges of the maxillary buccal cusps posteriorly.[64] But there are cases that can only be created and coordinated on a fully adjustable articulator upon which the centric, protrusive, and right and left lateral positions of the mandible can be registered accurately. In these cases it is important that they show a complete disclusion of posterior teeth in the protrusive excursion with even distribution on as many anterior teeth as possible (only the maxillary central incisors may be

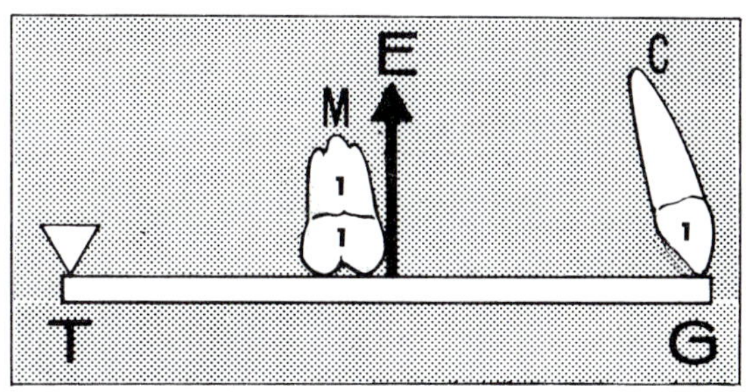

Fig. 7-113. *TG* is a diagrammatic representation of the mandible as a lever as it projects from the temporomandibular joint fulcrum *(T)*. Disposed along the mandible is a maxillary second molar *(M)*, a maxillary cuspid *(C)*, and an arrow representing the force vector of the bruxing muscles. In computing mechanical advantages, the arrow represents the effort and the *M* and *C* represent resistance. (Courtesy Niles F. Guichet.)

contacted), complete disclusion of posterior teeth on the nonfunctioning side in lateral or lateral-protrusive excursions, and "working side" contact or mutual protection as deemed necessary by the dentist.

Semiadjustable articulator

Again, I wish to emphasize that if a semiadjustable articulator is used correctly, it has a very definite place in the treatment of many cases. By correctly I mean not only the mechanics of its use but also its limitations, some of which have already been pointed out. Remember that a semiadjustable articulator is capable of only a simple laterotrusion.

The information of the patient's occlusion can be obtained not only from a study of the clinical and roentgenographic findings, but also from a careful study of correctly oriented diagnostic casts on a semiadjustable articulator. Its adequacy for a preliminary occlusal diagnosis is good. The casts should be mounted correctly in the hinge position using an arbitrary transverse axis which is as close as possible to the true transverse axis location. Also the casts should be mounted accurately in centric position at the properly determined vertical dimension. The centric position records should be kept as thin as possible without tooth interference. A semiadjustable articulator is used which approximates mandibular movements closely and which can be set to accommodate check-bite records made by the patient. Not only is an arbitrary transverse axis location used, but also an adjustable horizontal condylar guidance, an adjustable lateral condylar guidance on the horizontal axis, and an adjustable anterior guide table.

A careful study of the mounted casts will reveal areas causing deflection of terminal hinge jaw closure and interferences with free multidirectional gliding movements. This will allow us the opportunity to accurately judge what corrections are necessary as we are planning the indicated restorations.

The face-bow allows the operator to gain estimated axis-orbital relations for the upper cast. An ear-type face-bow (Whip-Mix*) for mounting the maxillary cast is not too difficult to master. The external auditory meati are used for the condylar or posterior reference points, and the nasion is used as the anterior reference point. This is an arbitrary transverse axis location and, in many instances, it is fairly accurate even when compared to the kinematic location of the transverse axis technique.[65] Stuart designates this ear-type face-bow as a self-centering caliper which eliminates the added time required to center and align the articulator to other types of face-bows (Fig. 7-114).

The anterior stop pin is removed from the articulator, and the condyle balls are set to the S, M, or L position, as indicated when the ear face-bow was in place. The fossae are likewise set with the proper spacers to agree with the condyle positions. The depressions on the medial side of the plastic projections on the face-bow are placed over the pin projec-

*Whip-Mix Corp., Louisville, Ky.

A 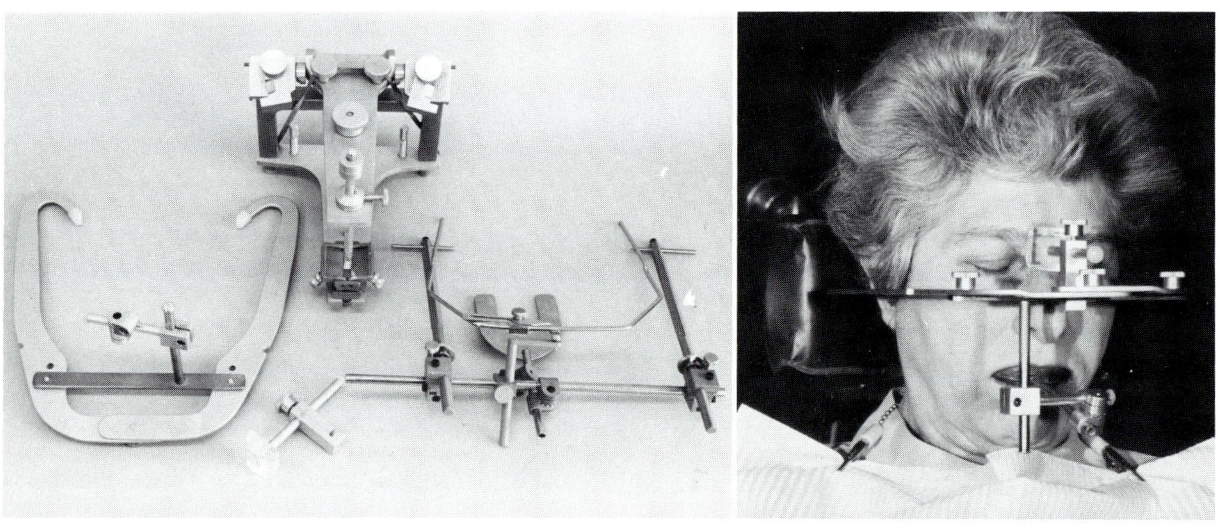 B

Fig. 7-114. A, The ear-type face-bow (a self-centering caliper which eliminates the added time required to center and align the articulator to other types of face-bows), the Whip-Mix Articulator, and the hinge-bow set up that can also be used. **B,** The application of the ear-type face-bow.

tions on the outside of the fossae elements. The front of the upper articulator frame will then rest on the cross bar of the face-bow. Again the three screws on the upper surface of the face-bow are tightened. The upper cast to be mounted is placed in the depressions in the upper surface of the bite fork, and stone is applied between the cast and the upper mounting plate. This will complete an estimated axis-orbital transfer. The lower cast is mounted next by making use of the centric bite after placing the anterior stop pin in its holder at the desired opening (Fig. 7-115). It is necessary to lower the anterior stop pin or incisal pin slightly so as to compensate for the thickness of the wax record in mounting the mandibular cast. This allows for the upper and lower members of the articulator to be more nearly parallel when the record is removed and the casts brought together. The condylar spheres are locked in the retruded position by the Bennett angle guides after the Bennett angle guides are turned to the negative position, and the articulator is inverted on the bench top. I am in the habit of holding the mandibular cast in the imprints of the record until

A

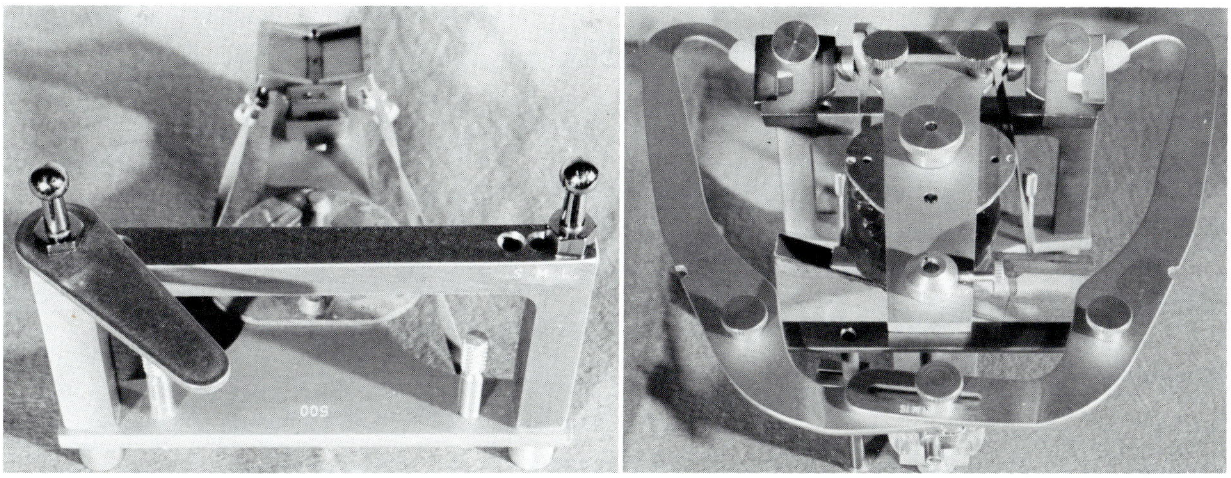

B

Fig. 7-115. A, Anterior stop pin is removed and condyle balls set to S, M, or L position as indicated when ear face-bow was in place. **B,** The ear face-bow lined up on the articulator.

A

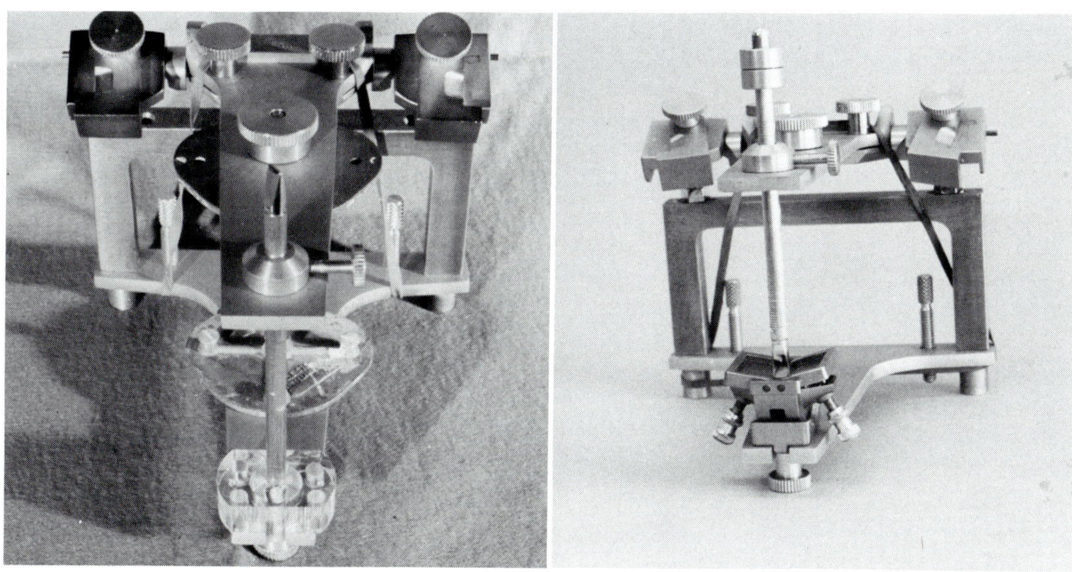

B

Fig. 7-116. A, The Whip-Mix Articulator with plastic anterior stop table. **B,** The Whip-Mix Articulator with adjustable anterior table.

the stone sets, and I always check the accuracy of the interocclusal record by use of the split-cast method. (Refer to Chapters 3 and 4 for a detailed discussion of the split-cast method.)

The Whip-Mix Articulator* is designed as a mechanical likeness of the human jaws. The condyle balls are mounted on the lower frame and can be spaced from large (124 mm.) to medium (110 mm.) to small (96 mm.), according to the size of the head. The adjustment is made by changing the condyle balls to the S, M, or L holes according to the scale on the front of the face-bow when applied to the face. This articulator has all condyle guidance on the upper frame as in the human masticatory system. The anterior stop pin is graduated in 1 mm. increments above and below the parallel of the bows. The anterior stop table is plastic and can be adjusted to any case by adding plastic or grinding. An adjustable anterior table is also available (Fig. 7-116).

For precise transverse axis location, the Whip-Mix Articulator is provided with center marks on the outer side of the fossae. These indicate the axis of opening and closing of the instrument. A mounting fixture (Whip-Mix No. 8700 mounting fixture) allows the lower frame to be used as a mounting jig. Calibrated condylar axis indicator pins can then be extended to meet the axis indicator points of the hinge-bow. Elevating screws are provided in the lower frame to facilitate this alignment (Fig. 7-117).

Positional wax records (centric, protrusive, right and left laterals) do not require too much time to execute and to set the articulator with them. Prior to making the protrusive record, both horizontal condylar inclination guidances are set to an average value of 35 degrees and the Bennett angle guides are set at 0 degrees. To set the condylar inclination and side shift, be sure to release the rubber band on the articulator so that the casts can rest freely in the interocclusal records. The protrusive record is made with the mandible positioned in a 5 mm. straight protrusive position. To set the articulator for protrusive position rotate the horizontal condylar guidance until it lightly touches the top of the condylar sphere and tighten the thumb or holding screw. Always support the casts in the positional records rather firmly.

Lateral wax records are made to establish horizontal inclination of the nonworking condylar path, and to adjust the Bennett angle guide for the Bennett movement of the working condyle.[64] The extent of the lateral movement used in obtaining the record is approximately 5 mm. To set the condylar inclination and side shift, one lateral bite is placed between the mounted casts with the condyle path guide and side-shift guide loosened on the advancing condyle side. With the upper cast seated firmly in the check bite, the angle of the condyle path is set by bringing the guide down to contact the condyle ball and tightening the holding screw. Then the side-shift guide is brought in contact with the condylar element. While applying

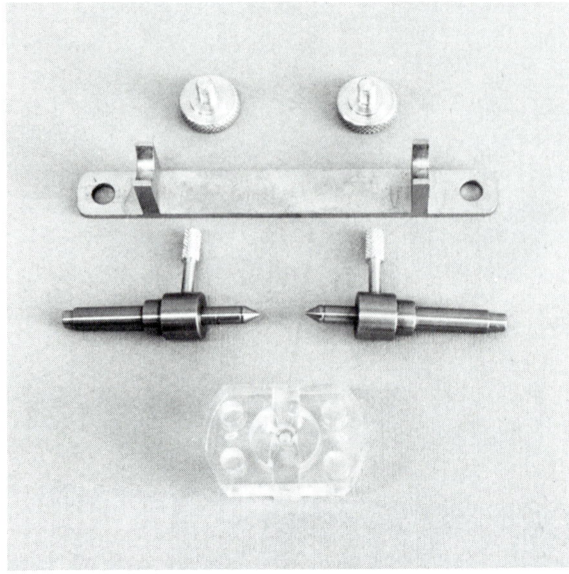

Fig. 7-117. Mounting fixture for precise transverse axis location.

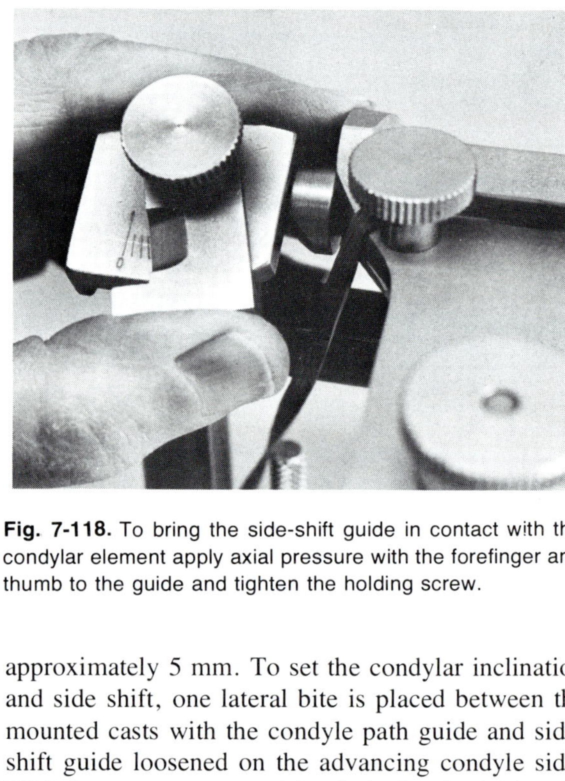

Fig. 7-118. To bring the side-shift guide in contact with the condylar element apply axial pressure with the forefinger and thumb to the guide and tighten the holding screw.

*Whip-Mix Corp., Louisville, Ky.

axial pressure with the forefinger and thumb to the guide, the dentist tightens the holding screw (Fig. 7-118). By using this pressure in setting the side-shift guides, possible errors in recording the Bennett movement can be avoided. This procedure is repeated for the opposite lateral bite. All articulator settings are marked on the patient's record card.

The plastic incisal table or guide can be moved anteriorly or posteriorly so that the rounded end of the incisal guide pin will be centered in the depression of the guide. The plastic is then ground to the proper contour to provide the correct incisal guidance.

If the adjustable incisal table or guide is used in place of the plastic guide, the customary procedure is followed to set the adjustments, using the chisel-shaped end of the incisal guide pin.

Side-shift guides are now available for each side calibrated for an immediate side shift of 0.25 to 1 mm. in 0.25 mm. intervals. A spring-operated arm on the lower member of the articulator engages a notch on the posterior edge of the upper member. Pressure from the spring returns the upper member to the centric position when the upper member is released.

With these settings we will be greatly helped in making proper cast analysis, such as prematurities, the why of wear facets, cusp pathways during the excursive movements, etc., and they will be of great importance in planning the execution of any selective grinding and necessary restorative procedures. Selective grinding (and charting) of the articulator-mounted casts will reveal the interferences which are causing improper relationships.

Ramfjord[66] has said that the most common occlusal interference acting as a trigger mechanism for bruxism and functional disturbance of the temporomandibular joints is located in the range of mandibular movement between centric relation and centric occlusion. Positional records do not provide information concerning the shapes of the mandibular fossae as precise as that obtained with pantographic tracings of mandibular movement. However, this method is good for cast analysis and simple or less complex procedures.

An important objective that should not be overlooked in our efforts to obtain a satisfactory end result is to make certain that the patient's intercuspation has even pressure on both sides, and that the bicuspids close simultaneously with the molars. We want mesiodistal as well as bilateral equal closure. The finished occlusion should have the maximum intercuspation with the jaw rearmost, midmost, and uppermost; any other contact between the upper and lower teeth is

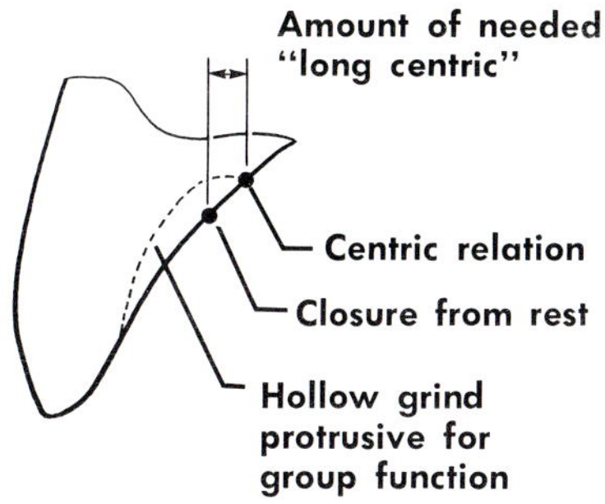

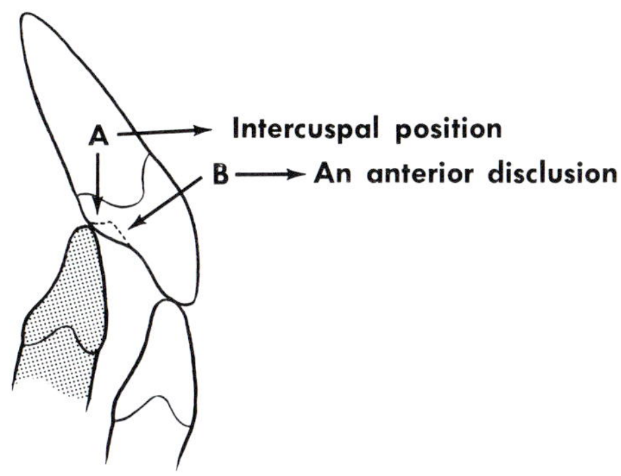

Fig. 7-119. "Centric relation" and "long centric." (Adapted from Dawson, Peter: Steps in harmonizing the anterior guidance, and Lundeen, Harry: Occlusal morphologic consideration for fixed restorations, Dent. Clin. N. Am., pp. 649-661, July, 1971.)

relegated to the anterior teeth outside the chewing cycle.

After the bicuspids and molars are relieved of eccentric contacts, the centric relation intercuspation can be made because the eccentric relations have been consulted. In waxing or any occlusal adjustment, we must test the eccentric relations first to make sure that our centric relation contacts are not destroyed in the eccentric excursions.[67]

Another important objective in our efforts to obtain good end results that is not to be overlooked is a clear understanding of what is meant by "centric relation" and "long centric." Dawson[68] expresses it very clearly: "*Centric relation is a precise point. The term 'long centric' refers to permitting the patient to close either in centric relation or slightly anterior to it (protrusive) at the same vertical dimension.* Some patients require no 'long centric.' Their centric relation closure and their closure from rest position are identical. Most patients require from .1 mm. to .5 mm. of anterior freedom from centric relation. Centric relation is used in swallowing and heavy chewing, and rest closure is used for light chewing and part of the heavy chewing cycle'' (Fig. 7-119).*

Amsterdam[69] has said: ''Conceptually, centric relation must be slightly anterior to the extreme condylar position as ultimately determined by the distensibility of ligaments. The distance between the extreme, strained terminal condylar position and the one in which the musculature and the ligaments are in a state of balance is usually not clinically measurable. The conceptual difference between the strained and the unstrained position must be kept in mind when one is attempting to locate the ideal harmonious relation between the temporomandibular articulation and the maximum intercuspation of the teeth.''†

Bellanti, [70] in my opinion, gives us an important reason why the semiadjustable articulator cannot be used in some cases. ''The semi-adjustable articulator is capable of reproducing intercondylar width in small and medium range with only a small error, but the large adjustment did not allow adequately for the possible range of patient variation, and this error would require more than minimal intraoral adjustment of a prosthesis in eccentric positions.''‡

So, in cases that call for rather large intercondylar width, we need an articulator with a wide range of intercondylar width adjustment and with posterior, medial, and superior fossa walls that can be adjusted. In order to accurately ''set'' such an instrument it is necessary to resort to pantographic tracings (Fig. 7-120).

Before a discussion of pantographic tracings is undertaken, a few important points should be brought out. Observations are that the action of the mandible is movement in three planes:—horizontal, vertical, and sagittal—and that these movements cause rotation about three different centers—horizontal (transverse axis), vertical, and sagittal. During function, movement in these planes and rotation about these centers occur simultaneously. If the rotational centers can be located and registered, these registrations could then be transferred to a mechanical counterpart, an articulator, whose mandibular member is so constructed that it would also move in the same three planes, with rotation about the same three centers.[71]

Location of the transverse axis orients the axis in one plane, the location of the center of rotation orients the axis in another plane. If we can locate the two axes, we automatically locate the third (sagittal) axis; the three axes coincide at a point center (Fig. 7-121).

We must differentiate between two terms which are often used—a ''changing axis'' and a ''moving axis.'' Granger[72] has said that (1) a ''changing axis'' is not the same as a ''moving axis''; the opening axis and the closing axis are ''changing axes''—they are different every time they operate, and (2) the transverse axis is a ''moving axis,'' always moving with the mandible, yet unchanging in its relation to tooth closures.

''In engineering, it is axiomatic to say that a hinge always dictates the mathematics of motion. Therefore, all rotating joints, whether they be associated with a biologic entity or a mechanical device, are responsive to and governed by the laws of motion. A basic requisite in contending with the mathematics of rotary motion is the determination of the center of rotation and its relation to the involved parts.

''It can be stated that the determination of axial centers is essential in order that the opening and closing arc of motion of the mandible together with the angle of the arc be identical in the articulator, as it is in the skull.''*

It is the individual's musculature which directs and places the condyle in its firmest fulcral bearing in the fossa. Centric relation denotes both condyles in their firmest bracing contact, and the only motion possible in this relationship is vertical rotation. Aside from the necessity of employing centric relation as a constant reference point is its value in the pivotal rotation of the condyle from eccentric relation to centric relation. The end of this movement should find all the posterior teeth contacting simultaneously. This act enables the masticatory forces to be dissipated over the greatest supporting area, thereby reducing traumatic impact of tooth closure.[73]

Clinically, it has been found that when difficulty is encountered in locating the axial centers, the certainty of registering centric relation will be equally troublesome. No centric relationship record should be trusted unless it is obtained under load.

All the paths of motion of the mandible are circular paths, and properly articulated teeth with their parabolic cusp form follow these paths, as dictated by the temporomandibular joint.

There are no flat planes of mandibular motion, and there are no flat planes on the cusps designed by

*From Dawson, Peter E.: Personal communication.

†From Amsterdam, Morton: Personal communication.

‡From Bellanti, Neal D.: The significance of articulator capabilities, J. Prosthet. Dent. **29**(3):269-275, 1973.

*From Dykins, William R.: Lecture notes and personal communication.

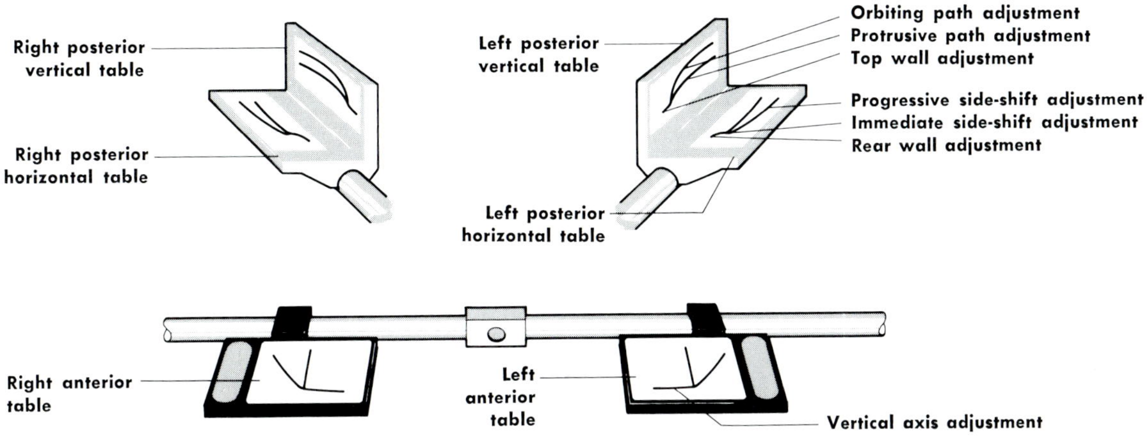

Fig. 7-120. Correlation of pantographic scribings to excursive movements. (Courtesy Denar Corp., Anaheim, Calif.)

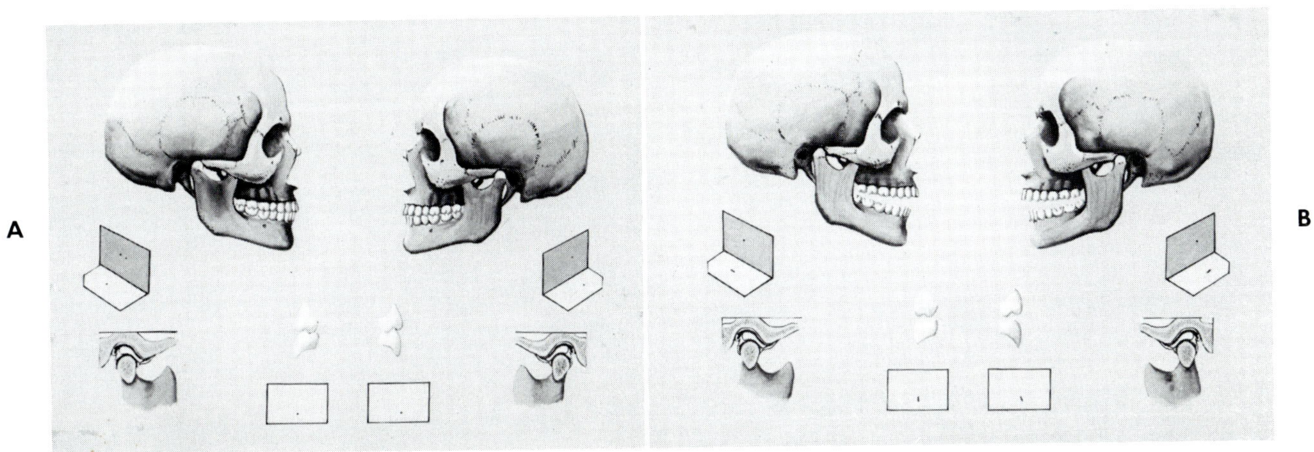

Continued.

Fig. 7-121. Axial centers of rotation. These composite drawings show the relationship of the head of the condyles to the recording plates and the teeth. Illustrated is **A,** centric position, **B,** when a pure hinge movement is performed the heads of the condyles rotate in the glenoid fossa. The maxillary and mandibular teeth move away from one another, and four of the six tracing plates record movement. Only the vertical plates, on which is registered the condylar curvature and angulation, show pure rotation, **C,** straight protrusive movement—maxillary and mandibular incisors are in an edge-to-edge position. A pure protrusive movement is a two-dimensional movement—mandible moves forward (horizontal) and downward (vertical) with no lateral (sagittal) movement, **D,** left lateral movement, **E,** right lateral movement. We notice in these movements that the balancing condylar element becomes the working condyle, and the working condylar element becomes the balancing condyle (and vice versa), and thus there are two condylar elements capable of both rotation and translation in two and three planes. Through this combination are produced the varied and complex movements of the mandible, and **F,** arrow indicates the diagonal arcuate surface of the medial aspect of the condyle that articulates in a lateral movement. The resultants of this diagonal surface are the vertical and sagittal centers of rotation. (Courtesy A. J. De Pietro.)

C D E F

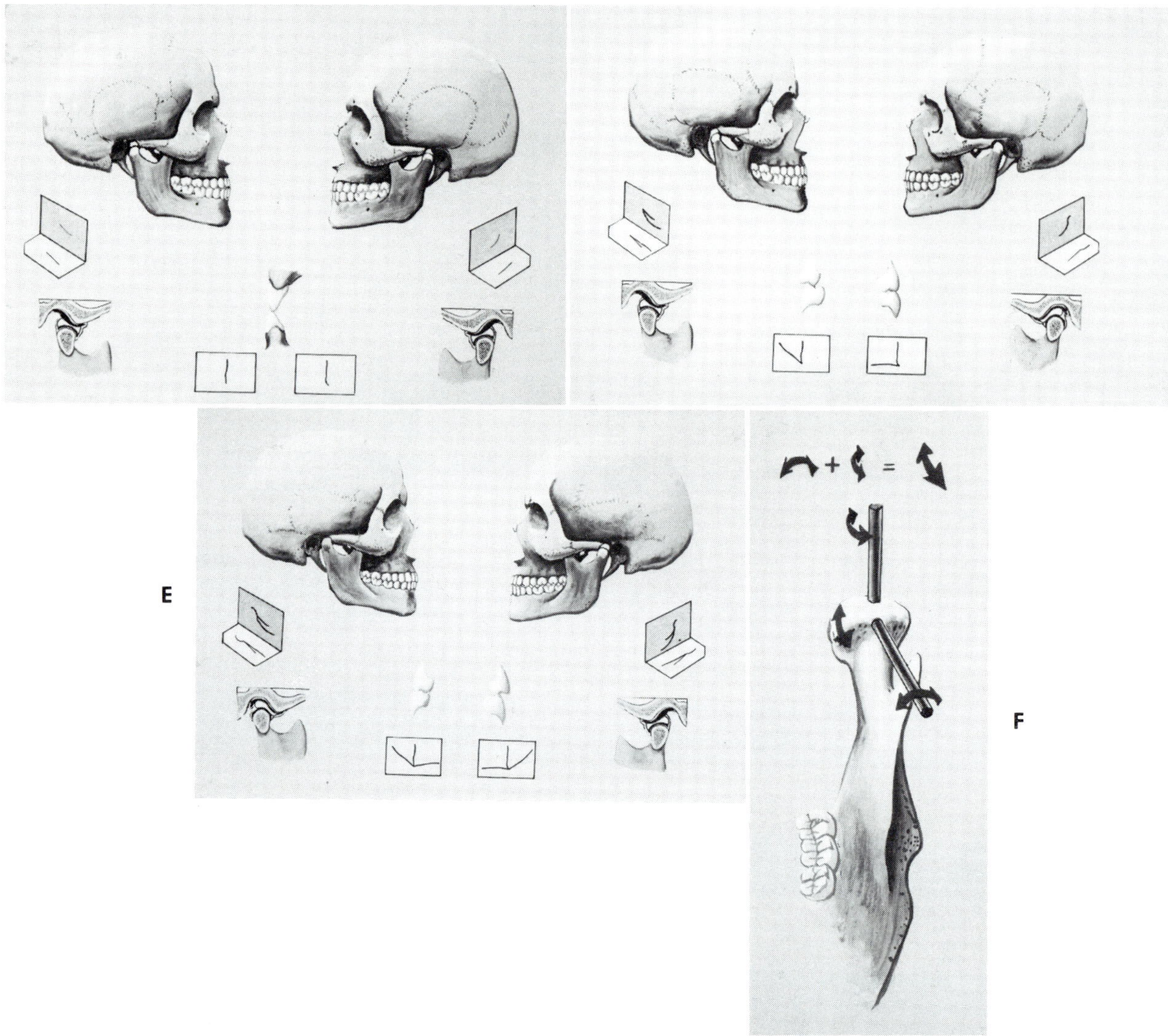

Fig. 7-121, cont'd. For legend see p. 327.

nature to harmonize with this type of motion. The appearance of flat planes on any cusp is a result of abnòrmal wear and is an indication of a lack of harmony between that cusp and the path of mandibular motion as dictated by the temporomandibular joints. Properly formed and properly related cusps travel around each other to masticate food efficiently and to maintain the direction of force through the long axes of the teeth. Our ability to treat and save mouths is directly related to our ability to capture and transfer jaw function to the restoration. And, as so aptly put by Stein,[74] cuspal design of restorations should be recognized as a directive for tissue response, and not as a matter of mechanistic creation.

Pantographic tracings graphically reflect anatomic characteristics of the temporomandibular articulations which influence mandibular paths of movement.

The fact of the envelope of motion has been proved. The pantograph can, if properly handled, scribe the anterior, posterior, and lateral limits of that envelope. It can also scribe the sequence of the motion from one position to another.[75] The positional wax records leave unknown that position of the movement between points (Fig. 7-122).

Pantographic tracings are possible to achieve within a reasonable amount of time. Anything less than a pantograph has the potential of compromise in many cases, and the articulator being used must be capable of

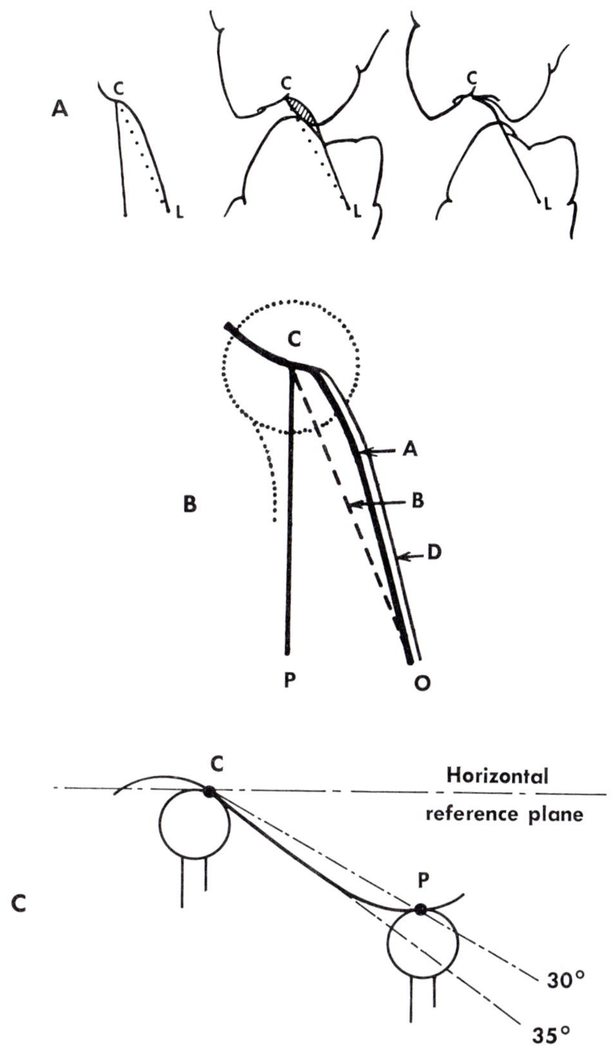

Fig. 7-122. A, Positional records leave unknown that position of the movement between points. Dotted line shows result of positional record, heavy line the properly scribed area, and the hashed area represents the amount of occlusal irritation introduced. **B,** Path *A* represents the orbiting condylar path of a patient. An articulator can be adjusted to (1) simulate the border movement (path *A*), (2) simulate a path within the border movement (path *B*), or (3) simulate a path beyond the border movement (path *D*). **C,** The condyle is in centric relation at point *C* and in a protrusive position at point *P*. Bold line *CP* represents the protrusive condylar path of the patient. Dotted line *CP* represents the straight protrusive condylar path guide of an articulator set to checkbite records. (Courtesy Denar Corp., Anaheim, Calif.)

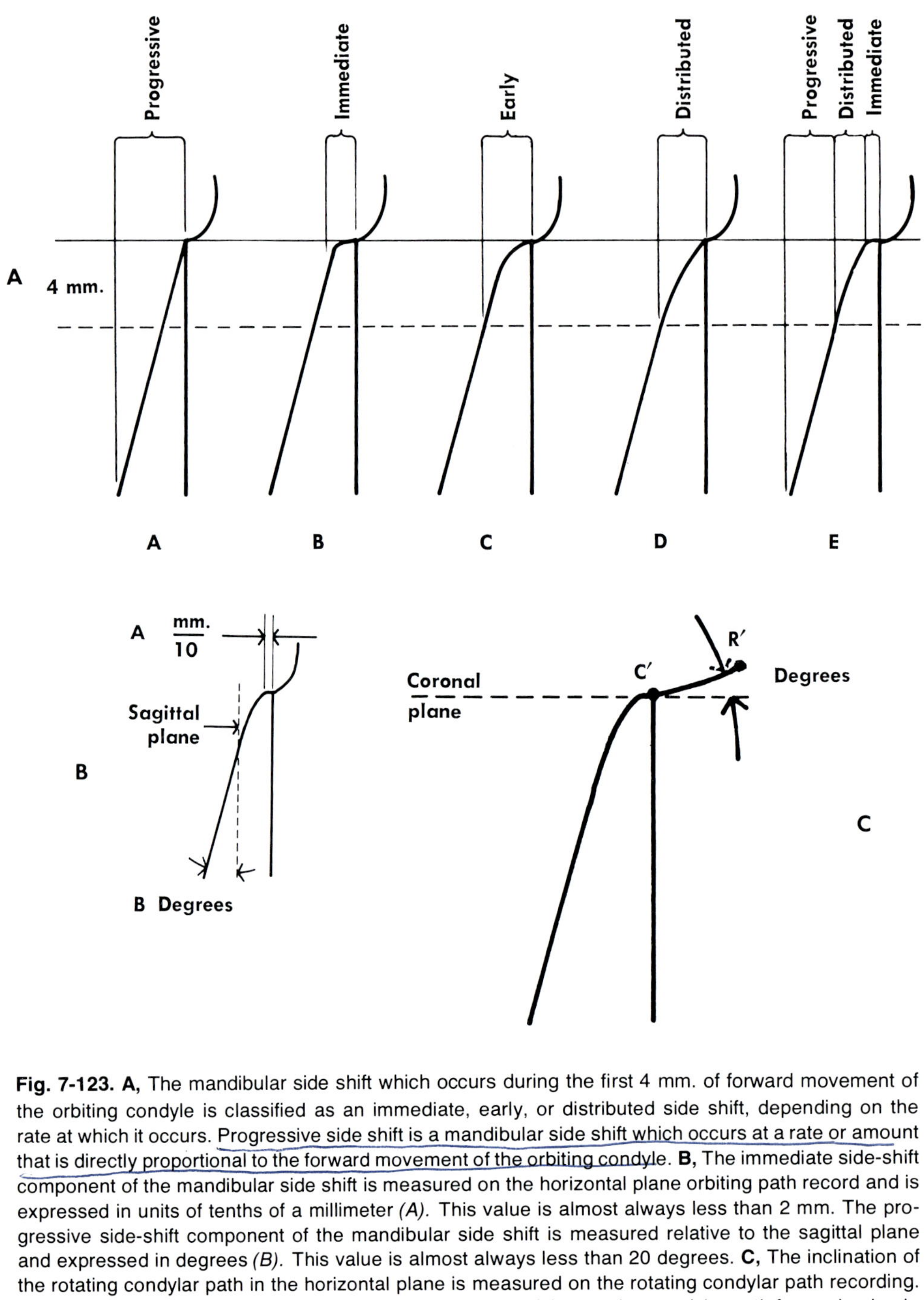

Fig. 7-123. A, The mandibular side shift which occurs during the first 4 mm. of forward movement of the orbiting condyle is classified as an immediate, early, or distributed side shift, depending on the rate at which it occurs. Progressive side shift is a mandibular side shift which occurs at a rate or amount that is directly proportional to the forward movement of the orbiting condyle. **B,** The immediate side-shift component of the mandibular side shift is measured on the horizontal plane orbiting path record and is expressed in units of tenths of a millimeter *(A)*. This value is almost always less than 2 mm. The progressive side-shift component of the mandibular side shift is measured relative to the sagittal plane and expressed in degrees *(B)*. This value is almost always less than 20 degrees. **C,** The inclination of the rotating condylar path in the horizontal plane is measured on the rotating condylar path recording. This measurement is expressed as degrees of inclination of the rotating condylar path forward or backward relative to the coronal plane. (Courtesy Denar Corp., Anaheim, Calif.)

adjusting for those essential elements of the determinants of mandibular movement which are of clinical importance. (For a discussion of determinants of occlusion refer to Chapter 17.)

A dentist who is knowledgeable of the initial or immediate side shifting of the mandible and its influence on occlusal anatomy appreciates that this motion must be recorded and reproduced in laboratory equipment upon which the occlusal restoration is to be constructed. Without this recording and reproduction, the restoration may require extensive occlusal correction in the mouth to avoid possible resultant disease. Therefore, the recording of this sideshift of the mandible is essential to a proper approach of recording jaw motion[63] (Fig. 7-123).

In summation, we can say that the existence of a transverse axis in the condyles is an important factor in diagnostic and restorative procedures. This axis can be located and transferred to an instrument for the accurate study and diagnosis of occlusal patterns. Casts mounted on any instrument without the hinge-bow transfer reveal little of the dictating influence of the temporomandibular joints. Unless casts can be occluded by closing them on the same arc of closure as that exhibited by the patient, erroneous conclusions may be drawn concerning existing occlusal patterns and the need for restorative procedures for the patient.

Always keep in mind that another important factor is the influence of the proprioceptors in the supporting tissues of the teeth, with their resultant neuromuscular patterns.

Destructive influences of abnormal occlusal patterns and their pathologic sequelae go unnoticed for the simple reason that the dentist does not recognize what he sees, and, in my opinion, a person sees only what he knows.

The necessity of proceeding in each step of the chosen technique with caution and extreme attention to detail cannot be overemphasized. Only by observing the utmost care in making measurements, casts, mountings, etc. can there be any hope of success in the outcome of the case at hand. The possibility of reestablishing the original contours and function of the mouth is entirely up to us—our willingness to study, observe, reflect, and work hard. Welter[19] has expressed it so well: "Minimal effort, in the accomplishment of good work, is secured only through maximal knowledge and its appropriate application."*

*From Welter, Charles J.: Personal communication.

In accepting new techniques and higher ideals, we do so only at the expense of greater vision and vigilance. Clinical evidence is the best criterion by which any technique, philosophy, or procedure can be evaluated.

CONCEPT OF MODERN DENTISTRY*

William R. Dykins, D.D.S., F.A.C.D., F.I.C.D.**

A concept of dentistry must be developed first in order to envision a comprehensive view of dentistry that reflects its needs, values, and associated problems. This concept must be responsive to and judged in relation to the involved biologic, anatomic, physiologic, and mathematical facts. In general, dentistry has been interpreted as being represented by tooth decay, tooth eruptions, extractions, restorations, orthodontic corrections, and periodontal bone loss. Yet the quest for knowledge of the stomatognathic system has advanced the role of factors such as genetic variables, condyle-fossa fulcral potential, the neuromuscular defensive mechanism, fossa remodeling, and the biochemistry of nutrition, and these must be evaluated.

The dominant problem

For the most part, dentistry may be looked upon as a biomechanical art, for it is universally agreed that an important function of teeth is to bite and chew food. An analysis of this fact leads to the conclusion that the dissipation of forces produced by mastication or other jaw movement is the dominant problem to be considered.

The reduction of a bolus of food to a state for swallowing demands the use of force. The effect of force upon a human being is expressed by the word trauma. In turn, trauma is interpreted as an enemy of cell life since the disturbance of a nucleus of a cell will either cause the death of the cell or alter its form. Force is defined as power directed against resistance, and it is as effective in the mouth as anywhere else. Somehow this fact seems to be absent or overlooked in developing a dental concept.

Development of the concept

MATHEMATICAL VIEW

The idea that mastication can be evaluated mathematically is questioned by many dentists inasmuch as a

*From J. Prosthet. Dent. **29**(2):191-194, 1973.

**Former President and Secretary, Pennsylvania State Board of Dental Examiners; Research Senior Instructor, Hahnemann Medical College and Hospital.

human being has the quality of life. They believe that, due to its biologic nature, the act of mastication cannot be construed in a mathematical light. Nevertheless, nature must respect and respond to mathematical laws or no law would have validity.

Since force is an integral part of all functions, the development of a dental concept should be directed to the problems inherent with its use and abuse. Reducing this to simple enumeration, the masticatory mechanism is made up of a fixed and a movable jaw, a sliding hinge, teeth, musculature, ligaments, tongue, lips and cheeks; the anatomic parts which can be controlled are the teeth and temporomandibular joints.

With the thought that consistent and identical answers in mathematics demand the employment of constants, within the boundaries of practicality, the teeth and their position in bone could be classified as a constant; and again, with the thought of striving for constants, a study of the joints both clinically and physiologically is revealing.

CLINICAL OBSERVATIONS

Clinically, the temporomandibular joints will function with any occlusal surface known to dental science whether or not the condyles are braced solidly in the fossae. Due to the second phenomenon, a difference of opinion will always exist among the various clinical disciplines relative to accepting the idea of maximum bracing of the condyle in the fossa for fulcral potential, as well as initiating the constant in the mathematics of function.[1] However, if the therapy of all the clinical disciplines demanded the elimination and replacement of the occlusal surfaces of the teeth, all would be faced with the same problem of relating two jaws to each other. All disciplines would understand that it is essential to strive for a constant—a repeatable and identical condyle-fossa occlusion-tooth relationship, generally referred to as centric relation. The fact that this relationship does not respond to the five senses suggests that it is not considered an anatomic entity.

Clinical experience has shown that roughly 20% of the temporomandibular joints can consistently return to an identical condyle-meniscus-fossa relationship by free closure, while around 65% need the assistance of an anterior fulcrum to register the maximum bracing relationship. The remaining joints never return to a consistent and identical relationship by any technique.

The conclusions reached by Fountain,[2] in his study of condyle-fossae relations on dry specimens, confirm these observations. His research also provides a probable explanation for some of our clinical failures.

HISTOLOGIC CONSIDERATIONS

There is no awareness of dissipation of force in the joint. The bearing surface of the interposed meniscus is composed of dense avascular connective tissue which is not capable of registering force.[3] Histologically, only the thickened borders of the meniscus are rich in vascularity. Consequently, when these borders are infringed upon in function and the hinge is compelled to dysfunction, various pain syndromes are manifested. Usually, relief from pain is obtained when the control of the condyle-meniscus-fossa relationship is not dictated solely by the occlusion of the teeth. Clinical therapy, such as the placement of an occlusal splint, interarch occlusal equilibration, and complete occlusal rehabilitation, has confirmed this fact.

CONCEPTS OF PHYSICS

LEVER PRINCIPLE

The mandible is considered a third-class lever. In the act of mastication, the demands for the degree of fulcral effect are governed by (1) the quality and nature of the food, (2) the size of the bolus of the food, and (3) the resistance to breakdown of the food.

To utilize the lever principle, it is necessary to employ a fulcrum. Clinically, nature insured the application of the fulcrum by providing the physical contact of both the condyle and the disc with the posterior articular lip of the fossa[4] and by mandibular suspension with muscles and ligaments.

Unfortunately, there is no repeatable constancy in registering a jaw relationship with muscles and ligaments. Fortunately, however, the physical contact within the joint initiates the constancy upon which the mathematics of function must be predicted. Occlusions based upon this premise subscribe to the engineering practice of dissipating forces over the greatest area possible.

TYPES OF MOTION

In mechanics, a fixed hinge always dictates the path of motion of a moving part, and the same mathematical laws prevail for a sliding hinge, such as the temporomandibular joints. In function, these joints rotate in the vertical, horizontal, and sagittal planes and at any point of translatory movement. In addition, these joints are capable of a bodily side shift (the Bennett movement) which adds another motion to the complexity of our interpretation of joint physiology.

Only a biologic entity could comply to all mathematical determinants and blend them into one fluid motion.

Dental articulators perform as mechanical equivalents of the chewing stroke, *but* they never demonstrate its fluidity.

Principles of basic engineering

The basis of all engineering design and performance originates with either a point or a plane and, in the case of a moving body, with the form and direction of movement. These principles lead to the need for understanding and appreciation of the axial centers of rotation, the hinge axis, the curve and slant of the condylar path, the curve of Spee, the Wilson curve, and the parabolic cusp form.

RATIONALE FOR PARABOLIC CUSP FORM

Analyzing the why of parabolic cusp form indicates that nature responds to the disciplines of mathematics and physics and that motion is the primary determinant of the shape of the contacting occlusal surface. Physics teaches the scissor principle as being the most efficient and as requiring the least amount of effort to produce work. The application of the theory of the scissors can be observed in the occlusal surface of a newly erupted, well-formed posterior tooth. This surface is a series of slightly raised ridges on a parabolic surface (the cusp) and is opposed by a concavity (the fossa) with sides having similar raised ridges.

MECHANICAL ANALOGY

Additional confirmation supporting the response of nature to the influence of mathematics and physics is seen in the application of the mechanical axiom which states that the working surface of any moving object must be compatible to the form of motion. The reciprocating motor illustrates this fact. In the bearing crankshaft, the contacting surfaces are circular, thus harmonizing with the rotary form of the motion. In the piston block, the contacting planar surfaces are compatible to the translatory behavior of the piston. Since the chewing stroke is a composite of rotary and translatory movement, nature adhered to the mechanical principle by creating the parabolic form of the cusp. The working surfaces of the posterior teeth are neither planar nor circular, but lend themselves to both forms of movement. In fact, it can be said that motion is the dominant determinant for the need of the cuspal type of occlusion.

Summary

The knowledge of the factors related to adequate dissipation of force is not complete. Present-day sophisticated occlusal systems have contributed to this goal. Yet, in the end, the age-old problem of bringing two jaws together accurately at the right place still remains.

REFERENCES

1. Dykins, W. R.: A consideration of centric relation, J. Prosthet. Dent. **20:**494-497, 1968.
2. Fountain, J. W.: The temporomandibular joints—a fulcrum, J. Prosthet. Dent. **25:**78-84, 1971.
3. Sicher, H.: The temporomandibular joint, Springfield, Ill., 1951, Bannerstone House, p. 6.
4. Sicher, H.: The temporomandibular joint, Springfield, Ill., 1951, Bannerstone House, p. 7.

OCCLUSION, ARTICULATION AND THE DEVELOPMENT OF A FUNCTIONAL MASTICATORY APPARATUS

Charles J. Welter, B.A., B.S., D.D.S., F.A.C.D., F.I.C.D.*

What do you need in an occlusion?

MINIMUM

1. We need some cusps to engage and chew food.
2. We need an occlusal table upon which to place food.
3. We need centric contacts to maintain posterior vertical support.

GOAL—OPTIMUM OCCLUSION

An occlusal design that is compatible and acceptable to the patient which will conserve remaining tissue, conserve energy, and will be functionally efficient.

Do Not Want

Lack of harmony, overload, torque, less efficiency than possible practically, damage to tissue (supportive, muscular, or solid). Briefly, anything which leads to pain, damage, or destruction.

Need to Know

Resistance capabilities of the tissues we are working with (the more delicate the situation, the more delicate the work).

a. Condition of ridge
b. Condition of bony support
c. Amount of bony support
d. Condition of abutment teeth, (length, quality, vital, nonvital, etc.)
e. Condition of opposing teeth or restorations

* Assistant Clinical Professor, Department of Occlusion, University of Minnesota School of Dentistry.

f. Condition of remaining teeth
g. Tongue size
h. Vertical dimension
i. Musculature type
j. Movement range and pattern of mandible in relation to maxilla
k. General host condition
l. *General Occlusal Examination*

1. *Midline*

MAXILLARY

_______ ideal
_______ to right _______ mm.
_______ to left _______ mm.

MANDIBULAR

_______ ideal
_______ to right _______ mm.
_______ to left _______ mm.

2. *Deflection of jaw on opening*

_______ none
_______ to right _______ mm.
_______ to left _______ mm.
_______ angular deviation
_______ confluent deviation

3. *Maximum opening:* _______ mm.
4. *Anterior overbite:* _______ mm.
5. *Anterior overjet:* _______ mm.
6. *Anterior slide:* _______ mm.
7. *Lateral slide*

_______ none
_______ to right _______ mm.
_______ to left _______ mm.

8. *Occlusal classification (first molar relationship)*

_______ class I
_______ class II (_______ mm.)
    _______ division 1
    _______ division 2
    _______ subdivision R
    _______ subdivision L
_______ class III (_______ mm.)

9. *Skeletal facial type*

_______ open bite
_______ deep bite
_______ class I
_______ class II
_______ class III

10. *Teeth in crossbite*

L _______________________ R

11. *Teeth in lateral guidance*

L _______________________ R

12. *Teeth in protrusive guidance*

L _______________________ R

13. *Heavy facets of wear*

L _______________________ R

14. *First contact in centric relation*

L _______________________ R

15. *Posterior fulcrums (balancing contacts)*

L _______________________ R

16. *Marginal ridge discrepancies*

L _______________________ R

17. *Periodontal breakdown areas*

L _______________________ R

18. *Jaw manipulation*

_______ easy
_______ normal
_______ difficult

19. *Presence of crepitus*

_______ right TMJ
_______ left TMJ
_______ with stethoscope
_______ without stethoscope

20. *Ear palpation*

_______ negative
_______ soreness
_______ right TMJ
_______ left TMJ

21. *Curve of Spee (anteroposterior)*

_______ normal
_______ exaggerated
_______ reversed
_______ flat
_______ distorted

22. *Curve of Wilson (transverse)*

_______ normal
_______ exaggerated
_______ reversed
_______ flat
_______ distorted

23. *Suspected bruxism*

_______ yes
_______ no

24. *Suspected oral habits*

_______ tongue thrust
_______ nail biter
_______ pipe smoker
_______ pencil chewer

25. *Patient awareness of clenching teeth*

_______ daytime
_______ upon awakening in morning
_______ in sleep (as told by others)
_______ part of mouth sore from clenching

26. *Presence of temporomandibular pain*

_______ none
_______ right side
_______ left side

27. *Presence of muscular pain*
    ________ none
    ________ neck muscles
    ________ masticatory muscles
    ________ bilateral
    ________ right side
    ________ left side
28. *Presence of headaches*
    ________ none
    ________ infrequently
    ________ occasionally
    ________ regularly
    ________ mild
    ________ severe
    ________ migraine type
29. *Tenderness to palpation*
    ________ masticatory muscles
    ________ temporal area
    ________ neck area

TERMS FOR CONSIDERATION

simplicity is achieved by eliminating all that is unnecessary. To accomplish this with success one must first know all the conditions or specifications relative to the case, and then the requirements for an optimum result relative to the particular patient. Only then can we eliminate those items which are excessive and unnecessary.

success is a term which is relative to the criteria of the evaluators.

optimum means all that is practically necessary in the simplest manner applicable to achieve success as evaluated by the patient as well as the dentist.

occlusion is a term which vaguely connotes a relationship of upper and lower teeth in some kind of contact. This relationship is evaluated as good, bad, or indifferent, depending on the evaluators' concept of what is optimum. It is the collective end result of the development and function of nerves, muscles, supportive structures, and teeth. It is a study of the statics and dynamics of form and functional relationships.

articulation relative to teeth is the fit or mesh of the teeth of one arch as they contact the opposite arch. It is generally visualized as a tooth arrangement without regard for the pertinence of the structures which bear the teeth. The patterns visualized are usually divided into the following: (1) cuspless (flat occlusals) and (2) cusped (anything other than flat).

cuspid rise is arch separation accomplished by virtue of an inclined plane on the lingual of the upper cuspid which is steep enough to make separation of the posterior teeth immediate and mandatory from centric relation. This is done without regard for movement patterns or capability of the mandible and is an arbitrary inclusion of design by the operator based usually upon a conception rather than a specification.

cuspid protection is an effective separation of mandibular and maxillary teeth (disclusion) accomplished by incorporating the curvatures, angulations, quantities, and sequence of motion into the design of the lingual surface of the upper cuspids in a manner which enhances the likelihood of forces being directed parallel to their long axes as the lower cuspid moves across them. It is a design which is relative to the functional capabilities of the individual patient and not a preconceived design of the operator.

group function means several teeth brought into contact simultaneously. This is a nonspecific description of a condition. The effectiveness of the situation is relative to its method of application. When used in ramping style the design could be of questionable value. When used to distribute forces in a direction compatible with and beneficial to the teeth involved, it is effective and often desirable. (Lateral forces should be minimal—vertical force or loads are preferable.)

working bite is that side toward which the mandible moves to gain a buccal cusp–to–buccal cusp relationship necessary for the application of chewing forces. The articulation of teeth in a working bite relationship is a contact of the inner slope of the upper buccal cusps with the outer slope of the lower buccal cusps. Problems arise usually from the difficulty surrounding ordinary methods of set up of teeth because the technician has no means of determining quantity or quality of contacting surfaces relative to the patient's muscular and movement capabilities. This lack of quantitative and qualitative specification introduces lateral forces into the restoration of an uncontrolled as well as unpredictable nature. Many operators rely upon adjustment in the mouth to correct for these discrepancies on the erroneous basis that the mouth is the best articulator. The unpredictable ability of the neuromuscular mechanism to respond correctly to the command of the dentist along with the surrounding limitations for vision, the difficulty encountered in achieving a mutually comprehensive method of communication between patient and dentist, plus a generally confused and misunderstood knowledge of the art of equilibration, would seem to create some speculation as to the predictable level of success.

balancing contacts are those contacts made by cusps along lateral routes other than the working contacts. Balancing contacts on either the working side of the mouth or the balancing side of the mouth are generally accepted as injurious.

cross-tooth balance occurs when both working and balancing (Bu and Li) cusps are brought into contact during the total excursive movement. True cross-tooth balance would be of an equalized nature; however, as in the working bite situation, it becomes a matter of successful measurement and architecture, exceedingly difficult to achieve with security. It is doubtful, if it should be accomplished, that it would be desirable. Cross-tooth and cross-arch balance means that all teeth remain in contact constantly in all movements of the mandible except when separation occurs upon deliberate opening. Many men claim patients become tooth conscious through constant contact. It also seems to promote excessive wear.

balance is an inappropriate term since balance should mean a vertical, precise loading. It has come to be a term which implies a lateral force on an inclined plane of unfavorable nature, particularly when dealing with natural teeth. Balance in its pure form is a contact thought to be desirable and necessary by contrast when dealing with full dentures.

curve of Wilson is the combination of the motions about the vertical axis and the sagittal axis which occur simultaneously, that is, their timing or sequence and amount or degree develop the curve of Wilson. This curve is the curvature or slant from the tip of the buccal cusp to the tip of the lingual cusp on the posterior teeth on one side, but is not necessarily a continuous, single curve from one side of the arch to the other.

curve of Spee is an anteroposterior curve which is developed in harmony with the curvature of the eminence and the anterior guidance. It should be designed in such a way as to maintain an even quantity of separation between upper and lower teeth as the mandible moves protrusively or laterally. Since this portion of the design is a combination of posterior and anterior guidance segments, one of which is fixed and the other variable depending on esthetics and tooth position, the curve of Spee is the most arbitrary portion of the occlusal design.

Principal elements of motion in the development of an acceptable, functional, masticatory apparatus (occlusion)

HINGE AXIS AND CENTRIC RELATION

The first consideration is to achieve a comfortable, even closure capability which will preclude excessive stress in any direction to the teeth or supportive structures. It is a diagnostic consideration, in fact a necessity, for the dentist to determine whether this is to be coincidental with an existing centric occlusion or in harmony with the hinge axis. The relevancy of the hinge axis becomes more obvious and necessary with the increase of replacement area as well as with the increase of traumatic and pathologic symptoms involved. Its use is a matter of degree of involvement. Not all patients exhibit a Bennett movement; many patients have an intercondylar distance close to that of fixed post articulators, many cases do not call for meticulous customizing of an instrument because of an unusual movement capability, but every one has a centric relation of some sort and every one exhibits tolerance or intolerance to it. Hinge axis is a center of rotation easily locatable. An approximation of hinge location is even easier.

The securing of accurate "centric relation bites" is technique which requires practice, experience, and the application of knowledge and reason. This is more difficult because it requires desire of a sincere nature, patience, and hours of practice. Nothing we desire, no compensatory short cut or rationalization, will change the fact. An accurate centric relation is a necessary, inviolate fact from which we cannot escape. The use of the hinge axis is synonymous with it, inseparable and inescapable. Modification is usable only to the limit of tolerance, and this is a speculative, immeasurable hope. To use less than accuracy is a crossed fingers approach. In this category I would place all the compensatory and/or quicky, or shotgun, techniques in dentistry. This is not condemnation or criticism of dentistry, but I believe it is a recognition of temptation and human nature. Until the operator has personally become convinced himself that failure or success is proportional to effort and knowledge, he will continue to have no change in his success ratio. Exactitude is precision and all else is wishful desire based on unfounded hope unless compensation is utilized and derived from the knowledge of the exact hinge axis. Centric relation is the first and most inviolate consideration. How you use it depends upon your understanding of it.

The second consideration in the development of a functional masticatory apparatus is the quantity of Bennett movement. In its absence most conventional techniques or styles of occlusion can have a measure of success providing that centric contact is accurate and the angulation of the cusps is not in excess of the patient's limitation. If, however, Bennett shift is present and not allowed for, the cusps become boxed in; lateral escape is impossible without severe lateral stress. Bennett movement is a lateral side shift bodily of the mandible which occurs immediately before and after centric contact is made in chewing excursions and bruxism motions. The wider the Bennett movement, the lower the cusp height. Bennett movement is peculiar to the individual and cannot be averaged. It can be duplicated accurately only through precise measurement. (Visualize the Bennett pathway as something similar to a straight driveway from the street to the garage. The farther from the street, the longer the driveway, and it may vary from house to house. If you do not use it but drive around it, something becomes damaged. If not the car [or the cusps] then the landscape [the supportive structures or musculature] must suffer. The pathway of Bennett shift may be horizontal; however, it can be an inclined pathway or curvature just as a driveway may be flat or an incline, or partly both, and may even include a curve. It can be compensated for but not guessed at. When designing a cusp and opposing groove relationship, the pathway and bulk or shape of the cusp must be considered along these lines. The extent and direction are a measurable and duplicate quantity.) Total Bennett range may be zero; however, I have seen it to be as much as ½ inch.

The third most important consideration is intercondylar distance or relative positions of the vertical axes. Intercondylar distance is the distance between the vertical centers of rotation of the right and left condyles. These centers of rotation determine the positions of the buccal and lingual cusps and groove direction of opposing teeth relative to one another in the same manner as the distance between the centers of two gears must be known to determine size, shape, and position of gear teeth of a harmonious nature. Think of a vertical center of rotation as a horizontal rotation of the body of the mandible from one side to another, parallel to the floor, with one condyle as the center of that motion. The opposite condyle would be the other center for the motion in the opposite direction. Since the teeth are borne upon the mandible, they scribe or follow arcs of curvature dependent upon the distance they are from the center of rotation and the location of one condyle relative to the other.

This fact is another reason for the use of a face-bow transfer. The face-bow will position the teeth at the proper distance from the condyle. It will not, however, provide intercondylar distance. If a marking or tracing of the motion were to be made, one motion would scribe one side of the Gothic arch tracing and the other side of the tracing would be the arc of the second condyle. To determine the location of the vertical axis, we place the respective condyle as the center of the motion which created the particular arc. The effect upon the anatomy of the teeth is to position the cusps relative to one another in such a manner as to allow an opposing cusp to pass between them. Its omission is comparable to assuming that two large posts were placed on either side of your driveway entrance, only to find that the turning capability of your car is such that you can only collide with the post.

Observe the positions of all cusps on a set of good models. Note the possibilities for free escape or entrance of the cusps of one tooth relative to its antagonist. Move the lower model left and right and note that there is relatively little freedom of choice. Examine the teeth of your patients in the areas of escape for wear facets and fracture. Take note of whether cusps ride over cusps, or through grooves. Observe freedom of muscular action where lack of harmony exists. Correlate muscular pain using the interfering areas as fulcrum points which would prohibit smooth and gradual muscular contracture but require abnormal spasm to get the teeth by one another. Note the sensitivity of the teeth involved, i.e., hot, cold, pressure, etc. Examine the actual bruxism path or pattern of the patient. Is he able to maintain contact upper to lower or does he involuntarily open and hop over to escape the interference? It is the intercondylar distance that determines precisely the mesiodistal position of the cusps relative to one another and their opponents. Intercondylar distance is widely variable from one patient to another, hence, it cannot be successfully averaged (varies from 4 to 5½ inches).

Sagittal displacement or rotation occurs about an imaginary axis which runs anteroposteriorly through each condyle. Think of sagittal rotation as a rise or fall of, for example, the right side of the mandible from the ceiling to the floor on an arc with the left condyle the center of this circular arc. It is relative to the centric position and is the quantity or distance of this up or down motion on either side. On the balancing side of the mandible it is the quantity of the downward displacement of the mandible as it travels from centric contact to the extreme of the stroke. Its rate is determined by the angle of the eminence. Its exact pathway is determined by the curvature or configuration of that eminence. On the working side the sagittal displacement is the directional deviation which occurs as the condyle rotates in the fossa. This can and does occur in spite of, and without regard for, the anterior guidance.

It is often found that while the anterior segment of the mandible is dropping down, the posterior segment is rising. If one imagines a cone in this area into which the rotating condyle would move, the direction taken (rise, fall, forward, or backward) could be anywhere within this area. It is, however, a specific pattern for each individual and therefore an item which must be measured. If, for example, the condyle should rise on its rotating movement the posterior teeth of the mandible would also rise. The effect, unless allowed for, would create a tendency for the lower teeth to dig into the opposing upper teeth as they leave centric relation and become fulcrums subject to great lateral force. Pathways or grooves might have to be deepened, the curve of Wilson made steeper, or cusps shortened in order to allow freedom of escape. If the condyle should drop, however, from centric position, the teeth also would drop and separation without lateral stress becomes much easier to accomplish. *This is the fourth most important consideration in the design of a "functional masticatory apparatus."*

The fifth consideration is not the least but is an integral part of all the preceding items: the timing or sequence of occurrence. It does no good to allow for any portion of the other items if the movement occurs before or after it should. It is the combination of the elements in proper sequence and harmony which will justify their inclusion into the analysis and subsequent fabrication.

The process of developing a functional occlusion is undertaken through the use of several methods and materials. Equilibration is the removal of interfering areas of tooth structure or restorations by selectively grinding upon them. Replacement or reorganization of teeth is done with wax and gold, porcelain or plastic, amalgam, and occasionally even steel. Gold should oppose either gold, amalgam, or natural tooth. Porcelain should oppose porcelain or natural tooth but not gold as a general rule. Teeth should have cusps to conserve energy and promote efficiency and should be designed to preserve tooth structure as well as supportive structures. The anatomy of the natural tooth is the objective in design. The placement of the parts is the result of functional demands. The occlusal anatomy is still only the occlusal portion and does not eliminate the requirements for proper design of vertical aspects of the tooth. Consideration for convexities, concavities, contacts, and dimension relative to the supportive structures is every bit as important, and perhaps even more important in some ways, than elimination of occlusal stress. A good occlusal design with bad gingival contour will negate all effort.

I believe that the easiest method of learning what constitutes occlusal design incorporates the following steps:

1. The individual analysis of jaw motion must be made via a pantographic tracing so that the movements can be visualized in the mind. Three-dimensional spatial configurations during motion of the mandible relative to the maxilla must be seen and understood.
2. The development in wax of teeth must be designed in harmony with these configurations of motion. This is best learned and appreciated through the add-on technique of waxing. It is essential to the dentist to know, for unless he does he can neither direct nor analyze the results of the fabrication of any restoration. It is easier to learn by add-on than carving simply because it is much more controllable and deliberate.
3. Equilibration provides the opportunity to see the results of the removal of interferences and enhances the respect for the effect of improper relationship.
4. The last step is the "set up" of prefabricated teeth, for this will show the variable modifications necessary to achieve the goals you have now learned to respect with reason.

The preceding explanations are pointed out in particular not to impress upon you a degree of complexity, for they are indeed simple to record, but rather as basics for understanding on how to simplify an occlusal design. Optimum occlusion requirements are not the discovery and addition of new restrictions upon design but rather the investigation of requirements and subsequent elimination of the unnecessary. Hinge axis location is an essential under certain circumstances. Slides from centric relation to centric occlusion should be eliminated under certain conditions. The greater the number of teeth being replaced, the more important these items become. The longer the saddle area of a distal extension partial denture, be it mucostatic base with precision attachment or acrylic with clasps, the greater the potential for the partial restoration to become a lever arm with increased chance of destruction to ridge and abutments. Anyone can design an occlusion. Anyone can make a mucostatic based partial denture. The trick is to increase the odds for success. The more you know about your patient's movement patterns, the more you can anticipate in design. Most often heard is the question—"What articulator should I buy?" The answer, once we know what potentials of motion and design there are, should be obvious. It is the same in any trade, profession, or general occupation. You use whatever instrument is needed to most practically and efficiently do the job. To my knowledge there are no instruments which will accommodate 100% of the situations encountered, just as there is no one occlusal design which is best for everyone. Every case is a custom job. Some instruments come very close in versatility. Some occlusal designs are more frequently used. It becomes necessary for your success to be able to know and apply. I believe that check-bites have gross inadequacies. Chew-in techniques are loaded with potential inaccuracies, are not readily readable or repeatable, and depend upon great skill and sense of feel for setting an instrument, with results of questionable accuracy. A pantographic tracing is readily readable, reproducible, and transferable and can be secured more rapidly than any check-bite or "chew-in" technique which is done with care. An average, nonrushed pantograph can be secured in not too long a time from start to finish and can save hours of future difficulty when applied where needed. Unfortunately almost everyone wishes for a simplified technique which excludes doing more than a minimal amount of preparation and procedure. I submit that minimal effort is secured only through maximal knowledge and its appropriate application. This is simplicity.

By this time you will realize, if you have read carefully, that I have not been writing about the process of reconstruction of the total mouth, but rather rehabilitation of the total mouth, even though the reconstructed area may be a partial denture, a three-tooth bridge, a single crown, thirty-two crowns, or perhaps no restoration at all. This is what constitutes the development of a functional masticatory apparatus. I have not discussed techniques but rather components and objectives. Techniques are readily available in many texts and postgraduate courses. It does no good to teach technique until after a reason for learning them has been developed. The effects of the dynamics of occlusion are multitudinous. I have touched on only a few. My intentions were to point out the components involved in the design of a functional occlusion, suggest how they might be planned for and recognized, and illustrate that the cure for a problem is related to the cause. I also realize that this is not "light" reading, but then the subject carries an equally heavy implication.

Pertinent points of analysis of a pantograph

GOALS

We are seeking to find the maximal directional movement possibilities of the mandibular body with special emphasis on its timing and spatial contours of motion relative to the maxillary body, which remains in a fixed position as an antagonist.

To accomplish this we must utilize positive anatomic relationships, find provable geometric centers of rotation relative to the individual, and assemble them on a controllable instrument which is then customized for sequence or timing of movement. The models of teeth are then attached to the instrument (articulator) relative to those same positive anatomic relationships and geometric centers of rotation. We then have an exact, but lifeless, *duplication of relationship* of the dental arches with both static and dynamic capabilities of the life form specially relative to the basic bony structures. The teeth are analyzed as tools placed in or upon the basic supportive structures, and their functional efficiency is judged with regard to form and harmony relative to one another, i.e., neighbor and antagonist, the supportive structures, and the timed, spatial limitations of the dynamic movement capabilities of the patient.

The method therefore requires an initial spatial orientation which both dental arches share in common with the skull of the patient. This orientation utilizes the hinge axis and a relocatable anterior point such as the infraorbital notch or a measured reference point on the side of the nose. The cast of the upper teeth is then transferred to an instrument and attached to the upper member utilizing these spatial coordinates (face-bow transfer). The mandible shares spatial relationship with the maxilla through the hinge axis. The lower member of the articulator also shares spatial relationship with the upper member through its hinge axis. Since the upper cast is mounted relative to the hinge axis of both the patient and instrument, the lower cast can be accurately related to the upper cast through the use of a bite registration taken with the mandible positioned at any vertical opening desired, so long as the body of the mandible is revolving only about its hinge axis position.

(1) Since teeth are tools of function, subject to stress or force, and (2) since that stress can be transferred to supportive structures with demonstrable damage, and (3) since muscular pain and spasm can be triggered by unbalanced resistance to these forces, and (4) since the temporomandibular joint mechanism can also be made to express pain through excessive strain placed upon them, and (5) since movements may occur within the limits imposed upon the mandible by ligaments and capability of the musculature, and (6) since forces placed upon teeth are the results of capability of contraction of musculature, the speed and direction of tooth contact, as well as duration and frequency, it would seem logical to measure and duplicate the perimeters of motion capability along with the timing factors so that restorative design within these perimeters may be accomplished, with control of force the primary objective. Since the motion of the mandible is a three-dimensional occurrence, a three-dimensional recording would be most desirable if it is repeatable, provable, and readable. A pantographic tracing fills this requirement with regard to the condylar elements. The anterior segment can be varied by the design of the teeth; however, compatibility with the posterior segment is the desire of design and hence dictates that design. The relevancy of a pantograph comes with its readability and subsequent usability (i.e., spatial transformation to an instrument). The analysis of the tracings provides the information necessary for articulator selection on the basis of a visual demonstration of the patient's capability of motion. The design of the occlusal surfaces follows as a matter of the combination of the dentist's philosophy of objectives coupled with the patient's three-dimensional movement capabilities and the selected instrument limitation. (It should be understood that unless the technician's knowledge of these areas is equal to and in agreement with that of the dentist, a totally incompatible product is inevitable. Not having this requirement fulfilled is similar to asking a drugstore clerk to fill a prescription, anticipating that because the clerk works in a drugstore he automatically is a pharmacist.)

LOGIC OF THE APPROACH

Virtually every item or object in our world which serves any type of usable function has placed upon it fundamental requirements of design relative to the function it is called upon to perform. Facial tissues must meet requirements for absorption and wet strength, tires must be able to withstand forces of abrasion, pressure, temperature, etc., heart pacemakers must control heart rate in the environment in which they are placed. Silver points must be trimmed to length, be compatible within the tissue, and be sterile and adequate to seal the canals in which they are placed. Stone of the dental variety must be dimensionally stable and of sufficient strength and texture to be used for duplication of tissues. The items are made to serve the function, and quality becomes obvious.

It is illogical to assume anything, particularly if there is the possibility that the assumption, if incorrect, can cause harm. It is impractical to assume, if it is within the realm of practical capability to know. The dentist would not function today if he consistently was denied the use of radiographs, even though there are other diagnostic tools available. One could hardly deny that the evaluation of character of tissues, vertical dimension, esthetic requirements, host condition and resistance, speech analysis, psychologic involvement, nature of the disease (i.e., analysis of condition) are portions of diagnosis and necessary to the determination of treatment. It should be equally obvious that to deprive the patient the advantage of an adequate analysis of his functional potential is illogical, for if restorations are made for him they should be designed with his functional potential in mind. I believe this cannot be accomplished without a recording of that functional range potential which is duplicable and repeatable.

The question of the use of a pantographic tracing seems to revolve about the words "practical, difficult, adequate, functional analysis, recording, duplicable, repeatable, functional range, normal, border movements, necessary," etc. Briefly stated, the fact of the envelope of motion has been proved. The pantograph can, if properly handled, scribe the anterior, posterior, and lateral limits of that envelope. It also can scribe the sequence of the motion from one position to another. Check-bites leave unknown that position of the movement between points. "Chew-ins" do not demonstrate that border movement capability has actually been accomplished and, depending upon how it is used, utilize many more compromises. Pantographic tracings are today possible to achieve quickly and practically. Less than a pantograph has the potential of compromise, which seems foolish. The debate of words then becomes irrelevant, for what is adequate, normal, and necessary is prepared for by knowing the borders and proving it.

PERTINENT POINTS OF ANALYSIS OF A PANTOGRAPH

1. Rate and relative angle of drop of condyle in protrusive as well as lateral movement
2. Intercondylar distance
3. Quantity of Bennett movement
4. Working condyle—vertical shift and anteroposterior shift
5. Quantitative and sequential (timing) analysis individually and collectively of 1 through 4

PURPOSE

To determine instrument requirements based upon capability requirements of the patient.

Figs. 7-124 to 7-134 will complement some areas of Dr. Welter's treatise.*

*These illustrations courtesy Dr. Niles F. Guichet, The Denar Corp., Anaheim, Calif.

Figs. 7-124 to 7-134. The illustrations in this series (Figs. 7-124 to 7-134) courtesy Denar Corp., Anaheim, Calif.

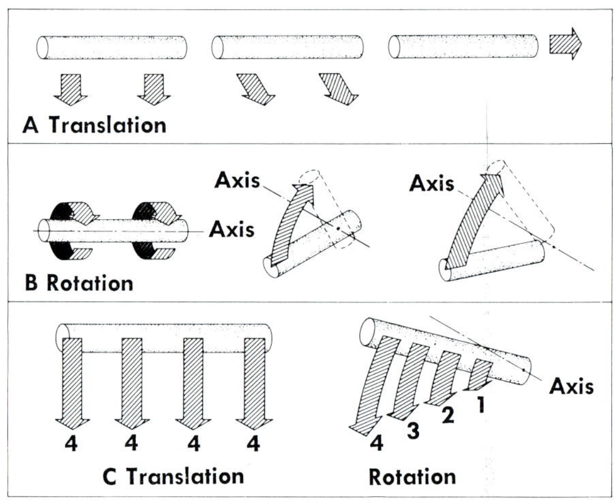

Fig. 7-124. Translation (the motion of a body which occurs when all points within the body are moving in the same direction at the same rate of speed) and rotation (the motion of a body which occurs about an axis).

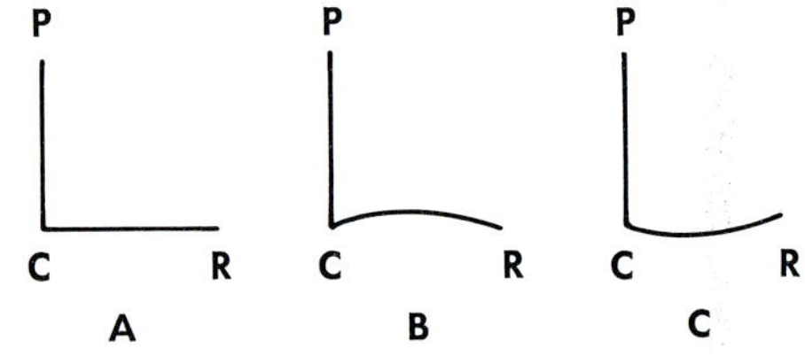

Fig. 7-125. Various basic configuations of the medial leg of a right anterior Gothic arch recording. When there is no forward or backward displacement of the rotating condyle, the medial leg is straight *(A)*. If forward displacement of the rotating condyle occurs, the medial leg *CR* is bowed posteriorly *(B)*. If backward displacement of the rotating condyle occurs, the medial leg will be bowed anteriorly *(C)*.

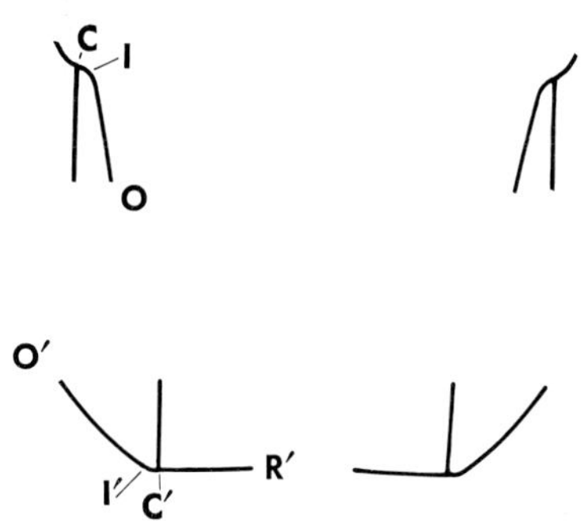

Fig. 7-126. As the patient moves from centric relation to left lateral position, the left posterior vertical stylus records line *CIO* while the left anterior stylus records line *C′I′O′*. The immediate side shift occurs as the styli move from *C* to *I* and from *C′* to *I′*. The progressive side shift occurs as the styli move from *I* to *O* and from *I′* to *O′*.

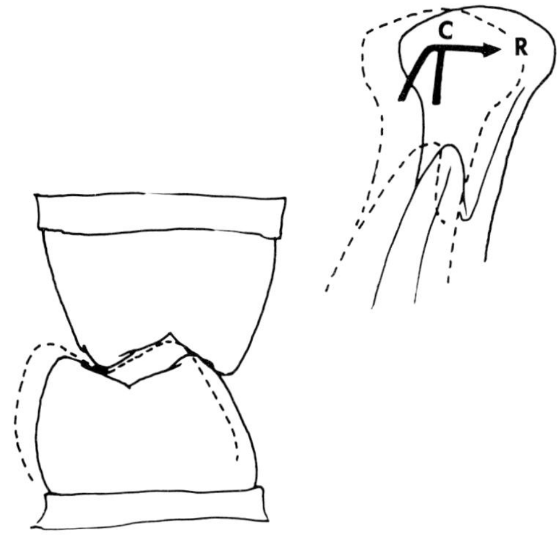

Working contacts

Fig. 7-128. By studying this illustration and simultaneously visualizing condylar paths of movement during a left lateral excursion, one can readily appreciate the relationship between the inclination of the rotating condylar path in the coronal plane and the mediolateral inclination of working bite inclines of posterior teeth.

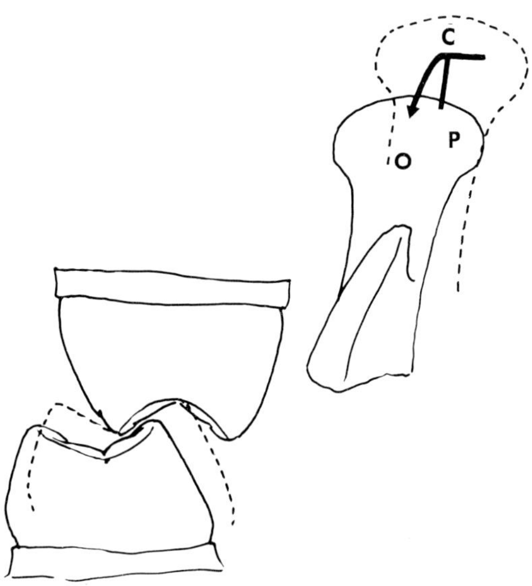

Orbiting contacts

Fig. 7-127. By studying this illustration and simultaneously visualizing condylar paths of movement during a right lateral excursive movement, one can readily appreciate the relationship between the immediate side shift and the width of the central groove of the teeth. Also, as the orbiting condyle traverses the progressive side-shift portion of the orbiting condyle path *CO,* one can appreciate why the progressive side shift has a primary influence on the buccolingual inclination of the balancing inclines of maxillary lingual and mandibular buccal cusps on the orbiting side.

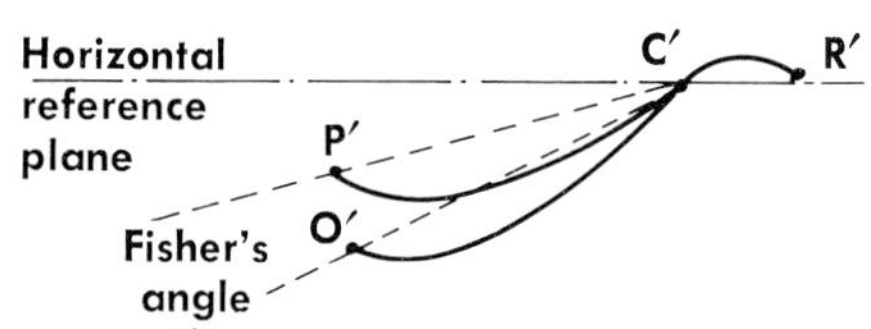

Fig. 7-129. The angle formed by the inclinations of the protrusive and orbiting condylar paths is known as Fisher's angle.

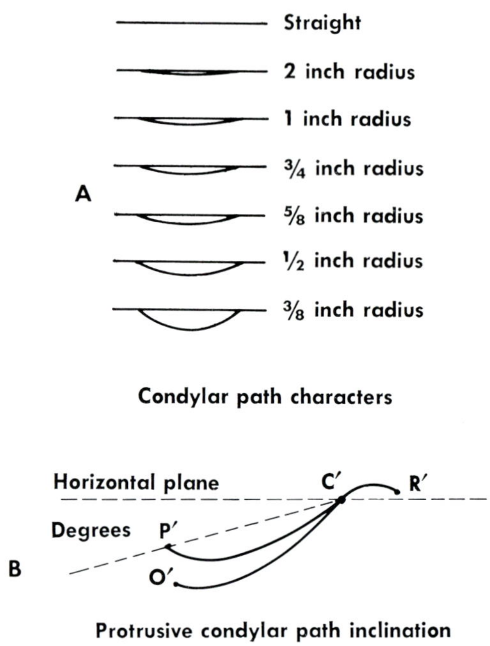

Fig. 7-130. A, The protrusive condylar path is generally convex in nature with the convexity facing downward. The character of the curvature of the path is generally flatter in that segment of the path nearest centric relation and becomes increasingly convex as the condyle advances. The character of segments of the protrusive condylar path as viewed in the sagittal plane may range from a straight line to the arc of a circle of ⅜ inch radius. The protrusive condylar path is inclined downward from the horizontal plane. **B,** The protrusive condylar paths are classified according to their convexity and are measured relative to their degree of inclination from the horizontal plane.

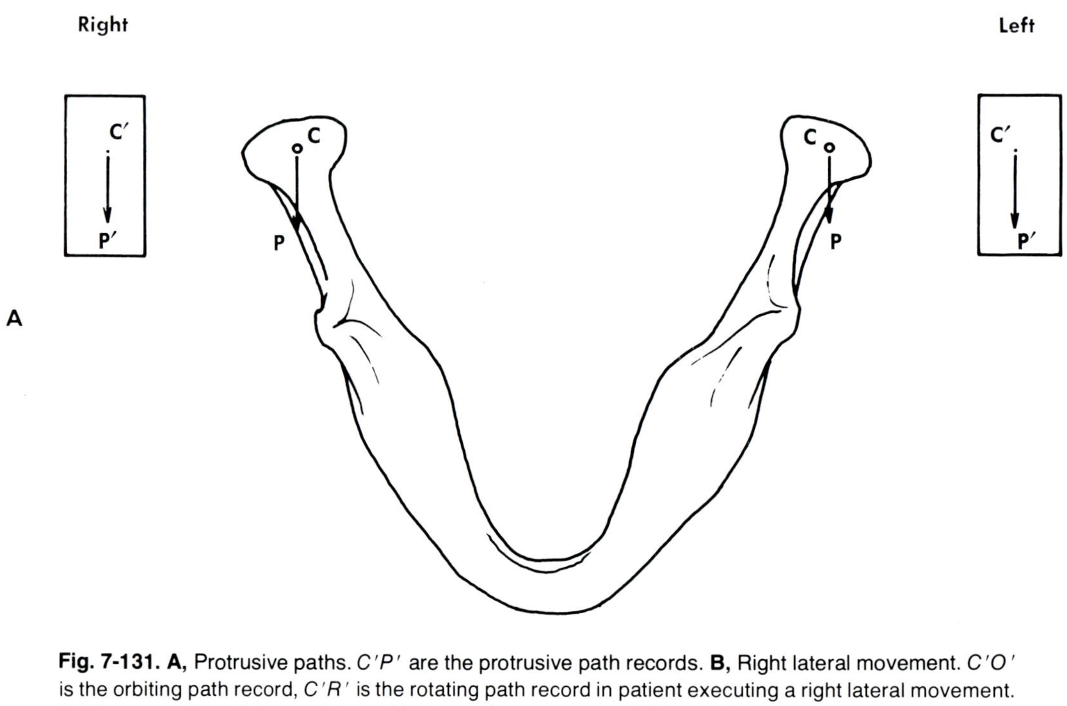

Fig. 7-131. A, Protrusive paths. *C′P′* are the protrusive path records. **B,** Right lateral movement. *C′O′* is the orbiting path record, *C′R′* is the rotating path record in patient executing a right lateral movement. **C,** The recording of the vertical and horizontal movements of the condyles simultaneously.

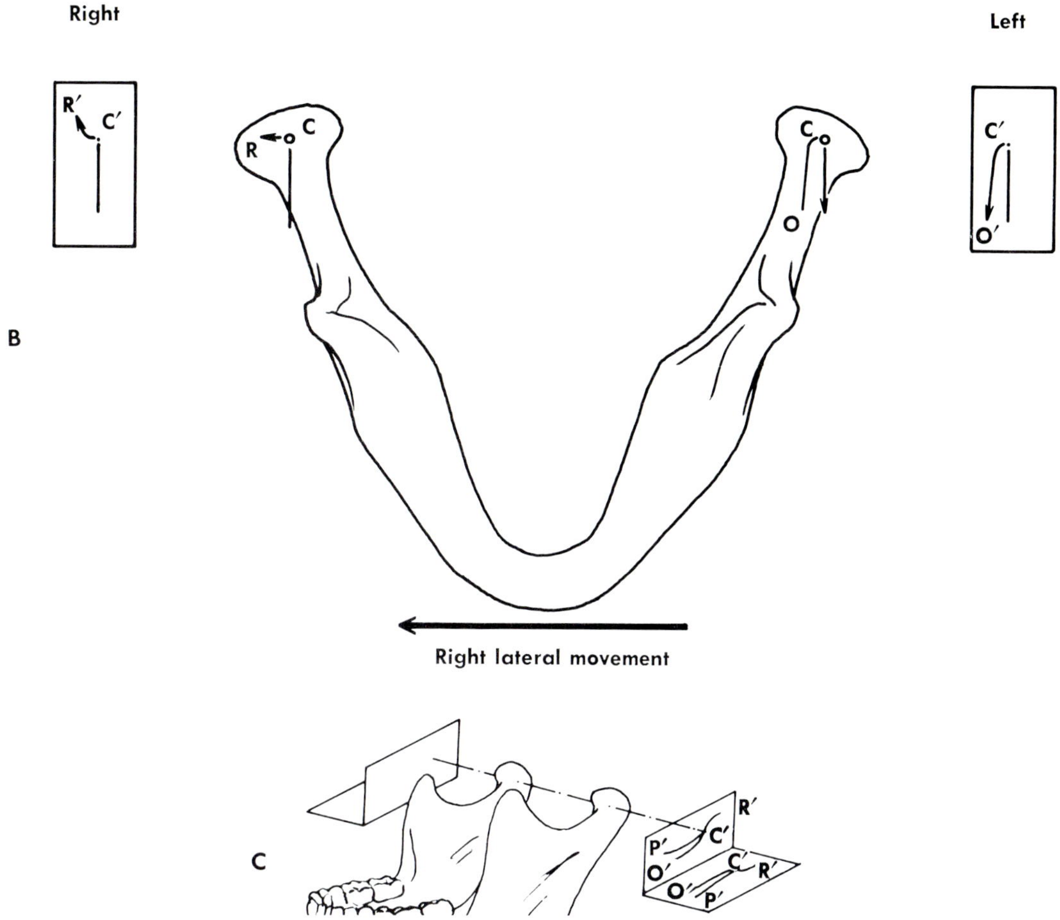

Fig. 7-131, cont'd. For legend see opposite page.

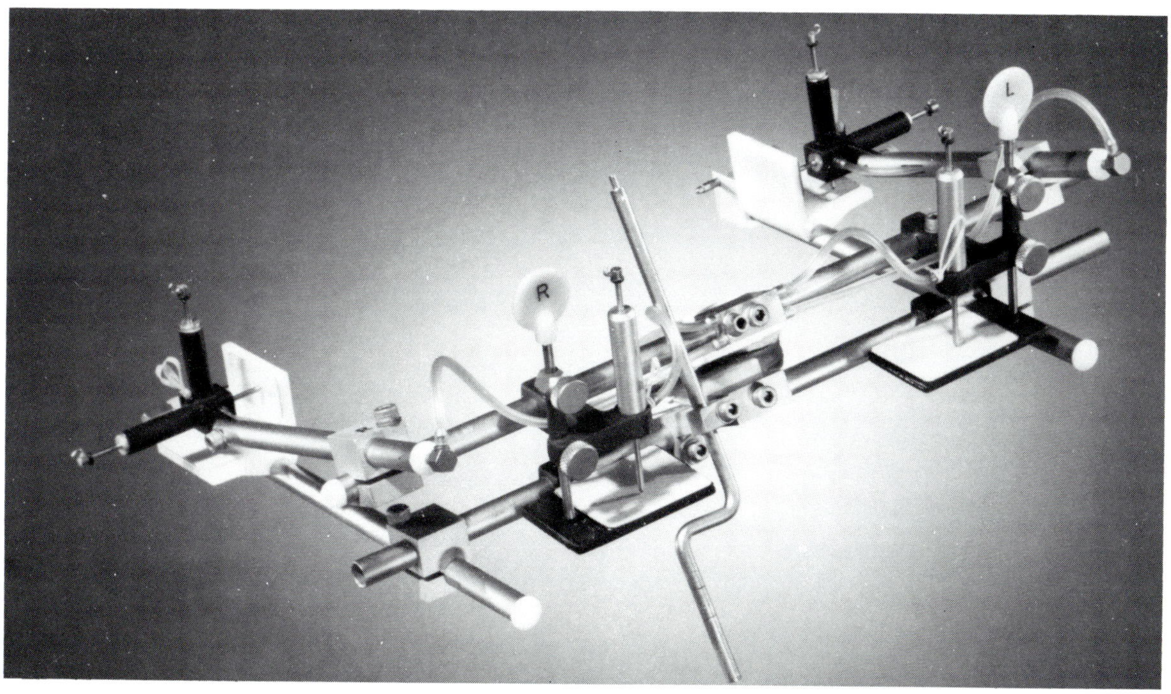

Fig. 7-132. Denar Pantograph.

A
B

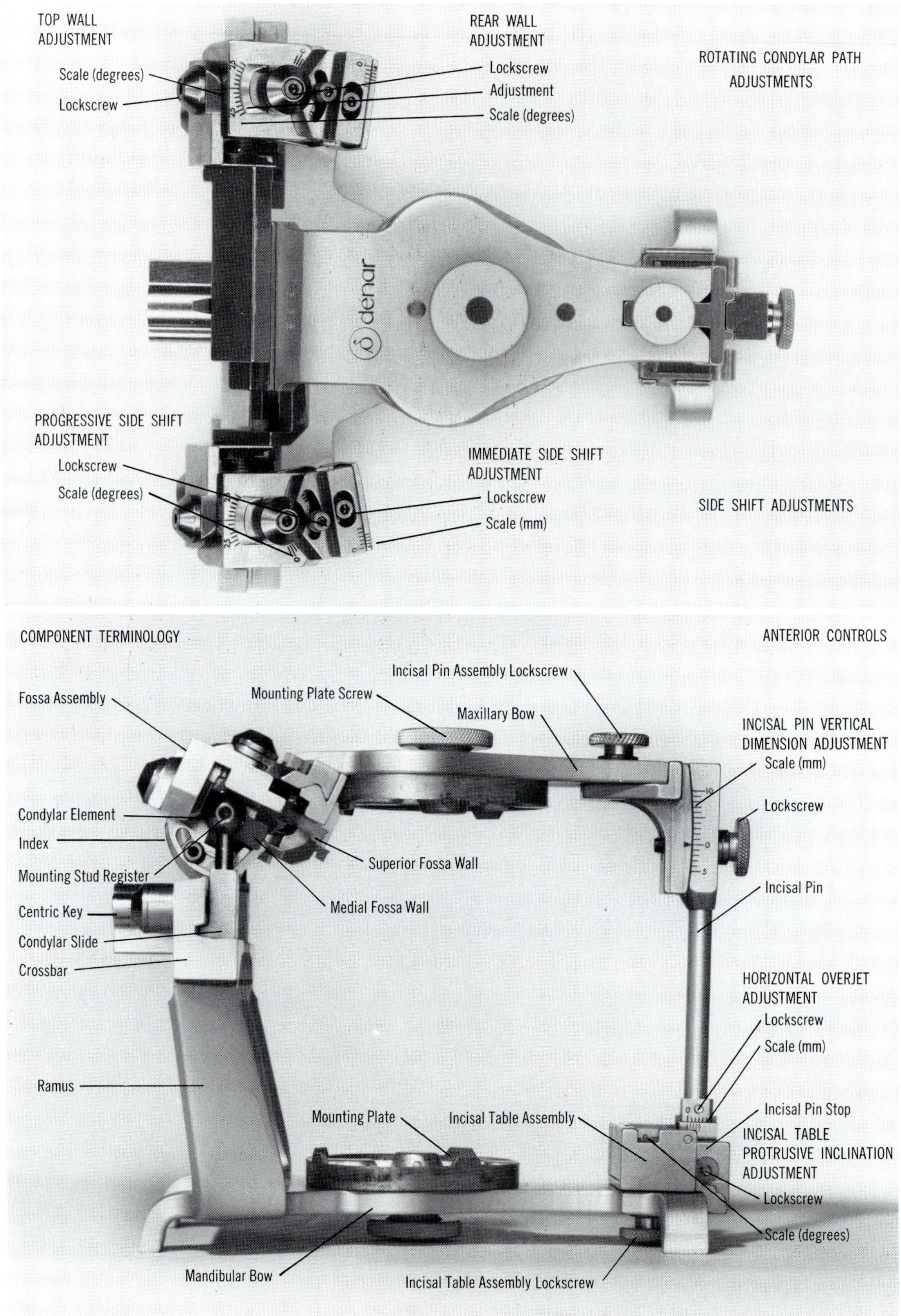

Fig. 7-133. Denar Articulator. **A,** Top view adjustments and scales. **B,** Right side view component terminology and anterior controls. **C,** Posterior view adjustments and scales.

C

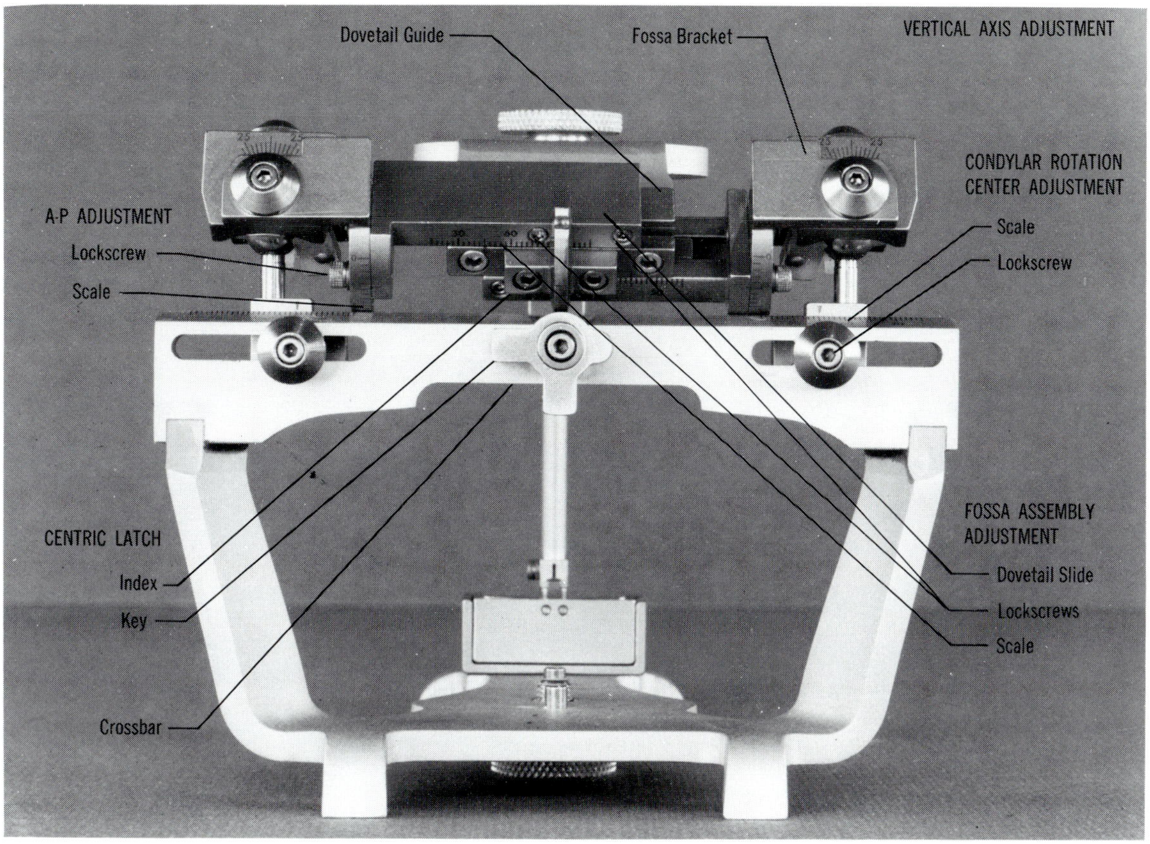

Fig. 7-133, cont'd. For legend see opposite page.

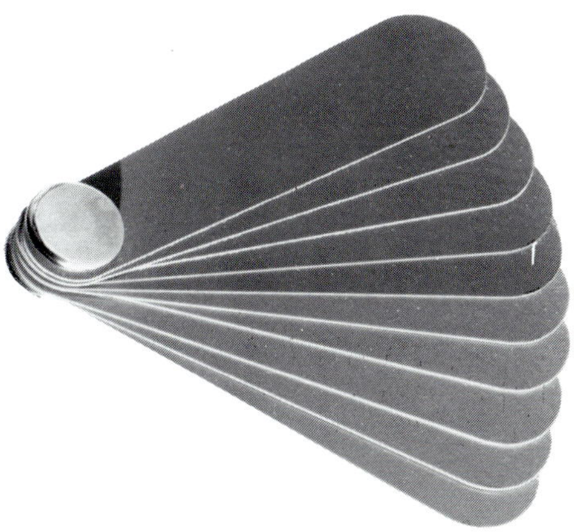

Fig. 7-134. The Leaf Gage consists of 10 leaves of .010 inch plastic and is useful in occlusal equilibration techniques.

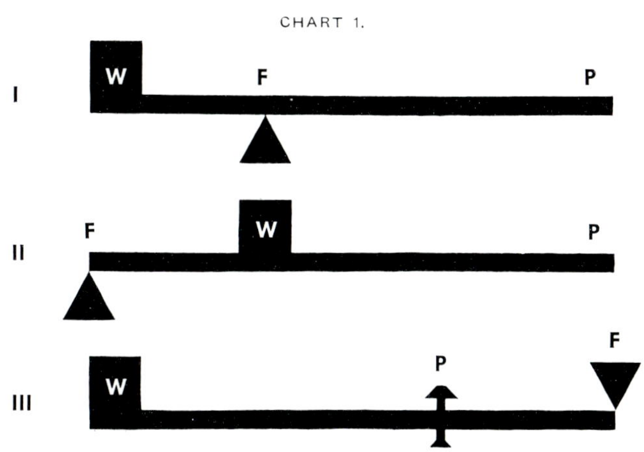

Fig. 7-135. The three classes of levers. *F* is the fulcrum, *W* is the work, and *P* is the power.

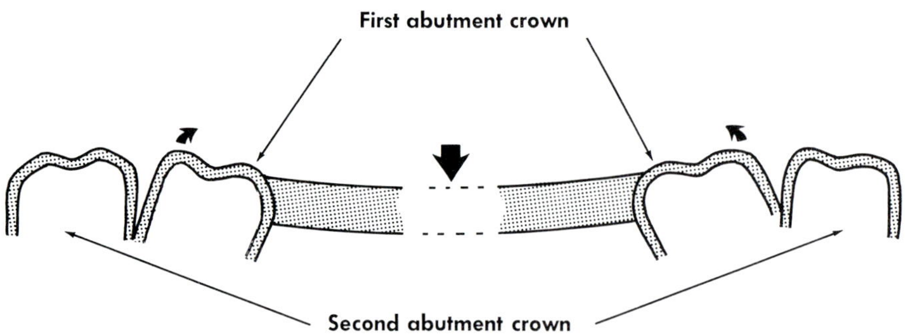

Fig. 7-136. Effect of occlusal stress on a long span bridge. The first abutment acts as a fulcrum or pivot for a force applied on the pontic section of the bridge, thus imposing a shearing stress on the connection between first and second abutment. To withstand this force be sure that this connection area is made as large and strong as possible. (Adapted from Thermalite instruction manual, ed. 2, East Orange, N. J., 1966, American Thermocraft Corp.)

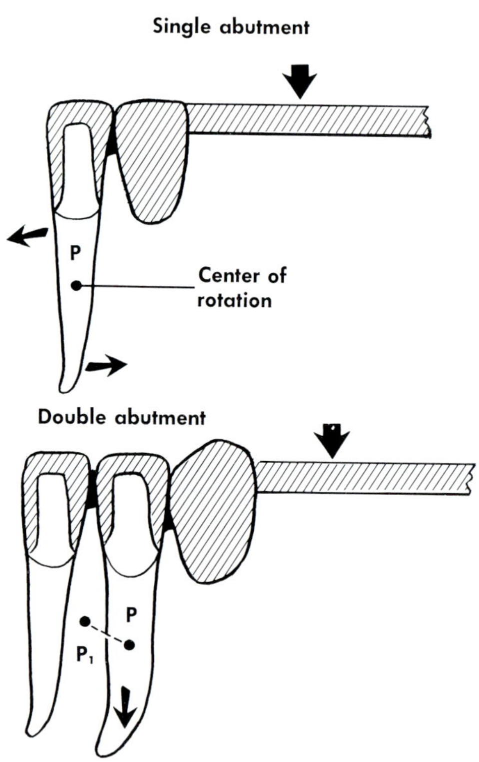

Fig. 7-137. A diagrammatic representation which shows that in a fixed partial denture with a single abutment, occlusal stress can produce a torque or twisting effect upon the root of the abutment tooth, which can be damaging to the supporting structures. By the splintage action of two abutments the center of rotation shifts to a more favorable position. (Courtesy American Thermocraft Corp., East Orange, N. J.)

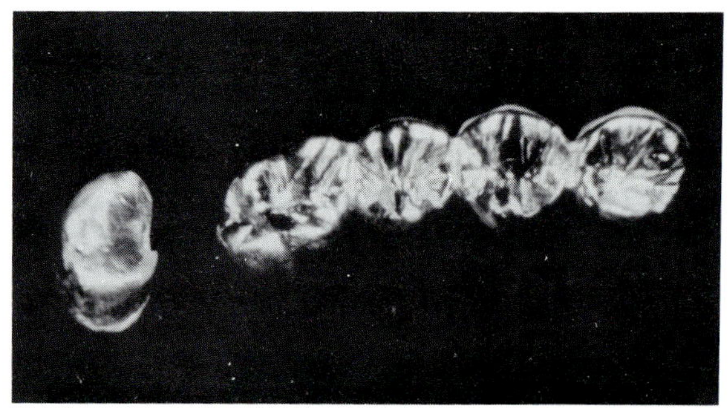

Fig. 7-138. A fixed partial denture necessitating a coping on the molar abutment for parallelism.

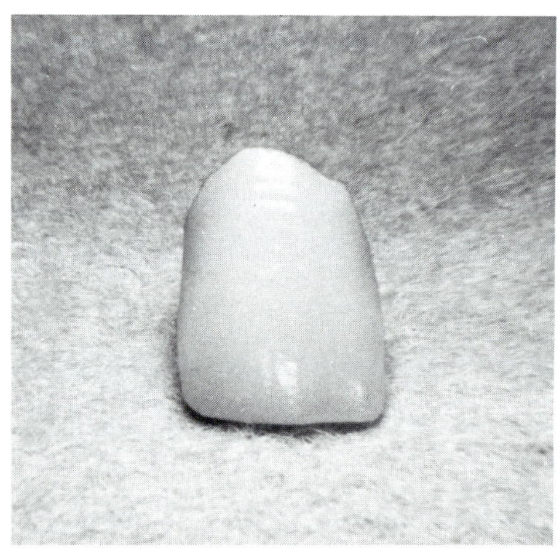

Fig. 7-139. A porcelain-fused-to-gold restoration showing good coronal form.

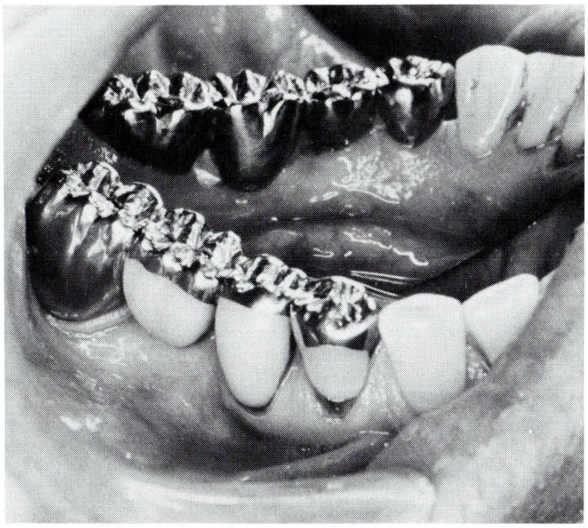

Fig. 7-140. A mirror view of a fixed partial denture in service for many years showing good form and periodontal health.

Stern[76] has called attention to the fact that certain patient-learned movements of the mandible can be reproduced on an articulator, but that these are not normal masticatory movements nor do they form even a small part of the infinite number of movement pathways of which the mandible is capable. He is of the opinion that the condyles are important, but that they are no more than vehicles for muscular movements of the mandible. And this is in spite of the fact that most dentists have heretofore looked upon the temporomandibular articulation as being the key to the occlusion of the teeth. He thinks that the movement path of the cusps of the teeth is from a lateral to a centric position as the jaws close—a spiral arc.

In other words, in his opinion, the temporomandibular joint must be considered as secondary, and the motivating neuromuscular complex of the mandible must be considered as the primary factor in directing the movement of the mandible.

REFERENCES

1. Faust, Homer E.: Anterior fixed bridgework, J. Mo. State Dent. Assoc. **28**(10):356-360, 1948.
2. Myers, George E.: Textbook of crown and bridge prosthodontics, St. Louis, 1969, The C. V. Mosby Co., pp. 11-13.
3. Reynolds, J. Marvin: Abutment selection for fixed prosthodontics, J. Prosthet. Dent. **19**(5):May, 1968.
4. Ante, I. H.: The fundamental principles of abutments, Mich. Dent. Soc. Bull. **8:**14, 1926.
5. Glickman, Irving: Clinical periodontology, Philadelphia, 1972, The W. B. Saunders Co., p. 432.
6. Brumfield, R. C.: Load capacities of posterior dental bridges, J. Prosthet. Dent. **4**(4):530-547, 1954.
7. Dental gold structures—analysis and practicalities, J. F. Jelenko & Co., Inc., 1949, p. 23.
8. Tuccillo, J. J.: Load carrying capacities of dental alloys, Thermotrol Technician **24**(2):4, 1970.
9. Structural investigation and design of dental bridges, Brumfield, R. C. In Tylman, Stanley D.: Theory and practice of crown and bridge prosthodontics, ed. 5, St. Louis, 1965, The C. V. Mosby Co., p. 1172.
10. Smyd, E. S.: The role of torque, torsion, and bending in prosthodontic failures, J. Prosthet. Dent. **11**(1):95-111, 1961.

10a. Smyd, E. S.: Role of mechanical stress in dentistry, N. Y. J. Dent. **28:**227-235, 1958.

11. Smyd, E. S.: Dental engineering, J. Dent. Res. **27:**649, 1948.
12. Peyton, F. A., and Craig, R. G.: Restorative dental materials, ed. 4, St. Louis, 1971, The C. V. Mosby Co., p. 61.
13. Reed, R. R.: The application of mechanical laws to bridge construction, Northwest Dent. **21:**191, 1943.
14. Jones, Walter E.: The scientifically designed partial veneer crown, J.A.D.A. **86**(6):1337-1343, 1973.
15. James, Allison G.: Crown and bridge restorations in periodontics, J. Periodontol. **27:**36-39, 1956.
16. Smyd, E. S.: Mechanics of dental structures, J. Prosthet. Dent. **2**(5):668-692, 1952.
17. Lorey, Robert E., and Myers, George E.: The retentive qualities of bridge retainers, J.A.D.A. **76**(3):568-572, 1968.
18. Amsterdam, Morton, Goldman, Henry M., and Cohen, D. Walter: Periodontal therapy, ed. 5, St. Louis, 1973, The C. V. Mosby Co.
19. Welter, Charles J.: Personal communication.
20. Reynolds, J. Marvin: Occlusal wear facets, J. Prosthet. Dent. **24**(4):367-372, 1970.
21. Prime, James M.: Dental physiology, J.A.D.A. **16**(10):1850-1865, 1929.
22. Shillingburg, H. T., Jr., Kaplan, M. J., and Grace, C. S.: Tooth dimensions—a comparative study, J. S. Calif. Dent. Assoc. **40**(9):830-839, 1972.
23. Courtade, Gerard L.: Pin pointers. I. New instruments, J. Prosthet. Dent. **16**(4):748-750, 1966.
24. Courtade, Gerard L.: Pin pointers. II. Venting and cross pinning, J. Prosthet. Dent. **16**(5):978-980, 1966.
25. Courtade, Gerard L.: Pin pointers. III. Self-threading pins, J. Prosthet. Dent. **20**(4):335-338, 1968.
26. Moffa, J. P., Razzano, M. R., and Folio, J.: Influence of cavity varnish on microleakage and retention of various pin-retaining devices, J. Prosthet. Dent. **20**(6):541-551, 1968.
27. Moffa, J. P., Razzano, M. R., and Doyle, M. G.: Pins—a comparison of their retentive properties, J.A.D.A. **78**(3):529-535, 1969.
28. Weiss, Arthur B.: The bolt inlay: a new method of repairing and modifying cemented fixed prostheses, J. Prosthet. Dent. **23**(3): 296-309, 1970.
29. Timmermans, John J., and Courtade, Gerard L.: Nonparallel threaded pin retention of fixed prosthesis, J. Prosthet. Dent. **19**(4):381-392, 1968.
30. Linkow, Leonard I., and Cherchene, Raphael: Theories and techniques of oral implantology, vols. 1 and 2, St. Louis, 1970, The C. V. Mosby Co.
31. Skinner, E. W., and Phillips, R. W.: The science of dental materials, ed. 6, Philadelphia, 1965, W. B. Saunders Co., pp. 516-544.
32. Tuccillo, Joseph J.: Thermal and firing effects in porcelain,

Thermotrol Technician **22**(5):1-4, Nov.-Dec., 1968; **23**(2):1-4, Mar.-Apr., 1969.
33. Katz, Sigmund: Factors affecting the strength of dental prostheses fabricated from porcelain fused to metal, Thermocraft Techn. Bull. **2**(3):1-3, 1968.
34. Mumford, George: The porcelain fused to metal restoration, Dent. Clin. N. Am., pp. 241-249, March, 1965.
35. Tuccillo, Joseph J.: Why a porcelain-gold "matched pair"? Thermotrol Technician **18:**1, 4, Nov.-Dec., 1964.
36. J. M. Ney Co.: The perfect combination for structurally sound and esthetically perfect restorations, Ney Technical Bulletin, No. 77, 1963.
37. Shelby, David S.: Practical considerations and design of porcelain fused to metal, J. Prosthet. Dent. **12**(3):542-548, 1962.
38. Shillingburg, H. T., Hobo, S., and Fisher, D. W.: Preparation design and margin distortion in porcelain fused to metal restorations, J. Prosthet. Dent. **29**(3):276-284, 1973.
39. Hobo, S., and Shillingburg, H. T., Jr.: Tooth preparation and coping design, J. Prosthet. Dent. **30**(1):28-36, July, 1973.
40. Berman, Martin Henry: Cutting efficiency in complete coverage preparation, J.A.D.A. **79**(5):1160-1167, 1969.
41. J. M. Ney Co.: Ney Technical Bulletin, No. 90, 1968.
42. Purcell, Fred: How to avoid warpage in a long-span bridge, Thermotrol Technician **26**(2):3-4, 1972.
43. Weinberg, L. A.: Personal communication.
44. J. M. Ney Co.: Ceramic golds with super micro-grain, Ney Technical Bulletin, Nos. 88 and 89, 1967.
45. Andrew, J., and Goodsir, L.: Advantages of Ceramco "O" to the user, Thermotrol Technician **25**(1):3, Jan.-Feb., 1971.
46. Tuccillo, Joseph J.: 50/50, Thermotrol Technician **27**(3):1, May-June, 1973.
47. Hoffman, E. J.: How to utilize porcelain fused to gold as a crown and bridge material, Dent. Clin. N. Am., pp. 57-64, March, 1965.
48. Tuccillo, J. J., and Nielsen, J. P.: Interfacial stress measurements in bonded porcelain-gold alloy systems, Int. Assoc. Dent. Res., abstract, p. 131, 1971.
49. Straussberg, George, Katz, Gerry, and Kuwata, Masahiro: Design of gold supporting structures for fused porcelain restorations, J. Prosthet. Dent. **16**(5):928-936, 1966.
50. Shell, John S., and Nielsen, J. P.: A study of the bond between gold alloys and porcelain, J. Dent. Res. **41**(6):Nov.-Dec., 1962.
51. Waltke, Robert: Glazing, Ceramco Technigraph **4**(1):1-4, Aug., 1972.
52. Billmeyer and Saltzman: Principles of color technology, New York, 1966, John Wiley & Sons, Inc.
53. Sproull, Robert C.: Color matching in dentistry. Part I. The three-dimensional nature of color, J. Prosthet. Dent. **29**(4): 416-423, 1973.
53a. Sproull, Robert C.: Color matching in dentistry. Part II. Practical applications of the organization of color, J. Prosthet. Dent. **29**(5):556-566, 1973.
54. Munsell, A. H.: A color notation, ed. 11, Baltimore, 1961, Munsell Color Co., Inc.
55. Ceramco, Inc.: Ceramco Color System, 1968.
56. Goodsir, Leonard: Creating illusions of tooth size by varying tooth form, Thermotrol Technician **25**(2):1, Mar.-Apr., 1971; **25**(3):May-June, 1971.
57. Hildebrand, G. Y.: Studies in masticatory movements, Skand. Arch. Physiol., p. 31, 1931.
58. Kornfeld, Max: Mouth rehabilitation—clinical and laboratory procedures, ed. 2, St. Louis, 1974, The C. V. Mosby Co., Chap. 15.
59. Bellanti, Neal D.: The significance of articulator capabilities, J. Prosthet. Dent. **29**(3):269-275, 1973.
60. Celenza, Frank: Personal communication.
61. Fox, Lewis: The occlusal factor in periodontal disease, Alpha Omegan **43:**124-133, 1949.
62. Amsterdam, Morton: Personal communication.
63. Guichet, Niles F.: Occlusion, The Denar Corp., 1970, Anaheim, Calif.
64. Lundeen, Harry C.: Crown and bridge occlusal considerations in restorative dentistry, In Goldman, Henry M., and others: Current therapy in dentistry, vol. 3, St. Louis, 1968, The C. V. Mosby Co., p. 207.
65. Teteruck, W. R., and Lundeen, H. C.: The accuracy of an ear facebow, J. Prosthet. Dent. **16**(6):1039-1046, 1966.
66. Ramfjord, Sigurd P., and Ash, Major M., Jr.: Occlusion, ed. 2, Philadelphia, 1971, W. B. Saunders Co.
67. Stuart, Charles E.: Personal communication.
68. Dawson, Peter E.: Personal communication.
69. Amsterdam, Morton: Personal communication.
70. Bellanti, Neal D.: The significance of articulator capabilities, J. Prosthet. Dent. **29**(3):269-275, 1973.
71. J. M. Ney Co.: The technic of articulation, Ney Technical Bulletin, No. 82, pp. 1-4, 1965.
72. Granger, E. R.: Principles of obtaining occlusion in occlusal rehabilitation, J. Prosthet. Dent. **13:**714-718, 1963.
73. Dykins, W. R.: Lecture notes and personal communication.
74. Stein, R. Sheldon: Personal communication.
75. Welter, Charles J.: Personal communication.
76. Stern, Ralph H.: An approach to the understanding of mandibular movement, J. S. Calif. Dent. Assoc. **28**(7):205-206, July, 1960.

CHAPTER 8

FUNCTIONAL PREPARATIONS

GENERAL CONSIDERATIONS

In considering functional preparations the type and form of tooth preparation will depend to a great degree upon the relationship of the teeth to each other and to their opposing members. Some of the problems are (1) cross-bite relations, (2) relations of the long axes of the teeth, and (3) insufficient overjet of posterior teeth, extruded teeth, tipped teeth, versions, and rotations.

The type of retainer to be used depends on the functional demands of the case on hand, and this implies that an accurate set of study casts must be oriented correctly upon an adjustable articulator so that a complete study can be made of the cuspal relationship necessary to make the mouth function properly.

This study also will allow for a visualization of the finished articulation, which enables one to develop a harmonious interplay of cooperating cusps that constitutes function and equitable stress distribution. A study of function and stress distribution is impossible without casts correctly mounted on an articulator that reproduces the mandibular movements of the individual (Figs. 8-1 to 8-3).

It is well worth the time and effort to prepare and mount a second set of casts and to prepare the plaster teeth with burs and stones. Then the occlusal surfaces are worked out in wax, determining in advance not only the type of preparation necessary for all of the involved teeth, but also which areas are to be removed or built up, which teeth have to be warped for proper interdigitation with opposing teeth, the position of the cusps, etc. The problem of esthetics, especially in the anterior part of the mouth, also can be evaluated properly. Above all, by these means it usually is possible to determine in advance if the case can be successfully corrected.

Always remember that the functions of a tooth are contained in its dynamic anatomy and its position in the jaw, and also that its cusps must cooperate harmoniously to produce efficient function with equitable stress distribution. Time spent in preoperative study before starting extensive rehabilitative treatment pays big dividends.

Proper cavity preparation is of prime importance. We must always keep in mind not only definitive retentive form and marginal outline, but also proper tooth form and function. An understanding of the fundamental principles of cavity design is of the utmost importance. From the beginning of the preparation to the completion of the restoration, the procedures involved are governed by surgery, engineering principles, art, and good workmanship.

One of the most common causes of small type casting failures is haphazard cavity preparation. It is not necessary to cut the cavities very deeply, especially since experience has taught that parallel walls, judicious use of pits, wells, or pin anchorage, and proper selection of the gold alloy will give adequate retention and will maintain as much frictional adaptation as possible with less probability of degenerating pulps.

The extent and depth of an abutment cavity should

Figs. 8-1 to 8-3. Casts correctly mounted on adjustable articulator.

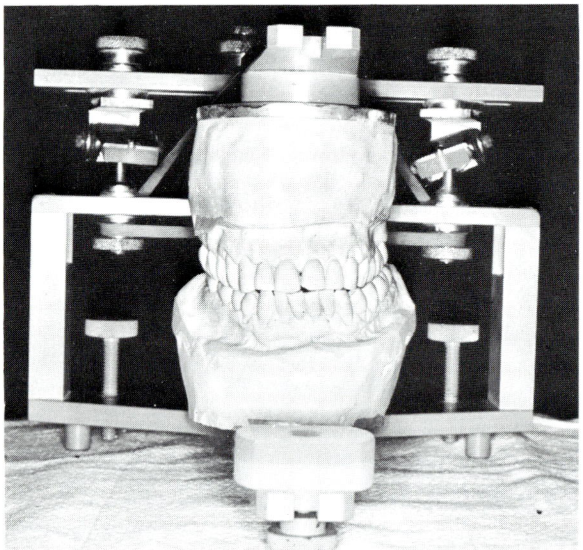

Fig. 8-1. Relation of teeth—anterior view.

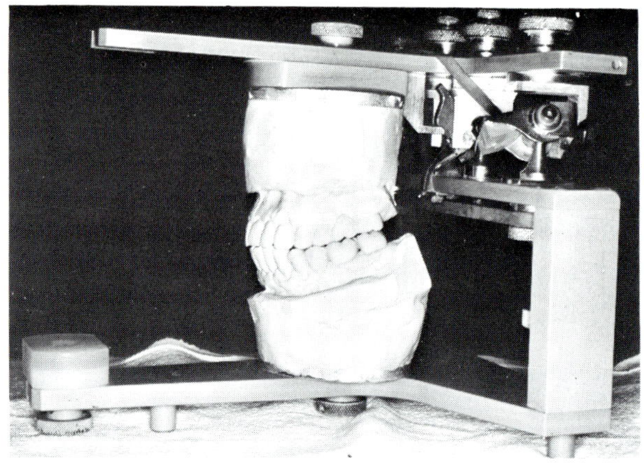

Fig. 8-2. Relation of teeth—right side.

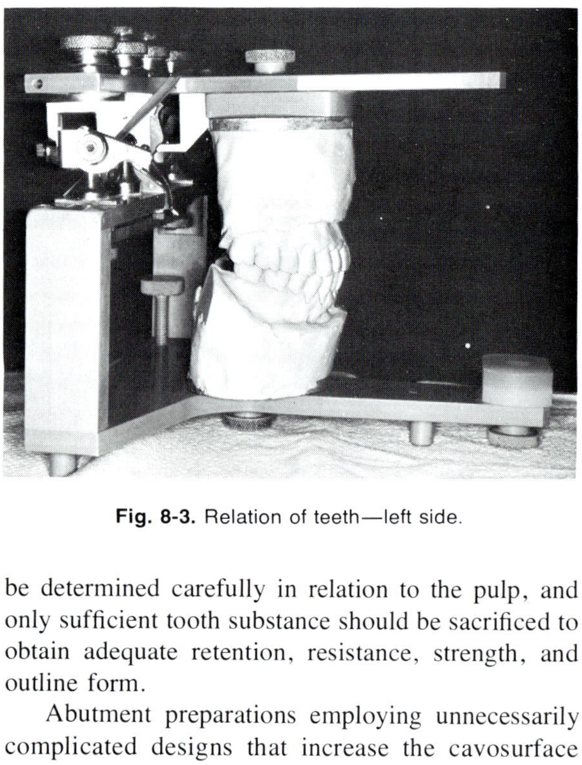

Fig. 8-3. Relation of teeth—left side.

be determined carefully in relation to the pulp, and only sufficient tooth substance should be sacrificed to obtain adequate retention, resistance, strength, and outline form.

Abutment preparations employing unnecessarily complicated designs that increase the cavosurface length, which in turn increases the hazard of poor margins, should be avoided. The amount of retention and strength required in a retainer varies with, and under, different conditions. The degree of torque and strain to which a retainer will be subjected depends upon the length of the span, the occlusion, the mobility of abutment teeth, the musculature of the individual, etc. Retainers should be self-retentive since the function of cement is to hermetically seal it to the prepared tooth.

The question of what constitutes an ideal retainer is asked frequently. An ideal retainer requires the least amount of destruction to the abutment tooth, least destroys the outline form of the tooth, can be finished about its periphery with great accuracy, will be so rigid that it will withstand the requisite load without distortion and will have frictional adaptation, least destroys the cervical marginal ridge, can be prepared without trauma to the pulp or surrounding tissues, is an accurate complement to the lost tooth structure, and fulfills the requirements of esthetics.

What requirements must be observed when preparing teeth for retainers? A few requirements will be given now, and more will be listed as the types of retainers used in mouth rehabilitation are discussed. Retainers should offer a series of angles and surfaces best suited to resist stress or the tendency to fracture the tooth, Black's principle of extension for prevention should be observed, they should present margins so prepared as to conserve the enamel structure of the tooth and not expose it to injury during stress of occlusion, and they should offer a retentive receptacle.

Keys[1] has shown with photomicrographs and diagrams from well-known texts on metallography and physical metallurgy that sharp corners and acute angles in castings tend to produce planes of weakness and areas of porosity because of their influence on the rate of cooling of the cast metal as it freezes. From this he concluded that in small type castings results can be improved by modifying the cavity preparation so that all sharp and abrupt angles are eliminated and a cove effect at all lines and points within the cavity is formed.

It can be added that modifications in cavity preparation that reduce the detrimental effect of failure to balance the variables in casting include beveling of margins, maintaining as nearly as possible uniformity in thickness of the various parts of the casting, and avoiding irregular angles and sharp curves.

Amsterdam[2] has listed the following criteria for successful utilization of abutment teeth: (1) the gingiva should be pink, firm, well attached, have good architectural form, and exhibit minimum crevicular depth; (2) tooth should be firm or become so following therapy, there should be no objective symptoms, periodontal ligament should be thin and lamina dura distinct, supporting bone should be dense and well trabeculated, there should be no cemental tears and root resorption; (3) coronal contours should be conducive to gingival health and allow force dissipation within the root support area of the tooth; (4) periodontal structures should be in a state of health, and remain so; home care and oral physiotherapy program should be followed; (5) endodontic climate should be satisfactory; and (6) considering all the factors, the tooth should be able to function in health, and contribute to the health of the entire dentition.

A repertoire of designs for cavity preparation must be available, and the one best adapted to meet the requirements of the case under consideration should be selected. Types of retainers that do not encroach upon the terrain of the marginal gingiva must be used, when at all possible. The more we can stay away from the attachment apparatus, the more favorable will be the end result. Some of us have one type of preparation for all teeth, which, despite the precision used in its preparation, is a definite handicap.

Fox[3] has made the following pertinent statements:

"Clinical evidence clearly demonstrates that subgingival extensions of full coverage margins produce an environment unfavorable to the health of the marginal gingiva. In the area adjacent to full coverage, it is difficult to maintain marginal gingiva which are thin and acceptably contoured for physiologic function and flood flow.

"In contrast to the maintenance of healthy gingiva around enamel and cementum of natural tooth substance, the gingival tissues around full coverage seem to be more thickened, more rolled, and generally more inflammatory in character.

"Even with the most careful techniques of tooth preparation and tissue handling during preparation of tooth, impression taking, temporization, and final cementation, the full coverage extended subgingivally limits the opportunity for the marginal gingiva to achieve maximum patterns of health.

"This is not an indictment of full coverage. There has, however, been a tendency to utilize this procedure without definitive indication. Where indicated and demanded in the therapeutics of restorative dentistry, it can be utilized to advantage. Where full coverage is therapeutically utilized with finesse and understanding and precision technique, it offers much in many clinical circumstances."*

TRIPODAL STABILIZATION

All of my retainers, with the exception of some full coverage, have a basic retentive feature in common, the principle of the tripod. Tripodism is the most stable system in mechanics. It has been found that this principle, when carefully followed, simplifies tooth preparations and at the same time gives maximum stability and retention.

The tripod principle is applied by placing three pin retention areas or grooves (or combinations of the two) at strategic points not in the same line. When possible, they are placed equidistant from each other. Thus, by joining them, an equilateral triangle would be formed. (See Fig. 8-4.)

Retainers having these three points, when cemented on the abutment teeth, effectively resist torque and thrust. These three locking devices further serve to prevent the slightest displacement of the castings on the abutment teeth in taking the impression and bite registration.

Stabilization is best effected by a minimum of three points, as in the case of a common three-legged stool. Then, too, the surface on which a three-legged stool rests does not necessarily have to be smooth, as in the case of a four-legged one. It is very likely that only three points ever are useful.

Pin retention is one of the strongest retentive forces, mechanically, that can be used in dentistry.

Frictional wall retention (parallel walls) and the interlocking of the cement between the prepared surface of the tooth and the casting also should be considered. It is the opinion of a number of excellent dentists that the surfaces of the prepared tooth should not be polished, with the exception of the margin area, and that all castings within 1 mm. of the margins

*From Fox, Lewis: Letters to the editor, Dent. Times **3**:6, 1961.

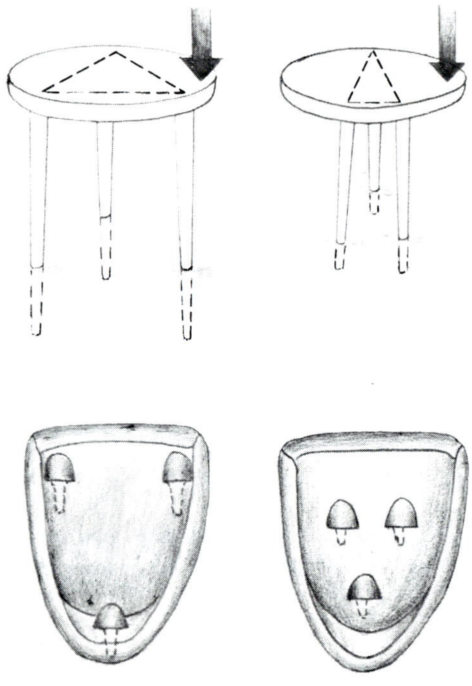

Fig. 8-4. Principle of tripodism. The larger the boundary of the triangle created by connecting the pins, the more retentive the retainer.

should be roughened with a small bur before cementation.

In other words, retention is obtained by the use of grooves (regular and locked), pins, and close adaptation to nearly parallel walls, with the variation from absolute parallelism being sufficient only to permit the withdrawal of the wax pattern and the subsequent seating of the restoration.

The Kyprie tapered keyed groove, or lock groove, is one whose inner diameter is larger than the entrance to it (Fig. 8-5).

It is sound practice to remove all old fillings and cement bases. Experience has shown in a high percentage of cases that this operation is justified because of conditions found under these circumstances, and therefore it is highly desirable that the restorations be placed on teeth that are known to be absolutely free of caries and that every effort be put forth to preserve the pulp in a normal healthy condition.

However, there is no danger in leaving some solid amalgam filling in the tooth if it is roentgenographically and clinically sound of galvanic currents between the two dissimilar metals, provided the gold restoration completely covers the amalgam. Even when this is not fully accomplished, it is unusual for the subsequent galvanic action to have any clinical significance.

PULPAL CONSIDERATIONS

Another important factor to take into consideration during tooth preparations is the avoidance of permanent injury to the pulp. The maintenance of vital

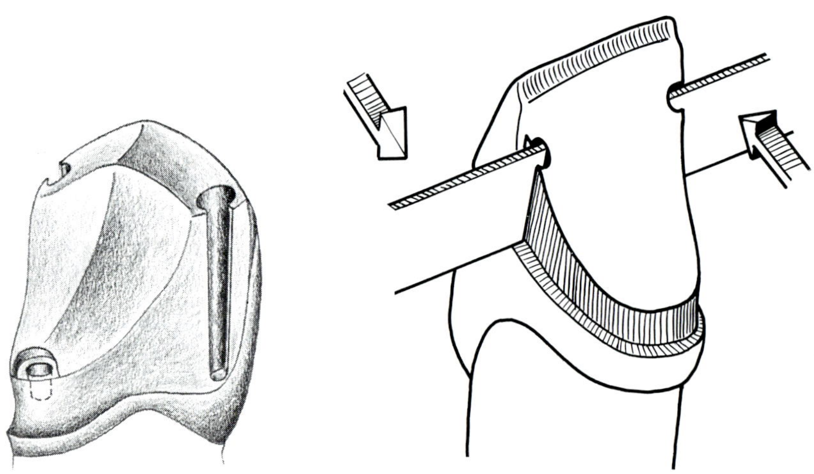

Fig. 8-5. Kyprie tapered keyed groove or lock groove, a great aid in resistance to displacement both faciolingually and mesiodistally.

functional teeth is to be desired, as is the conservation of tooth structure and preciseness in cavity preparation. The teeth being prepared should never be overheated. A coolant should be used copiously, with warm water either as a spray with air or as a stream, to reduce frictional heat. The coolant must always be directed where needed, and adequate aspiration should be available. It is not the amount of water coming from the outlet, but the water arriving at the actual site of contact between bur and tooth structure that is decisive. As a rule, an air-water spray is preferable. If any operation cannot be covered in its entirety by the air-water spray, administer extra water spray from the unit with the help of the dental assistant. Quantity as well as intensity of heat applied to the pulp is important.

What must be uppermost in our minds during tooth preparation is conservatism, being sure not to overcut the teeth and realizing that the damage inflicted on the pulp is not always reversible—it can be irreversible. Also, a thorough study of the speed, type, and handling of the cutting tools used in tooth preparation should be made. For gross reduction of tooth structure the ultrahigh-speed equipment is used with very light pressure, and for the preparation of wells, pits, pinholes, tapered keyed grooves, and the finishing of margins the conventional lower speed equipment is used. Diamond stones and carbide burs should be kept free of debris for greater cutting efficiency, and they should run true and be kept under control at all times.

In a study which considered the question of whether an air-turbine handpiece can be used to finish a cavity preparation, Cantwell, Alpin, and Mahler, came to the conclusion that the answer was "yes," providing this procedure is done at the "stallout zone."[4] "The *stall-out zone* is that condition in which the air pressure to the air-turbine handpiece is reduced to the point at which a very small amount of operating force will stall the bur."* In other words, where both speed and cutting efficiency are reduced to a minimum, surface smoothness results. A plane fissure bur will, in most instances, produce a smoother surface than a cross-cut fissure bur. By using the "stall-out zone" and a white polishing stone, I have been able to finish the margins of my preparations to a very smooth surface. However, for finishing the margins of gold restorations I use a conventional handpiece.

Unfortunately, in many instances pulpal damage cannot be detected through clinical signs of pain and discomfort until months or years later. Trauma can be the cause of this trouble, and the main source of this trauma is heat. In these cases, there is probably a hastening of evaporation of fluid from the dentinal tubules, and in turn this serves to suck dentin odontoblasts into the tubules. This certainly points up the importance of avoiding heat damage.

Shallow preparations, intermittent periods of drilling on teeth with a washed-field technique for cooling the tooth and the cutting tool, and the proper treatment and protection of the cut dentinal surfaces, with the minimum use of chemical agents, will reduce the amount of irritation to a point where the chance of pulp degeneration is almost negligible.

A review of the research work of Weiss[5] is in order at this time:

(1) "Histologically there are three zones of the dental pulp which are affected by injury (Fig. 8-6).

"The most superficial zone affected is the odontoblastic layer which is in reality an extension of the dentin. The mildest reaction is the disarrangement of those cells and aspiration of the nuclei into the dentinal tubules (Fig. 8-7).

"If only a few of these odontoblastic cells are affected, the pulp will recover in about 14 days with the regeneration of new cells, provided the tooth does not sustain any further injury such as thermal shock.

"A protected pulp will differentiate new odontoblasts from the embryonic mesenchymal cells that are present in the pulp.

(2) "More traumatic injury will extend the damage to the zone of Weil which is normally a cell-free zone (Fig. 8-8). Histologically, cells of inflammation and new capillaries are seen in this area. This type of injury is still reversible if proper sedative protection is given to the pulp. Recovery time is approximately thirty (30) days.

(3) "Irreversible damage is sustained by the dental pulp when the injury takes the form of a massive invasion of cells of inflammation into the pulp, thrombosed blood vessels and hemorrhage (Fig. 8-9, *A*). The climax is either a necrotic pulp or abscess formation which may occur over a long period of time with few clinical symptoms to signify that it is occurring."*

Pulpal insult must be kept to a minimum.

Another important factor to keep in mind is that periodontal disease can have a profound influence on

*From Cantwell, K. R., Alpin, A. W., and Mahler, D. B.: Cavity finish with high-speed handpieces, Dent. Progr. **1**(1):42-46, Oct., 1960.

*From Weiss, Marvin B., Massler, Maury, and Spence, John M.: Operative effects on adult dental pulp, Dent. Progr. **4**:10-19, 1963.

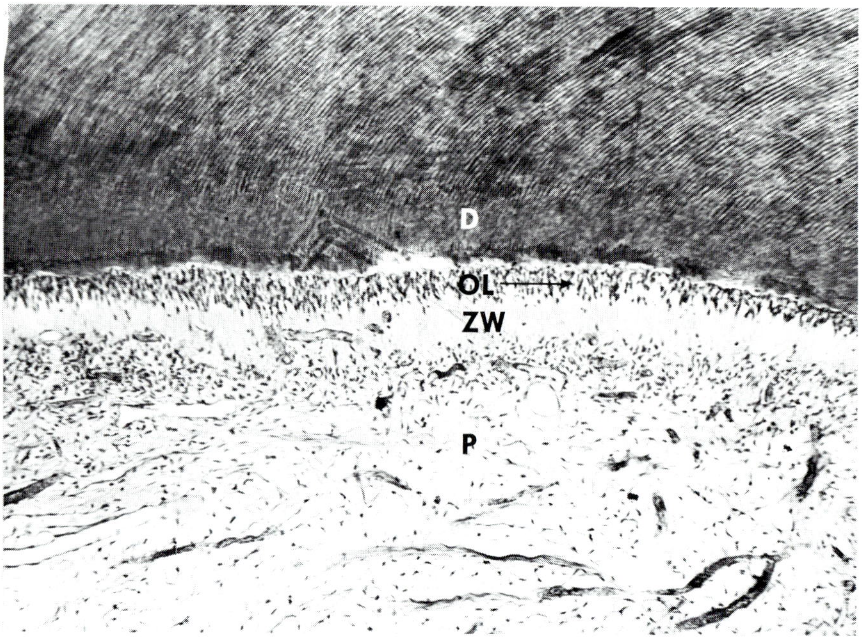

Fig. 8-6. No reaction to operative procedures is seen in section 48 hours after cavity preparation by carbide bur revolving at 250,000 r.p.m. with water-spray coolant. The three levels of pulp inspected for changes are indicated. (1) *D* plus *OL,* dentin plus odontoblastic layer, considered as one level, (2) *ZW,* the cell-free zone of Weil, and (3) *P,* main body of pulp. (From Weiss, Marvin B., Massler, Maury, and Spence, John M.: Dent. Progr. **4**:10-19, 1963.)

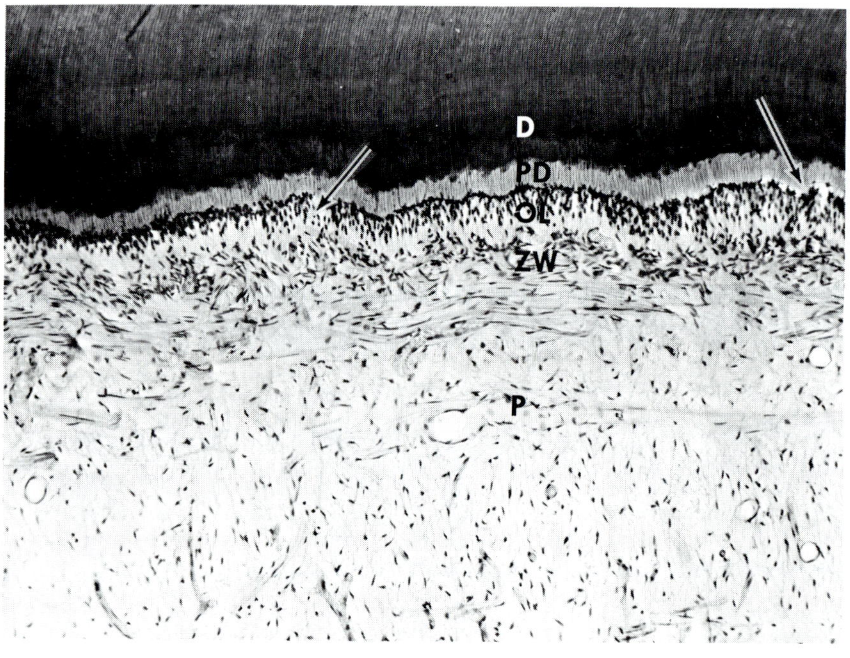

Fig. 8-7. A mild reaction in which disarrangement of odontoblasts has persisted for 35 days. Note displaced nuclei (black) and small vacuoles (white) indicated by arrows near predentine border (*PD*). Remainder of section appears normal. Cavity cut with carbide bur at 30,000 r.p.m., water-spray coolant. (From Weiss, Marvin B., Massler, Maury, and Spence, John M.: Dent. Progr. **4**:10-19, 1963.)

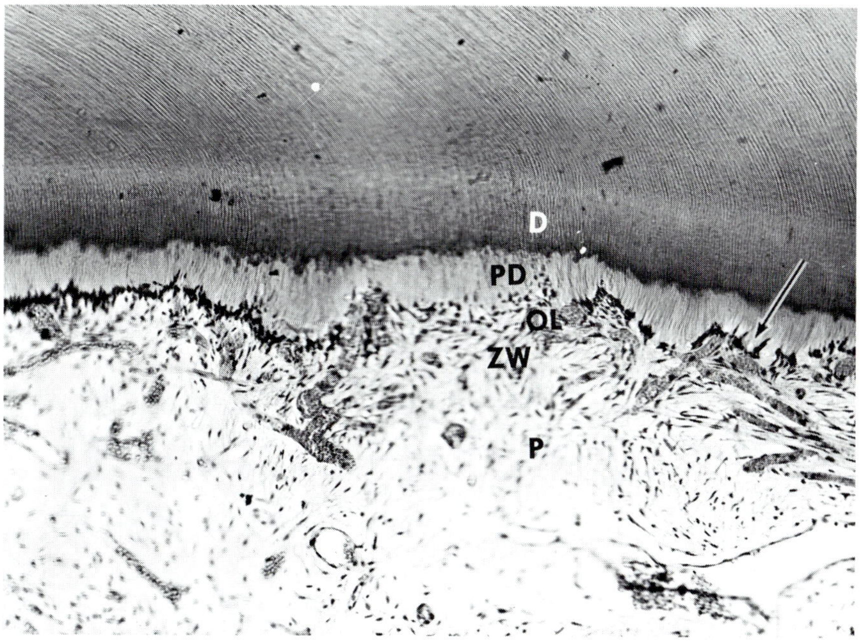

Fig. 8-8. A moderate reaction seen 9 days after cutting with new steel bur at 3,000 r.p.m. without use of coolant. Odontoblastic layer is greatly disturbed and invaded by capillary loops (dark gray streaks, arrow). The zone of Weil also is infiltrated by blood, but main pulp level *(P)* remains normal. (From Weiss, Marvin B., Massler, Maury, and Spence, John M.: Dent. Progr. **4:**10-19, 1963.)

A

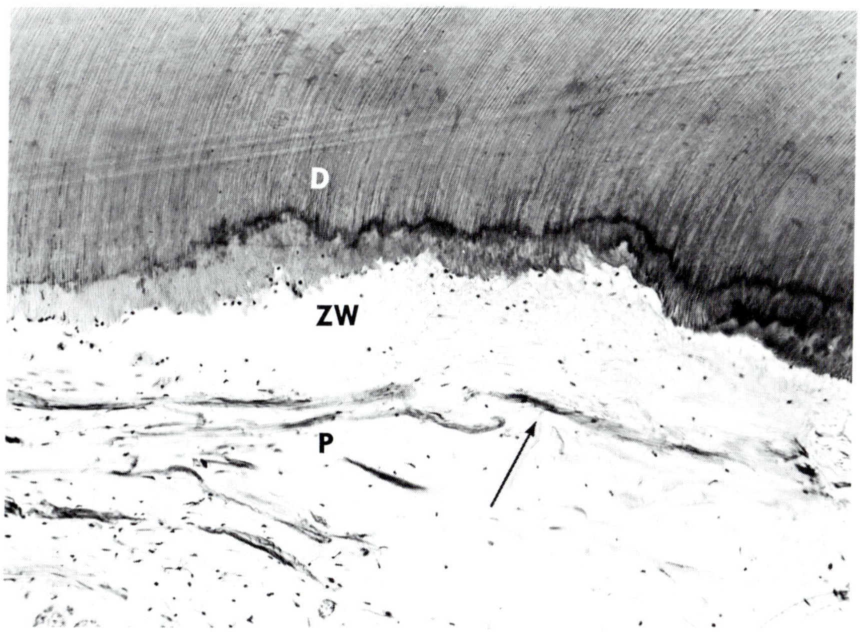

Continued.

Fig. 8-9. A, Severe reaction produced by cutting at 70,000 r.p.m. with steel bur under dry conditions, seen 48 hours postoperatively. Few odontoblasts are present, and these are shrunken so that only the nuclei are seen, scattered among large vacuoles and coagulated material that stained eosinophilic. The zone of Weil shows heavy influx of cellular material from pulp. At both this level and in deeper pulp appear enlarged blood vessels (gray streaks, arrow), largely filled with coagulum. **B,** Periapical pulpo-osteosclerosis. Note the radiopaque change in the roentgenogram, which appears as a radiopaque area of varying configurations. (**A** from Weiss, Marvin B., Massler, Maury, and Spence, John M.: Dent. Progr. **4:**10-19, 1963; **B** courtesy Dr. Peter Simon.)

B

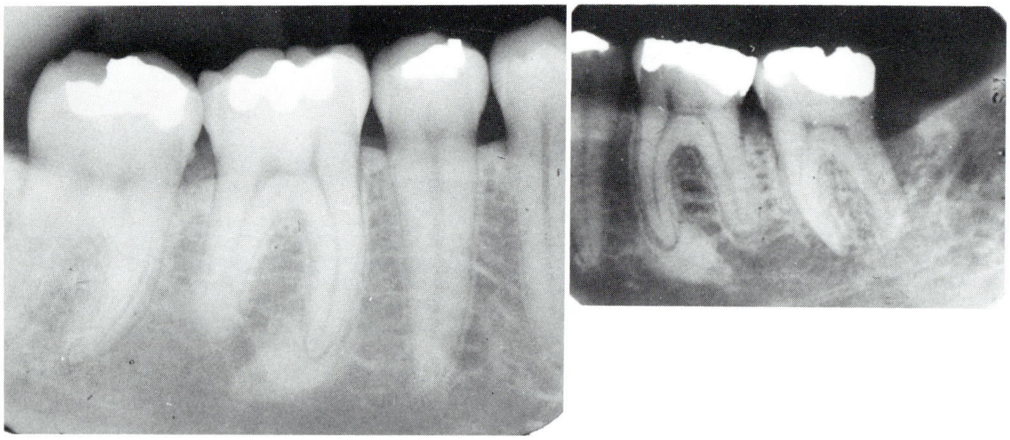

Fig. 8-9, cont'd. For legend see p. 355.

pulp integrity. Conversely, a necrotic pulp can, through an accessory canal, cause disease of the periodontium. This interrelationship between the pulpal and periodontal diseases is further exaggerated by their communicating blood supply.

For a long time I believed that an exposed pulp meant a lost pulp, even in noninfected, accidentally exposed pulps in younger individuals. However, for a number of years I have preserved a number of such pulps with proper pulp capping. The fact that defense cells have been recognized in the pulp, and that in many instances dentin is formed at the site of the exposure, forming a dentin barrier or bridge allowing the pulp to remain vital, caused a change in my approach to this problem.

We must also be on the alert for retrogressive changes that occur in the dental pulp. These changes may be mild or severe. Bevelander[8] has cautioned that clinical pulp testing has not yet reached the state of refinement which permits the detection of these pulpal changes.

Bone changes as seen in the roentgenogram are always important to the clinician. The dentist's curiosity should always be aroused by a variation in osseous architecture or density. Some of the differences can be diagnosed as variations of the normal; however, others are definitely associated with pathosis. Equal importance should be associated with the pathologic changes, regardless of whether they appear radiopaque or radiolucent. Perhaps there is a tendency to place greater significance upon the radiolucent changes. In an effort to balance that tendency, Peter Simon,[9] an excellent endodontist from Fort Worth, Texas, presents a clinical condition which exhibits a radiopaque change in the roentgenogram. He refers to it as "periapical pulpo-osteosclerosis," and he is of the opinion that it is a more precise term than "condensing osteitis." In its incipiency, periapical pulpo-osteosclerosis is not under the stimulating influence of osteoclasia, but rather under the influence of an irritated pulp. The periapical pulpo-osteosclerotic lesion appears as a radiopaque area of varying configurations (Fig. 8-9, *B*).

MARGIN PLACEMENT

Where to place the margin of the restoration in relation to the gingival sulcus is a controversial subject.

Whenever possible, it is advantageous to lay the peripheral margins on sound enamel with a definite abrupt bevel and slightly above the gingival margin, since it not only facilitates accurate marginal adaptation of the gold, but also prevents gingival tissue irritation.

However, the need for a longer retainer on short abutment teeth and the periodontally involved tooth poses a problem of margin placement quite different from a normal noncarious tooth.

The finalized position of the gingival margin of the preparation and, in turn, the crown margin must never be determined until a healthy gingival sulcus is present. This is especially important for teeth that have undergone extensive periodontal treatment. In other words, pocket elimination must be completed, and the tissue must be returned to a state of health before the final marginal placement position is made. When this is done, be sure that any rough marginal areas created by high-speed instrumentation are made

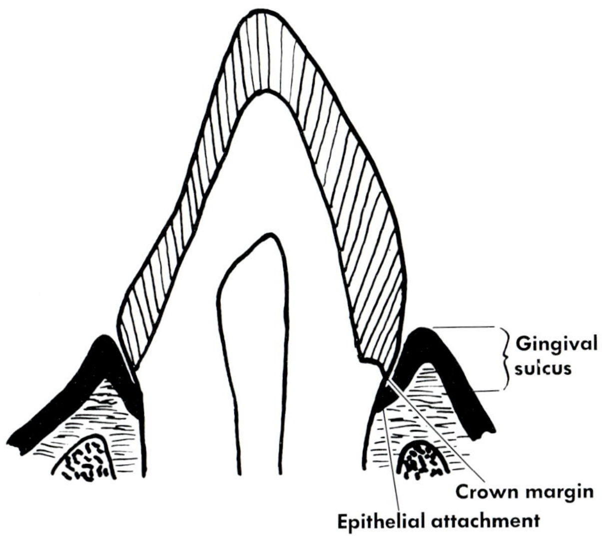

Fig. 8-10. Crown margin should finish short of epithelial attachment, which means that it should not be more than 1 to 1.5 mm. subgingival, depending upon depth of sulcus. (Courtesy Dr. Irving Gordon, Miami Beach, Fla.)

smooth for accurate impression taking, resulting in good fitting restorations.

Many times, because of the importance of esthetics, especially in the region of the upper right bicuspids around the arch to the region of the upper left bicuspids and the lower anterior teeth, and also because of carious, decalcified, or highly sensitive spots in the gingival area, the margin must be positioned in the gingival sulcus.

The answer to the question of how far subgingivally should the crown margin be placed would be that it should finish short of the epithelial attachment—in most cases approximately 1 or 1.5 mm. in the sulcus. Usually this would mean an extension of the finished margin of the retainer slightly more than halfway into the gingival sulcus, which also will cover all prepared tooth structure. If the proper form is given to the cervical third of the restoration, gingival health maintenance is assured also. (See Fig. 8-10.)

Stein[6] has this to say: "Ideally the margin of the crown should be located at the base of the sulcus at the coronal level of the epithelial attachment. Otherwise we can get involved in an area which is not self-cleansing and vulnerable to caries because of plaque accumulation at the margin of the restoration."*

*From Stein, R. Sheldon: Periodontal-prosthetic interrelationships. In Glickman, Irving: Clinical periodontology, Philadelphia, 1964, W. B. Saunders Co., p. 756.

Certainly we should not go subgingivally into areas where the gingival tissues would not be receptive to this transgression.

BEVELS

Proper bevels should be used to enhance the life of the restorations. Bevels protect the enamel rods and facilitate marginal adaptation of the gold.

A butt joint is most difficult to cast to precisely. The end result is a cement line, which eventually washes out, leading to plaque formation and its sequelae—decay and gingival irritation. Therefore, a slight bevel is needed on all shoulder preparations, with the exception of the porcelain jacket crown.

PARALLELISM

Parallelism is another acute problem in extensive restorative work. Its need is very obvious, but its accomplishment is not executed as easily as it is verbally expressed.

In some instances minor orthodontic tooth movement may be needed. In other cases gold copings on some strategic teeth paralleled to themselves or to other preparations around the arch may be very helpful.

Excellent equipment such as the Parallaid, the Pontostructor, and the Chayes Loma Linda paralleling device has been a great help in solving this problem (Fig. 8-11). Learning to be proficient in the use of these tools makes a difficult task much easier.

In the preparation of teeth, definite requirements in self-retention and draw of the restoration must be fulfilled. The term "parallelism," according to Jermyn,[7] is used in place of the correct terminology "ease of path of insertion." With the Parallaid machine (Fig. 8-11, *A*) preparations can be made in a way to conserve tooth structure and still allow parallel cutting of the teeth with proper draw and retention.

If one desires to do paralleling of teeth freehand, a few simple rules must be observed. First, paralleling of slices as well as grooves or pinholes can be obtained by using some line or plane such as the plane of occlusion as a guide. If the operator holds the handpiece parallel to this definite plane, then any slice on any tooth, regardless of its inclination or rotation, will be parallel to any other slice on any tooth at any inclination or degree of rotation. Watch the plane of the straight handpiece or the head of the contra-angle.

I was told a number of years ago to follow a rule borrowed from elementary geometry—two lines perpendicular to the same plane are parallel.

A

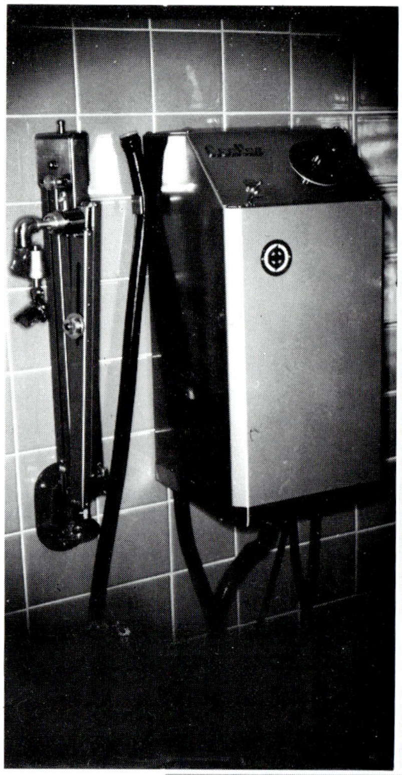

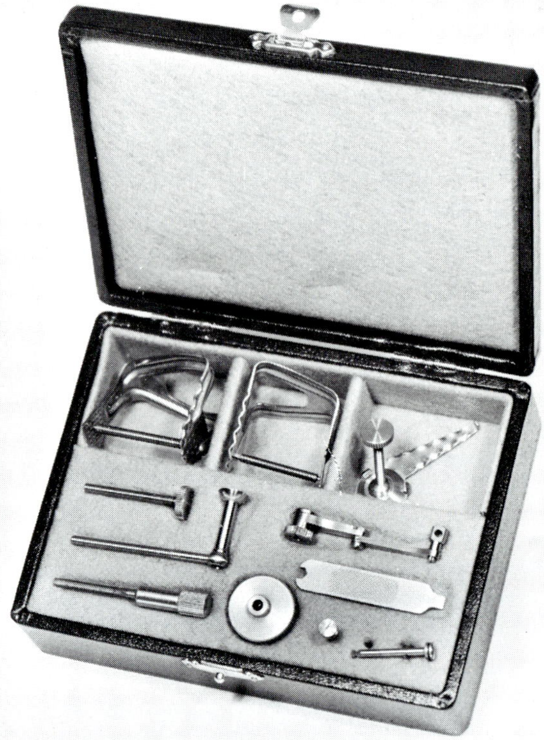

B

C

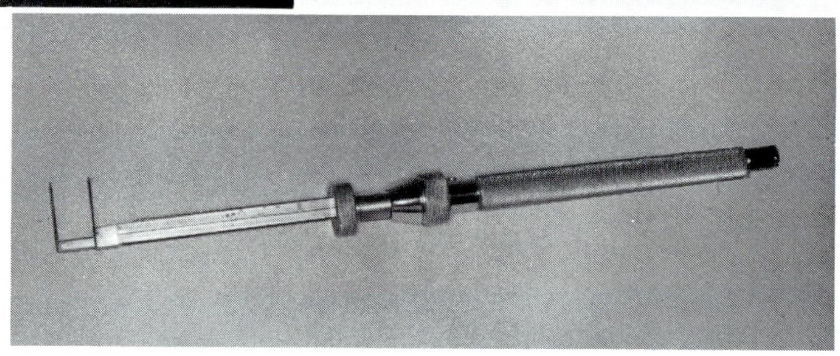

Fig. 8-11. Paralleling aids. **A,** Parallaid. **B,** Instruments composing the Pontostructor set. **C,** Evslin Bridge-o-Meter.

Another good point to remember in paralleling abutments is to keep the fingers, wrist, and forearm rigid. The handpiece then can be held constantly in the determined line of shed. Principles of parallelism must be adhered to when anterior and posterior teeth are to be included in the same fixed bridge or splint.

SIT-DOWN DENTISTRY

A book of this nature should record a few remarks of the ways and means of making the very difficult tasks encountered in this type of work as easy and as least fatiguing as possible to both the dentist and the patient.

First, the auxiliary personnel must be well trained, and the office should have properly designed equipment, especially for operating room efficiency. Learning to work in the correct seated position on a comfortable and properly designed operating stool will lead to more production with less physical and emotional effort. Kilpatrick[10] has pointed out that under these circumstances production can continue over a longer lifespan.

Making use of preoperative sedation medication, modern anesthetics, good lighting facilities, pre-prepared instrument tray set ups, a good contour chair or correct positioning of the patient, comfortable seating and properly designed equipment for the dentist and his carefully trained assistant, high-speed cutting

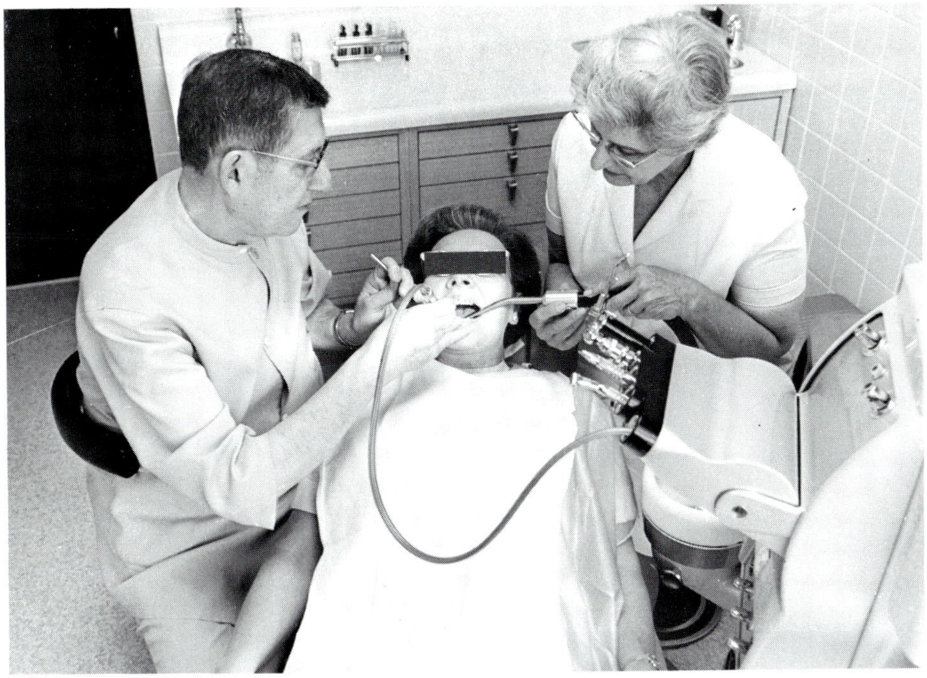

Fig. 8-12. Sit-down dentistry leads to less fatigue, frustration, and extended lifetime of practice.

tools with washed field techniques, etc. will create the proper climate for less fatigue and frustration to all concerned in the performance of concentrated dental procedures. It also will lead to an extended lifetime of practice. (See Figs. 8-12 and 8-13.)

Anderson[11] has told us not to be afraid to change habit patterns. What I have discovered—that has proved to be very beneficial—is changing bad postural operating habits for good ones.

And, above all, the dentist must be in good health—both physically and emotionally.

CAVITY DESIGN AND PREPARATION

As I have said previously, we must have at hand a repertoire of designs for cavity preparation (basic and modifications of the basic form) in this type of work, and a discussion of these preparations now will be undertaken in much detail. This section will deal with procedures of cavity design and preparation that have been proved satisfactory and stable in my hands.

It is essential that the finished product be visualized before operating and that close attention be paid to detail from start to finish. Use must be made of sharp burs, clean true-running diamond points, and well-sharpened hand instruments. The cutting of sound tooth structure should be limited to the amount of substance required for a proper outline form, retention, resistance form, and parallelism of the walls of the

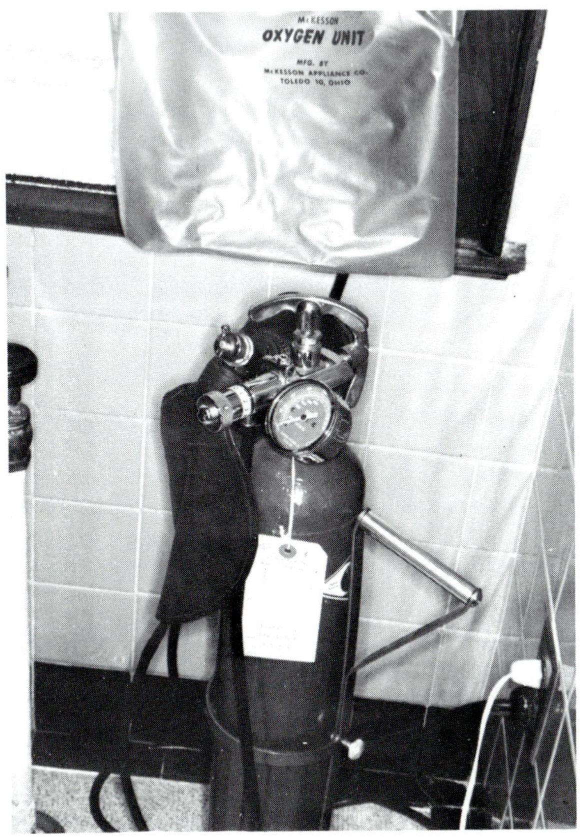

Fig. 8-13. An essential aid in operatory.

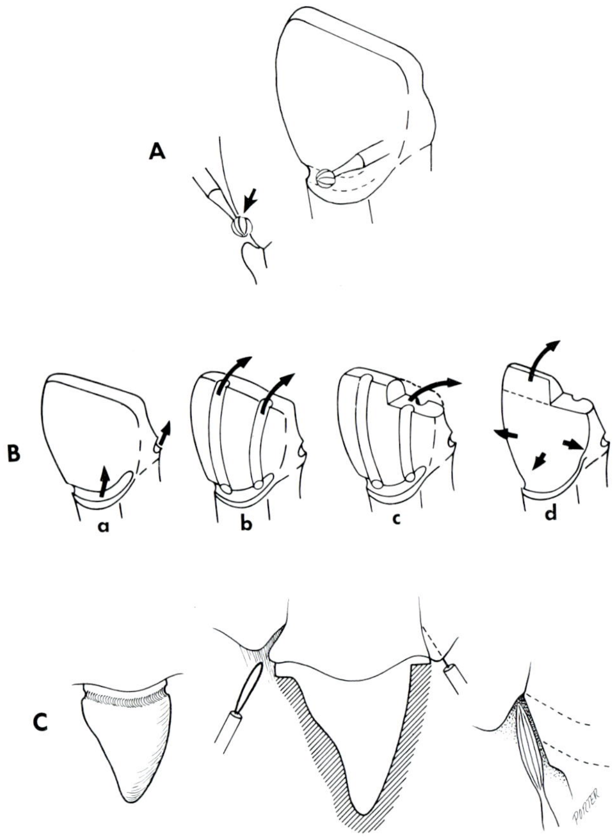

Fig. 8-14. A, Utilizing a No. 6 round bur, a trough is made just above the crest of the gingival tissue, to the depth of the shank. **B,** This is done labially and lingually *(a)* with no attempt to go interproximally. Two vertical troughs are made in the center of mesial and distal thirds of the involved tooth both lingually and labially *(b)*. Then 1½ mm. is removed from half of the incisal edge *(c)*. In *d* we see the result after removal of the tooth structure between the troughs. This reduction procedure is repeated on the lingual and the remaining one-half of the incisal edge. Mesial and distal reduction is made in the usual manner. Adequate reduction of the surfaces have been accomplished, providing for the necessary thickness of metal and porcelain. **C,** Gingival margins are refined and properly beveled. (**A** and **B** courtesy J. M. Ney Co., Hartford, Conn.).

abutment teeth of 2 to 5 degrees from the perpendicular to permit the placing of the retainers from a common direction and also to give the right amount of draft so that retention is not affected. All preparations must have smooth walls and polished margins. A roentgenogram of the tooth or teeth involved must be in full view.

Dento-Metric system

I use the Starlite Dento-Metric sized system, as developed by Amsterdam, and diamond points used in the various types of preparation will be designated by this system.

This system for straight cylinders, tapered cylinders, and flamed shaped diamonds introduces (1) uniform progression of lengths and diameters to encompass exactly any surface length of any crown or cavity, (2) uniform shank length, (3) a numbering system that indicates shape, head length, and diamond form of the instrument, and (4) tapered cylinders having uniform tapers, permitting one instrument to follow another without altering the cutting angle.

In the numbering system the scale below illustrates how Starlite Dento-Metric numbers indicate a full description of the instrument:

Instrument No. 700 – 7 P

Shape	Head length	Diamond form
(Like a No. 700 bur)	(7 mm.)	(P: Prestressed)

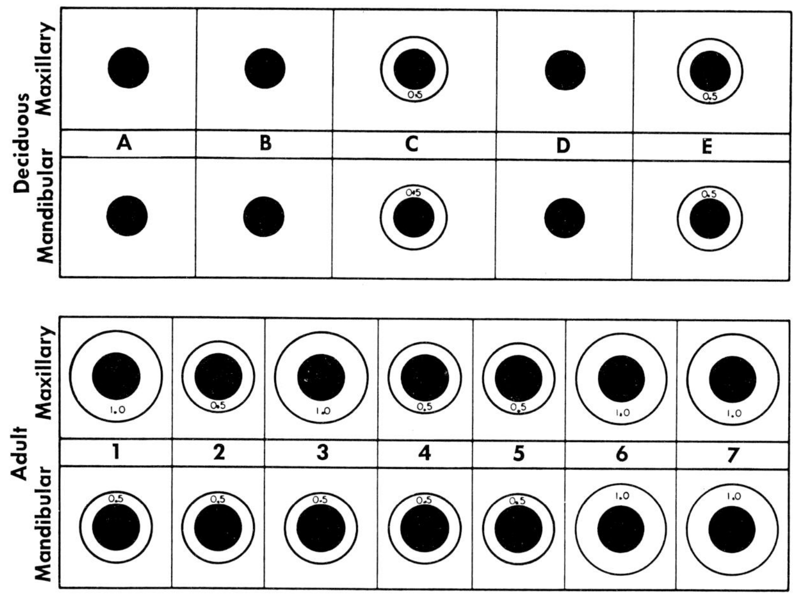

Fig. 8-15. *Safety zones.* The depth to which dentin may be excised safely, measured from the dentinoenamel junction pulpally, is indicated in millimeters by the numerals within the circles. If the depth of a cavity preparation does not exceed the figure within the circle, there will always be at least 0.5 mm. of dentin between the cavity floor and pulpal wall. There is an exception to this rule on the lingual surface of the maxillary lateral incisor where as little as 0.8 mm. dentin has been found between the tip of the pulp horn and the dentinoenamel junction. The figures are based on the least amount of dentin ever found, not on the average. (Courtesy Dr. Sumter S. Arnim.)

In the diamond form there is also available the micro-grain (M) and the superfinishing (F) that indicates the fineness of the diamond particles, which in turn determines the speed of cut.

Arnim[12] has called attention to the fact that there is a limited amount of dentin available for safe cutting in any tooth. Since dentin is deposited rhythmically, there is a relatively constant amount around the pulp of each tooth. The dentinoenamel junction is a stable guideline from which the dentist can measure the depth of the preparation (Fig. 8-14). A safety zone can be formulated for groups of teeth (Fig. 8-15). "Cavities prepared within the limits of the safety zones seldom cause pulp injury. One cannot cut dentin without cutting thousands of living cells of the dental pulp. Each odontoblast has a process extending from the cell through a tubule to the dentinoenamel junction."* Coolants do not always prevent heat production and pulp damage during cavity preparations. Pulpal tissue is traumatized if its temperature is raised as much as 10° F. Arnim[12] is also of the opinion that the customary practice of using local anesthetic for cavity preparation on all patients contributes, more than any other single factor, to a careless disregard of basic principles. And this in spite of the fact that the human dental pulp is not seriously or permanently damaged by local anesthesia.

It would be amiss not to delve into the significant research work done by Craig, M. Kamal El-Ebrashi, Peyton, Farah, Tillitson, and Nally on experimental stress analysis of dental restorations[13] at this time. These experiments included (1) inlays, (2) crowns, (3) proximal margins, (4) axial walls, (5) occlusal reduction and pins, (6) proximal reduction in compound restorations, (7) fixed partial dentures, (8) gold and chromium fixed partial dentures, (9) porcelain-bonded-to-gold crowns, (10) stress distribution in porcelain-fused-to-gold crowns and preparations constructed with photoelastic plastics, and (11) reflection photoelastic stress analysis of a dental bridge.

All models were constant two-dimensional, photoelastic, cataline resin designs, and all measurements were made on a very intricate recording device.[14]

The conclusions drawn from these experiments and some illustrations are given here (with the permission of the authors) for the reader's perusal and consideration. In spite of the fact that I have had many

*From Arnim, Sumter S.: Conservation of the dental pulp—cavity preparation, J. Prosthet. Dent. **9**(6):1017-1036, 1959.

years of extensive clinical experience and have observed the end results very closely over a period of years, I have learned a number of important facts from these experiments, which in turn have cleared up a number of misconceptions in my own mind.

INLAYS

1. Compressive stresses were reduced near the pulpal surface of M.O.D. restorations, when the load was applied either mesially or distally to it.

2. The rate of change of compressive stresses is relatively higher in tilted teeth compared with teeth in normal occlusion, under similar test conditions.

3. The M.O.D. box preparation with rounded axiopulpal line angles has lower stress concentration in comparable areas to the shoulderless slice preparation.

CROWNS

1. The maximum compressive stresses on the interior of crowns were generally found to be on the reduced cusp surface of the restorations. Maximum tensile stresses were observed in the central fossa and along the axis of symmetry of the crown, when the crowns were loaded bilaterally, or with two-point contact along the axis of symmetry to simulate oral conditions.

2. It is desirable to have multiple point contact when an antagonistic tooth occludes with the abutment crown, to reduce stress concentrations near the central fossa of the restored tooth.

3. Full shoulders (or their equivalent) on complete crowns are recommended, and in instances of proximal caries, proximal boxes and bevels are suggested in order to increase the bulk in the critical cervical margin, thus redistributing the tensile stresses developed.

4. Reduced cusps should be rounded on the preparation to avoid the development of high compressive stresses on the interior surface of the crown, which may induce postoperative pain.

5. Deep developmental grooves carved near the center of the tooth should be avoided, since they will tend to produce deleterious stress concentrations. This consideration is also important if cusps of teeth are reduced and then protected in occlusal rehabilitation.

PROXIMAL MARGINS

1. The chamfer and rounded-type preparations were the optimum designs in proximal occlusal posterior restorations. They showed the lowest stress concentration when loaded vertically.

2. Rounding the axiogingival line angle in shoulder geometry experiments reduced the stress concentration factor up to 50%.

3. The gingival area of proximal shoulders was a critical location for stress concentration. Extraretentive features (pins or grooves) should not be placed in this area.

PARALLELISM OF AXIAL WALLS

1. Sloping the two axial walls of the proximal portion increased the stress concentration factor in restorations with axial walls. The optimum convergence angle was between 2.5 and 6.5 degrees. The stress concentration factor increased slightly from 0 to 15 degrees, and increased sharply at 20 degrees.

2. The tensile stress at the axiogingival line angle was small when the occlusal load was applied on the opposite occlusoaxial line angle.

OCCLUSAL REDUCTION AND PINS

1. Buccal and lingual cusps on posterior teeth to be used as abutments in restorative dentistry should be protected with gold on the occlusal surface if the cusp length exceeds the breadth of the cusp as measured at the base.

2. The stress concentration factor computed for a flat reduction of cusps was 40% less than that for anatomic reduction of cusps because of the increase in the thickness of the restoration (pulpal configuration must permit).

3. A definite relationship was found between the extent of cuspal protection and stress concentration factors. Increasing the thickness of gold on the occlusal surface decreases the stress concentration factor.

4. In two-point loading of the occlusal surface of posterior restored teeth, the stresses in the restoration in the region of the central fossa were tensile in nature. Deep developmental grooves in this region should be avoided.

5. The tensile stress at the central fossa was small in magnitude and could be reduced by decreasing the corresponding cuspal angles.

6. Nontapered vertical occlusal pins did not alter the distribution of stress in posterior restorations or in the residual tooth structure. Long pins had a higher stress concentration than the short pins.

PROXIMAL REDUCTION IN COMPOUND RESTORATIONS

1. No significant structural differences were found between the slice restoration, proximal boxes with parallel walls, and proximal boxes with walls of 45

degree inclination. These three designs showed the same stress concentration factor.

2. If minimization of tensile stresses in the slice restoration is desired, it may be accomplished by additional reduction of tooth structure at the proximo-linguo-occlusal point angles, which would increase the bulk of gold at these critical surfaces.

3. Proximal boxes with parallel walls result in concentration of stress at the junction of the parallel wall with the remainder of the restoration.

FIXED PARTIAL DENTURES

1. Fixed partial dentures do not function in bending as a symmetrical beam. Alternate areas of tension and compression were demonstrated when multiple contact loading was used.

2. The weakest part in posterior fixed partial dentures is the fixed joint (soldered area), since it exhibited high concentration of tensile and shear stresses.

3. V-shaped grooves at the fixed joints should be avoided and should be replaced by regular U-shaped grooves. Through isochromatics, U-shaped grooves show twice as much strength as V-shaped grooves. The ratio of the radius of the groove to its depth (r/d) should be as large as possible to reduce the tensile and shear stresses at these critical locations.

4. Cantilever fixed partial dentures had much higher stresses at the fixed joint than fixed partial dentures that were attached at both ends.

PORCELAIN-BONDED-TO-GOLD CROWNS

1. In a crown restoration the cement functions as a stress distributor.

2. The gold part of the crown also acts as a stress distributor and absorbs most of the stress put on the crown.

3. A restricted occlusal surface provides a more favorable stress distribution.

4. A shoulder type preparation with rounded internal line angles seems to be the best geometry for the porcelain-bonded-to-gold crown restorations.

5. Sharp grooves should be avoided in carving the occlusal surface of the porcelain.

REFLECTION PHOTOELASTIC STRESS ANALYSIS OF A FIXED PARTIAL DENTURE

The stress distribution on the surface of a four-unit bridge was determined by reflection photoelasticity. The highest stress concentration was at the soldered joints. The distribution of stress was a function of the support of the abutment teeth. Good support caused the bridge to function as one that was fixed at both ends, whereas poor support caused it to function as a cantilever beam.

STRESS DISTRIBUTION IN PORCELAIN-FUSED-TO-GOLD CROWNS AND PREPARATIONS

1. The gold-porcelain joint near the shoulder should be 30 degrees from the horizontal.

2. Porcelain supported by gold is superior to a porcelain jacket crown.

3. A bulk of gold in the gingival region reduces the state of stress.

4. The porcelain-gold joint on the lingual shoulder should be as far as feasible from the site of loading.

5. Complete porcelain coverage of metal is not superior to providing a bulk of gold on the lingual shoulder* (Figs. 8-16 to 8-25).

Modified onlay preparation

In many cases of mouth rehabilitation the lower mandibular first premolar is only in need of a modified type of onlay—a D.O. type, with a slight mesial bevel above the contact area, provided the mesial surface is not carious or filled and has a good contact area.

The first premolar is a particularly difficult tooth to prepare, and conservation of tooth structure must be stressed. The occlusal floor of the preparation should not be too deep; it must be sloped lingually to avoid pulpal encroachment and the path of withdrawal is usually in a linguo-occlusal direction. A shallow box preparation is made distally after the occlusal surface has been dressed down properly, keeping in mind a reduced reproduction of the anatomic form of this surface instead of a flat one, with buccal and lingual extensions in the form of a reverse bevel. A slight mesial bevel is incorporated in this preparation to avoid a ''bunchy'' or grotesque effect to the finished restoration and to give the necessary aid sometimes needed in the development of a cusp-fossa occlusion. Two pin retentions are made in the point angles of the distal box, one at the gingivobuccoaxial angle and the other at the gingivolinguoaxial angle. These pin retentions are made with a No. 700 tapered fissure bur, not more than 0.5 mm. deep. During this operation,

*From Craig, Robert G., and others: Experimental stress analysis of dental restorations (Parts I through IX), J. Prosthet. Dent. **17**:277-291, 1967; **17**:292-302, 1967; **22**:333-353, 1969; **22**:565-577, 1969; **22**:663-670, 1969; **23**:177-186, 1970; **24**:174-180, 1970; **25**:307-316, 1970; J. Dent. Res. **50**(5):1253-1259, 1278-1283, 1971.

Figs. 8-16 to 8-25. The illustrations in this series (Figs. 8-16 to 8-25) courtesy R. G. Craig, University of Michigan, Ann Arbor, Mich.

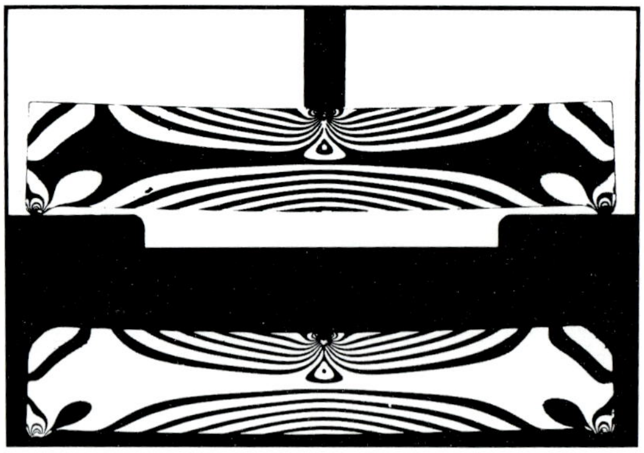

Fig. 8-16. A beam in bending. *Above:* A dark-field isochromatic fringe pattern. *Below:* A light-field isochromatic fringe pattern.

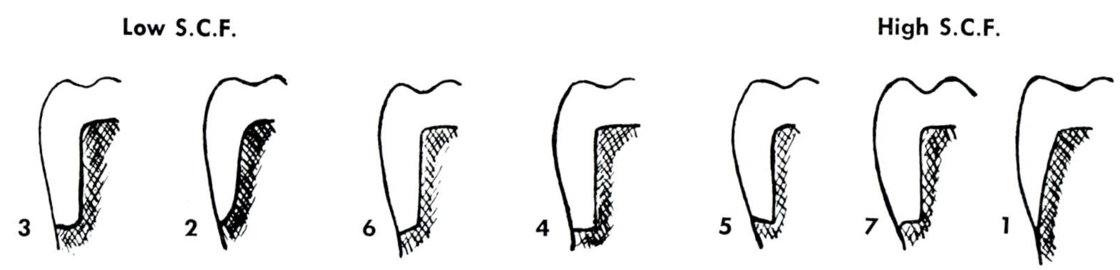

Fig. 8-17. Shoulder geometry models are arranged in order of their stress concentration factor (S.C.F.).

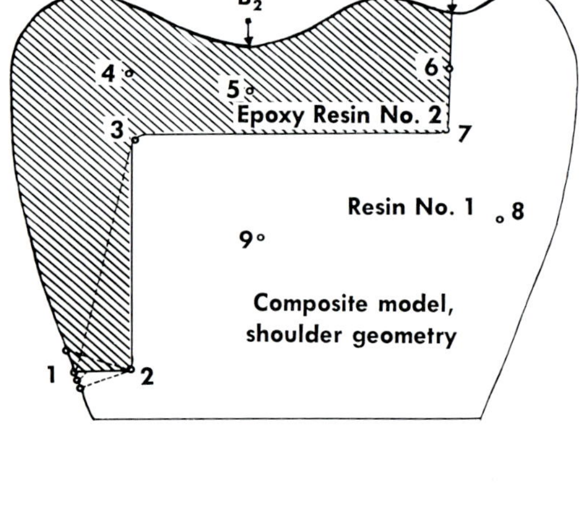

Fig. 8-18. Different loading sites of shoulder geometry models. Points 1 to 9 are of interest in the final stress analysis.

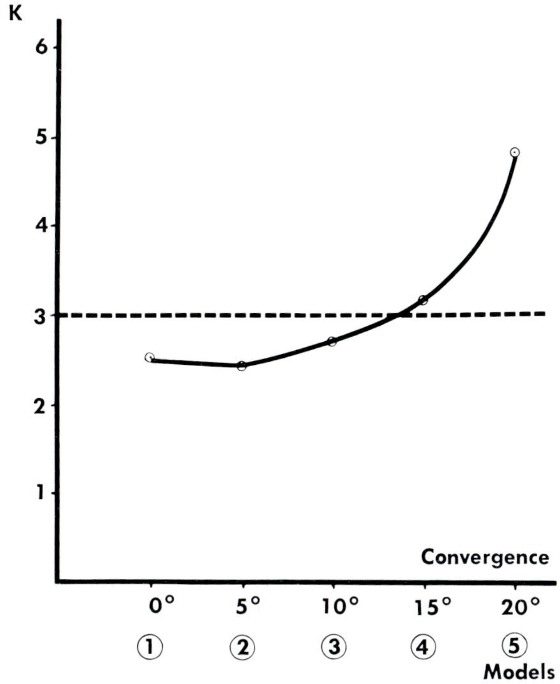

Fig. 8-19. Stress concentration factors for models with various convergence angles of the axial walls.

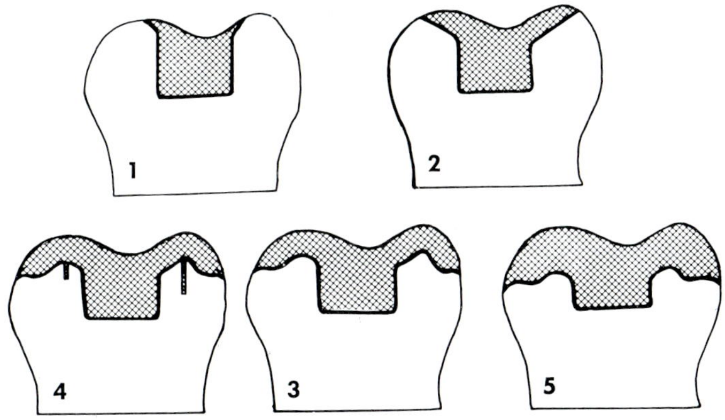

Fig. 8-20. The type of occlusal reduction is depicted for models 1 through 5.

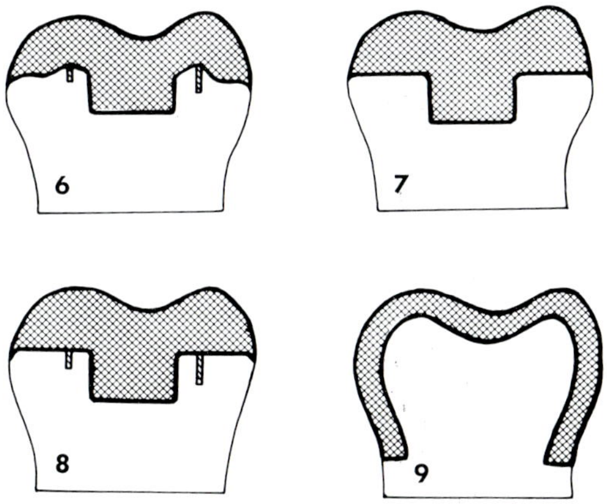

Fig. 8-21. The type of occlusal reduction is depicted for models 6 through 9.

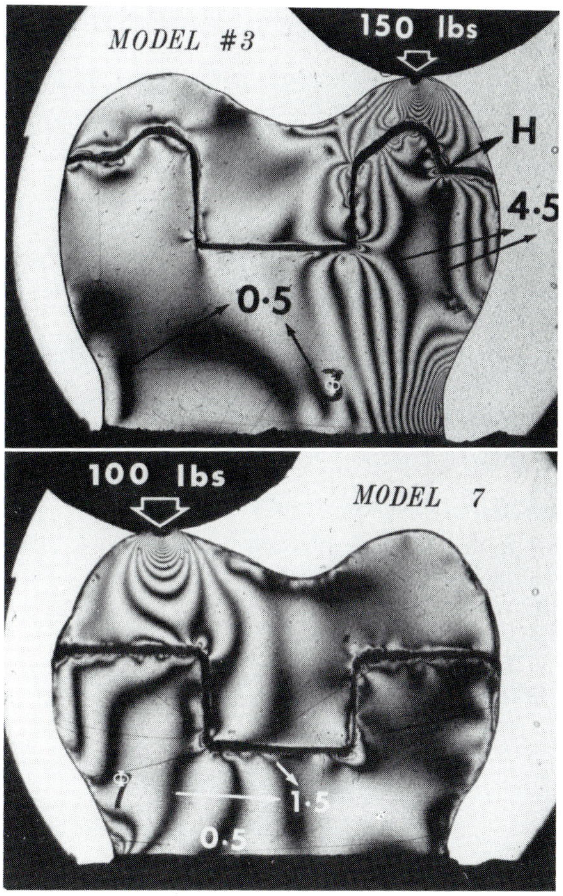

Fig. 8-22. Light-field views of isochromatics of two models resulting from a 150 pound load on the lingual cusp and a 100 pound load on the buccal cusp.

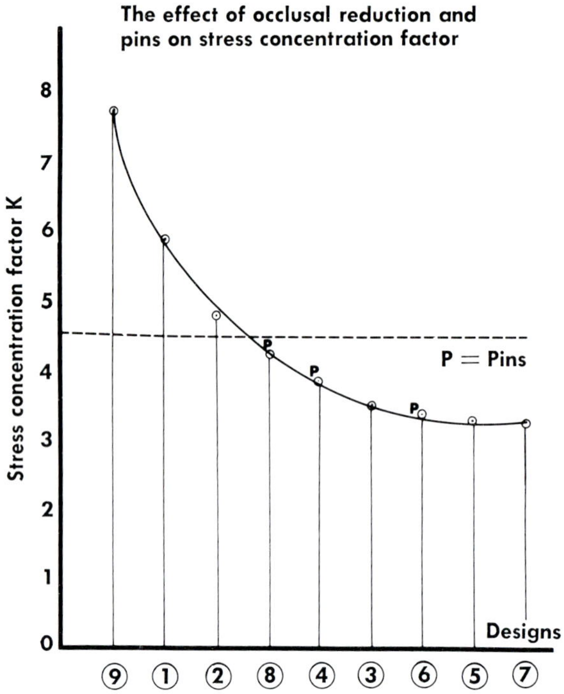

Fig. 8-23. Stress concentration factors for models with various modification of occlusal reduction of tooth structure.

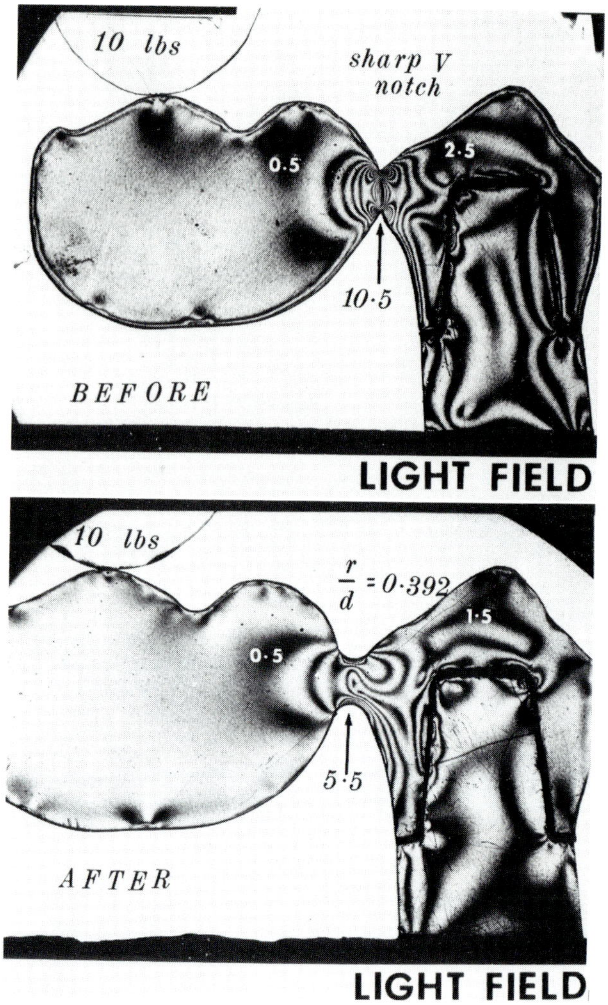

Fig. 8-24. Cantilever model with a sharp V notch (top) is contrasted with the same model with U notches (bottom). Both models were loaded with 10 pounds to produce a bending moment of 21 pound–inches.

grooves also are being made on the buccal and lingual walls. A well is developed in the mesial fossa to a depth of 0.5 to 2 mm., or a pinhole can be made with the same No. 700 tapered fissure bur to the depth of 1.5 to 2 mm. for greater retention. This gives the basic tripodal balance that was discussed previously (Fig. 8-26).

The gingival margin is finished with sharp gingival trimmers, being sure that a definite gingival bevel has been established (Fig. 8-27). An axial undercut should be avoided because it is impossible to make a casting fit accurately in a cavity with axial undercuts. The axial and gingival margins should join in a graceful curve and all margins finished and polished very carefully.

Onlays

In the preparation of a tooth for an M.O.D. onlay, all functioning surfaces should be covered or "shoed" completely so that fracture or shearing of a cusp is prevented. This is accomplished by covering the occlusal surface with buccal and lingual extensions (giving the shingle-roof effect) beyond the functioning range of contact with the opposing teeth, which also allows the restoration to blend harmoniously into the remaining contours of the tooth, thereby negating an otherwise grotesque effect. The buccal and lingual walls are contained, the buccal and lingual extensions are beyond any occlusal facets, and some portion of the outer walls always remains, which acts as an excellent guide to a more nearly correct anatomic reconstruction. Because of these guidelines, we can do a better job in developing our functional carvings. (See Fig. 8-28.)

The occlusal surface should not be dressed down flat, for in so doing the pulp horns are approached unnecessarily. The reduction, following the cusp planes, should be sufficient to provide adequate metal protection and strength in all mandibular excursions when the restoration is completed (at least the equivalent of the thickness of two pieces of blotter paper) (Fig. 8-29).

A

B

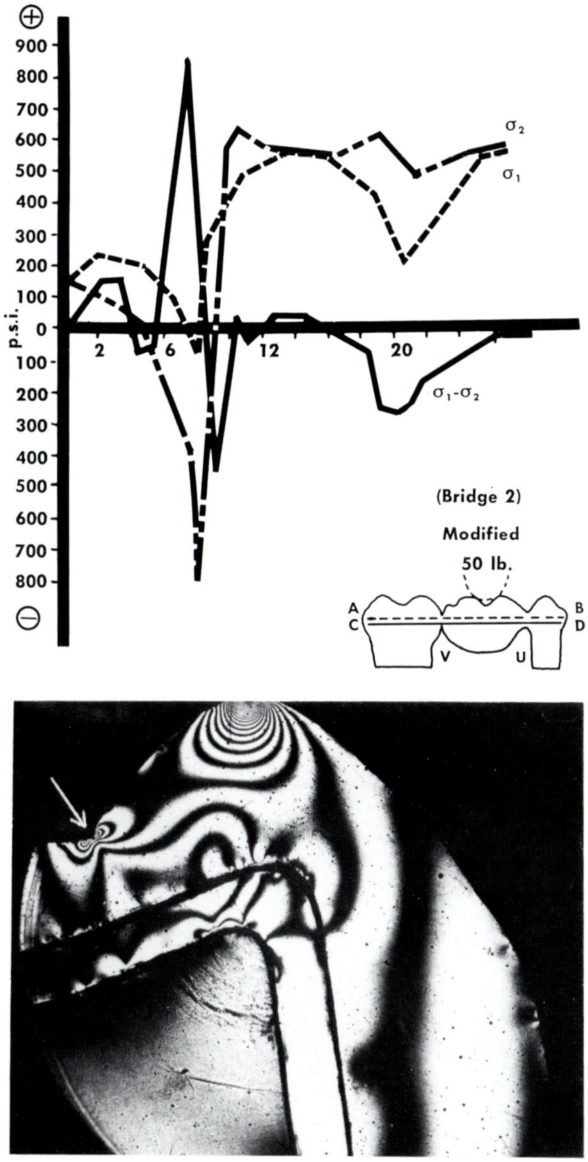

Fig. 8-25. A, The principal stresses are indicated along a line midway between *AB* and *CD* in modified model when loaded on the pontic with a 50 pound load. The difference between the principal stresses ($\sigma_1 - \sigma_2$) is shown as the solid-line curve, σ_1 is denoted by the dashed line curve, and σ_2 is denoted by the interrupted black line curve. **B,** Isochromatics are shown in above model under 150 pounds of load on the lingual cusp. Note the stress concentration around the sharp groove on the occlusal surface (white arrow). (From Craig, R. G., El-Ebrashi, M. K., Peyton, F. A., and others: J. Prosthet. Dent. 1967, 1969, 1970.)

The convergence of the mesial and distal walls from gingival surface to occlusal surface should be in the area of 2 degrees from the perpendicular if possible. If a group of teeth are to be splinted and the M.O.D. onlay is the restoration of choice, the walls of the preparation may need a taper of slightly more than 2 degrees from the perpendicular.

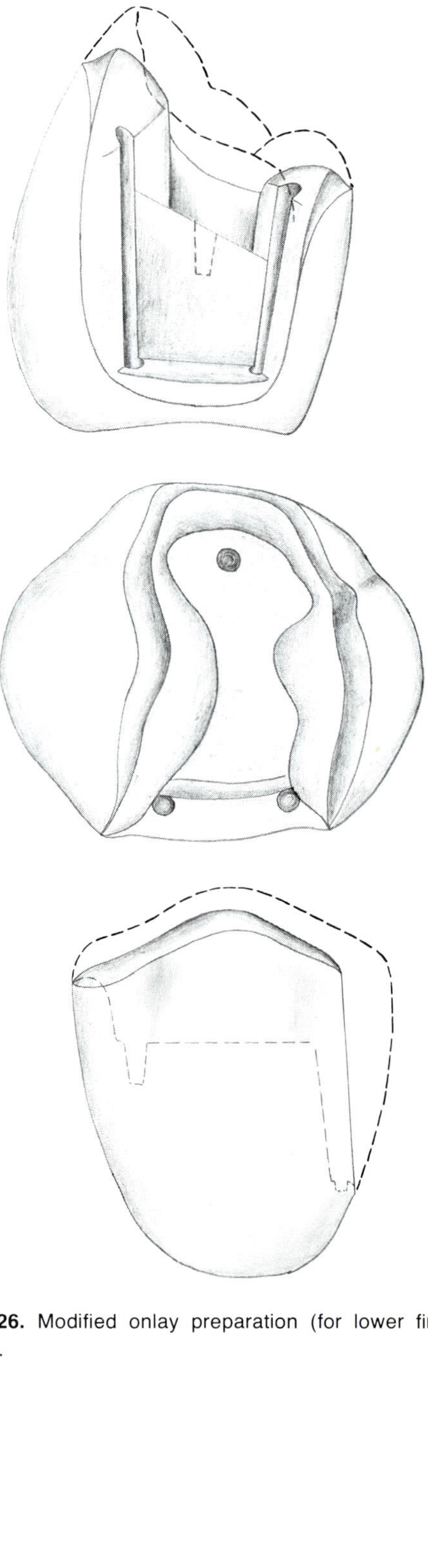

Fig. 8-26. Modified onlay preparation (for lower first premolars).

The occlusal depth should be at least 1 mm. into the dentin, and the floor of the cavity should be flat and rather wide. Shallow modified box retention with flat or axially inclined gingival seats, square walls, and properly beveled gingival margins, both mesially and distally, is essential. The axiopulpal line angles should be slightly coved to strengthen the casting. The use of grooves mesiobuccally and mesiolingually as well as distobuccally and distolingually with pin retentions made in the point angles to the depth of 0.5 mm., one at the gingivobuccoaxial angle, the other at the gingivolinguoaxial angle (mesially and distally), and of an auxiliary pin positioned on the occlusal surface either buccally or lingually to the depth of 1.5 to 2 mm. is indicated many times especially in teeth that are shorter than normal. (See Fig. 8-30.)

A

B

C

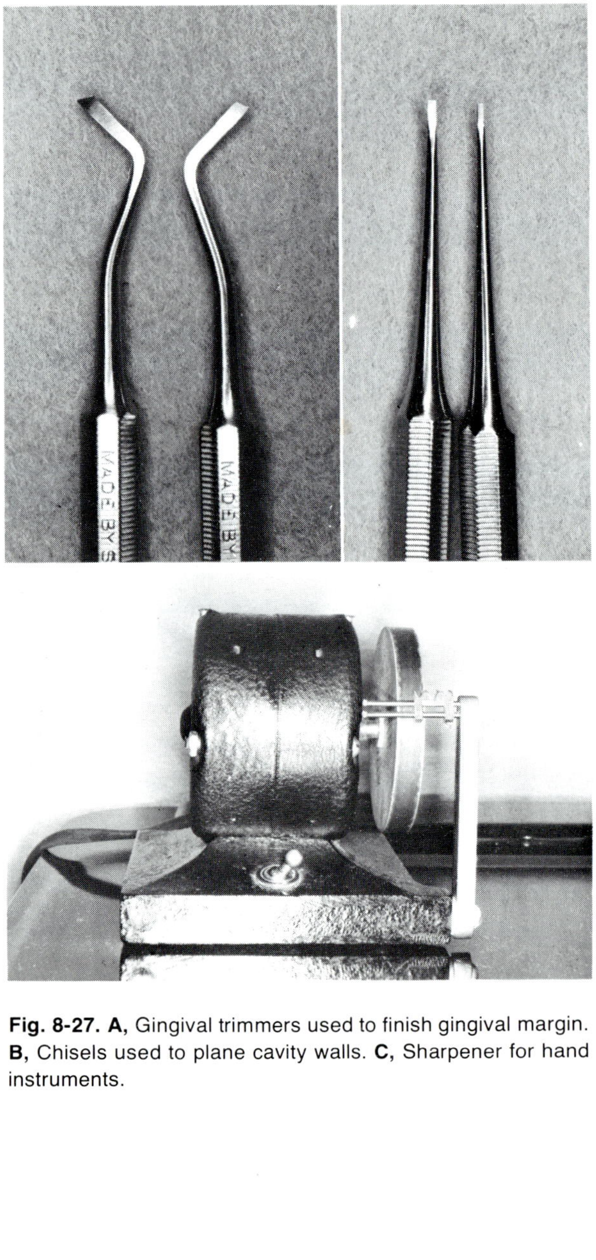

Fig. 8-27. A, Gingival trimmers used to finish gingival margin. **B,** Chisels used to plane cavity walls. **C,** Sharpener for hand instruments.

Undercuts, which result from removal of last traces of decay, are avoided by leaving the caries until the impression is made, after which the carious dentin is removed while the anesthesia is still effective.

Finish the gingival margin with sharp gingival trimmers and be sure that a definite gingival bevel has been established. Avoid an axial undercut because it is impossible to make a casting fit accurately in a cavity with axial undercuts. The axial and gingival margins should join in a graceful curve. Finish cavity walls by a final planing with freshly sharpened instruments, cuttle disks, and fine diamond points, which results in smooth walls and polished margins.

The principle of tripodism also has been carried out in this type of preparation with resultant stability. (Fig. 8-31).

Three-quarter crowns

The veneer type of retainer can withstand heavy functional stresses. It ties the structural elements of the crown more tightly together, thus preventing fractured walls and cusps.

Willey[15] has aptly told us that in the veneer type of retainer the entire functioning surface, incisal or occlusal, should be covered.

"By the use of long bevels, the margins are carried out beyond the facets of wear, to achieve three definite ends:

"(a) grinding or wear is never allowed to exert destructive force on the margin between metal and tooth;

Text continued on p. 373.

A

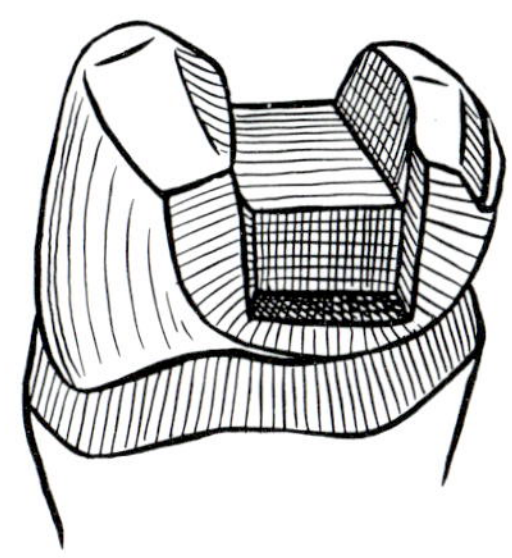

B

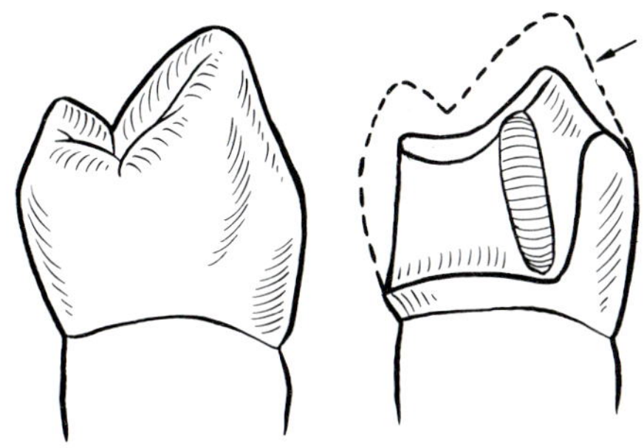

C

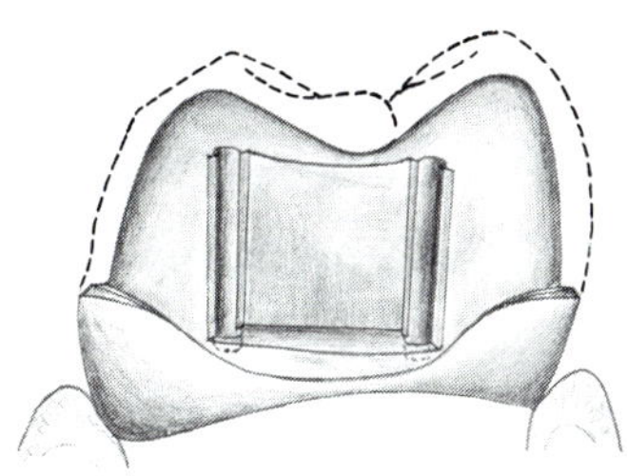

Fig. 8-28. Outer walls (unprepared) act as excellent guidelines in developing functional carvings. **A,** M.O.D. onlay. **B,** Three-quarter crown (shingle-roof effect). **C,** Modified onlay preparation.

A

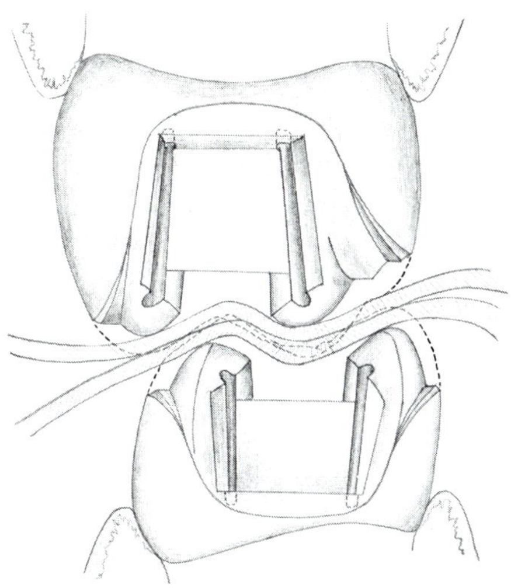

B

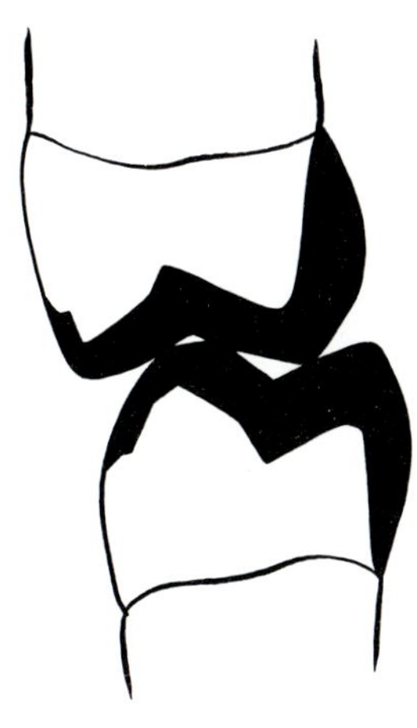

Fig. 8-29. A, The thickness of two pieces of blotter paper is used to provide adequate metal protection. **B,** Adequate metal protection and correct placement of facial margins.

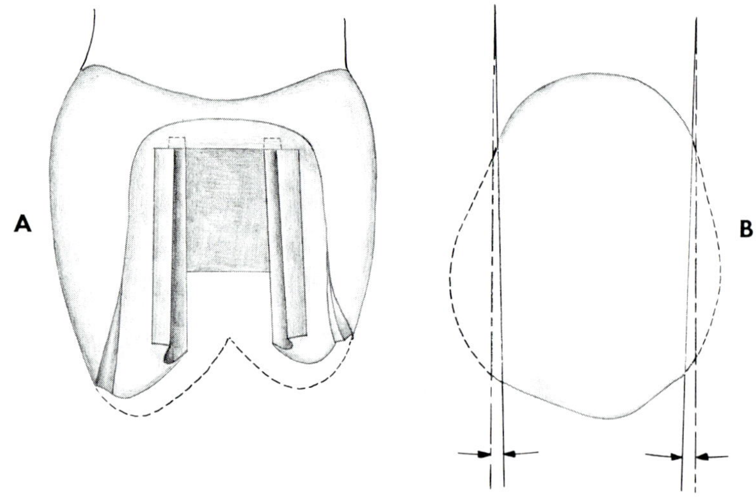

Fig. 8-30. A, Floor of cavity should be flat and rather wide. Shallow modified box retention, use of grooves mesiobuccally and mesiolingually, as well as distobuccally and distolingually with pin retention in point angles to at least depth of 0.5 mm. **B,** Convergence of mesial and distal walls from gingival to occlusal surface should be in the area of 2 degrees from the perpendicular if possible.

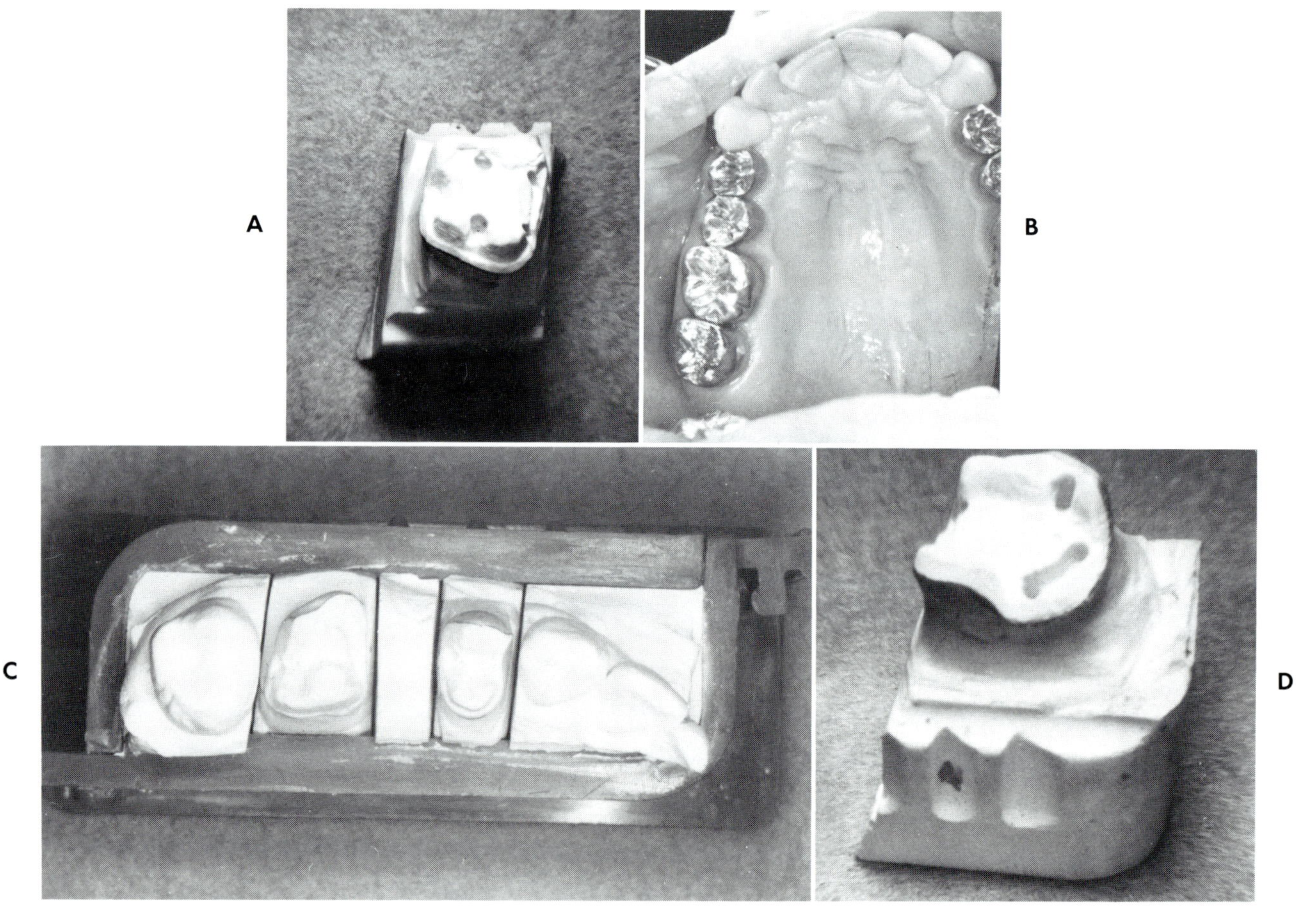

Fig. 8-31. A, Various preparations from practice illustrating principle of tripodism with resultant stability. **A** and **B,** Preparation and view of finished restoration in mouth. **C,** Preparations for a fixed partial denture. **D,** A modified preparation. $\mathbf{E}_1$ and $\mathbf{E}_2$, Electro-Torque Handpiece Selection (Kerr Dental Mfg. Co., Detroit, Mich.). $\mathbf{E}_3$, Titan High-Torque Handpiece System (Star Dental Mfg. Co., Inc., Conshohocken, Pa.).

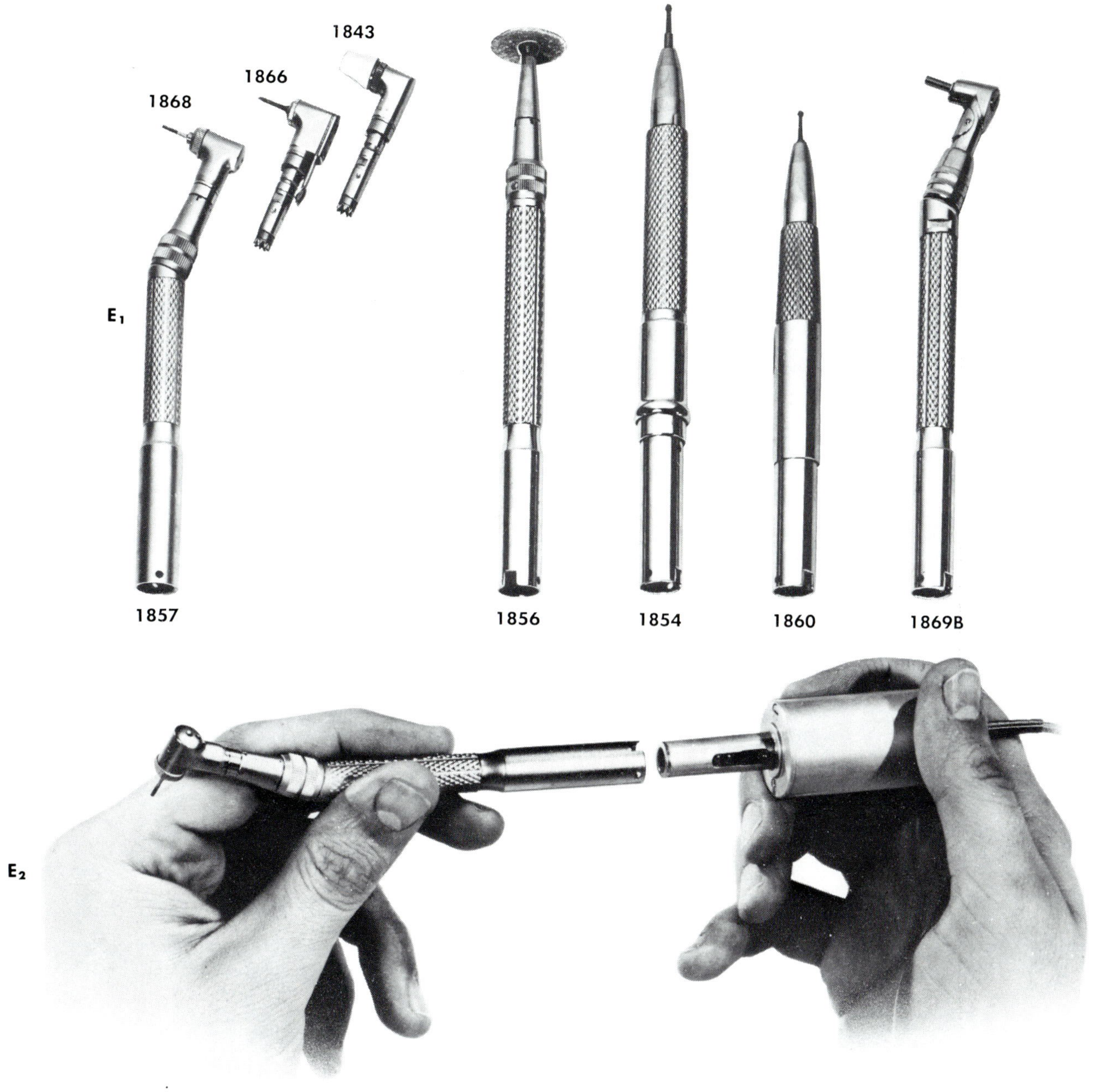

Fig. 8-31, cont'd. For legend see opposite page.

E₃

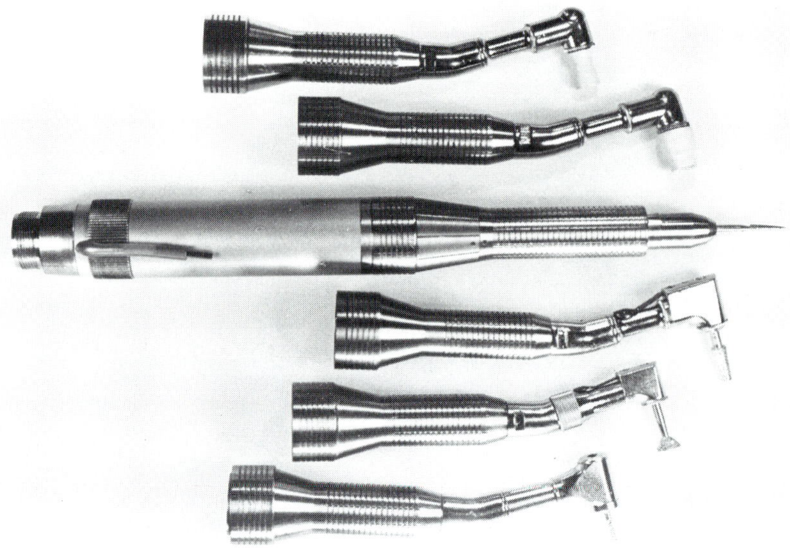

Fig. 8-31, cont'd. For legend see p. 370.

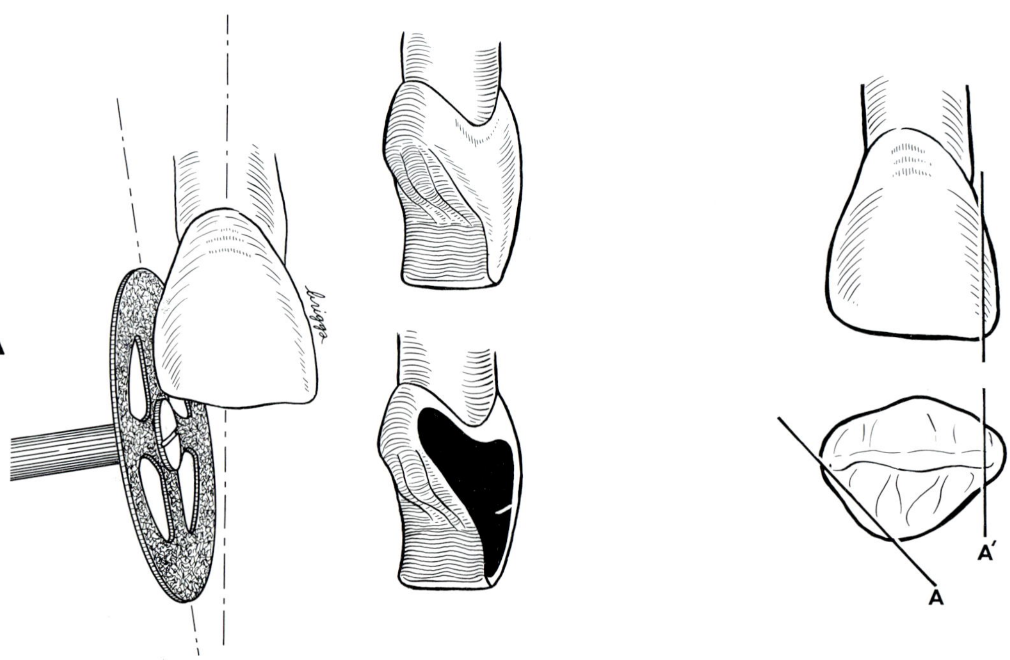

Fig. 8-32. A, Mesial and distal slices are made from lingual approach, allowing for full mesiodistal width of labial surface and thereby almost invisible gold margins. **B,** Correct *(A)* and incorrect *(A')* methods of preparing mesial and distal slices.

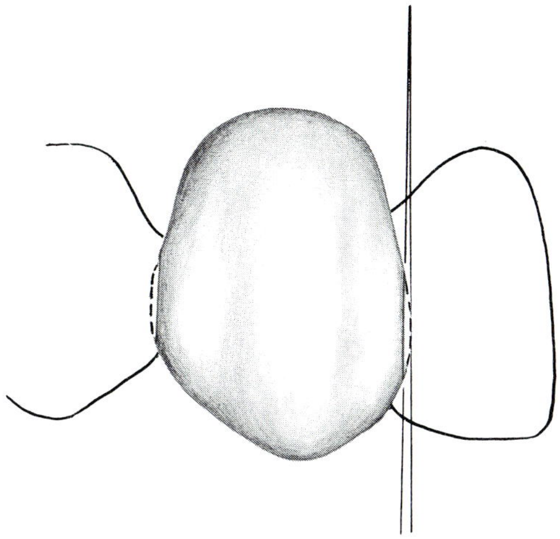

Fig. 8-33. Convergence of mesial and distal walls from gingival to incisal surface should be from 2 to 5 degrees from perpendicular—the closer to 2 degrees the better.

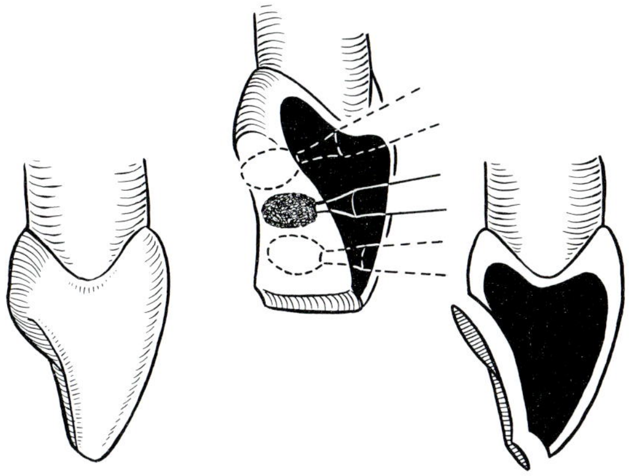

Fig. 8-34. Reduction of lingual surface of upper anterior tooth.

"(b) the sweep of food over this margin during function is similar to the shedding of water by a shingle roof; the action tends to close the margin rather than open it; and

"(c) the structural elements of the tooth are held together."*

The three-quarter crown gives maximum retention with a minimum loss of tooth structure. By preserving the facial enamel surfaces of both anterior and posterior teeth, not only is a pleasing esthetic appearance obtained, but also the vulnerable gingival tissues remain healthy.

The mesial and distal slices are made from the lingual approach extending to the labial surface only enough to include areas vulnerable to decay. The full mesiodistal width of the labial surface should be retained, providing casting margins that are practically invisible. The convergence of these walls from the gingival to the incisal surface should be from 2 to 5 degrees from the perpendicular, and the closer to the former the better the end result will be. (See Figs. 8-32 and 8-33.)

In the reduction of the lingual surface of upper anterior teeth (Fig. 8-34) the cut extends from the crest of the cingulum to the incisal edge, leaving the cingulum intact because of its retentive value. Enough tooth structure must be removed to provide clearance in the centric position and the eccentric excursions (allow for a thickness of metal of about 0.75 to 1 mm.).

The incisal area on the lingual surface is beveled to a 45-degree angle to the long axis of the tooth and is hollow ground for a greater bulk of metal at this vulnerable area, so that the gold is prevented from becoming work hard, brittle, and opening up or lifting away at the margin (Fig. 8-35).

The grooves on the proximal surfaces, running from the incisal bevel to the gingival limit of the preparation, are started with a No. 701 or 701L tapered crosscut fissure bur or its equivalent, and then are followed with a No. 700 or 700L tapered crosscut fissure bur, moving the bur in a labiolingual direction, thereby creating a tapered keyed groove or lock groove. The depth of the groove should extend into the dentin and its diameter in proportion to the size and bulk of the tooth. Round grooves can be used if the tooth is large and the demands are not too great, but the interlocking groove is best because it is effective whether the demands are great or not so great and the tooth is small or large. With a groove of this type the tooth is engaged actively in grasping the casting, which practically obviates the possibility of the casting opening up at the cervical margin. The direction of the groove is in a plane closely parallel with the incisal two thirds of the labial surface (Fig. 8-36). This is the longest distance obtainable, which is a "must," and the grooves should be parallel to each other. If the mesial or distal surface is carious or contains restorations, a shallow box–type preparation with lateral interlocking or tapered keyed grooves and a gingival floor ditch or inclincation is indicated. Walls and grooves of proper convergency and adequate

*From Willey, Robert E.: The preparation of abutments for veneer retainers, J.A.D.A. **53:**141-154, 1956.

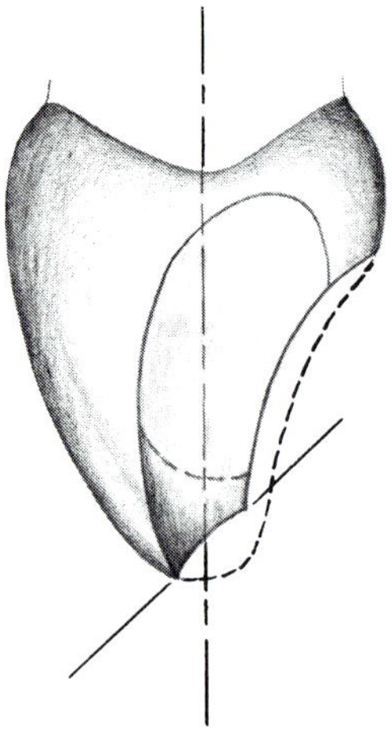

Fig. 8-35. Incisal area on lingual surface beveled to 45 degree angle to long axis of tooth and hollow ground.

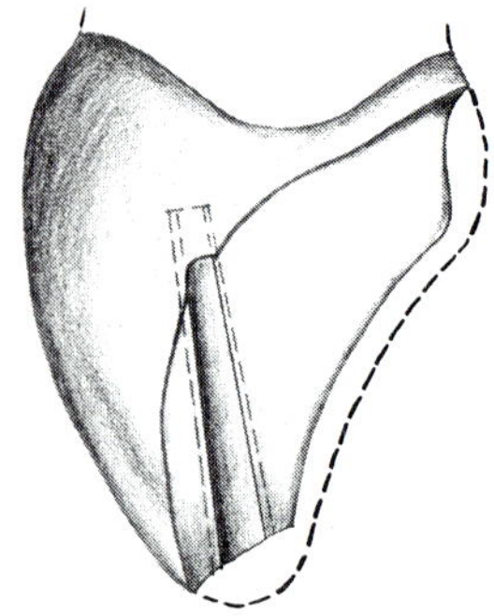

Fig. 8-36. Direction of groove is in plane closely parallel with incisal two thirds of labial surface. This is the longest distance obtainable.

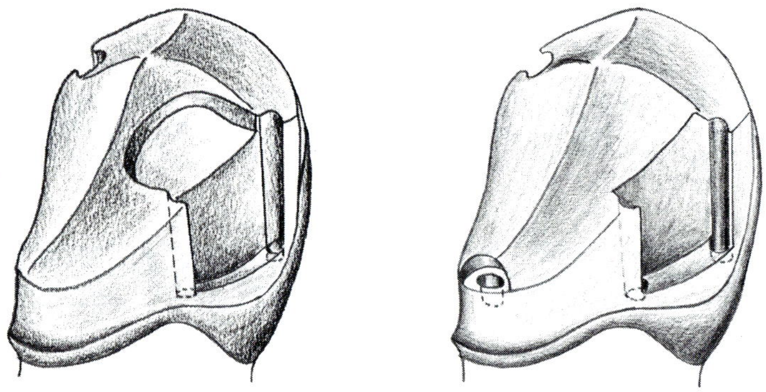

Fig. 8-37. A, Filled or carious mesial or distal surface is prepared with shallow box with lateral interlocking or tapered keyed grooves. **B,** Additional pin retention in region of cingulum also can be used.

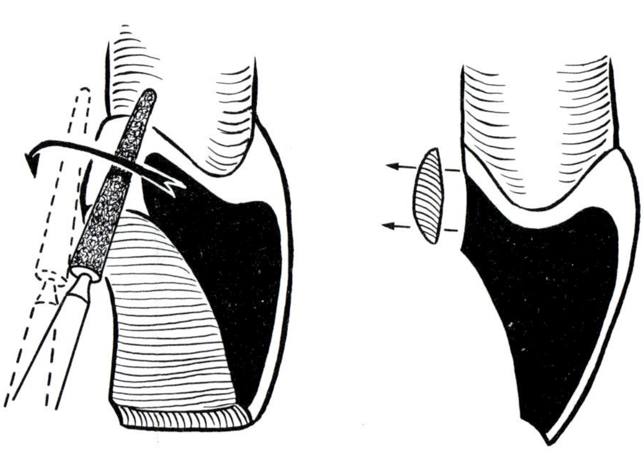

Fig. 8-38. Removal of small amount of tooth structure from around cingulum.

length give the needed frictional retention to the casting. (See Fig. 8-37.)

The next step in the preparation is to remove a small amount of tooth structure from around the cingulum, keeping this surface as nearly parallel to the mesial and distal walls and grooves as possible for retention (Fig. 8-38).

Willey[15] has shown that the development of properly convergent walls result in various formations of the finishing line region. This principle, as applied to the cingula of anterior teeth, develops a collarlike form, which is a retentive factor (Fig. 8-39). On the lingual surface of the lower molar a knife-edge finish line ensues, whereas on the buccal surface a shoulder or chamfer that is incidental to the paralleling of the walls of the preparation may be developed (Fig. 8-40).

The island of tooth structure in the area of the

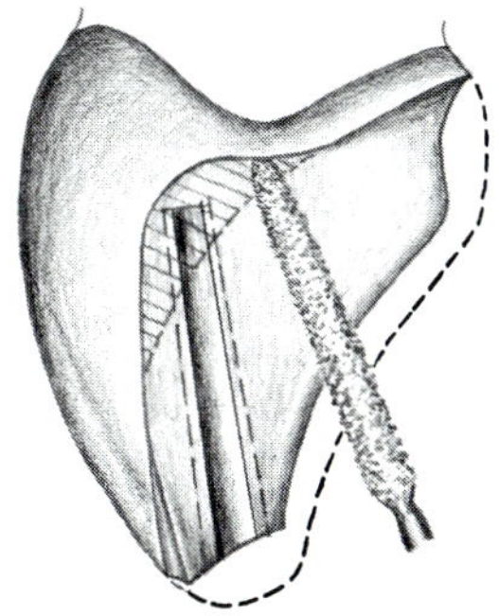

Fig. 8-39. Development of properly convergent walls gives a collarlike form in cingulum area of anterior teeth, which is retentive factor.

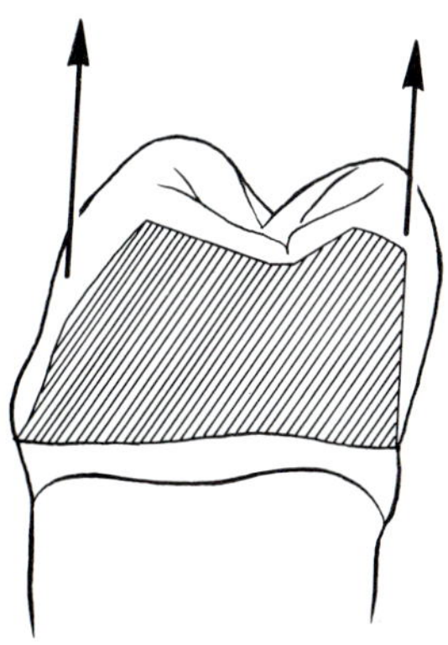

Fig. 8-40. On lingual surface of lower molars a knife-edge finish line usually results, and on buccal surface a shoulder or chamfer results when paralleling walls of preparation.

interproximal slice and the end of the groove is removed using a small diamond flame stone with high speed and very light pressure, thereby establishing a definite finish line.

A pin is used in the cingulum area for added retention. The pinhole, made with a twist drill (0.024 or 0.027), must be made parallel to the retention grooves. The pinhole also can be made with a No. ½ round bur, followed with a No. 700 tapered fissure bur, extending to the depth of 1.5 to 2 mm. The pinhole must be made in sound dentin (See Fig. 8-41.)

A slight reverse bevel is given to the incisal edge. This is done with a xx fine garnet disk coated with petroleum jelly. This procedure bevels the labioincisal enamel rods and protects them against chipping during fabrication of the restoration (Fig. 8-42).

In the preparation of posterior teeth for three-

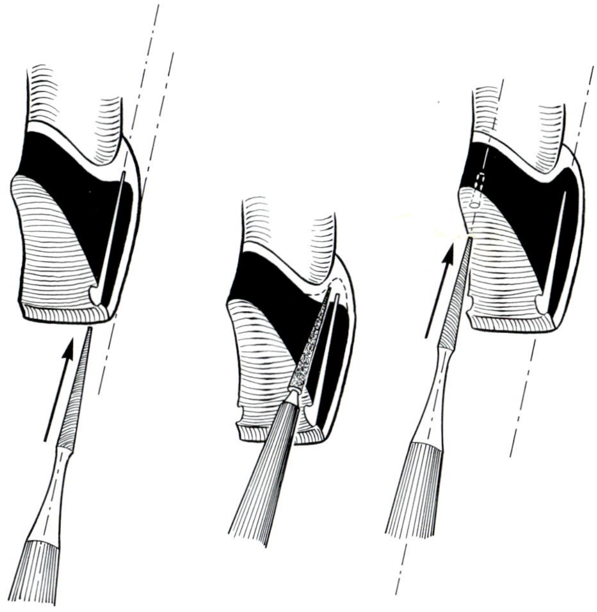

Fig. 8-41. A, Development of lock groove. **B,** Removal of island of tooth structure in area of interproximal slice and end of groove. **C,** Added pin retention in cingulum area.

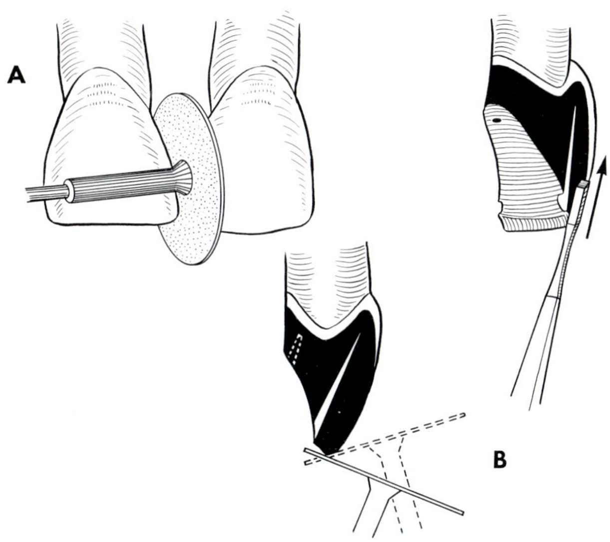

Fig. 8-42. A, Use of sandpaper and chisels for finishing and planing of margins. **B,** Slight reverse bevel given to incisal edge to bevel the labioincisal enamel rods and protect it against chipping.

A

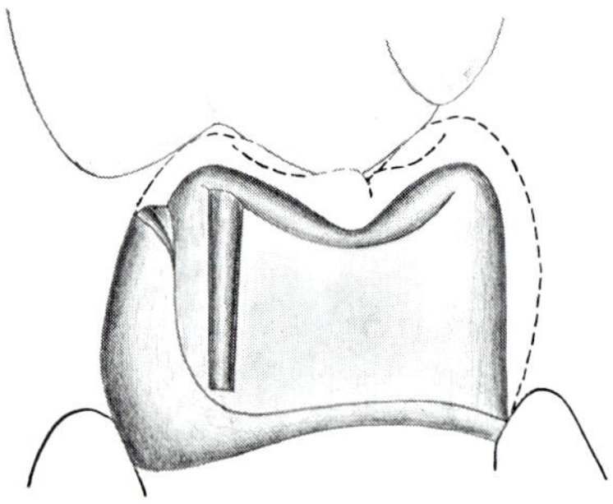

B

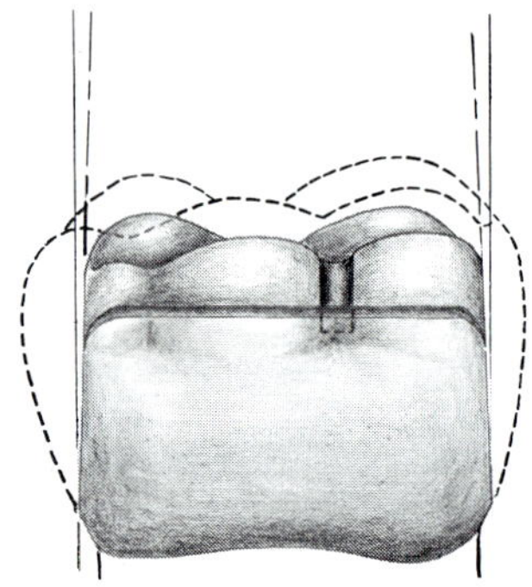

Fig. 8-43. A, Occlusal surface is a reduced reproduction of anatomic form. B, Mesial and distal slices made parallel to each other with a convergence toward occlusal surface of 2 to 5 degrees from perpendicular.

quarter crowns the occlusal surface is a reduced reproduction of the anatomic form instead of a perfectly flat surface, and the mesial and distal slices are made parallel to each other with a convergence toward the occlusal surface of 2 to 5 degrees from the perpendicular (Fig. 8-43).

For bicuspids two grooves are placed on the distal surface and one groove is placed on the mesial surface. The mesial groove is placed as far buccally as possible, permitting at the same time a sliced lap beyond for seal, and the distal grooves are placed at the buccoaxial

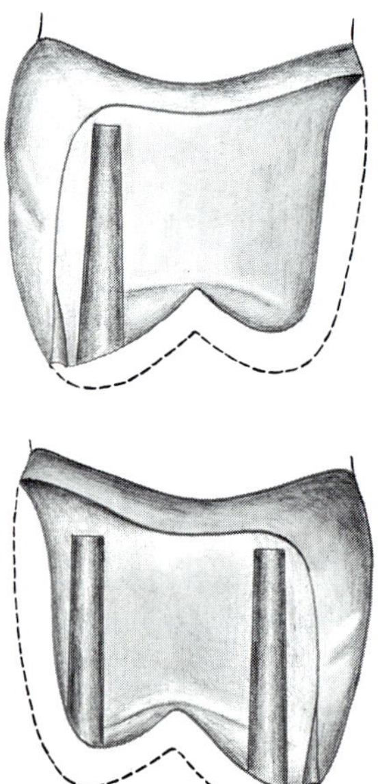

Fig. 8-44. For posterior three-quarter crowns (keeping to principle of tripodism) one groove is placed on mesial surface as far buccally as possible, and two grooves are placed on distal surface.

A

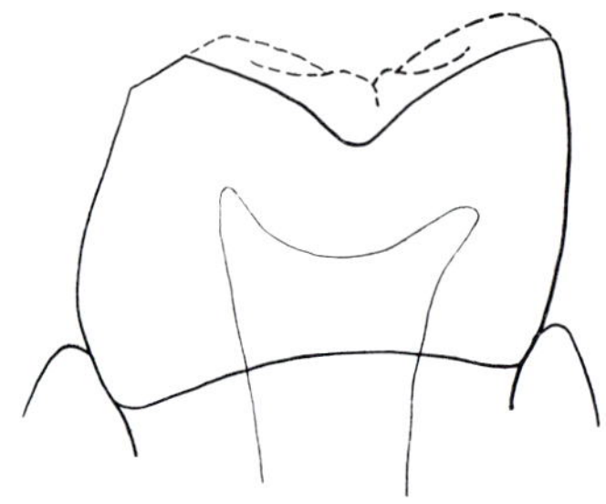

B

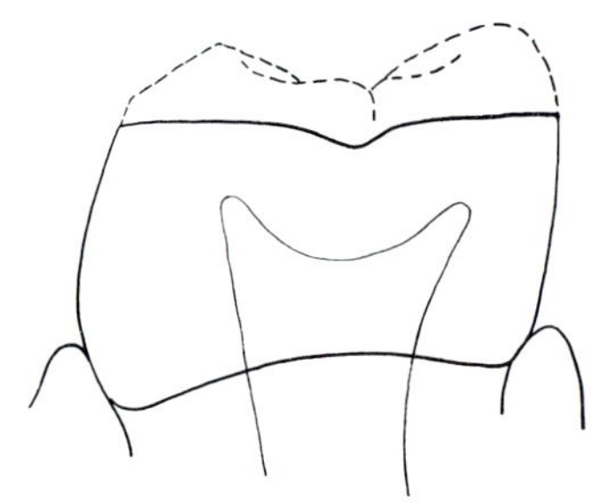

C

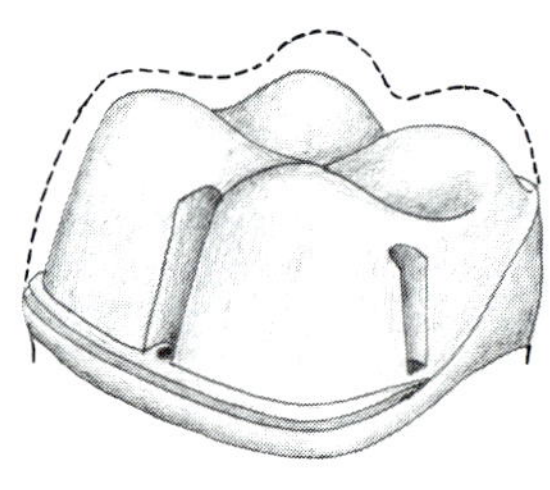

D

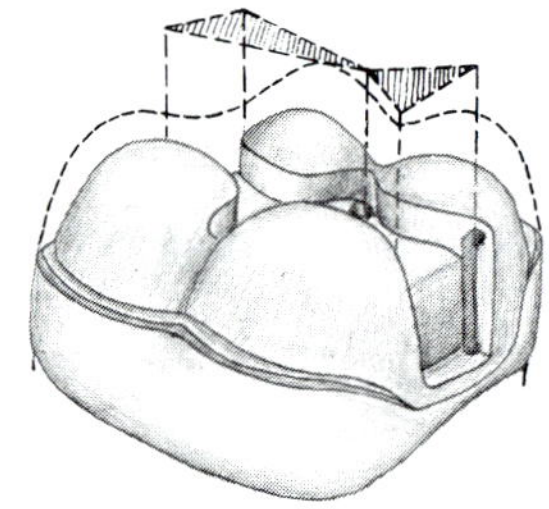

Fig. 8-45. A, Correct occlusal reduction. B, Incorrect occlusal reduction. C and D, Use of grooves, locked grooves, and pins in solid dentin (not cement), fulfilling principle of tripodism for added retention against displacement.

and linguoaxial line angles (Fig. 8-44). In upper molars, after occlusal, proximal, and lingual reduction, and also a buccal extension or modified reverse bevel, one groove can be placed on the mesial surface, one groove in the lingual groove, one groove in the buccal groove, and a slight groove on the distal surface to facilitate the handling of the wax pattern. In mandibular posterior teeth, because of their functional relations with the maxillary teeth and their lingual inclinations, a collarlike formation or shoulder is created on the buccal surface, which must be beveled. A groove is placed on the mesial, distal, and buccal surfaces.

A combination of pins and grooves also are used, and locked grooves must be in solid dentin not less than 2 or 3 mm. in length (Fig. 8-45).

Vale[16] says that the grooves in posterior three-quarter crowns should be parallel in a buccolingual direction and slightly convergent mesiodistally. These grooves should be positioned toward the buccal edge of the slice and directed parallel to the occlusal third of the buccal surface, rather than parallel to the long axis of the tooth, since this enables greater length to be established.

Binocular loupes are used for the final inspection of all preparations. Care must be taken that all margins are smooth, no undercuts exist, all flares are polished, and the axial and gingival margins join in a graceful curve.

Correct step-by-step procedures for the preparation of a three-quarter crown have been considered and fully illustrated, but an understanding of the principles that make the three-quarter crown stay in position during functional and afunctional uses and abuses should also be a matter of great concern to the practitioner of dentistry. In other words, the application of mechanistic and engineering principles to the three-quarter crown preparation and casting.

We must prevent any undesirable effects of forces and machines, especially on the relationship between the casting and its supporting tooth. Forces produced on the bearing surface of the anterior teeth by the actions of the jaw are generally from the incisal toward the gingival. Forces produced on the bearing surface of the posterior teeth are generally from the buccal to the lingual or vice versa.

A *machine* is a device that is able to transmit work on other objects only when work is done on it. Four of the six simple machines are encountered in partial veneer construction—*the wedge, the inclined plane, the lever,* and *the wheel and axle.*[17]

Mesial and distal surfaces of all teeth prepared for partial veneer crowns converge, as previously stated

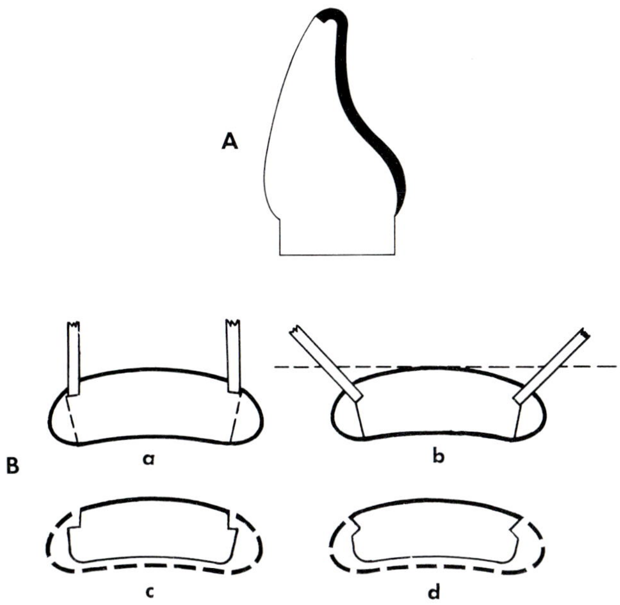

Fig. 8-46. A, Incisal step or groove and correct waxing of incisal aspect. **B,** *a,* incorrect angle for cutting lateral grooves. *b,* correct angle. *c,* Incorrect angle tends to waste tooth structure and to show more gold than does correct angle, *d.* (Adapted from Jones, Walter E.: J.A.D.A. **86:**1337-1343, June, 1973.)

and illustrated, toward the lingual aspect giving the tooth a *wedge shape,* and anterior and posterior teeth, as a rule, have their facial and lingual surfaces converging toward the incisal or occlusal aspect *forming an additional wedge.*

To stop this wedging action, Jones[17] has shown and used for many years (as I have over a period of years in many cases involving the upper and lower cuspids, bicuspids, and molars and a number of upper incisors) gold over the functional edge of the wedge, the labioincisal of anterior teeth, and occlusal surfaces of posterior teeth, going over the bucco-occlusal angle in a hooklike manner. This is accomplished by developing a step (0.5 × 0.5 mm.) at the labioincisal or bucco-occlusal angle or edge of the tooth (Fig. 8-46). This design also stops the effects of the shearing forces developed on the bearing surface of anterior teeth and posterior teeth (moving of gold alloy from incisal toward gingival aspect and from buccal to lingual or vice versa). Any movement of material in any other direction is taken care of by the walls of the casting. The forces of mastication produce tangential forces on the bearing surface of all teeth, giving that surface the effects of an *inclined plane.*

Forces of mastication cannot be eliminated, but undesirable effects of these forces on the machines present, the wedge and the inclined plane of the tooth and the lever and the wheel and axle of the bridge (on the crown, on the underlying cementation, and on the relationship of the crown to its supporting tooth) must be stopped.[17]

"When a partial veneer crown becomes a bridge abutment, the forces of mastication acting on the bridge cause it to act as a *lever* and a *wheel and axle*. Both machines (*lever* and *wheel and axle*) produce movement that subjects the cementation to shear and changes the relation of the casting to its supporting tooth.

"The *bridge becomes a lever* when one end is depressed, one end being in occlusion and the other out of function. This action tends to rotate the casting around the labiolingual or buccolingual axis, clockwise or counterclockwise. The effects of this force are stopped by the wrench-like engagement of a rigid casting engaging the mesial and distal surface of the tooth. The slight movement that is involved must not

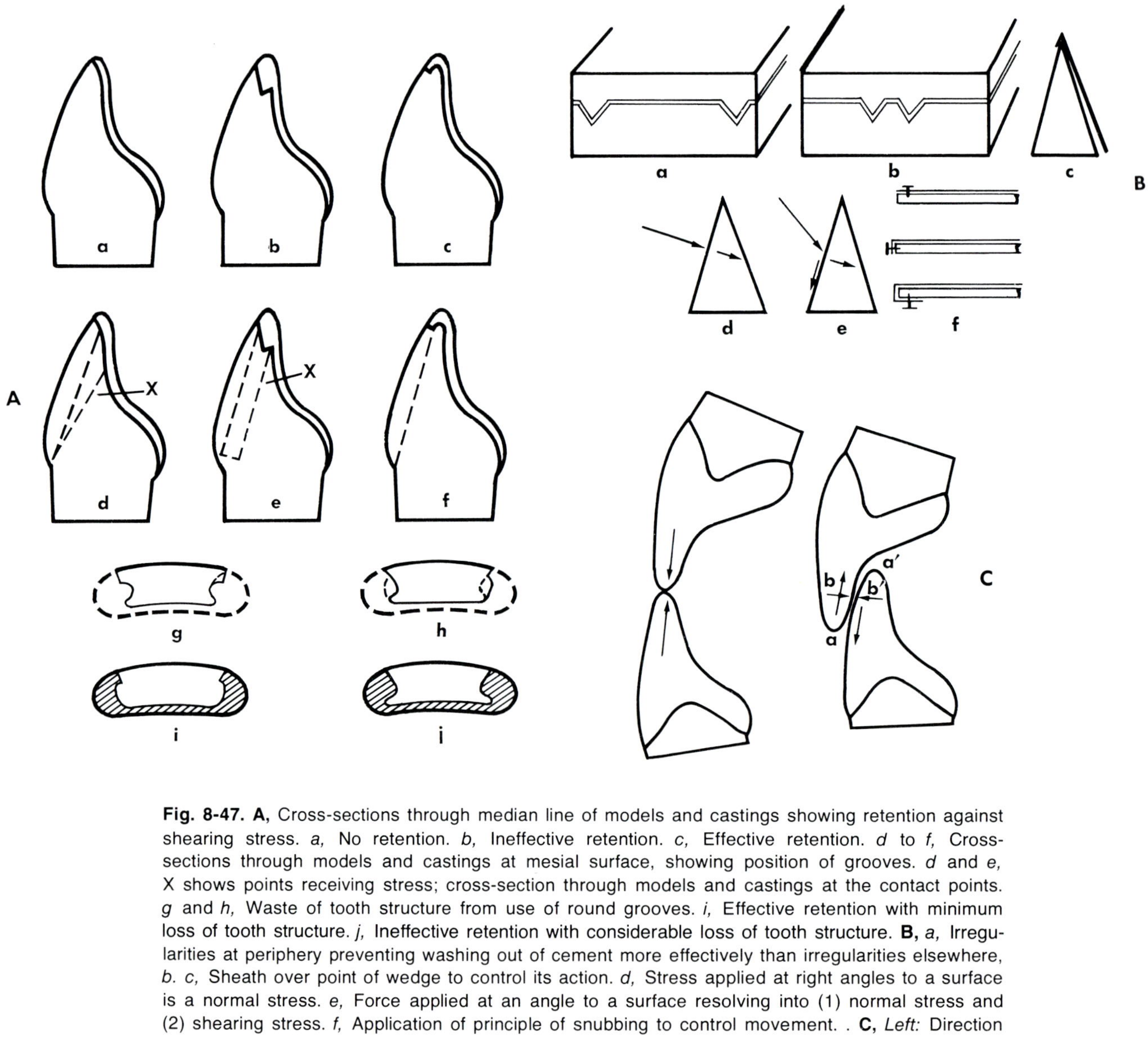

Fig. 8-47. A, Cross-sections through median line of models and castings showing retention against shearing stress. *a,* No retention. *b,* Ineffective retention. *c,* Effective retention. *d* to *f,* Cross-sections through models and castings at mesial surface, showing position of grooves. *d* and *e,* X shows points receiving stress; cross-section through models and castings at the contact points. *g* and *h,* Waste of tooth structure from use of round grooves. *i,* Effective retention with minimum loss of tooth structure. *j,* Ineffective retention with considerable loss of tooth structure. **B,** *a,* Irregularities at periphery preventing washing out of cement more effectively than irregularities elsewhere, *b. c,* Sheath over point of wedge to control its action. *d,* Stress applied at right angles to a surface is a normal stress. *e,* Force applied at an angle to a surface resolving into (1) normal stress and (2) shearing stress. *f,* Application of principle of snubbing to control movement. . **C,** *Left:* Direction of stress in initial act of incising. *Right:* Direction of stress during remaining act of incising. *a* and *a'*, Shearing stresses; *b* and *b'*, normal stresses. (Adapted from Jones, Walter E.: The scientifically designed partial veneer or three-quarter crown [its technic, analysis, and comparison], Minneapolis, 1952, Burgess Publishing Co.)

take place between the casting and its supporting tooth, but between the tooth and its supporting tissues.

"Whenever a force is applied in a labiolingual or buccolingual direction or vice versa, on a point on a bridge, a torsional (twisting shear) force is developed—*the wheel and axle at work.* This force tends to rotate the crown around the long axis of its supporting tooth breaking up the relationship between them, and subjecting the cement to shear. The most effective way to stop this action is to engage the tooth at its greatest mesiodistal width at right angles to the direction of the force to obtain the greatest possible leverage. The tooth, being smooth, should be grooved in the general direction of its long axis. It will be remembered that the tooth was grooved in that general direction and position to take care of the shedding action of one of the wedges of the tooth.

"Another rotating force is present when the pontics are set in an arc, as in a bridge in the anterior part of the mouth, and a force is applied to the incisal edge of a pontic in this arc. The result is to rotate the crowns around the mesiodistal axes of the supporting teeth (abutment teeth), and the gingival portion of the pontics to move lingually. The surfaces of the abutment teeth next to the edentulous area diverge toward the labial. This, the divergence of the surfaces of the abutment teeth next to the edentulous area toward the labial, in conjunction with the lateral grooves, stops the tendency to rotate. The more nearly that the walls of the prepared tooth can be kept parallel to the line of withdrawal or insertion, the more resistance will be obtained to prevent the results of tension on the crown."*

A few salient facts in regard to the partial veneer crown are in order:

1. *Rigidity of the casting,* a most desired property, is obtained in partial veneer crowns (especially) by giving the gold an *inverted channel iron shape* as it extends slightly over the incisal or buccal edge of the tooth in a hooklike manner (Fig. 8-47). This gives the gold casting a structural shape (I-beam, the angle iron, the channel iron, and others are structural shapes) which prevents deformation of the casting, and the channel iron shape stops the wedging action of the tooth.
2. Keep in mind that hardness of an alloy is not rigidity; the use of the proper material, correctly shaped and disposed in a proper manner with respect to the direction of the load, is the way to obtain rigidity.
3. The tooth must be so prepared and designed so that it imparts a structural shape to casting to give it rigidity, and it also must be so designed that the cementation is subjected to compressive forces only.

If all steps are executed properly, the three-quarter crown, when started to place, should slide in frictional resistance from the time that the gingival ends enter the incisal openings until the crown is seated in position—cement being merely the material used to hermetically seal the joint. Here again the principle of tripodism has been carried out with its resultant stability. (See Fig. 8-48.)

Pinledges

Pin retention is one of the strongest retentive forces, mechanically, that can be used in dentistry. Retention is gained primarily by means of the length as well as the judicious placement of the pins. Other advantages of pinledges as individual restorations or retainers are the conservation of tooth structure and good esthetics.

It is now possible to parallel any number of walls and pinholes in any number of teeth, especially in the construction of fixed periodontal splints or extensive fixed partial dentures, by the use of the rules of freehand paralleling or with the aid of the recently developed paralleling devices such as the Parallaid, the Pontostructor, and the Chayes Loma Linda paralleling device. Only true-running handpieces should be used, being careful to run them at comparatively low speeds.

The advent of a new type of drills and sized nylon bristles, as developed by E. D. Shooshan, gives us the tools whereby great accuracy in the preparation of pinholes and their duplication, with extreme fidelity, by the indirect impression technique is possible (Fig. 8-49).

Before starting a pinledge preparation a roentgenogram of the tooth should be studied very carefully for the size and position of the pulp. Not only must the pulp be avoided, but also a perforation of a side of the tooth must be prevented.

In cases in which the pinledge is to be used on upper anterior teeth for corrective purposes in occlusal reconstruction, the interproximal surfaces need not be involved. After the proper lingual reduction from the crest of the cingulum and the correct treatment of the cingulum area, a bracing effect and rigidity are given to the casting by grooving the mesial and distal areas in the marginal ridges by means of

*From Jones, Walter E.: The scientifically designed partial veneer crown, J.A.D.A. **86**(6):1337-1343, 1973.

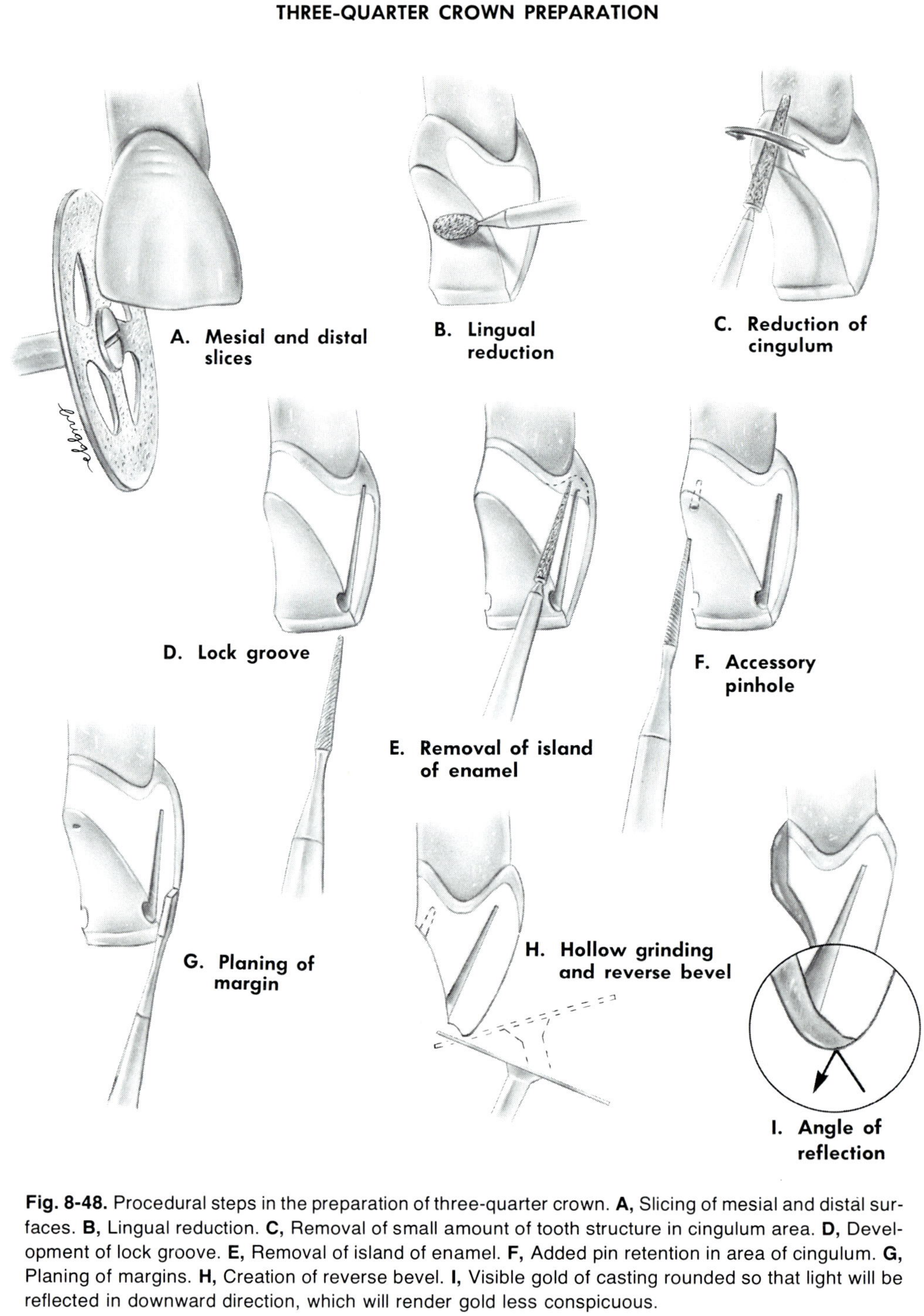

Fig. 8-48. Procedural steps in the preparation of three-quarter crown. **A,** Slicing of mesial and distal surfaces. **B,** Lingual reduction. **C,** Removal of small amount of tooth structure in cingulum area. **D,** Development of lock groove. **E,** Removal of island of enamel. **F,** Added pin retention in area of cingulum. **G,** Planing of margins. **H,** Creation of reverse bevel. **I,** Visible gold of casting rounded so that light will be reflected in downward direction, which will render gold less conspicuous.

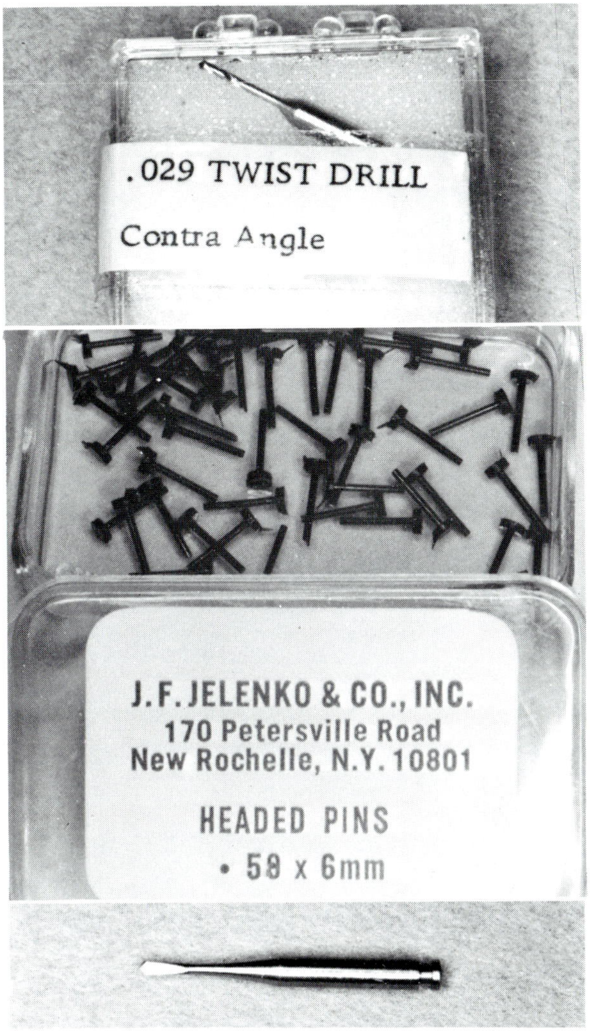

Fig. 8-49. A, Twist drill. **B,** Sized headed pins (Perlon). **C,** Bibeveled carbide center drill.

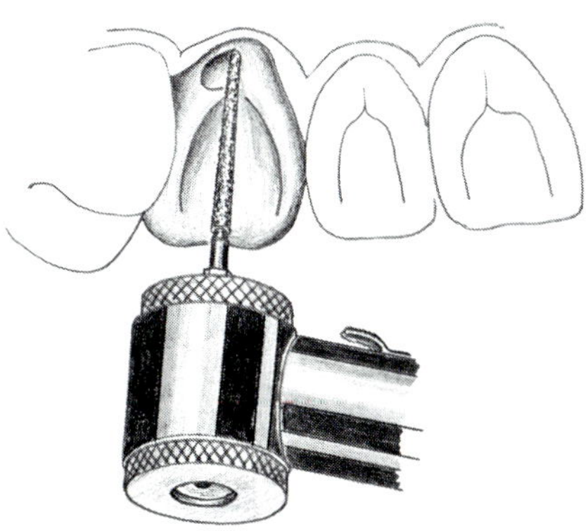

Fig. 8-50. Reduction of cingulum area in pinledge preparation.

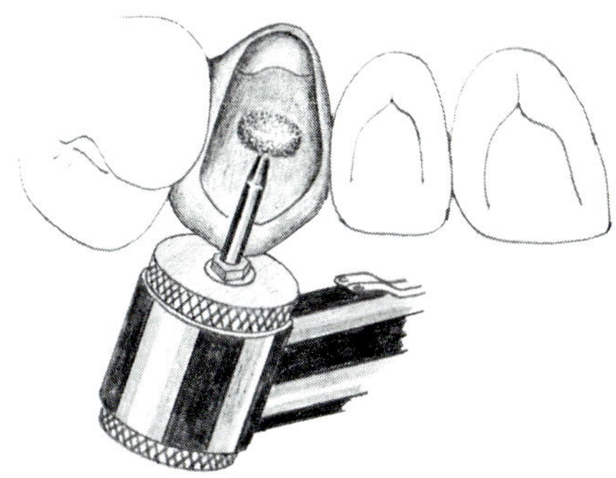

Fig. 8-51. Proper lingual reduction.

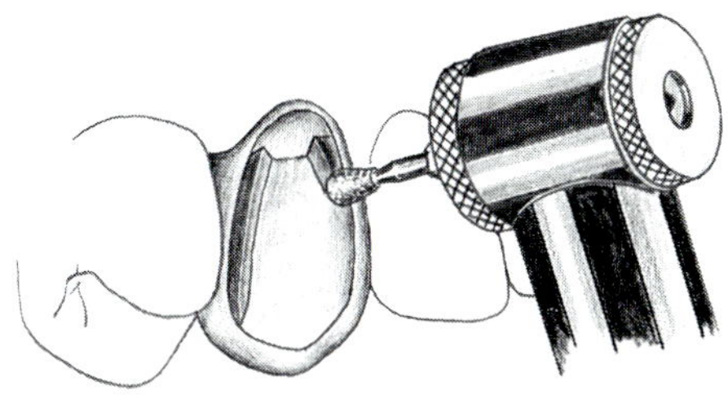

Fig. 8-52. Grooving of mesial and distal areas in marginal ridges creating V-shaped wedge grooves for bracing and rigidity.

V-shaped wedge grooves. Then the incisal edge is beveled to a 45 degree angle to the tooth's long axis, or this area can be hollow ground. Small flat ledges or seats are prepared in appropriate positions for starting the pinholes. The pinholes must be drilled parallel to each other to a depth of 2 to 3 mm. I drill the cingulum area hole or holes first because of the pulpal factor and drill the others parallel to this first pinhole. By the use of the twist drill the pinholes can be made small in diameter, permitting adequate frictional resistance and retention without extensive cutting. A very slight incisal reverse bevel then is created to complete the preparation. (See Figs. 8-50 to 8-53.)

The first step in the preparation of a pinledge type of retainer for a fixed splint or bridge is to slice the proximal surface very carefully, using the lingual approach and bringing the labial margin to a self-cleansing area (Figs. 8-54 to 8-56). In many instances one of the proximal surfaces need not be prepared, ending the preparation with a V-shaped wedge groove in the marginal ridge area of this surface (Fig. 8-57).

A proximal surface that is adjacent to a pontic area must have a concave surface to allow for more bulk of metal for the avoidance of the warpage of margins during the soldering operation (Fig. 8-58).

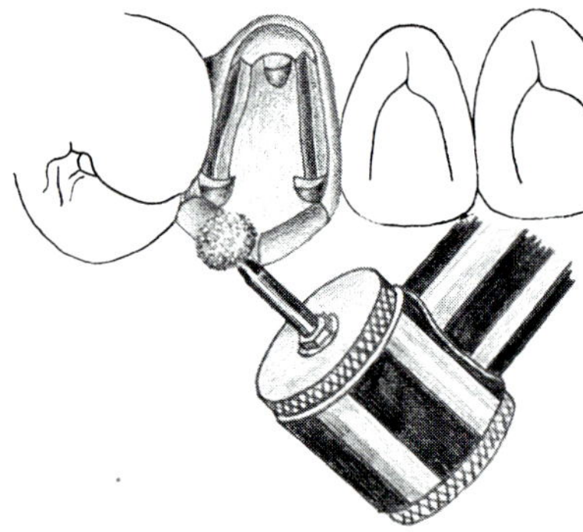

Fig. 8-53. Preparation of small flat ledges to receive pinholes and treatment of incisal edge (bevel to 45-degree angle to long axis of tooth and hollow grind). Follow with slight reverse bevel.

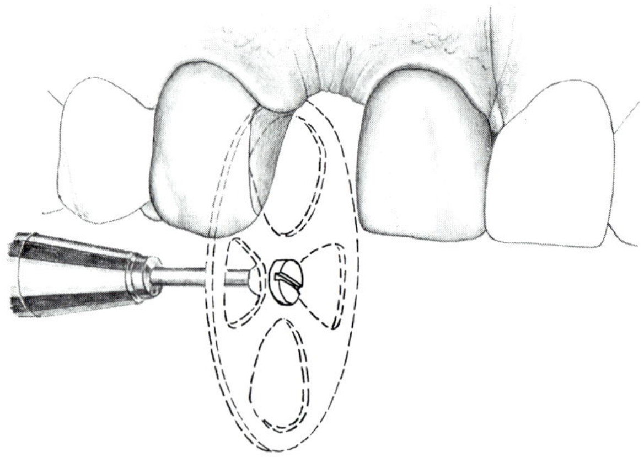

Fig. 8-54. Slicing of proximal surface for preparation of pin-ledge retainer with disk.

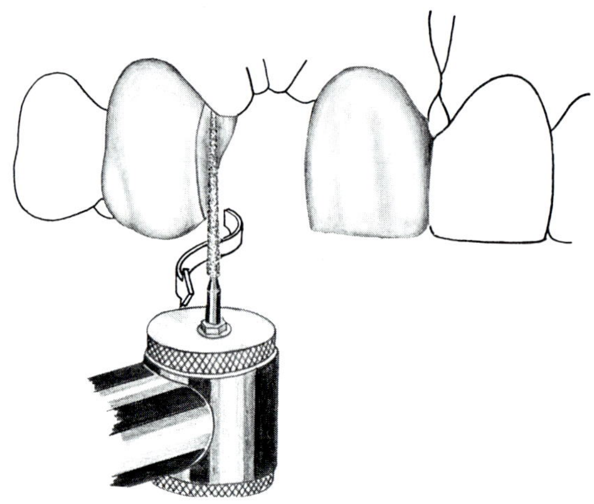

Fig. 8-55. Slicing of proximal surface with small flame-shaped diamond stone (proximal surface must be concave).

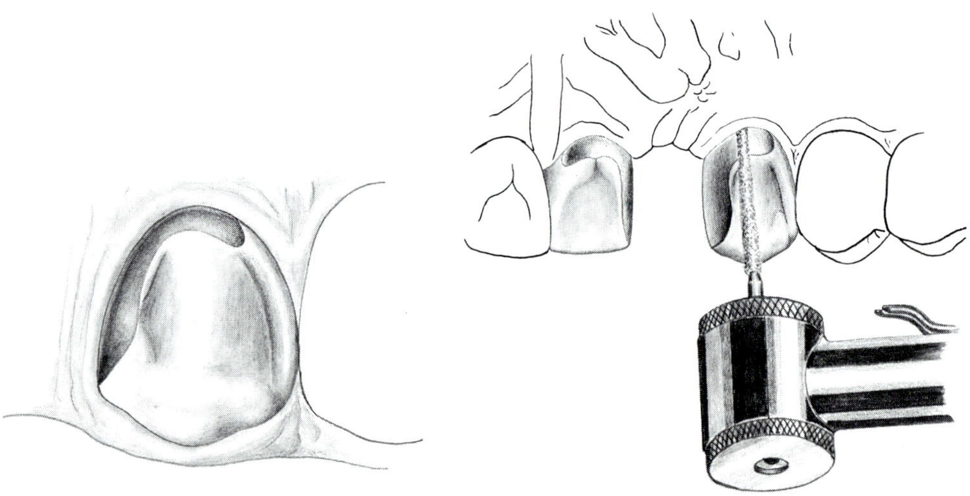

Fig. 8-56. Treatment of cingulum area.

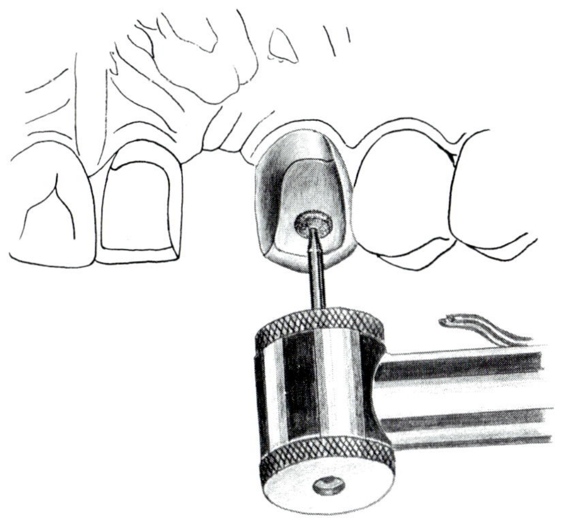

Fig. 8-57. Reduction of lingual surface and ending preparation of this surface with V-shaped wedge groove in marginal ridge area of opposite proximal surface.

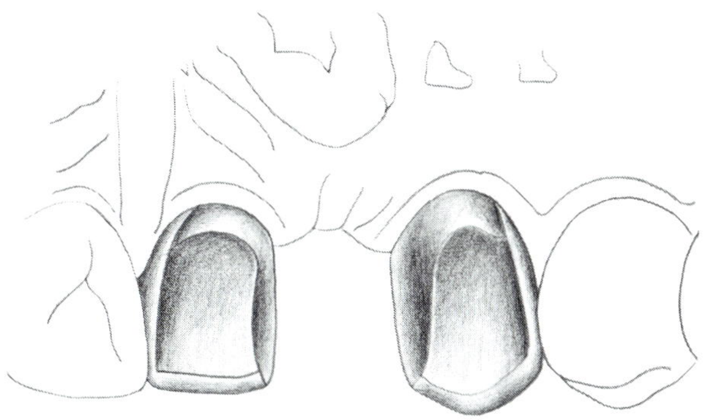

Fig. 8-58. Proximal surface adjacent to pontic area must have concave surface to allow for more bulk of metal to avoid warpage of margins during soldering.

Where rotational stresses are likely to be great, a tapered keyed groove or locked groove should be used on that side where the pontic is to be soldered, thereby breaking the rotational stress at its inception and keeping it off the pins, which so often results in the loosening of our pinledge retainers. The utilization of a groove in combination with the pins results in a very adequate retainer in short span cases.

The reduction of the lingual surface to the crest of the cingulum is the next step in the procedure, followed by the removal of a small amount of tooth structure from the area around the cingulum producing a definitive gingival margin—a chamfer or modified collarlike formation with very little taper (Fig. 8-59). Because of this vertical surface, the retentive factors of the preparation is enhanced greatly.

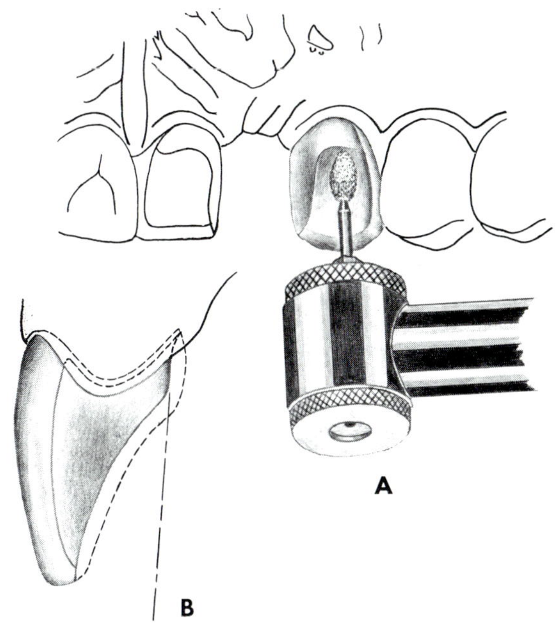

Fig. 8-59. A, Reduction of lingual surface to crest of cingulum followed by removal of small amount of tooth structure in area around cingulum. **B,** Above procedure produces a gingival margin that is chamfered or modified collarlike formation with very little taper.

The incisal area is then reduced, creating a 45 degree angle to the long axis of the tooth, and it is also slightly hollow ground (Fig. 8-60). In lingual reduction care must be exercised to provide for adequate thickness of metal when the teeth are in centric and eccentric occlusal relations.

Shallow recesses or ledges are cut toward the labial surface with a small cylindrical diamond stone —one at the mesioincisal edge, one at the distoincisal edge, and one in the cingulum area. The ledges for the pinhole openings are made with sharp angles. The formation of ledges throws the occlusal stress on the tooth rather than on the pins, which merely hold the attachment in position. The shank of the diamond stone should be kept parallel to the face of the tooth viewed labiolingually and parallel to the long axis of the tooth viewed mesiodistally. (See Fig. 8-61.)

The positioning of the pinholes is next in order. Pencil marks can be made at the spots where a small round bur or a special carbide center drill will penetrate any remaining enamel and facilitate the accurate positioning of the holes. This is followed with a Spirec drill or a twist drill or a tapered fissure bur sized to the round bur (if a No. ½ round bur is used, the corresponding sized tapered fissure bur used to finish the

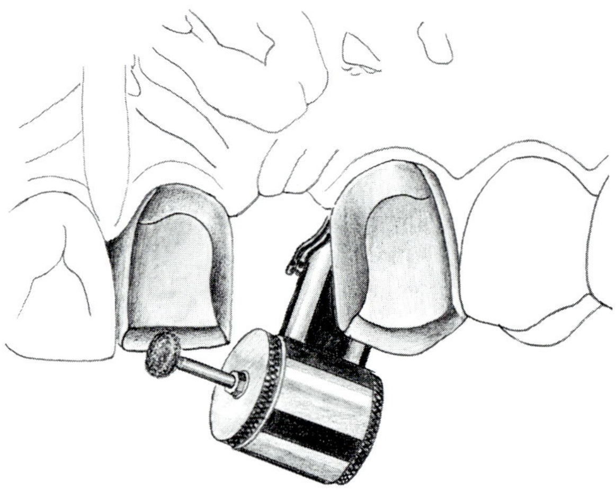

Fig. 8-60. Reduction of incisal area. Hollow-ground incisal area is end result.

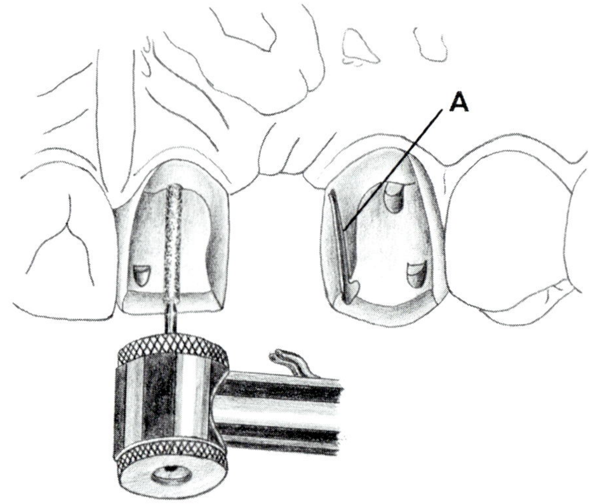

Fig. 8-61. Ledges prepared for pinhole openings. Utilization of lock groove *(A)* in combination with pins makes for retentive retainer.

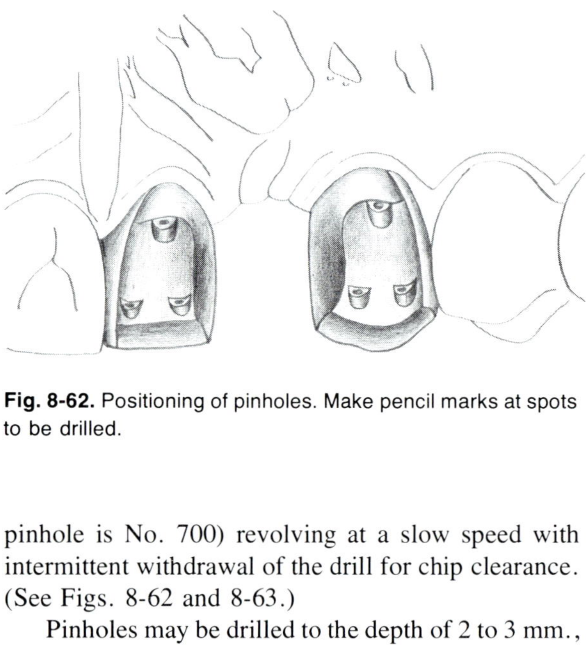

Fig. 8-62. Positioning of pinholes. Make pencil marks at spots to be drilled.

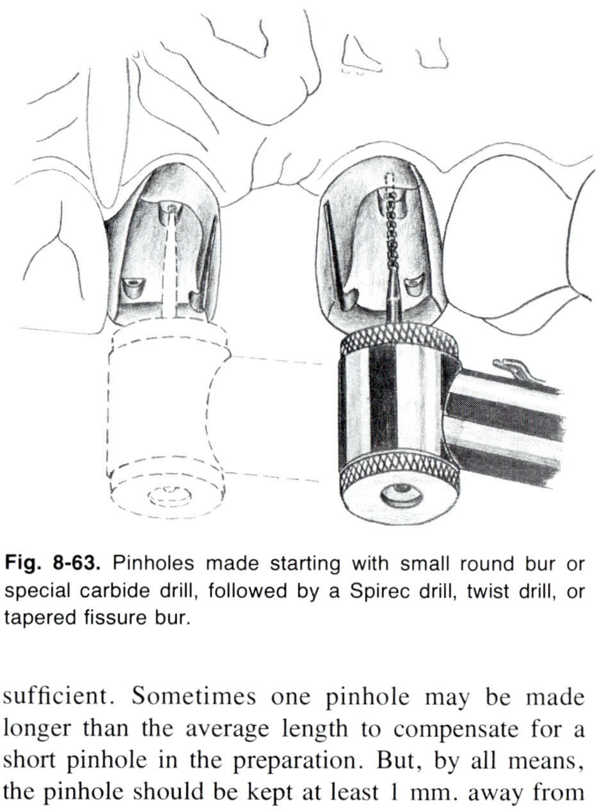

Fig. 8-63. Pinholes made starting with small round bur or special carbide drill, followed by a Spirec drill, twist drill, or tapered fissure bur.

pinhole is No. 700) revolving at a slow speed with intermittent withdrawal of the drill for chip clearance. (See Figs. 8-62 and 8-63.)

Pinholes may be drilled to the depth of 2 to 3 mm., provided the holes fall mesially, distally, or lingually to the pulp chamber. If a twist drill is used, the depth of penetration, be it 0.024, 0.027, or 0.029 inch, is determined, as a rule, by the collar on these twist drills. Circumstances may make it necessary to decrease this length. If, because of parallelism, one has to be carried directly toward the pulp, 1 mm. will be sufficient. Sometimes one pinhole may be made longer than the average length to compensate for a short pinhole in the preparation. But, by all means, the pinhole should be kept at least 1 mm. away from the pulp. (See Fig. 8-64.)

The gingival pinhole should be drilled first because of the delicate pulpal position, and the other pinholes made parallel to this one. The development of the twist drill allows for pinholes of small diameter, which at the same time permits adequate frictional resistance and retention.

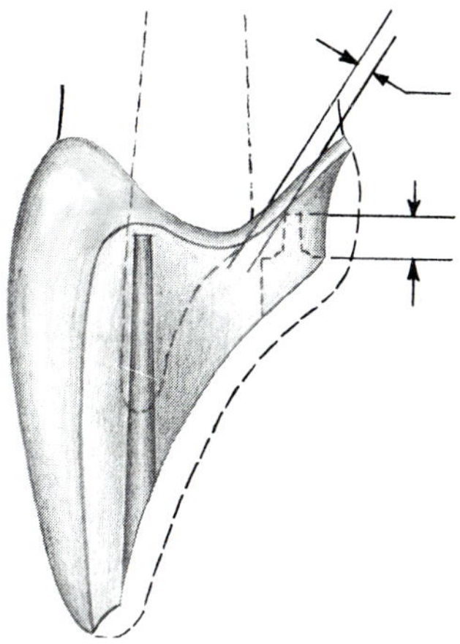

Fig. 8-64. If, because of parallelism, it is necessary to carry pinhole directly toward pulp, a depth of 1 mm. is sufficient.

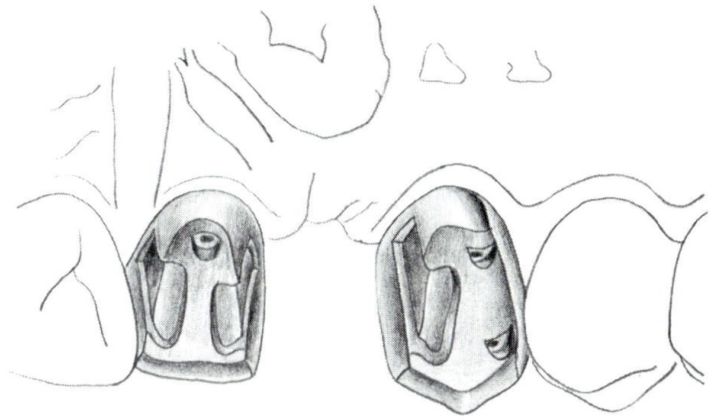

Fig. 8-65. Fillings or extensive caries on a proximal surface necessitates box preparation and two pins.

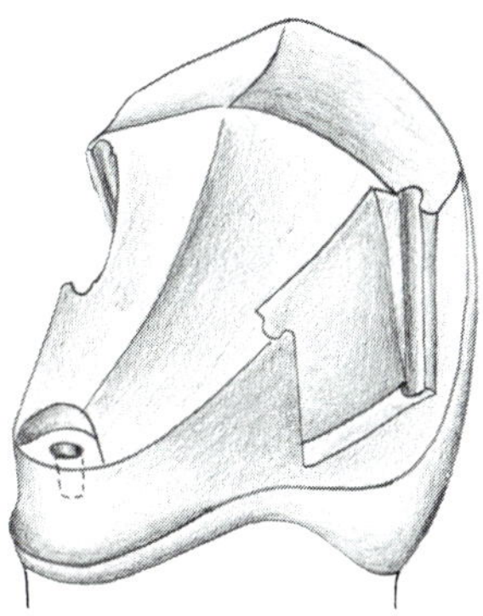

Fig. 8-66. If both proximal surfaces involved, use box preparation with pin retention in cingulum area, a somewhat modified three-quarter crown preparation.

Three or four pinholes are usually adequate, and they must be placed in sound dentin. Pins must be parallel with each other and the walls of the preparation, which gives us the retentive feature of the pins in sound dentin and also internal or external wall retention. Place pinholes inside the dentinoenamel junction and at least 1 mm. from the proximal wall of the preparation.

A proximal cavity or filling may be encountered on one or both sides of the tooth. In such a case a locked groove can be used if little decay or filling material is present and is well confined at the proper place, or it may be necessary to "box out" one or both sides. If one proximal surface is involved—that is, the distal surface—a box preparation with a labiodistal and a linguodistal groove is made on the distal surface with the addition of two pinholes, one at the mesioincisal area and one in the region of the cingulum. It also is possible that a locked groove would suffice on the involved distal surface. If both proximal surfaces are involved, the preparation calls for "boxed out" or locked groove preparations, both mesially and distally, with a pinhole in the cingulum area—really a three-quarter crown preparation, or at least a modified three-quarter crown type of cavity design. Pinholes or grooves should never be made in cement since it is not retentive. (See Figs. 8-65 and 8-66.)

The preparation is then smoothed with fine finishing diamond points and sandpaper disks. At this time, with the aid of binocular loupes, the incisal edge is given a slight reverse bevel. The visible gold of the casting in this area can be rounded in such a manner that light will be reflected in a downward direction, which will render the gold practically invisible (Fig. 8-67). We must remember that old law in physics regarding reflection: "The angle of reflection is equal to the angle of incidence, and the two angles lie in the same plane" (Fig. 8-68).

Before the casting is seated, the sharp edges around the top of each pinhole are beveled slightly with a suitably sized round bur. This permits the casting to go to place in its entirety with perfect adaptation and also allows some latitude in aligning the pins with their respective openings.

An effort should be made to fit the pins in the pinholes snugly, but this creates a problem in cementation. Some dentists think that the pins should be beveled slightly on a bias at the bottom of the pins, while others believe that a vent for the cement to escape during cementation should be made with the

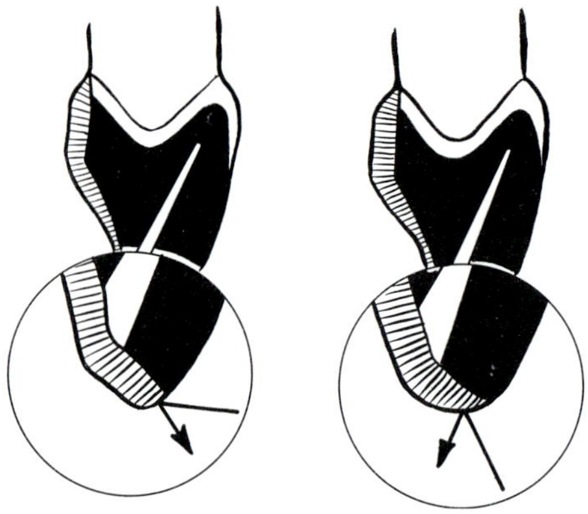

Fig. 8-67. Visible gold of casting rounded so that light will be reflected in downward direction to render gold practically invisible.

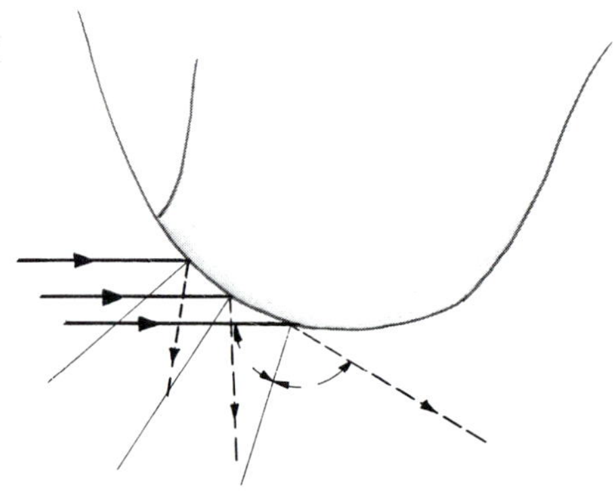

Fig. 8-68. Angle of reflection is equal to angle of incidence, and the two angles lie in same plane.

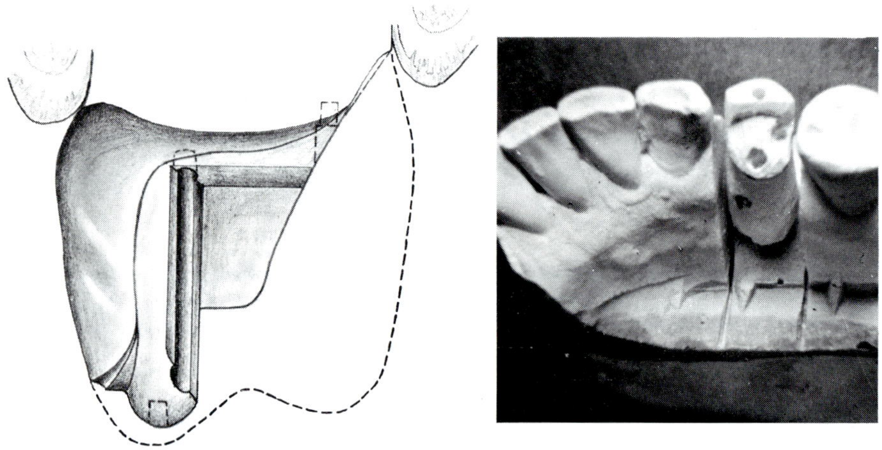

Fig. 8-69. Pins helpful in cases of badly broken down teeth or cases of buccal or lingual wall fracture.

smallest round bur available inserted into the bottom of the pinholes and withdrawn, a groove resulting which will counteract the plunger effect created by the act of cementation. The twist drill and sized nylon bristle technique compensates for this by giving us a finished pin that is slightly smaller in diameter than the pinhole. This allows for complete seating in cementation by counteracting the plunger effect, and it also gives ample retention and resistance to displacement.

Pins also are useful in the restoration of badly broken down teeth or in cases of fractures of the buccal or lingual plates of posterior teeth (Fig. 8-69).

It has been clearly shown that pins should be distributed as in a tripod, and not bunched together on one side of the tooth (Fig. 8-70).

Pulpless teeth

In mouth rehabilitation procedures the endodontist is a very important member of the team. Pathology may result from the necessary extensive tooth preparation, impression taking, temporization, cementation, etc., weeks, months, or even years later. This may call for conservative treatment or surgical procedures such as hemisection and apicoectomy. In other words, it will need the expert help of the endodontist.

In diagnosis and treatment planning the conclusions reached may call for the use of elective endodontics to effect parallelism, a better plane of occlusion, a modification of crown-to-root ratios and tooth contours, and the problems of extruded and tipped teeth, versions, and rotations. Also, success-

PINLEDGE PREPARATION

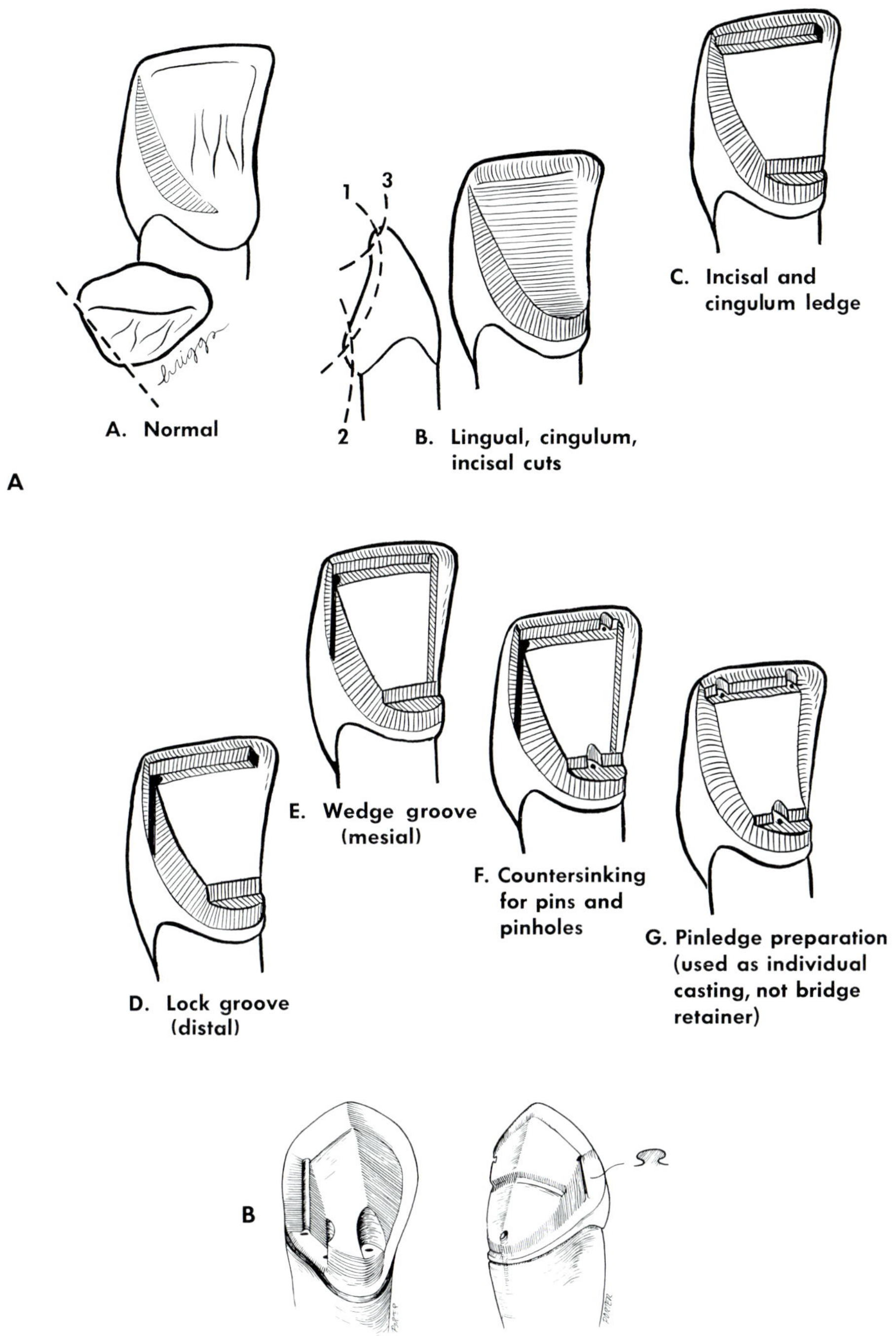

Fig. 8-70. A, Coordinated steps in preparation of pinledge and pinledge bridge retainer. *A,* Removal of proximal surface (make concave). *B,* Lingual, cingulum, and incisal edge reduction. *C,* Creation of ledges for pinhole openings. *D,* Preparation of lock groove. *E,* V-shaped wedge groove in marginal ridge area made. *F,* Pinholes paralleled to lock groove. *G,* In pinledge preparation, as individual casting, same preparation as above with exception of lock groove. Instead use V-shaped wedge grooves in both marginal ridges and three pins for retention and rigidity. **B,** Slight variations in the preparation of a partial veneer crown for upper cuspid.

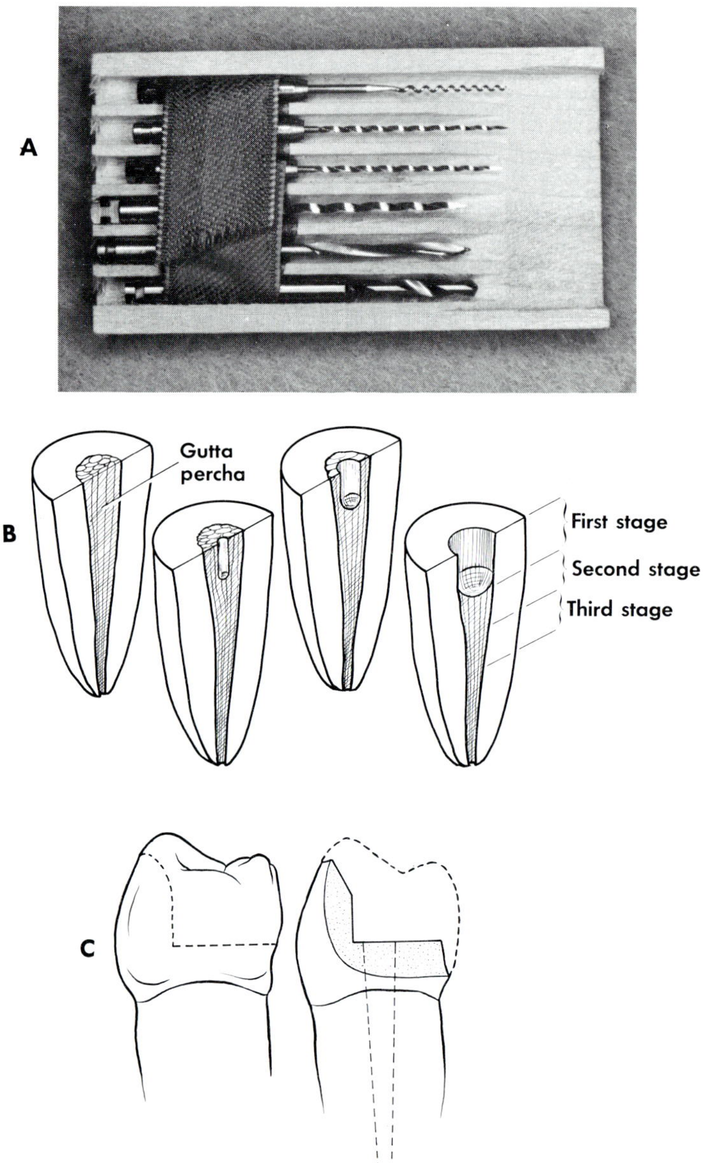

Fig. 8-71. A, Drills and reamers used in reaming and enlarging canals for posts. **B,** Stages of development of canal opening to receive post—round burs of various sizes, drills, and reamers are used. **C,** Length of post should be, if possible, two thirds the length of the root or equal to the length of the crown.

ful endodontic treatment sometimes can prevent the complete loss of a case by salvaging strategic abutment teeth or preventing the need for a removable prosthesis where the teeth could not stand the torque and stresses. Many patients cannot adjust themselves psychologically to even the best designed and constructed removable partial denture.

After endodontic treatment the remaining tooth structure must be given maximum strength and protection. Pulpless teeth are more brittle than vital teeth. Therefore, the complete "shoeing" of the cusps and the use of a post or dowel in one or more canals will give this additional strength and retention. The length of the post or dowel should be at least equal to the length of the coronal portion of the restoration. This may not be possible always because of the length and shape of the roots, periodontal involvements, etc. If this is not possible, then more than one post should be used, or an increase in the width of the walls of the canal is necessary. It has been determined that

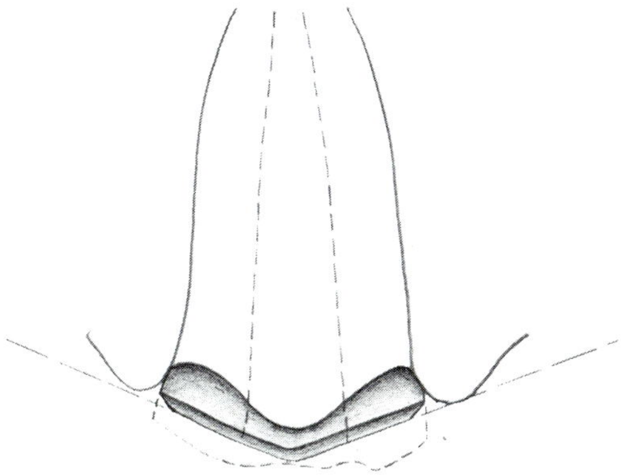

Fig. 8-72. Root face prepared to correspond to curvature of gingival tissue. Two planes are established—one facially and one lingually.

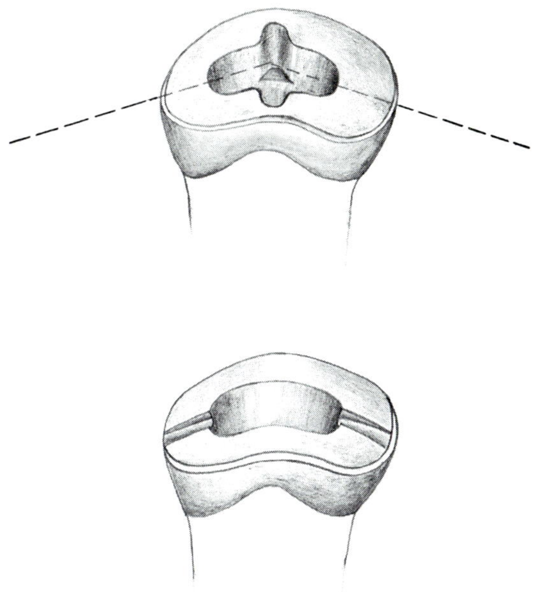

Fig. 8-73. Small shallow slot or lock is cut to facilitate accurate seating of casting. This prevents possibility of rotation.

there is a direct correlation between the lateral area of the dowel and the retention it affords, but the effort to achieve a post length of two thirds the length of a root or roots is the goal to be achieved (Fig. 8-71).

Even if endodontics is done in a tooth with full coverage, a post in the canal after treatment is a good policy because that can prevent the possibility of a shearing of the tooth at the gingival line. This holds true for all endodontically treated teeth.

The apical portion of the root canal can be sealed with a section of the silver point or gutta-percha point after the canal or canals have been reamed to enlarge them for the reception of a post or dowel. Many endodontists use the twist-off method of the silver point in the canal-filling operation to make it easier for more reaming and enlarging of the canal.

One must remember that the parallelism of the post or posts to the involved internal and external walls of the preparation must be observed carefully. Also, the enlargement of the canal to a point where a thin shell of dentin remains is contraindicated—it can lead to a lateral perforation.

In cases in which all coronal tooth structure is gone, dependence for survival of the tooth is placed upon the root and the root face. The root face is so prepared as to correspond to the curvature of the gingival tissue establishing two planes, one facially and one lingually (Fig. 8-72).

The post or dowel should be as long as possible, and the gingival portion of the post-anchorage cast gold core must not only contact the two planes of the root face, but also it must encircle the axial surfaces of the preparation. The retention furnished by the post and the additional support afforded by the encirclement of the axial surfaces of the preparation by an accurate fitting casting give longevity to the restoration and preclude the possibility of root fracture.

A small shallow slot or lock also should be cut facially or lingually so that the casting can be seated with ease and accuracy. It prevents the possibility of rotation (Fig. 8-73).

A cast gold or veneered crown is constructed to fit over this primary restoration. The crown has a subgingival apron of gold surrounding the entire circumference of the root, which not only acts as a support or brace, but also gives us the opportunity of removing this crown, if necessary, without taking the chance of fracturing the root or any other remaining tooth structure while trying to remove a post and core (Figs. 8-74 and 8-75).

In cases of "old root canal fillings," in which reentry into the canals is not feasible for one reason or another, "pulp chamber anchorage" with mesial and distal locked grooves or boxes is used (Fig. 8-76). The walls of the pulp chamber are kept parallel to each other and to the grooves or boxes, with little convergence, and go as deep as the particular case allows.

Where there is ample tooth structure to make a full coping unnecessary and at the same time not enough tooth length gingivo-occlusally or incisally, a post and casting extension should be used (Fig 8-77).

We try, however, to encircle the remaining tooth

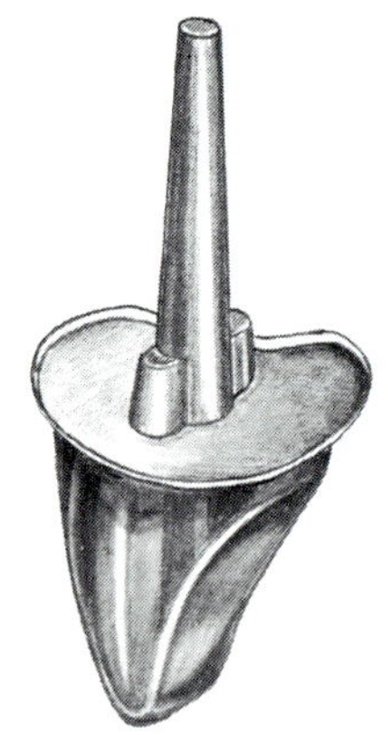

Fig. 8-74. Post anchorage cast gold core.

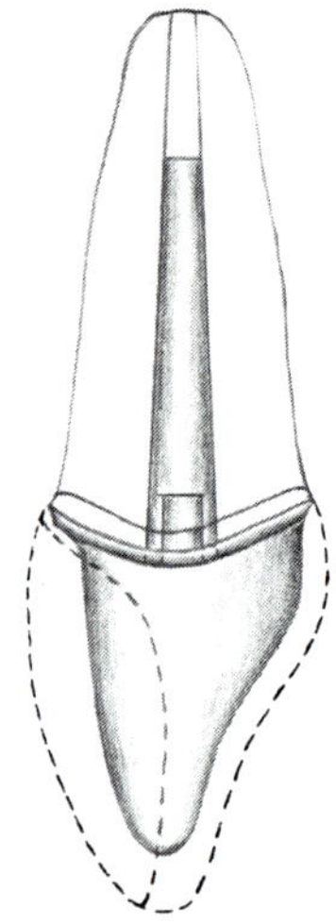

Fig. 8-75. Veneer crown fits over the post anchorage core restoration. It has subgingival apron of gold surrounding entire circumference of root for support and bracing.

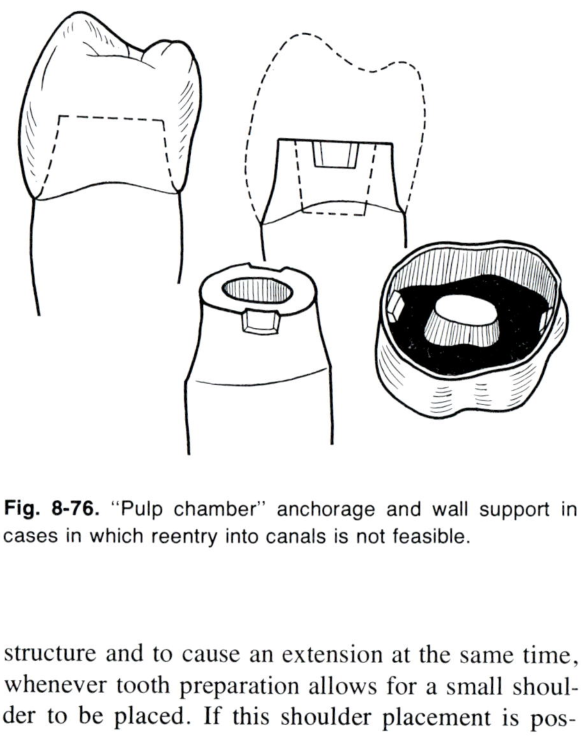

Fig. 8-76. "Pulp chamber" anchorage and wall support in cases in which reentry into canals is not feasible.

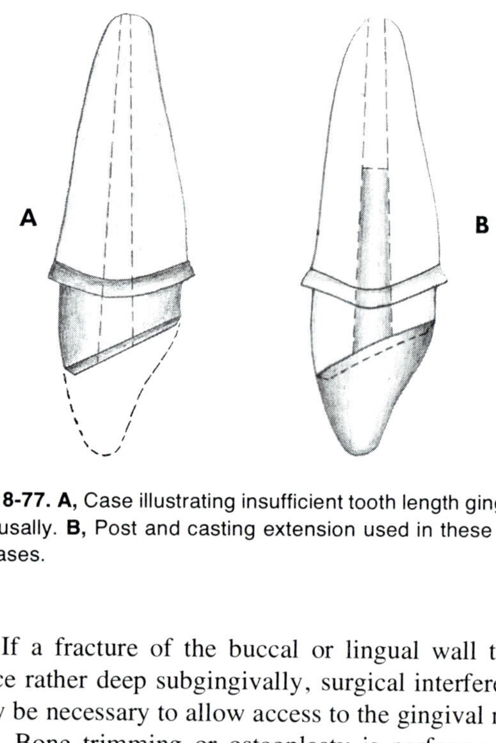

Fig. 8-77. A, Case illustrating insufficient tooth length gingivo-occlusally. **B,** Post and casting extension used in these type of cases.

structure and to cause an extension at the same time, whenever tooth preparation allows for a small shoulder to be placed. If this shoulder placement is possible, an oversized crown will not result.

The *"Para-Post System"** for endodontic parallel posts and cores is most worthy of consideration. The multiparallel pin channels are obtained with the miniature Para-Post jig, and the prefabricated pins and color coded parts facilitate the fabrication of posts and cores (Fig. 8-78).

If a fracture of the buccal or lingual wall takes place rather deep subgingivally, surgical interference may be necessary to allow access to the gingival margin. Bone trimming or osteoplasty is performed. A post-anchorage restoration is made, being sure to "shoe" the intact buccal or lingual cusp, using the principle of the "shingle-roof" or reverse bevel. If it is the buccal surface, it can be veneered. (See Fig. 8-79.)

Posts for multirooted teeth need not be as long as for anterior teeth. White[18] and Rosen[19] have shown how posts and cores for teeth with divergent roots are constructed in sections (Fig. 8-80). These are

*Whaledent, Inc., New York, N. Y.

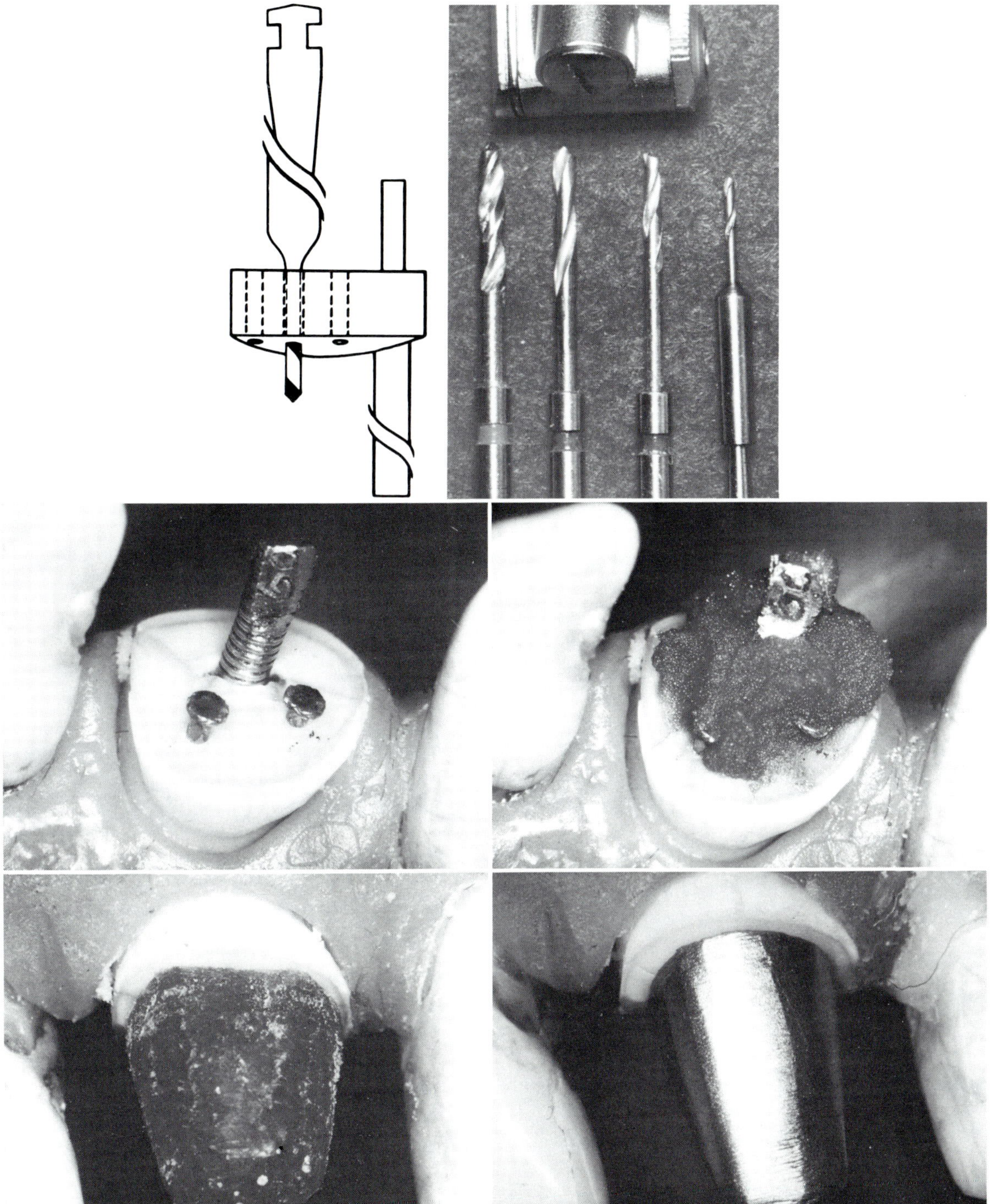

Fig. 8-78. Para-Post System for endodontic posts and cores. (Courtesy Whaledent, Inc., New York, N. Y.).

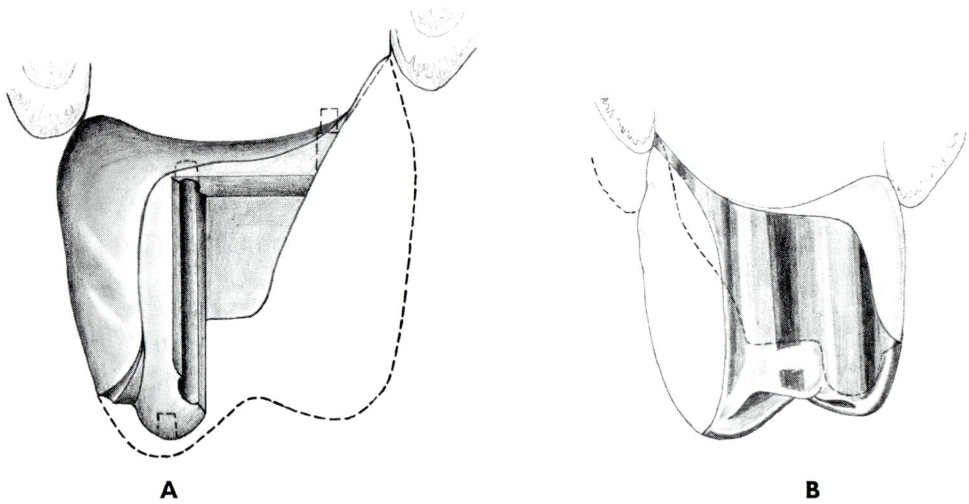

Fig. 8-79. A, Buccal or lingual wall fracture treated by "shoeing" the intact buccal or lingual cusp and making use of accessory pin or post-anchorage retention. **B,** Double deflecting curvature or contour at cervical third region in cases surgically treated, and "shoeing" of lingual cusp.

cemented in place independently and can be united with semiprecision locks (in the form of a dowel head) to provide additional strength. The lock in the section to be cemented or seated first must be prepared so that it will be parallel to the canal of the other section (Fig. 8-80, *A*).

A more recent development in this type of work has been the Kerr endo-post (Fig. 8-81). I have used the Kerr endo-post with much success and believe that it has a very definite place in the restoration of the pulpless tooth.

The endo-post technique works equally well on both anterior and posterior teeth, and narrow-diameter roots cause no problem with this method.

Hand instrumentation, instead of burs or engine reamers, is used to create the canal hole or holes. This obviates the necessity of removing excessive amounts of root structure and minimizes the danger of root splitting or root perforation.

Restorations are safer because two thirds to four fifths of the root length, rather than the root diameter, is used for retention and strength. Short tapered cast posts, even with increased lateral areas, will not withstand occlusal stresses as well as a post having at least the length of the coronal surface to be restored.

The endo-post has the same size and taper as the standardized file and/or reamer used to create the hole, and, because of this, the bearing stress and load are distributed uniformly over the entire length and diameter of the post. It has a high tensile strength, and it is said that it is two to four times that of a cast post.

Full coverage

The full crown is unquestionably the strongest and most retentive retainer we have in our repertoire of cavity designs. However, full-crown retainers should be used only when the circumstances demand it, after careful diagnosis and prognosis point to its requirement.

In health, the exposed part of the tooth in the mouth is surrounded by a periphereal seal (epithelial attachment) regardless of the gingival level or contour. Our operative and restorative procedures must try to preserve this protective feature.

It has been said many times that subgingival extensions of full coverage margins produce an environment that is unfavorable to the health of the marginal gingiva, giving tissues that are more rolled, more thickened, and more inflammatory in character.

This accusation cannot be denied, but does the fault lie with full coverage or the dentist? Can an understanding of tooth form and function, crown preparation, and the skillful and careful use of the necessary tools and materials prevent this catastrophe? I think it can.

The marginal finish lines used in the preparation of teeth for full coverage are (1) shoulder, (2) beveled-shoulder, (3) chamfer, (4) knife-edge or featheredge, and (5) McEwen's "chamferette"—a finish line between a chamfer and a featheredge (Fig. 8-87).

The full shoulder preparation is used only in the preparation of teeth for procelain jacket crowns. This type of crown preparation with its definitive shoulder

Text continued on p. 397.

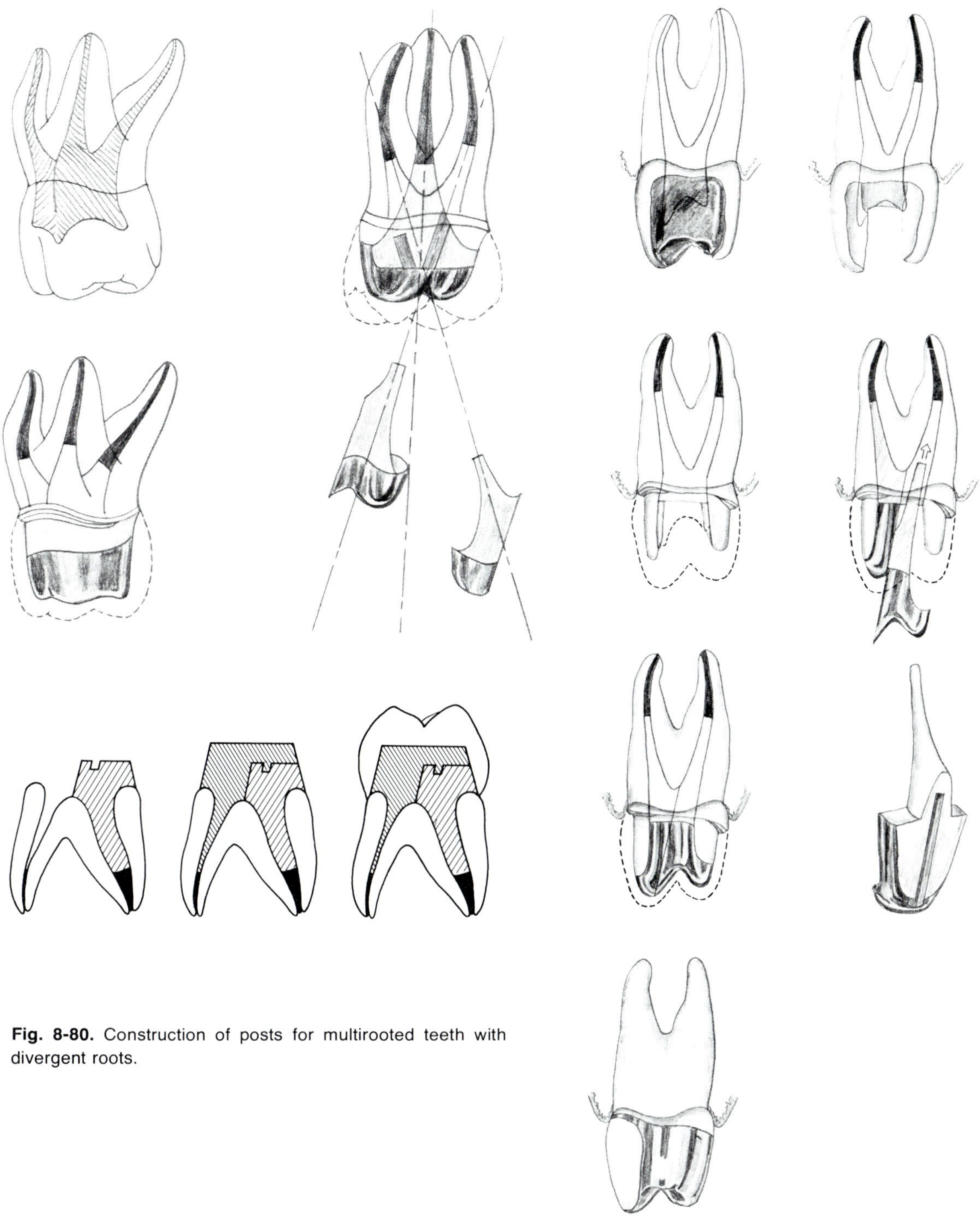

Fig. 8-80. Construction of posts for multirooted teeth with divergent roots.

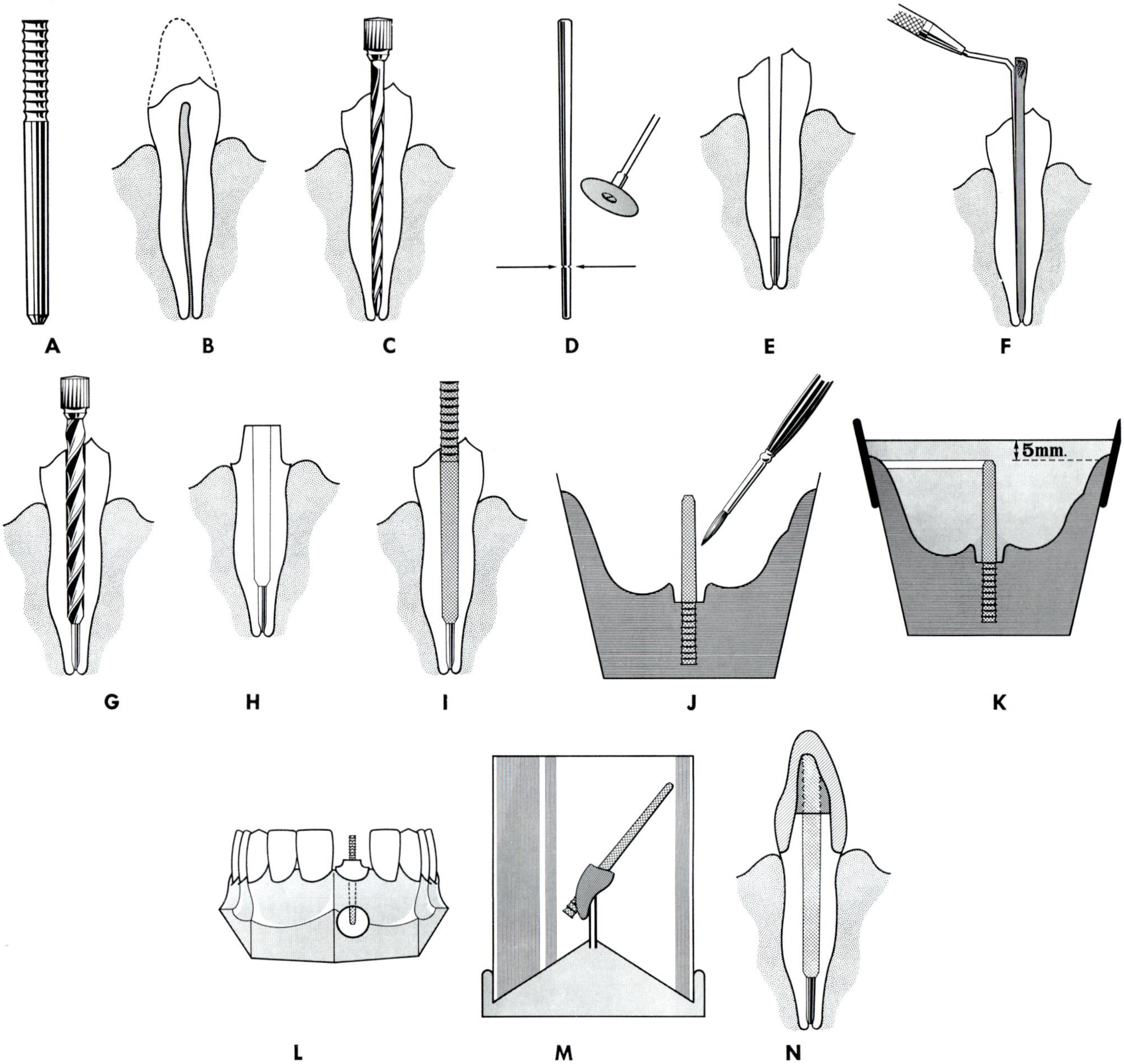

Fig. 8-81. Endo-post technique. **A,** Endo-post. **B.** Tooth to be treated and restored. **C,** Clearing and enlarging root canal. **D,** Notch silver point with a disk around its circumference at its apical third or less. Tip of silver point cemented into place. **E,** Point twisted gently until it breaks where notched. **F.** Gutta-percha points may be used to seal apical third. Standardized files and reamers used to remove gutta-percha from midportion and coronal portion of canal. **G,** Remainder of canal enlarged with files and reamers. As little tooth structure as possible removed. **H,** Tooth prepared, leaving as much of the crown portion as possible. **I,** Endo-post inserted and impression taken. Permlastic, Elasticon, or copper tube–modeling compound can be used. **J,** Root end of the endo-post lubricated with Kerr microfilm. **K,** Plastic toothpick or banker's pin luted to periphery of impression and to side of endo-post at its root end extremity. Stone model poured to level of 5 mm. above end of post. **L,** After removal of model from impression, plastic toothpick or pin removed and hole enlarged to form window that enables one to check seat of post after it has been removed and reinserted into model. Any stone that forms seat at end of endo-post should not be cut away. **M,** Wax coronal part of core, sprue and invest in luster cast investment (type of investment that must be used in casting metal to metal to avoid contamination and oxidation of embedded metal). **N,** Casting trimmed and seated in model. Veneer crown constructed and cemented over post-anchorage cast core, which had been previously cemented. (Courtesy Kerr Dental Mfg. Co., Detroit, Mich.)

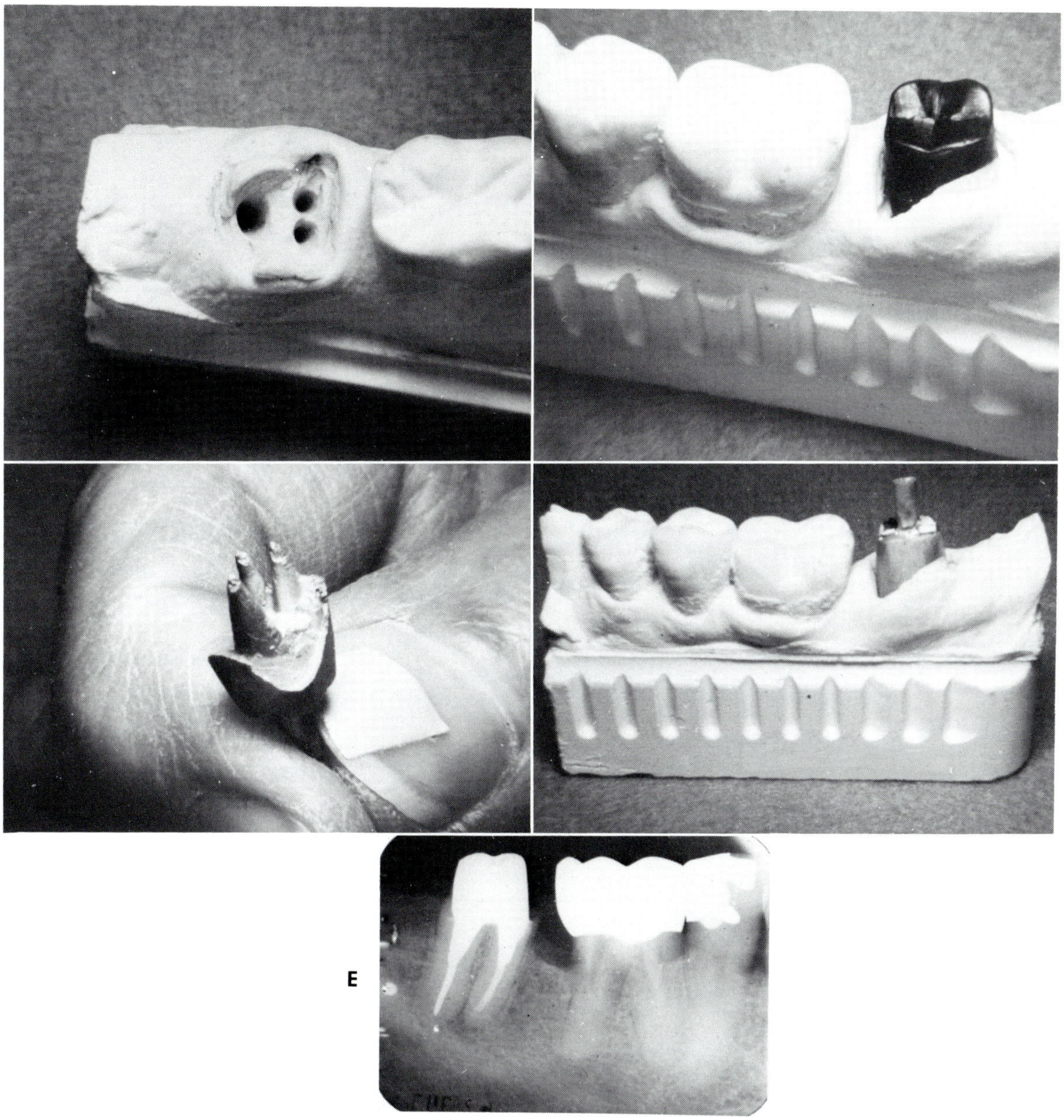

Fig. 8-82. A case of a lower left second molar treated by Kornfeld.

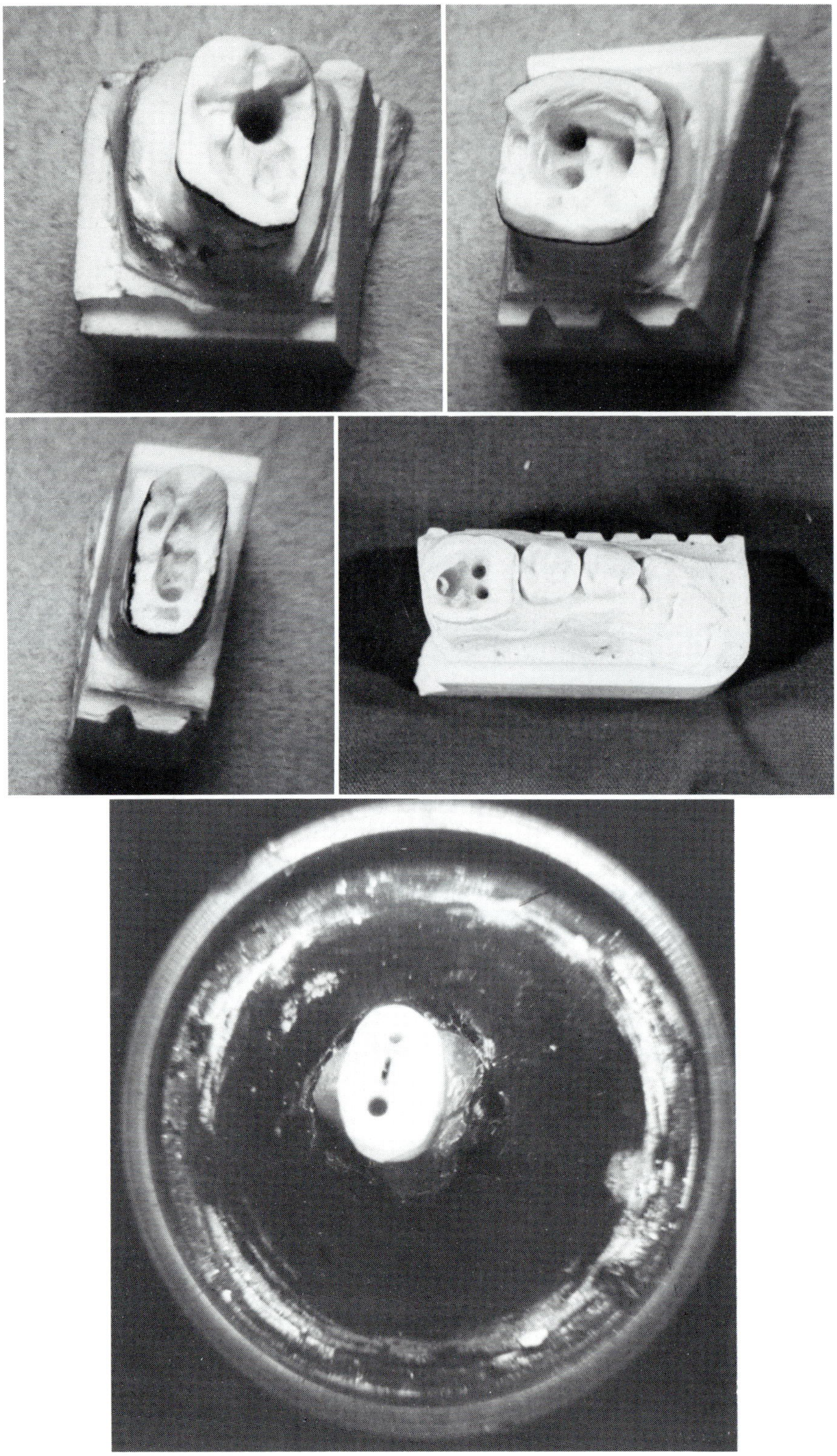

Fig. 8-83. Stone dies (made from hydrocolloid impressions) of endodontically treated teeth.

makes use of a butt joint, which cannot be used in the construction of cast crowns—all metal or veneer.

The prepared tooth that will give the maximum support to a porcelain jacket crown will conform closely in outline to the natural form of the dentin. Its proximal surfaces will be almost parallel, the variations from the parallel being sufficient only to permit the removal of the impression without distortion.

The surfaces intended to support porcelain under direct pressure will be perpendicular to the direction of the applied forces. The shoulder will form a right angle or a slightly acute angle with the axial surfaces, the form of the angle being more important than the width of the shoulder.

In determining the length as well as other dimensions of the prepared tooth, the dominant thought should be that we are preparing a support for the porcelain rather than for its undue thickness.

It is impossible to cast precisely to a butt joint, and it is difficult to seat a casting adequately to this kind of joint. The process of cementation will verify this statement, and the end result is a cement line that eventually leads to a "wash-out" and subsequent plaque formation and its sequelae—decay and gingival irritation. Therefore a short bevel is needed on the shoulder whenever a cast veneer crown is to be constructed.

In the preparation of average length or short teeth for full coverage, when a veneering material is to be used for esthetics, a facial, mesial, and distal "beveled-shoulder" finishing line is indicated so that room is allowed for the porcelain or acrylic facing and for better periodontal health such as the avoidance of impingement or strangulation of the interseptal tissue. The shoulder width in these cases should be 1 to 1.5 mm., which also allows for the proper contouring of the crown at the cervical third.

This beveled-shoulder marginal finish line gradually will fade into a chamfer finish line as it ap-

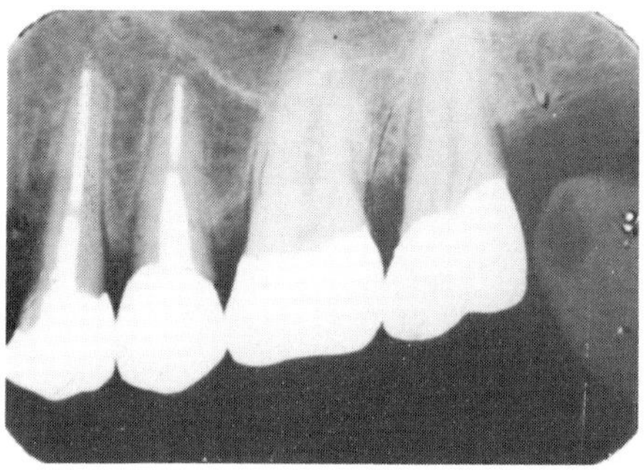

Fig. 8-84. A case of endodontically treated premolars treated by the author 20 years ago. Radiograph taken in 1974.

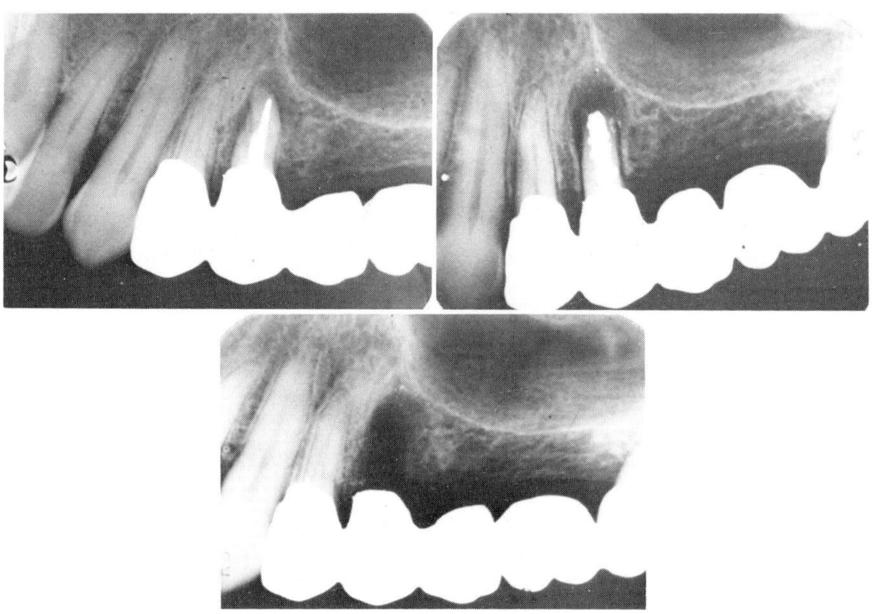

Fig. 8-85. A case treated endodontically. Apparently the root was fractured, because an acute infection ensued in less than a year. Part of root end was removed and filled with amalgam alloy apically. It failed shortly thereafter and the root was removed surgically. Fixed partial denture is still serviceable.

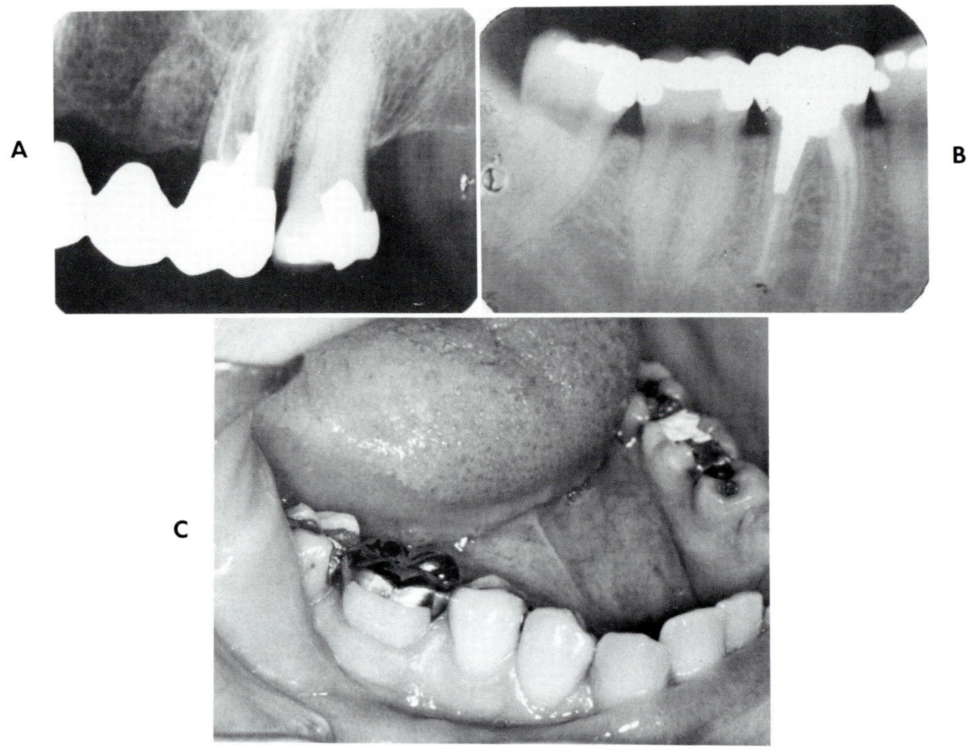

Fig. 8-86. A, An endodontically treated tooth became infected because the root had been perforated and not detected at time of insertion of post anchorage cast gold core. By hard and soft tissue curettage and surgical interference the fixed bridge has, so far, remained in service for 7 years. B, C, Radiograph and restoration of an endodontically treated tooth executed by the author.

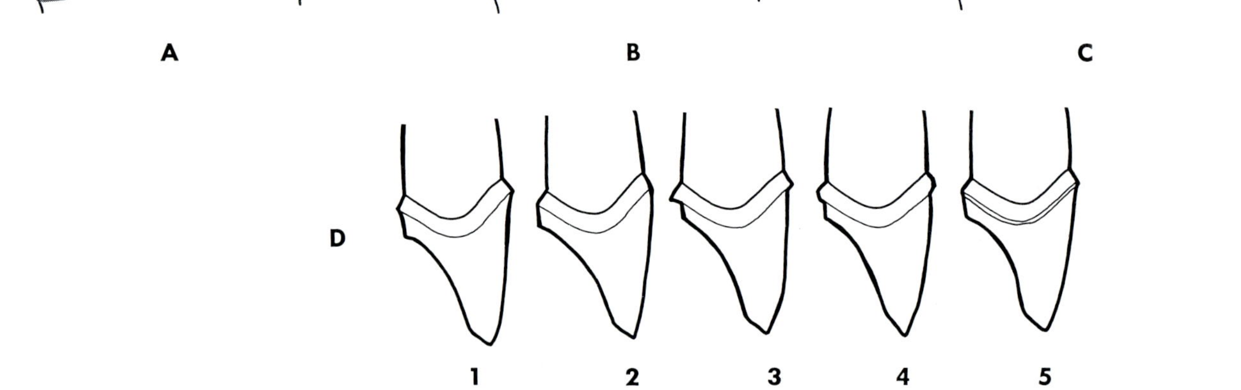

Fig. 8-87. Marginal finish lines. A, Shoulder. B, Beveled shoulder. C, Chamfer. D, Chamfer, featheredge, shoulder, beveled shoulder. D, *1* to *5* are different views of what one sees in A to C with the addition of featheredge *(2)* and another view of the beveled shoulder *(4)*.

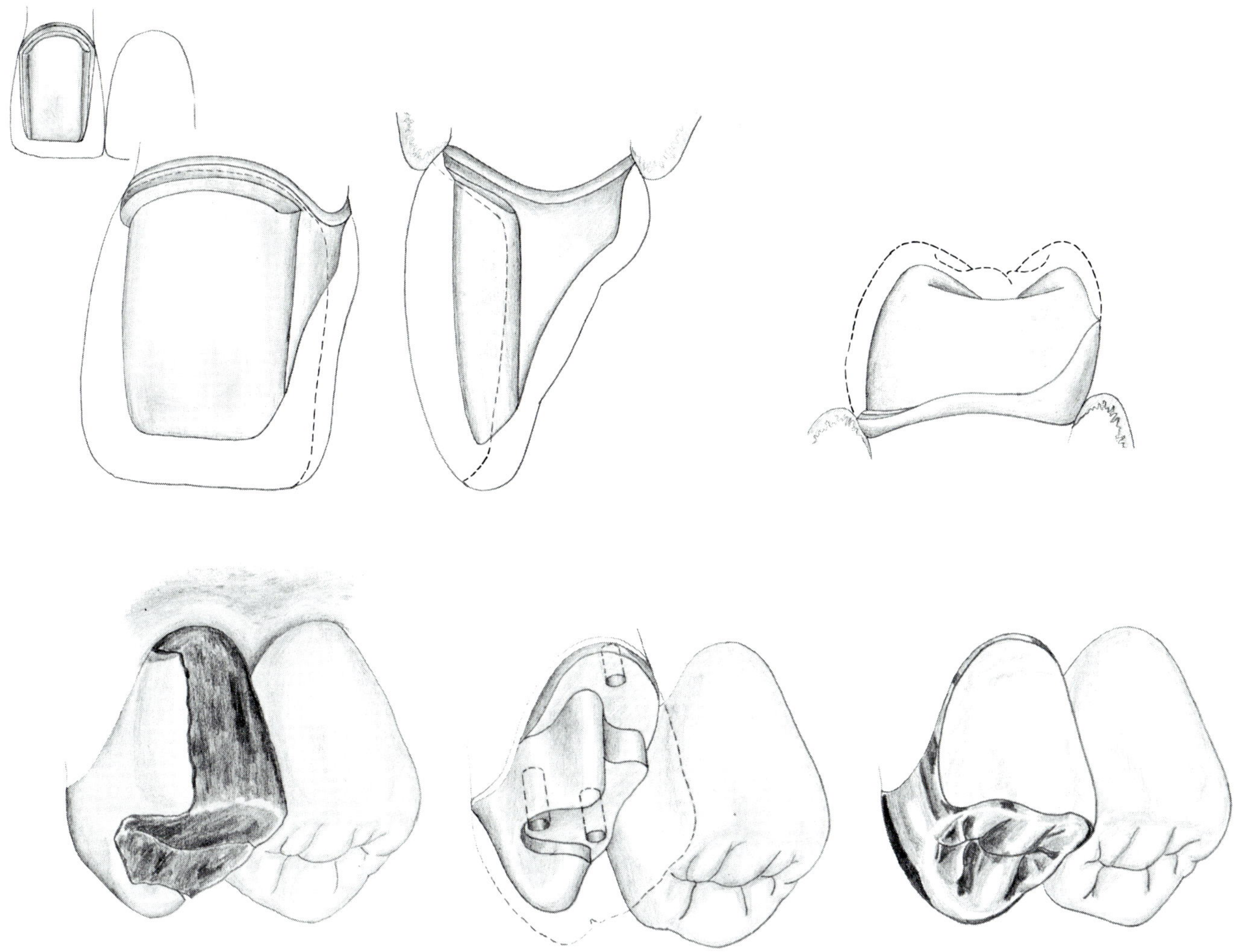

Fig. 8-88. Beveled-shoulder marginal finish line gradually fades into chamfer finish line as it approaches lingual surface.

proaches the lingual surface, which has a finish line in the form of a chamfer from the mesial and distal aspects (Fig. 8-88).

The taper of this type of preparation should be 2 degrees from the perpendicular, which allows for a tighter frictional grip of the casting to the tooth, and the axial line angles should be reduced sufficiently, which allows more room for the veneering material. If teeth with short or average sized coronal lengths are to be splinted, the preparations should be tapered 2 to 5 degrees from the perpendicular for ease of positioning and correct marginal fit of the restorations.

For teeth with lengthened clinical crowns and large open interdental embrasures, the aftermath of bone loss and periodontal treatment, the "chamferette" finish line is indicated (Fig. 8-89). In these cases, where a number of teeth have to be splinted to reduce mobility patterns, etc., the taper is at least 5 degrees from the perpendicular. This allows for ease of seating of the finished restoration, less chance of pulp involvement, and excellent marginal fit of castings, thereby avoiding the dreaded subgingival cement line.

The technique and instrumentation that are used in the preparation of teeth for full coverage will be considered now (Fig. 8-90).

Before considering technique and instrumentation used in the preparation of teeth for full coverage, let us review the characteristics a finished full veneer crown should embody:

1. A properly supported foundation filling (gold, alloy, or composite), if one is indicated.

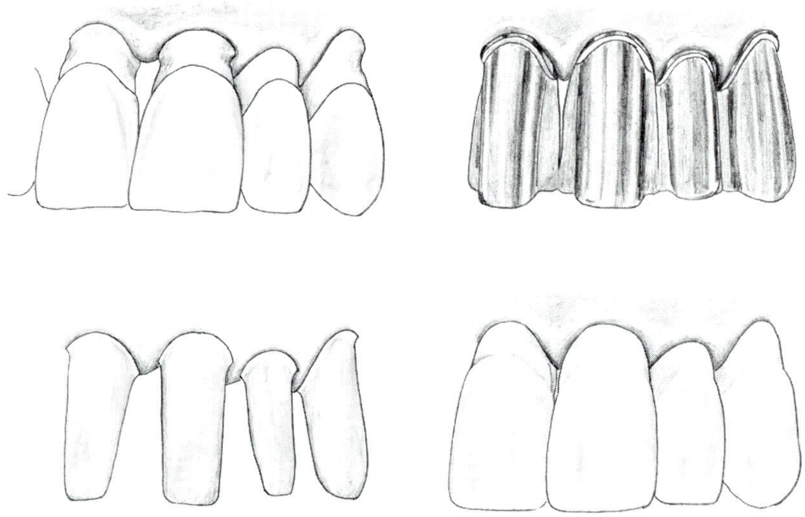

Fig. 8-89. "Chamferette" finish line indicated with lengthened clinical crowns and large open interdental embrasures. (Suggested by Dr. R. A. McEwen, Atlanta, Ga.)

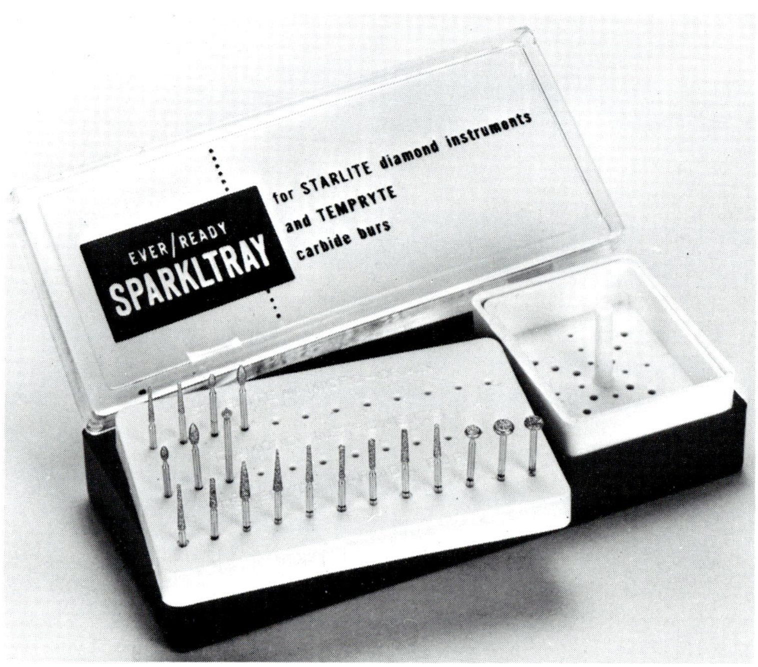

Fig. 8-90. Types of diamond points that I use.

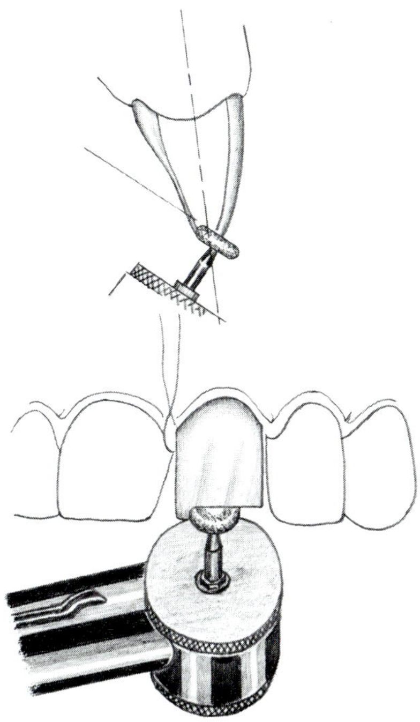

Fig. 8-91. Reduction of incisal area in full coverage preparation.

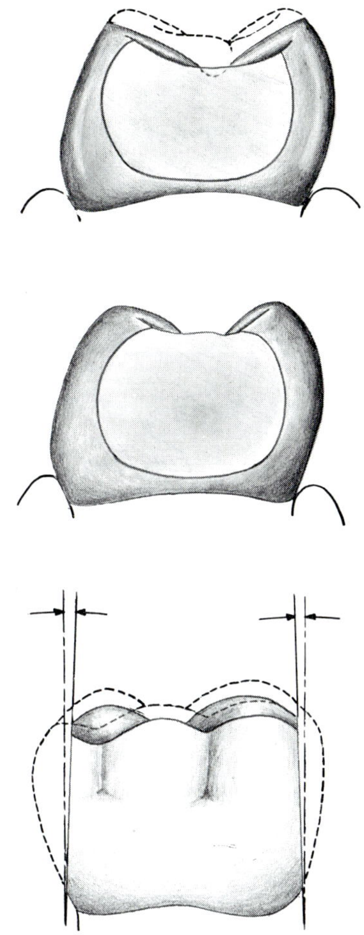

Continued.

Fig. 8-92. A, Occlusal reduction of posterior teeth for full-coverage preparation. Occlusal architecture is followed. **B,** Proximal surfaces reduced tapering slightly toward occlusal surface. **C,** Amount of taper in preparation for full coverage should be within the range of 2 to 5 degrees from the perpendicular. **D,** Procedural steps in preparation of a posterior tooth for full coverage.

2. Smooth, properly tapered (2 to 5 degrees) proximal, facial, and lingual surfaces devoid of undercuts.
3. An even reduction of the occlusal surface following cuspal contours with sufficient clearance (2 mm.) to avoid thin spots in the finished casting. The reduction of the occlusal by 2 mm. should be a clearance of 2 mm. created with all pathways of movement (eccentric excursions) considered, observed, duly noted, and allowed for, in addition to clearance for correct centric position.
4. If possible, 2 mm. of bulk reduction where there is to be a veneer of acrylic or porcelain placed.
5. A well-defined finishing line placed under the gingival tissue crevice.
6. Vertical grooves and pins (especially if needed for added retention), good boxes for housing precision attachments or dowels, and room for the casting to ''draw'' in relation to itself and some adjacent tooth or teeth.

The incisal area is reduced, as a rule, about 2 mm. following the lingual plane at a 45 degree angle to the long axis of the tooth. In the lower anterior teeth the incisal plane is inclined toward the labial surface (Fig. 8-91).

The general fundamentals of occlusal reduction are similar for both mandibular and maxillary posterior teeth. The occlusal architecture should be followed, making the occlusal cut in two planes, sloping from the height of the buccal and lingual cusps toward the central groove and following the inclines and slopes of the cusps, at the same time comparing with the opposing occlusion as we go along to gain a uniform reduction of the surfaces involved. We try for a replica of the original occlusal surface at a reduced level, creating sufficient clearance from articulating contacts in every direction, and thereby allowing for an adequate thickness of gold. (See Fig. 8-92.)

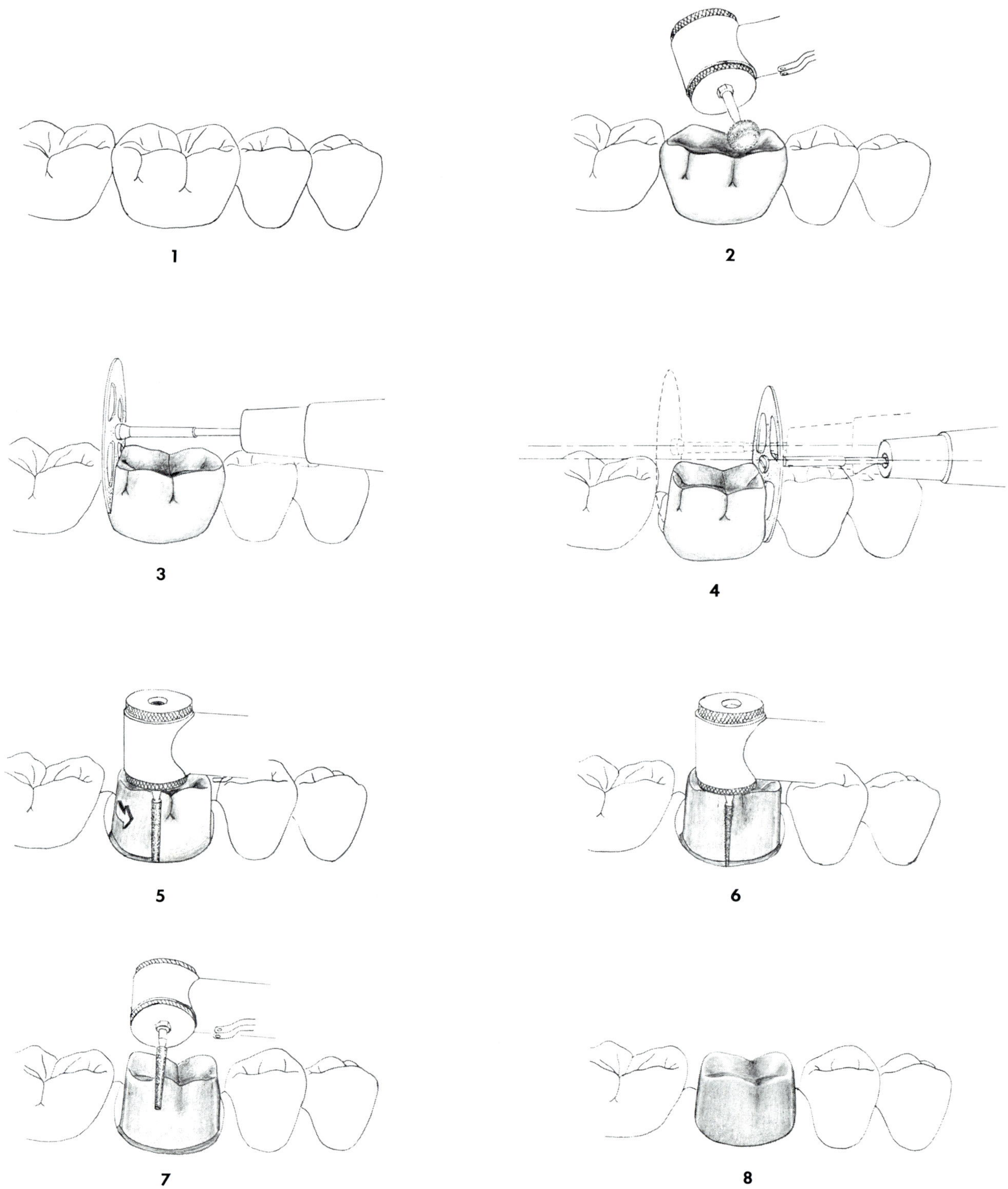

D

Fig. 8-92, cont'd. For legend see p. 401.

The proximal surfaces are reduced next, tapering slightly toward the occlusal surface.

The facial and lingual surfaces are then reduced with the cutting tool in a rapid, brushlike movement, starting at the distal surface and working gently and carefully in a mesial direction. This is done with an instrument running axially with the tooth, being sure to emphasize its action around the axial line angles to reduce them sufficiently and to round them off.

In average length or short teeth, when veneering material is to be used either in the form of a porcelain jacket crown or a cast veneer crown, a slight taper has not only been given to the tooth, but also a shoulder has been developed. Then the shoulder outline should be extended below the free margin of the gum and its definition and smoothness improved. If the cast veneer crown is the one being prepared, then the shoulder is beveled with a very fine flame-shaped diamond stone.

For teeth with lengthened clinical crowns and showing a bone loss, the facial and lingual surfaces are reduced with a diamond instrument, starting at the distal surface and working with rapid brushlike movements, in an axial direction, to the mesial surface, at the same time emphasizing its action around the axial line angles for sufficient reduction. A taper is given to the tooth, at the same time creating a chamfer finish line, which is extended under the free margin of the gum with a flame-shaped diamond point. The point of this instrument, when carried below the free gum margin, will produce a minimal cut, giving the "chamferette" finish line, whereas the wider portion of the instrument will engage that part of the tooth where maximal removal for correct taper and parallelism is required.

Preparation of an anterior tooth for a porcelain jacket crown

1. Break the contact areas with a very small flame-shaped diamond stone, No. 265-8P, making sure to avoid abrading the proximal surfaces of the adjacent teeth (Fig. 8-93). A flat diamond disk, running at conventional lower speeds, can be used if desired. The mesial and distal slices, extending from the incisal surface to the gingiva, will establish slight interproximal shoulders (Fig. 8-94).

2. Reduce the incisal surface about 2 mm., following the lingual plane at a 45 degree angle to the long axis of the tooth (Fig. 8-95). In lower anterior teeth the incisal plane is inclined toward the labial surface (Fig. 8-96). All three cutting surfaces of Starlite No. 34P or 110SP are employed to undercut as well as reduce the incisal edge to a proper depth and to establish incisal bevel.

3. Reduce labial surface and area around the cingulum with a No. 556-7P or 558-7P, running the instrument axially with the tooth with rapid, light strokes in a brushlike manner (the labial and lingual enamel bulk also can be removed by using the rounded edge of No. 110SP) (Fig. 8-97). With a No. WM-1

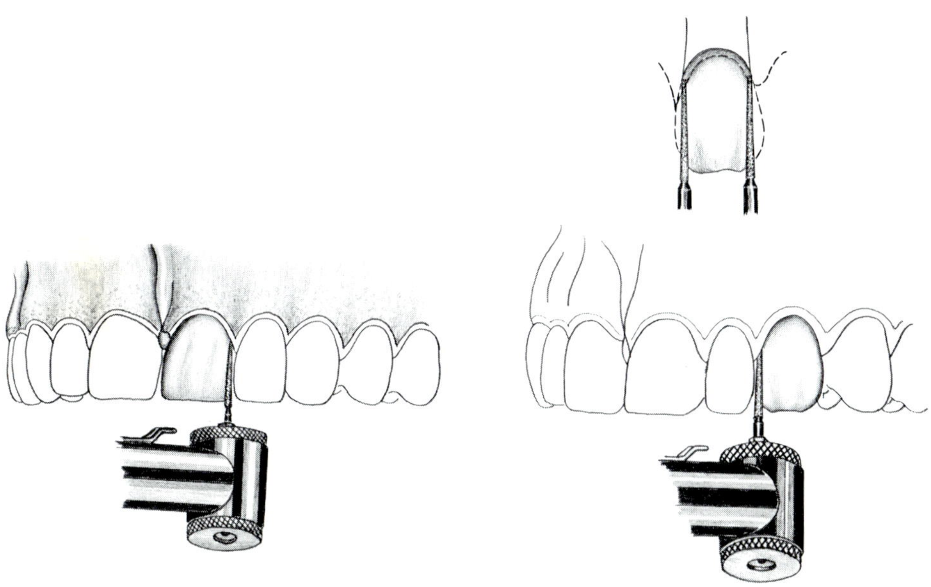

Fig. 8-93. Breaking contact area with small flame-shaped diamond stone in preparation of anterior tooth for porcelain jacket crown.

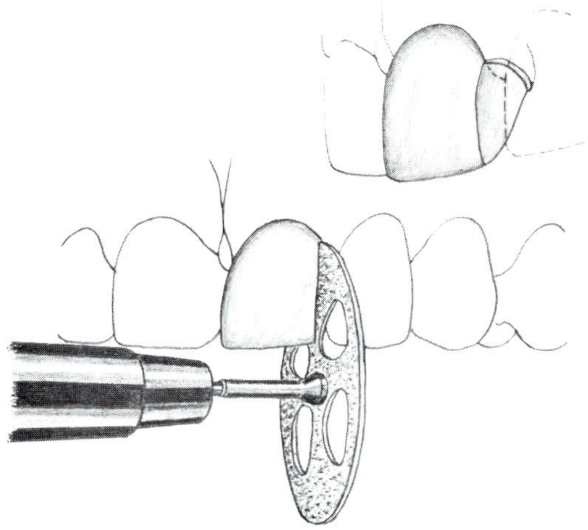

Fig. 8-94. Breaking the contact area with a disk (alternate method).

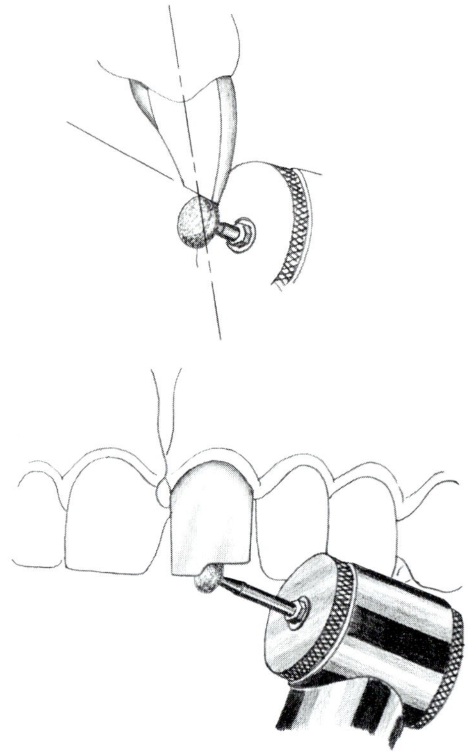

Fig. 8-95. Reduction of incisal surface following lingual plane at 45 degree angle to long axis of tooth.

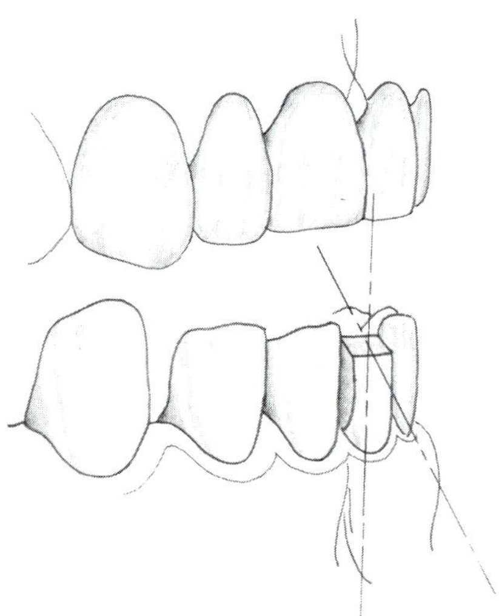

Fig. 8-96. In lower anterior teeth incisal plane is inclined toward labial surface.

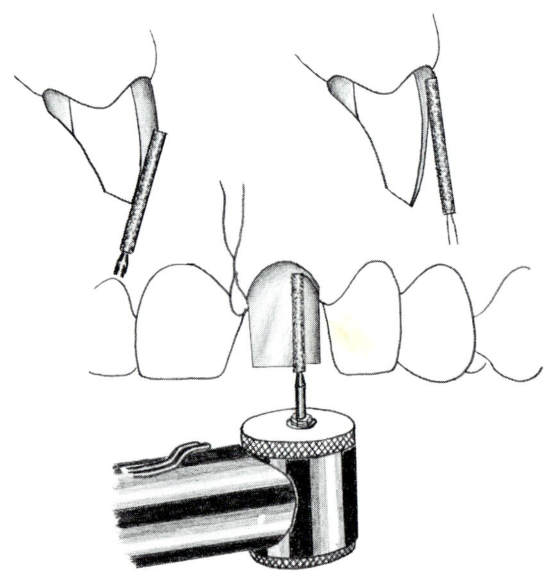

Fig. 8-97. Reduction of labial surface with No. 556-7P or 558-7P diamond stone. Labial and lingual enamel bulk also can be removed by using rounded edge of No. 110SP.

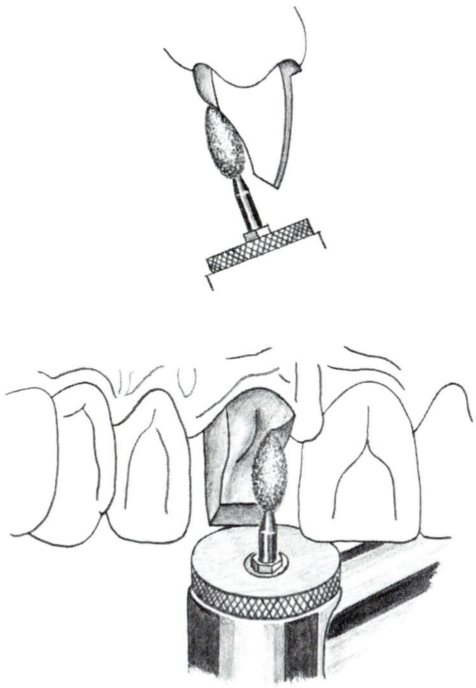

Fig. 8-98. Removal of lingual tooth structure from incisal edge to upper border of cingulum area with a special functionally shaped diamond instrument—No. WM-1 or WM-2.

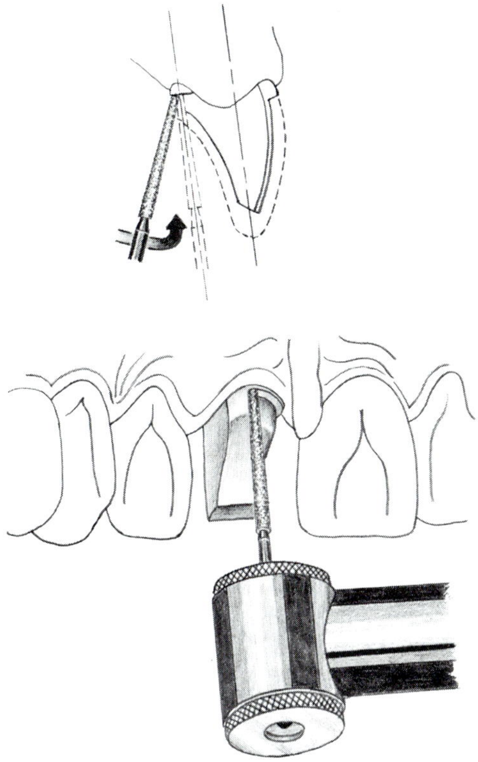

Fig. 8-99. Removal of tooth structure in cingulum area and creation of shoulder.

or WM-2, which is a special functionally shaped instrument, remove lingual tooth structure from the crest of the cingulum to the incisal edge by planing from proximal to proximal. This instrument will preserve the lingual concavity, assuring uniform removal of bulk, and it also assures an even thickness of porcelain in the finished crown (Fig. 8-98).

4. Follow with a No. 700-7P or 700-8P, which is a tapered diamond stone that is 0.8 mm. wide at its tip. This point establishes uniform depth, and the curvature of the cut is oriented to the curvature of the tissue. (At no time should we traumatize tissue.) Make the cut away from tissue, the diamond point first being tipped away to establish a shoulder and then angled parallel to the long axis of the tooth (Fig. 8-99). This imparts proper taper and establishes a shoulder of desired depth or thickness. (If a wider shoulder is desired, use No. 701-8P, which is 1.1 mm. wide at its tip.)

This instrument follows around from the labial surface to the mesial surface and then around the linguocingulum area to the distal proximal surface, creating an even width of shoulder automatically, which is required especially for a porcelain jacket crown.

5. The shoulder should be extended carefully below the free gum margin and developed fully with cutting tools used at conventional lower speeds (Fig. 8-100). This may be done with a No. 900 or 901 end-cutting bur, which can be used without danger of undercutting the axial walls of the preparation because its axial surface is smooth. The plane of the shoulder is squared and placed at right angles to the axial surfaces of the preparation, and the shoulder can be planed smooth by using a hoe (S.S.W. No. 6-2-6 or 8-3-6) and special Bastian or Krause files.

A shoulder that forms a slightly acute angle with the axial surface, thus transmitting the induced forces toward the interior of the tooth, gives us a most favorable condition. A shoulder that forms a right angle with the axial surface absorbs all the transmitted force, but a shoulder that forms an obtuse angle with the axial surface gives rise to a horizontal component of force, which is likely to cause fracture of the crown. (Fig. 8-101).

The preparation is then treated with superfinishing

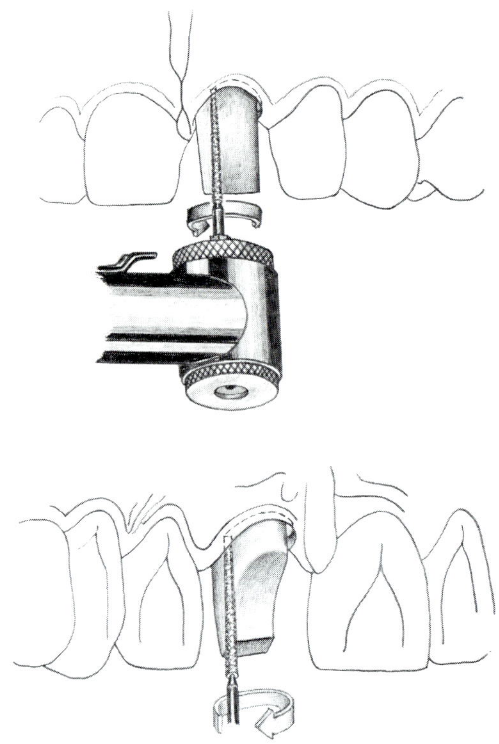

Fig. 8-100. Extending shoulder below free gum margin—developed with cutting tools used at conventional lower speeds (stones, end-cutting burs, etc.).

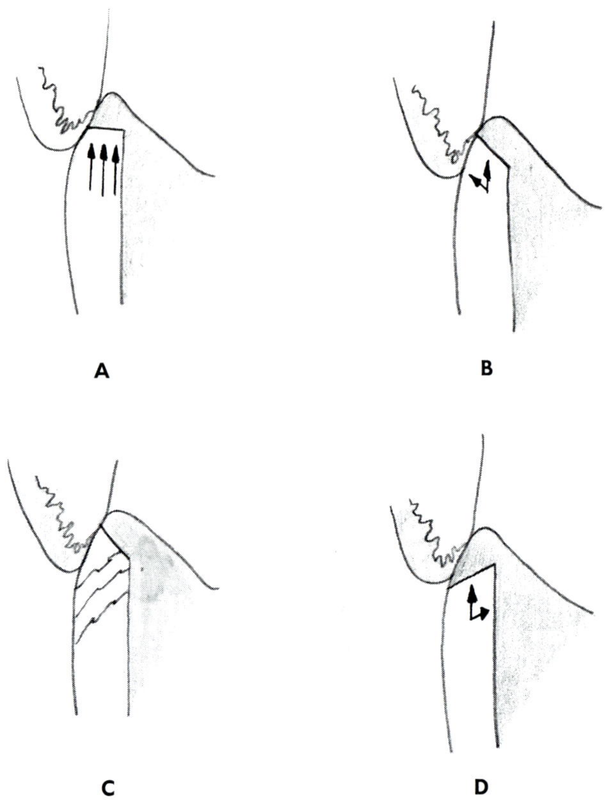

Fig. 8-101. A, Shoulder that forms right angle with axial surface absorbs all the transmitted force. B, Shoulder forming an obtuse angle gives rise to horizontal component of force, which is likely to cause fracture of crown, as in C. D, Most favorable condition exists when shoulder forms slightly acute angle with axial surface, thus transmitting induced forces toward interior of tooth. (Redrawn from Conod, H. In Grubb, H. D.: Basic procedures essential for successful porcelain restorations, Proceedings of the Dental Centenary Celebration, 1940.)

diamond stones—No. 700-8F and No. WM-1F or WM-2F—after which it is carefully examined, using binocular loupes and a light stream of warm air, for undercuts or roughness (Figs. 8-102 and 8-103).

Preparation of an anterior or posterior tooth for a cast veneer crown

1. Break the contact areas with a very small flame-shaped stone No. 265-8P, making sure to avoid abrading the proximal surfaces of the adjacent teeth. McEwen[20] accomplishes this by following the contour of the proximal surface of the adjacent tooth, creating a concavity and then establishing the proper taper to the preparation. A flat diamond disk, running at conventional lower speeds, can be used if desired. The mesial and distal slices, extending from the incisal edge to the gingiva, will establish slight interproximal shoulders.

For posterior teeth the mesial surface is reduced, using a straight safeside diamond disk from the occlusal surface to the gingiva, and a cup-shaped diamond disk is used for the distal surface reduction.

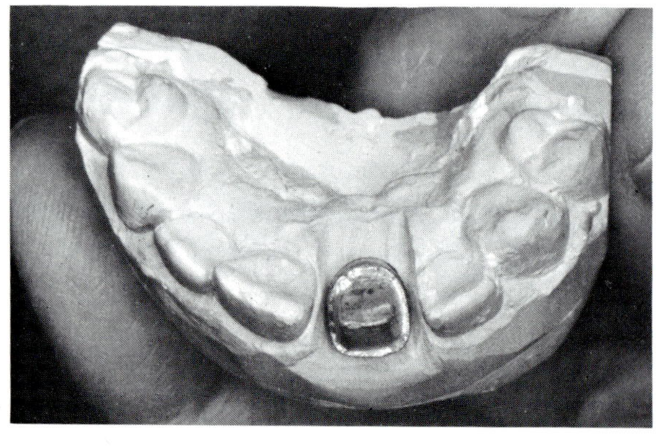

Fig. 8-102. Die of completed preparation from practice.

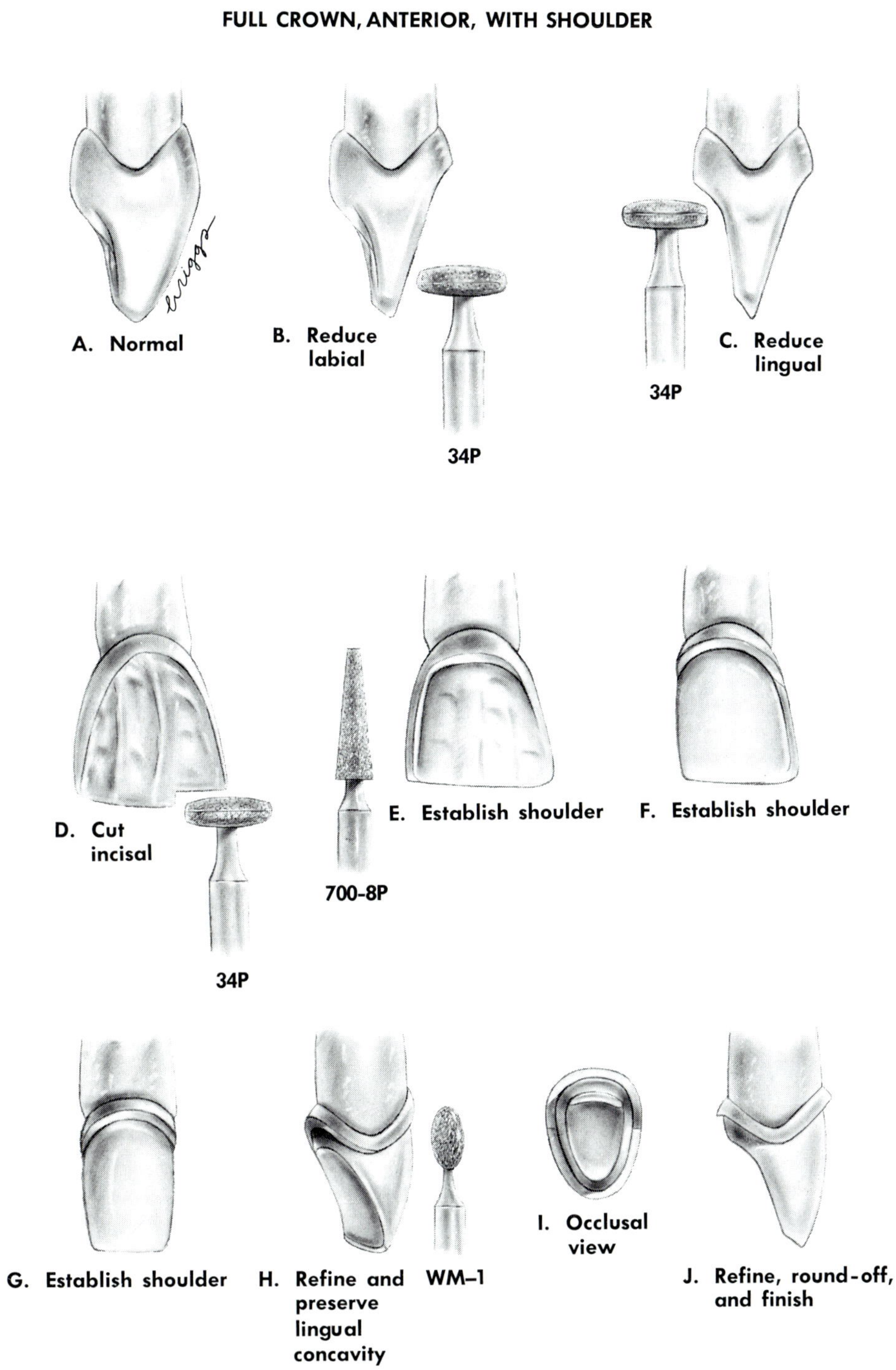

Fig. 8-103. Procedural steps in preparation of anterior tooth for porcelain jacket crown.

2. All three cutting surfaces of No. 110SP are employed to undercut as well as reduce incisal edge to proper depth and to establish incisal bevel.

For posterior teeth reduce occlusal surface with No. 110SP, removing enamel into dentin, following the occlusal architecture. Make the occlusal cut in two planes—sloping from the height of the buccal and lingual cusps toward the central groove and following the inclines and slopes of the cusps.

3. Facial gross enamel reduction just into the dentin is accomplished with No. 556-7P or 558-7P or with the rounded edge of No. 110SP, moving the stone in an axial relation to the tooth with rapid, light strokes in a brushlike manner.

Gross lingual enamel reduction of posterior teeth and the cingulum area of anterior teeth is reduced with No. 556-7P or 558-7P or with the rounded edge of No. 110SP.

With a No. WM-1 or WM-2, which is a special, functionally shaped stone, remove lingual tooth structure of anterior teeth from the crest of the cingulum to the incisal edge by planing from proximal to proximal surface. This instrument will preserve lingual concavity, assuring uniform removal of bulk.

4. Follow this planing with a No. 700-7P or 700-8P, which is a tapered diamond stone 0.8 mm. wide at its tip. This point establishes uniform depth, and the curvature of the cut is oriented to the curvature of the tissue (instrument must not contact soft tissue).

Make the cut away from the soft tissue, the diamond point first being tipped away to establish shoulder and then being angled parallel to the long axis of the tooth. This imparts proper taper and establishes shoulder of desired depth or thickness. (If a wider shoulder is desired, use No. 701-8P, which is 1.1 mm. wide at the tip.)

This diamond stone is used on the facial surface and then is followed around from the facial surface to the mesial surface and from the facial surface to the distal surface, the shoulder preparation gradually fading out proximally to the shoulderless lingual surface.

The linguocingulum area of anterior teeth and the lingual surface of posterior teeth are then tapered with No. 770-7P or 770-8P. The lingual finish line in these cases can be featheredge or a slight chamfer.

5. Refine shoulders and axial line angles using No. 700-8F, a superfinishing diamond stone. Use No. WM-1F or WM-2F to finish or smooth lingual concavity above crest of cingulum of anterior teeth, and use No. 103SP to round or bevel occlusal line angles of posterior teeth and to establish buccal and lingual grooves.

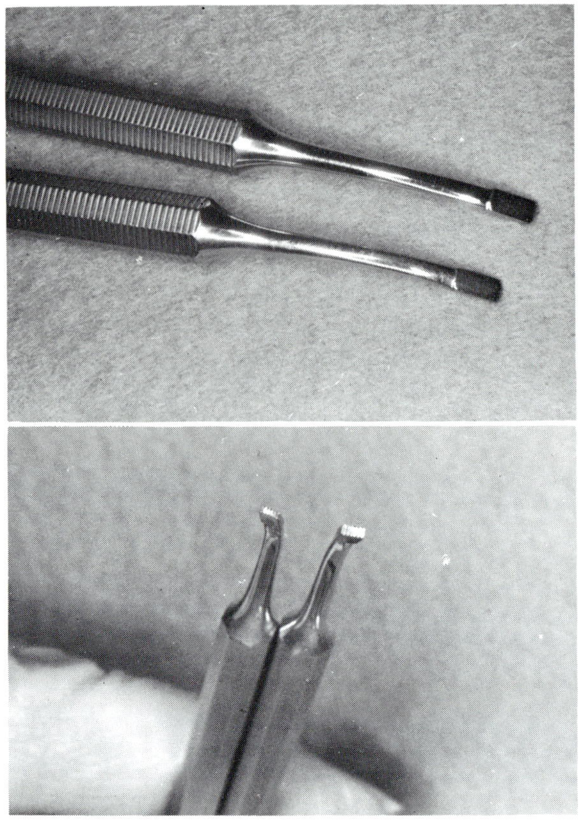

Fig. 8-104. Bastian files used to plane shoulder smooth.

6. The facial, mesial, and distal shoulder should be extended carefully below the free gum margin and developed fully with cutting tools used at conventional lower speeds. This may be done with a No. 957 or 958 end-cutting bur, which can be used without danger of undercutting the axial walls of the preparation because its axial surface is smooth. The plane of the shoulder is squared and placed at right angles to the axial surfaces of the preparation, and the shoulder can be planed smooth by using a hoe (S.S.W. No. 6-2-6 or 8-3-6) and special Bastian or Krause files (Fig. 8-104).

7. The preparation is completed with a beveling of the shoulder, using the tip of a small flame-shaped diamond point.

In cases in which short clinical crowns are present, increased retention may be obtained by introducing accessory anchorage, grooves and pits, in accordance with the principles of tripodism.

For the all-metal posterior crown use a chamfer marginal finish line.

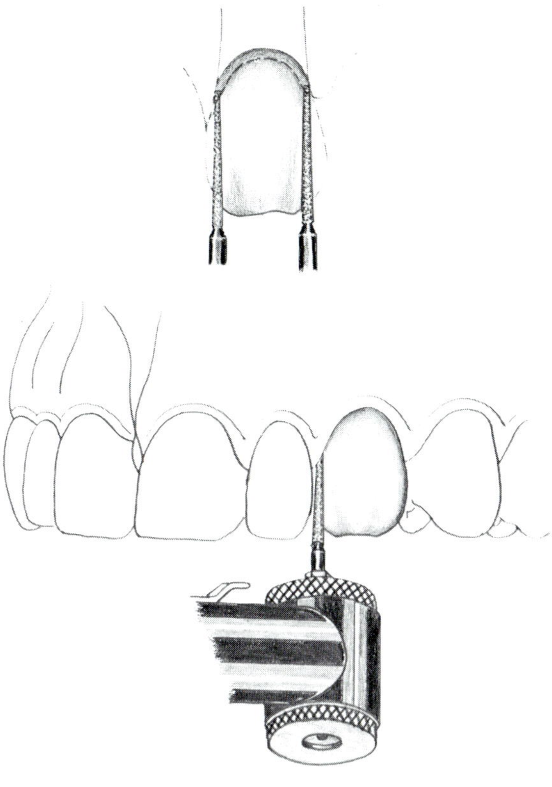

Fig. 8-105. Break contact areas with flame-shaped diamond stone.

Preparation of anterior or posterior teeth with lengthened clinical crowns for cast veneer crowns

The following procedural steps are used in the preparation of teeth that have lost a great deal of supporting bone for cast veneer crowns.

1. Break the contact areas with a very small flame-shaped stone, No. 265-8P (Fig. 8-105). (See also Fig. 8-106.)

2. All three cutting surfaces of No. 110SP are employed to undercut as well as reduce incisal edge to proper depth and to establish incisal bevel (Fig. 8-106, *D*).

For posterior teeth reduce occlusal surface with No. 110SP, removing enamel into dentin, following the occlusal architecture. Make the occlusal cut in two planes—sloping from the height of the buccal and lingual cusps toward the central groove and following the inclines and slopes of the cusps (Fig. 8-112, *D*).

3. Facial gross enamel reduction just into dentin is accomplished with the rounded edge of Starlite No. 110SP (Fig. 8-107). Move the handpiece from the incisal or occlusal edge to the gingival edge with short, rapid, light strokes. Continue the use of No. 110SP for bulk lingual reduction of posterior teeth and the cingulum area of anterior teeth (Fig. 8-106, *C*). With a No. WM-1 or WM-2 (Fig. 8-108), which is a special, functionally shaped stone, remove lingual tooth structure of anterior teeth from the crest of the cingulum to the incisal edge by planing from proximal to proximal surface. This instrument will preserve lingual concavity, assuring uniform removal of bulk.

4. Beginning at facial gingival line with a No. 770-7P stone, penetrate to width of instrument (0.8 mm. wide at tip, and tip is rounded), creating chamfer at gingiva. Then begin to establish taper of preparation by holding diamond stone parallel to long axis of tooth. Carry stone around interproximally and lingually. Continue to refine taper of tooth and chamfer and to contour it into bifurcation and trifurcation areas where indicated.

For a tooth with a longer clinical crown, select a diamond stone with a longer cutting head, No. 770-8P or 10P (No. 771-7P will inscribe more deeply than No. 770-7P). In other words, choose the cutting length of this instrument to agree with the length and accessibility of the tooth (Fig. 8-109).

5. With a No. 210-10P stone, placing the tip of this instrument carefully under the tissue, begin subgingival extension, narrowing chamfer slightly and carrying preparation onto the root surface. Only the tissue adjacent to the tooth is touched at this time (Fig. 8-106, *F*).

6. Continue subgingival extension, using same No. 210-10P stone (Fig. 8-110). The functional taper of this diamond stone imparts proper taper to the preparation. Also, this instrument will remove undercuts at this time (Fig. 8-106, *G*).

7. Use diamond point No. 769-9P (Fig. 8-111), which does the most delicate and least amount of reduction, for the final finishing. It establishes the finishing line subgingivally, the "chamferette," rounds the axial line angles, and refines occlusal contours. Follow with No. 769-9F, which is a superfinishing diamond stone, to removal striations, rough areas, and smooth all surfaces (Fig. 8-106, *H*). (See also Fig. 8-112.)

Upon completion of crown preparation a careful rotary curettage of existing pockets is executed. Minker[21] uses the diamond point No. 769-9P for soft tissue curettage when needed. Using an abundant stream of water, the dentist slightly tilts the instrument against the tissue and moves it around the

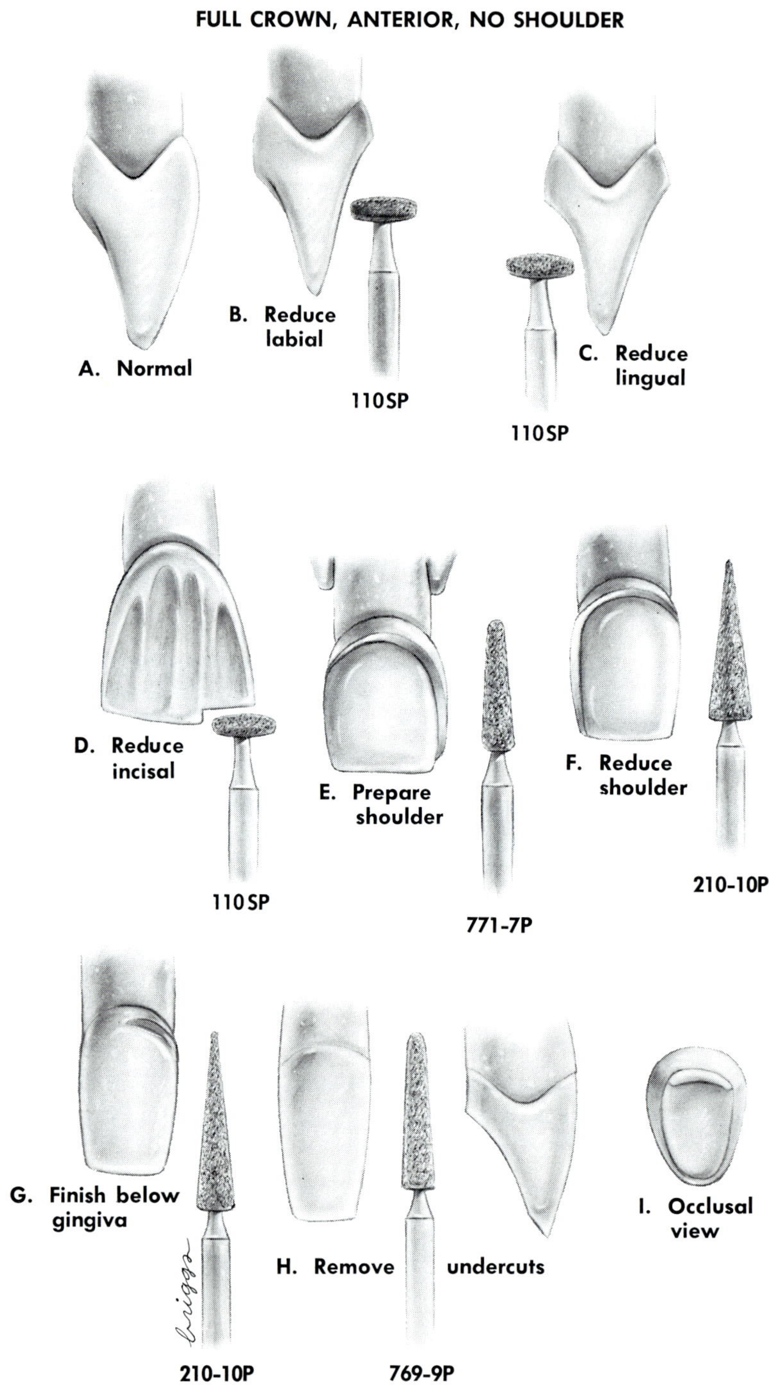

Fig. 8-106. Procedural steps in preparation of anterior tooth with lengthened clinical crown for cast veneer restoration.

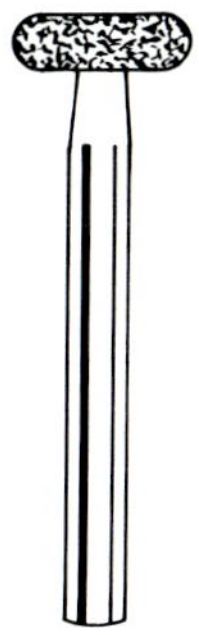

Fig. 8-107. Diamond point No. 110SP.

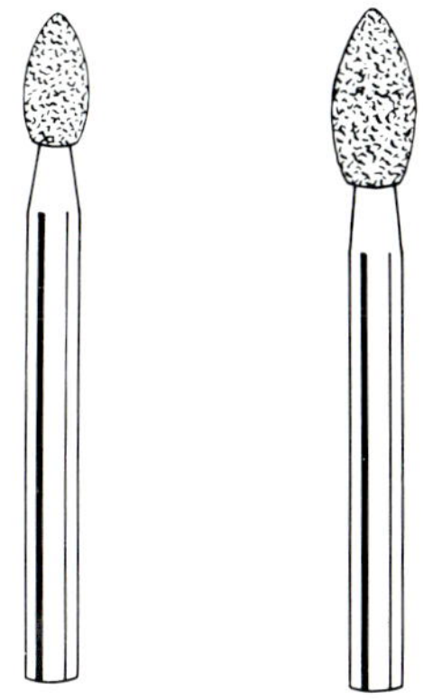

Fig. 8-108. Starlite No. WM-1 or WM-2—special, functionally shaped stone for removal of lingual tooth structure.

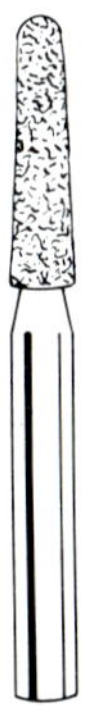

Fig. 8-109. Diamond instrument (Nos. 770-8P and 771-8P or 770-10P and 771-10P) used to create chamfer at gingiva and taper to preparation both facially and lingually.

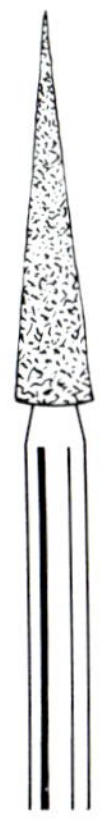

Fig. 8-110. Cutting instrument (No. 210-10P) used for subgingival extension—narrows chamfer slightly and carries preparation onto root surface. Functional taper of this diamond stone imparts proper taper to preparation and removes undercuts.

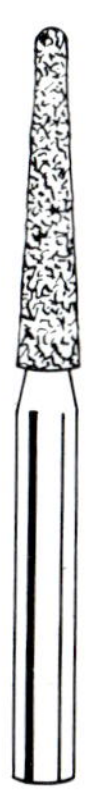

Fig. 8-111. Diamond point No. 769-9P for final finishing of preparation. Rounds axial line angles, establishes finishing line, and refines occlusal contours. Follow this procedure with stone 769-9F (superfinishing diamond stone) to remove striations, rough areas, and smooth all surfaces.

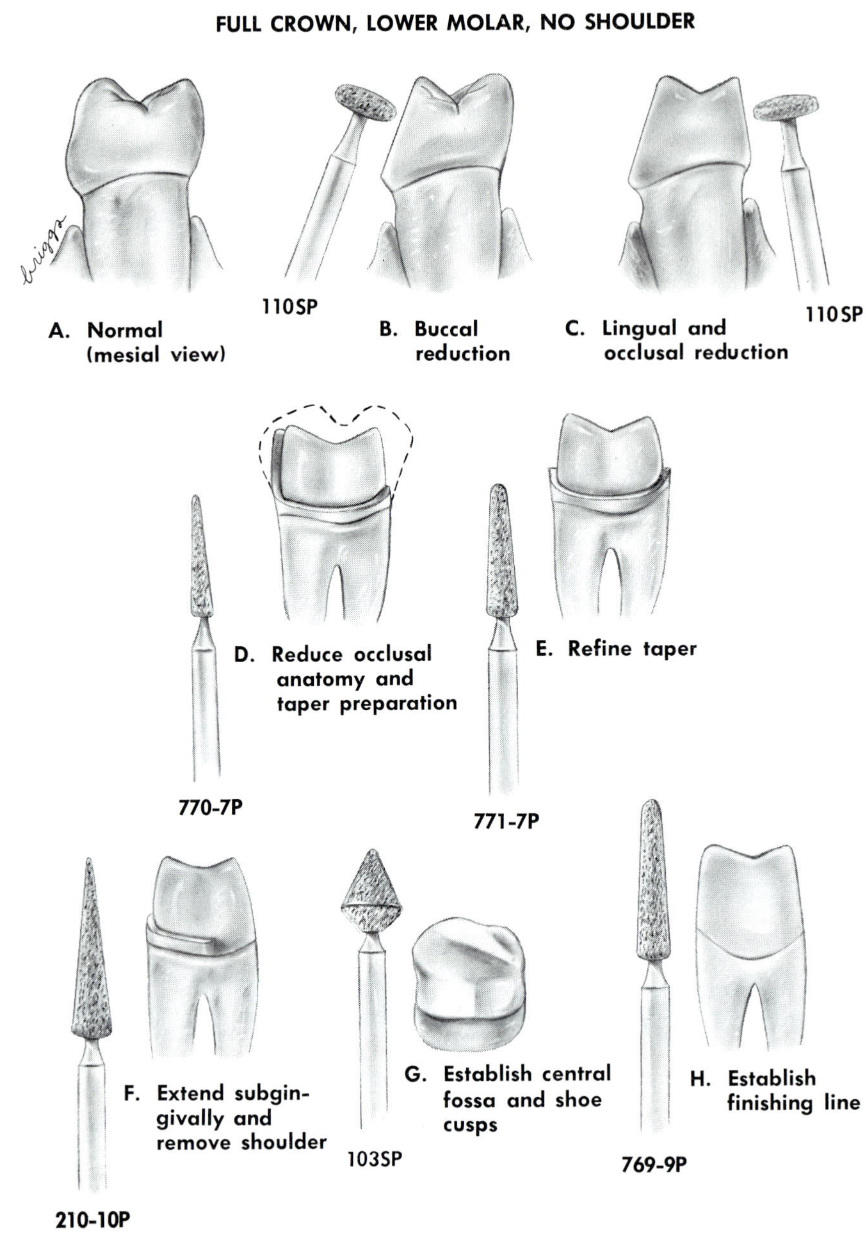

Fig. 8-112. Various steps in preparation of posterior tooth with lengthened clinical crown for cast veneer restoration.

tooth, removing the epithelial lining of the pocket.

Berman[22] describes an excellent method of cutting efficiency in complete coverage preparation (which I have used extensively since November, 1969) that has improved cutting efficiency because of bulk removal of tooth structure to depths controlled by the instrument itself.

Berman[22] emphasizes the following important facts: (1) the torque-speed relationship is fundamental to the evaluation of cutting efficiency of dental instruments, (2) the mechanism that retains the cutting instrument in the contra-angle influences not only the possibility of slippage during work and loss of torque but also concentricity and end-whipping, especially when long shanks are used; effective chucking also reduces the annoyance of vibration, and (3) he suggests that all diamond instruments be examined under magnification (five to ten times) to ascertain their quality before acceptance.

"In complete coverage, the usual method of sur-

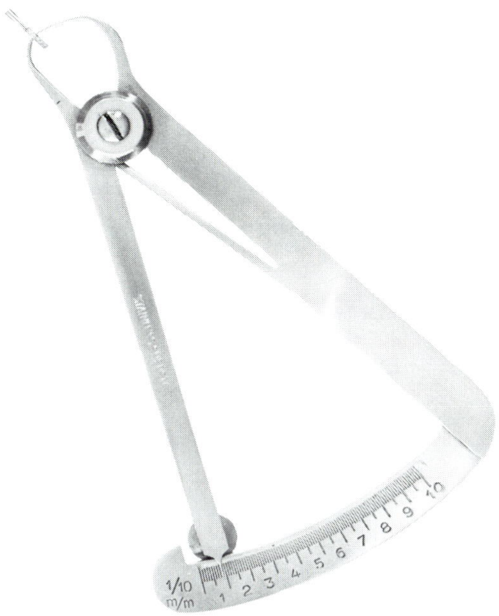

Fig. 8-113. Actual caliper measurement of the diamond stone is important. Note that my caliper measurement shows slightly less than 1 mm., which was originally its measurement before usage. It is now discarded.

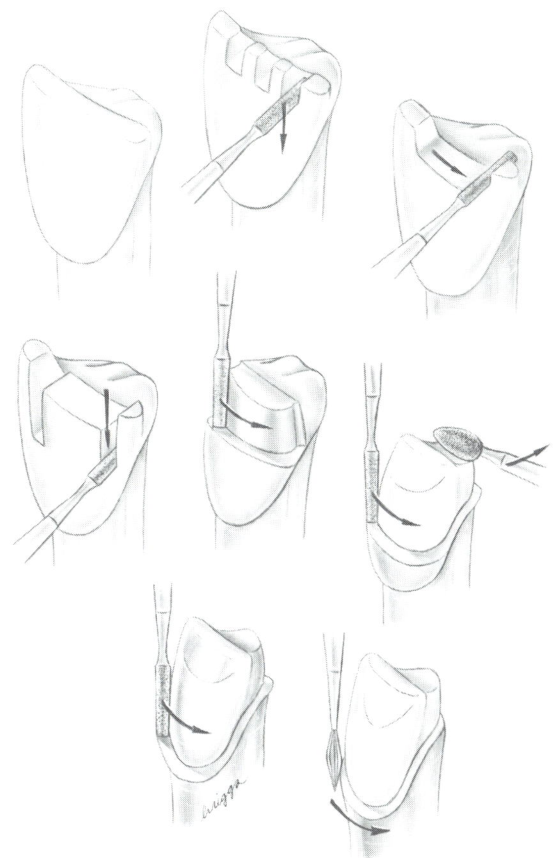

Fig. 8-114. Various steps in the preparation of an anterior tooth using the Berman depth control measurement technique as executed by the author.

face abrasion is by wiping. However, improved cutting efficiency may be achieved by using a method that permits the bulk removal of tooth structure in depth, to depths that are controlled by the dimensions of the instrument. In other words, the slow method of wiping or gradual abrasion is replaced by cutting to controlled depth with calibrated instruments. The selection of the instrument should be based on the actual caliper measurement of the instrument, and this should be related to the specific work intended for the instrument. The selection of rotary tools on the basis of dimension is basic for any toolmaker, diemaker, or technical person who uses rotary force.

"In selecting the armamentarium of cutting instruments, the use of cylindrically shaped diamonds instead of tapering shapes is recommended, because the diameter of a cylindrical shape is constant throughout its entire length. Also, a cylinder stone properly aligned will produce a more retentive straight-walled preparation and conserve tooth structure (less conical in shape and therefore more retentive). The walls of a complete coverage preparation should have minimum convergence. If 1 mm. of tooth structure is to be removed, the cylindrical diamond stone should have the same diameter and this should be determined by actual caliper measurement of the diamond stone. If 1.5 mm. of tooth structure is to be removed, the same is true. The diamond instrument selected should be just long enough to reach the area of work. Extra-length diamond stones should be avoided, if possible, because they are more prone to end-whipping and eccentricity."*

With Berman's method a definite and visible amount of tooth structure is removed at each step, eliminating the need for repetition of previous steps and advancing the work with precision (Figs. 8-113 to 8-115).

SALIENT FACTS

For expediency the teeth should be prepared in quadrants, using the necessary instruments in sequence for efficiency in tooth structure reduction,

---

*From Berman, Martin Henry: Cutting efficiency in complete coverage preparation, J.A.D.A. **79**(5):1160-1167, 1969.

finishing completely with one cutting tool before changing to another.

Remember how the finished preparations should appear when coupled with any necessary, modified relationship to the plane of occlusion, curve of Spee, etc.

Multiple tooth preparations may be accomplished in the following four basic steps: (1) incisal or occlusal reduction, (2) axial reduction, (3) retention and resistance form placement, and (4) correct margin placement.

When it is judged that the teeth have been ade-

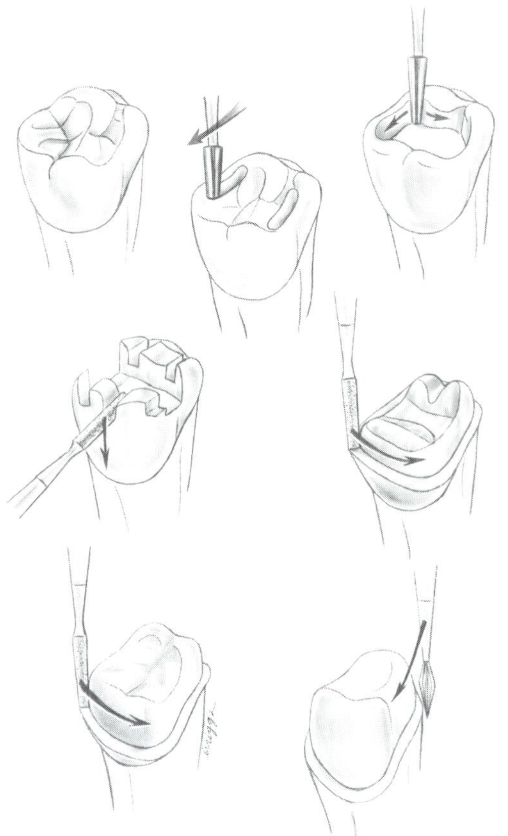

Fig. 8-115. Various steps in the preparation of a posterior tooth using the Berman depth control measurement technique as executed by the author.

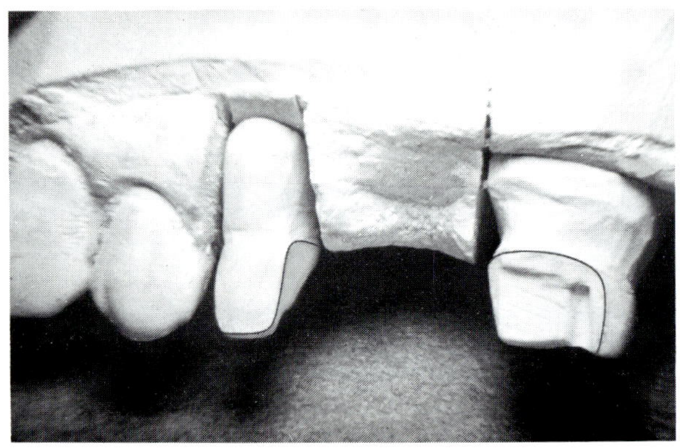

Fig. 8-116. Use of half-crown on an upper second molar.

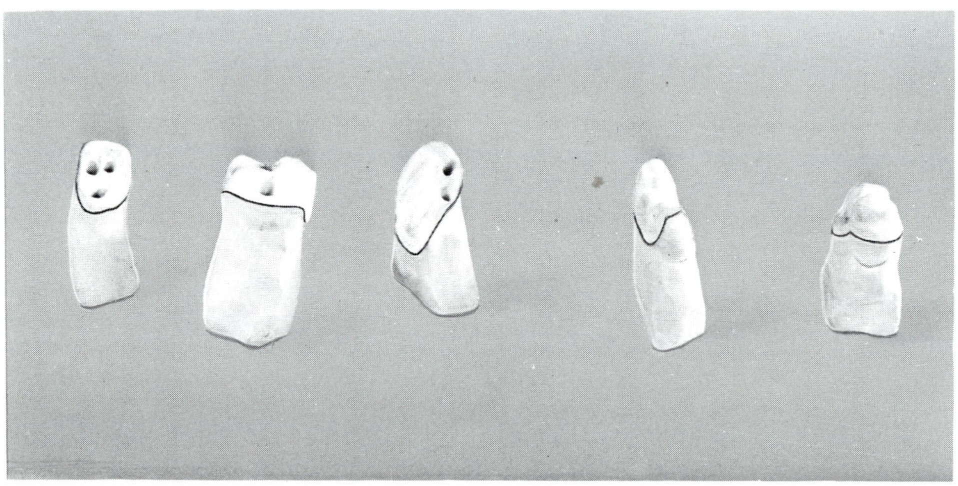

A B C D E

Fig. 8-117. A group of preparations made from previously prepared and badly decayed and broken-down teeth. **A,** Pinledge with concavity on distal surface for establishment of contact area. **B,** Short coronal surface necessitating accessory anchorage. **C,** Treatment of distal-incisal preparation of cuspid with badly broken-down distal surface. **D** and **E,** M.O.D. onlay on upper and lower bicuspids (note treatment of buccal surfaces by pencil outlines).

quately prepared, dry each area with a warm-air syringe, which will also reflect the gingival tissue, and subject it to a critical inspection for (1) length and parallelism of walls, pins, and grooves, (2) absence of undercuts, (3) smoothness of walls and margins, and (4) delineation of marginal finish lines. Also recheck clearance in centric position and eccentric excursions. Binocular loupes should be used during this inspection.

Avoid the use of strong drugs, and make use of liners or bases to protect the pulp from irritating restorative materials.

Cover the teeth immediately following preparation; this allows the pulps to recuperate from the trauma and irritation of the preparation.

Preparations must be made so as to accept a completed restoration and meet the requirements of good form and function. (See Figs. 8-116 to 8-163.)

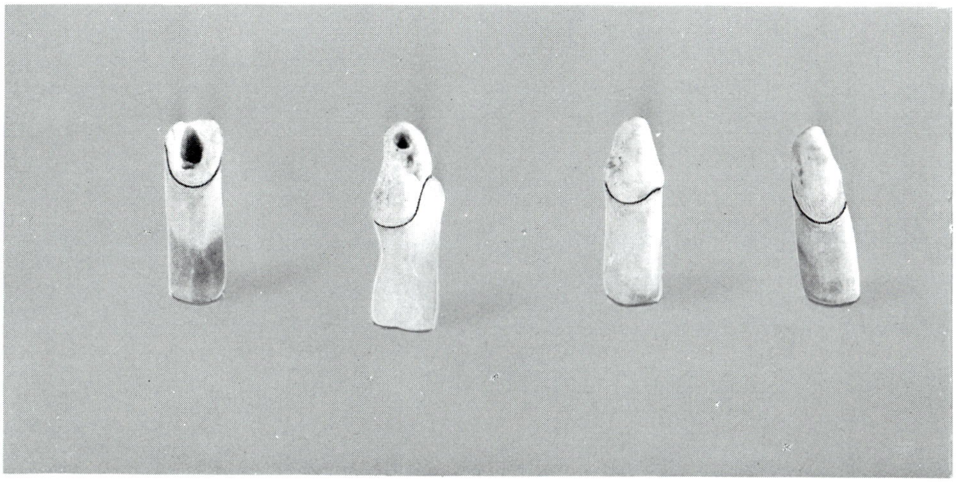

A B C D

Fig. 8-118. Preparations showing treatment of previously prepared and decayed teeth. **A,** Treatment of tooth for post anchorage support. **B,** Use of auxiliary pin in full coverage with fractured lingual wall. **C** and **D,** Treatment of carious and previously prepared teeth for full coverage.

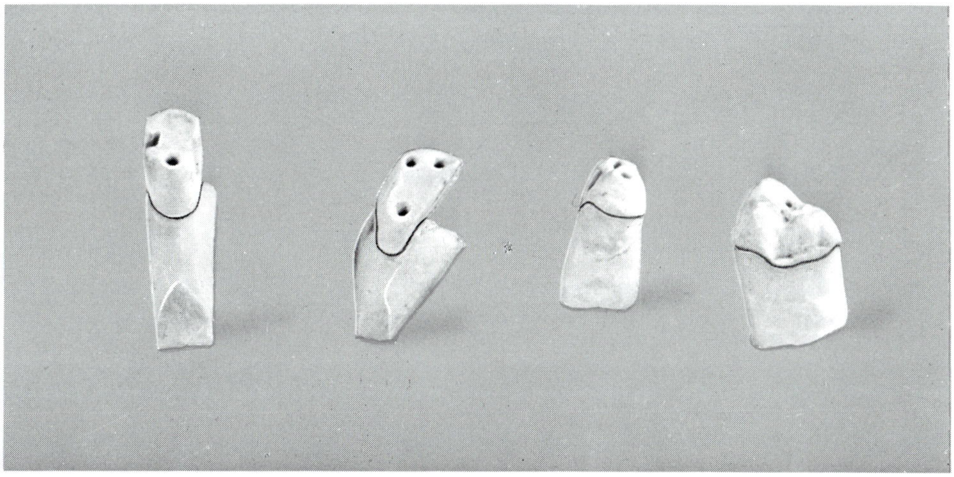

A B C D

Fig. 8-119. Preparations made from previously filled teeth. **A,** Use of lock groove and auxiliary pin in three-quarter crown preparation. **B,** Shallow groove (distal) and pinholes for modified pinledge preparation for restoration of correct contact area. **C** and **D,** Use of groove-pin accessory anchorage in short and broken-down teeth for full coverage.

A B

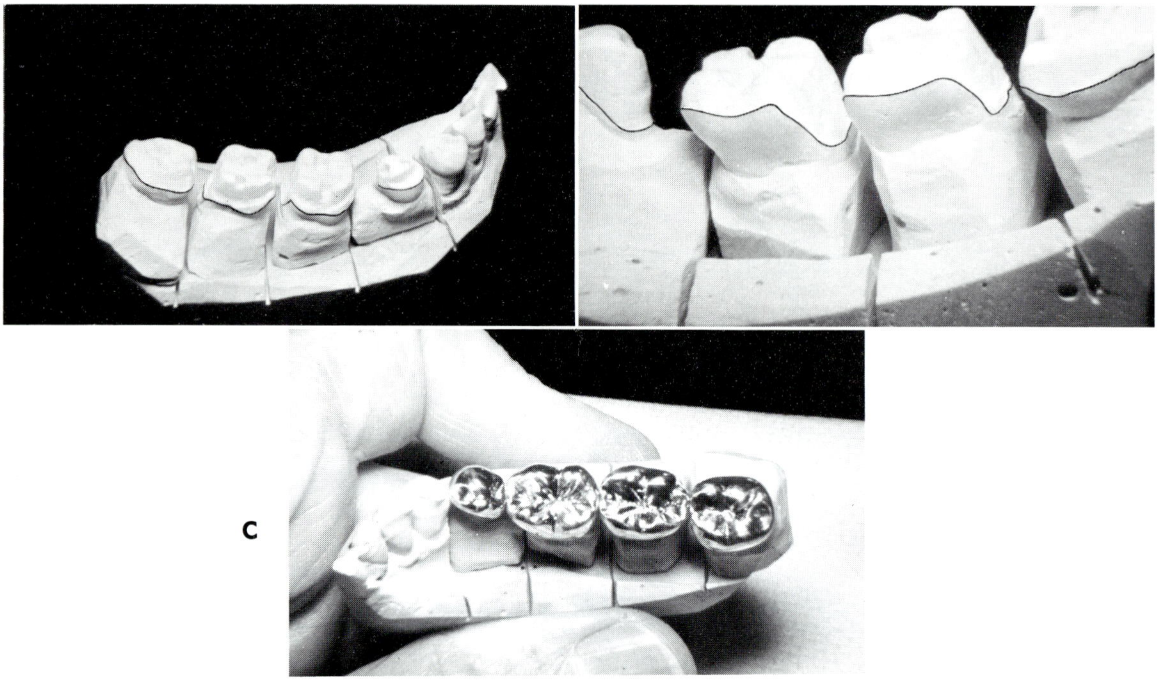

C

Fig. 8-120. Modified onlay preparations. A, Buccal view. B, Lingual view. C, Occlusal view of castings.

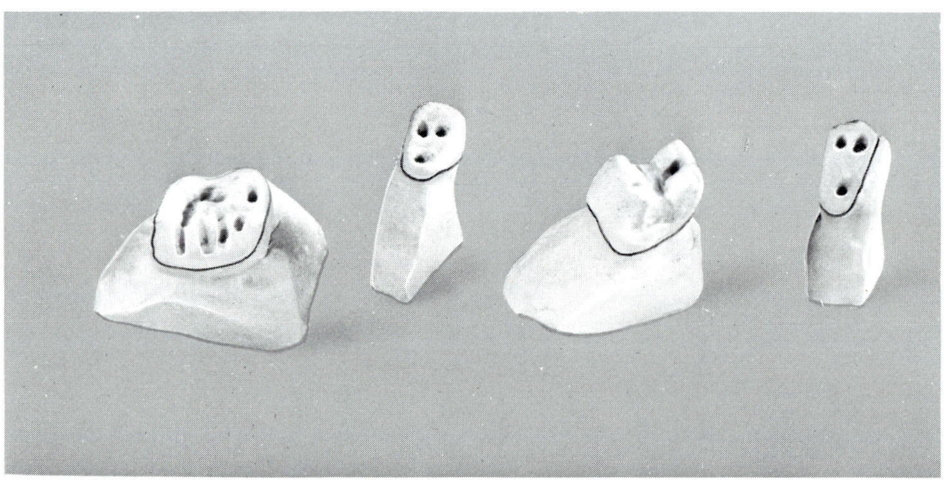

A B C D

Fig. 8-121. Some atypical preparations. A, Use of pin and groove retention for modified onlay. Carious areas sometimes lend themselves to placement of these grooves and pins for added retention without encroachment on pulp. B and D, Pinledge preparations for establishment of correct contact area and for corrective purposes in occlusal reconstruction. C, Three-quarter crown preparation with accessory anchorage.

A B C, D E F

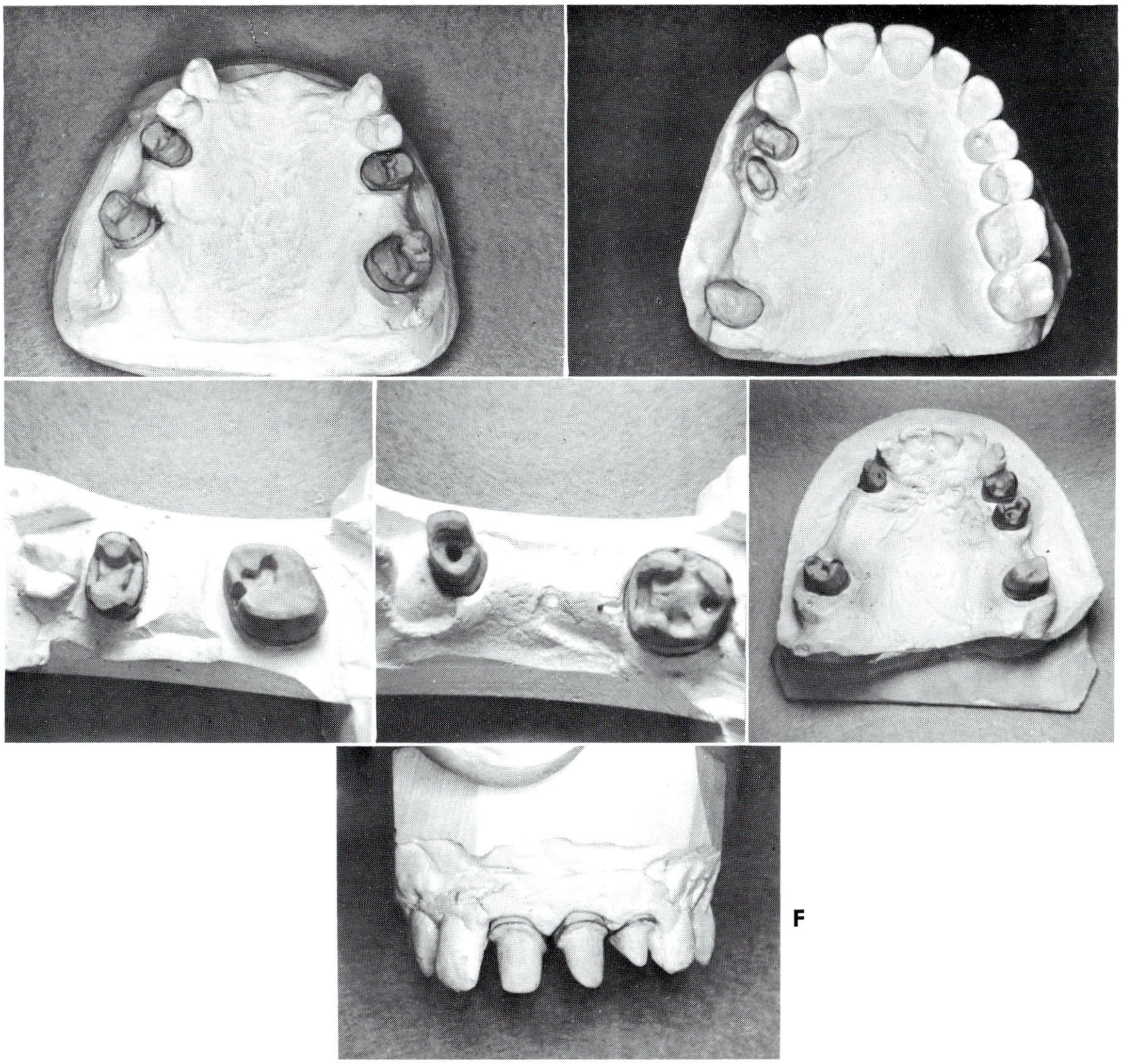

Fig. 8-122. A, Caries and "old" fillings necessitate various modifications in preparation of teeth for three-quarter crown retainer. **B,** Rotated teeth require establishment of enough shoulder for proper coronal form and solder joint to avoid impinging upon interdental papilla. **C** to **E,** Showing treatment of teeth (preparations) requiring onlay, post anchorage, and full coverage. **F,** In preparation of teeth for veneer crowns create ample shoulder facially and interproximally to midline.

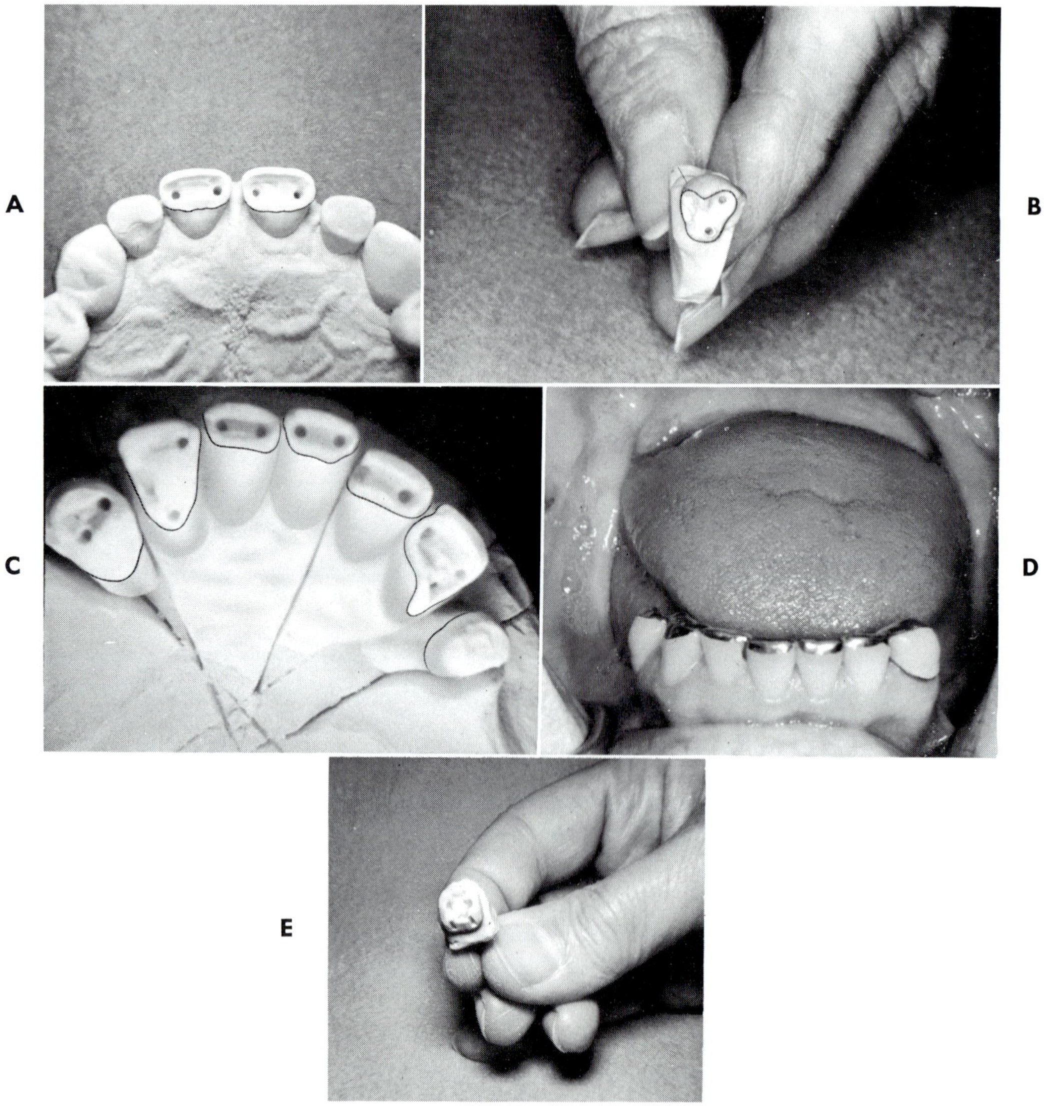

Fig. 8-123. A and **B,** Use of pin retention to gain resistance to displacement and avoid excessive tooth destruction. **C,** Pinlay preparations in lower anterior teeth and full coverage on bicuspids. **D,** Note double deflecting curvature on buccal veneer surfaces of bicuspids for maintenance of gingival health. **E,** Use of mesial lock grooves and occlusal pin anchorage for onlay on lower third molar.

A B C D E F G H

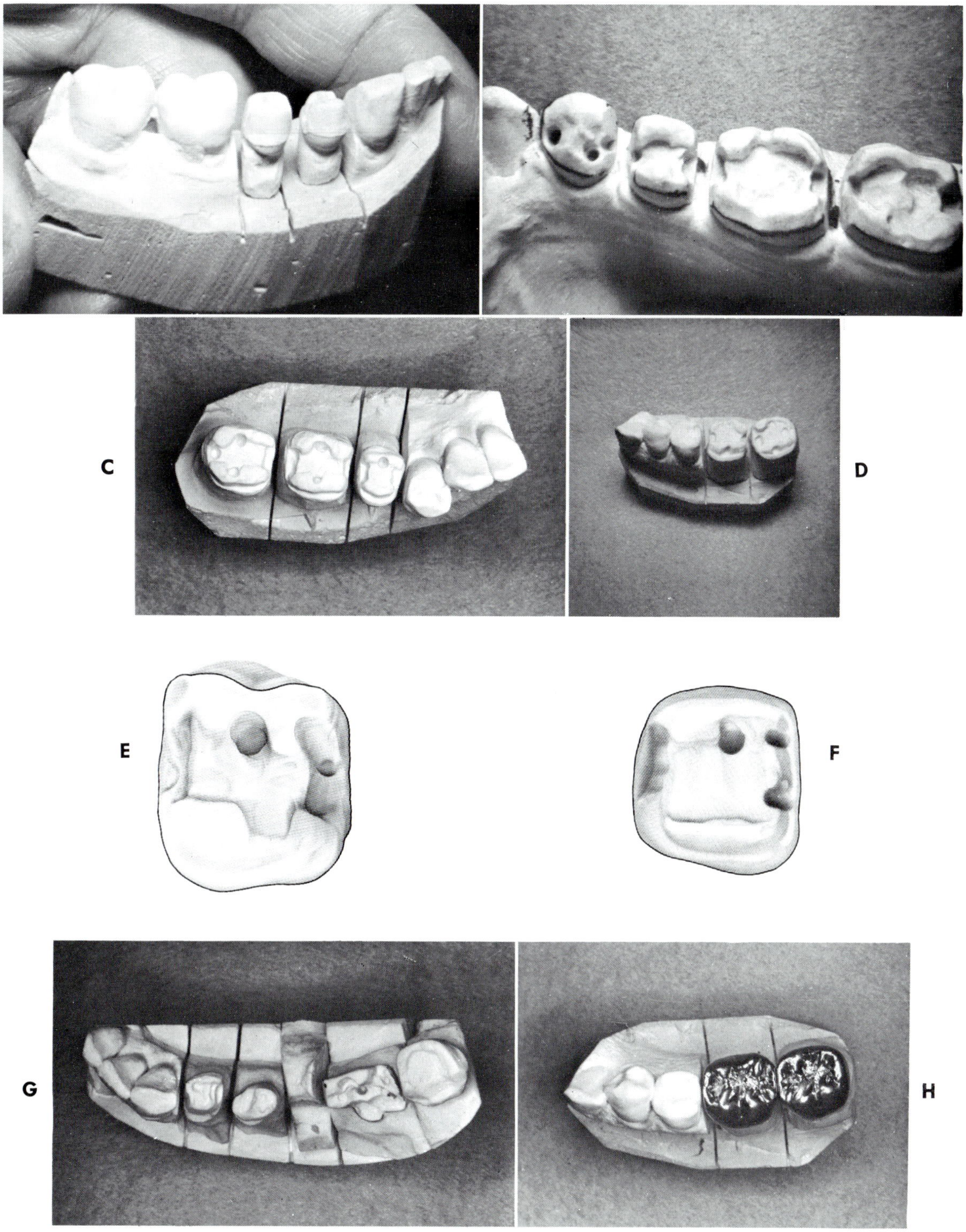

Fig. 8-124. A to **G,** Modified onlay preparations—every effort should be made to avoid need of restoring the cervical third. **H,** Occlusal view of castings for preparations, **D.**

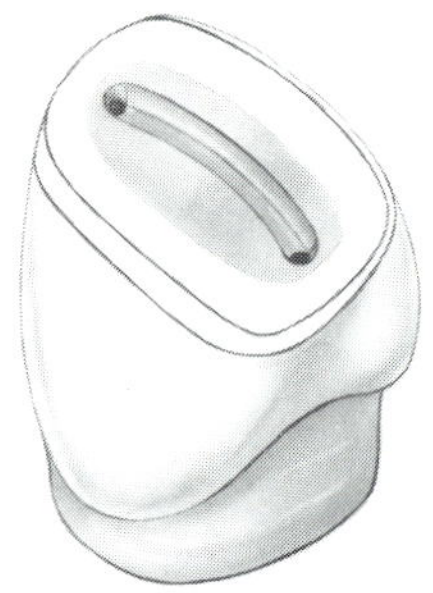

Fig. 8-125. A central incisor depicting attritional wear with a cupping out of the dentin and some chipping. Illustration shows completed preparation with incisal trench and pinholes.

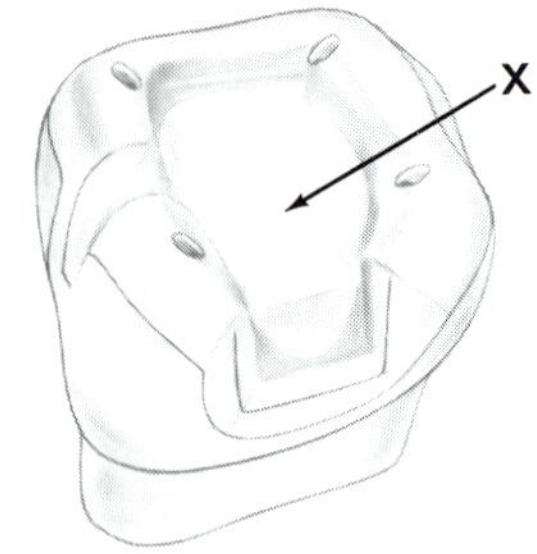

Fig. 8-126. Preparation showing multiple pinhole preparation and a large cement base *(X)*.

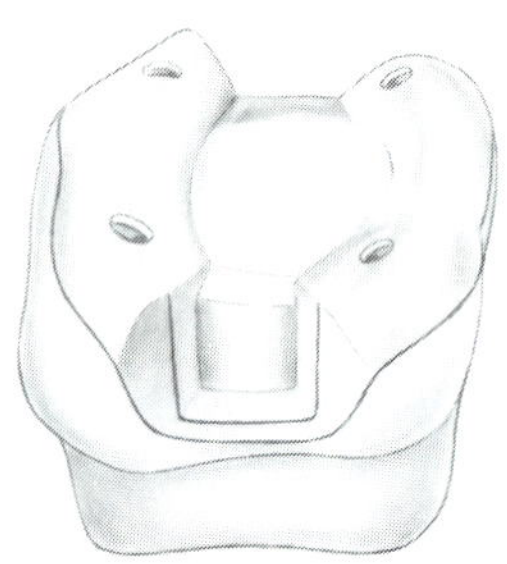

Fig. 8-127. Multiple pinholes cut by a twist drill in M.O.D. preparations for weakened teeth.

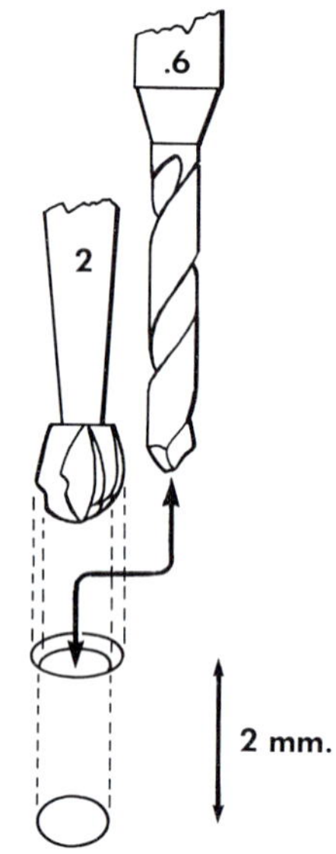

Fig. 8-128. Pinholes are cut by a 0.6 mm. twist drill, and the lip of each hole is beveled by a No. 2 bur. (From Sturdevant, Clifford M., Barton, Roger E., Brauer, John C., and Harrison, M. Lamar: The art and science of operative dentistry, New York, 1968, McGraw-Hill Book Co.)

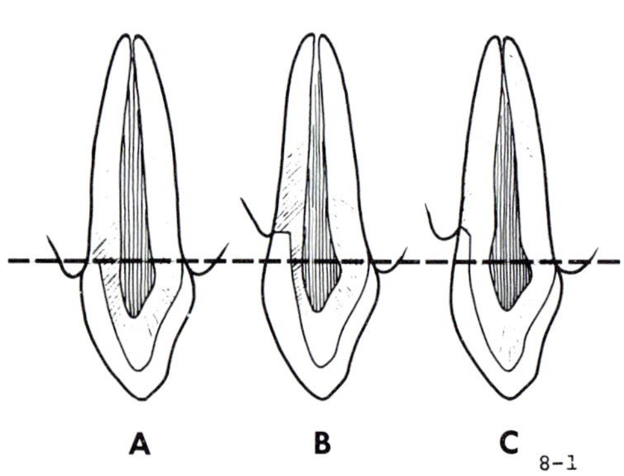

Fig. 8-129. A, Correct shoulder preparation to minimize injury to the pulp. **B,** Incorrect shoulder treatment. When a labiogingival recession is present, the preparation of an orthodox shoulder on the labial aspect of the tooth will remove too much tooth structure for pulpal safety. **C,** Correct treatment of labial recessions. A narrow bevel or chamfer is prepared at the labiogingival area, thus less tooth structure is removed and the health of the pulp is better protected.

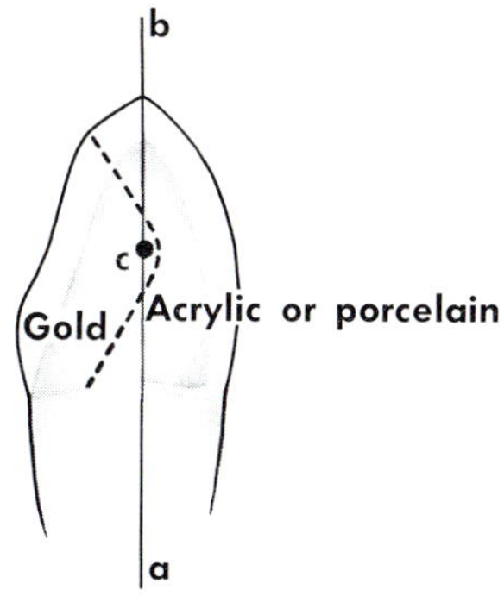

Fig. 8-130. Schematic drawing to illustrate the preparation of the shoulder, carrying it to the lingual of the interproximal area. *a-b,* Line of interproximal relationship to an adjacent tooth. *c,* The approximate contact area. (Courtesy Dr. Louis Alexander Cohn.)

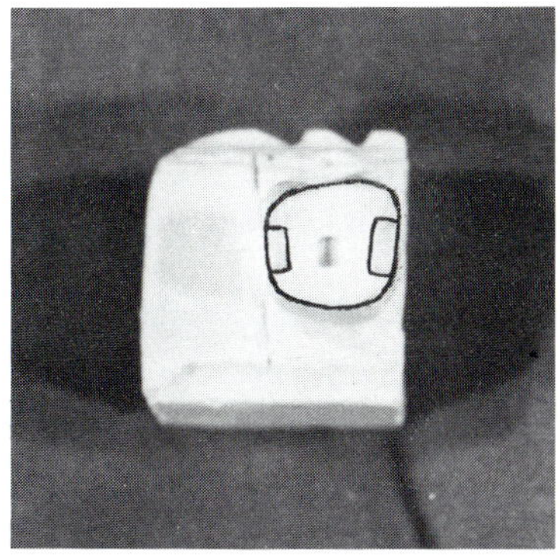

Fig. 8-131. Preparation of a post anchorage cast gold core to receive a modified onlay restoration or a full cast crown.

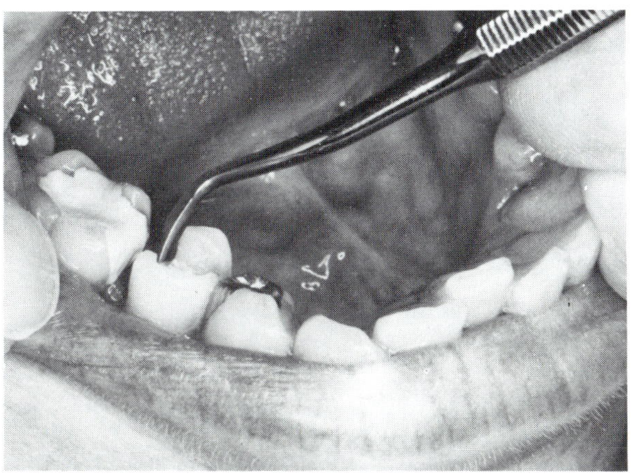

Fig. 8-132. The use of the gingival marginal trimmer in the preparation of inlays, onlays, and partial veneer crowns.

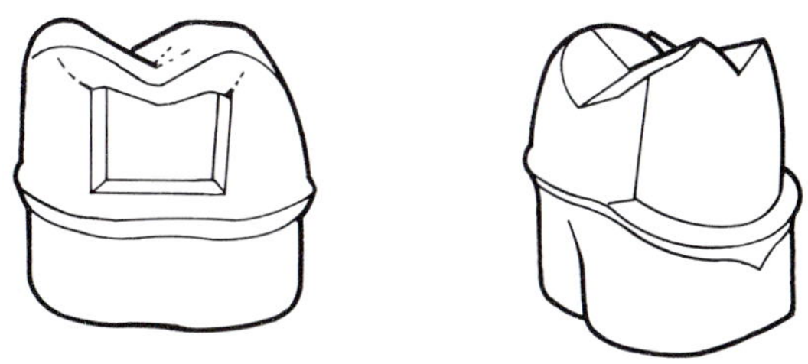

Fig. 8-133. The full crown preparation utilizing interproximal box form for housing dowel or precision attachments and when needed vertical grooves for added retention.

Figs. 8-134 to 8-163. A series of typical and atypical preparations selected from my practice over the past number of years. The cases in which these preparations were used, and their respective restorations, have been inspected and x-rayed periodically over a number of years, and the percentage of successes has been rather high.

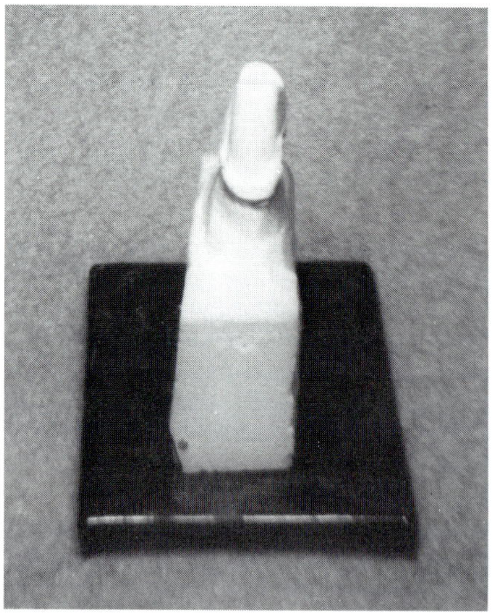

Fig. 8-134

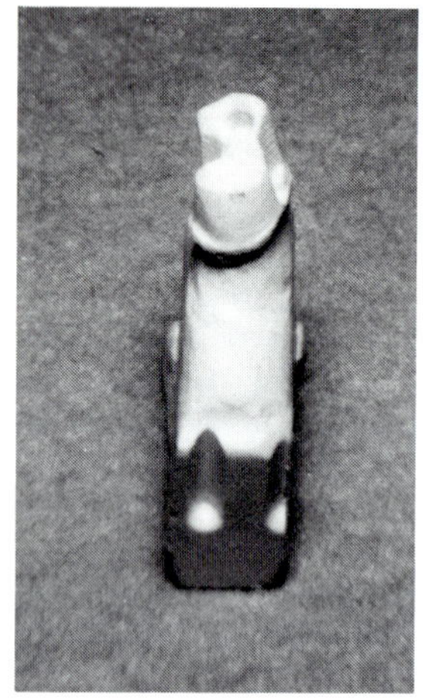

Fig. 8-135

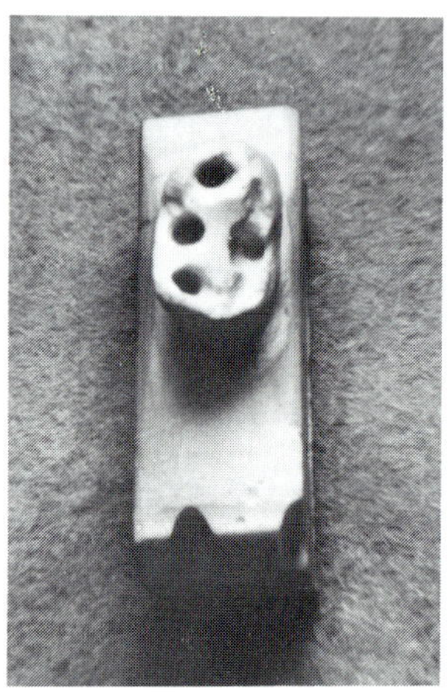

Fig. 8-136

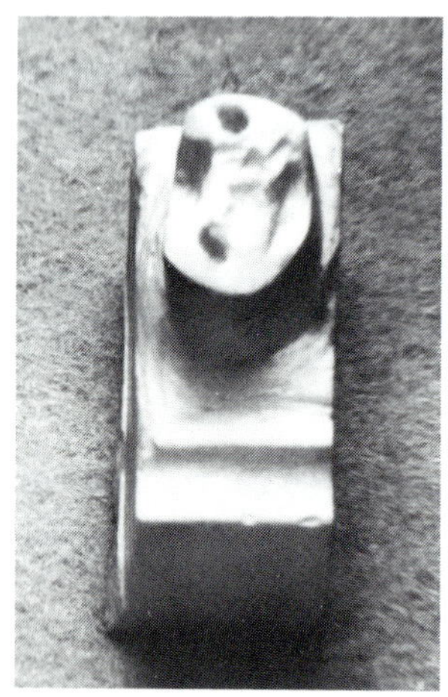

Fig. 8-137

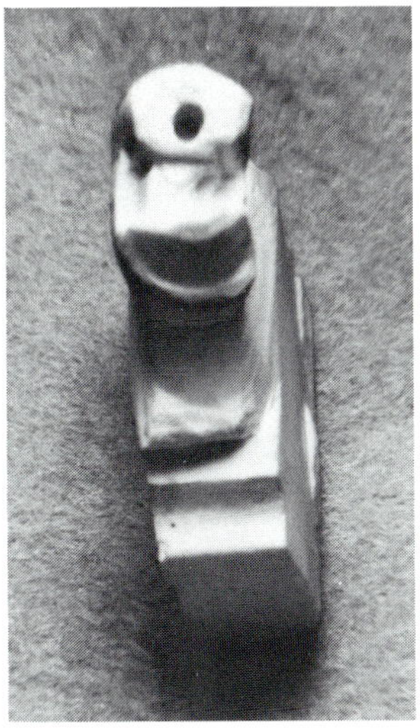

Fig. 8-138

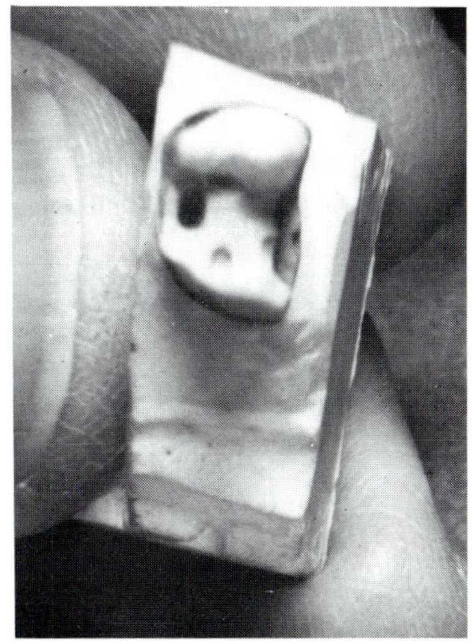

Fig. 8-139

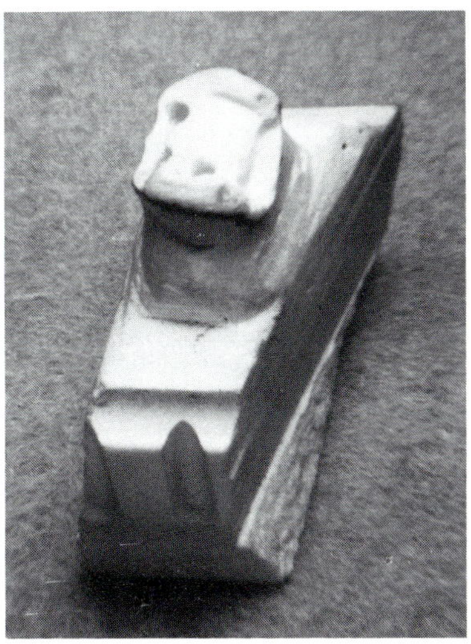

Fig. 8-140

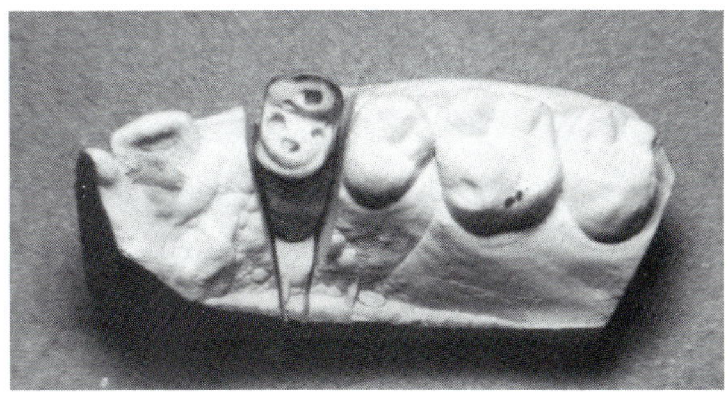

Fig. 8-141

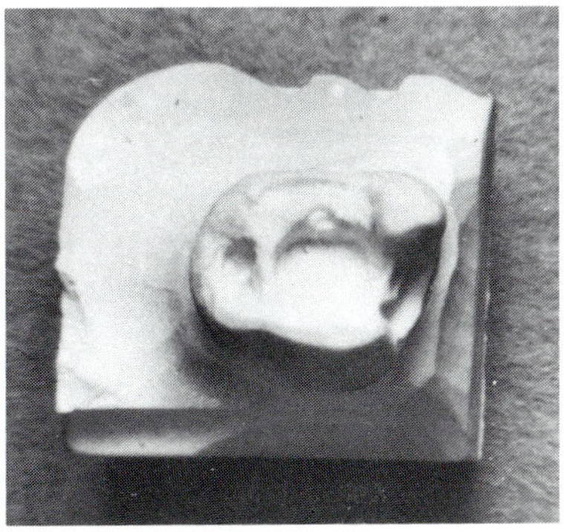

Fig. 8-142

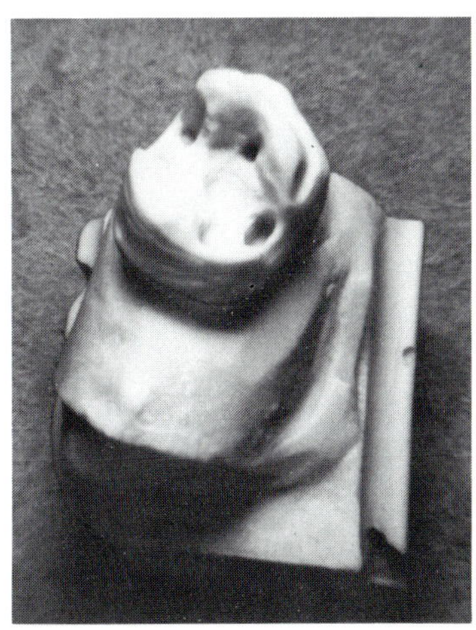

Fig. 8-143

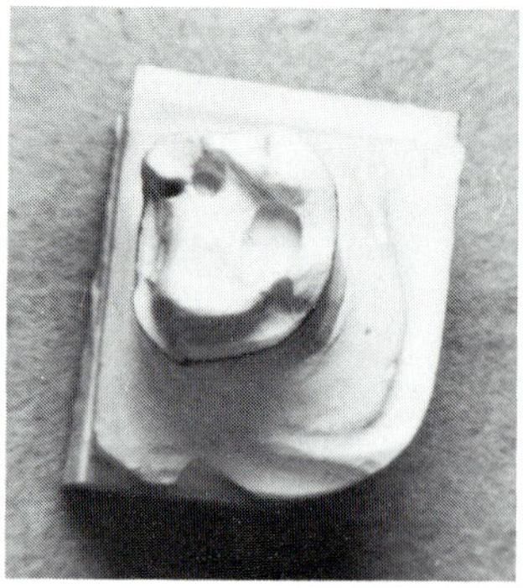

Fig. 8-144

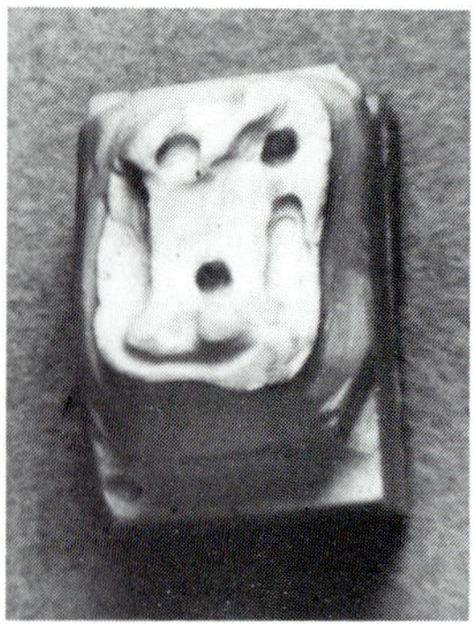

Fig. 8-145

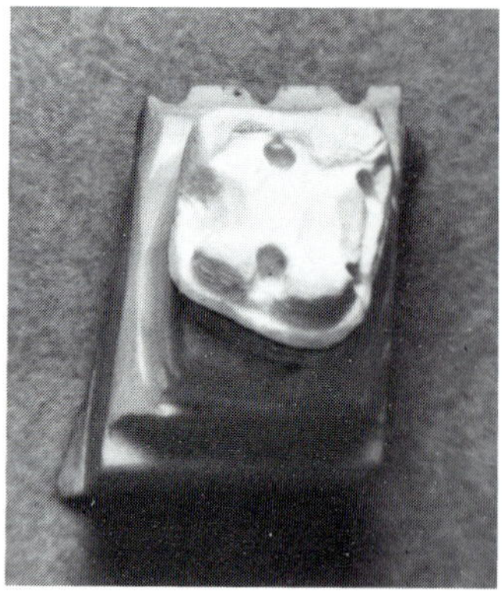

Fig. 8-146

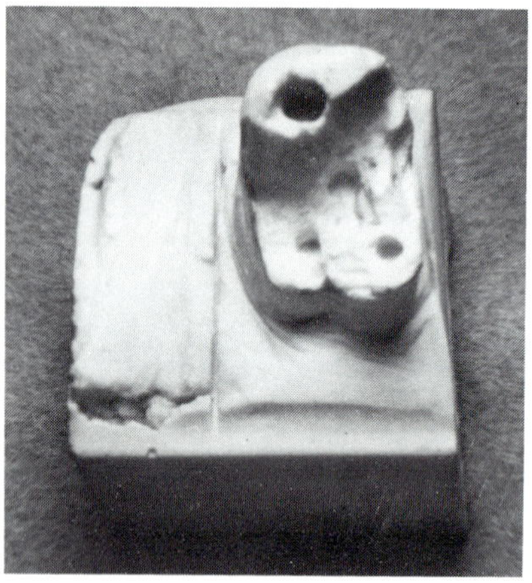

Fig. 8-147

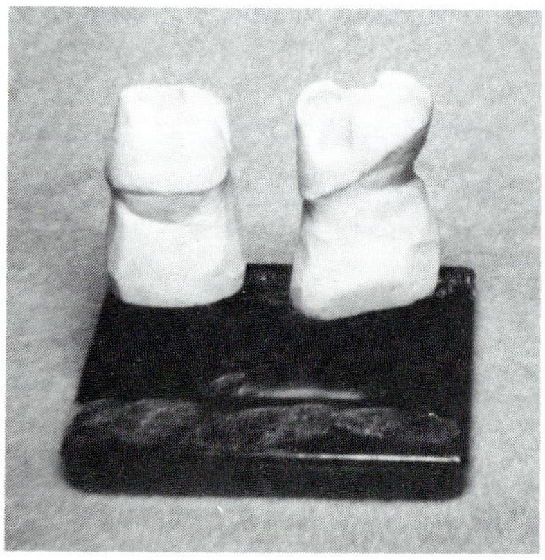

Fig. 8-148

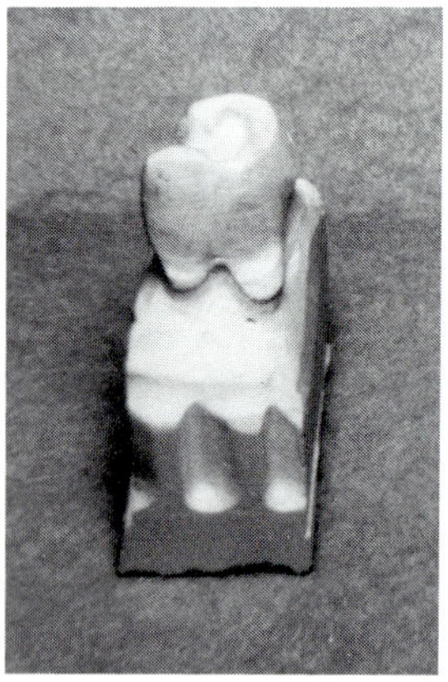

Fig. 8-149

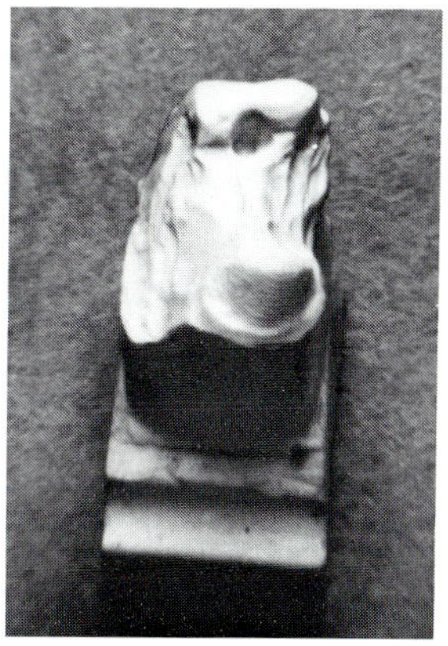

Fig. 8-150

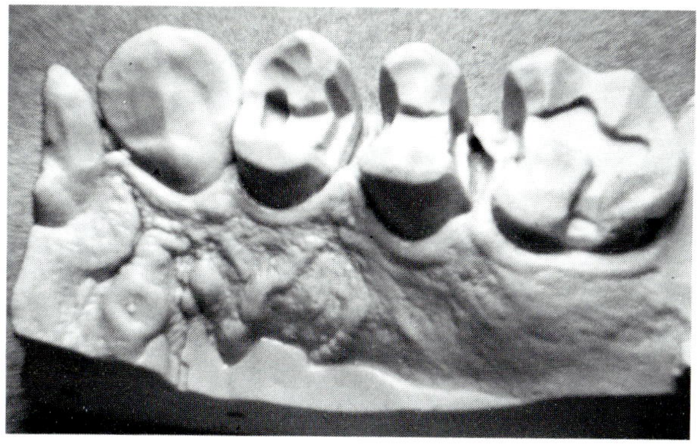

Fig. 8-151

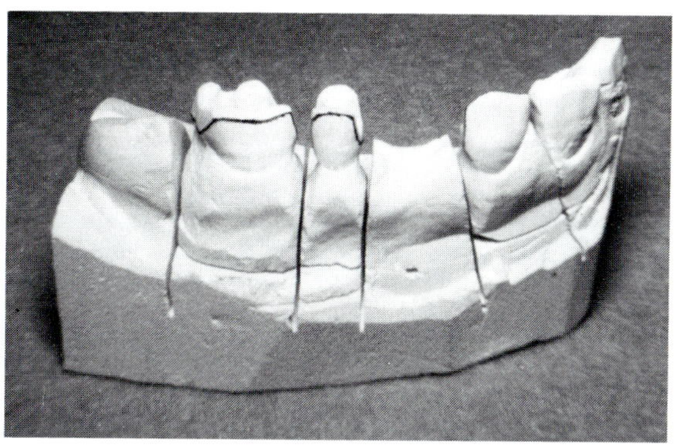

Fig. 8-152

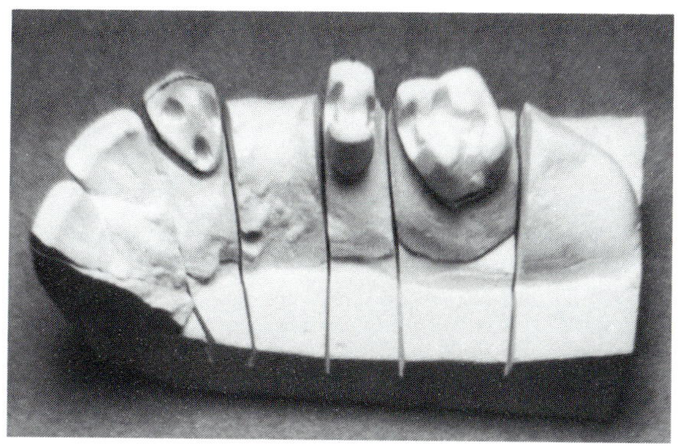

Fig. 8-153

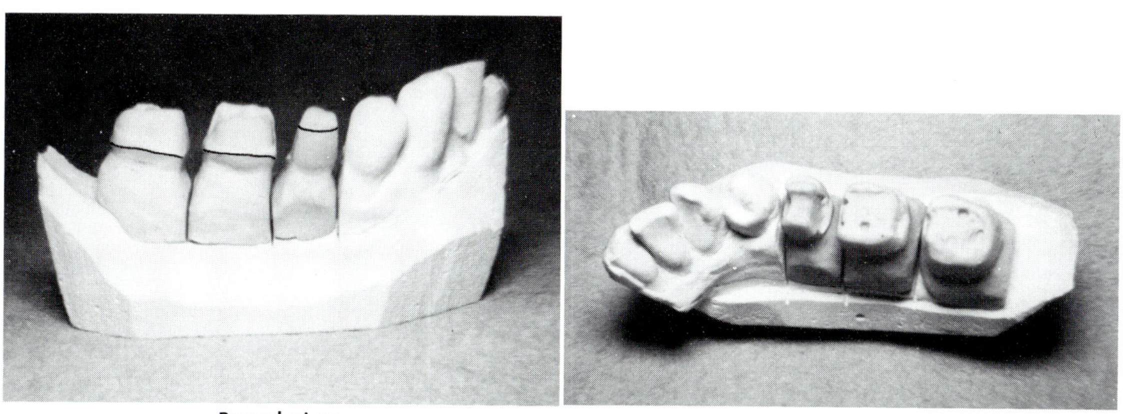

Buccal view

Occlusal view

Fig. 8-154

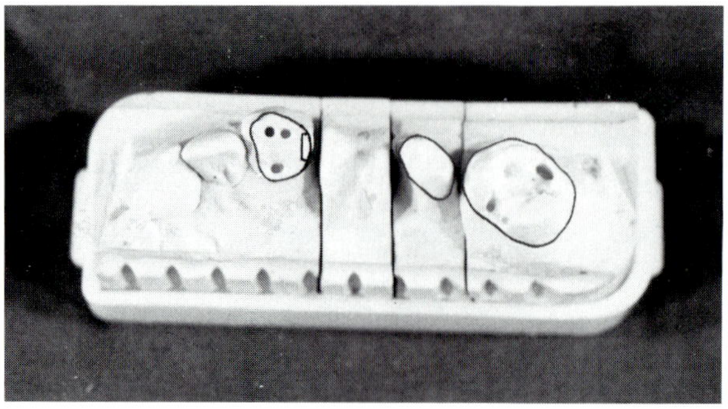

Fig. 8-155

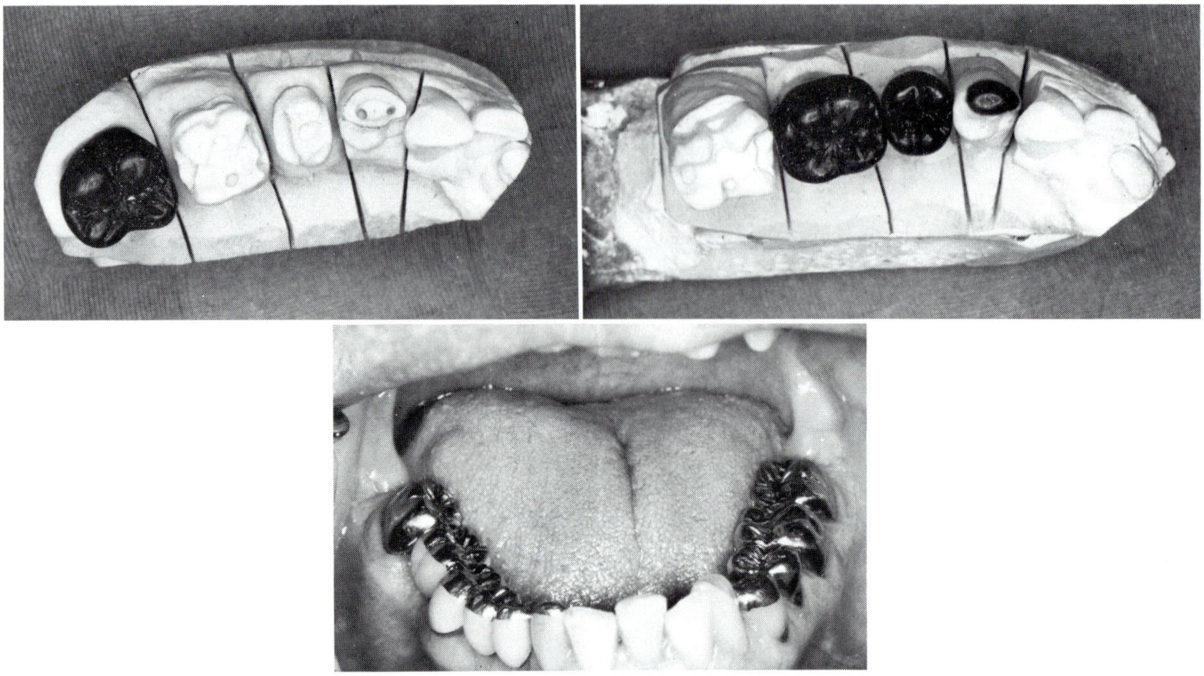

Fig. 8-156

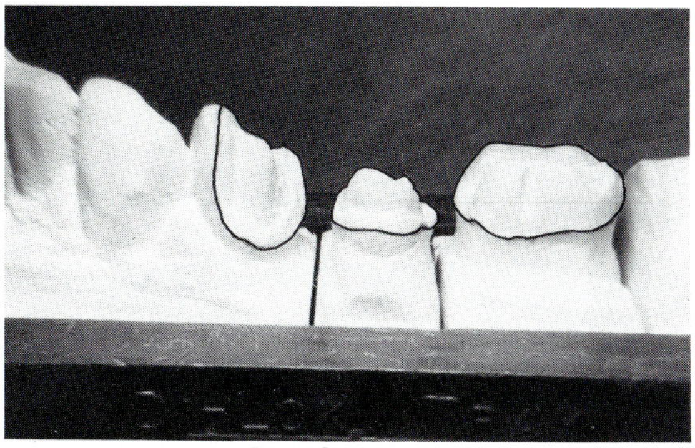

Buccal view

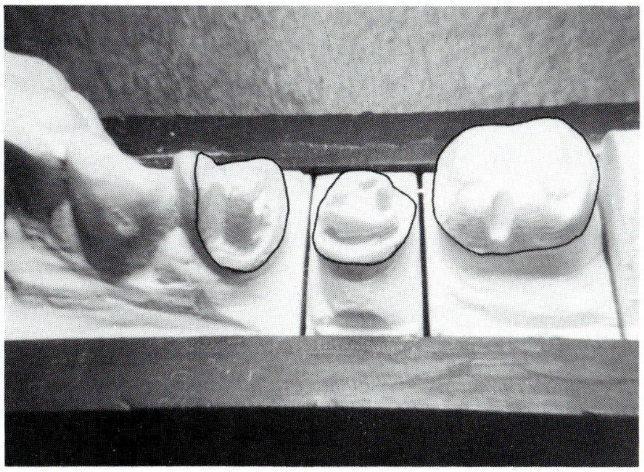

Bucco-occlusal view

Fig. 8-157

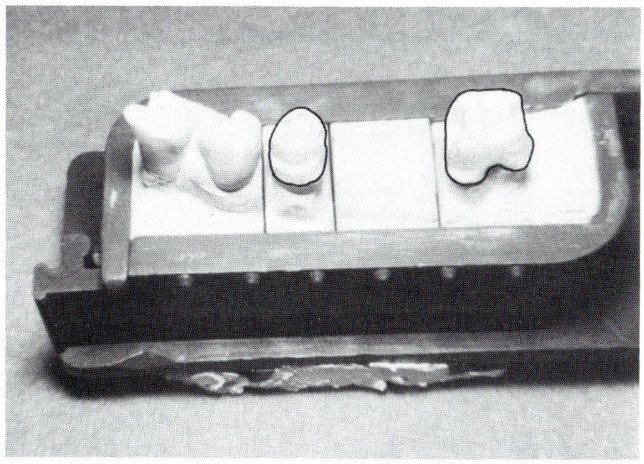

Fig. 8-158

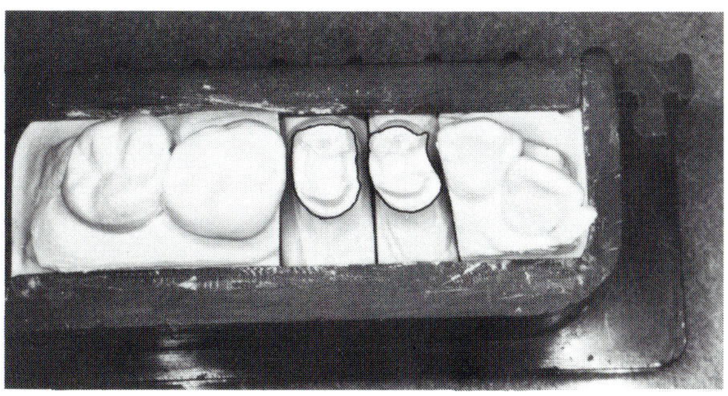

Fig. 8-159

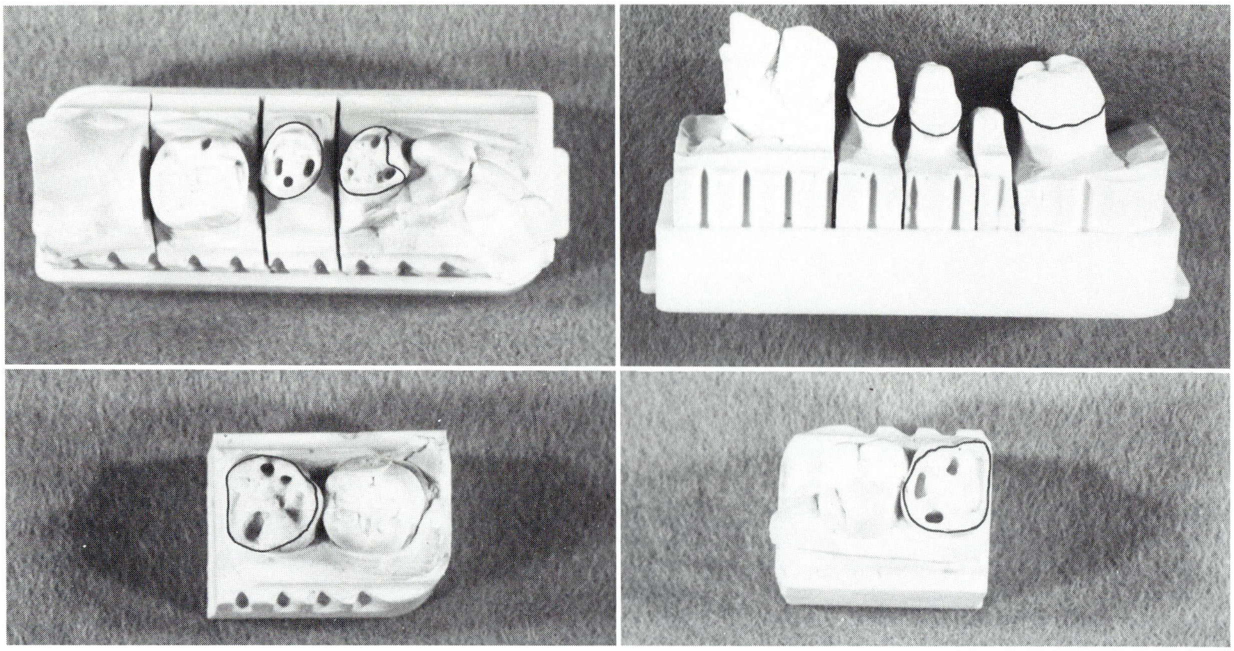

Fig. 8-160

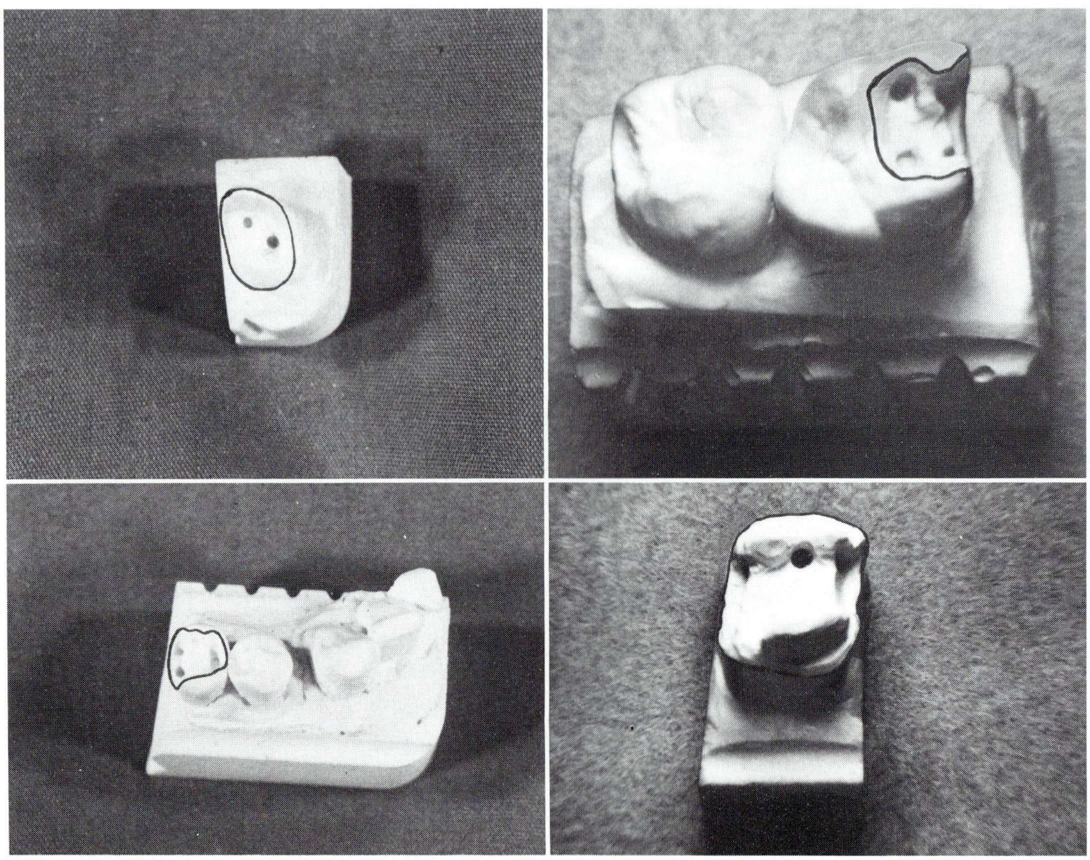

Fig. 8-161

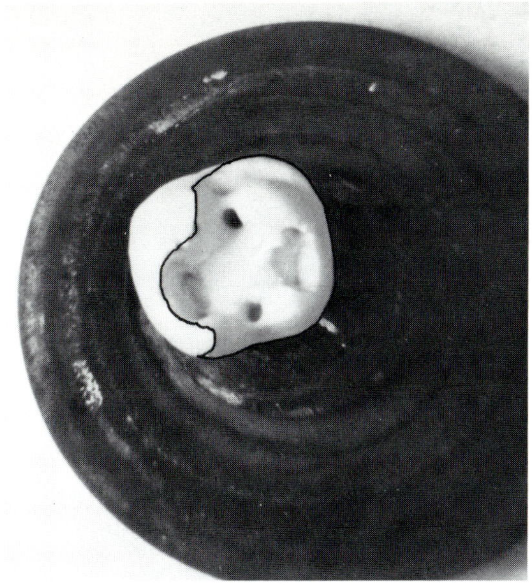

Fig. 8-162

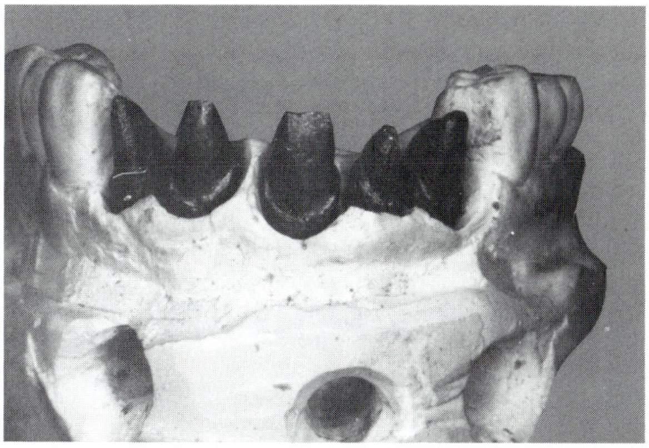

Copper plated dies

Fig. 8-163

REFERENCES

1. Keys, Donald A.: Effect of cavity and pattern design on structure, stress, strain and density of castings, J.A.D.A. **30:**1432-1437, 1943.
2. Amsterdam, Morton: Personal communication and lecture notes.
3. Fox, Lewis: Letters to the editor, Dent. Times **3:**6, 1961.
4. Cantwell, K. R., Alpin, A. W., and Mahler, D. B.: Cavity finish with high-speed handpieces, Dent. Progr. **1**(1):42-46, Oct., 1960.
5. Weiss, Marvin B., Massler, Maury, and Spence, John M.: Operative effects on adult dental pulp, Dent. Progr. **4:**10-19, 1963.
6. Stein, R. Sheldon: Periodontal-prosthetic interrelationships. In Glickman, Irving: Clinical periodontology, Philadelphia, 1964, W. B. Saunders Co., p. 756.
7. Jermyn, Arthur C.: Machine-controlled tooth preparation for inlays and bridgework, Dent. Dig. **68:**454-459, Oct. 1962.
8. Bevelander, G.: Retrogressive changes in dental pulp, J. S. Calif. Dent. Assoc. **28**(4):139, 1960.
9. Simon, Peter: Periapical pulpo-osteosclerosis, Dent. Radiogr. Photogr. **39:**75-82, 1966.
10. Kilpatrick, Harold C.: Work simplication in dental practice, Philadelphia, 1964, W. B. Saunders Co.
11. Anderson, John A.: The selection and use of operator's stools and contour chairs, Dent. Clin. N. Am., pp. 303-318, July, 1965.
12. Arnim, Sumter S.: Conservation of the dental pulp—cavity preparation, J. Prosthet. Dent. **9:**1017-1036, 1959.
13. Craig, Robert G., and others: Experimental stress analysis of dental restorations, J. Prosthet. Dent. **17:**277-302, 1967; **22:**333-353, 1969; **22:**565-577, 1969; **22:**663-670, 1969; **23:**177-186, 1970; **24:**174-180, 1970; **25:**307-316, 1970; J. Dent. Res. **50**(5):1253-1259, 1278-1283, 1971.
14. Danielson, Gerald L.: Stress analysis related to tooth preparation and fixed partial denture design, J. S. Calif. Dent. Assoc. **40:**928-933, 1972.
15. Willey, Robert E.: The preparation of abutments for veneer retainers, J.A.D.A. **53:**141-154, 1956.
16. Vale, W. A.: Abutment preparations for fixed bridgework, Dig. Dent. Sci. **2:**360-363, 1953.
17. Jones, Walter E.: The scientifically designed partial veneer crown, J.A.D.A. **86:**1337-1343, 1973.
18. White, Jesse D.: Personal communication.
19. Rosen, Harry: Operative procedures on mutilated endodontically treated teeth, J. Prosthet. Dent. **11:**973-986, 1961.
20. McEwen, R. A.: Efficient restorative procedures, Dent. Clin. N. Am., pp. 343-354, July, 1965.
21. Minker, Jules S.: Simplified full coverage preparations, Dent. Clin. N. Am., pp. 355-372, July, 1965.
22. Berman, Martin Henry: Cutting efficiency in complete coverage preparation, J.A.D.A. **79:**1160-1167, 1969.

CHAPTER 9

IMPRESSIONS; CASTS AND DIES

IMPRESSION MATERIALS

Several types of impressions are involved in the process of mouth rehabilitation. In this chapter impressions for the dentulous and the semidentulous as well as prepared teeth for the construction of microscopically accurate dies will be discussed.

A consideration of both the irreversible (alginate) and reversible (hydrocolloid) impression materials will be undertaken.

Alginates

PREPARATION OF MATERIAL FOR A FULL CAST

The alginate gels used in the dental alginate impression materials change from the liquid, or sol, phase to the solid, or gel, phase as the result of a chemical reaction. Once gelation is completed the material cannot be reliquefied.

The alginate impression products have good elastic properties and compare well with the agar materials. Important factors to consider in choosing an alginate impression material are flow and elasticity. Ideally, an impression material should have constant flow during manipulation and a clearly marked set point. Also, the rate at which elasticity develops after the material is set is of the utmost importance, because it can affect the accuracy of the result. A number of the alginates improve in elasticity with time; therefore, leave the alginate impression material in the mouth for from 2 to 4 minutes after the end of flow in order to allow maximum elasticity to develop. The importance of this fact certainly must be considered when large undercuts are to be recorded.

Preparation for use requires only the mixing of measured quantities of water and powder (Fig. 9-1). Careful attention must be paid to the details of handling this type of material. The manufacturer's instructions should always be followed. The water-powder ratio and the temperature of the water must be observed. If this is done, the resulting mix will flow well and register fine surface detail accurately. Some manufacturers have this material available in small sealed packets containing a quantity suitable

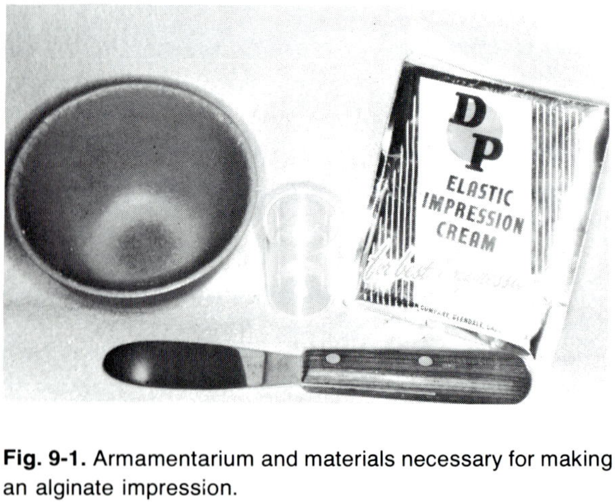

Fig. 9-1. Armamentarium and materials necessary for making an alginate impression.

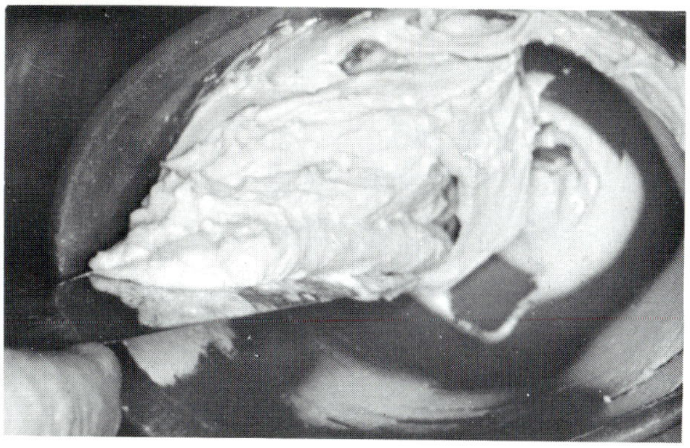

Fig. 9-2. Mix of alginate is made in rubber bowl using spatula with broad and stiff blade. Mixing time is exactly 1 minute.

for one impression and ready for mixing with a measured quantity of water. In most instances this is the best method for greater accuracy.

The use of alginate impression material requires a precise step-by-step procedure that must be followed exactly. If this is done, the impression is accurate, and it is axiomatic that accurate impressions are a prime requisite for forming accurate casts.

The proper proportioning of the powder and water before mixing is critical if consistent results are to be obtained. Changes in the water-powder ratio will alter the consistency and setting times of the mixed material and also the strength and quality of the impression. The manufacturers usually provide suitable containers for proportioning the powder and water by volume, which are sufficiently accurate for clinical use. Distilled water is recommended for use with all alginate mixes, because it will eliminate contamination of the mix with calcium and other minerals often found in tap water.

The mix usually is made in a rubber bowl using a spatula having a broad and stiff blade (Fig. 9-2). The mixing time for the alginate materials is 1 minute (mix the alginate vigorously for exactly 1 minute), and it is most important that this should be timed since undermixing and overmixing are both detrimental to the strength of the set impression. The mix also can be made under vacuum. Vacuum mechanical spatulation of the alginate mix will produce smooth air-free mixes, which is helpful in the avoidance of air entrapment in critical parts of the impression. It requires approximately 15 seconds of mixing with about 28 pounds of vacuum.

The setting time of the alginate products is determined and established by the manufacturer. Variation in the temperature of the mixing water will give some modification and control of setting time. High temperatures speed the set, and low temperatures prolong the setting time. It is not advisable to use water that is cooler than 65° F., nor warmer than 75° F. *The temperature of the water is important. Do not attempt to modify the setting time of a given product to individual needs. Follow the manufacturer's instructions.*

The strength of the alginate type of materials is adequate if they are manipulated correctly. This requires spatulation for the correct time, correct water-powder ratio, and retention in the mouth for the recommended time after loss of surface tackiness. Although the alginate materials have higher compressive strength values than does the agar type and are sufficiently elastic or flexible for all clinical purposes, they tear more readily in thin sections than do the agar hydrocolloids. The alginates recover well following compression or bending.

The impression tray should never be removed prematurely nor left in the mouth too long. It has been shown that if the impression is left in the mouth too long after gelation, a definite distortion results.

PREPARATION OF IMPRESSION TRAY FOR A FULL CAST

In the taking of an accurate alginate impression, one of the important problems encountered is the distortion that is caused by excessive deformation of the material in removing the jelled impression over deep undercuts. The greater the bulk of material and the smaller the percentage of deformation that is required for removal, the less danger of distortion there will be in the finished impression. Therefore, a tray large enough to hold an adequate bulk of material and one that is rim-locked is necessary. In some instances impression trays have to be custom-made because of arch size, tooth positions, etc. (Fig. 9-3). These can be constructed of acrylic or cast aluminum.

It is important also to prevent the overseating of the impression tray and to prevent the tray from showing through the material. A palatal stop is made of wax or modeling compound in the vault of the upper tray to create less bulk of material in this area, and a post dam is placed across the posterior boundary to confine the material (Fig. 9-4).

The rim-locked lower tray, provided it is carefully positioned and as much room lingually as buccally is provided between the teeth and the tray, works well for the fully dentulous mouth. In the semidentulous mouth it usually is necessary to rim the periphery of the tray with a low-heat compound. The compound should not be carried down into the tray

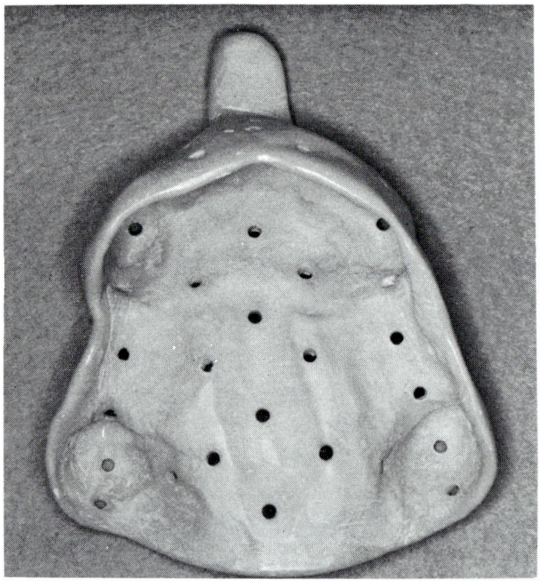

Fig. 9-3. Custom-made acrylic tray to accommodate arch size.

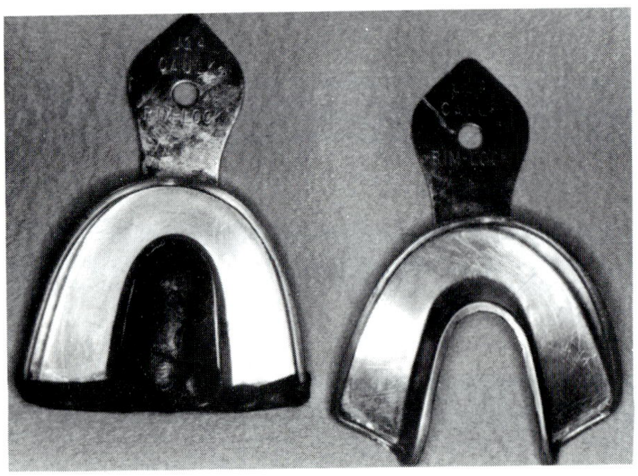

Fig. 9-4. Preparation of tray to confine material and create less bulk of material in vault area.

to fill the area between the tray and the teeth, nor should the compound be placed in any area where there is a possibility of becoming locked into an undercut.

All these precautions prevent the overseating of the tray and the showing of the tray through the material and make proper confinement of the impression compound possible.

TECHNIQUE FOR A FULL CAST

The trays, having now been prepared for impression taking, are again tested by fitting them in the mouth. The impression material and other necessary equipment are checked for completeness and readiness.

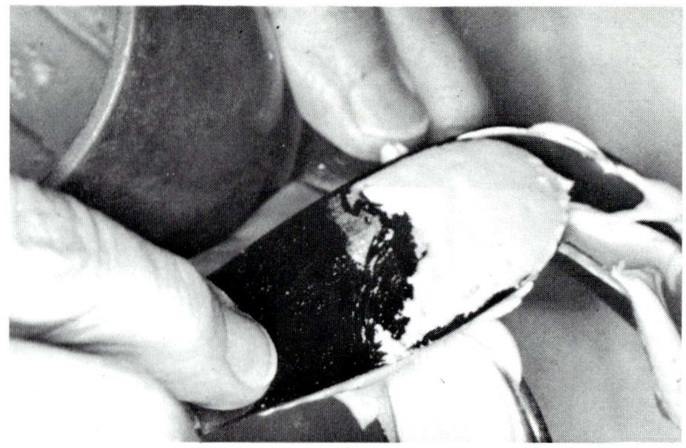

Fig. 9-5. Load tray carefully, avoiding trapping of air.

At this time, it is appropriate to call attention to an important fact that I learned from Dr. Kenneth D. Rudd. It is very important that the alginate impression material does not adhere to tooth surfaces upon removal of the impression, because if it adheres to critical parts the impression is useless. Therefore, before taking the impression polish teeth with a prophylactic paste to remove food plaques. Rudd[1] suggests a paste made of 50 gm. of silicone compound (Dow Corning Silicone 555*), 50 drops of oil of peppermint (U.S.P.), 20 drops of liquid petrolatum, and 40 gm. of flour of pumice. Then the excess paste is flushed away with a strong stream of air and water.

After the teeth have been coated with silicone, be sure that the teeth and soft tissues are relatively free of saliva—isolate arch with gauze packs until ready to insert filled tray. A nondrying silicone material applied to tooth surfaces helps to assure the release of impression material intact.

The proper proportions of water and powder are placed in the bowl, and the material is mixed well for 1 minute. Then the tray is loaded carefully, avoiding the trapping of air (Fig. 9-5). The occlusal surfaces of the teeth are dried with a gentle blast of air, and a small amount of the alginate material is picked up with the finger and wiped over the occlusal surfaces of the teeth to prevent air from being trapped in the sulci and grooves (Fig. 9-6). In the placement of some of the mix on the occlusal surfaces with the fingertips, do not rub it on, since it will remove the silicone coating. Also place some of the mix from the bowl along the borders, the heels, and the palate.

*Dow Chemical Co., Midland, Mich.

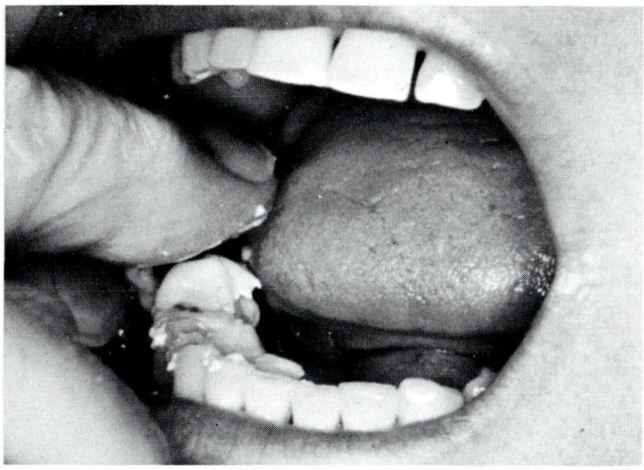

Fig. 9-6. After drying occlusal surfaces of teeth with gentle blast of air, wipe small amount of the alginate material over these surfaces, thereby preventing air from being trapped in sulci and grooves.

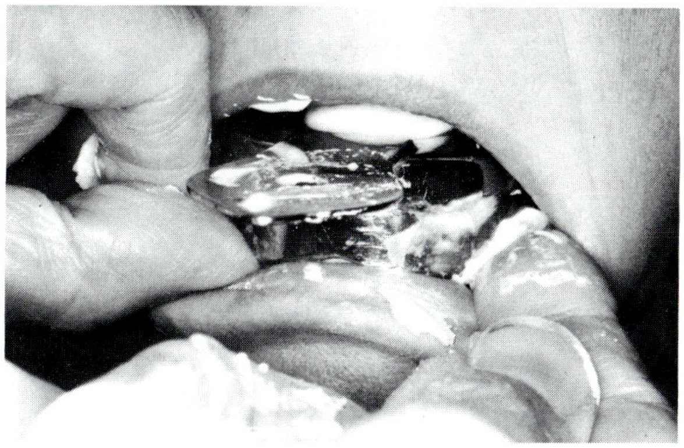

Fig. 9-7. In tray removal never grasp handle of tray and pull. Place finger on the periphery of the tray on each side in region of premolars and remove with rapid, vertical pull.

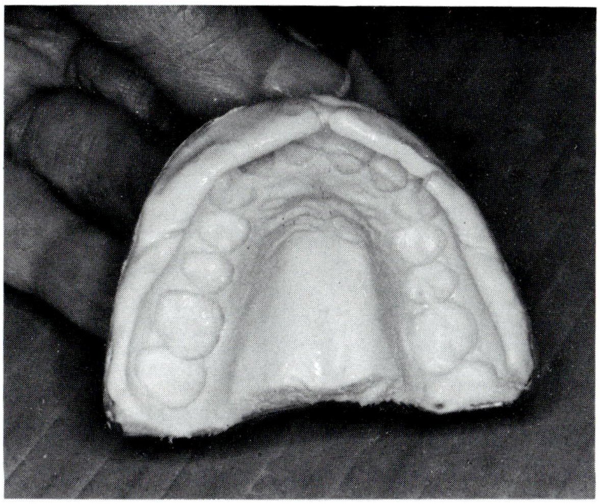

Fig. 9-8. Completed upper impression.

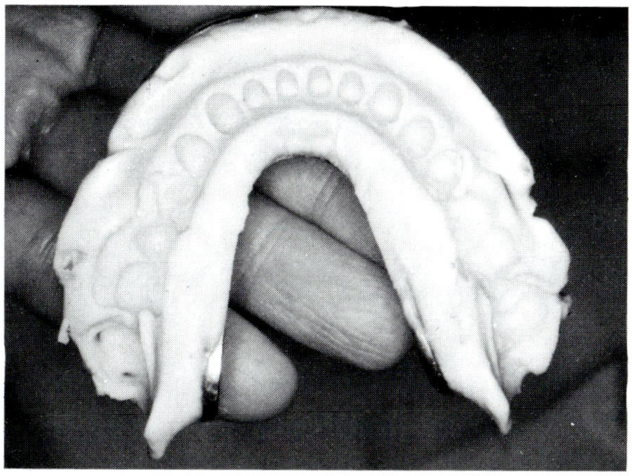

Fig. 9-9. Completed lower impression.

Then the loaded tray is carried carefully to position and held passively and steadily for 3 minutes until gelation has taken place. In other words, seat the tray by gently jiggling it into place or with a slight rocking motion. Be sure not to force the tray into contact with the teeth, and by all means avoid moving the tray until after complete gelation. By holding the tray passively and steadily it is impossible to apply pressure to the tray while the alginate material is setting. If pressure is applied the impression will set under strain, and on removal of the tray from the mouth under these conditions, the strains will be released, resulting in a distorted impression and an inaccurate cast.

In removing the impression do not take hold of the handle and pull, but grasp the periphery of the tray on each side in the region of the premolars and remove with a quick, straight, vertical pull (Fig. 9-7). Never twist, rock, or slowly remove an impression tray—it will cause distortion. (See Figs. 9-8 and 9-9.)

With the modern alginates control solutions are not necessary. The impression should be poured immediately, and, if for some reason it must be left for 5 or 10 minutes before pouring, it is best stored in a humidor or wrapped in a wet towel.

Since the alginates lose water to the air on standing, they shrink, and impressions left on the bench

Figs. 9-10 to 9-14. Correct method of pouring stone into impression to make good cast.

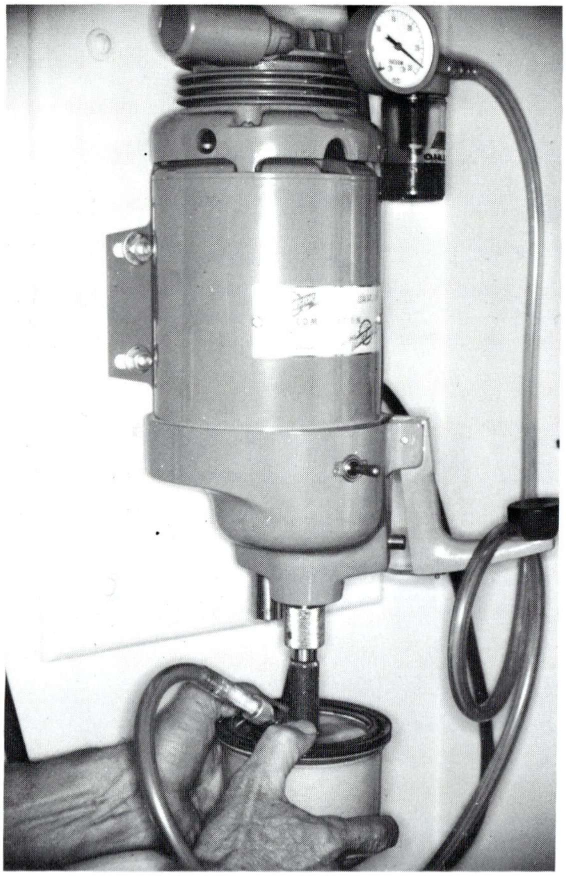

Fig. 9-10. Proper water-powder ratio and mechanical mixing.

for as short a time as 30 minutes may become inaccurate. If the impression is then placed in water, it will absorb moisture, but it does not return to its previous contours exactly—a similar phenomenon to that observed with the agar hydrocolloids.

Also, if the impression is left uncovered on the bench for a period of time, the alginate will lose moisture to the air and subsequently may absorb moisture from the surface of the stone during setting, with a detrimental effect on the surface quality of the cast.

If maximum accuracy is to be derived from the use of elastic impression materials, be sure and pour impressions very soon after their removal, and in the office of the dentist. Even the most stable materials show considerable dimensional change in 1 hour. The greater the time lapse between the taking and pouring of the impression, the greater will be the inaccuracy.

The impression is rinsed well in cold water to remove saliva, and then all free water is eliminated before pouring the cast. If free water is left on the surface, it tends to accumulate in the deeper parts of the impression and to dilute the stone. Such areas on the cast are chalky and friable. In other words, the impression should not be completely dry. Although it should remain shiny, it should have no visible liquid film droplets at the time the stone mix is poured. Do not box an alginate impression or even fill in the tongue space in the mandibular tray, because distortion will result.

If ropy saliva is encountered, then a thin wash of

A

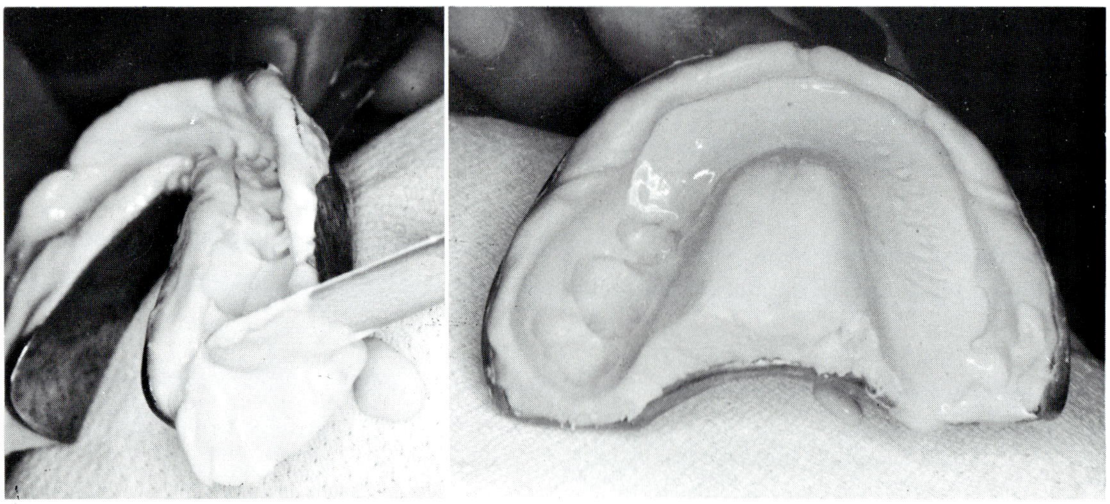

B

Fig. 9-11. Gently vibrate impression material into impression to eliminate air bubbles, pouring stone at one end of impression and flowing it around to the other end. **A,** Pouring lower impression. **B,** Pouring upper impression.

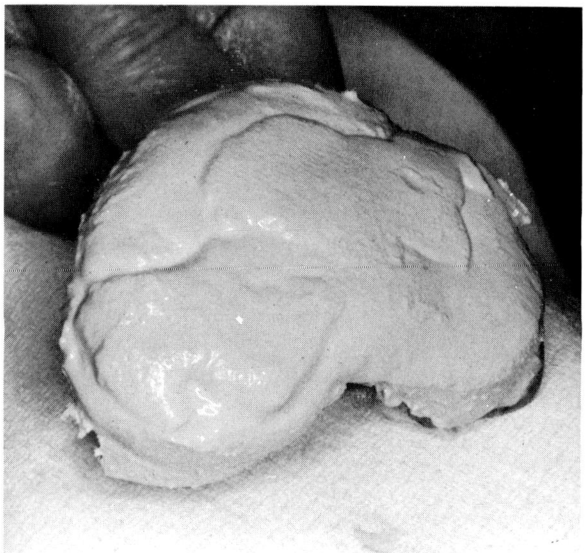

Fig. 9-12. Never invert poured impression onto a slab—weight of stone will pull it away from impression.

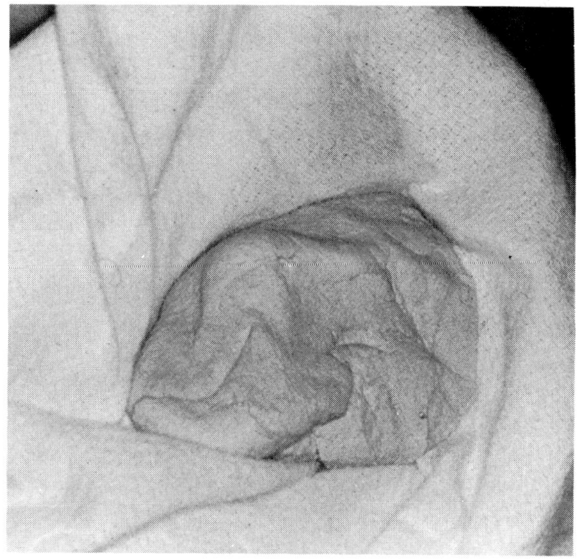

Fig. 9-13. A harder stone cast results if, after pouring mix into imprints proper, the remaining stone in bowl is partially dried by compressing in towel.

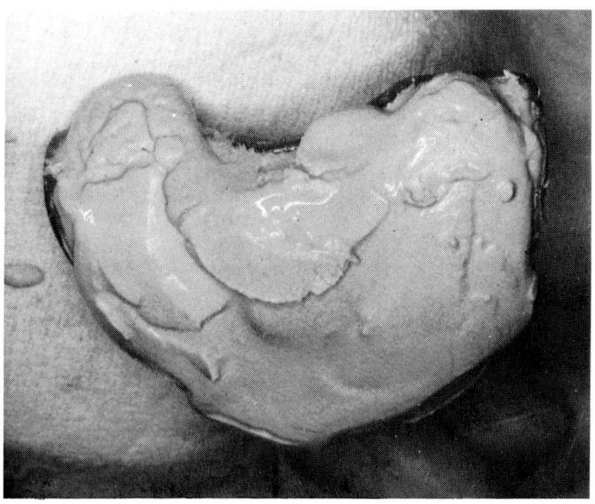

Fig. 9-14. Place compressed material on top of softer material in impression and lightly vibrate for few seconds to create union of the two parts.

plaster or stone is used for removal of this debris. A small amount of powdered stone, the same as will be used for the cast, is placed in the impression, and the inside is scrubbed gently with a soft, wet brush to cut the saliva and debris and to produce a better cast. The impression then is washed out very carefully.

After the free moisture is removed with a gentle blast of air, the mixed stone, using the correct water-powder ratio (weigh the stone accurately, and use a precisely measured amount of distilled water—100 gm. of powder to 24 ml. of distilled water), is poured into the impression and vibrated gently to eliminate air bubbles (Figs. 9-10 and 9-11). Never invert the poured impression onto a glass or plastic slab because the weight of the stone will pull it away from the impression (Fig. 9-12). (See also Figs. 9-13 and 9-14.)

The poured impression should be placed in an atmosphere of high relative humidity. This is best achieved by the use of a humidor, but, when one is not available, the impression can be wrapped in a wet towel (Fig. 9-15).

After 45 to 60 minutes the cast may be separated from the impression and trimmed to the desired shape (Fig. 9-16).

If the poured impression remains in the humidor longer than 1 hour, the alginate can affect the surface of the stone cast, making it rough and pitted.

Rudd[2,3] recommends pouring of the impression in two stages:

1. Pour the anatomic portion of the impression until covered—this surface will be rough and have irregularities with undercuts. Put in humidor at 100% humidity.
2. After the initial set, while stone is still warm due to heat of crystallization, submerge impression and stone in slurry water for 3 to 5 minutes. (*Slurry water* is a supersaturated liquid made by allowing discarded artificial stone casts to set in a container of water for 48 hours.) Excess water is blown away, and

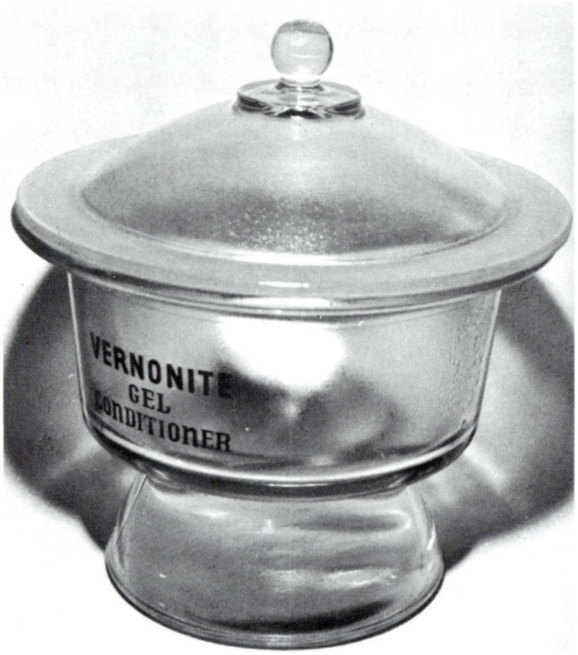

Fig. 9-15. Poured impression in humidor (atmosphere of high relative humidity).

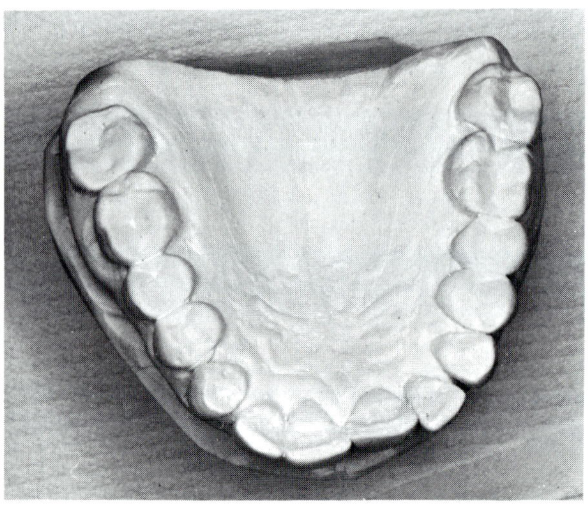

Fig. 9-16. Cast properly trimmed and debubblized.

a base of the same kind of stone and the same water-powder ratio is made.

An important fact to keep in mind is that certain brands of artificial stone are not compatible with certain brands of alginate impression material. Inquire of manufacturers of these products for assurance of compatibility.

Do not wash or trim cast after separation from impression for at least 1 hour, and preferably 3 hours or more. In trimming of the cast do not soak it in tap water, because artificial stone is soluble in plain water and the surface of the cast will be etched. Use only slurry water, because this solution, being saturated with stone, cannot dissolve anymore. Soak cast in slurry water for a few minutes, trim, and, while trimming, rinse the cast in a pan of slurry water from time to time. When trimming is completed also rinse in slurry water. Any sludge that still remains on the cast can be removed with a soft camel's-hair brush.

If the removal of gross undercuts in the first impression is feasible without any chance of distorting it or losing some important details, then it is possible to pour a second cast with fairly accurate results. This second cast can be used for preoperative wax ups, construction of clutches, etc.

Agar hydrocolloids

When a standardized and sound procedure is followed, reversible hydrocolloid is unexcelled as an impression material. This material produces accurate results with a minimum of effort.

The problem involved in taking accurate hydrocolloid impressions is distortion that is caused by excessive deformation of the material in removing the gelled impression over deep undercuts. The danger of impression distortion upon removal can be minimized by using ample bulk of material and creating conditions that lessen the possibility of deformation. Experimental evidence[4] has shown that the degree of accuracy of the hydrocolloid impressions was improved when using a tray permitting a bulk of 6 mm. of material as compared to trays permitting only 3 mm.

TRAY SELECTION

A water-jacketed tray with no perforations should be used. A large enough impression tray should be selected so that an adequate bulk of material can be used, eliminating the possibility of deformation, especially in the molar areas.

The tray must be centered accurately so that the impression material on the buccal and lingual surfaces will be equal in amount, thereby avoiding distortion caused by the larger mass of material on one side shrinking more than the small mass on its opposite side. This particular problem sometimes necessitates the construction of custom-built acrylic or cast aluminum trays, allowing for the use of a minimal amount of impression material, equal in amount both buccally and lingually, thereby giving maximum accuracy.

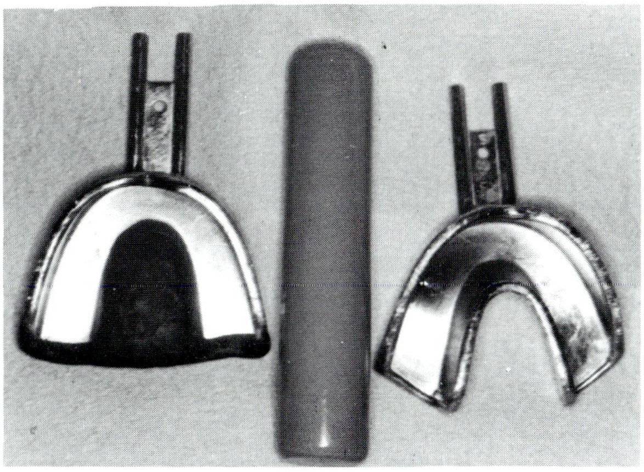

Fig. 9-17. Upper tray properly prepared for agar hydrocolloid impression to confine material, to prevent it from flowing out of the back of tray, and to create less bulk in vault area.

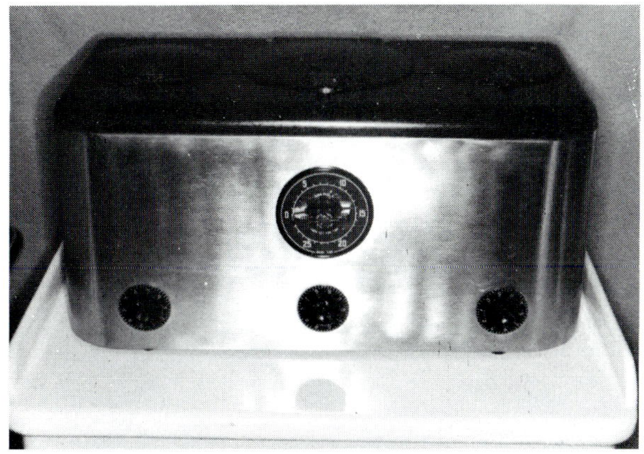

Fig. 9-18. Thompson agar hydrocolloid conditioner—thermostatically controlled.

The trays should be rim-locked to retain the material mechanically. It also is important to prevent the overseating of the tray and to prevent the tray from showing through the material.

In full upper mouth impressions with agar hydrocolloid a post dam should be used across the posterior boundary to prevent the material from flowing out of the back end of the tray, and the tray should be built up in the palatal area with modeling compound to ensure a uniform thickness of material. These procedures not only confine the material to the tray, but also prevent movement and distortion during the gelation period (Fig. 9-17). It prevents overseating of the tray and the possibility of the tray showing through the material.

In a fully dentulous mouth the lower tray, which is rim-locked, must have an equal amount of space both buccally and lingually between the tray and the teeth, and it must be seated carefully when taking the impression. The labial, buccal, and lingual flanges of the tray assist in holding it in position.

A requirement in taking an impression of a semidentulous mouth is the rimming of the periphery of the try in the edentulous area with a low-heat modeling compound. Care must be exercised not to carry the compound beyond the peripheral seal area, and definitely not into an area where there is a possibility of becoming locked into an undercut, such as in wide embrasure spaces, under pontics, or overcontoured restorations. Also, remember the need to prevent the overseating of the tray and the showing of the impression tray through the material.

PREPARATION OF MATERIALS

The trays, having now been prepared for impression taking, are again tested by fitting them in the mouth. The impression material and other necessary equipment are checked for completeness and readiness.

The agar hydrocolloid impression material should be prepared each morning by boiling it for 8 to 10 minutes in a thermostatically controlled water bath and then by transferring the material to the storage compartment (Fig. 9-18). This bath or conditioner contains three compartments—one for boiling of the material, one for storage of the melted material at 150° to 155° F., and one for tempering of the material at 115° F.

The boiled material in the small syringes and large jacketed tubes is stored in chamber 3 of the hydrocolloid conditioner at a temperature of 150° to 155° F. until ready for use. The minimum cooling period before use is 5 minutes.

After the hydrocolloid material has been ejected into the rim-locked water-jacketed tray, it is put into the tempering chamber of the hydrocolloid conditioner at a temperature of 115° F. to lower the temperature of the tray material and to condition it. The material should be held at that temperature between 10 and 15 minutes to obtain the most desirable consistency and body. The temperature also should be checked by insertion of a small thermometer into the impression material in the tray—a precaution that can prevent serious and aggravating mouth tissue burns (Fig. 9-19).

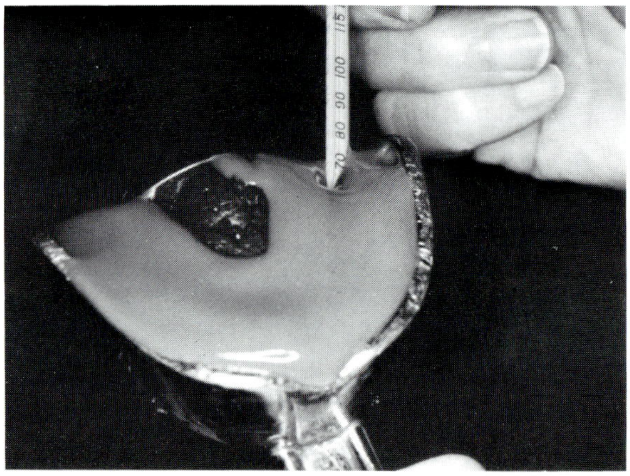

Fig. 9-19. Checking temperature of material in tray before insertion into mouth to prevent tissue burns.

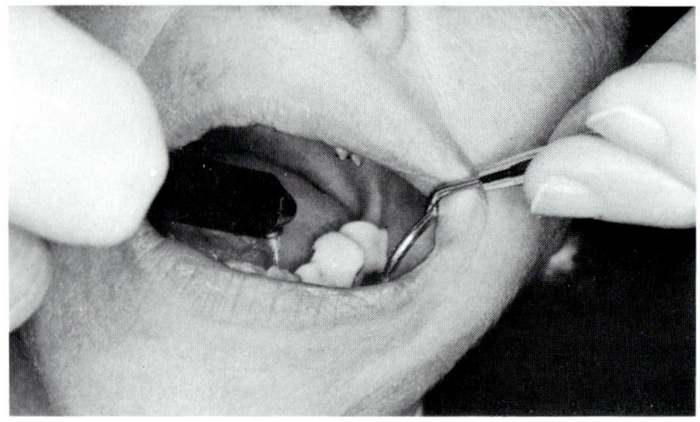

Fig. 9-20. Injection of fluid hydrocolloid onto incisal and occlusal surfaces using a small syringe. This procedure prevents trapping of air in sulci and grooves.

A

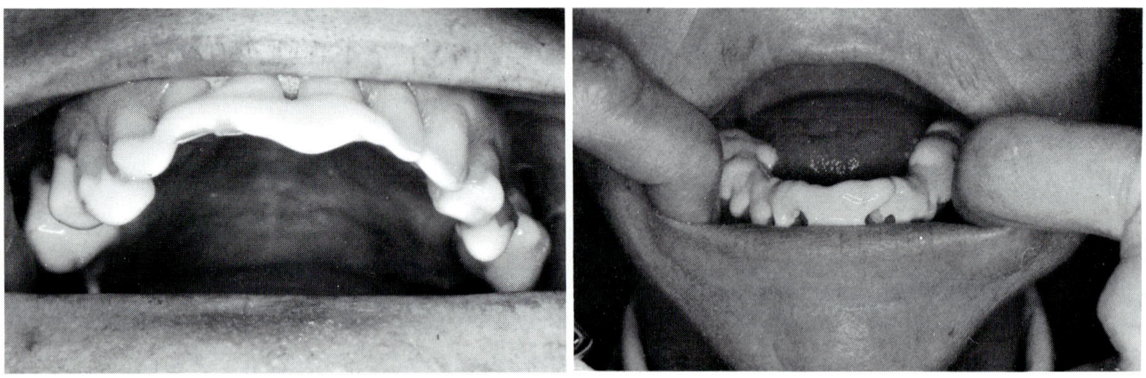

B

Fig. 9-21. Incisal and occlusal surfaces of entire arch is so treated. **A,** Upper arch. **B,** Lower arch.

The cheeks are retracted and the excess saliva blown from the teeth with a gentle blast of air. The fluid hydrocolloid is injected onto the occlusal surface of the teeth by means of a small syringe. This procedure prevents air from being trapped in the sulci and grooves. (See Figs. 9-20 and 9-21.)

The tray is removed from the tempering bath, the temperature checked, the hoses to the tray and water line connected, the contaminated, water-covered surface material scraped away, thereby exposing fresh hydrocolloid, and the tray centered gently and accurately into place, holding passively and steadily for a full 5 minutes of continuous chilling until gelation has taken place (Fig. 9-22). If the tray moves or jiggles in the mouth during this period, distortion will occur.

The chilling of the agar hydrocolloid material is important and critical. As aforementioned, the material must be chilled for 5 full minutes (Fig. 9-23), with water running through the jacketed tray, changing the sol into the gel by circulating water at 50° to 60° F. Too cold or too rapid a chilling will produce distortion, and inadequate chilling will leave the material in a somewhat softened condition with incorrect registrations of the desired areas.

After proper and adequate cooling the impression is removed by placing a finger on the periphery of the material on each side of the tray and then quickly pulling the tray vertically away from the teeth without hesitation.

After the tray has been removed from the mouth it must be examined carefully for sharpness of outline or distorted and ruptured areas. If satisfactory, the impression is washed gently in water at room temper-

A

B

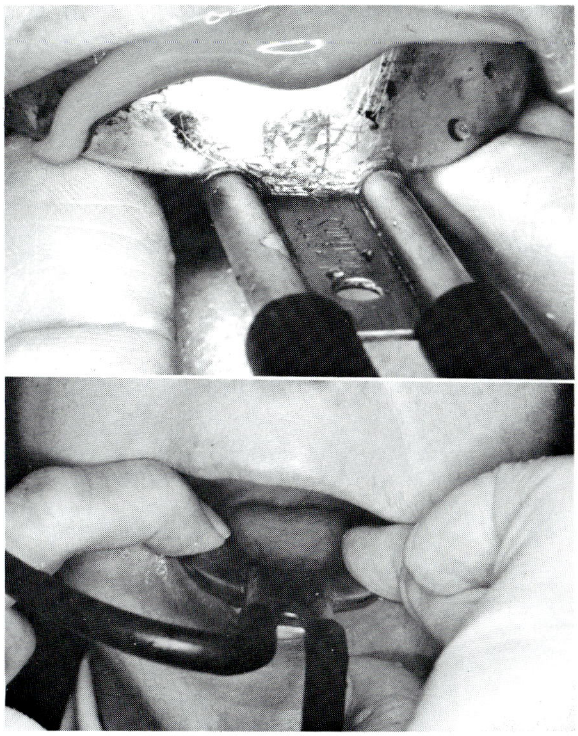

Fig. 9-22. Tray properly centered and passively held during chilling process. **A,** Upper tray. **B,** Lower tray.

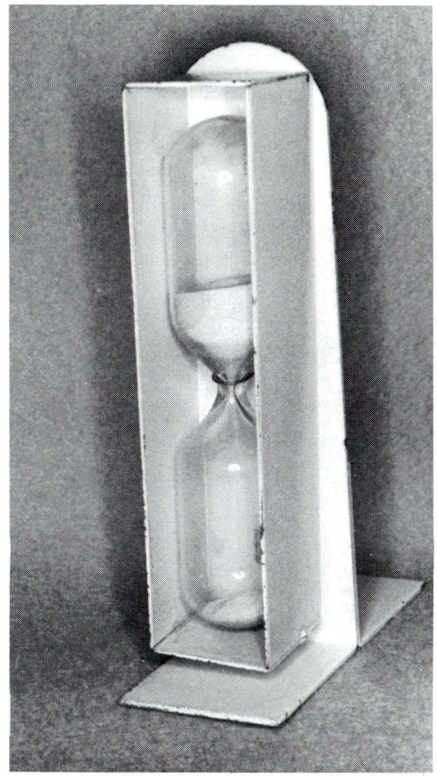

Fig. 9-23. Apparatus for exact timing for proper gelation of hydrocolloid material—5 minutes.

A

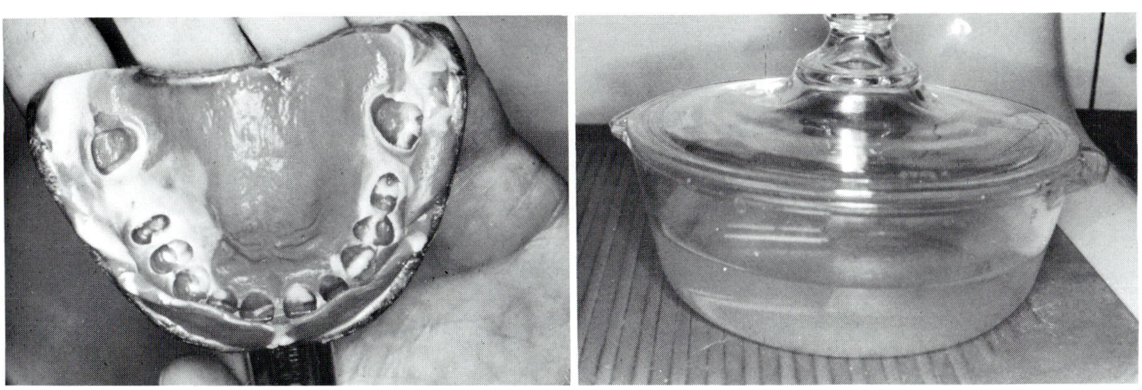

B

Fig. 9-24. A, Impression is examined for sharpness of outline and definitiveness. **B,** Impression is placed in container of 2% aqueous solution of potassium sulfate to accelerate setting of stone and to give smooth and dense surface to stone.

ature to remove the saliva and any small particles of material and then is placed immediately in a 2% aqueous solution of potassium sulfate (Fig. 9-24).

If a thick or ropy saliva is encountered, the impression should be washed thoroughly and carefully with a very thin mix of plaster of Paris or stone before placing it into the potassium sulfate bath. A small amount of powdered stone, the same as that to be used for the cast, or a fine plaster of Paris is placed in the impression, and the inside is scrubbed gently with a soft, wet brush to cut the saliva and debris and thereby produce a better cast. Then the impression is washed out very carefully and placed into the potassium sulfate bath.

All impressions should be poured within 10 to 15 minutes after removal from the mouth. It must be remembered that no hydrocolloid impression should be left exposed in air longer than 2 to 3 minutes. If an impression is allowed to dehydrate, subsequent immersion in water before pouring does not produce an accurate cast. The hydrocolloid will imbibe the amount of water lost, but it will be done at the expense of a distorted cast, which is caused by the release of stresses within the impression.

The impression is placed in a 2% aqueous solution of potassium sulfate to accelerate the setting of the stone, which is poured into the impression, and to give a smooth, dense surface to the stone.

Before pouring the impression all excess and droplets of potassium sulfate solution are blown out of the impression carefully. Do not dehydrate the hydrocolloid surface; otherwise the gel will adhere to the surface of the cast upon its removal. The surface of the impression should have a moist appearance.

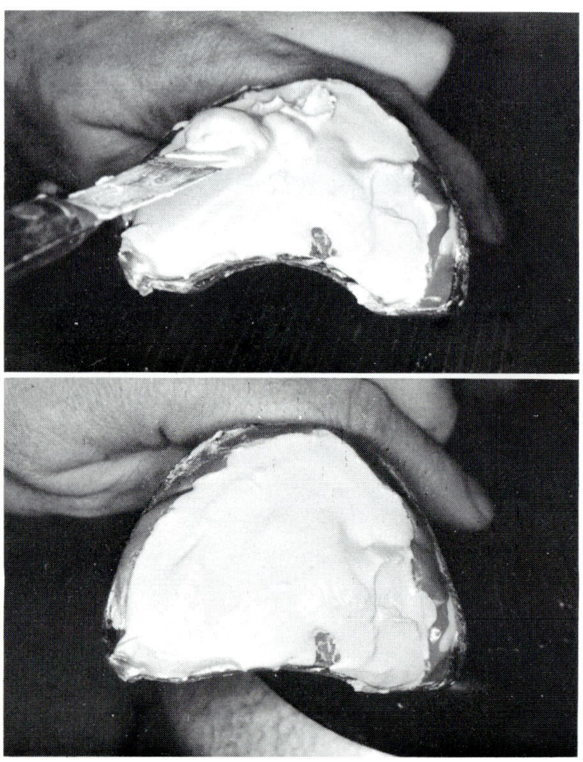

Fig. 9-25. Pouring full hydrocolloid impression.

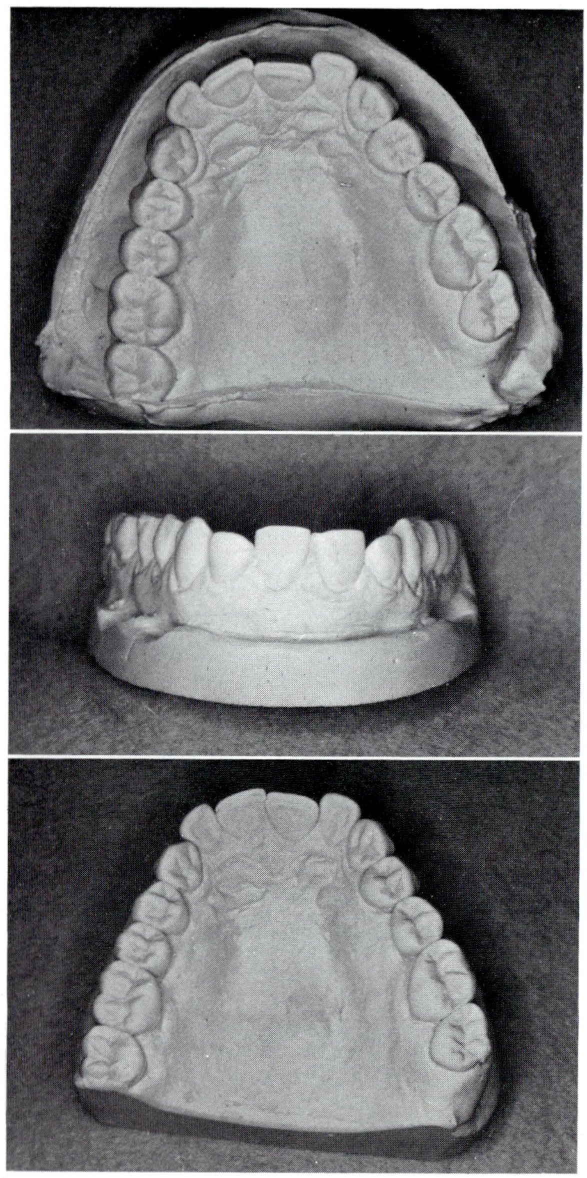

A

B

C

Fig. 9-26. A, Cast separated from impression. **B** and **C,** Trimmed to desired shape.

Following the use of the correct water-powder ratio the mixed stone is poured into the impression and is vibrated gently so that air bubbles are eliminated. The poured impression should never be inverted because the weight of the stone will pull it away from the impression (Fig. 9-25).

The poured impression should be placed in an atmosphere of high relative humidity. This is best achieved by the use of a humidor, but, when one is not available, the impression can be wrapped in a wet towel. After 45 to 60 minutes the cast may be separated from the impression and trimmed to the desired shape (Fig. 9-26). The cast is trimmed with the use of slurry water, as described fully in the section on alginates.

TISSUE DISPLACEMENT

Necessity for tissue displacement

That the indirect technique has been accepted by the profession as a whole in the reconstructive phases of dentistry is due primarily to the development of materials that can reproduce accurately all areas and types of preparations and retain their dimensional accuracy upon removal from the mouth.

When a standardized and sound procedure is followed, reversible hydrocolloid is unexcelled as the impression material of prepared teeth for the construction of microscopically accurate dies. My clinical and laboratory experiences over a number of years verify this statement.

Impression materials such as Dietrich's or modeling compound, when properly manipulated, are capable physically of pressing away the gingiva and creeping into the crevice, thus reproducing the margin. The hydrocolloid gels, however, do not possess this ability to displace soft tissue adequately; therefore, the margins must be exposed before the impression is attempted. Failure to retract or remove interfering gingival tissue prior to impression taking has led to more failures with hydrocolloid than all other causes combined. It is imperative that the margin of the preparation and about 0.5 mm. beyond it must be visible, or the hydrocolloid cannot reproduce the margin accurately. Tissue displacement should be done very carefully so that the membrane is not detached from the tooth.

The dentist must possess a thorough understanding of periodontal tissues if gingival retraction is to be accomplished routinely without unfavorable sequelae.

It is most important to remember, before preparation of the teeth or tissue displacement for impression taking, that the gingiva must be healthy, not swollen or inflamed, and that its position on the tooth must be established.

Manipulation of the gingiva to expose finish lines may produce an alteration in its coronal height. Anatomic variations of the periodontium dictate the amount of recession found postoperatively.

Also it must be remembered that a mechanical vehicle always is necessary to carry a medicament into the sulcus area for effective exposure of the cavity margin, to which must be added the factors of time and pressure.

TECHNIQUE OF CHOICE

In the tissue displacement technique that I use, the first step is to spray into the gingival crevice a 3% solution of hydrogen peroxide under pressure with a spray bottle for a period of 2 or 3 minutes, at which time the tissue adjacent to the gingival seat turns white or blanched because of the absorption of free oxygen. Bassett and Ingraham, who introduced this method, believe that "it is the most advantageous method of inhibiting hemorrhage and preparing the tissue for retraction by additional methods. And also there ensues an elimination of a large percentage of pathogenic bacteria in the area, and better tissue tone and improved healing post-operatively."*

The area that has been sprayed with the 3% solution of hydrogen peroxide then is isolated from the cheek with cotton rolls or Fiber-Lint.† A chemically

*From Bassett, R. W., Ingraham, Rex, and Koser, J. R.: An atlas of cast gold procedures, Buena Park, Calif., 1964, Uni-Tro College Press, p. 48.

†S. S. White Dental Mfg. Co., Philadelphia, Pa.

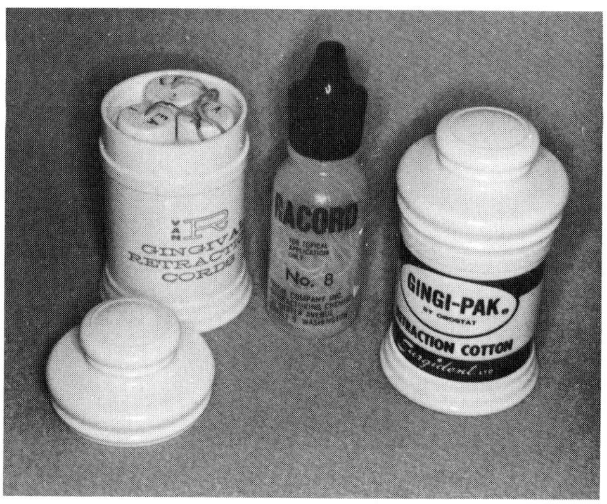

Fig. 9-27. Chemically impregnated string for tissue displacement.

impregnated string is used to cause the tissue displacement in the area of the subgingival margins and also to arrest any remaining hemorrhage or seepage that is present (Fig. 9-27).

For interproximal inlays, onlays, pinledges, or crowns a few pieces of tightly twisted strands of Van R retraction cord No. 1* (or Racord No. 8† or Gingi-Pak retraction cotton‡) are tucked into the gingival crevice, stepping it apically from the margin with the aid of a gingival retraction instrument, which has serrated ends and is designed for this purpose. The tissue is forced away from the tooth and is not depressed. The pressure is directed obliquely against the long axis of the tooth rather than toward the apex of the root. The strands mechanically deflect the tissue from the margin and chemically constrict the small blood vessels.

The next step in the procedure, following the method advocated by La Forgia,[5] is the enlargement of the sulcus and the arrest of any slight hemorrhage and seepage (Fig. 9-28). This is accomplished by using a number of tightly twisted strands of Van R retraction cord No. 3 stepped into the sulcus to and not below the margin. This step allows for greater accuracy and convenience in registering marginal detail during the impression taking.

The Van R retraction strands No. 3 are removed after 5 to 10 minutes, but the Van R retraction strands No. 1, positioned apically from the margin, are allowed to remain.

*Van R Dental Products, Inc., Los Angeles, Calif.
†Pascal Co., Inc., Seattle, Wash.
‡Surgident, Ltd., Los Angeles, Calif.

The enlargement or Van R No. 3 strands are replaced with three to six strands of dried alum string, which absorbs all moisture and keeps the sulcus open until all is in readiness for impression taking (Fig. 9-29). At this time the Van R retraction cord No. 1 below the gingival margin and the alum string in the enlarged sulcus are removed. The area is flushed and dried with a gentle stream of warm air, allowing for a quick inspection of the margins and surrounding field just before the impression is taken.

A word of warning must be given at this time. The use of a string for tissue displacement containing an 8% solution of epinephrine calls for some careful consideration. In many instances, patients with cardiac involvements, hypertension, hyperthyroidism, etc. cannot tolerate this procedure very well. In cases in which the tissues are abraded and two, three, or more subgingivally prepared teeth need tissue displacement, the absorption into the general circulation can cause a severe reaction. It is advisable to consult with their physician and, if necessary, use a string containing a decreased concentration of epinephrine or one without this particular medicament.

Displacement using aluminum shells

Another good procedure for tissue displacement for full and three-quarter crowns is one that utilizes aluminum shells.

The aluminum shells are selected slightly larger than the prepared teeth and are contoured gingivally with crown and bridge shears and left long enough to allow the edge of the shell to enter the gingival crevice. The shells are checked then for length under biting stress. They now are filled with soft, warm, temporary stopping and forced into place, first with finger pressure and then under biting stress, to clear the occlusion. Then the filled shells are removed with

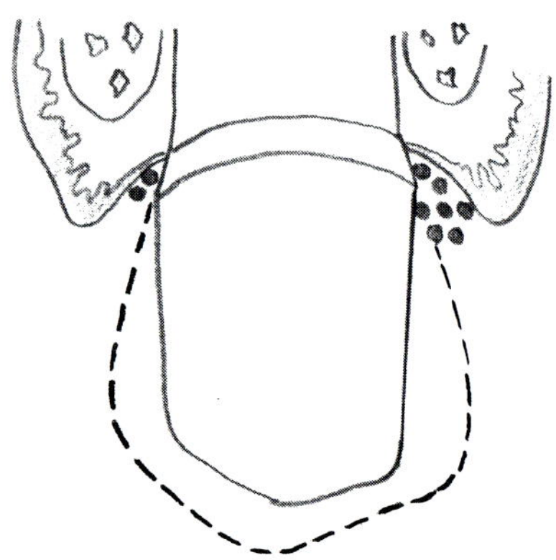

Fig. 9-28. Enlargement of sulcus follows tucking of retraction cord apically from margin. Small blood vessels are constricted.

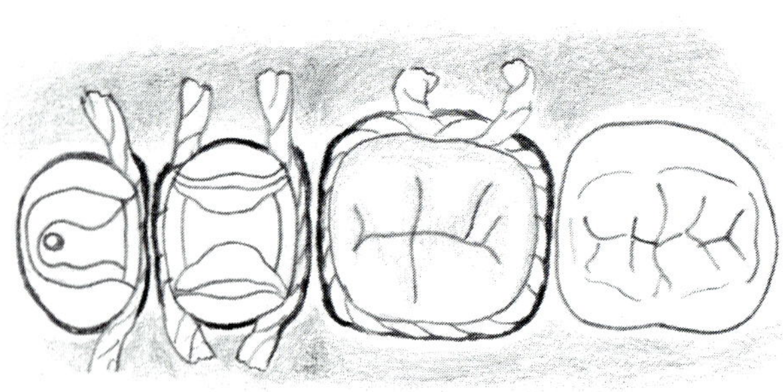

Fig. 9-29. Enlargement strands are replaced with strands of dried alum string, which absorbs the moisture and keeps sulcus open. This is method advocated by La Forgia that I use in practice.

a curved serrated hemostatic forceps, and the excess stopping is trimmed away.

Two lengths of Van R retraction cord No. 1 or Gingi-Pak that are long enough to loop around the tooth are cut. One length is looped around the tooth and twisted tightly with curved serrated forceps; then the gingival retraction instrument is used to gently tuck it down into the gingival crevice. The second length of cord is looped over the crevice that was created by the first length and packed into position. The prepared aluminum shell or shells now are placed on the teeth and forced to place under biting stress for 4 or 5 minutes. Thus the cord is held snugly in the crevice while the medicament is at work relaxing the tissue. Tissue displacement occurs while bleeding is controlled simultaneously (Fig. 9-30). When you are ready to take the impression, remove the aluminum shell, carefully remove the cord or pack, and flush, isolate, and dry the area with a gentle stream of warm air.

A slightly overextended temporary acrylic crown, bridge, or splint also can be used to force the retraction cord against the tissue for further displacement (Fig. 9-31).

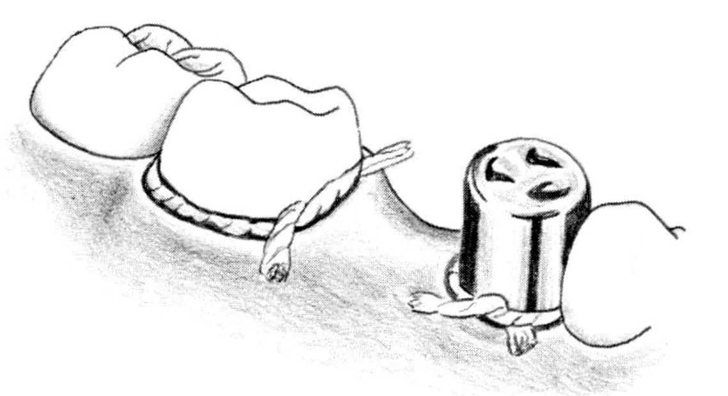

Fig. 9-30. Tissue displacement by means of impregnated string and filled aluminum shells.

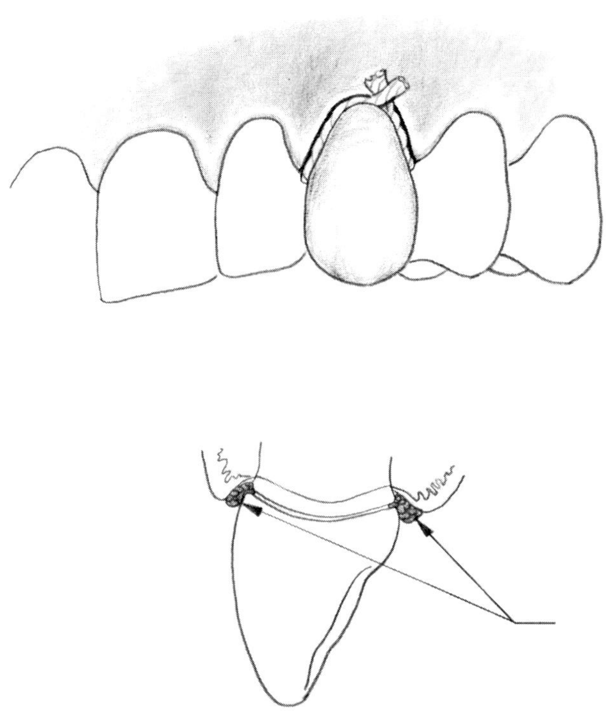

Fig. 9-31. A slightly overextended temporary acrylic crown can be used to force retraction cord against tissue for further displacement.

DISPLACEMENT USING A RADIO KNIFE

In a certain percentage of cases the tissue displacement problem cannot be handled by the methods already discussed. These are usually the cases in which a large bulk of inflammatory edematous tissue interferes with making a good preparation and/or taking a good hydrocolloid impression. When confronted with this problem, we must resort to the least desirable way of attaining access to the margins of the preparations, that is, with surgery or the radio knife. The electrodental scalpel or radio knife must be used with skill and great care because, if it touches the interproximal septa of bone, a sequestrum can result (Fig. 9-32).

Tissue displacement, by whatever means, should be carried out with care and understanding of principles so that irreparable damage to the gingival tissues is avoided.

IMPRESSIONS OF TOOTH PREPARATIONS

Choice of material

After the retraction of the gingival tissue has been accomplished, the next procedure is the taking of the impression. The material of choice for the construction of the small type casting is a reversible dental hydrocolloid, which allows for accuracy, simplicity, speed, and versatility.

REVERSIBLE HYDROCOLLOIDS

ARMAMENTARIUM IN SMALL TYPE CASTINGS

The armamentarium necessary for the reversible hydrocolloid method of impression taking is a conditioner that is thermostatically controlled and contains water baths for the liquefaction, storage, and tempering of the impression material, small and large syringes, individual jacketed hydrocolloid, rim-locked water-cooled trays, and tubing for the cooling water supply (Figs. 9-33 to 9-35). With such equipment it is possible to liquefy the hydrocolloid impres-

A

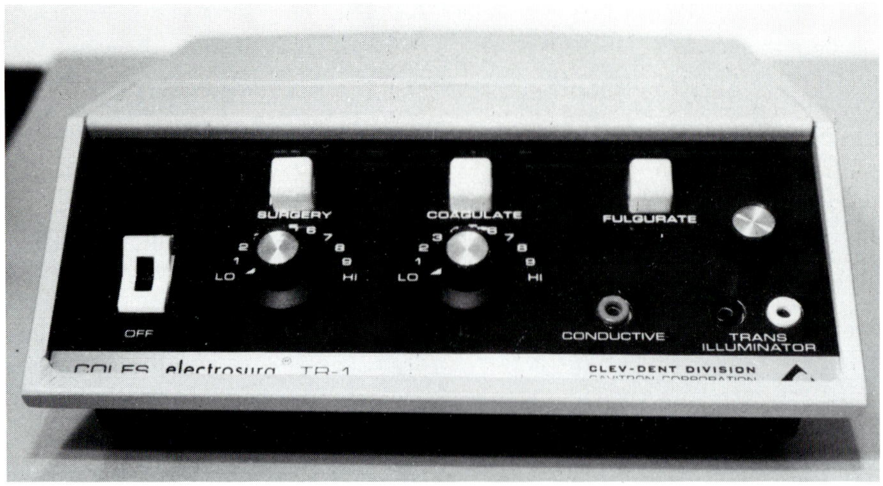

B

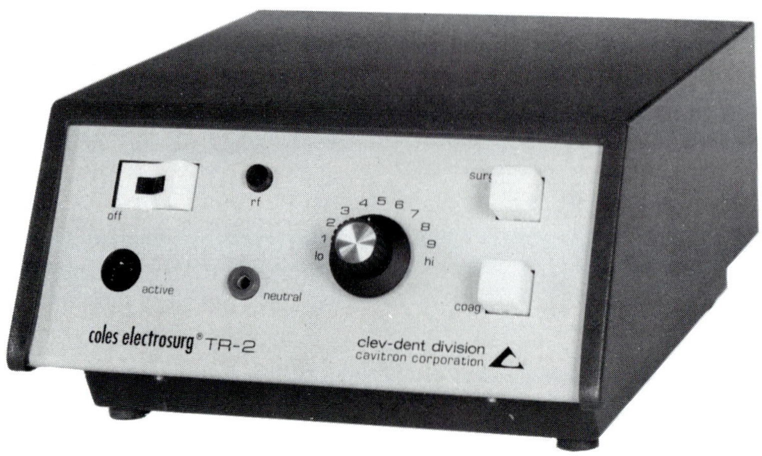

Fig. 9-32. A, and **B,** Radiosurg scalpel used when confronted with a large bulk of inflammatory edematous tissue, and routinely used for elastic impression taking. If used with knowledge, skill and great care, it can be used routinely with great success. **C** illustrates various electrosurg tips. $\mathbf{D_1}$ shows use of the electrosurg scalpel. In $\mathbf{D_2}$ we see the needle placement for the treatment of a lingual pocket. The cross-hatched area represents the tissue that will be affected by the desiccating current; the heavy curved line shows the approximate postoperative tissue level. **E,** Direction of wire scalpel for creating gingival space (in long axis of tooth) for obtaining an accurate hydrocolloid or rubber base impression.

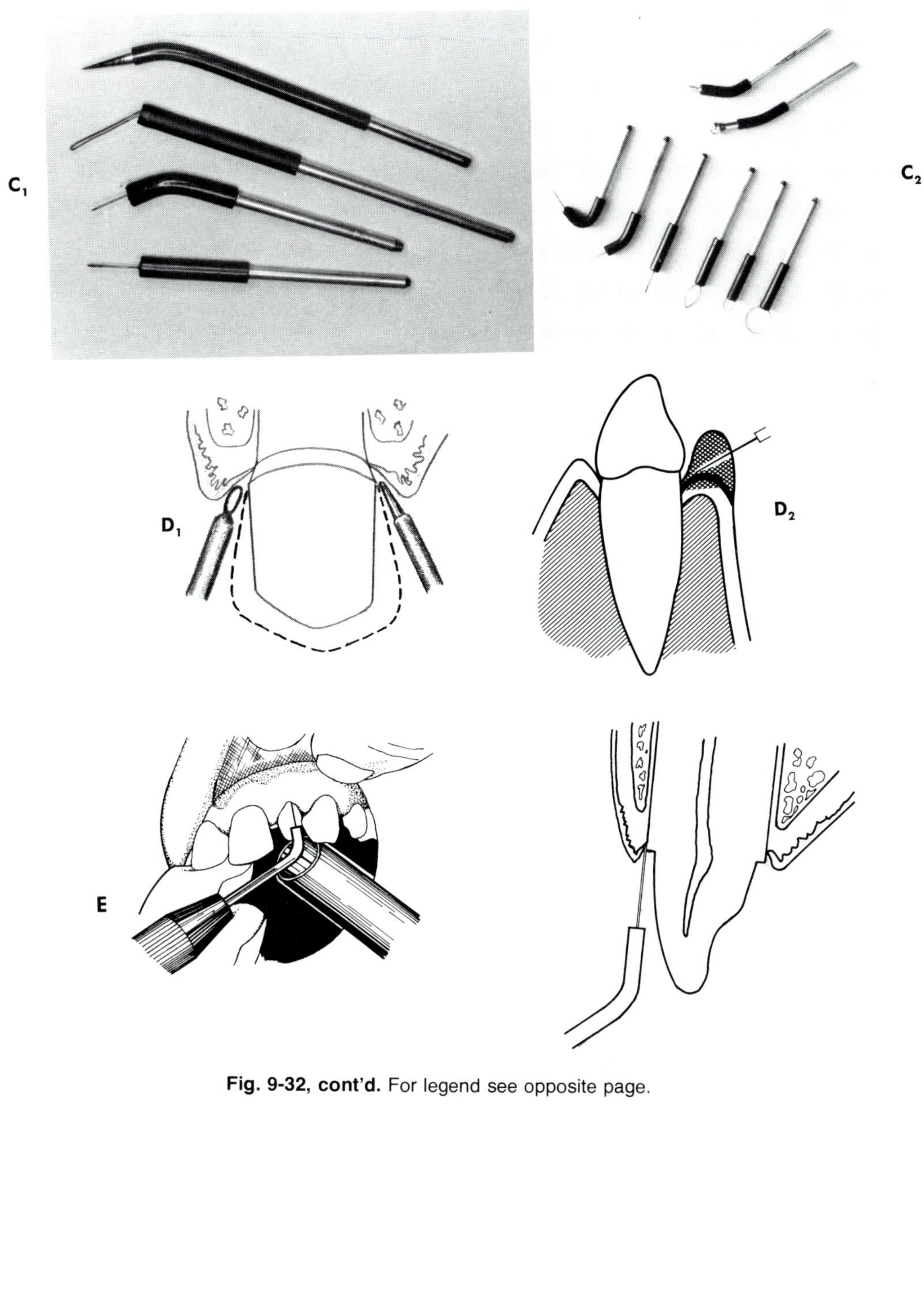

Fig. 9-32, cont'd. For legend see opposite page.

Figs. 9-33 to 9-35. Armamentarium necessary for agar hydrocolloid impressions in crown and bridge procedures.

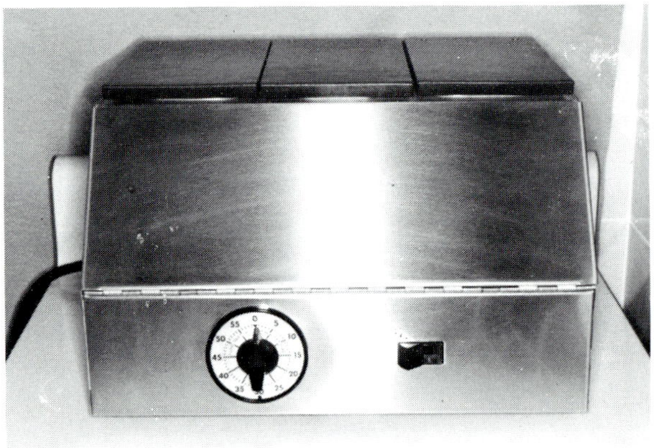

Fig. 9-33. Van R hydrocolloid conditioner.

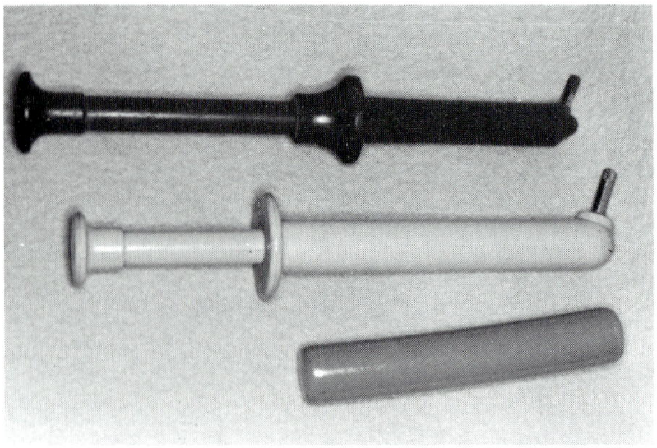

Fig. 9-34. Small syringes (different gauge needles) and small jacketed tubes of hydrocolloid.

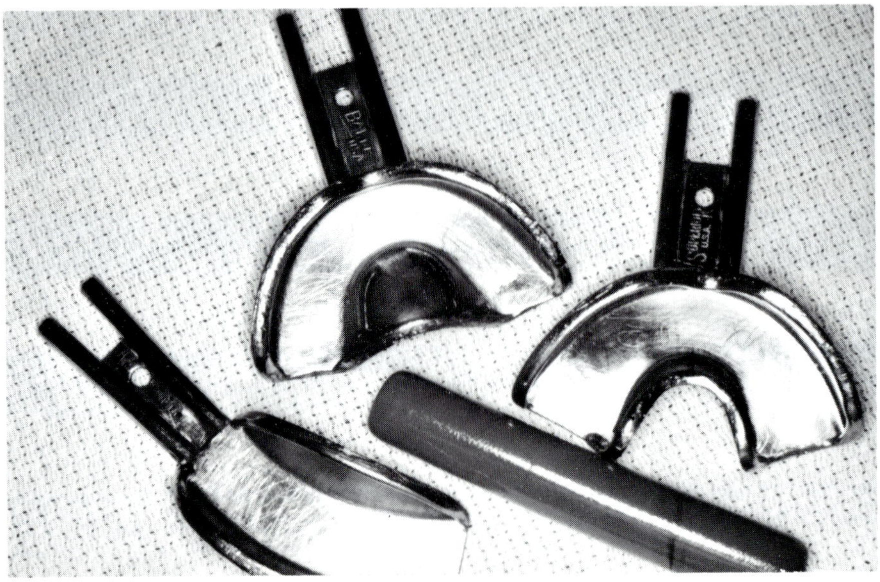

Fig. 9-35. Small water-cooled trays for different quadrants of mouth.

sion material to the proper temperatures and to place it into the mouth without injuring the tissues.

TECHNIQUE

Before taking the impression make sure that the prepared teeth are clean and dry, free of blood and saliva.

The impression is taken in a tray of sufficient size to provide a bulk of material so that, if undercuts are present, there will be sufficient bulk of impression material to allow for passing these areas without permanent distortion. The hydrocolloid should be able to be stretched or compressed without crushing or fracturing the material. Stops, either of wax or modeling compound, should be placed at each end of the tray beyond the prepared teeth to allow for sufficient thickness of the impression material over the occlusal area of the prepared teeth and to restrict and confine the material in the tray when the impression is taken. These steps also aid in maintaining stability during the critical period of gelation.

The procedure of using reversible hydrocolloid can be divided into the following steps:

1. Liquefaction of the material by boiling for 8 to 10 minutes (4 to 5 minutes for junior jacketed tubes).

2. Storage of the boiled material in the small syringes and jacketed tubes in storage chamber at a temperature of 150° to 155° F. until ready for use. This maintains the material in a colloidal state.

3. Placement of the tray material in tempering chamber at a temperature of 115° F. and holding that temperature between 5 and 15 minutes. The temperature of the tray material is lowered so that it is not too hot when introduced into the mouth and it has the desired degree of stiffness or body.

4. Filling of the prepared teeth with the fluid hydrocolloid (reproduces the cavity details more accurately) in the small syringe taken from storage chamber.

5. Removal of the tray with its tempered material from the tempering bath and carrying it to the mouth, after scraping off the top layer, which was exposed to the water.

6. Careful location of the tray, followed by changing the sol into the gel by circulating water at 50° to 60° F. through it. The tray must be held immovable until gelation is completed.

7. Rapid removal of the impression from the mouth, which prevents distortion, and pouring of the dies or casts in artificial stone.

Boiling water is a convenient means of liquefying the material. A minimum boiling time of 8 minutes is essential, and longer periods of boiling are not harmful. Phillips[6] calls attention to the fact that "whenever the material is reliquefied after a previous use it is more difficult to break down the agar lattice-work, so approximately three minutes should be added each time the material is reboiled."*

After the liquefaction process the syringes and tubes of material in the sol condition are stored in the water bath at a temperature of 150° to 155° F. until ready for use.

After the preparations are completed and before the displacement of the gingival tissue is started, the tray is filled and placed immediately in the tempering bath at 115° F. for about 10 minutes (Fig. 9-36). The purpose of tempering is to increase the viscosity of the impression material so that it will not flow out of the tray and also to reduce the temperature to prevent discomfort to the patient.

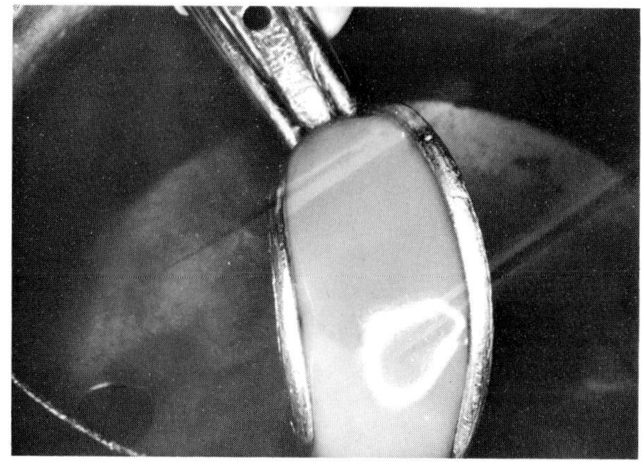

Fig. 9-36. Tray filled with agar hydrocolloid and placed immediately in tempering bath at 115° F. for about 10 minutes.

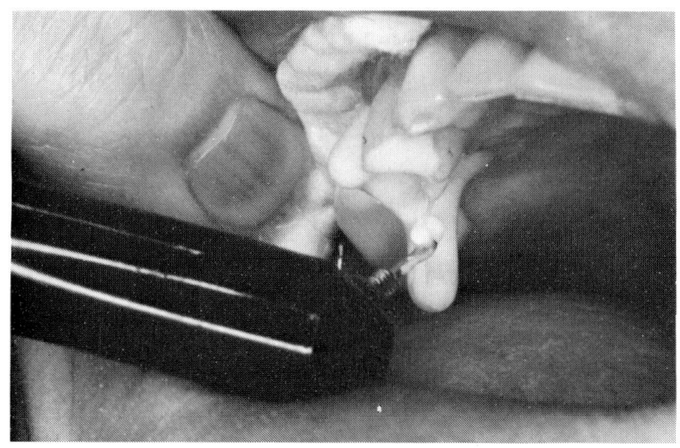

Fig. 9-37. Injecting fluid hydrocolloid from small syringe into preparations.

By the time the hydrocolloid material has been conditioned properly, the toilet of the cavity preparation and displacement of the gingival tissue have been completed, and all is in readiness for taking the impression of the prepared teeth. The small syringe is removed from the storage bath, and the portion of the colloid within the needle is expelled in an area outside of the cavity before the sol is first ejected at the gingival portion of the preparation and then carried distomesially over the cavity (Fig. 9-37). The needle must be held close to the tooth, beneath the surface of the ejected material, to prevent a trapping of air bubbles.

*From Phillips, R. W.: Hydrocolloid impression materials; technical consideration. In Skinner, E. W., and Phillips, R. W.: The science of dental materials, Philadelphia, 1960, W. B. Saunders Co.

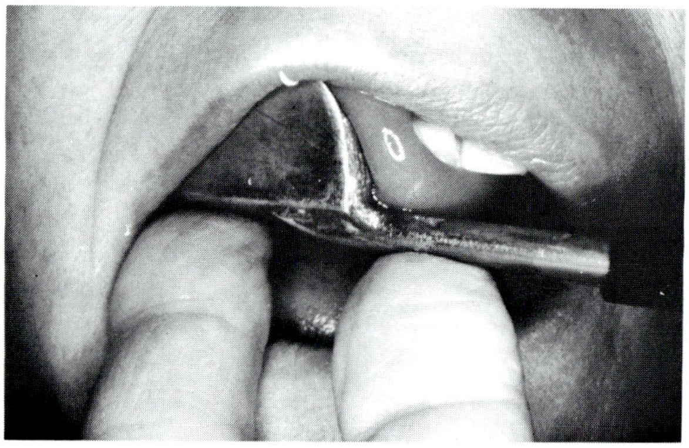

Fig. 9-38. After water-soaked outer layer of hydrocolloid is removed, tray properly positioned and held with passive pressure.

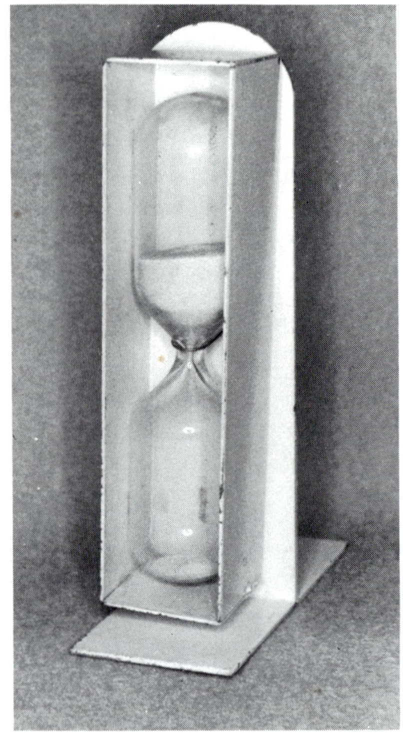

Fig. 9-39. Complete gelation requires 5 minutes of chilling.

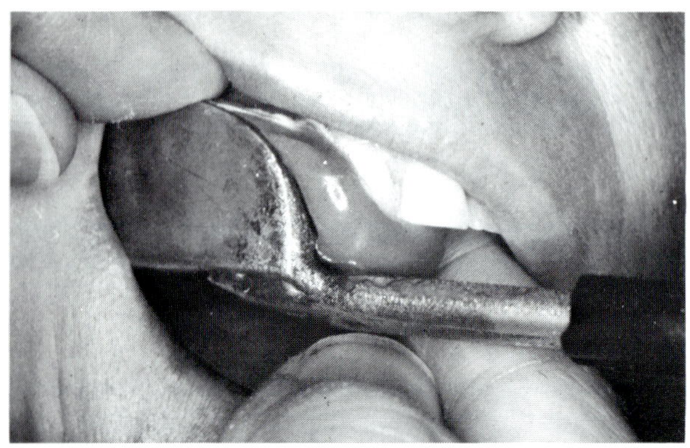

Fig. 9-40. Correct removal of impression—placing finger on periphery of tray on each side and quickly pulling tray vertically away from teeth.

After the preparations and adjoining teeth have been covered with a bulk of hydrocolloid to prevent premature chilling, the tray material, which has been tempering, is removed, and the water-soaked outer layer of hydrocolloid is scraped off. Failure to remove that layer may prevent a firm union between the tray material and the hydrocolloid, which has been injected previously into the cavity preparation.

The tray is brought immediately into position and completely seated with passive pressure (Fig. 9-38). The tray, with the water circulating very slowly, must not be allowed to move in any direction during the gelation period. Gelation is accomplished by circulating water at a temperature of approximately 50° to 60° F. for not less than 5 minutes (Fig. 9-39). It is not advisable to use ice water.

The impression must not be removed before complete gelation has taken place because, if the hydrocolloid material is incompletely gelled, there will be a distortion of the impression, and an inaccurate die or cast will result. Gelation depends on coordinating the factors of time and temperature—time is as important a factor as the temperature of the water used.

After the gelation process the impression is withdrawn by placing a finger on the periphery of the material on each side of the tray and then by quickly pulling the tray vertically away from the teeth (Fig. 9-40). Removing the tray with a rocking motion will result in distortion; also, fracture is more likely to occur.

"The brush-heap structure of the gel is of such a nature that a sudden force is always resisted without distortion or fracture more successfully than a force which is applied slowly. Consequently, when the impression is removed, it is necessary to remove it suddenly, with a jerk rather than to tease it out. The removal is accomplished in a direction as nearly as possible parallel to the long axes of the teeth."*

After the tray has been removed from the mouth it must be examined carefully for sharpness of cavity

*From Skinner, E. W., and Phillips, R. W.: The science of dental materials, Philadelphia, 1960, W. B. Saunders Co.

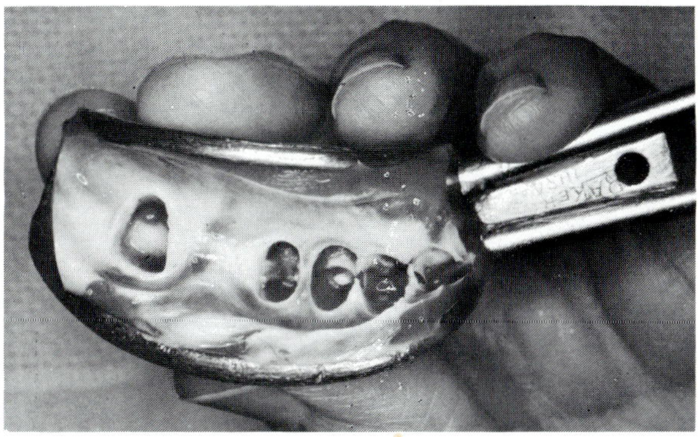

Fig. 9-41. Examine impression for definitiveness of detail—sharpness of cavity outline and absence of distorted or ruptured areas.

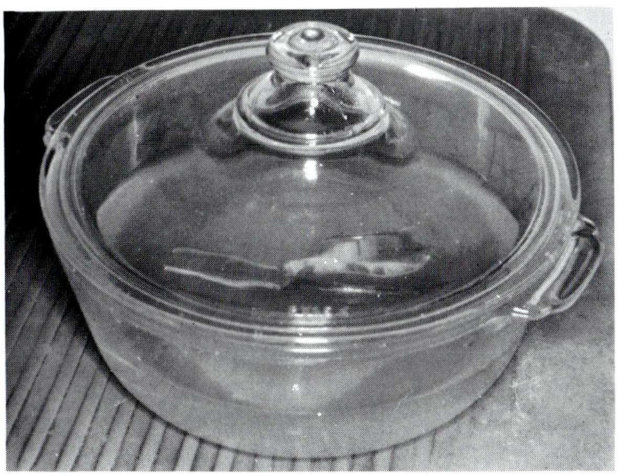

Fig. 9-42. Impression placed immediately in 2% aqueous solution of potassium sulfate.

outline or distorted and ruptured areas (Fig. 9-41). If satisfactory, the impression is washed gently in water at room temperature to remove the saliva and small particles and placed immediately in a 2% aqueous solution of potassium sulfate (Fig. 9-42).

ROPY SALIVA

If a thick or ropy saliva is encountered, the impression should be washed thoroughly and carefully with a very thin mix of plaster of Paris or stone before placing it into the potassium sulfate solution.

A small amount of powdered stone, the same as that to be used for the cast, or a fine plaster of Paris is placed in the impression, and the inside is scrubbed gently with a soft, wet brush to cut the saliva and debris and thereby to produce a better cast. Then the impression is washed out very carefully and is placed into the potassium sulfate bath.

PINLEDGES AND PINLAYS

The technique developed by Shooshan,[7] together with new types of drills and the use of graded nylon bristles, has simplified the reproduction of the cavity preparation by the indirect impression method and the construction of the wax pattern.

The reversible hydrocolloid impression material is the material of choice in the taking of pinledge or pinlay impressions.

Sized Perlon pins* or nylon bristles are fitted, prepared, and positioned in the pinholes of the preparation with a special inserting pliers, prior to the taking of the impression.

Perlon pins are of a nylon material and because of their uniformity of size, especially in roundness and consistency of diameter size, are the impression pin material of choice. They afford a more precise result with regards to strength and fit of the finished cast pin.

The Perlon pins with flat heads are available in three sizes (Nos. 6, 7, and 8) to correspond with the drill sizes (5 mm. and 6 mm. lengths) and are color coded:

Drill size		*Perlon pin*			
mm.	*Inches*	*No.*	*mm.*	*Inches*	*Color*
0.6	0.024	6	0.58	0.023	Lavender
0.7	0.028	7	0.68	0.027	Orange-red
0.8	0.032	8	0.78	0.031	Lime-green

The Perlon pins are slightly smaller in size than the corresponding drill and give a snug fit (Fig. 9-43).

The Perlon pins are placed in the prepared pinholes, making sure that they do not bind on being removed and also that the impression tray does not contact any of these pins. Contact of the tray with any of the pins will place them under tension, and release of this tension upon removal of the impression will cause a displacement of the Perlon pins.

The water-jacketed tray, which has been prepared with wax or modeling compound stops for seating and stability, is loaded with agar hydrocolloid and placed in the tempering bath. The fluid hydrocolloid from a small syringe is ejected around each headed Perlon pin, and the pins are held in place with the tip of the index finger (of the hand not controlling the small syringe) until they are covered with the hydrocolloid material, at which time the index finger is moved away carefully at a right angle so that

*J. F. Jelenko & Co., Inc., New Rochelle, N. Y.

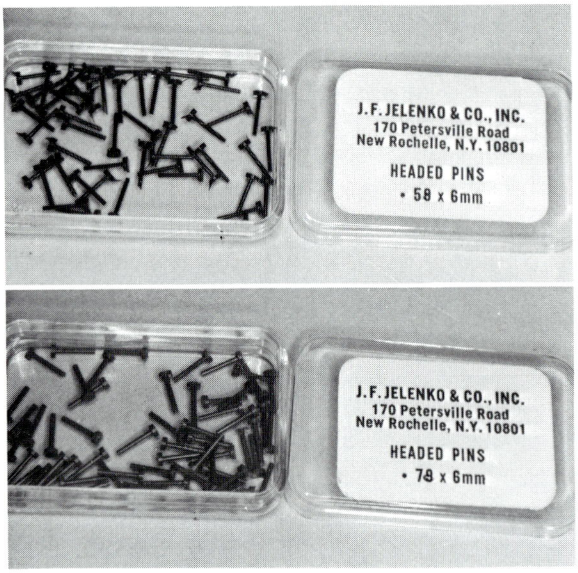

Fig. 9-43. Sized Perlon pins with flat heads.

the pins are not dislodged.[8] This operation should be rapid and deliberate.

To avoid premature chilling, when all the pins and the remainder of the preparation are covered with a liberal amount of impression material, the tempered tray with the water-soaked outer layer of hydrocolloid scraped off is positioned and held passively and steady for a full 5 minutes to chill it adequately. It then is removed with a quick snap and examined carefully for detailed reproduction of the preparation and correct position of the pins, making sure that there has not been any displacement of the pins. Now it is washed gently in water at room temperature to remove the saliva and any small particles and is placed immediately in a 2% aqueous solution of potassium sulfate.

SALIENT FACTS ABOUT AGAR HYDROCOLLOIDS (REVERSIBLE)

1. Inaccurate hydrocolloid impressions may be caused by the following:
   a. Movement of tray during gelation
   b. Removing impression from mouth too soon
   c. Teasing out of impression rather than removal with a quick snap
   d. Storage of impression before pouring
   e. Chilling with water at very low temperatures
2. Rough or chalky surfaced casts are caused by the following:
   a. Impression not treated with a 2% aqueous solution of potassium sulfate
   b. Incorrect water-powder ratio for stone
   c. Cast or die removed from impression before 30 to 45 minutes or cast or die left too long before separation
   d. Excess water or solution not blown from mold
   e. Too much vibration during pouring

RUBBER BASE—TWO-MIX TECHNIQUE

PRELIMINARY PREPARATIONS

The technique for impression taking with Thiokol and silicone is very similar. I use the Elasticon* and Citricon* material, which is furnished in two viscosities—a tray type and a syringe type. The syringe type is of a lower viscosity so that it will inject readily into the prepared teeth. (See Fig. 9-44.)

A custom-made tray is constructed, making use of a study cast of the case at hand. Two layers of Thin-Wax† are adapted over the teeth of the study cast, extending at least a tooth beyond the ones to be included in the impression. The unprepared tooth or soft tissue acts as an anterior and posterior stop in positioning the tray properly during impression taking. The tray is made with Forma-tray,* which is a quick-setting acrylic material.

After the tray has been prepared, the Elasticon adhesive is applied lightly to all inner and peripheral surfaces and permitted to dry (Fig. 9-45).

After the syringe is prepared (Figs. 9-46 to 9-50), which is used to apply the thinner material, the tray, Elasticon mixing pads, spatulas, and dappen dish are laid out (Fig. 9-51).

Tissue displacement has been accomplished, and cotton roll or Fiber-Lint is positioned to absorb moisture.

TECHNIQUE

1. Heavy-bodied Elasticon material is dispensed on a mixing pad—4 inches for a small bridge tray. Use 2 drops of heavy-bodied Elasticon accelerator (red) per inch of heavy-bodied Elasticon base material. (See Fig. 9-52, *A*.)

2. Syringe Elasticon material is dispensed on another mixing pad—4 inches for a small bridge tray. Use 1 drop of syringe Elasticon accelerator (yellow) per inch of syringe Elasticon base material. (See Fig. 9-52, *B*.)

The mixing pads should be of heavy stiff paper, and the spatulas should be slightly flexible and should have straight sides.

---

*Kerr Dental Mfg. Co., Detroit, Mich.

†Modern Materials Mfg. Co., St. Louis, Mo.

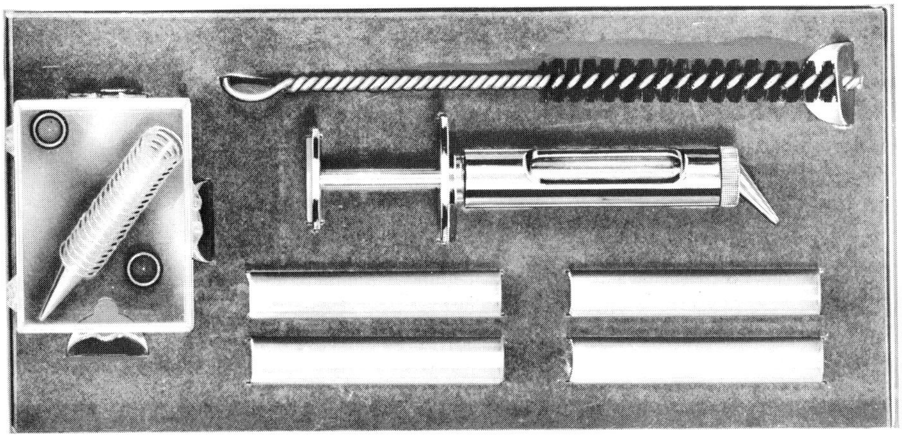

Fig. 9-44. Versatile syringe for all rubber base impression materials.

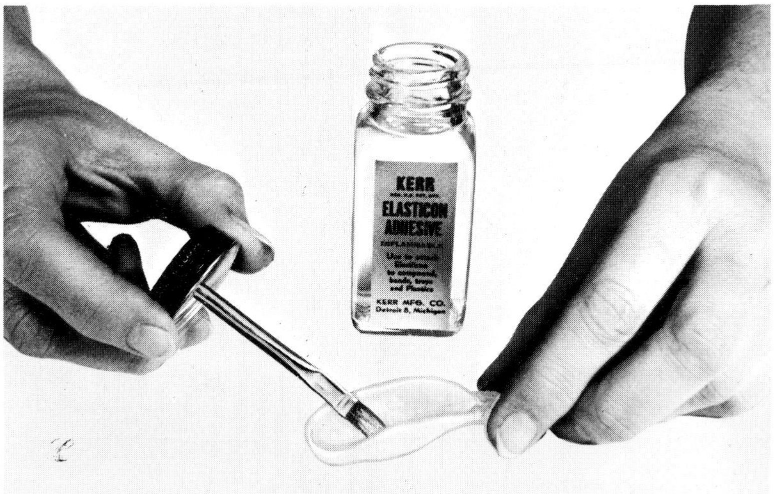

Fig. 9-45. Apply Elasticon adhesive lightly to all inner and peripheral surfaces of tray and permit to dry. (Courtesy Kerr Dental Mfg. Co., Detroit, Mich.)

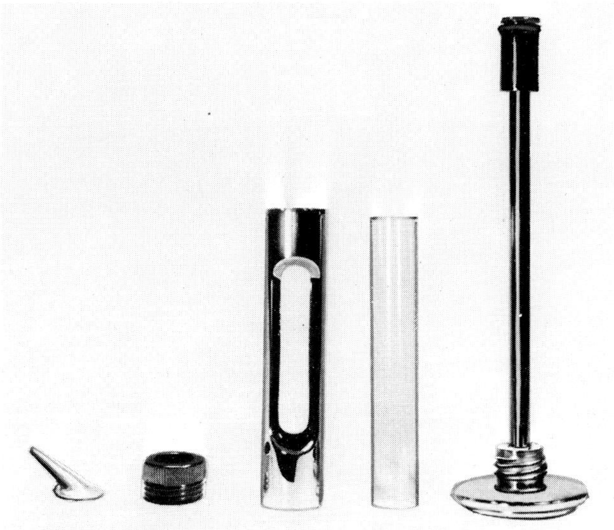

Fig. 9-46. Syringe completely disassembled. (Courtesy Kerr Dental Mfg. Co., Detroit, Mich.)

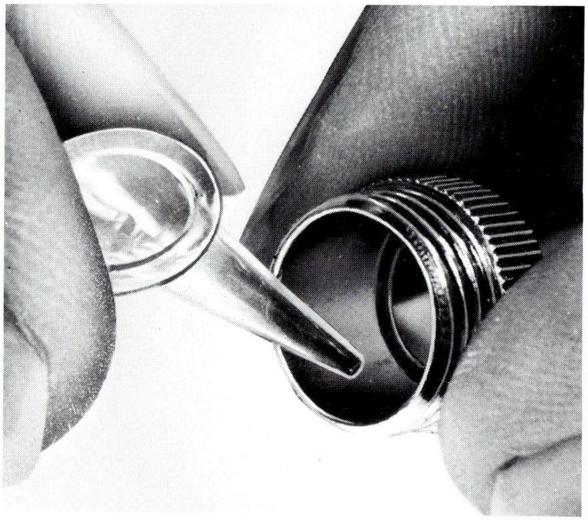

Fig. 9-47

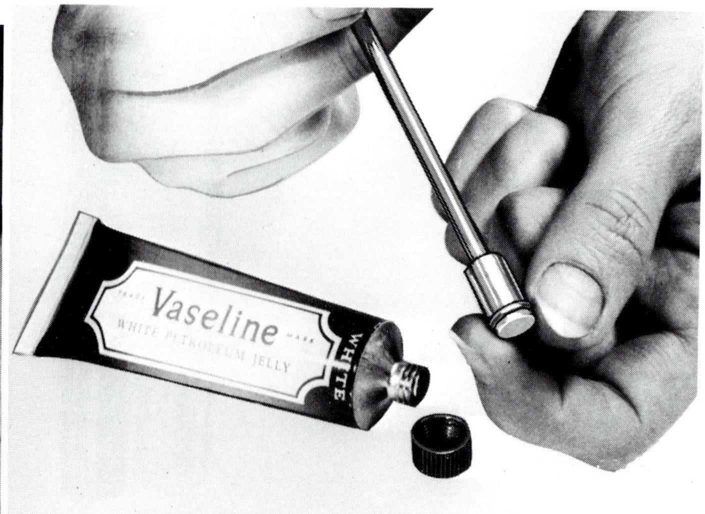

Fig. 9-48

Fig. 9-47. Insert plastic tip into tip retainer and screw retainer into metal barrel. (Courtesy Kerr Dental Mfg. Co., Detroit, Mich.)

Fig. 9-48. Lightly lubricate rubber ring washer with petroleum jelly and wipe off excess with tissue. (Courtesy Kerr Dental Mfg. Co., Detroit, Mich.)

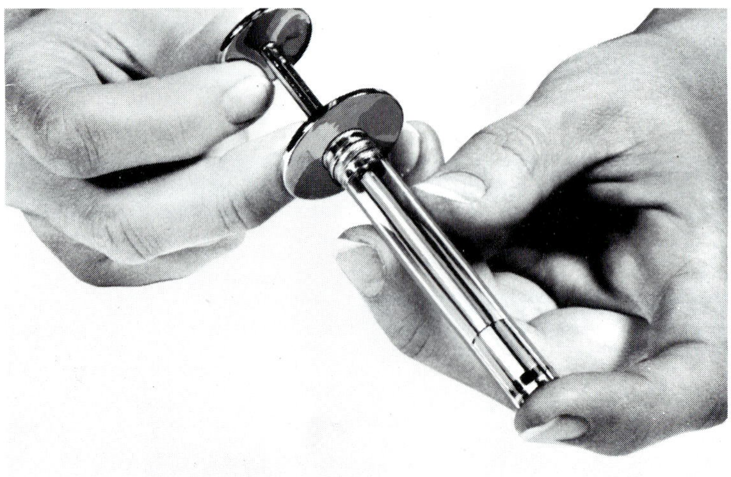

Fig. 9-49. Insert plunger into plastic sleeve and press forward until flush with end of plastic sleeve. (Courtesy Kerr Dental Mfg. Co., Detroit, Mich.)

3. Mix syringe Elasticon base and accelerator a maximum of 30 seconds. Thorough mixing is necessary if the accelerator is to be impregnated throughout the mass. Mixing and loading of syringe must be completed in 1½ minutes (Fig. 9-53).

4. Pick up the entire mix of syringe Elasticon and transfer it to a dappen dish. Load the syringe from the dappen dish. (See Figs. 9-54 to 9-58.)

5. Mix heavy-bodied Elasticon base and accelerator. Thorough mixing is necessary if the accelerator is to be incorporated completely throughout the mass. Complete the mix within 40 to 45 seconds (Fig. 9-59). The tray must be loaded with heavy-bodied Elasticon and seated in the mouth within 2 minutes.

6. Spread heavy-bodied Elasticon over all adhesive-covered surfaces of the tray and set tray aside (Fig. 9-60).

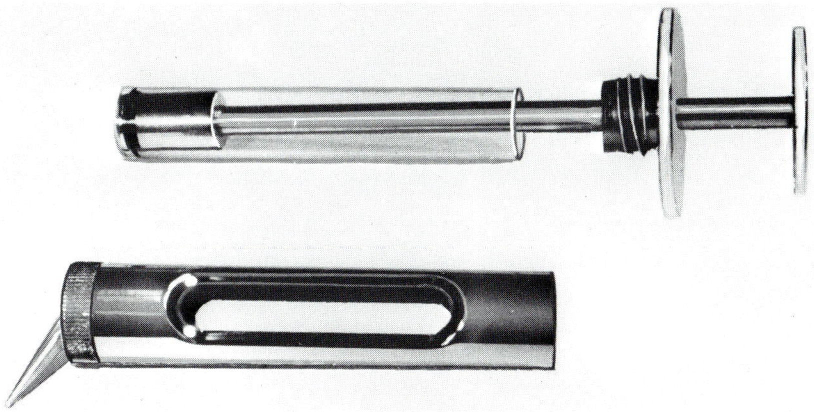

Fig. 9-50. Prepared syringe set aside until syringe Elasticon has been mixed. (Courtesy Kerr Dental Mfg. Co., Detroit, Mich.)

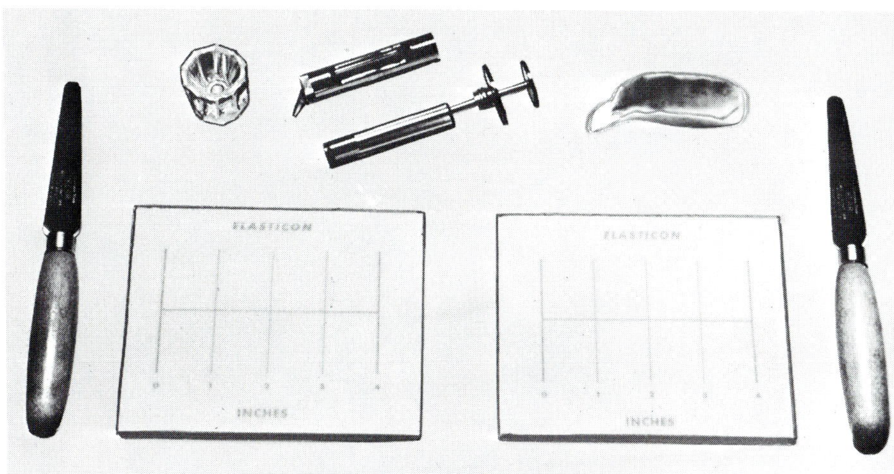

Fig. 9-51. Elasticon mixing pads, spatulas, and dappen dish laid out. (Courtesy Kerr Dental Mfg. Co., Detroit, Mich.)

7. Dry prepared teeth and gingival crevices, and with the syringe inject syringe Elasticon into the subgingival crevices and the preparations, being careful not to trap air between the preparation and the material.

8. Pick up the tray that is loaded with the heavy-bodied material, and seat to place with a rocking motion, holding the tray firmly in position until impression material has completely set—approximately 10 minutes from beginning of syringe mix.

9. Remove impression, rinse, and dry with a gentle blast of air.

Examine the impression carefully for preparation details, being sure that all margins and at least 0.5 mm. beyond have been copied accurately. Pour immediately to avoid any possibility of dimensional change. (See Figs. 9-61 and 9-62.)

This impression technique is best accomplished by two persons mixing simultaneously—the assistant mixing the syringe material and the dentist the heavy-bodied material.

Treatment of impression before and after pouring of stone

All impressions should be poured within 10 to 15 minutes after removal from the mouth. It must be remembered that no hydrocolloid impression should be left exposed in the air for longer than 2 or 3 minutes. If an impression is allowed to dehydrate, subsequent immersion in water before pouring does

Text continued on p. 458.

A 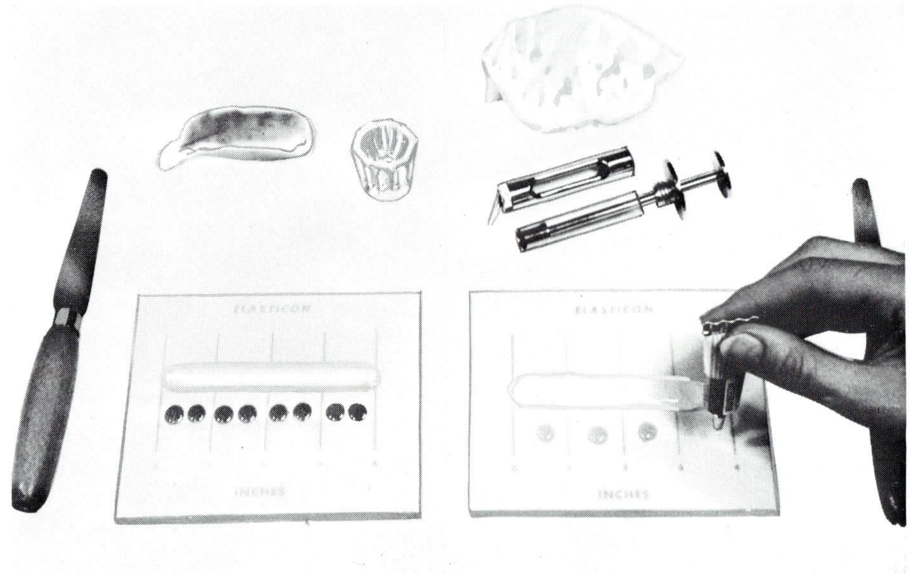 B

Fig. 9-52. A, Heavy-bodied Elasticon material dispensed on mixing pad—4 inches for a small bridge tray. Use 2 drops of heavy-bodied Elasticon accelerator (red) per inch of heavy-bodied Elasticon base material. **B,** Syringe Elasticon material is dispensed on another mixing pad—4 inches for a small bridge tray. Use 1 drop of syringe Elasticon accelerator (yellow) per inch of syringe Elasticon base material. (Courtesy Kerr Dental Mfg. Co., Detroit, Mich.)

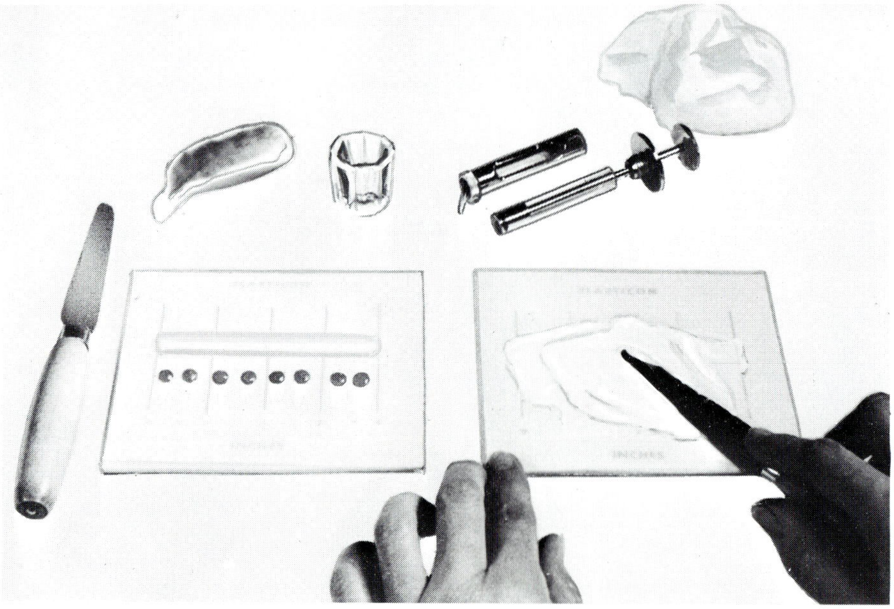

Fig. 9-53. Mix syringe Elasticon base and accelerator a maximum of 30 seconds. Mixing and loading of syringe completed in $1^1/_2$ minutes. (Courtesy Kerr Dental Mfg. Co., Detroit, Mich.)

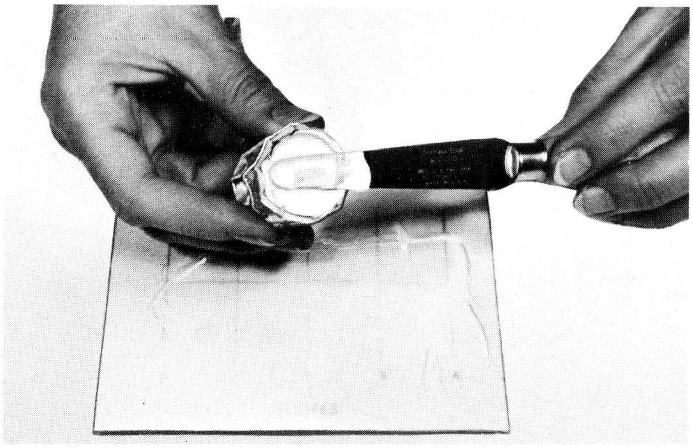

Fig. 9-54. Pick up entire mix of syringe material and transfer to dappen dish. (Courtesy Kerr Dental Mfg. Co., Detroit, Mich.)

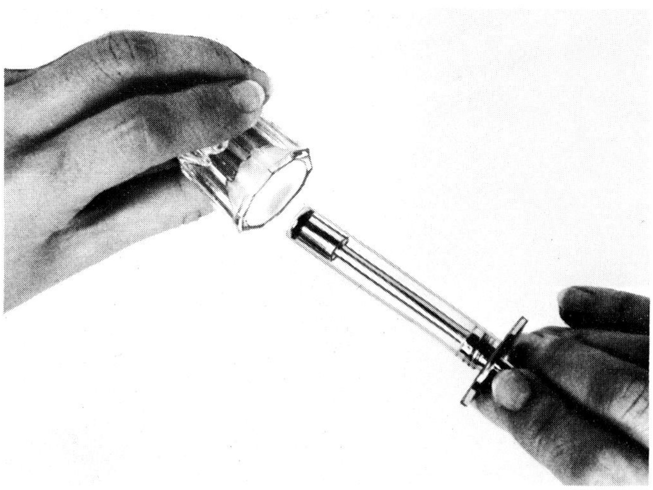

Fig. 9-55. Insert plastic sleeve of syringe with plunger into filled dappen dish. (Courtesy Kerr Dental Mfg. Co., Detroit, Mich.)

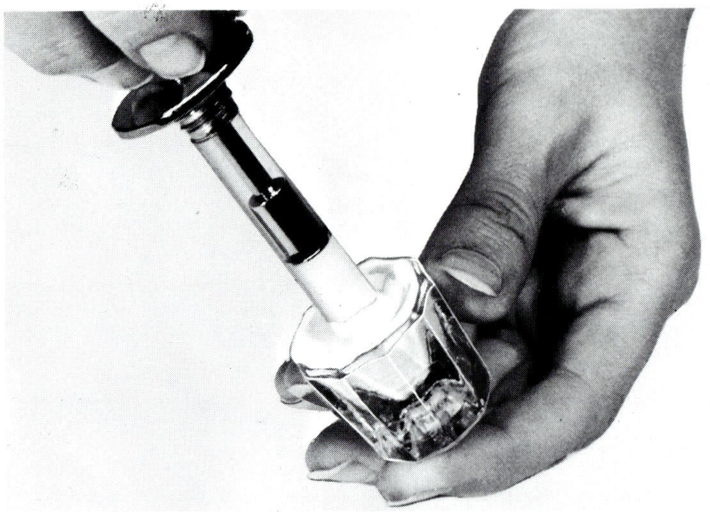

Fig. 9-56. With locking disk forced against plastic sleeve, draw plunger back slowly to fill sleeve. (Courtesy Kerr Dental Mfg. Co., Detroit, Mich.)

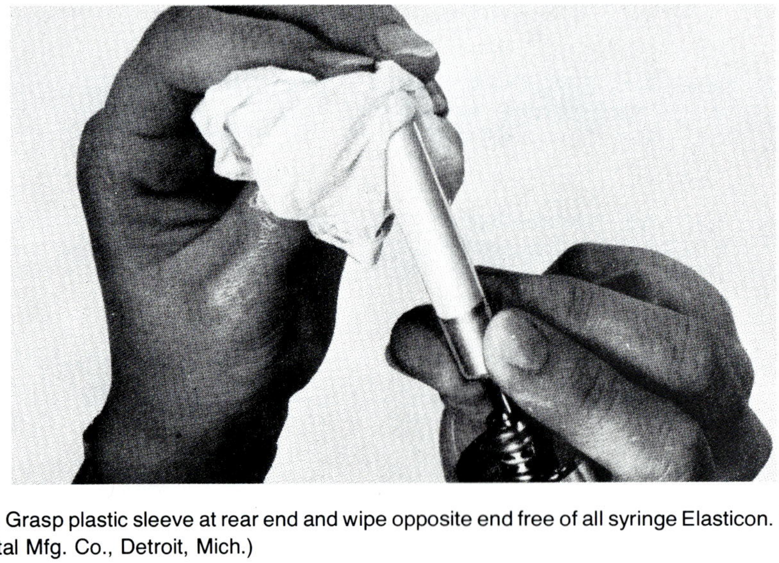

Fig. 9-57. Grasp plastic sleeve at rear end and wipe opposite end free of all syringe Elasticon. (Courtesy Kerr Dental Mfg. Co., Detroit, Mich.)

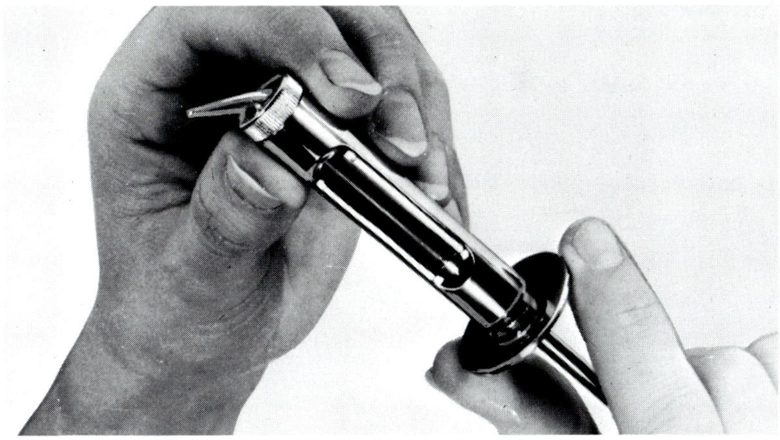

Fig. 9-58. Place filled plastic sleeve into metal barrel of syringe and screw locking disk down as far as possible. Tighten securely. (Courtesy Kerr Dental Mfg. Co., Detroit, Mich.)

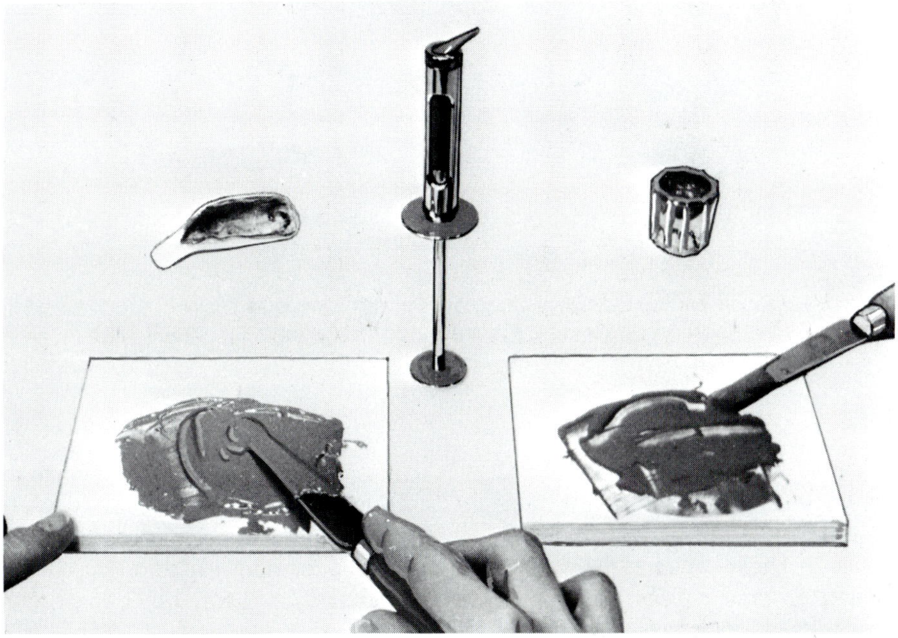

Fig. 9-59. Mixing of heavy-bodied Elasticon base and accelerator. Complete the mix within 40 to 45 seconds. (Courtesy Kerr Dental Mfg. Co., Detroit, Mich.)

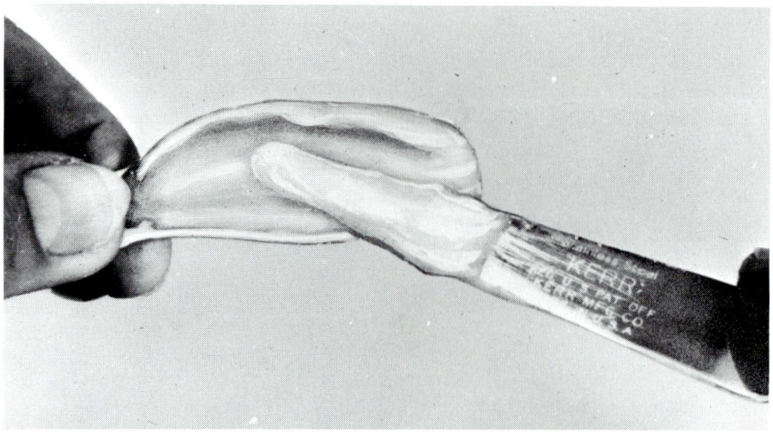

Fig. 9-60. Spreading of heavy-bodied Elasticon over all adhesive-covered surfaces of tray. (Courtesy Kerr Dental Mfg. Co., Detroit, Mich.)

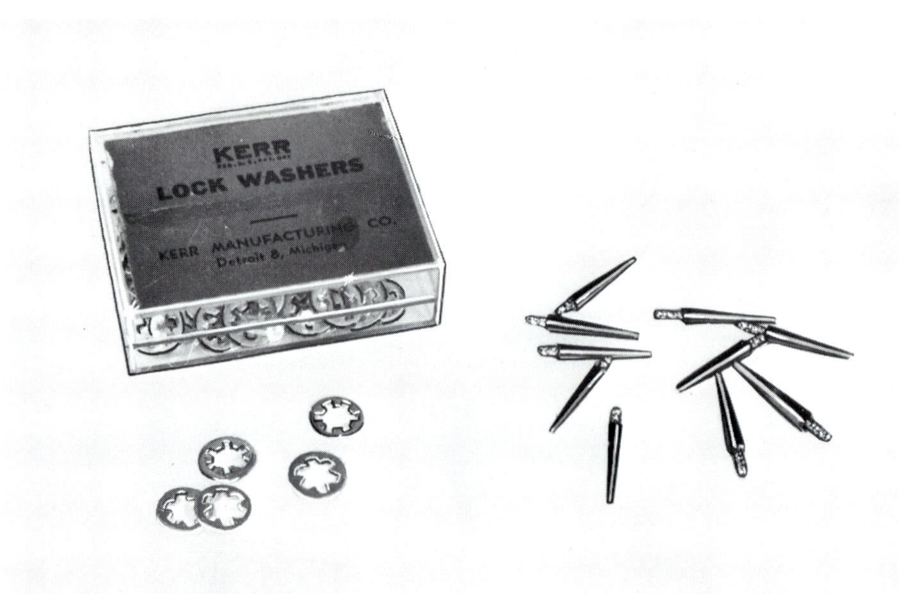

Fig. 9-61. Lock washers provide necessary anchorage between two pours of stone, and dowel pins are used to produce individual removable dies. (Courtesy Kerr Dental Mfg. Co., Detroit, Mich.)

not produce an accurate die. The hydrocolloid will imbibe the amount of water lost, but it will be done at the expense of a distorted die or cast, which is caused by the release of stresses within the impression. Phillips[6] sums it up thus: "Consequently, the dental stone cast should be constructed as soon as possible after the impression has been obtained, not only to prevent troublesome effects due to imbibition and syneresis, but also to minimize the possible distortions due to relaxation of stress."*

The impression was placed in a 2% aqueous solution of potassium sulfate to accelerate the setting of the stone die or cast, which is poured in the impres-

*From Skinner, E. W., and Phillips, R. W.: The science of dental materials, Philadelphia, 1960, W. B. Saunders Co., pp. 103, 105, 106.

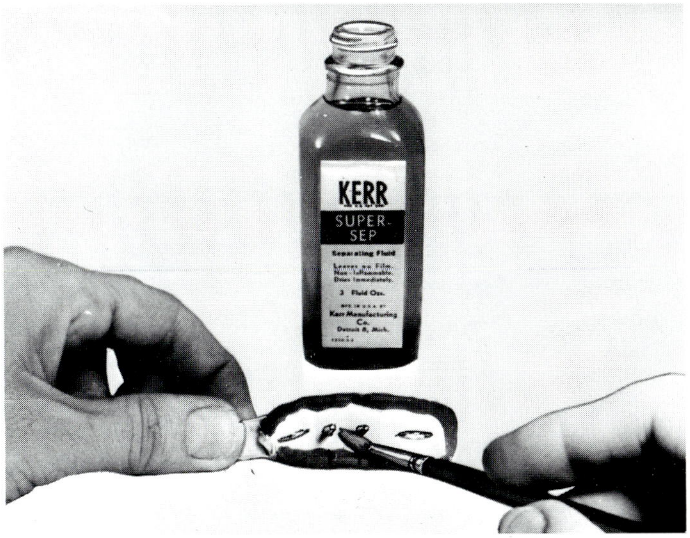

Fig. 9-62. Allow first pour of stone to set; then apply one or more coats of separating medium (Super Sep) over areas of dies that are to be removable. (Courtesy Kerr Dental Mfg. Co., Detroit, Mich.)

sion, and to give a smooth, dense surface to the stone. The impression can be poured after 5, 10, or 15 minutes in the potassium sulfate solution, but the period of time must not exceed 15 minutes. "It has been shown that the hardening solution may affect the dimensional stability of the hydrocolloid impression. This effect varies with the chemical employed, its concentration, and the composition of the gel. For this reason, the hydrocolloid impression should not be immersed in the hardening solution for more than 10 to 15 minutes since only the surface layer of the gel need be saturated with the solution. Usually, a period of five minutes is sufficient to provide such a saturation."*

While the impression is undergoing this treatment, preparation is being made for the stone mix. Before pouring the cast all excess and droplets of potassium sulfate solution are blown carefully out of the impression. Do not dehydrate the hydrocolloid surface, or the gel will adhere to the surface of the cast upon its removal. The surface of the impression should have a moist appearance (Fig. 9-64).

POURING THE CAST

TYPES AND CORRECT USE OF STONE

The type of stones to be used for the dies and casts are the newer Hydrocal stones, which have been specially prepared for the indirect technique; these stones possess a minimum amount of setting expansion and a maximum amount of surface hardness and smoothness.

Routine fabrication of dense, smooth dies and casts is very essential and can be accomplished by following the manufacturer's directions and adhering to a careful, standardized procedure.

The water-powder ratio always should be measured correctly, following the manufacturer's directions, because a variation influences surface smoothness as well as strength and setting expansion (Fig. 9-65). I advocate and use distilled water in all mixes to be poured into alginate and hydrocolloid impressions.

Mechanical spatulation, preferably under vacuum, is valuable in assuring a smoother, denser, and stronger die or cast (Fig. 9-66).

Powder and water also may be combined by hand mixing as well as by mechanical mixing under vacuum, and both these methods produce satisfactory results if properly carried out. In mechanical mixing care must be taken that the mixing time be comparatively short. Overmixing produces too rapid a set and also tends to increase slightly the setting expansion.

Phillips[9] has shown that the rate at which stone is flowed into the impression has a very significant effect upon the surface of the die, as does the amount of vibration that accompanies the flowing of the stone into the impression. Use mild agitation or vibration.

*From Skinner, E. W., and Phillips, R. W.: The science of dental materials, Philadelphia, 1960, W. B. Saunders Co., pp. 103, 105, 106.

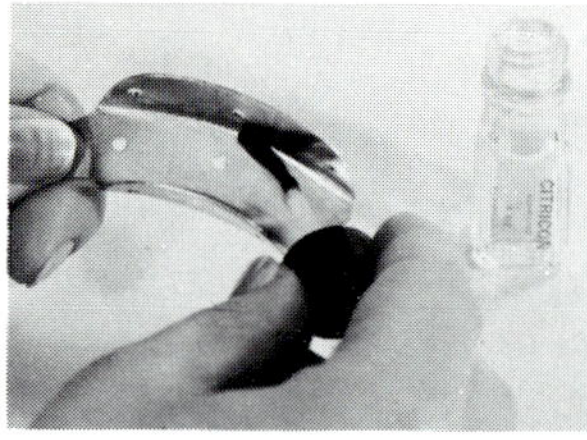

Select a close fitting perforated stock tray (Kerr Kwik-Tray). Apply Kerr Citricon Adhesive to all inner and peripheral surfaces of tray. Allow to dry.

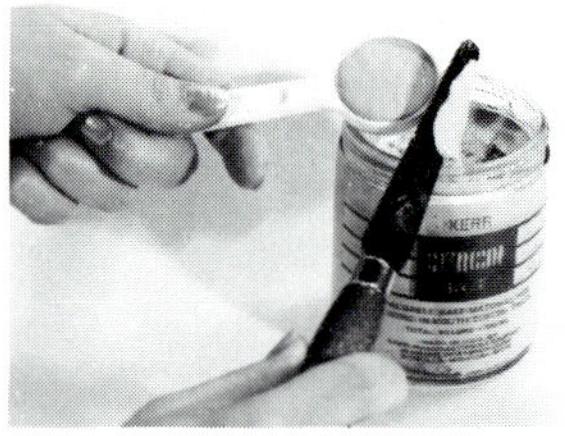

Dispense one (1) level scoop Citricon (putty) Base and place on mixing pad. For full mouth impressions 2 or 3 scoops may be necessary.

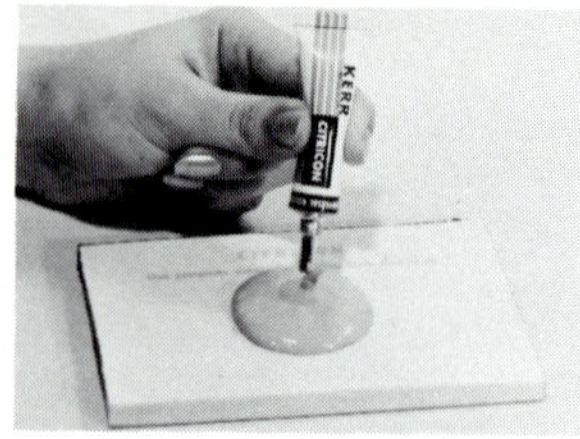

Add 6 to 8 drops Citricon Universal Accelerator

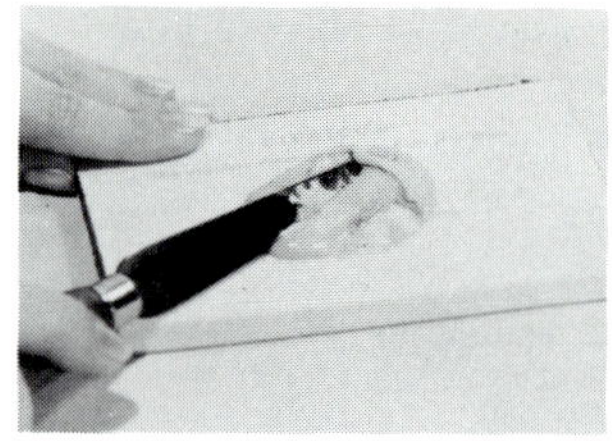

Incorporate on pad for 10 seconds.

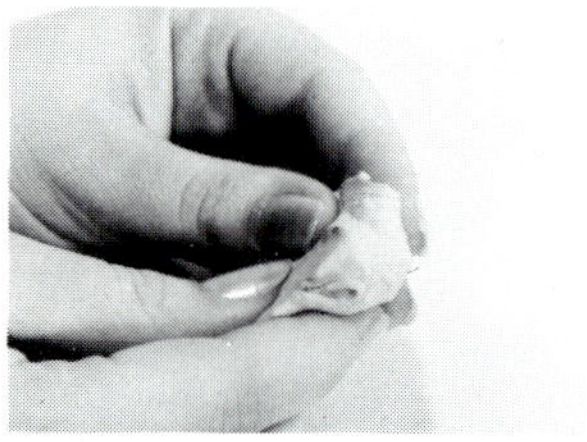

Transfer (putty-like) Base to hands and knead for 20 seconds, until streak-free.

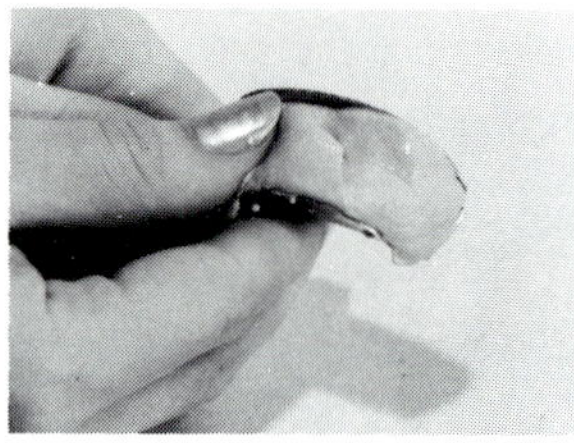

Place kneaded, putty-like base in stock tray to form your own custom tray.

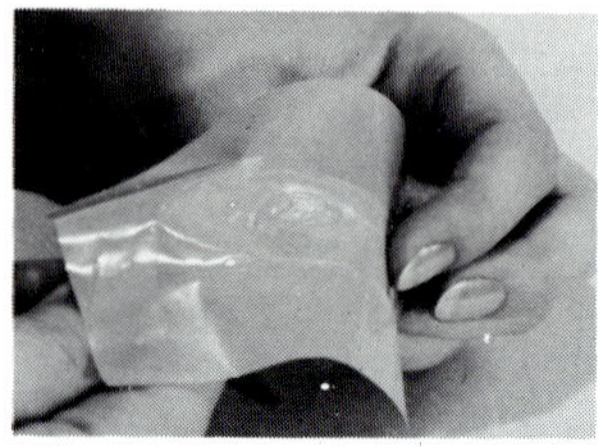

Cover with spacer and seat in mouth with **rocking motion.** **Note:** To insure that sufficient space is created, perform above procedure prior to cutting preparations.

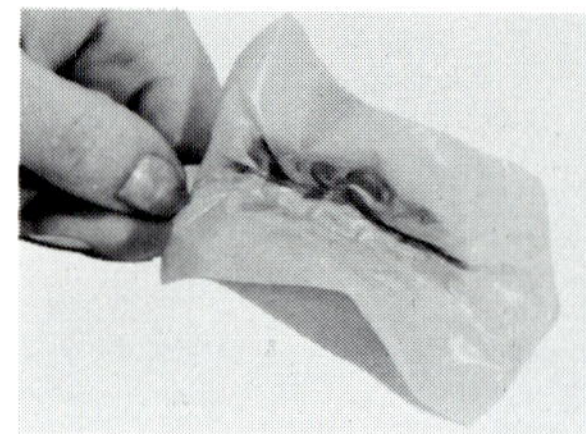

Remove from mouth after initial set (approximately 1 minute).

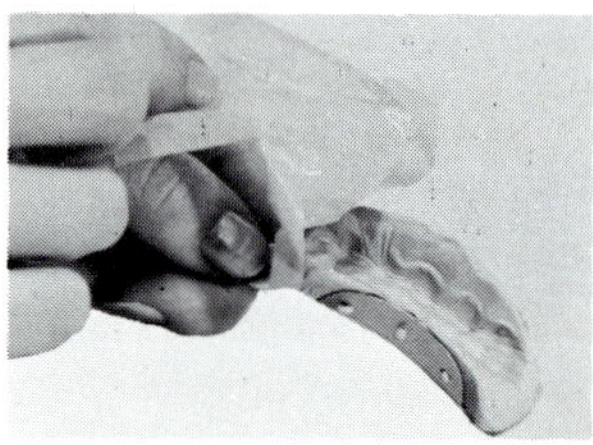

Strip spacer and reduce periphery with sharp blade. YOU HAVE NOW CREATED YOUR OWN CUSTOM TRAY.

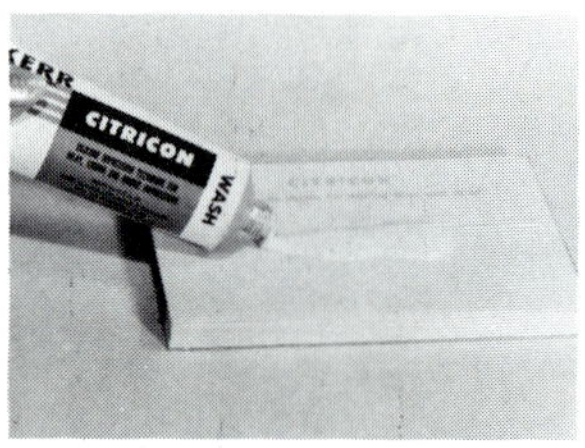

Extrude 2" of Citricon Wash (if a syringe is utilized, then a 3" mix should be used.)

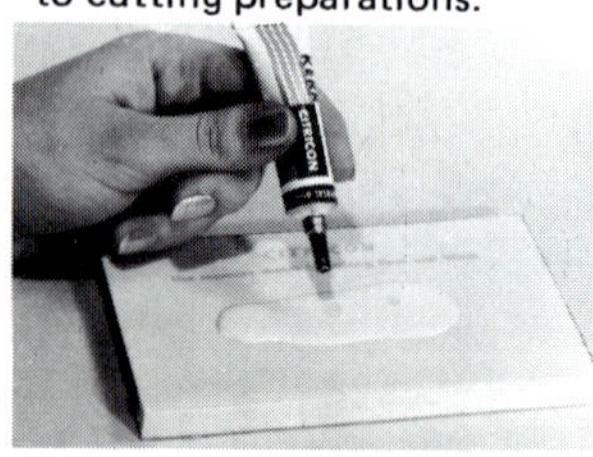

Add 1 drop of Citricon Universal Accelerator for each inch of extruded Citricon Wash.

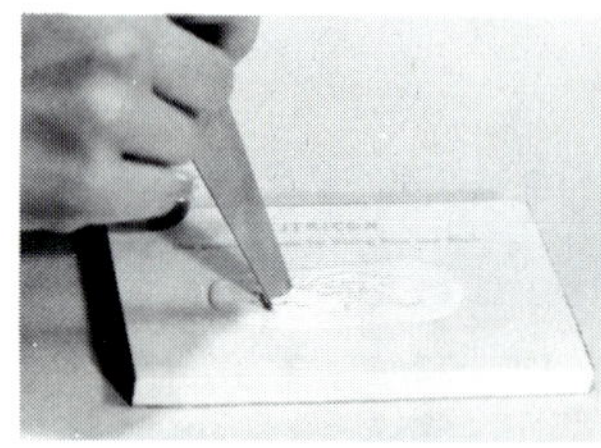

Mix with stirring motion until thoroughly incorporated.

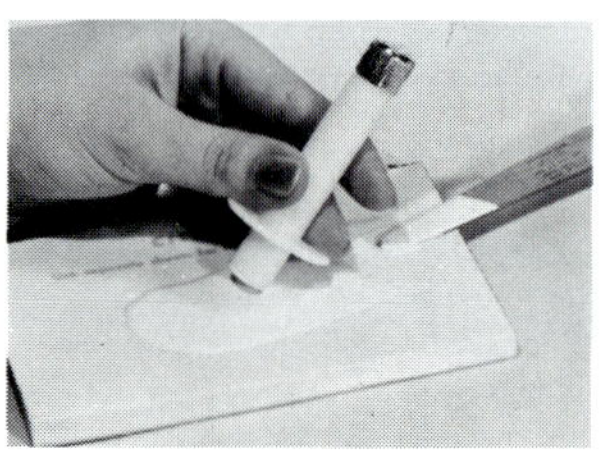

Fill syringe by scraping barrel through impression material at approximately 45° angle. Insert plunger and inject into preparations. Place remainder of wash material into custom tray.

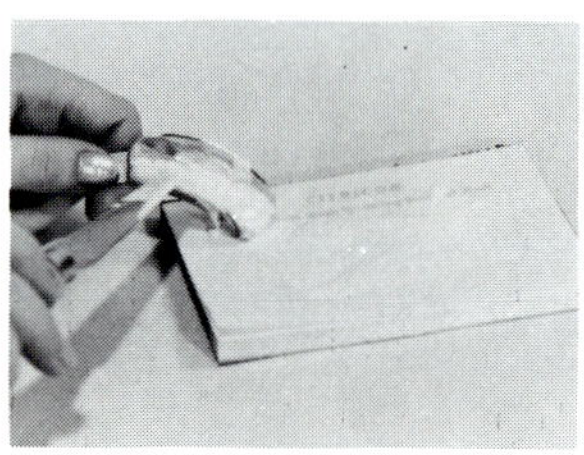

ALTERNATE FINAL IMPRESSION PROCEDURE FOR FULL CROWN PREPARATIONS W/TAPERED WALLS & NO SUBGINGIVAL INVOLVEMENT: Place mixed Citricon Wash into tray in the area of preparation & insert in mouth. Hold without pressure until set (3-4 minutes).

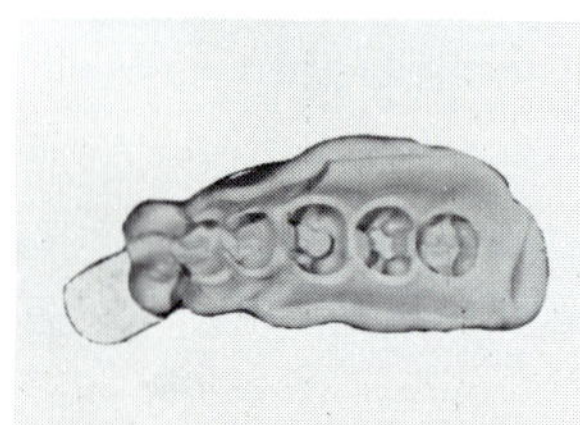

FINAL, ACCURATE CITRICON IMPRESSION.

CITRICON APPLICATIONS

- Crown and Bridge impressions (quadrant or full mouth)
- Partial denture impressions
- Full denture impressions
- Copper band impressions and
- Citricon putty for bite registration.

Fig. 9-63. The Citricon Technique for inlay, crown and bridge impressions. (Courtesy Kerr Dental Mfg. Co., Detroit, Mich.)

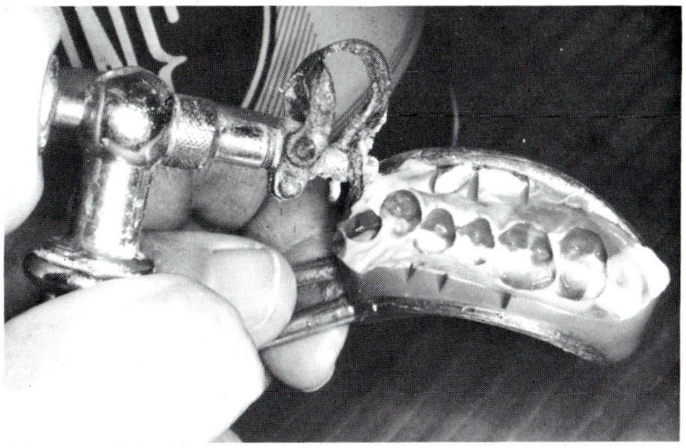

Fig. 9-64. Do not dehydrate surface of impression. Surface must have moist appearance to avoid adherence of gel to cast surface.

It also is important that the stone be added slowly and in small quantities. Put the stone in one section of the impression, and allow the stone to flow into the other parts of the impression from this initial point of application. (See Figs. 9-67 to 9-70.)

While the stone is setting, the poured impression is placed into a humidor in an atmosphere of 100% humidity.

The poured impression should never be put in the same solution as that used to immerse the impressions coming from the chair. It is thought that the salt from the stone comes out in the solution and very soon enriches the solution so that succeeding impressions are warped.

Another method that is used by some for pouring up the hydrocolloid impression is to vibrate gently the properly mixed stone into the impression, using small increments of stone until the cavity portion is filled completely. A portion of the remaining stone is dried partially by compressing it in a towel, placing it on top of the softer material in the impression, and lightly vibrating for a few seconds to create a union of the two parts. This results in a very hard stone die or cast.

A

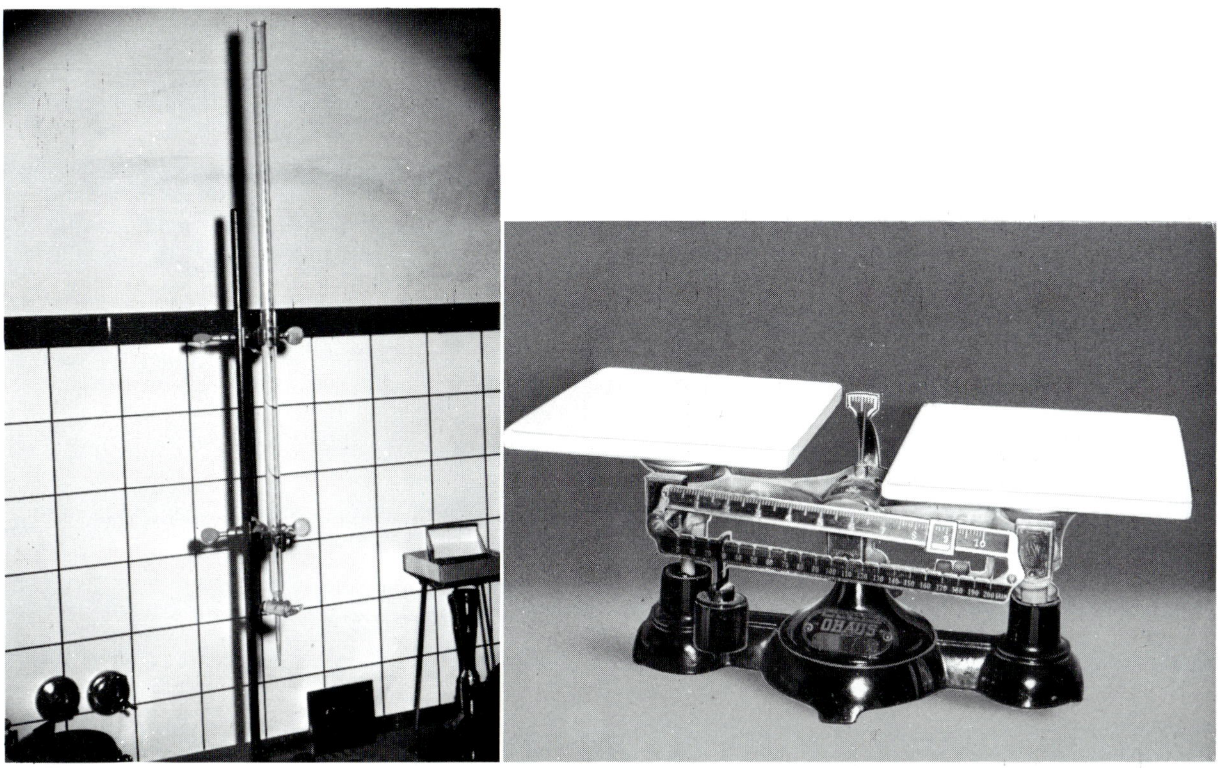

B

Fig. 9-65. Accurate measuring devices for water-powder ratio. **A,** Burette; **B,** scale.

A 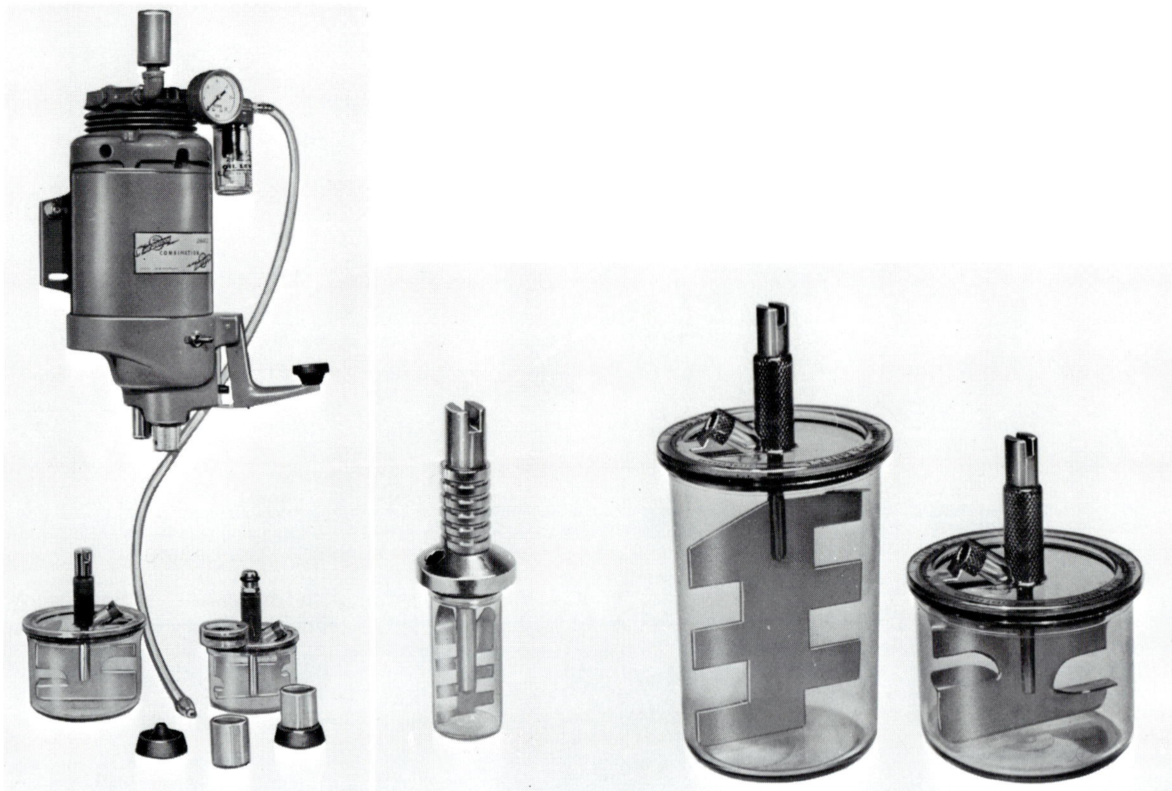 B

Fig. 9-66. Means of mechanical spatulation. A, Power mixer and Vac-U-Spat. B, Die mixer and Vac-U-Mixer. (Courtesy Whip-Mix Corp., Louisville, Ky.)

DOWEL PINS

Before the impression is poured, if removable stone dies are desired, dowel pins may be suspended in position by means of straight banker's pins and sticky wax or use can be made of the Mann paralleling instrument (Figs. 9-71 to 9-73), or they may be placed in position, after the initial pour, in previously marked areas (Figs. 9-74 and 9-75). The Di-Lok technique is also very good.

After the poured impression has been in the humidor for 30 minutes, a second mix of stone (if dowel pins are used) of a different color but with identical physical properties is added to the first mix and is returned immediately to the humidor for another 30 minutes (Figs. 9-76 to 9-78). This step is very useful in die separation because, when the saw cut reaches the stone of the second color, we know that the cut has been completed.

After being in the humidor for 60 minutes from the time of the initial pour, the cast is separated from the impression (Fig. 9-79). Premature separation will cause a rough surface. No attempt should be made to work on the die or cast (such as waxing and carving) until the stone has hardened fully, approximately 24 hours later.

Trim the dies while still damp, if possible, to avoid chipping. Properly trimmed dies give good access to all cavity margins; therefore the proper removal of stone bulk around the root portion is necessary. This allows for the proper use of the carving tool while contouring the margins of the wax patterns.

IMPORTANT FACTORS IN USE OF GYPSUM PRODUCTS

Docking[10] points out some very important factors to consider when gypsum products are used:

1. "Particle size, setting time, expansion and strength are the important physical factors, and some manufacturers furnish this data on the product label.

Fig. 9-67

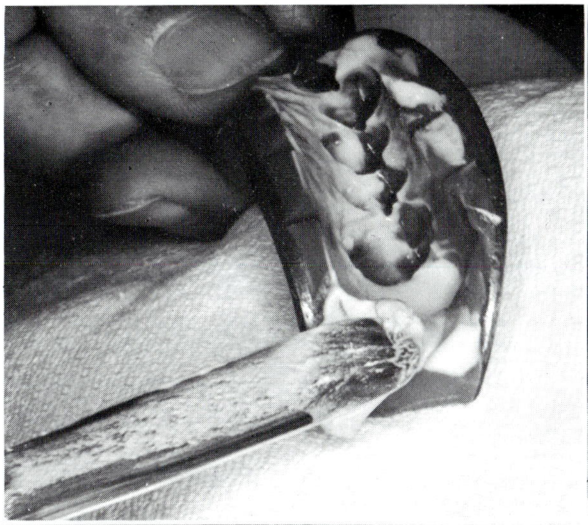

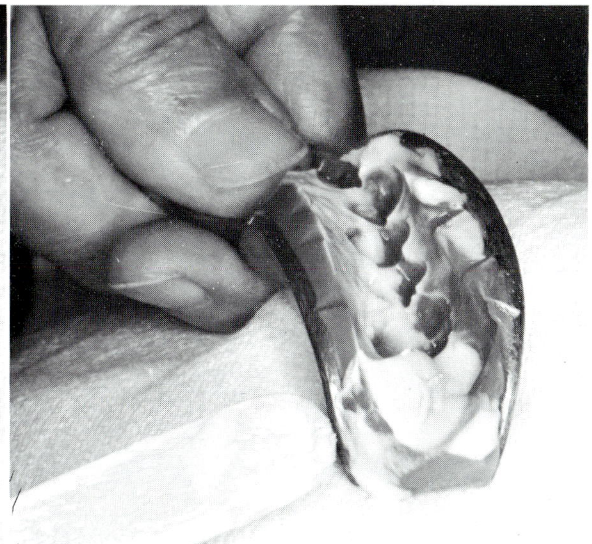

Fig. 9-68

Fig. 9-69

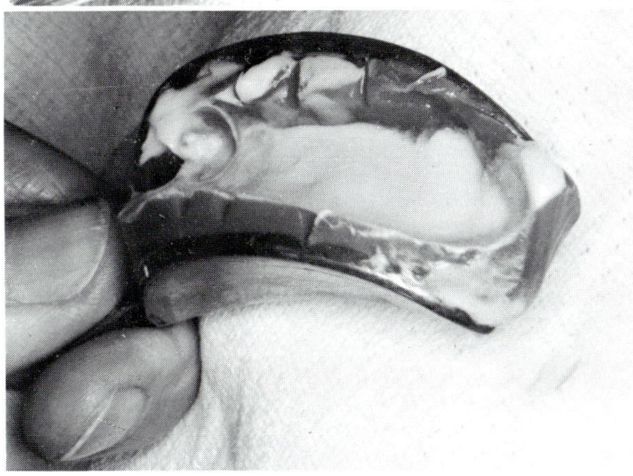

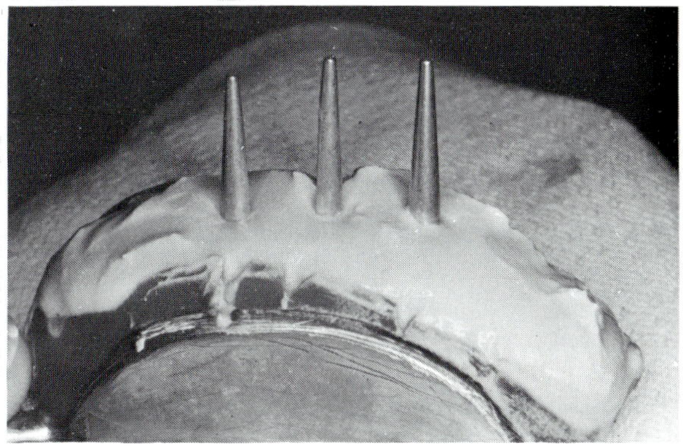

Fig. 9-70

Figs. 9-67 to 9-70. Correct pouring of small elastic impression. Put stone in one section of impression and allow it to flow to other parts of impression, using mild vibration and adding stone slowly and in small quantities. Position dowel pins and place immediately in a humidor.

2. "The mixing ratio is the key to the proper use of gypsum products. Plaster, artificial stone, and the extra strength die stones differ physically, but are based on the same chemical entity—calcium sulfate hemihydrate. Their chief physical difference lies in the compactness and uniformity of the crystals. With an artificial stone, less water is required for a given consistency than with plaster. The water-powder ratio recommended by the manufacturer usually can be relied upon to give the optimum properties for a particular product.

3. "One of the ways of producing relatively gross distortion of the impression is to invert the filled impression and press it firmly down into a heap of stone on the bench.

4. "Soaking in water, glycerin, or oil was not found to improve the surface hardness or abrasion resistance, and it definitely reduced the crushing strength of the stones investigated.

5. "Although plasters and stones are commonplace materials, they require care in handling for best results. This entails the selection of suitable products for the work in hand, correct proportioning for optimum strength and hardness, careful spatulation and pouring to minimize porosity, and adequate precautions concerning any impression materials and separating media that come into contact with them."*

---

*From Docking, Allan R.: Plaster and stone, Dent. Clin. N. Am., pp. 727-735, Nov., 1958.

Figs. 9-71 to 9-73. Mann paralleling instrument is excellent for suspending dowel pins into position.

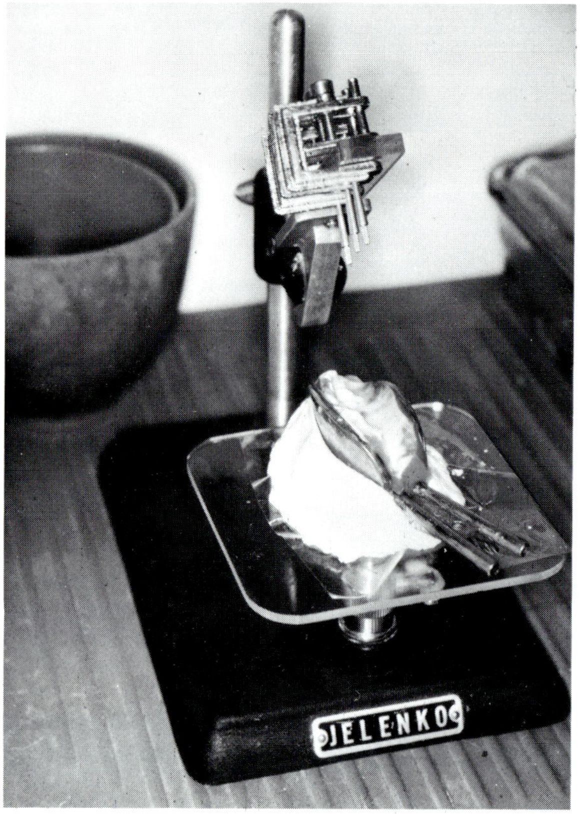

Fig. 9-71. Impression (with moist cotton in cavity area) is positioned on base of paralleling instrument by means of quick-setting impression plaster.

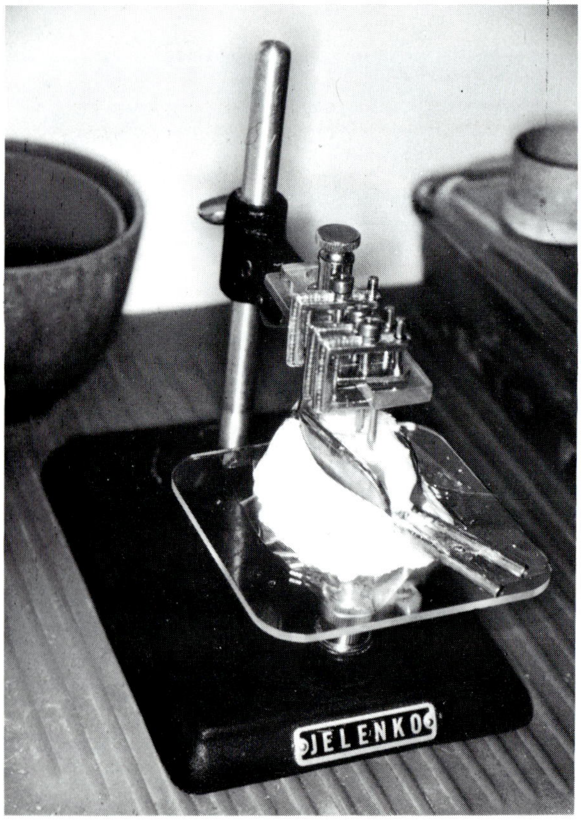

Fig. 9-72. Dowel pins aligned so that they center correctly in each preparation area and are parallel to each other. Stone poured and pins lowered into position.

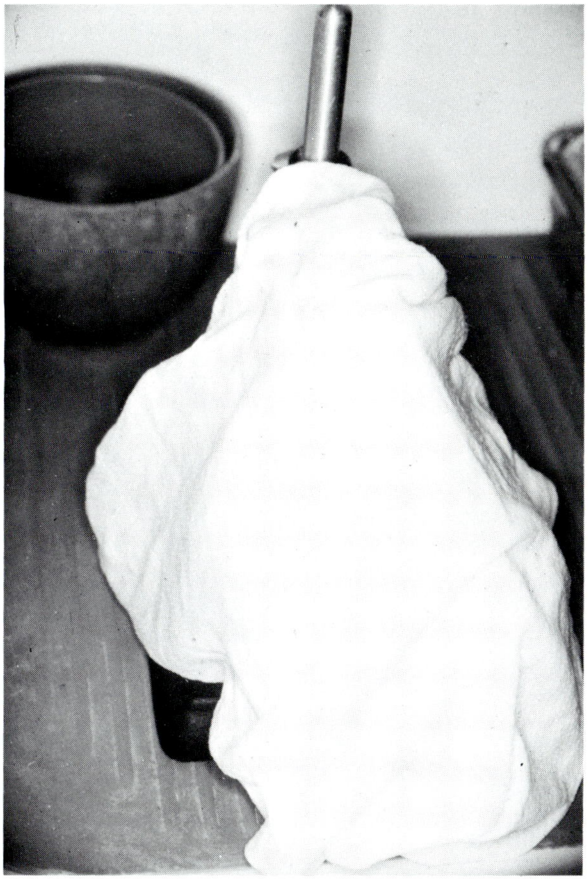

Fig. 9-73. Whole assembly is covered with a wet towel to obtain an atmosphere close to 100% humidity.

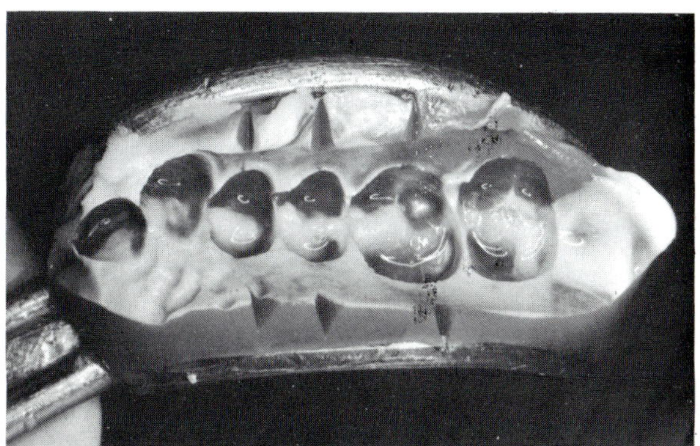

Fig. 9-74

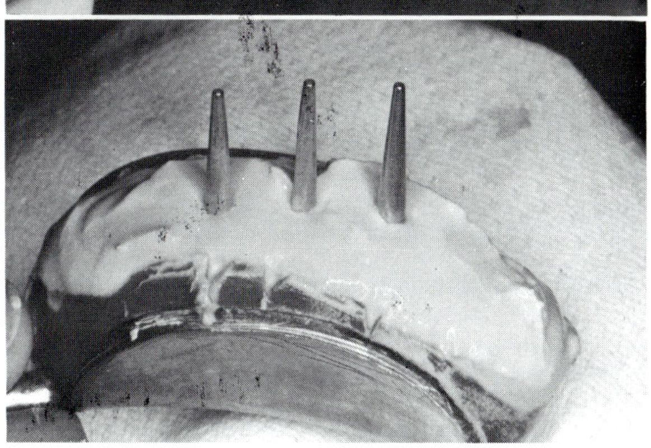

Fig. 9-75

Figs. 9-74 and 9-75. Dowel pins can be placed in position, after initial pour, in previously marked areas (small V-shaped "cutouts").

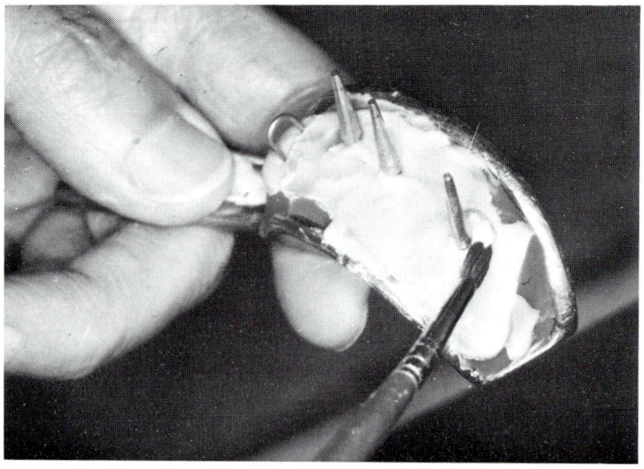

Fig. 9-76

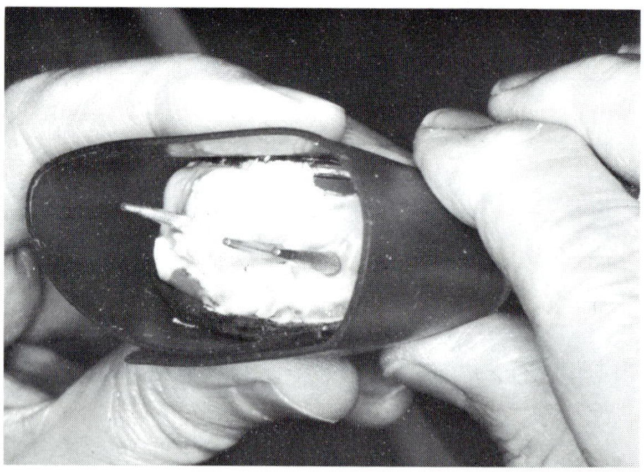

Fig. 9-77

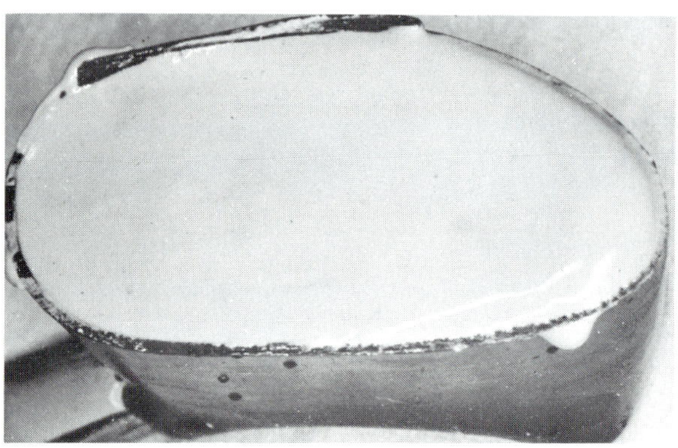

Fig. 9-78

Figs. 9-76 to 9-78. After poured impression has set, a coat of separating medium is applied over areas of dies that are to be removable, the impression is boxed and poured with a stone of a different color but identical physical properties. A stone of different color for this second pour is necessary for convenience in die separation.

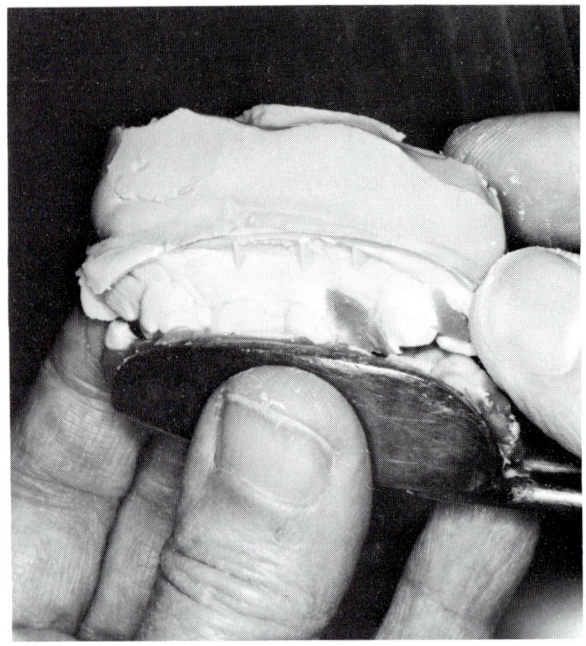

Fig. 9-79. Carefully separate cast from impression after it has been in humidor for 45 to 60 minutes. Premature separation causes rough surfaces.

COPPER TUBE–MODELING COMPOUND IMPRESSION

WHEN TO USE

I use the copper tube–modeling compound impression when retraction of the gingival tissue to take a hydrocolloid or rubber base impression is impossible without radical procedures. This applies only to full veneer crowns.

TECHNIQUE

An annealed copper band is selected as soon as the peripheral outline of the preparation has been established. The band should fit the cervical margin snugly and should be festooned to fit slightly over the shoulder or chamfer. In other words, slip the copper band over the prepared tooth until it reaches the gingival crest of the interdental papilla and mark its overtension with a pencil. Remove the band and festoon with a contouring scissors, following the pencil mark. Remove rough cut edges with a stone, and keep repeating the process of fitting the band, pencil marking overextensions, festooning, and smoothing the cut edges until the band extends approximately 1 mm. beyond the peripheral outline of the preparation. Burnishing all around the gingival collar of the band with a plastic instrument, espe-

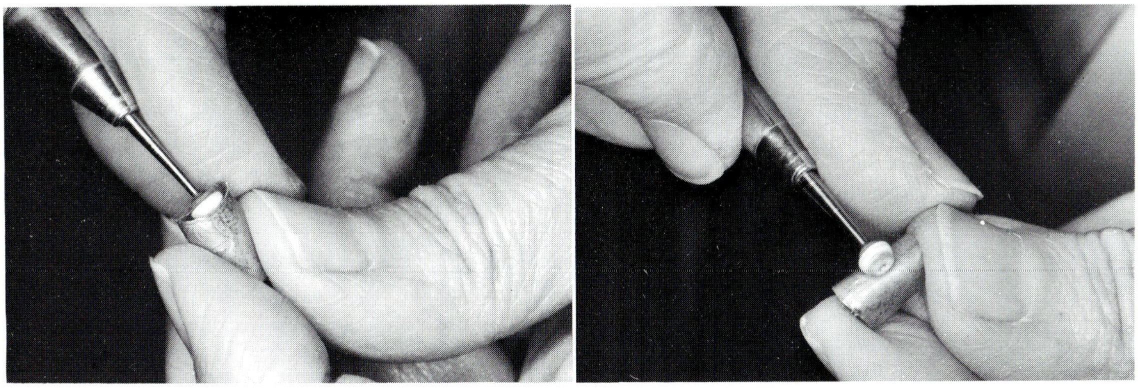

Fig. 9-80. Copper band prepared to fit cervical margin snugly, going slightly over shoulder or chamfer. Smooth edges, stone inner surface of band at gingival edge for 2 to 3 mm. to get a positive seal of compound to band, and mark facial surface for identification.

cially when confronted with barrelled teeth, is worthy of consideration.[11] Square out the occlusal end of the band with a contouring pliers. When I have reached this stage of the operation, and before I fill the band with modeling compound, I take a preliminary impression of the prepared tooth with a beading or carding wax to view for any possible undercuts and sharpness of the preparation, as suggested by Dr. I. F. Miller. If necessary, further festooning may be accomplished before completion of the modeling compound impression. Be sure to smooth the edges of the band, to stone the inner surface of the band at the gingival edge for about 2 mm., ensuring a positive seal of the compound to the band, and to have the band parallel to the long axis of the tooth. Be sure that the festooned band will stay firmly in place when tested for rocking with finger pressure. Mark the labial or buccal surface of the band for identification. (See Fig. 9-80.) The above procedure must be executed with great care so that the gingival tissue is not damaged.

Soften the compound by means of dry heat, tempering the surface which will contact the tooth in hot water. Seat the filled band carefully on the prepared tooth, which has been slightly lubricated with petroleum jelly, and when it is in position, which will be evident when a little compound is forced out at the cervical area, put pressure on the impression material with a finger. Chill with tepid water, or hold without chilling for 3 minutes, and remove the band with a steady vertical pull after all excess compound has been removed subgingivally and occlusally. The impression also can be removed with the aid of a

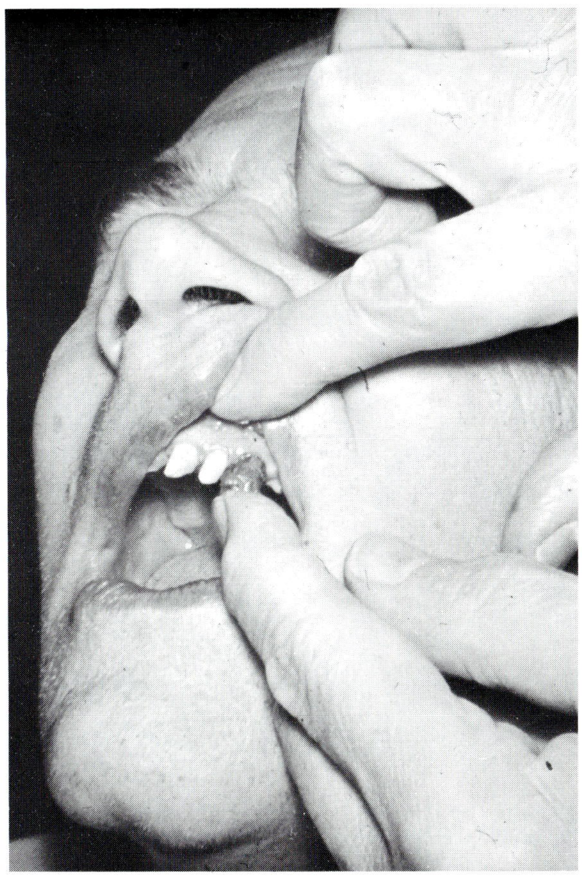

Fig. 9-81. Position copper tube–modeling compound impression with great care. Chill with tepid water or hold without chilling for 3 minutes. Remove with steady vertical pull after excess compound has been removed subgingivally and occlusally.

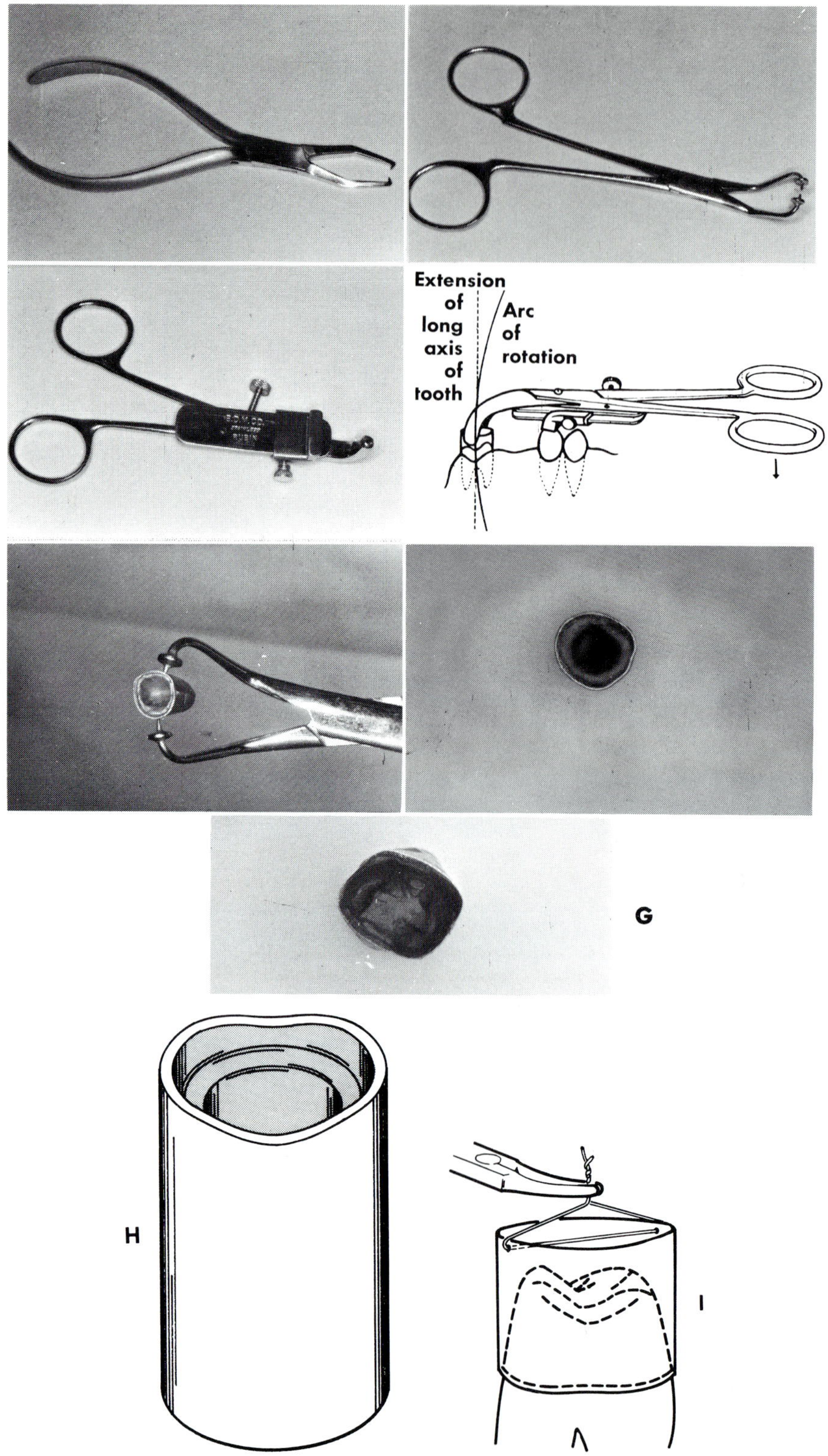

Fig. 9-82. A to **G,** Special pliers such as Rubin and Baade can be used in removal of copper tube–modeling compound impressions. **H,** A properly developed copper tube–modeling compound impression. **I,** A wire of 25 to 28 gauge is threaded through small holes made in the occlusal end of the copper band and twisted to form a "bale," which will ensure the removal of the band with the finished impression in the proper line of withdrawal with the least possibility of distortion. (Suggested by E. David Shooshan.) (**D** courtesy Buffalo Dental Mfg. Co., Brooklyn, N. Y.)

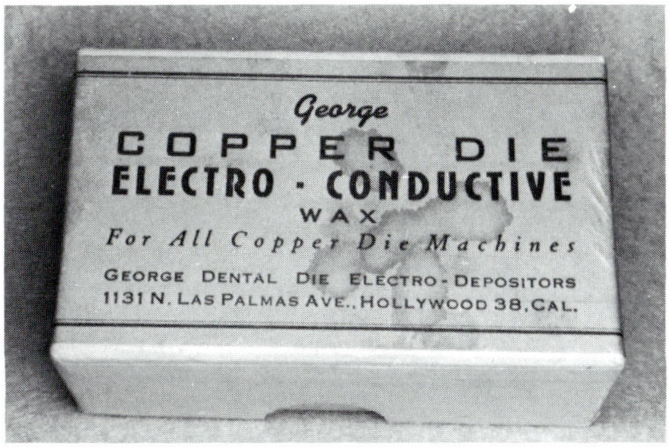

Fig. 9-83. Copper tube–modeling compound impression rebasing material for greater accuracy.

Baade pliers or the Rubin copper tube impression remover in the long axis of the tooth. Never rock or twist the band impression when removing it from a tooth. (See Figs. 9-81 and 9-82.)

Examine the impression very carefully for all preparation details. In some instances the impression is rebased with George copper die electroconductive wax (Fig. 9-83). This particular type of wax does not harden completely when it sets, so that care must be taken to prevent distortion. Impressions taken with copper bands can temporarily detach the gingiva from the root, but the removal of all particles of impression material from this area will be followed by a healing of the gingival margin.

Introduction of a new instrument, the Starlite Feinberg Bandlever,* and of a new method for installing and removing copper bands has resulted in modeling compound impressions free of warpage and distortion, achieved with extraordinary operational ease.

INSTRUMENTATION AND TECHNIQUE

1. Select a properly annealed copper band to fit tooth. Contour gingival portion to fit (Fig. 9-84, *A*).

2. Use a bur or hand-punch pliers to place a small hole in the buccal surface and another in the lingual surface, as near to occlusal edge of copper band as possible (Fig. 9-84, *B*).

3. Cut a straight portion of wire from a paper clip. Make a loop 3 to 4 mm. long on one side. Pass the wire through holes in band so that the loop end is on the buccal side. Leave enough clip wire to extend 3 to 4 mm. past the lingual edge of band (Fig. 9-84, *C*).

*Star Dental Mfg. Co., Inc., Philadelphia, Pa.

4. Grasp the lingual end of the wire with a hemostat so that the loop end will be drawn firmly against the band. The hemostat should be placed firmly against band on lingual side as shown in Fig. 9-84, *D*. The band cannot move or turn while held in position over the flame. The compound is heated evenly and is soft throughout entire copper band, with proper flowability, giving increased working time (Fig. 9-84, *D*).

5. Take from flame, remove the hemostat, and, using fingers greased with petroleum jelly, grasp the band with one finger on the buccal wire loop, the other on the occlusal ridge of the copper band. Place over the tooth, pressing toward the gingiva to make the impression. Hold in place while compound is chilled with water spray, and then trim away excess compound with a Starlite MG Columbia 2 L or 2 R Curette* (Fig. 9-84, *E*).

6. Using a Starlite Feinberg Bandlever, remove the band. This instrument automatically exerts firm pressure parallel to the long axis of the tooth, to break the seal between tooth and compound without distorting or warping the impression. Starlite Bandlever is used in this fashion:

   a. Removable arms are locked in two of the four holes in the Bandlever to fit under wire extending on the buccal and lingual sides of band (Fig. 9-84, *F*).
   b. Place a wooden tongue depressor on an adjacent tooth, which will provide a fulcrum upon which to operate the Bandlever (Fig. 9-84, *G*).
   c. Gently, using lever action, move handle of Bandlever toward gingiva, breaking seal between compound and prepared tooth. Band on an upper tooth will fall off. A band on a lower tooth may be lifted off easily after seal is broken.

MAKING THE DIE

The die from this impression can be copper-plated, or a die can be made of stone.

POURING THE IMPRESSION IN STONE

Wrap the band with a piece of 30 gauge casting wax extending 8 to 10 mm. beyond the cervical margin.

Again, remembering the need of following the manufacturer's instructions as to the recommended water-powder ratio, carefully spatulate the mix and introduce small increments of stone into the impression by the use of mild vibration, thereby avoiding any

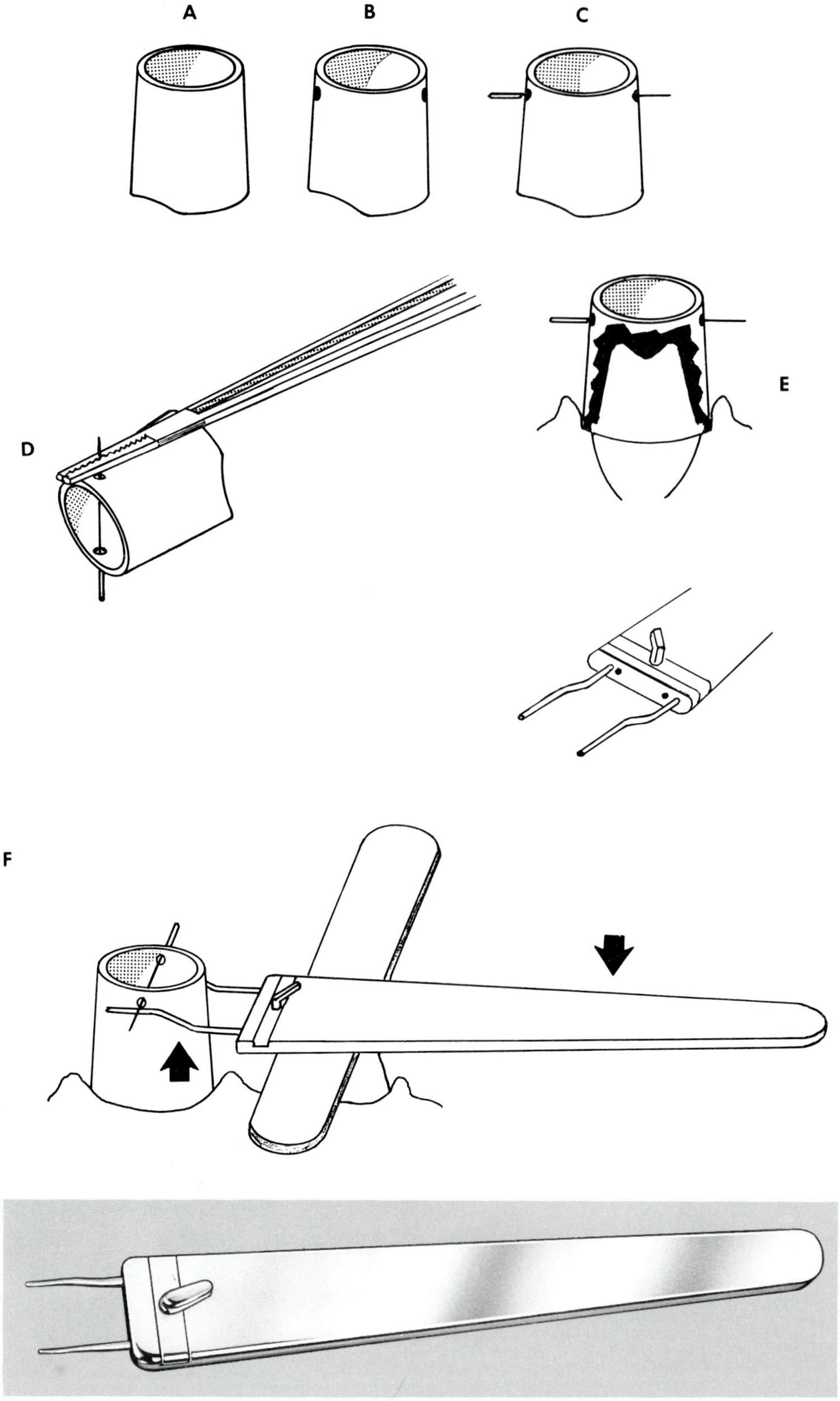

Fig. 9-84. Starlite Feinberg bandlever technique. Correlate illustrations with text. (Courtesy Star Dental Mfg. Co., Philadelphia, Pa.)

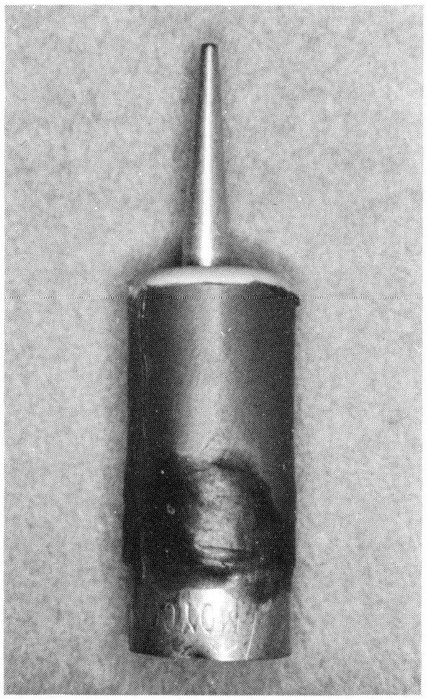

Fig. 9-85. Copper tube–modeling compound impression wrapped with a piece of 30 gauge wax extending 8 to 10 mm. beyond cervical margin. Fill with stone and insert brass dowel.

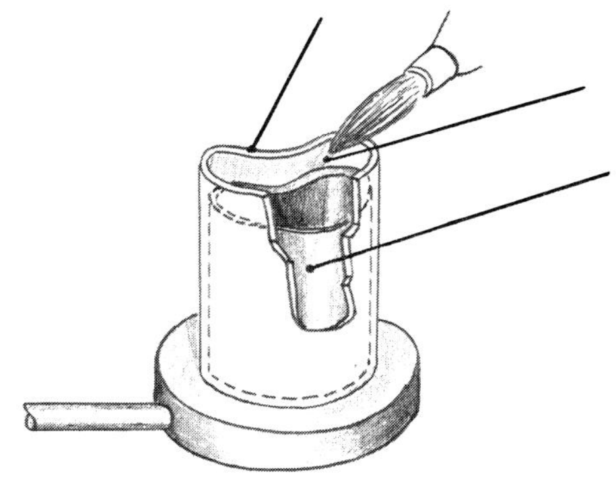

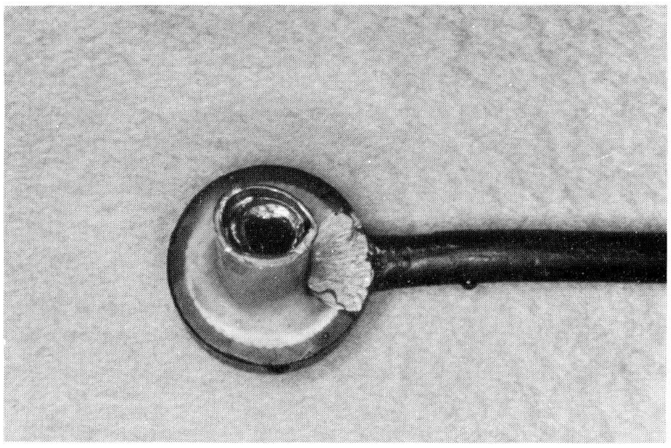

Fig. 9-86. Tube impression attached to cathode platform. It has a 2 mm. collar of wax (protection skirt), which is metallized with the impression.

imperfections or voids in the finished die. When the impression has been filled with stone, insert a Jelenko or Ney brass dowel pin to ensure a good handle when the pattern is being waxed (Fig. 9-85).

COPPERPLATING THE IMPRESSION

Copperplated dies offer dimensional accuracy and edge strength, making it possible to obtain fine margins. They offer good surface strength and therefore may be swaged against; they will not contaminate precious metals.

For proper contact, trim any excess compound or wax at the closed end of the band to expose the edge of the copper band and ensure metal-to-metal contact with the cathode platform. Wash the impression, dry it thoroughly, and attach it to the cathode platform with sticky wax. Cover the joint of the holder and platform with wax.

Adapt the usual 28 gauge wax chimney closely to the band after it is attached properly to the cathode platform, as previously described. Trim the wax to within 2 mm. of the band, and metallize this 2 mm. collar of wax with the impression, using Flash* or Aqua Dag.† In other words, the impression is made conductive by metallizing it with graphite (Fig. 9-86). Apply this with a small brush, using a rotary motion and making sure that every surface and angle is metallized thoroughly and is extended to the 2 mm. collar of 28 gauge casting wax. The metallized 2 mm. chimney plates a copper protection skirt,[12] this added area obviating the possibility of the dentist or technician marring the definitive marginal area of the die by the accidental slip of the stone, disk, or bur that is used in its trimming. Use compressed air very carefully to force all excess graphite from the impression and to dry the surface.

Over this metallized 2 mm. chimney adapt another layer of 28 gauge wax in the usual way, leaving it unmetallized. Wind this layer of wax tightly around the band and lute it together securely, forming one waxed unit with the cathode platform and covering all metal surfaces. The metallized impression is now ready for the tank.

Wet the impression in copper electrolyte, retaining a little of the electrolyte in the impression, and sprinkle control powder over the impression so that

---

*Hanau Engineering Co., Inc., Buffalo, N. Y.

†Acheson Colloid Corp., Port Huron, Mich.

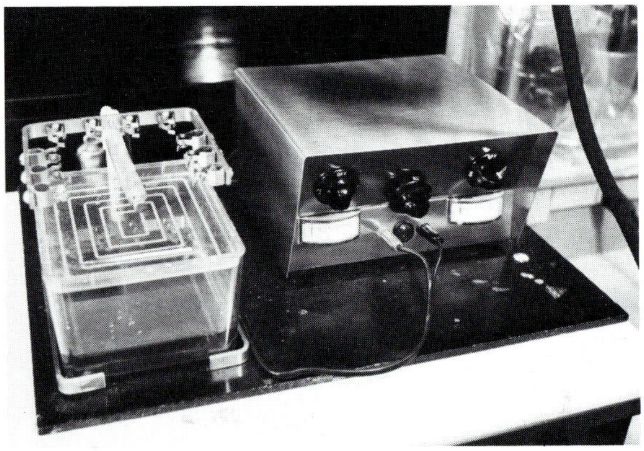

Fig. 9-87. Metallized impression on cathode platform is lowered into electroforming unit. Cathode holder is inserted into cathode clip of unit.

all metallized areas are covered thinly with this powder. With a medicine dropper containing some copper electrolyte, mix control powder by playing the liquid back and forth from the dropper to the impression until the blue of the electrolyte has disappeared and a copper-colored sludge has been created.

Wash the impression under the tap or, if necessary, use a forced stream of water, since the impression must be clean of all sludge. Insert the cathode holder into the cathode clip of the electroforming unit, avoiding trapped air. To eliminate the possibility of air entrapment it is advisable to fill the impression with some electrolyte such as ethyl alcohol before the cathode is lowered into the bath. (See Fig. 9-87.)

Start the electroplating at one half of $^1/_{10}$ (0.05) ampere and allow the impression to remain in the bath at this amperage for about 20 minutes, after which it should be removed and examined to see that the electroplating is being uniformly deposited. If so, replace it in the copper sulfate bath for 8 to 10 hours or overnight, raising the current to 0.1 ampere.

With the latest model Hanau Electroformer (Fig. 9-87), 50 milliamperes is recommended for the average single tooth impression in copper. The copper deposit must at all times be a "salmon pink" color. Darker deposits indicate excessive current which must be reduced immediately. I have had very good results using between 20 and 30 milliamperes for one or two impressions, with the new model Hanau Electroformer, overnight.

With this model for one or two average single tooth impressions, the *Low,* 0-100 Milliameter is used, and for three to ten impressions the *High,* 0-1 Ammeter is used—with Rheostat Knob adjusting current.

After completion of the deposit, remove the impression from the cathode support and wash under the tap, neutralize with sodium bicarbonate, wash again, and dry with air. Box with wax or Mystik tape to receive the stone, clear plastic, or low-fusing metal for a base or root. If a low-fusing alloy such as Dialoy* is used, coat the surface of copper with a film of 50% zinc chloride, which acts as a flux and permits a union of the low-fusing alloy with the copper.[13] Lucia[14] advocates reinforcing the plated band with soft solder and attaching a metal stem to the solder, thus ensuring a crush-proof die.

When this base material has set, warm the impression and remove the die, which should be cleaned to remove all traces of debris. Then the base can be trimmed to the desired shape. (See Fig. 9-88.)

TEMPORARY COVERAGE

NECESSITY FOR TEMPORARY RESTORATIONS

After the teeth have been prepared and the impressions taken, the next step is the construction of well-made temporary restorations.

Good "temporaries" are a must because of the importance to seal freshly cut areas, especially the cervical finish lines, and to obviate the possibility of forces being introduced that would cause positional tooth changes to take place. This type of coverage, provided coronal contours, embrasures, contact areas, margins, and occlusal form are executed properly, will maintain the necessary positional relationships in the interval between preparation and placement of the permanent restoration. Also it will allow hyperemic pulps, which were caused during tooth preparation, to recover and possibly to form secondary dentin because of the temporary sedative cement used. It also serves to test parallelism of abutment preparations and to determine the correct vertical dimension, esthetic possibilities, minor tooth movements, status of temporomandibular joint disorders, questionable teeth, and state of health of the periodontal tissues before the construction of the final restoration.

I believe that one cannot compromise this phase of the operation. The consumption of time and nervous energy is costly, economically and physically, if inadequate temporary restorations are constructed because of breakage, displacement, gingival irritation, positional changes, etc. Gold or gold-acrylic

*J. M. Ney Co., Hartford, Conn.

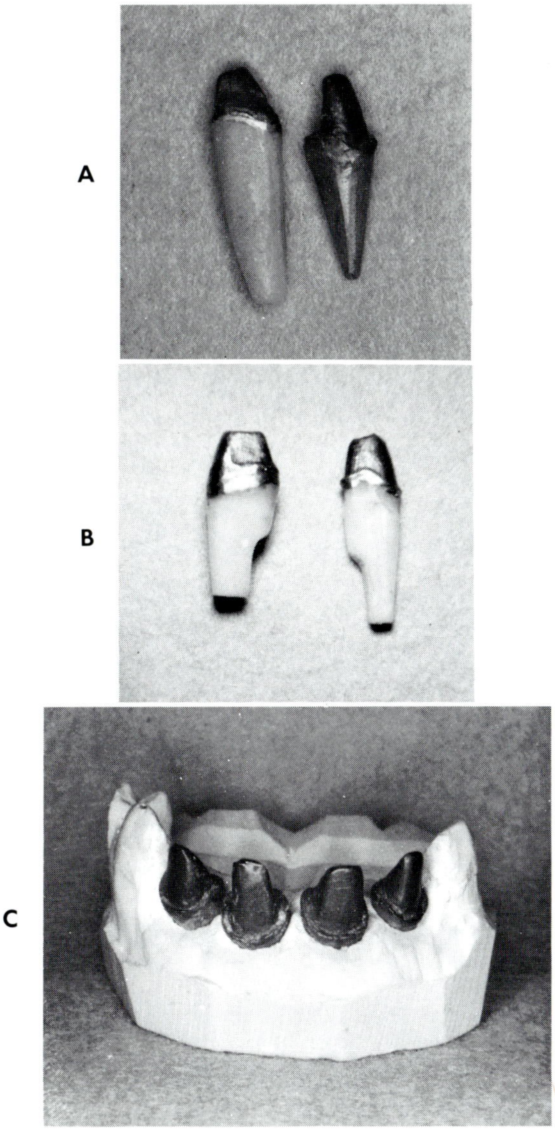

Fig. 9-88. A and **C,** Base or root of copperplated die can be made of plastic or low-fusing metal. **B,** Properly prepared roots or stems of copper plated dies.

temporary restorations should be made for all patients except the ones that can be completed in a very short span of time. (See Fig. 9-89.)

CONSTRUCTION OF TEMPORARY RESTORATIONS

TECHNIQUE 1 (ACRYLIC TEMPORARIES)

1. An alginate impression is taken of each arch, hinge-bow transfer made, and centric bite taken for mounting on an anatomic articulator. This allows for the making of the acrylic splints before any tooth preparations have been started in the mouth.

2. Mounted casts are equilibrated for gross discrepancies, and the teeth on the casts are prepared to conform approximately to the anticipated preparation in the mouth. Slight underpreparation allows for an easier seating of the acrylic splint shell (Fig. 9-90).

3. The cast tooth preparations are lubricated with a die lubricant, and the case is waxed with great care. Attention is given to coronal contours, embrasures, occlusal form, and replacement of missing teeth (Fig. 9-91).

4. The wax form is removed from the cast and processed in acrylic, being sure to use one of proper shade. After processing, the acrylic form is returned to the mounted casts and occlusal and other adjustments are made, including an intracoronal reaming of each restoration with a suitable bur leaving a form of eggshell thickness (Fig. 9-92).

5. Holes are punched with a suitable bur all along the lingual surface, which later (see step 8) will allow for a correct seating of the filled splint because of the problem of hydraulics (Fig. 9-93, *A*).

6. The abutment teeth in the mouth are prepared, and the acrylic splint is tried in to test for complete seating. The acrylic shell usually is thin enough and flexible enough to fit over any prepared tooth, but, if it binds, the internal surface causing the interference is reamed out. Also make sure that there is no displacement of the splint shell in centric closure. If so, make necessary occlusal adjustments.

7. Preannealed, soft gold bands,* developed by Amsterdam,[15] are fitted carefully and festooned to the cervical finish line. Do not extend any part of the band into bifurcation or trifurcation undercut areas. After gingival adaptation the bands are removed and trimmed so that the occlusogingival height of the band does not exceed 1 mm. on the facial surface and 4 mm. on the proximal and lingual surfaces. Serrations are cut around the occlusal periphery of each band for retention of these bands in the acrylic.[15]

8. The prepared teeth are dried and lubricated with Splint Lube,† as are the soft tissues, the gold bands are reseated, and the processed acrylic splint is filled with a mix of "quick-cure" plastic‡ and is seated over the prepared teeth contacting the serrated festooned bands. The patient is instructed to close the teeth slowly in centric relation, and excess acrylic is molded around the gingival margins of the teeth,

---

*J. M. Ney Co., Hartford, Conn.

†Williams Gold Refining Co., Buffalo, N. Y.

‡Lang Dental Mfg. Co., Chicago, Ill. (Jet); Kerr Mfg. Co. Detroit, Mich. (Temp-Span).

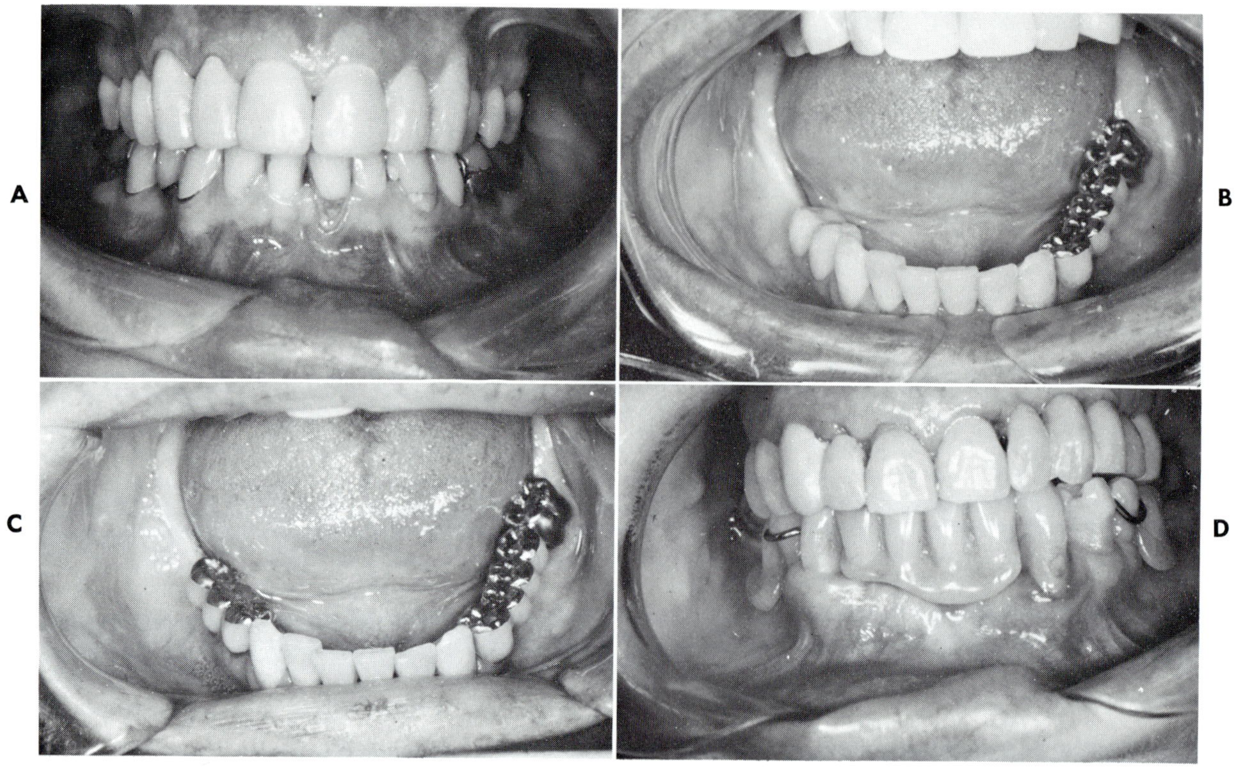

Fig. 9-89. Temporary restorations must be adequate and gingival irritation should not occur. A, Adequate upper temporary acrylic resin splint extending from right second bicuspid to left cuspid. B, Well-formed acrylic resin splint (lower right side) that did not cause gingival irritation and allowed placement of permanent restoration in a healthy environment, C. D, Inadequately constructed temporary acrylic resin splint caused gingival irritation—upper right lateral, cuspid area, and left central, lateral area.

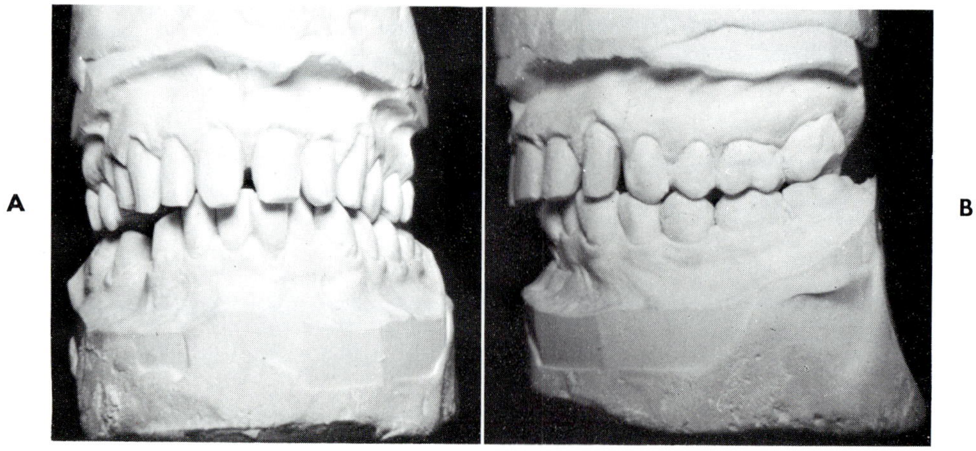

Fig. 9-90. Underpreparation of teeth on mounted casts to conform approximately to anticipated preparations. A, Anterior view. B, Side view.

A 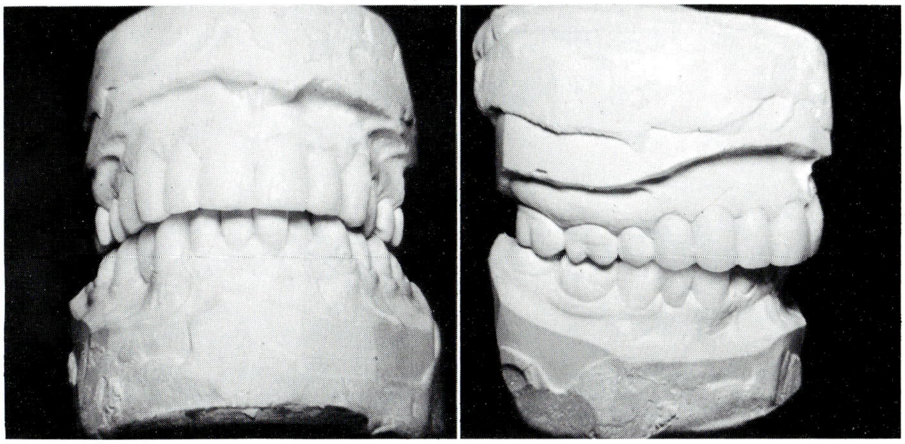 B

Fig. 9-91. Case waxed with great care, giving attention to coronal contours, embrasures, and occlusal form. **A,** Anterior view. **B,** Side view.

A
B
C
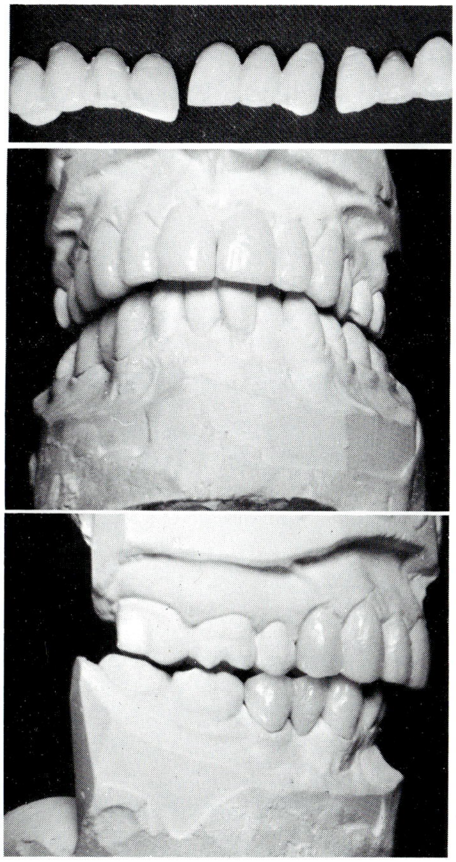

Fig. 9-92. Processed wax forms returned to mounted casts; adjustments made, including an intracoronal reaming of each restoration leaving a form of eggshell thickness. **A,** Processed forms. **B,** Anterior view after adjustments and intracoronal reaming. **C,** Side view.

making sure that no gold bands are exposed. Excess flash on the lingual surface, where holes were punched, is removed while it is soft. After a short wait of approximately 1 minute, the bridge or splint is lifted slightly away from the gingival margin several times while the lining acrylic is setting in order to prevent binding when it is fully set. This is repeated several times during the setting process, the patient always closing in centric position after each slight lifting of the splint. The shell is cooled with water to prevent overheating.

9. After the final set the complete acrylic splint is removed. This procedure may necessitate gentle taps from a mallet on a gold plugger or the use of a reverse hammer crown remover moving from one area to another until the splint is released.

10. The gold bands must be attached firmly to the acrylic and in correct position. A thin mix of quick-cure acrylic is brushed around the exposed margins of the gold bands, care taken to keep any part of this mix out of the internal surfaces of the crowns.

11. The excess acrylic should be trimmed away, a recheck made in the mouth for correct form and fit, and the splint removed and polished.

12. It is ready now for cementation. This procedure can be used for full-arch or quadrant splints.

TECHNIQUE 2 (ACRYLIC TEMPORARIES)

Acrylic splint shells also can be made directly from alginate impressions taken of stone casts that were formed from the impressions taken in the mouth. In this technique rearrangement of coronal and occlusal forms is not as accurate as in technique 1.

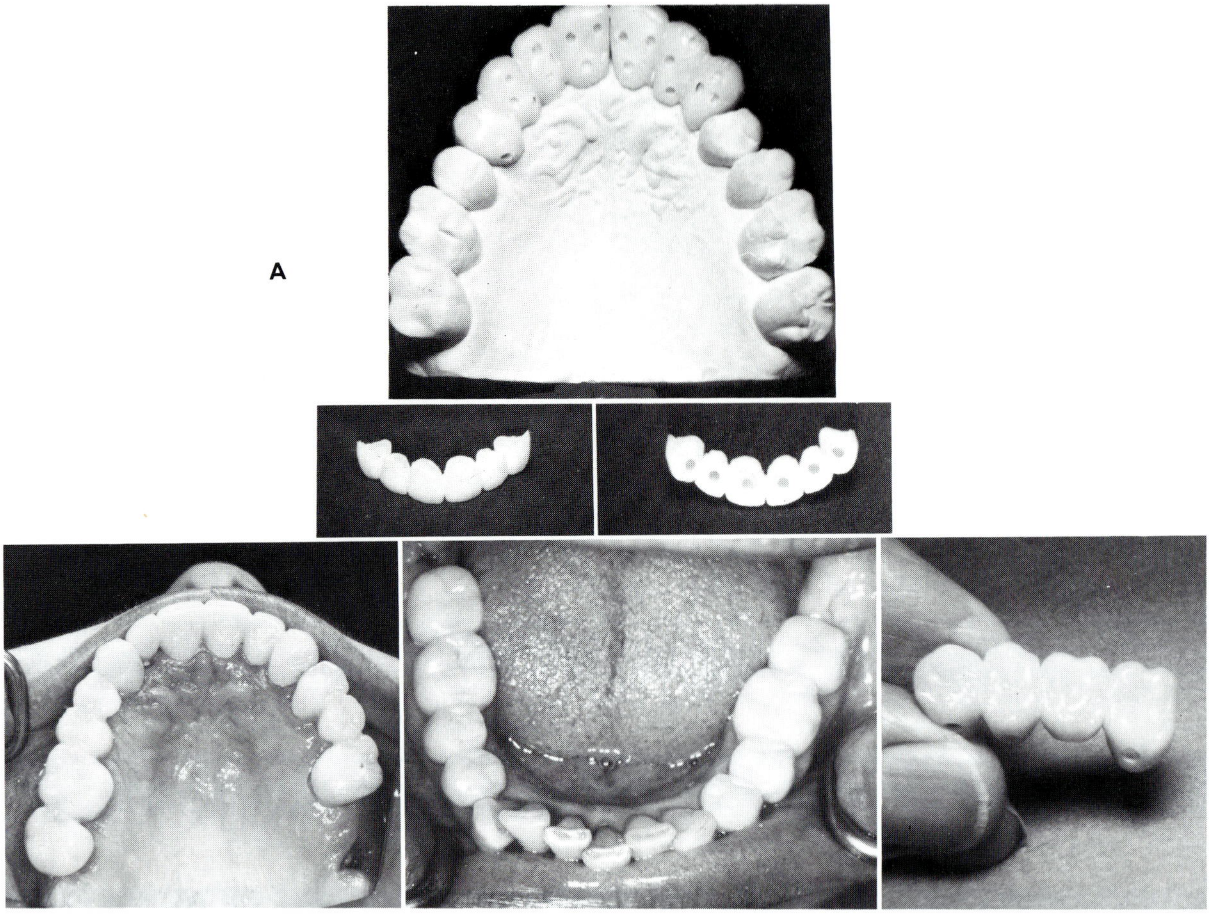

A

B C D

Fig. 9-93. A, Holes punched (with suitable bur) on lingual surface that subsequently will allow for correct seating during rebasing because of problems of hydraulics. **B** to **D,** Temporary acrylic splints constructed for a patient undergoing mouth rehabilitation.

1. An alginate impression is taken of each arch prior to tooth preparations. Hard stone casts are formed from these impressions.

2. Edentulous areas, if any, are filled in with acrylic teeth or properly molded wax, undercuts are waxed in, and the desired form on the abutment teeth is made by the addition of wax.

3. An alginate impression of the prepared cast is taken.

4. The next step is the construction of a thin shell of acrylic. Excess moisture is removed from the impression with a gentle blast of air, and the desired shade of acrylic, or preferably one of a shade lighter, is painted into the impression with a small sable brush. The brush is dipped into a dappen dish containing the liquid or monomer, and then a generous amount of powder is picked up by the moistened brush from a second dappen dish and is applied in the impression so that a uniform layer of acrylic will result. This process is continued, using a gentle blast of warm air after each layer is painted on and also tilting the impression to move the soft acrylic evenly and to prevent the formation of very thick sections. Amsterdam[15] flows a comparatively loose mix of "quick-cure" acrylic into a gently warmed alginate impression.

5. When set, the acrylic shell is removed carefully from the alginate impression. Any thin overextensions are removed with a small pair of scissors, and thick areas inside the shell are reamed out intracoronally with a suitable round bur, leaving a form of eggshell thickness. Holes are punched all along the

lingual surface, which later (see step 8) will allow for a correct seating of the filled splint because of the problem of hydraulics.

6. The abutment teeth in the mouth are prepared, and the acrylic splint is tried in to test for complete seating. The acrylic shell usually is thin enough and flexible enough to fit over any prepared tooth, but, if it binds, the internal surface causing the interference is reamed out. A check should be made to be sure that there is no displacement of the splint shell in centric closure. If so, the necessary occlusal adjustments should be made.

7. Preannealed, soft gold bands, developed by Amsterdam,[15] are fitted carefully and festooned to the cervical finish line. No part of the band should extend into bifurcation and trifurcation undercut areas. After gingival adaptation, the bands are removed and trimmed so that the occlusogingival height of the band does not exceed 1 mm. on the facial surface and 4 mm. on the proximal and lingual surfaces. Serrations are cut around the occlusal periphery of each band for retention of these bands in the acrylic.[15]

8. The prepared teeth are dried and lubricated with Splint Lube, as are the soft tissues; the gold bands are reseated, the processed acrylic splint is filled with a mix of "quick-cure" plastic and is seated over the prepared teeth contacting the serrated festooned bands. The patient is instructed to close the teeth slowly in centric position, and excess acrylic is molded around the gingival margins of the teeth, making sure that no gold bands are exposed. Excess flash on the lingual, where holes were punched, is removed while it is soft. After a short wait of approximately 1 minute the bridge or splint is lifted slightly away from the gingival margin several times while the lining acrylic is setting in order to prevent binding when it is fully set. This is repeated several times during the setting process, the patient always closing in centric occlusion after each slight lifting of the splint. The shell is cooled with water to prevent overheating.

9. After the final set the complete acrylic splint is removed. This procedure may necessitate gentle taps from a mallet on a gold plugger or the use of a reverse hammer crown remover moving from one area to another until the splint is released.

10. Make sure that the gold bands are attached firmly to the acrylic and are in correct position.

A thin mix of "quick-cure" acrylic is brushed around the exposed margins of the gold bands, care being taken to keep any part of this mix out of the internal surfaces of the crowns.

11. The excess acrylic should be trimmed away; a recheck in the mouth should be made for correct form and fit, and the splint removed and polished.

If a change in vertical dimension is indicated, make use of an anterior acrylic stop to determine and hold the desired dimension, and add soft pads of acrylic to the occlusal surfaces of the splint or splints, and have patient close placing a piece of tinfoil, which prevents adherence to the opposing splint, or the opposing restoration during the set of the acrylic. In many instances more trimming and carving is necessary for the establishment of correct form and function with this method than with technique 1.

12. The splint is ready now for cementation. This procedure can be used for full-arch or quadrant splints.

FABRICATION OF OMNIVAC SHELL

1. After the cast to be used for the fabrication of the Omnivac shell has been properly trimmed so that it fits within the confines of the platform of the Omnivac Precision Vacuum Adapter anteroposteriorly and laterally with a flat smooth base (so that it will not rock), fill in any edentulous areas with denture teeth set in Omnivac clay. This clay can also be used to change coronal contours, contact areas, etc. to the desired form.

2. Place a strip of Mortite around the entire cast slightly apical to the desired gingival line on both the buccal and the lingual surfaces. This procedure allows for the removal of the splint from the cast with greater ease (Fig. 9-94, *A*).

3. Center the cast on the vacuum plate (Fig. 9-94, *B*).

4. Grasp both handles of the hinged frame and raise until it clicks into the heating position approximately 3 inches above the vacuum plate (the heating unit had been swung to the rear and the heating element switch turned on—it requires approximately 3 minutes to preheat).

5. Open the hinged frame using handle provided, and place a sheet of Omnidental Resin Material (5 × 5 inches) on the lower frame. Center the sheet carefully (Fig. 9-94, *C*).

6. Close the frame and secure with the frame latch knob. Swing the heating unit into position squarely over the material. Do not leave machine unattended when heating material prior to adaptation —material heats quickly and will be useless if allowed to droop excessively.

7. Watch the material as it heats (1 to 2 minutes depending on the thickness of the material). When

A B C D

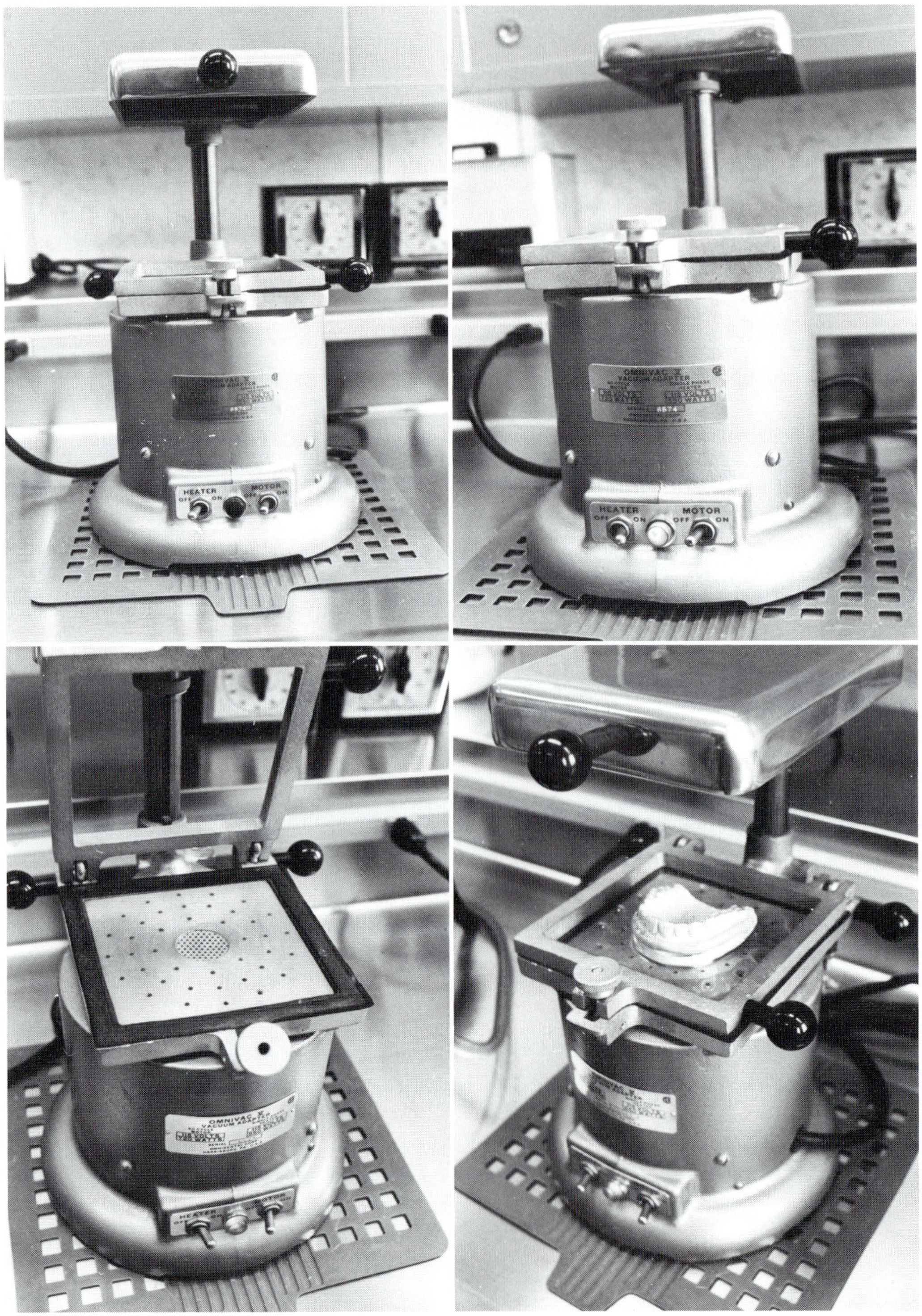

Fig. 9-94. Fabrication of Omnivac shell. Correlate illustrations with text.

the material begins to sag appreciably (approximately ½ inch) or slightly beyond the bottom of the hinged frame, the frame should be lowered to make the adaptation (Fig. 9-94, *D*).

8. Grasp both handles at the rear of the hinged frame and lower it into position over the vacuum plate. The material will be draped over the cast. Turn on the motor switch to complete the adaptation. Leave the heating unit in place over the cast until you are sure the adaptation process is complete (10 to 15 seconds) (Fig. 9-94, *E*).

9. Swing the heating unit out of the way, and allow cooling of the adaptation for at least 30 seconds with the motor running. Turn off heating unit if no more adaptations are to be made.

10. Turn off motor, release hinged frame knob, and open frame to remove Omnivac shell (Fig. 9-94, *F*).

E
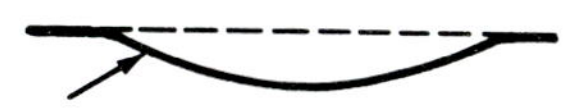

F G H I J
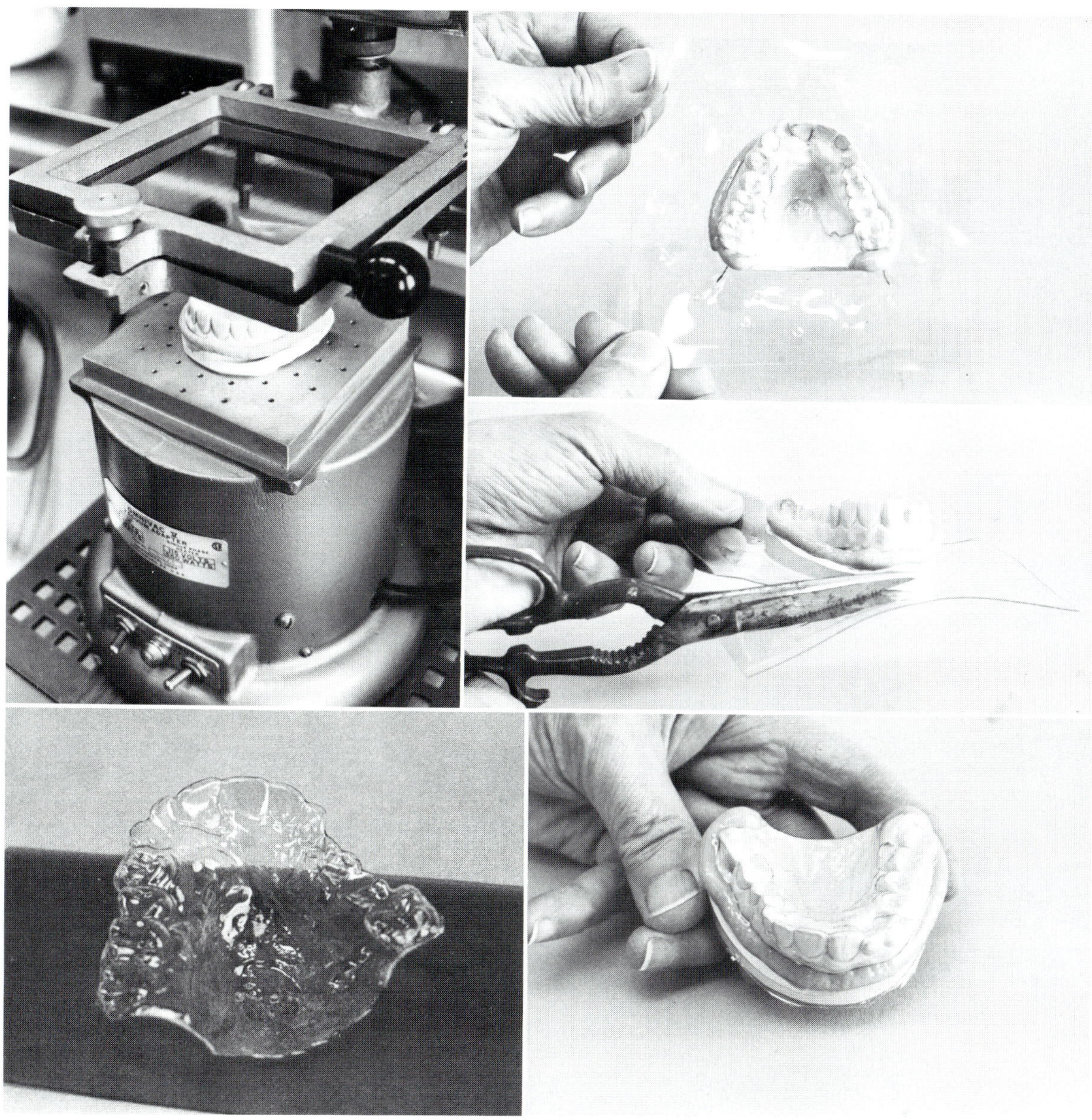

Fig. 9-94, cont'd. For legend see opposite page.

11. With a sharp instrument cut through the plastic sheet directly into the Mortite strip, and carefully push or pry the entire plastic splint off the cast.

12. Trim gross excess of the shell with scissors. The finished shell should extend about 2 to 3 mm. beyond the gingival margin (Fig. 9-94, *G*).

13. Rebase the shell on the prepared teeth with "quick-cure" acrylic.

14. Contour the temporary splint properly, and adjust occlusion ("centric position" and "excursive movements").

15. Polish and cement with temporary cement (Fig. 9-94, *H* to *J*).

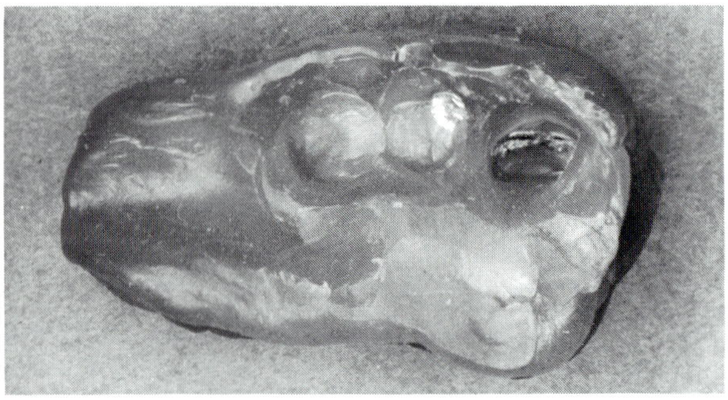

Fig. 9-95. Rebased wax bite, which will allow for great accuracy of duplication of coronal surfaces of teeth as they were before preparation. This method is excellent in construction of temporary acrylic crowns in many instances.

GOLD AND GOLD-ACRYLIC TEMPORARY RESTORATIONS

These restorations are used for mouths that are not seriously involved periodontally and are free of temporomandibular joint disturbances. This type of a mouth can be prepared one quadrant at a time.

Technique. The first quadrant to be prepared is the lower right posterior region. Before preparations are started a rebased Thin-wax* bite is taken for the construction of "temporary temporaries" made of acrylic.

The Thin-wax is softened in a water heater or a bunsen burner, and a piece of tinfoil (0.002 inch thickness) is placed between two thicknesses of the wax like a sandwich. The "bite sandwich" is adapted on the lower right posterior teeth (in this particular instance), and the patient is told to close in centric position. After chilling, the bite is removed and dried. The upper portion of this bite is completely "candled" with a rope of Thin-wax, that is, in each tooth depression, and then the lower part of the bite (which has not been candled as yet) is seated on the lower teeth, and again the patient is instructed to close in centric position. This is chilled, removed, and dried with a blast of air, and the surplus wax on the upper part is trimmed. The lower part of the bite is now completely "candled" with a rope of Thin-wax, the rebased upper portion seated carefully, and the patient told to close in centric position. It is chilled, removed, and dried, and the surplus wax trimmed. Some wax is removed in the gingival finish line area to allow for a greater bulk of acrylic for proper finishing purposes. We now have a rebased wax bite, which will allow for great accuracy of duplication of the coronal surfaces of the teeth before preparation (Fig. 9-95).

Preparations, partial or full coverage, are completed and elastic impressions taken. If possible at this time, two impressions are taken, one (and a bite) for the gold "temporaries" and one for the "finish dies" in the construction of the permanent restorations at the proper time. If indicated, copper tube–modeling compound impressions are taken for the construction of "finish dies."

The rebased Thin-wax is used now for the construction of the fast-curing acrylic "temporary temporaries." The prepared lower teeth and surrounding soft tissues are dried and lubricated with Splint Lube. A doughy mix of fast-curing acrylic (Temp-Span or Jet) is placed, in this case, in the lower section of the rebased bite, and the top of the acrylic mass is lubricated lightly with Splint Lube. The upper section of the rebased bite is seated carefully and accurately, and the patient is told to close. Excess acrylic that seeps out of the bite is removed and used as a guide to the setting of the acrylic. When the final set has taken place, the wax bite is removed, and the lower acrylic splint is removed making use of a reverse hammer crown remover or gentle taps from a mallet on a gold plugger. The excess acrylic is trimmed away, and embrasures and cervical finish lines are established properly.

The acrylic splint is reseated to be sure that it seats accurately, without a rock. The occlusion is checked, after which it is removed, polished, and cemented with a temporary cement. This method is excellent for the construction of full crowns, three-quarter crowns, onlays, or other variations in the preparations.

One of the casts made from the elastic impression is mounted on a simple Crescent articulator* making

*Modern Materials Mfg. Co., St. Louis, Mo.

*Crescent Dental Mfg. Co., Chicago, Ill.

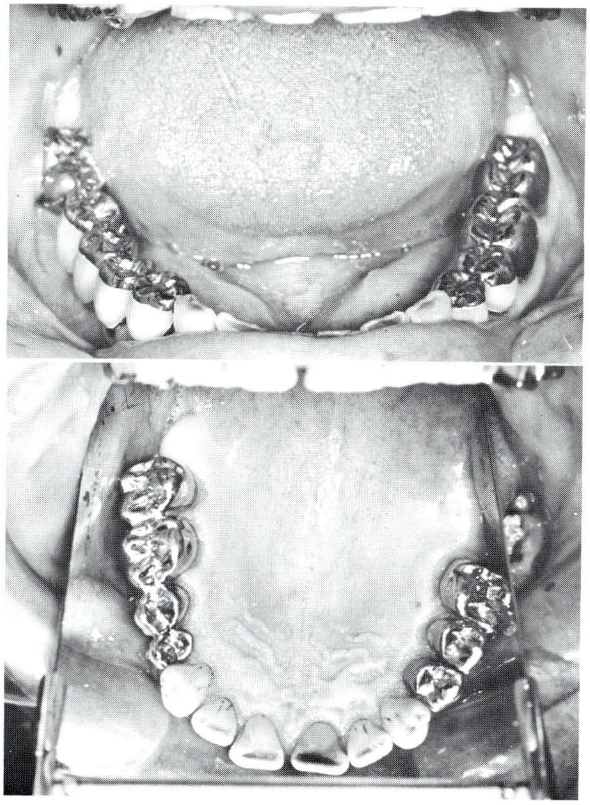

Fig. 9-96. Completed and cemented (zinc oxide–eugenol) temporary gold and gold-acrylic veneer restorations.

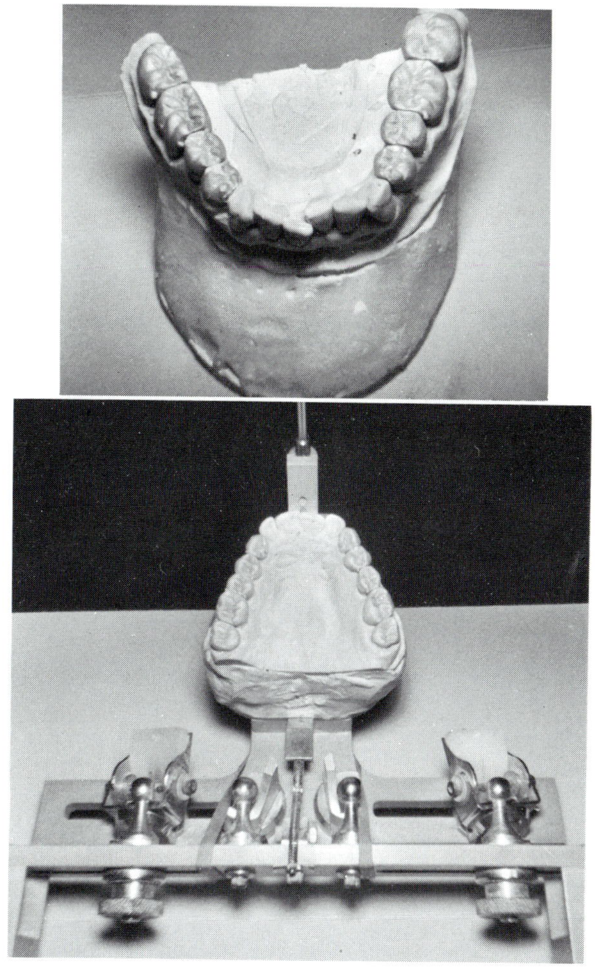

Fig. 9-97. Castings on mounted casts after first remount in case with temporomandibular joint disturbance.

use of the bite taken after the preparations were completed.

Any gross irregularities on the opposing model are cut away, and the gold temporaries are made to this newly established relationship. If possible, this temporary restoration is made in the form of a fixed splint for ease of removal and recementation during the various procedures used in mouth rehabilitation. The processing of acrylic veneers is completed in areas where indicated.

At the next appointment the gold temporaries are cemented with temporary cement. The upper teeth in the right posterior quadrant are prepared as indicated by the lower gold restorations. A temporary acrylic splint is made for the upper right quadrant, using the rebased wax technique as previously described.

The same procedure is followed for the quadrants on the left side.

At this stage of the operation the gold temporaries have been cemented with temporary cement on the lower right and left posterior quadrants, and temporary acrylic splints have been cemented temporarily on the upper right and left posterior quadrants.

The upper acrylic restorations are removed, the prepared teeth are cleaned, and a full elastic impression is taken of the upper arch. Also a full elastic impression is taken of the lower arch with the gold temporaries in place. A hinge-bow transfer and centric relation bite (the patient is guided back into a centric bite as the upper gold temporaries will be made in correct centric) are taken. The upper and lower stone casts are mounted on an anatomic articulator with the use of this bite and transfer. The upper gold temporary restorations are made and cemented with temporary cement (Fig. 9-96). The case is checked out for centric position and, if necessary, is equilibrated for lateral excursions directly in the mouth.

All restorations, although temporary, should be

Text continued on p. 486.

Figs. 9-98 to 9-102. Series of illustrations showing various phases of construction of restorations for pulpless teeth, using agar hydrocolloid as impression material.

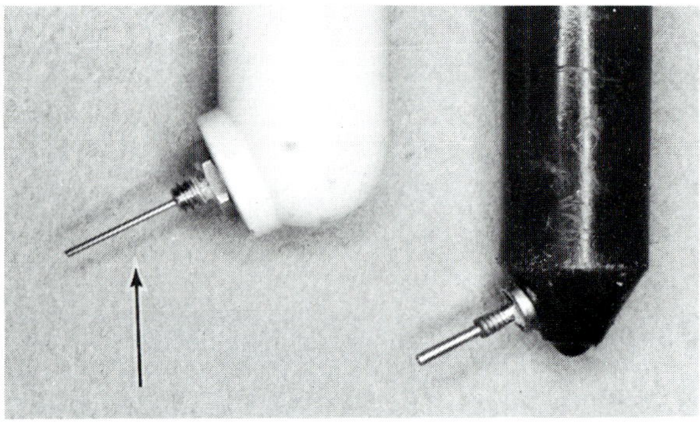

Fig. 9-98. Syringe with a special long needle for obtaining impression of prepared canals.

A B C D

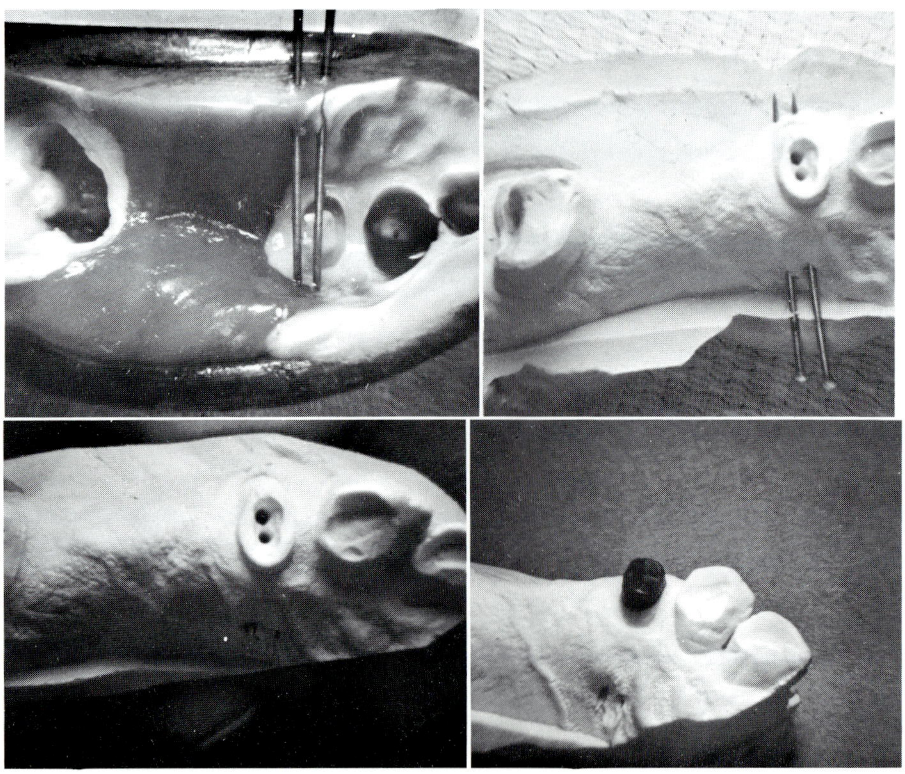

Fig. 9-99. A, Impression. **B** and **C,** Die and cast (one with banker pins still in position, other with pins removed). **D,** Wax-up. **E,** Post anchorage cast gold core. **F,** Post anchorage cast gold core shown on cast. **G,** Post anchorage cast gold core in patient's mouth. **H,** Complete bridge in patient's mouth.

E F G H

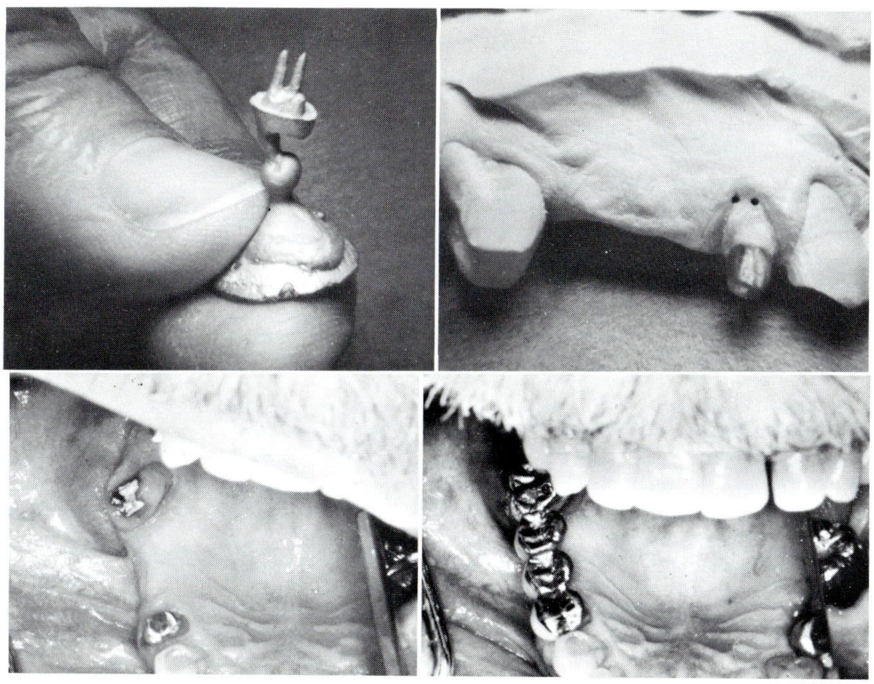

Fig. 9-99, cont'd. For legend see opposite page.

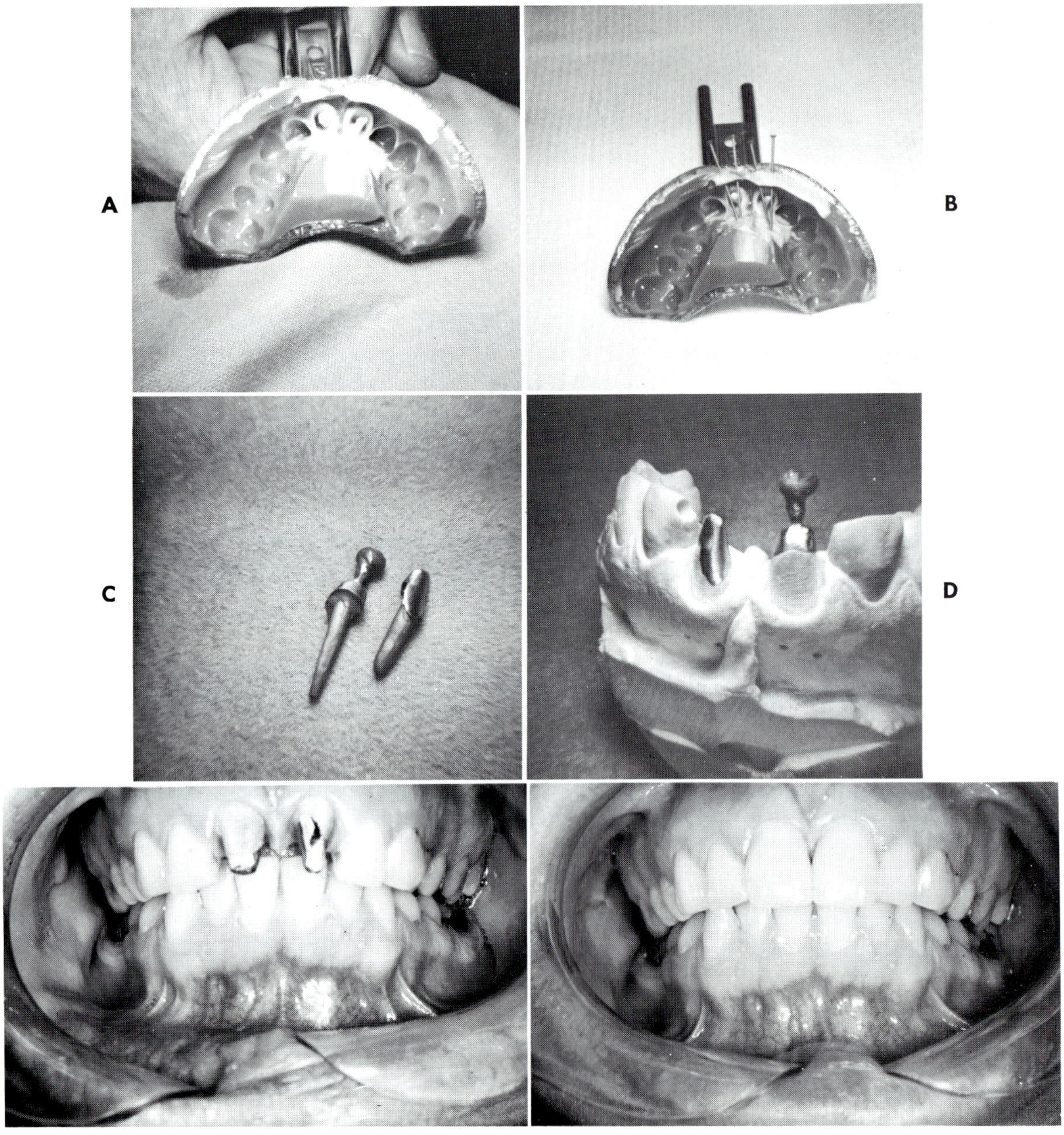

A B C D E F

Fig. 9-100. Case of pulpless central incisors. **A,** Impression. **B,** Treatment of impression with banker pins before pour up. **C,** Post anchorage cast gold cores. **D,** Cores on cast. **E,** Cemented cores. **F,** Completed case in mouth.

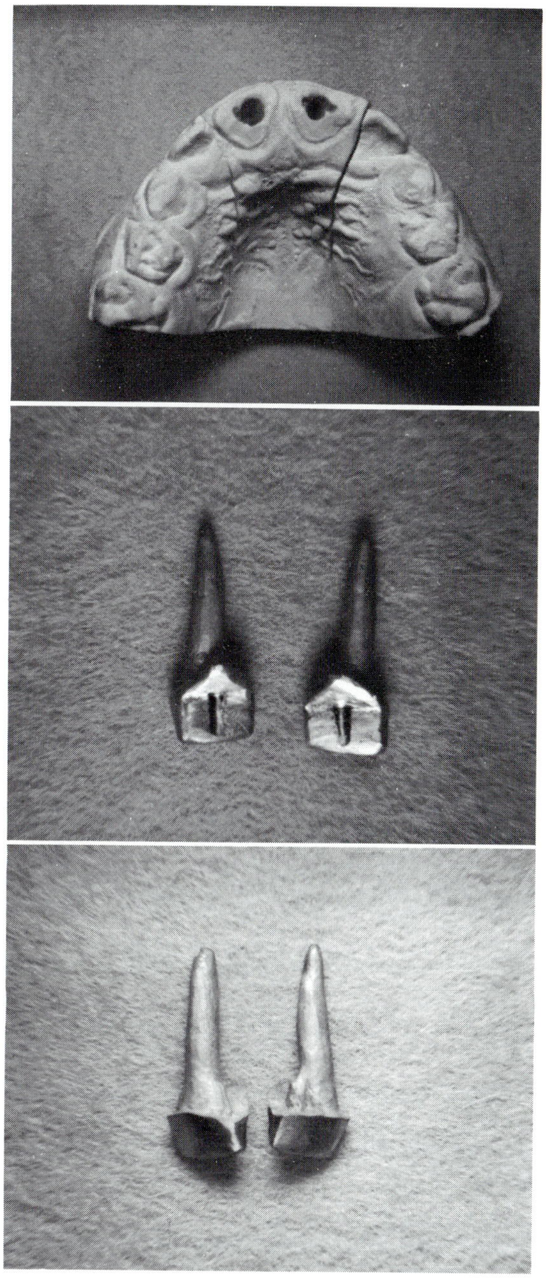

A

B

C

Fig. 9-101. Case of child 10 years old, involving upper central incisors. **A,** Cast. **B** and **C,** Labial and lingual views of post anchorage cast gold cores.

A

B

C

D

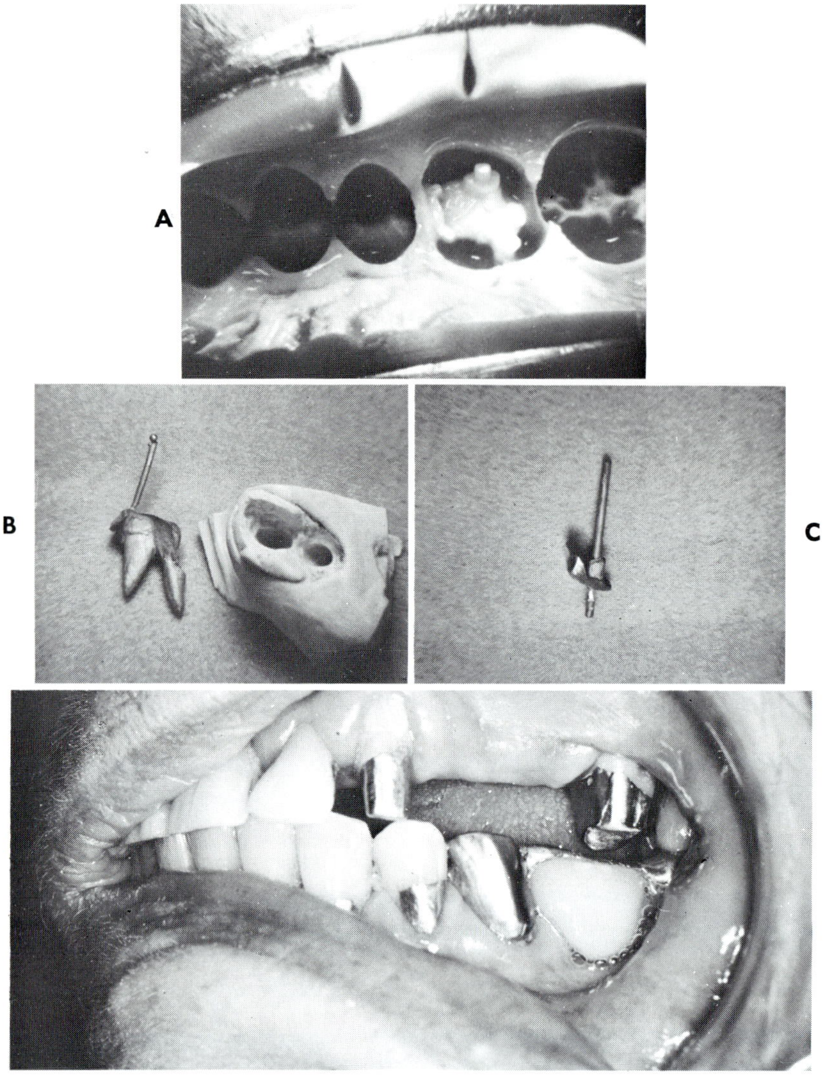

Fig. 9-102. A, Impression of pinholes with agar hydrocolloid. **B,** Post anchorage cast gold core for an upper molar. **C,** Post anchorage core making use of an endo-post. **D,** Cemented post anchorage cast gold cores—cuspid and second molar.

checked for accuracy of marginal fit, absence of rock or spring, correct relationship of coronal contours and embrasure patterns to gingival tissues to avoid "wash-outs" (leading to sensitivity and caries), and gingival irritations resulting in inflammation. We must not recreate pathology after it has been cured.

MOUTHS WITH SERIOUS PERIODONTAL INVOLVEMENTS AND TEMPOROMANDIBULAR DISTURBANCES

In mouths with more serious periodontal involvements and temporomandibular joint disturbances or muscle spasm, the temporary restorations must be constructed with the best occlusion possible to obtain at this particular stage of rehabilitation. It must be done on a completely adjusted anatomic articulator. The carvings and castings are made as accurate as possible, and at least one remount for adjustment is made before temporary cementation (Fig. 9-97).

Why all this painstaking work for a temporary or treatment restoration? By these means we have a better chance of obtaining correct interocclusal records, intermaxillary relations, and intra-arch relations. A better centric relation than the patient presented at the beginning of treatment allows healing and changes in the right direction to take place. As more remounts are made at various intervals and as changes occur, more stability and better occlusal relations are attainable. Periodontal tissues are brought within physiologic limits, temporomandibular joint symptoms subside, and joint stability is achieved.

A stable relationship must be obtained before permanent restorations are made. Temporary partial dentures, in conjunction with fixed restorations, also are constructed, when indicated, in cases of mouth rehabilitation. Care and thought in design and technical execution are most important.[16] (See Figs. 9-98 to 9-102 for treatment of the pulpless tooth.)

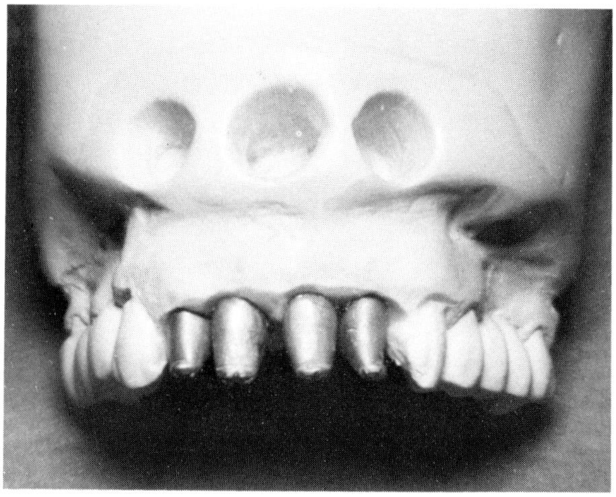

Fig. 9-103

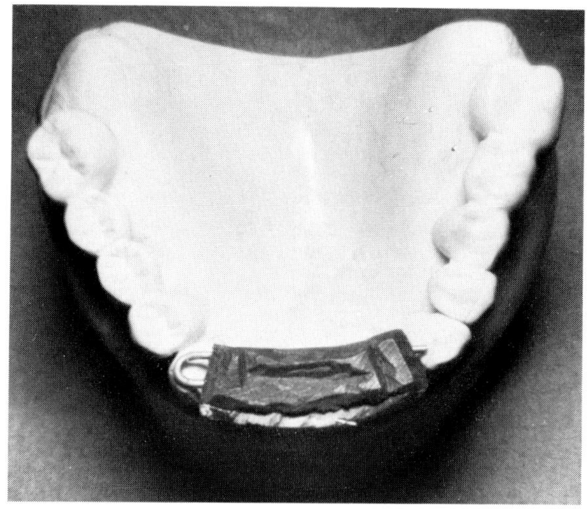

Fig. 9-104

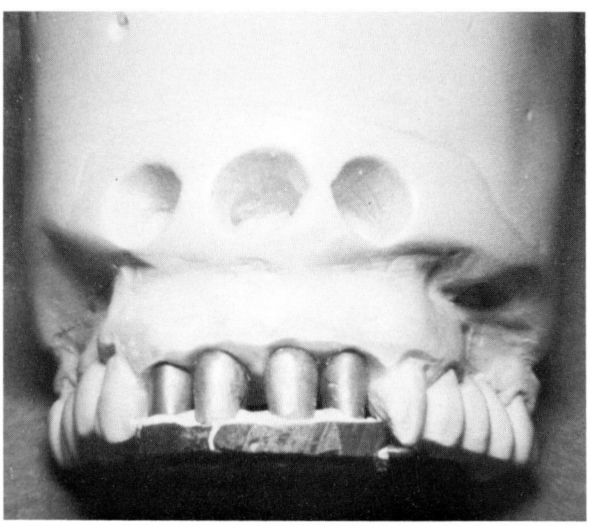

Fig. 9-105

Figs. 9-103 to 9-112. Correct positioning (for anterior or posterior restorations) of copper plated dies or individual stone dies as to faciolingual, mesiodistal, and incisogingival or occlusogingival dimensions by means of cast copings, modeling compound, or acrylic index forms rebased with Kerr's Temp-bond and an overall alginate impression which is then poured with stone. (For a detailed description of the use of this method in "remount" procedures, refer to Chapter 17.)

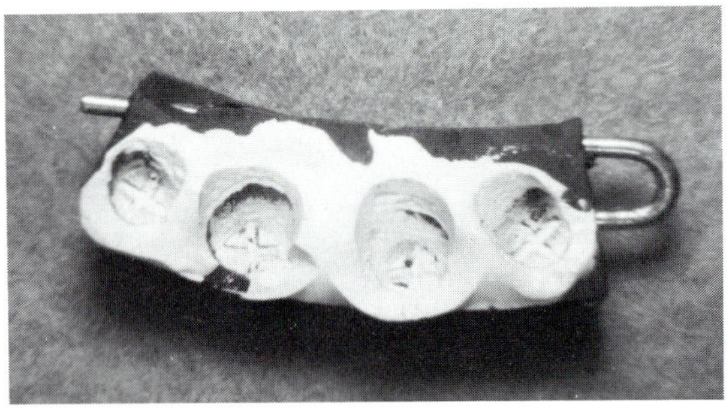

Fig. 9-106

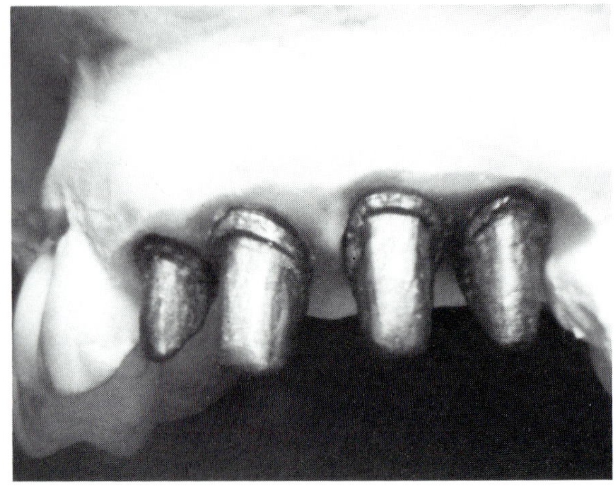

Fig. 9-107

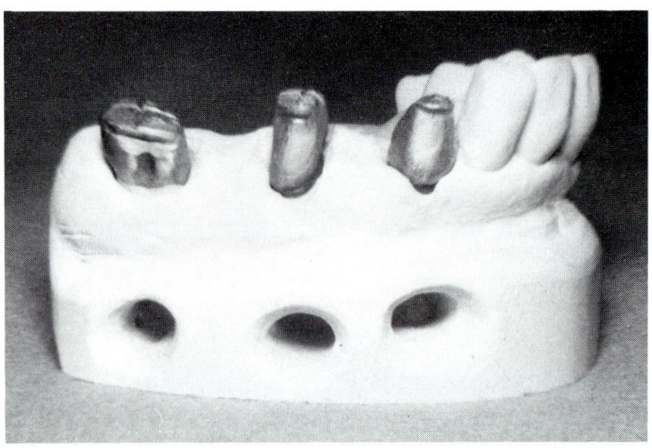

Fig. 9-108

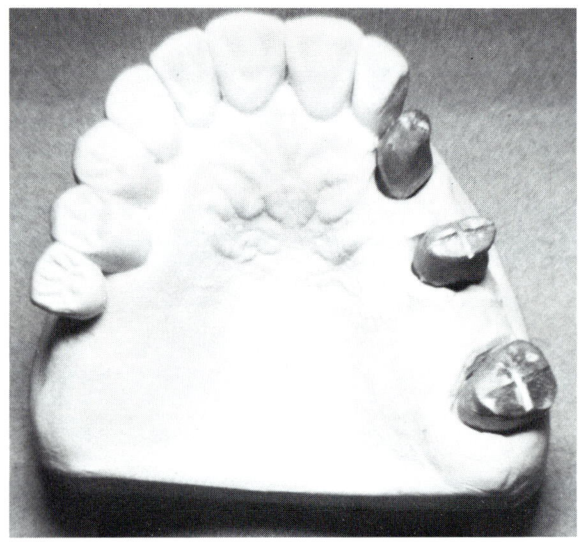

Fig. 9-109

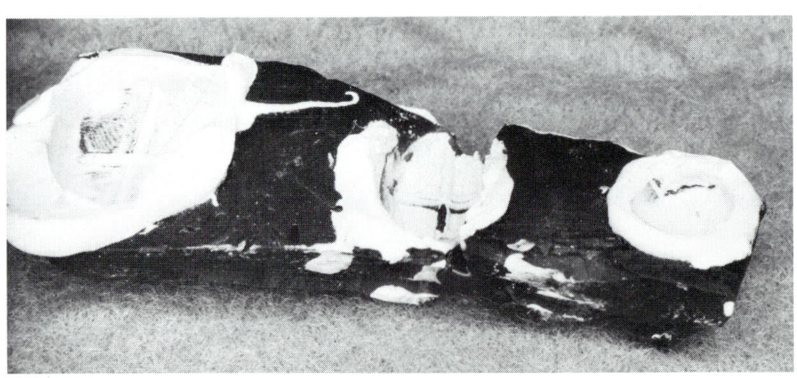

Fig. 9-110

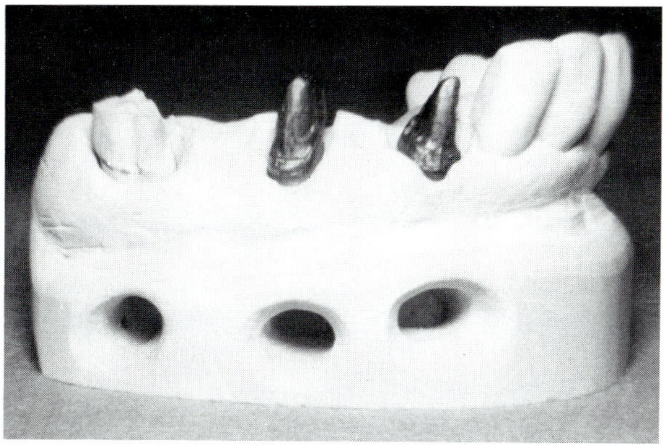

Fig. 9-111

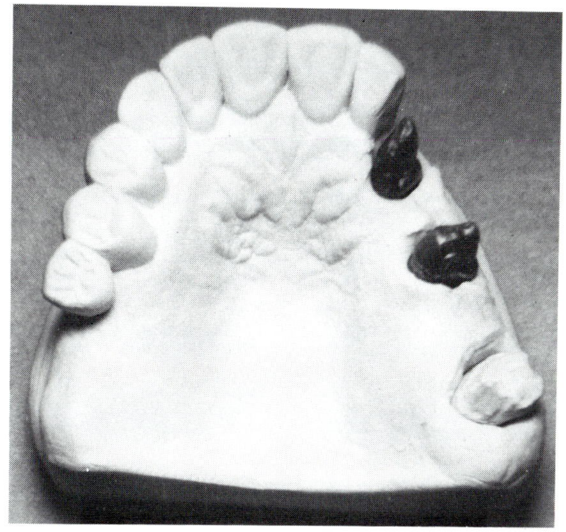

Fig. 9-112

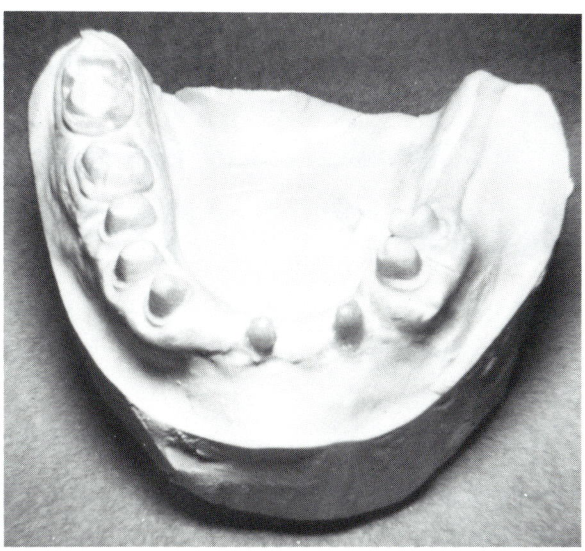

Fig. 9-113

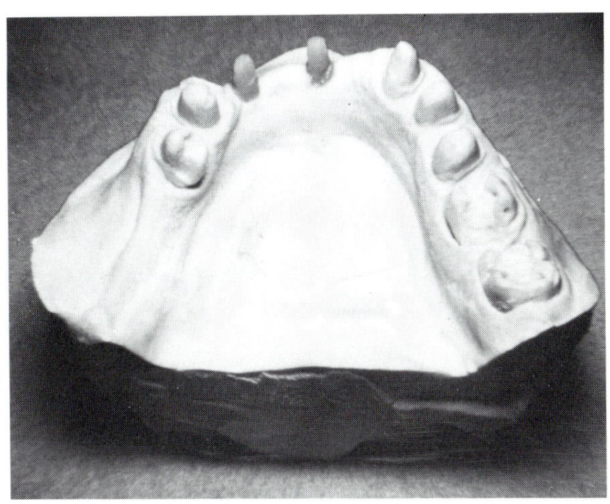

Fig. 9-114

Figs. 9-113 and 9-114. Cast of a case (two views) showing "acrylic buttons" inserted in anterior region for the construction of a temporary acrylic splint in preparation of the insertion of an anterior implant.

REFERENCES

1. Rudd, K. D., Morrow, R. M., and Strunk, R. R.: Accurate alginate impressions, J. Prosthet. Dent. **22**(3):294-300, 1969.
2. Rudd, K. D., Morrow R. M., and Bange, A. A.: Accurate casts, J. Prosthet. Dent. **21**(5):545-554, 1969.
3. Rudd, K. D.: Lecture notes, Washington University School of Dental Medicine, Postgraduate course, St. Louis, 1971.
4. Bassett, R. W., Vander Heide, J. D., and Smith, D. D.: Clinically oriented tests comparing accuracy of elastic impression materials, J. S. Calif. Dent. Assoc. **37**(2):47-57, 1969.
5. La Forgia, Anthony: Mechanical-chemical and electrosurgical tissue retraction for fixed prosthesis, J. Prosthet. Dent. **14:** 1107-1114, 1964.
6. Phillips, R. W.: Hydrocolloid impression materials; technical considerations. In Skinner, E. W., and Phillips, R. W.: The science of dental materials, Philadelphia, 1960, W. B. Saunders Co., pp. 103, 105, 106.
7. Shooshan, E. David: A pin-ledge casting technique—its application in periodontal splinting, Dent. Clin. N. Am., pp. 189-206, Mar., 1960.
8. Courtade, Gerard L.: Creating your own "dentin," Dent. Clin. N. Am., pp. 805-822, Nov., 1963.
9. Phillips, R. W., and Ito, B. Y.: Factors affecting the surface of stone dies poured in hydrocolloid impressions, J. Prosthet. Dent. **2:**390, 1952.
10. Docking, Allan R.: Plaster and stone, Dent. Clin. N. Am., pp. 727-735, Nov., 1958.
11. Stern, Noah: Atraumatic adjustment of copper bands in fixed prosthodontics, Alpha Omegan **63:**171-174, Dec., 1970.
12. Weinberg, Lawrence A.: Atlas of crown and bridge prosthodontics, St. Louis, 1965, The C. V. Mosby Co., p. 35.
13. Bassett, R. W., Ingraham, Rex, and Koser, J. R.: An atlas of cast gold procedures, Buena Park, Calif., 1964, Uni-Tro College Press, pp. 48, 130.
14. Lucia, Victor O.: Modern gnathological concepts, St. Louis, 1961, The C. V. Mosby Co., p. 368.
15. Amsterdam, Morton, and Fox, Lewis: Provisional splinting-principles and technics, Dent. Clin. N. Am., pp. 73-99, Mar., 1959.
16. Granger, E. R.: Practical procedures in oral rehabilitation, Philadelphia, 1962, J. B. Lippincott Co., pp. 260-265.

INDEX

D

E

G

H

N

P

Q

R

T